General Dilution Chart (mg to mcg)							
Amount of Drug Required in Grams	Amount of Diluent						
	1,000 ml	500 ml	250 ml	125 ml	100 ml	50 ml	25 ml
	mcg/ml	mcg/ml	mcg/ml	mcg/ml	mcg/ml	mcg/ml	mcg/ml
20 mg	20	40	80	160	200	400	800
19 mg	19	38	76	152	190	380	760
18 mg	18	36	72	144	180	360	720
17 mg	17	34	68	136	170	340	680
16 mg	16	32	64	128	160	320	640
15 mg	15	30	60	120	150	300	600
14 mg	14	28	56	112	140	280	560
13 mg	13	26	52	104	130	260	520
12 mg	12	24	48	96	120	240	480
11 mg	11	22	44	88	110	220	440
10 mg	10	20	40	80	100	200	400
9 mg	9	18	36	72	90	180	360
8 mg	8	16	32	64	80	160	320
7 mg	7	14	28	56	70	140	280
6 mg	6	12	24	48	60	120	240
5 mg	5	10	20	40	50	100	200
4.5 mg	4.5	9	18	36	45	90	180
4 mg	4	8	16	32	40	80	160
3.5 mg	3.5	7	14	28	35	70	140
3 mg	3	6	12	24	30	60	120
2.5 mg	2.5	5	10	20	25	50	100
2 mg	2	4	8	16	20	40	80
1.5 mg	1.5	3	6	12	15	30	60
1 mg	1	2	4	8	10	20	40
0.5 mg	0.5	1	2	4	5	10	20
0.25 mg	0.25	0.5	1	2	2.5	5	10

To use chart:

1. Find mcg/ml desired, track to amount of diluent desired and amount of drug in mg required.
2. Find amount of drug in mg required, track to diluent desired and/or mcg/ml desired.
3. Find amount of diluent required, track to amount of drug in mg and/or mcg/ml desired.

Formula: Substitute any number for X

X mg diluted in 1,000 ml = X mcg/ml (1 mg in 1,000 ml = 1 mcg/ml)
X mg diluted in 500 ml = 2 X mcg/ml (1 mg in 500 ml = 2 mcg/ml)
X mg diluted in 250 ml = 4 X mcg/ml (1 mg in 250 ml = 4 mcg/ml)
X mg diluted in 125 ml = 8 X mcg/ml (1 mg in 125 ml = 8 mcg/ml)
X mg diluted in 100 ml = 10 X mcg/ml (1 mg in 100 ml = 10 mcg/ml)
X mg diluted in 50 ml = 20 X mcg/ml (1 mg in 50 ml = 20 mcg/ml)
X mg diluted in 25 ml = 40 X mcg/ml (1 mg in 25 ml = 40 mcg/ml)

Some variation occurs from manufacturer's overfill or if the drug is in liquid form. If absolute accuracy is required, these variations can be avoided by withdrawing an amount in ml from the diluent equal to manufacturer's overfill and/or an amount equal to the amount in ml of the drug. Consult the pharmacist for specific information on manufacturer's overfill of infusion fluids used in your facility.

How to Use This Book

STEP 1

Refer to the index at the back of the book. You can find any drug by any name in less than 5 seconds. All drugs are cross-indexed by generic and all known trade names. The index is easily distinguished by a printed blue bar at the edge of the pages. Drugs are also indexed by pharmacological action. With one turn of the page, all drugs included in the text with similar pharmacological actions and their page numbers are available to you. Everything is strictly alphabetized; you will never be required to refer to additional pages to locate a drug.

STEP 2

Turn to the single page number given after the name of the drug. All information about the drug is included as continuous reading. You will rarely be required to turn to another section of the book to be completely informed. Specific breakdowns of each drug (Usual Dose, Pediatric Dose, Dose Adjustments, Dilution, Compatibility, Rate of Administration, Actions, Indications and Uses, Precautions, Contraindications, Drug/Lab Interactions, Side Effects, and Antidote) are consistent in format and printed in boldface type. Subheadings under these categories are in boldface. Scan quickly for a Usual Dose check, Dose Adjustment, Drug/Lab Interaction, Side Effect, or Antidote or carefully read all included information. The choice is yours. A quick scan will take 5 to 10 seconds. Even the most complicated drugs will take less than 2 minutes to read completely. Read each monograph carefully and completely before administering a drug to a specific patient for the first time and review it any time a new drug is added to the patient's drug profile.

That's it! A fast, complete, and accurate reference for anyone administering intravenous medications. The spiral binding is specifically designed to lie flat, leaving your hands free to secure needed supplies, prepare your medication, or even ventilate a patient while you read the needed information.

Develop the "look it up" habit. Clear, concise language and simplicity of form contribute to quick, easy use of this handbook. Before your first use, read the preface; it contains lots of helpful information.

Check out the *NEW Intravenous Medications* website for monographs for selected diagnostic agents and other useful IV medication information:

http://evolve.elsevier.com/IVMeds

INTRAVENOUS MEDICATIONS

A Handbook for Nurses and Allied Health Professionals

BETTY L. GAHART, RN
Nurse Consultant in Education
Napa, California
Former Director, Education and Training
Queen of the Valley Hospital
Napa, California

ADRIENNE R. NAZARENO, PharmD
Clinical Coordinator, Department of Pharmacy
Queen of the Valley Hospital
Napa, California

TWENTIETH EDITION

Mosby
An Affiliate of Elsevier Science

Mosby
An Affiliate of Elsevier Science

11830 Westline Industrial Drive
St. Louis, Missouri 63146

INTRAVENOUS MEDICATIONS ISBN 0-323-02413-0

NOTICE

Pharmacology is an ever-changing field. Standard safety precautions must be followed, but as new research and clinical experience broaden our knowledge, changes in treatment and drug therapy may become necessary or appropriate. Readers are advised to check the most current product information provided by the manufacturer of each drug to be administered to verify the recommended dose, the method and duration of administration, and contraindications. It is the responsibility of the licensed prescriber, relying on experience and knowledge of the patient, to determine dosages and the best treatment for each individual patient. Neither the publisher nor the authors assume any liability for any injury and/or damage to persons or property arising from this publication.

THE PUBLISHER

TWENTIETH EDITION
Previous editions copyrighted 1973, 1977, 1981, 1984, 1988, 1989, 1990, 1991, 1993, 1994, 1995, 1996, 1997, 1998, 1999, 2000, 2001, 2002, 2003

Executive Publisher: Darlene Como
Senior Developmental Editor: Barbara Watts
Publishing Services Manager: Deborah L. Vogel
Senior Project Manager: Jodi M. Willard
Book Design Manager: Bill Drone

Printed in the United States of America

Last digit is the print number: 9 8 7 6 5 4 3 2 1

Nursing and Pharmacology Consultants

CHARLOTTE DENEEN, BSN, MPA
Quality Improvement Consultant
San Ramon, California

KIM HUBER, PharmD
Clinical Pharmacist
Memorial Hospitals Association
Modesto, California

GREGORY D. NAZARENO, PharmD
Clinical Pharmacist
Sutter Solano Hospital Pharmacy
Vallejo, California

MERRILEE NEWTON, RN, MSN
Administrative Director of Quality, Service, and Clinical Resource Management
Alta Bates/Summit Medical Center
Berkeley, California

To my husband,

Bill,

for his patience, support, and many hours of much needed and appreciated assistance, and to our children, **Marty, Jeff, Debbie, Rick,** and **Teresa;** their spouses, **Sally, Terri, Jim, Suzanne,** and **Bill;** and our grandchildren, **Meghan, Laurie, Alex, Anne, Kathryn, Lisa, Benjamin, Matthew, Claire, Neil, Scott,** and **Alan** for their encouragement and understanding.

BLG

To my husband,

Greg,

for his loving support and encouragement and to my children, **Danielle, Bryan, Emily,** and **Mark,** for allowing me the freedom to pursue my professional practice.

ARN

Preface

This Year 2004 edition marks the thirty-first year of publication of *Intravenous Medications.*

In this twentieth edition, 6 new drugs approved by the FDA for intravenous use are included. In addition, many new uses have been approved for established drugs. There is, however, a major change in the way we are addressing compatibilities and incompatibilities. **In response to your many requests, our primary focus has changed from incompatibilities to compatibilities.** This section has been completely revised throughout this edition. This was a difficult decision for us to make because of the numerous criteria that can impact compatibility. Just because a drug is listed as compatible doesn't mean it can be administered in any concentration. Temperature, pH, and time together in solution, as well as other parameters, must all be considered. It is imperative that you refer to the section on Compatibilities in the Format and Content section on p. xvi. Because today's hospital units are very specialized (e.g., cancer care, intensive coronary care, various intensive care units, transplant units, and orthopedic units to name just a few), nursing staff in each of these areas most likely administer similar combinations of drugs to their patients. **Take the initiative and research the drug combinations that are most frequently used on your unit. Then consult with the pharmacist and make your own compatibility chart for additives, Y-site, and syringe (if applicable).** By creating a chart specific to your unit, you will limit the number of consults required with the pharmacist to combinations that fall outside of the parameters you have researched. This approach will save time for every nurse on your unit and will give each of you the necessary compatibility information to administer the IV drug combinations specific to your unit. **The Solution Compatibility Chart on the inside back cover has been expanded and updated. Diluents that are not identified in Dilution will be listed in this chart.**

We are all aware that the **Joint Commission on Accreditation of Healthcare Organizations (JCAHO)** and the **Institute for Safe Medication Practices (ISMP)** have strongly emphasized various ways to reduce errors in drug ordering and administration. One of their suggestions is to refer to a drug by both its generic and its trade name. ***Intravenous Medications* is the only reference that has consistently used both names since its first publication.** They also recommend that symbols (e.g., <, >, ≤, ≥) be spelled out. **Although we have always spelled out most of them, they are now all spelled out. The only exception is in charts, where there isn't room for the spelled out version.** The symbols are included in the Key to Abbreviations (p. xix) if you need a refresher. **Some of the other ways we assist in safe administration** is to spell out the word *units;* we use Gm instead of gm so it is not confused with mg, use mcg instead of µg, and drop all trailing 0's (as in 1.0) to prevent overdoses. **JCAHO, ISMP, the American Pharmaceutical Association, and several other organizations have identified "High-Alert Medications" (a list of medications with the highest risk of injury when misused).** The websites of these organizations contain considerable information and identify common risk factors and suggested strategies. The top five high-alert medications are insulin, opiates and narcotics, injectable potassium chloride (or phosphate) concentrate, IV anticoagulants, and sodium chloride solutions above 0.9% (NS). Others listed are adrenergic antagonists, aminophylline-theophylline, benzodiazepines, IV calcium, cardioplegic solutions, chemotherapeutic agents, colchicine, IV digoxin, dextrose solutions greater than 10%, lidocaine, IV magnesium sulfate, neuromuscular blockers, thrombolytics, and vasoactive drugs. From the authors' viewpoint, **all drugs given by the IV route should be considered high-alert medications.** They have an immediate effect, are irretrievable, and can cause life-threatening side effects with incorrect usage.

Also in response to your many requests, Mosby is publishing an electronic version of *Intravenous Medications* for personal digital assistants (PDAs). This "handheld" electronic version is a convenient and portable supplement to the book. Although the handheld version is easy to carry, keep in mind that only a few lines of text are available at any one time. It is the user's responsibility to be familiar with the complete monograph and ***all*** aspects of each drug before administration.

Health care today is an intense environment. The speed of change is overwhelming, but the authors and publisher of *Intravenous Medications* have a commitment to provide all health care professionals who have the responsibility to administer IV medications with annual editions that incorporate complete, accurate, and current information in a clear, concise, accessible, and reliable tool. FDA websites are monitored throughout the year and provide many important updates, such as dose changes, new pediatric doses, additional disease-specific doses, refinements in dosing applications, new indications, new drug interactions, additional precautions, updates on postmarketing side effects, and new information on antidotes. Most drugs currently approved for intravenous use are included. Exceptions are opaque dyes used in radiology, some general anesthetics used only in the OR, and a few rarely used drugs (see Appendix C). To stay within the confines of the spiral binding, selected diagnostic agents, muscle relaxants intended for use only in the OR, and several other rarely used drugs have been moved to the Mosby website: http://evolve.elsevier.com/IVMeds. (See p. xxiv for a listing.) Helpful charts for dilution and/or rate of administration are incorporated in selected monographs. A General Dilution Chart to simplify calculations is found on the inside front cover. Front matter material provides a Key to Abbreviations and Important IV Therapy Facts.

Intravenous Medications is designed for use in critical care areas, at the nursing station, in the office, in public health and home care settings, and by students and the armed services. Pertinent information can be found in a few seconds. Take advantage of its availability and quickly review every intravenous medication before administration.

The nurse is frequently placed in a variety of difficult situations. While the physician verbally requests or writes an order, the nurse must evaluate it for appropriateness, prepare it, administer it, and observe the effects. Intravenous drugs are instantly absorbed into the bloodstream, leading, it is hoped, to a prompt therapeutic action, but the risk of an inappropriate reaction is a constant threat that can easily become a frightening reality. It will be the nurse who must initiate emergency measures should adverse effects occur. This is an awesome responsibility.

If, after reviewing the information in *Intravenous Medications,* you have any questions about any order you are given, clarify it with the physician, consult the pharmacist, or consult your supervisor. The circumstances will determine whom you will approach first. If the physician thinks it is imperative to carry out an order even though you have unanswered questions, never hesitate to request that the physician administer the drug, drug combination, or dose himself or herself. In this era of constant change, the physician should be very willing to supply you, your supervisor, and/or the pharmacist with current studies documenting the validity and appropriateness of orders.

All information presented in this handbook is pertinent only to the intravenous use of the drug and not necessarily to intramuscular, subcutaneous, oral, or other means of administration.

Our sincere appreciation is extended to Gregory Nazareno, Charlotte Deneen, Kim Huber, and Merrilee Newton for their ongoing participation in our efforts to bring you current, accurate, and relevant information; and to Darlene Como, Barbara Watts, Deborah L. Vogel, Jodi M. Willard, and Bill Drone, who are the editors, production staff, and design staff that make the publishing of *Intravenous Medications* happen each year. We also wish to thank you, the users of this reference. By seeking out this information, you serve your patients' needs and contribute to the safe administration of IV meds. We will continue to strive to earn your trust and confidence as we look forward together to an exciting future for health care.

Betty L. Gahart

Adrienne R. Nazareno

WE NEED TO HEAR FROM PROFESSIONALS LIKE YOU!

Congratulations on your purchase of the 2004 edition of **Gahart & Nazareno: *Intravenous Medications!*** We hope that you will find it to be a trusted resource. With each new edition, we encourage our customers to provide comments and suggestions on how to make it a better and more useful reference. Since you are a valued customer, your opinion really matters to us!

Log on to http://evolve.elsevier.com/IVMeds and complete a brief survey to give us your suggestions.

Thank You!

Contents

General Dilution Charts, inside front cover and facing page

How to Use This Book, iii

Evolve website information, iv

Format and Content of *Intravenous Medications,* xv

Key to Abbreviations, xix

Important IV Therapy Facts, xxii

Resources, xxiv

IV Drugs, 1

Appendix A
Recommendations for the Safe Handling of Cytotoxic Drugs, 1142

Appendix B
FDA Pregnancy Categories, 1145

Appendix C
Alternate Choices for Infrequently Used Drugs, 1146

Appendix D
Information for Patients Receiving Immunosuppressive Agents, 1148

Appendix E
National Cancer Institute Common Toxicity Grading Criteria, 1149

Appendix F
Recently Approved Drugs, 1154

Index, 1157

Solution Compatibility Chart, last page and inside back cover

Format and Content of *Intravenous Medications*

Designed to facilitate quick reference, each entry begins with the generic name of the drug in boldface type. Drug categories follow. The primary category may be followed by additional ones representing the multiple uses of a drug. Associated trade names are under the generic name. Boldface type and alphabetical order enable the reader to verify correct drug names easily. The use of a Canadian maple leaf symbol (🍁) preceding a trade name indicates availability in Canada only. The pH is listed in the lower right-hand corner of the title section. While this information is not consistently available, it is provided whenever possible. It represents the pH of the undiluted drug, the drug after reconstitution, or the drug after dilution for administration.

Headings within drug monographs are as follows:

Usual Dose: Doses recommended are the usual range for adults unless specifically stated otherwise. This information is presented first to enable the nurse to verify that the physician order is within acceptable parameters while checking the order and before preparation. If there are any questions, much time can be saved in clarifying them.

Pediatric Dose: Pediatric doses are specifically stated if they vary from mg/kg of body weight or M^2 dose recommended for adults. Not all drugs are recommended for use in children.

Infant and/or Neonatal Dose: Included if available and distinct from Pediatric Dose.

Dose Adjustments: Any situation that requires increasing or decreasing a dose will be mentioned here. The range will cover adjustments needed for the elderly, debilitated, or patients with hepatic or renal impairment, to adjustments required in the presence of other medications or as physical conditions are monitored.

Dilution: Specific directions for dilution are given for all drugs if dilution is necessary or permissible. Sadly, extreme cost-consciousness has overtaken the health care system. Nurses are being requested not to dilute drugs unless specifically required by the manufacturer, in order to save the cost of a needle, a syringe, or a small vial of diluent. Always use your best judgment and keep the safety of the patient as your priority. Appropriate diluents are listed. The Solution Compatibility Chart on the inside back cover has been expanded and updated. Diluents that are not identified in Dilution will be listed in this chart. This is the only reference that provides calculation examples to simplify dilution and accurate dose measurement. Charts are available in selected monographs. If recommendations for pediatric dilutions are available, they are listed. In some situations mcg or mg/ml dilutions partially account for this variation. If there are any doubts, consult with the pharmacist and/or pediatric specialist. Generic dilution charts for grams to milligrams and milligrams to micrograms are featured on the inside front cover and facing page.

Storage: A subheading. Content here includes such items as stability, refrigeration versus room temperature, predilution versus postdilution.

COMPATIBILITIES

This section has been completely revised for this edition and is divided into three areas. In all three areas, drugs are alphabetized by generic name for ease in locating the drugs with which you are working. To make identification easier, common trade names accompany generic names, or examples are presented for drug categories. No other reference consistently provides this helpful information.

The ***first area*** is **COMPATIBILITY.** This heading is used when general information is all that is available. It may include the manufacturer's recommendation to administer separately from other drugs or the potential for reaction with some plastic infusion bags or tubing.

The ***second area*** is **INCOMPATIBLE WITH.** Incompatibilities are listed only when they are specifically identified by the manufacturer. Statements regarding the potential inactivation or inhibition of one drug on another will be listed here.

The ***third and primary area*** is **COMPATIBLE WITH.** It is further divided into **Additive, Syringe, and Y-site.** In this section you will find the statement ***Consult pharmacist; specific conditions may apply; see Compatibilities, p. xvi.*** Because compatibilities may be influenced by many factors (e.g., temperature, pH, concentration, time together in solution, a specific order of mixing), **it is imperative that you verify compatibilities with your pharmacist.** Knowledge is growing daily in this field, and your pharmacist should have current information on the pharmacy computer or access to extensive references. Many compatibility studies have been done by other parties for both additive and Y-site compatibilities, and some studies have been done for syringe compatibilities. Almost all are based on specific concentrations, which may or may not relate to usual doses or recommended concentrations.

Occasionally sources disagree on compatibility. If there is conflicting information about a compatibility, you will be referred to the Incompatible With section or told that this is not recommended by the manufacturer, or ***the individual drugs that may have a conflict will be underlined.***

What steps should you consider before administering any drug?

- If the drug you wish to administer is not listed in the **Compatible With** section, ***consider it to be incompatible.*** To administer, you must turn off the infusing IV (at the stopcock or with a clamp close to the Y-site), flush the line with a solution compatible to both drugs (and/or solutions), administer the required drug, and flush the line again before turning the previously infusing IV back on. If you are unable to discontinue the infusion IV, you must have another IV access (e.g., a multi-lumen catheter, a second, IV line, or a heparin lock). Some drugs actually require separate tubing.
- If compatibilities are included in the package insert from the manufacturer, it will be so stated. If the manufacturer lists drugs as compatible by additive, syringe, or Y-site and doesn't list concentrations, this is a good assurance of compatibility. If concentrations are listed, review the concentrations of both drugs to make sure they are within the defined parameters.
- If the drug you wish to administer is listed in the **Compatible With** section of the access you wish to use (e.g., **additive, syringe, or Y-site),** ***you must consult with the pharmacist to confirm any specific conditions that may apply.*** After your consultation, write the results of your con-

sultation regarding the specific directions for co-administering drugs on the patient's medication record or nursing care plan so others will not need to retrace your research steps when the medication is to be given again.

- When combining drugs in a solution (additives), always consider the required rate adjustments of each drug. Can each drug produce the desired effect at the suggested rate, or is continuous adjustment necessary for one drug, making the combination impractical?
- Y-site means that the specific drug in a specific monograph is compatible at its Y-site with an injection or an infusion containing one of the drugs listed under Y-site. The reverse Y-site compatibility may not be true.
- Although some drugs may be listed as compatible at the Y-site, some drugs can be administered at the Y-site only if they are further diluted in compatible solutions and given as an infusion (e.g., potassium concentrates [e.g., acetates, chlorides, phosphates], saline solution in concentrations greater than 0.9% or NS, amino acids, and dextrose solutions greater than 10% [unless in small amounts such as 50 ml dextrose 50% in insulin-induced hypoglycemia]).
- Because today's hospital units are very specialized (e.g., cancer care, emergency room, intensive coronary care, various intensive care units, transplant units, and orthopedic units to name just a few), nursing staff in each of these areas most likely administer similar combinations of drugs to their patients. ***Take the initiative and research the drug combinations that are most frequently used on your unit. Then consult with the pharmacist and make your own compatibility chart for additives, Y-site, and syringe (if applicable).*** By creating a chart specific to your unit, you will limit the number of consults required with the pharmacist to combinations that fall outside of the parameters you have researched. This approach will save time for every nurse on your unit and will give each of you the necessary compatibility information to administer the IV drug combinations specific to your unit.
- The Solution Compatibility Chart on the inside back cover has been expanded and updated. Diluents that are not identified in Dilution will be listed in this chart.

Rate of Administration: Accepted rates of administration are clearly stated. As a general rule, a slow rate is preferred. 25-gauge needles aid in giving a small amount of medication over time. Problems with rapid or slow injection rates are indicated here. Adjusted rates for infants, children, or the elderly are listed when available. Charts are available in selected monographs.

Actions: Clear, concise statements outline the origin of each drug, how it affects body systems, its length of action, and methods of excretion. If a drug crosses the placental barrier or is secreted in breast milk, it will be mentioned here.

Indications and Uses: Uses recommended by the manufacturer are listed. Unlabeled uses are stated as such.

Contraindications: Contraindications are those specifically listed by the manufacturer. Consult with the physician if an ordered drug is contraindicated for the patient. The physician may have additional historical information that alters the situation or may decide that use of the drug is indicated in a critical situation.

Precautions: The section on precautions covers many areas of information needed before injecting any drug. The range covers all facets not covered under specific headings. There is no prioritizing; each listing is as important as the next. To make it easier for spot checks (after reading the entire monograph), additional subdivisions are now included.

Monitor: A subheading that includes information such as required prerequisites for drug administration, parameters for evaluation, and patient assessments.

Patient Education: A subheading that addresses only specific, important issues required for short-term IV use. It is expected that the health professional will always review the major points in the drug profile with any conscious patient, side effects to expect, how to cope with them, when to report them, special requirements such as the intake of extra fluids, and an overall review of what the drug does, why it is needed, and how long the patient can anticipate receiving it.

Maternal/Child: A subheading that addresses FDA pregnancy categories (see Appendix B for a complete explanation), any known specifics affecting patients capable of conception, safety for use during lactation, safety for use in children, and any special impact on infants and neonates.

Elderly: A subheading that is included whenever specific information impacting this patient group is available. Always consider age-related organ impairment (e.g., cardiac, hepatic, renal, insufficient bone marrow reserve), history of previous or concomitant disease or drug therapy, and route of excretion when determining dose and evaluating side effects.

Drug/Lab Interactions: Drug/drug or drug/lab interactions are listed here. If a conflict with the patient's drug profile is noted, consult a pharmacist immediately. Increasing or decreasing the effectiveness of a drug can be a potentially life-threatening situation. Check with the lab first on drug/lab interactions; acceptable alternatives are usually available. After this consultation, notify the physician if appropriate. To facilitate recognition, common trade names accompany generic names or examples are presented for drug categories. No other reference consistently provides this helpful information.

Side Effects: Alphabetical order simplifies confirmation that a patient's symptom could be associated with specific drug use. Specific symptoms of overdose are listed where available or distinct from usual doses.

Antidote: Specific antidotes are listed in this section. In addition, specific nursing actions to reverse undesirable side effects are clearly stated—an instant refresher course for critical situations.

Within a heading there may be references to other sections within an individual monograph (e.g., see Precautions, see Monitor, see Dose Adjustments, see Maternal/Child). These references indicate additional requirements and should be consulted before administering the drug.

Key to Abbreviations

<	less than
>	more than
¼NS	one-fourth normal saline (0.2%)
⅓NS	one-third normal saline (0.33%)
½NS	one-half normal saline (0.45%)
ACE	angiotensin converting enzyme
ACT	activated coagulation time
AIDS	acquired immune deficiency syndrome
ALT	(SGPT) alanine aminotransferase
aPTT	activated partial thromboplastin time
AST	(SGOT) aspartate aminotransferase
AUC	area under the curve
BP	blood pressure
BUN	blood urea nitrogen
BWFI	bacteriostatic water for injection
C	Celsius
Ca	calcium
CBC	complete blood cell count
CHF	congestive heart failure
Cl	chloride
CNS	central nervous system
CO_2	carbon dioxide
CPK	creatine-kinase
CrCl	creatinine clearance
CRT	controlled room temperature (20° to 25°C [68° to 77°F])
CSF	cerebrospinal fluid
C/S	culture and sensitivity
CVP	central venous pressure
D10NS	10% dextrose in normal saline
D10W	10% dextrose in water
D5/¼NS	5% dextrose in one-quarter NS (0.2%)
D5/⅓NS	5% dextrose in one-third normal saline (0.33%)
D5/½NS	5% dextrose in one-half normal saline (0.45%)
D5LR	5% dextrose in lactated Ringer's solution
D5NS	5% dextrose in normal saline
D5R	5% dextrose in Ringer's solution
D5W	5% dextrose in water
DC	discontinued
dl	deciliter(s) (100 ml)
DNA	deoxyribonucleic acid
ECG	electrocardiogram
EEG	electroencephalogram
F	Fahrenheit
GI	gastrointestinal
Gm	gram(s)
gr	grain(s)
gtt	drop(s)
GU	genitourinary

Hb	hemoglobin
Hct	hematocrit
Hg	mercury
HIV	human immunodeficiency virus
hr	hour
HR	heart rate
IgA	immune globulin A
ÍL	microliters, µL, mm^3
IM	intramuscular
IU	international unit(s)
IV	intravenously
K	potassium
KCl	potassium chloride
kg	kilogram(s)
L	liter(s)
lb	pound(s)
LDH	lactic dehydrogenase
LR	lactated Ringer's injection or solution
M	molar
M^2	meter squared
MAO	monoamine oxydase
mcg	microgram(s)
mCi	millicurie(s)
mEq	milliequivalent
Mg	magnesium
mg	milligram(s)
MI	myocardial infarction
min	minute
ml	milliliter
mmol	millimole(s)
mm^3	cubic millimeters, µL, ÍL
Na	sodium
NaCl	sodium chloride
ng	nanogram (millimicrogram)
NS	normal saline (0.9%)
NSAID	nonsteroidal antiinflammatory drug
NSR	normal sinus rhythm
N/V	nausea and vomiting
PaO_2	arterial oxygen pressure
PCA	patient controlled analgesia
pH	hydrogen ion concentration
PO	by mouth/orally
PSVT	paroxysmal supraventricular tachycardia
PT	prothrombin time
PTT	partial thromboplastin time
PVC	polyvinyl chloride
R	Ringer's injection or solution
RBC	red blood cell
refrigerate	temperature at 2° to 8°C (36° to 46°F)
RNA	ribonucleic acid
SC	subcutaneous

SrCr	serum creatinine
S/S	signs and symptoms
SW	sterile water for injection
TNA	3-in-1 combination of amino acids, glucose, and fat emulsion
TPN	2-in-1 combination of amino acids and glucose; total parenteral nutrition
TT	thrombin time
μL	microliters, mm^3, ÍL
VF	ventricular fibrillation
VS	vital signs
VT	ventricular tachycardia
WBC	white blood cell
WBCT	whole blood clotting time

Important IV Therapy Facts

- Read the Preface and Format and Contents sections at least once. They'll answer many of your questions and save time.

USUAL DOSE

- Doses calculated on body weight are usually based on pretreatment weight and not on edematous weight.
- Normal renal or hepatic function is usually required for drugs metabolized by these routes.
- Formula to calculate creatinine clearance (CrCl) from serum creatinine value:

  males: $$\frac{\text{Weight in kg} \times (140 - \text{age in years})}{72 \times \text{serum creatinine (mg/dl)}} = \text{CrCl}$$

  females: 0.85 × male CrCl value calculated from above formula.

  children: $$K \times \frac{\text{linear length or height (cm)}}{\text{SrCr (mg/100 ml)}}$$

  K for children >1 year of age=0.55
  K for infants=0.45
- Lean Body Weight (LBW)
  males=50 kg + 2.3 kg for each inch over 5 foot.
  females=45.5 kg + 2.3 kg for each inch over 5 foot.
  children weighing 15 kg or less—Use actual body weight in kg.

DILUTION

- Check all labels (drugs, diluents, and solutions) to confirm appropriateness for IV use.
- Sterile technique is imperative in all phases of preparation.
- Use a filter needle when withdrawing IV meds from ampoules to eliminate possible pieces of glass.
- Pearls: 1 Gm in 1 Liter yields 1 mg/ml
  1 mg in 1 Liter yields 1 mcg/ml
  % of a solution equals the number of grams/100 ml
  (5% = 5 Gm/100 ml)
- Pediatric dilution: If you dilute 6.0 mg/kg in 100 ml, 1 ml/hr equals 1.0 mcg/kg/min
  If you dilute 0.6 mg/kg in 100 ml, 1 ml/hr equals 0.1 mcg/kg/min
- See charts on inside front cover.
- Do not use bacteriostatic diluents containing benzyl alcohol for neonates. May cause a fatal toxic syndrome. S/S include CNS depression, hypotension, intracranial hemorrhage, metabolic acidosis, renal failure, respiratory problems, seizures.
- Ensure adequate mixing of all drugs added to a solution.
- When combining drugs in a solution (additives), always consider the required rate adjustment of each drug.
- Examine solutions for clarity and any possible leakage.
- Frozen infusion solutions should be thawed at room temperature (25° C [77° F]) or under refrigeration. Do not force by immersion in water baths or in the microwave. All ice crystals must be melted before administration. Do not refreeze.

- Syringe prepackaging for use in specific pumps is now available for many drugs. Concentrations are often the strongest permissible, but length of delivery is accurate.
- Controlled room temperature (CRT) is considered to be 25° C (77° F). Most medications tolerate variations in temperature from 15° to 30° C (59° to 86° F).

INCOMPATIBILITIES

- Some manufacturers routinely suggest discontinuing the primary IV for intermittent infusion; usually done to avoid any possibility of incompatibility. Flushing the line before and after administration may be indicated and/or appropriate for some drugs.
- The brand of intravenous fluids or additives, concentrations, containers, rate and order of mixing, pH, and temperature all affect solubility and compatibility. Consult your pharmacist with any question, and document appropriate instructions on care plan.

TECHNIQUES

- Never hang plastic containers in a series connection; may cause air embolism.
- Confirm patency of peripheral and/or central sites. Avoid extravasation.
- Avoid accidental arterial injection; can cause gangrene.

RATE OF ADMINISTRATION

- Life-threatening reactions (time-related overdose or allergy) are frequently precipitated by a too-rapid rate of injection.

PATIENT EDUCATION

- A well-informed patient is a great asset; review all appropriate drug information with every conscious patient.

SIDE EFFECTS

- Reactions may be caused by a side effect of the drug itself, allergic response, overdose, or the underlying disease process.

Resources

PUBLICATIONS

The following publications have been used as a resource to assemble the information found in *Intravenous Medications.* Additional and more detailed information on drugs may be found in these publications:

American Heart Association: *Handbook of Emergency Cardiovascular Care for Health Care Providers, 2002.*

American Hospital Formulary Service Drug Information 2003, Bethesda, Md, 2003, American Society of Hospital Pharmacists (updated via website).

Facts and comparisons, St Louis, 2003, Facts and Comparisons Division, JB Lippincott (updated monthly).

Fisher DS et al: *The cancer chemotherapy handbook,* ed 5, St Louis, 1997, Mosby.

The Johns Hopkins Hospital: *The Harriet Lane handbook,* ed 15, St Louis, 2000, Mosby.

Manufacturers' literature.

Merck manual of diagnosis and therapy, ed 17, Rahway NJ, 1996, Merck Research Laboratories.

Physician's Desk Reference, ed 57, Montvale NJ, 2003, Medical Economics.

Tatro DS, editor: *Drug interaction facts,* St Louis, 2003, Facts and Comparisons Division, JB Lippincott (updated quarterly).

Trissel LA: *Handbook on injectable drugs,* ed 12, 2003, American Society of Hospital Pharmacists, Inc.

United States Pharmacopeia: *Drug information for the health care professional,* ed 23, Rockville, Md, 2003, Micromedex (updated via website).

WEBSITE RESOURCES

http://www.fda.gov/cder/approval/index.htm—Drug Approvals
http://www.fda.gov/cder/ogd/rld/labeling_review_branch.html—Labeling
http://www.fda.gov/medwatch/safety.htm—Safety Information
http://evolve.elsevier.com/IVMeds

ABCIXIMAB

(ab-six′ih-mab)

Platelet aggregation inhibitor
Antithrombotic
Monoclonal antibody

ReoPro

pH 7.2

USUAL DOSE

Premedication: In all situations, premedication with histamine H_2 antagonists (e.g., famotidine [Pepcid], ranitidine [Zantac]) may be appropriate; prophylaxis should be considered when certain conditions are present (e.g., patients with HACA antibodies, readministration of abciximab).

Percutaneous coronary intervention: 0.25 mg/kg administered 10 to 60 minutes before percutaneous coronary intervention (PCI). Follow with a continuous infusion of 0.125 mcg/kg/min (weight adjusted) to a maximum of 10 mcg/min (non–weight adjusted) for 12 hours. Used concurrently with ***heparin*** and ***aspirin.*** Establish a separate IV site for heparin. The initial bolus of ***heparin*** is based on the results of the baseline ACT according to low-dose weight-adjusted guidelines in the following chart, but not exceeding a total bolus dose of 7,000 units.

Guidelines for Heparin Dosing

Low-Dose Weight-Adjusted Heparin (*Target ACT ≥200 seconds*)			Standard-Dose Weight-Adjusted Heparin (*Target ACT ≥300 seconds*)		
Initial Bolus	**ACT (sec)**	**Heparin**	**Initial Bolus**	**ACT (sec)**	**Heparin**
Not to exceed 7,000 units in patients >100 kg	<150	70 units/kg	Not to exceed 10,000 units in patients >100 kg	<150	100 units/kg
	150 to 199	50 units/kg		150 to 225	75 units/kg
	≥200	No heparin		226 to 299	50 units/kg
				≥300	No heparin
Additional bolus every 30 min or a 7-unit/kg/hr continuous infusion	<200	20 units/kg	Additional bolus every 30 min or a 10-unit/kg/hr continuous infusion	<275	50 units/kg
	≥200	No heparin		275 to 299	25 units/kg
				≥300	No heparin

Check ACT (Hemochron instrument used to measure) a minimum of 2 minutes after the initial and each additional heparin bolus. Give additional bolus doses of 20 units/kg until the target ACT of 200 seconds is achieved before PCI (a target ACT of up to 300 seconds using standard weight-adjusted doses of heparin has been used [see preceding chart] but may increase the risk of severe bleeding). During the procedure administer additional bolus doses every 30 minutes to maintain the target ACT. Alternately, after the target ACT is reached, a 7-unit/kg/hr continuous infusion may be administered with no further measurement of ACT for the duration of the procedure. Unless contraindicated, administer ***aspirin,*** 325 mg, 2 hours before PCI and once daily thereafter. At the completion of the procedure it is recommended that the heparin be discontinued and that removal of the sheath be accomplished within 6 hours; see Monitor for specific criteria. If prolonged therapy or later sheath removal is clinically indicated, do not discontinue heparin, but continue the 7 unit/kg/hr heparin infusion. Check the aPTT in 6 hours and adjust rate of heparin based on a target aPTT of 60 to 85 seconds. See Precautions/Monitor.

Unstable angina not responding to conventional medical therapy with planned PCI within 24 hours: ***Heparin*** is started before the abciximab; use a separate IV line. Maintain the aPTT between 60 and 85 seconds during the abciximab and heparin infusion period. Recent recommendations suggest that the low-dose weight-adjusted doses of heparin and anticoagulation guidelines described on p. 1 are also appropriate for the planned PCI in unstable angina. The recommended dose of abciximab is 0.25 mg/kg as an IV bolus followed by a continuous infusion of 10 mcg/min for a minimum of 18 hours up to a maximum of 26 hours (PCI usually accomplished between 18 and 24 hours). Discontinue abciximab 1 hour after the PCI (i.e., removal of guidewire). Unless contraindicated, administer at least 250 mg of ***aspirin*** at the time heparin is begun and aspirin 50 to 500 mg daily through day 30. Oral or IV nitroglycerin may also be indicated throughout the course of treatment. The process after the completion of the procedure is the same as in percutaneous coronary intervention.

DILUTION

Available in 5-ml vials (2 mg/ml). Solution must be clear. Must be filtered with a nonpyrogenic, low-protein binding 0.2- to 0.22-micron filter before administering the bolus and the infusion. Filtering of the infusion may be done during preparation or at administration, using the appropriate in-line filter. Do not shake.

IV injection: Bolus injection may be given undiluted.

Infusion: Withdraw desired dose and further dilute with NS or D5W (5 ml [10 mg] diluted with 250 ml NS or D5W equals 40 mcg/ml).

Storage: Refrigerate before use. Do not freeze. Check expiration date on vial. Contains no preservative; discard any unused portion.

COMPATIBILITY

According to the manufacturer, no incompatibilities have been shown with IV fluids or commonly used cardiovascular drugs; however, administration through a separate IV line and not mixing with other medications is recommended. No incompatibilities observed with glass bottles or polyvinyl chloride bags and administration sets.

RATE OF ADMINISTRATION

IV injection: An initial dose as a bolus injection; filter at this point if not done when withdrawing from vial.

Infusion: See Usual Dose. Must be administered through an in-line, nonpyrogenic, low-protein-binding filter (0.2 or 0.22 microns), if not done during preparation, and controlled by a continuous infusion pump. A 40-mcg/ml solution (10 mg in 250 ml) at a rate of 10.5 ml/hr will deliver 7 mcg/min, and 15 ml/hr will deliver 10 mcg/min. Discard unused portion at the end of the infusion.

ACTIONS

The fab fragment of the chimeric human-murine monoclonal antibody, abciximab binds to the glycoprotein GPIIb/IIIa receptor of human platelets and produces rapid dose-dependent inhibition of platelet function. It inhibits platelet aggregation by preventing the binding of fibrinogen, von Willebrand factor, and other adhesive molecules to GPIIb/IIIa receptor sites on activated platelets. Inhibition of platelet function is temporary following a bolus dose, but can be sustained at greater than 80% by continuous IV infusion. Has prevented acute thrombosis and resulted in lower rates of thrombosis as compared to aspirin and/or heparin. Initial half-life is 10 minutes. Second phase half-life is 30 minutes. A bolus dose followed by an infusion produces approximately constant free plasma concentrations throughout the infusion. Median bleeding time increases to over 30 minutes as contrasted to a baseline average of 5 minutes before administration. After the infusion is ended, free plasma concentration falls rapidly for 6 hours, then more slowly. Platelet function generally recovers gradually over 48 hours. In most patients, bleeding time returns to less than 12 minutes within 12 to 24 hours. Some abciximab remains in the circulation for 15 days or more.

INDICATIONS AND USES

An adjunct to PCI for the prevention of cardiac ischemic complications in patients undergoing PCI and in patients with unstable angina not responding to conventional medical therapy when PCI is planned within 24 hours. Abciximab use in patients not undergoing PCI has not been studied. Used concurrently with aspirin and heparin. In selected situations, clopidogrel (Plavix) or ticlopidine (Ticlid) may also be used concurrently.

Unlabeled uses: Combined with low-dose alteplase or low-dose reteplase in the early treatment of acute MI. ■ Treatment of acute ischemic stroke.

CONTRAINDICATIONS

Active internal bleeding, administration of oral anticoagulants (e.g., warfarin [Coumadin]) within 7 days unless PT is at or less than 1.2 times control, aneurysm, arteriovenous malformation, bleeding diathesis, clinically significant GI or GU bleeding within 6 weeks, history of CVA within 2 years, history of CVA with significant residual neurologic deficit, history of vasculitis (presumed or documented), hypertension (severe and uncontrolled), intracranial neoplasm, known hypersensitivity to any component of abciximab or to murine proteins, major surgery or trauma within 6 weeks, thrombocytopenia (less than 100,000/mm^3), or the use of IV dextran before PCI or intent to use it during PCI.

PRECAUTIONS

Administered only in the hospital under the direction of a physician knowledgeable in its use and with appropriate diagnostic, laboratory, and surgical facilities available. ■ Frequently causes major bleeding complications (e.g., retroperitoneal bleeding, spontaneous GI and GU bleeding, bleeding at the arterial access site). ■ Incidence of major bleeding was reduced in clinical trials that used weight-adjusted dosing of abciximab and low-dose weight-adjusted doses of heparin, with adherence to stricter anticoagulation guidelines and early sheath removal. This was true in patients weighing less than 75 kg (165 lb) that had increased incidences of bleeding with standard weight-adjusted heparin doses. ■ Incidence of major bleeding is increased in patients with a history of prior GI disease, those over 65 years of age, and those receiving thrombolytics (e.g., alteplase

[tPA], anistreplase [Eminase], reteplase [rPA], streptokinase). Consider if benefits will outweigh risks, and proceed with extreme caution if use is considered necessary. ■ Incidence of major bleeding is also increased if PCI occurs within 12 hours of the onset of symptoms of an acute MI, if the PCI procedure is prolonged (lasting more than 70 minutes), or if PCI procedure fails. ■ Extreme care must be taken in accessing the femoral artery for femoral sheath placement. Only the anterior wall of the femoral artery should be punctured (use of a single-walled needle versus double-walled [Seldinger through and through technique] is important). If both walls are punctured, massive bleeding could occur. ■ Avoid concurrent sheath placement in the femoral vein if possible (sometimes used to access right coronary artery or administer large amounts of medication). ■ Use of heparin concurrently also increases the risk of bleeding. ■ Anaphylaxis can occur at any time (a protein solution). Emergency drugs and equipment must always be available. In addition, use may result in the formation of human anti-chimeric antibody (HACA). Can cause hypersensitivity reactions including anaphylaxis, thrombocytopenia, or diminished benefit if abciximab is readministered at another time or other monoclonal antibodies are administered. Consider premedication as outlined under Usual Dose. ■ See Drug/Lab Interactions.

Monitor: Before initiating, obtain results of baseline CBC, platelet count, PT, ACT, and aPTT. Type and cross-match would also be appropriate. ■ Monitor heparin anticoagulation (ACT or aPTT) and PT closely. ■ While a femoral sheath is in place, the patient must be on strict bed rest, head of the bed should be less than 30°, and the appropriate limb(s) restrained in a straight position. Monitor sheath insertion site(s) and distal pulses of affected leg(s) frequently while sheath is in place and for 6 hours after removal. Measure any hematoma and monitor for enlargement. ■ Monitor platelet count 2 to 4 hours following the bolus dose and at 24 hours or before discharge, whichever is first. More frequent monitoring may be indicated. ■ Monitor patient carefully and frequently for signs of bleeding; take vital signs (avoiding automatic BP cuffs), observe any invaded sites at least every 15 minutes (e.g., sheaths, IV sites, cutdowns, punctures, Foleys, NGs); watch for hematuria, hematemesis, bloody stool, petechiae, hematoma, flank pain, muscle weakness; and do neuro checks every hour. Continue until clotting functions move toward normal. ■ Use care in handling patient; avoid arterial puncture, venipuncture, and IM injection. Use extreme precautionary methods and only compressible sites if these procedures are absolutely necessary. Apply pressure for 30 minutes to any invaded site and then apply pressure dressings. Saline or heparin locks are suggested to facilitate blood draws. ■ Discontinue heparin at least 2 to 4 hours before femoral sheath(s) are to be removed. Sheath removal should not occur until aPTT at or less than 50 seconds or ACT at or less than 175 seconds (approaching normal limits). Discontinue heparin after PCI, and remove sheath no sooner than 2 hours and no later than 6 hours after heparin is discontinued and while the abciximab is still infusing (aPTT must be at or less than 50 seconds or ACT at or less than 175 seconds). After removal, apply pressure to the femoral artery for at least 30 minutes. When hemostasis is confirmed, apply a pressure dressing. Maintain strict bed rest for at least 6 to 8 hours after sheath removal and/or abciximab is discontinued or 4 hours after heparin is discontinued, whichever is later. ■ Throughout process medicate as needed for back or groin pain and nausea or vomiting. ■ Remove pressure dressing before ambulation. ■ If complications arise that indicate the need for surgery within 48 to 72 hours of treatment with abciximab, an Ivy bleeding time should be obtained. Platelet function may be partly restored with platelet transfusions. ■ See Precautions, Drug/Lab Interactions, and Antidote.

Patient Education: Compliance with all measures to minimize bleeding (e.g., strict bed rest, positioning) is imperative. ■ Avoid use of razors, toothbrushes, and other sharp items. ■ Use caution while moving to avoid excessive bumping. ■ Report all episodes of bleeding and apply local pressure if indicated. ■ Expect oozing from IV sites.

Maternal/Child: Category C: use only if clearly needed and with extreme caution. ■ Safety for use during breast-feeding not established. Not known if it is secreted in breast milk; use extreme caution; probably best to postpone breast-feeding until bleeding time approaches normal. ■ Safety and effectiveness for use in children not established. Incidence of side effects may be increased with a weight under 75 kg.

Elderly: Increased risk of major bleeding complications if weight less than 75 kg or age over 65 years; see Precautions. ■ Consider age-related organ impairment; may also increase risk of bleeding.

DRUG/LAB INTERACTIONS

Use with extreme caution with other drugs that affect hemostasis (e.g., thrombolytics [e.g., alteplase (tPA), anistreplase (Eminase), streptokinase, urokinase], oral anticoagulants [e.g., warfarin (Coumadin)], NSAIDs [e.g., ibuprofen (Advil, Motrin), naproxen (Aleve, Naprosyn)], clopidogrel [Plavix], dipyridamole [Persantine], ticlopidine [Ticlid], selected antibiotics [e.g., cefamandole, cefoperazone, cefotetan, ticarcillin]). ■ Dextran solutions increased the risk of major bleeding events when used concurrently with abciximab; see Contraindications. ■ HACA titer may precipitate an acute hypersensitivity reaction with other diagnostic or therapeutic monoclonal antibodies (e.g., muromonab CD3).

SIDE EFFECTS

May cause major bleeding incidents (e.g., femoral artery or other access site, intracranial hemorrhage, spontaneous gross hematuria and other GU bleeds, spontaneous hematemesis and other GI bleeds, retroperitoneal bleeding). Decreases in hemoglobin greater than 5 Gm/dl or intracranial hemorrhage were defined as major during trials. Thrombocytopenia is common and may require platelet transfusion. Abdominal pain, back pain, bradycardia, chest pain, headache, hypotension, nausea, peripheral edema, positive HACA response, puncture site pain, and vomiting may occur. Other side effects that may occur are anemia, arrhythmias (e.g., atrial fibrillation/flutter, bradycardia, complete AV block, supraventricular tachycardia, ventricular PVCs, tachycardia, or fibrillation), confusion, hyperesthesia, intermittent claudication, leukocytosis, limb embolism, pericardial effusion, pleural effusion or pleurisy, pneumonia, pulmonary embolism, pulmonary edema, and visual disturbances. Anaphylaxis has not been reported but may occur.

ANTIDOTE

Stop the infusions of abciximab and heparin if any serious bleeding not controllable with pressure occurs. Stop infusion in patients with failed PCIs. Stop infusion if a hypersensitivity reaction occurs and treat with epinephrine, dopamine (Intropin), theophylline, antihistamines (e.g., diphenhydramine [Benadryl]), and/or corticosteroids as indicated.

Keep physician informed. If an acute platelet decrease occurs (less than 100,000/mm^3 or a decrease of at least 25% from pretreatment value), obtain additional platelet counts in separate tubes containing ethylenediaminetetraacetic acid (EDTA), citrate, or heparin. This is to exclude pseudothrombocytopenia due to anticoagulant interaction. If true thrombocytopenia is verified, discontinue abciximab immediately. Platelet transfusions may be required. Heparin and aspirin should also be avoided if the platelet count drops below 60,000/mm^3.

ACETAZOLAMIDE SODIUM

(a-set-a-zole′a-mide so′de-um)

Antiglaucoma
Anticonvulsant
Diuretic
Urinary alkalinizer

Diamox **pH 9.2**

USUAL DOSE

Antiglaucoma agent: 250 mg to 1 Gm/24 hr. May be given as 250-mg doses at 4- to 6-hour intervals. To rapidly lower intraocular pressure, give initial single dose of 500 mg followed by 125 to 250 mg at 4-hour intervals. **Edema of congestive heart failure or drug therapy:** 250 to 375 mg or 5 mg/kg of body weight as a single dose daily; when loss of edematous fluid stops, reduce to every other day or give for 2 days followed by a day of rest. **Anticonvulsant:** ***Adults and children:*** Dose in epilepsy may range from 8 to 30 mg/kg/24 hr in divided doses every 6 to 12 hours. Reduce initial daily dose when given with other anticonvulsants.

Urinary alkalinization: ***Adults and children:*** 5 mg/kg/dose every 8 to 12 hours.

PEDIATRIC DOSE

Acute antiglaucoma agent: 5 to 10 mg/kg every 6 hours.

Edema of congestive heart failure or drug therapy: 5 mg/kg as a single dose daily or every other day; see comment under Usual Dose.

Slowly progressive hydrocephalus in infants 2 weeks to 10 months: 25 mg/kg/24 hr in equally divided doses every 8 hours (8.3 mg/kg every 8 hours). Up to 100 mg/kg/24 hr or a maximum dose of 2 Gm/24 hr has been used.

DOSE ADJUSTMENTS

Reduced dose required when introducing acetazolamide into a treatment regimen with other anticonvulsants.

DILUTION

Each 500 mg should be diluted in 5 ml SW. May then be given by IV injection or added to standard IV fluids.

Storage: Use within 24 hours of dilution.

COMPATIBLE WITH

(Underline Indicates Conflicting Compatibility Information)

Consult pharmacist; specific conditions may apply; see Compatibilities, p. xvi.

Additive: Cimetidine (Tagamet), ranitidine (Zantac).

Y-site: Diltiazem (Cardizem).

RATE OF ADMINISTRATION

500 mg or fraction thereof over at least 1 minute or added to IV fluids to be given over 4 to 8 hours.

ACTIONS

A potent carbonic anhydrase inhibitor and nonbacteriostatic sulfonamide, acetazolamide depresses the tubular reabsorption of sodium, potassium, and bicarbonate. Excreted unchanged in the urine, producing diuresis, alkalinization of the urine, and a mild degree of metabolic acidosis.

INDICATIONS AND USES

Glaucoma. ■ Epilepsy. ■ Urine alkalinization to treat toxicity of weakly acidic medications (e.g., phenobarbital, lithium, salicylates). See Drug/Lab Interactions. ■ No longer the drug of choice for congestive heart failure or drug-induced edema (e.g., steroids). ■ Used orally for acute mountain sickness and hypokalemia/hyperkalemia of familial periodic paralysis.

Unlabeled uses: Prevention or treatment of alkalosis following open-heart surgery, treatment of acute pancreatitis and gastric ulcers (inhibits pancreatic and gastric secretions).

CONTRAINDICATIONS

Depressed sodium and potassium levels, hyperchloremic acidosis, marked kidney or liver disease, adrenocortical insufficiency, hypersensitivity to acetazolamide or any of its components. Long-term use contraindicated in some glaucomas.

PRECAUTIONS

Chemically related to sulfonamides; may cause serious reactions in sensitive patients. ■ May be alternated with other diuretics to achieve maximum effect. ■ Greater diuretic action is achieved by skipping a day of treatment rather than increasing dose; failure in therapy may be due to overdose or too-frequent dosage. ■ Administration by IV injection is preferred. ■ Use with caution in impaired respiratory function (e.g., pulmonary disease, edema, infection, obstruction); may cause severe respiratory acidosis. ■ Potassium excretion is proportional to diuresis. Hypokalemia may result from diuresis or with severe cirrhosis. ■ Introduce or withdraw gradually when used as an anticonvulsant.

Monitor: Obtain baseline CBC and platelet count before use and monitor during therapy.

Patient Education: Consider birth control options.

Maternal/Child: Category D: avoid pregnancy; may cause premature delivery and congenital anomalies. ■ Discontinue breast-feeding or discontinue acetazolamide. ■ Safety for use in children not established, but no problems are documented.

Elderly: Use caution; no documented problems, but age-related renal impairment may be a factor.

DRUG/LAB INTERACTIONS

May cause hypokalemia with concurrent use of steroids. ■ Hypokalemia may cause toxicity and fatal cardiac arrhythmias with digitalis or interfere with insulin or oral antidiabetic agent response, thus causing hyperglycemia. ■ Alkalinization of urine potentiates amphetamines, ephedrine, flecainide (Tambocor), methenamine, procainamide, pseudoephedrine (Sudafed), quinidine, and tricyclic antidepressants (e.g., amitriptyline [Elavil]) by decreasing rate of excretion. ■ May decrease response to lithium, methotrexate, some antidepressants, phenobarbital, salicylates, and urinary antiinfectives by increasing rate of excretion. ■ Metabolic acidosis induced by acetazolamide may potentiate salicylate toxicity (anorexia, tachypnea, lethargy, coma, and death can occur with high-dose aspirin). ■ Alkalinity may cause false-positive urinary protein and possibly urinary steroid tests. ■ May depress iodine uptake by the thyroid.

SIDE EFFECTS

Minimal with short-term therapy. Respond to symptomatic treatment or withdrawal of drug: acidosis, anorexia, bone marrow depression, confusion, crystalluria, drowsiness, fever, hemolytic anemia, hypokalemia (ECG changes, fatigue, muscle weakness, vomiting), paresthesias, photosensitivity, polyuria, rash, renal calculus, thrombocytopenic purpura.

ANTIDOTE

Notify physician of any adverse effects and discontinue drug if necessary. Treat allergic reactions as indicated.

ACYCLOVIR

Antiviral

(ay-sye′kloe-ver)

Zovirax

pH 10.5 to 11.6

USUAL DOSE

In all situations for adults, adolescents, children, and neonates, do not exceed a maximum dose of 20 mg/kg every 8 hours.

Adults and adolescents (12 years of age and older):

Herpes simplex infections; Mucosal and cutaneous HSV infections in immunocompromised patients: 5 mg/kg of body weight every 8 hours for 7 days.

Severe initial clinical episodes of herpes genitalis: 5 mg/kg every 8 hours for 5 days.

Herpes simplex encephalitis: 10 mg/kg every 8 hours for 10 days.

Varicella zoster infections (shingles) in immunocompromised patients: 10 mg/kg every 8 hours for 7 days.

PEDIATRIC DOSE

Children under 12 years of age:

Herpes simplex infections; Mucosal and cutaneous HSV infections in immunocompromised patients: 10 mg/kg every 8 hours for 7 days.

Severe initial clinical episodes of herpes genitalis: 250 mg/M^2 every 8 hours for 5 days.

Herpes simplex encephalitis: ***Children over 3 months of age:*** 20 mg/kg every 8 hours for 10 days.

Varicella zoster infections (shingles) in immunocompromised patients: 20 mg/kg every 8 hours for 7 days.

NEONATAL DOSE

Neonatal herpes simplex virus infections: ***Birth to 3 months:*** 10 mg/kg every 8 hours for 10 days. Doses of 15 mg/kg to 20 mg/kg every 8 hours have been used; safety and efficacy have not been established.

DOSE ADJUSTMENTS

Calculate dose by ideal body weight in obese individuals. ■ Reduced dose may be indicated in the elderly based on the potential for decreased renal function. ■ In adults and children with impaired renal function, reduce dose and/or adjust dosing interval based on CrCl as indicated in the chart below.

Acyclovir Dosage Adjustments for Adults and Children With Renal Impairment		
Creatinine Clearance (ml/min per 1.73 m^2)	Percent of Recommended Dose	Dosing Interval (hours)
>50	100%	8
25-50	100%	12
10-25	100%	24
0-10	50%	24

Plasma concentrations decrease with hemodialysis; adjustment of the dosing schedule is recommended so that an additional dose is administered after each dialysis. No supplemental dose is indicated in peritoneal dialysis after adjustment of the dosing interval.

DILUTION

Initially dissolve each 500 mg with 10 ml SW for injection (1,000 mg with 20 ml). Concentration equals 50 mg/ml. Do not use bacteriostatic water for injection (BWFI); will cause precipitation. Shake well to dissolve completely. Withdraw the desired dose and further dilute in an amount of solution to provide a concentration less than 7 mg/ml (70-kg adult at 5 mg/kg equals 350 mg dissolved in a total of 100 ml of solution equals 3.5 mg/ml). Compatible with most standard electrolyte and glucose infusion solutions. Use reconstituted solution within 12 hours; high pH may result in etching of glass vial surface after 12 hours.

Storage: Use solution fully diluted for administration within 24 hours. Manufacturer will supply data showing stability for longer periods under specific conditions.

INCOMPATIBLE WITH

Bacteriostatic water for injection (BWFI). Dilution in biologic or colloidal fluids (e.g., blood products, protein solutions) is not recommended.

COMPATIBLE WITH **(Underline Indicates Conflicting Compatibility Information)**

Consult pharmacist; specific conditions may apply; see Compatibilities, p. xvi.

Additive: Fluconazole (Diflucan), meropenem (Merrem IV).

Y-site: Allopurinol (Aloprim, Zyloprim), amikacin (Amikin), amphotericin B cholesteryl (Amphotec), ampicillin, cefamandole (Mandol), cefazolin (Kefzol), cefoperazone (Cefobid), cefotaxime (Claforan), cefoxitin (Mefoxin), ceftazidime (Fortaz), ceftizoxime (Cefizox), ceftriaxone (Rocephin), cefuroxime (Zinacef), chloramphenicol (Chloromycetin), cimetidine (Tagamet), cisatracurium (Nimbex), clindamycin (Cleocin), dexamethasone (Decadron), diltiazem (Cardizem), dimenhydrinate (Dinate), diphenhydramine (Benadryl), docetaxel (Taxotere), doxorubicin liposome (Doxil), doxycycline (Vibramycin), erythromycin lactobionate (Erythrocin), etoposide phosphate (Etopophos), famotidine (Pepcid IV), filgrastim (Neupogen), fluconazole (Diflucan), gatifloxacin (Tequin), gentamicin (Garamycin), granisetron (Kytril), heparin, hydrocortisone sodium succinate (Solu-Cortef), hydromorphone (Dilaudid), imipenem-cilastatin (Primaxin), linezolid (Zyvox), lorazepam (Ativan), magnesium sulfate, melphalan (Alkeran), meperidine (Demerol), meropenem (Merrem IV), methylprednisolone (Solu-Medrol), metoclopramide (Reglan), metronidazole (Flagyl IV), morphine, multivitamins, nafcillin (Nafcil), oxacillin (Bactocill), paclitaxel (Taxol), penicillin G potassium, pentobarbital (Nembutal), perphenazine (Trilafon), piperacillin (Pipracil), potassium chloride (KCl), propofol (Diprivan), ranitidine (Zantac), remifentanil (Ultiva), sodium bicarbonate, sulfamethoxazole-trimethoprim (Bactrim), tacrolimus (Prograf), teniposide (VM-26, Vumon), theophylline, thiotepa (Thioplex), ticarcillin (Ticar), tobramycin (Nebcin), vancomycin (Vancocin), zidovudine (AZT, Retrovir).

RATE OF ADMINISTRATION

A single dose must be administered at a constant rate over 1 hour as an infusion. Renal tubular damage will occur with too-rapid rate of injection. Acyclovir crystals will occlude renal tubules. Use of an infusion pump or microdrip (60 gtt/ml) recommended.

ACTIONS

An antiviral agent that inhibits DNA replication in viruses (e.g., herpes simplex virus, varicella zoster virus, Epstein-Barr virus, and cytomegalovirus). Onset of action is prompt and therapeutic levels maintained for 8 hours. Widely distributed in tissues and body fluids. Excreted in the urine. Crosses placental barrier. Secreted in breast milk.

INDICATIONS AND USES

Treatment of initial and recurrent mucosal and cutaneous herpes simplex (HSV-1 and HSV-2) infections in immunosuppressed patients. ■ Severe initial clinical episodes of herpes genitalis in immunocompetent patients. ■ Herpes simplex encephalitis in patients over 3 months of age. ■ Neonatal herpes simplex virus infections. ■ Varicella zoster infections (shingles) in immunocompromised patients. ■ Oral acyclovir is used to treat varicella zoster (chickenpox).

Unlabeled uses: Cytomegalovirus and HSV infection after bone marrow or renal transplantation. ■ Disseminated primary eczema herpeticum. ■ Varicella pneumonia. ■ Various herpes simplex infections (e.g., erythema multiforme, ocular, proctitis).

CONTRAINDICATIONS

Hypersensitivity to acyclovir or ganciclovir.

PRECAUTIONS

Confirm diagnosis of herpes simplex virus (HSV-1 or HSV-2) through laboratory culture. Initiate therapy as quickly as possible after symptoms identified. ■ For IV use only; avoid IM or SC injection. ■ Use caution in patients with underlying neurologic abnormalities, those with serious renal, hepatic, or electrolyte abnormalities, or significant hypoxia. ■ Use caution in patients receiving interferon or intrathecal methotrexate, or with patients who have had previous neurologic reactions to cytotoxic drugs. ■ Incidence of CNS adverse events may be more common in the elderly or in patients with decreased renal function.

Monitor: Maintain adequate hydration and urine flow before and during infusion. Encourage fluid intake of 2 to 3 L/day. ■ Monitor renal function; abnormal renal function (decreased CrCl can occur), concomitant use of other nephrotoxic drugs, preexisting renal disease, and dehydration make further renal impairment with acyclovir more likely. ■ Confirm patency of vein; will cause thrombophlebitis. Rotate site of infusion.

Patient Education: Virus remains dormant and can still spread to others. ■ Avoid sexual intercourse when visible herpes lesions are present. Use condoms routinely.

Maternal/Child: Category B: use during pregnancy only if benefits outweigh risk to fetus. ■ Breast milk concentrations can be higher than maternal serum concentrations. Discontinue breast-feeding or evaluate very carefully. ■ 10 mg/kg and 20 mg/kg doses in children from 3 months to 16 years achieved concentrations similar to those in adults receiving 5 mg/kg to 10 mg/kg.

Elderly: Effectiveness is similar to younger adults. ■ Plasma concentrations are higher in the elderly compared to younger adults; may be due to age-related changes in renal function. ■ Duration of pain after healing was longer in patients 65 years or older. ■ Incidence of side effects (e.g., CNS adverse events [coma, confusion, hallucinations, somnolence], dizziness, nausea, renal adverse events, vomiting) was increased. ■ See Dose Adjustments and Precautions.

DRUG/LAB INTERACTIONS

See Precautions. May cause neurotoxicity (e.g., severe drowsiness and lethargy) with zidovudine. ■ Side effects increased by other nephrotoxic drugs. ■ Potentiated by probenecid. ■ Synergistic effects with ketoconazole and interferon have been noted. Clinical importance not established. ■ In one case report, a patient stabilized on phenytoin and valproic acid experienced seizures and a reduction in antiepileptic drug serum concentrations when acyclovir was added to the regimen.

SIDE EFFECTS

Acute renal failure, aggressive behavior, agitation, angioedema, ataxia, coma, confusion, delirium, diaphoresis, disseminated intravascular coagulation (DIC), dizziness, encephalopathy, hallucinations, headache, hematuria, hemolysis, hives, hyperbilirubinemia, hypersensitivity reactions (e.g., anaphylaxis), hypotension, inflammation at injection site, lethargy, nausea, obtundation, phlebitis, rash, seizures, transient increased SrCr levels, tremors, vomiting. Some patients (fewer than 1%) may have abdominal pain, anemia, anorexia, anuria, chest pain, edema, fever, hemoglobinemia, hypokalemia, ischemia of digits, leukocytosis, lightheadedness, neutropenia, neutrophilia, pulmonary edema with cardiac tamponade, rigors, skin reactions (e.g., erythema multiforme, Stevens-Johnson syndrome, toxic epidermal necrolysis), thirst, thrombocytosis, thrombocytopenia.

ANTIDOTE

Notify physician of all side effects. Discontinue drug with onset of CNS side effects. Treatment will be symptomatic and supportive. Adequate hydration is indicated to prevent precipitation of acyclovir in the renal tubules. A 6-hour session of hemodialysis will reduce plasma acyclovir concentration by approximately 60%. Hemodialysis is indicated in patients with acute renal failure and anuria. Treat anaphylaxis and resuscitate as necessary.

ADENOSINE

(ah-den′oh-seen)

Antiarrhythmic
Diagnostic agent

Adenocard, Adenoscan

pH 4.5 to 7.5

USUAL DOSE

Conversion of acute paroxysmal supraventricular tachycardia (PSVT) (Adenocard): 6 mg initially. If supraventricular tachycardia not eliminated in 1 to 2 minutes, give 12 mg. A third dose of 12 mg may be given in 1 to 2 minutes if needed. Do not exceed 12 mg in any single dose. Patients with central lines may respond to lesser doses; peripheral lines usually require standard doses. See Dilution.

Do not administer a repeat dose to patients who develop a high-level block on one dose of adenosine.

Adenosine is not blocked by atropine. Digitalis, quinidine, beta-adrenergic blocking agents (e.g., atenolol, esmolol), calcium channel blocking agents (verapamil [Isoptin]), angiotensin-converting enzyme inhibitors (e.g., enalapril [Vasotec]), and other cardiac drugs can be administered without delay if indicated because of the short half-life of adenosine. Repeat episodes may be treated with adenosine or calcium channel blockers (e.g., diltiazem, verapamil).

Noninvasive diagnosis of coronary artery disease with thallium tomography (Adenoscan [unlabeled]): 140 mcg/kg/min (0.14 mg/kg/min) as a 6-minute continuous infusion. Inject thallium at 3 minutes. Dose should be based on total body weight. ■ See Drug/Lab Interactions.

PEDIATRIC DOSE

Conversion of acute paroxysmal supraventricular tachycardia (PSVT) in children weighing less than 50 kg (Adenocard): 0.05 to 0.1 mg/kg. May increase dose by 0.05 mg/kg increments every 2 min until PSVT terminated or maximum dose reached (0.3 mg/kg or 12 mg). AHA guidelines recommend 0.1 mg/kg rapid IV push. Follow each dose with 5 ml NS flush. Double to 0.2 mg/kg if a second dose is required. Maximum first dose 6 mg. Maximum second dose and maximum single dose is 12 mg. ■ See comments in Usual Dose.

Children weighing more than 50 kg: Same as Usual Dose.

DOSE ADJUSTMENTS

Metabolism of adenosine is independent of hepatic or renal function. No dose adjustment indicated. ■ See Drug/Lab Interactions; alternative therapy (e.g., calcium channel blockers) may be indicated.

DILUTION

Solution must be clear; do not use if discolored or particulate matter present.

Conversion of acute PSVT (Adenocard): Give undiluted directly into a vein. If given into an IV line, use the closest port to the insertion site and follow with a rapid NS flush (+/– 50 ml) to be certain the solution reaches the systemic circulation. Discard unused portion.

Pharmacologic stress testing (Adenoscan): Dilute a single dose in sufficient NS to distribute over 6 minutes.

Storage: Store at room temperature; refrigeration will cause crystallization. If crystals do form, dissolve by warming to room temperature.

COMPATIBLE WITH

Consult pharmacist; specific conditions may apply; see Compatibilities, p. xvi.
Y-site: ***Adenocard:*** Specific information not available; see Dilution.
Adenoscan: Thallium.

RATE OF ADMINISTRATION

Conversion of acute PSVT (Adenocard): Must be given as a rapid bolus IV injection over 1 to 2 seconds. Follow each dose with NS flush; see Dilution.

Pharmacologic stress testing (Adenoscan): See Usual Dose.

ACTIONS

A naturally occurring nucleoside present in all cells of the body. Has many functions. When given as a rapid IV bolus, adenosine has antiarrhythmic properties, slowing cardiac conduction (particularly at the AV node), and it restores sinus rhythm in patients with PSVT. When used as a diagnostic aid and given as a continuous infusion, adenosine acts as a vasodilator. Adenocard and Adenoscan have the same molecular structure, same solvent, diluent, and concentration. The difference in their actions is in the rate of administration; however, the FDA has approved Adenocard for converting PSVT and Adenoscan for pharmacologic stress testing. Effective within 1 minute. Half-life is estimated to be less than 10 seconds. Adenosine is salvaged immediately by erythrocytes and blood vessel endothelial cells and metabolized for natural uses throughout the body (regulation of coronary and systemic vascular tone, platelet function, lipolysis in fat cells, intracardiac conduction).

INDICATIONS AND USES

To convert acute paroxysmal supraventricular tachycardia (PSVT) to normal sinus rhythm; a first-line agent according to AHA. Includes PSVT associated with accessory bypass tracts (Wolff-Parkinson-White syndrome). Effective in up to 92% of patients. ■ To convert wide-complex tachycardia (even if tachycardia may respond to lidocaine). ■ Adjunct in diagnosis of atrial flutter or fibrillation.

Unlabeled uses: Noninvasive diagnosis of coronary artery disease with thallium tomography. (Results are similar to IV dipyridamole or exercise stress testing.) ■ Studies of the use of adenosine with BCNU as an adjuvant to treatment of brain tumors and in the prevention of myocardial reperfusion damage are under way.

CONTRAINDICATIONS

Atrial flutter or fibrillation and ventricular tachycardia (not effective in converting these arrhythmias to normal sinus rhythm [NSR]). ■ Known or suspected bronchospastic or bronchoconstrictive lung disease (e.g., asthma). ■ Known hypersensitivity to adenosine. ■ Symptomatic bradycardia, sick sinus syndrome, and second- or third-degree AV block unless a functioning artificial pacemaker is in place.

PRECAUTIONS

Absolutely confirm labeling for IV use. Do not use adenosine phosphate, which is for IM use in the symptomatic relief of varicose vein complications. ■ Valsalva maneuver may be used before use of adenosine in PSVTs if clinically appropriate. ■ Emergency resuscitation drugs and equipment must always be available. ■ Could produce bronchoconstriction in patients with asthma. ■ Considered the emerging drug of choice by many investigators, especially for terminating narrow-complex PSVT;

others limit use to hemodynamically stable patients who do not require direct-current cardioversion but do require rapid conversion to a normal sinus rhythm. Also used in patients who have not responded to cumulative doses of verapamil 10 mg IV or those with congestive heart failure, concomitant beta blockade, hypotension, or left ventricular dysfunction when verapamil is relatively contraindicated. ■ Some slowing of ventricular response may occur if atrial flutter or fibrillation is also present. ■ Use with caution in patients receiving digoxin or digoxin and verapamil in combination. Appropriate resuscitative measures should be available. ■ Adenosine will not terminate arrhythmias not caused by reentry involving the AV node but may clarify the diagnosis by producing a transient AV or ventriculoatrial block. ■ Patients with unstable angina may be at greater risk for major side effects. ■ During pharmacologic stress testing, women, heavy to obese patients, and younger patients may be at greater risk for side effects.

Monitor: ***Conversion of acute PSVT:*** Must reach systemic circulation; see Dilution. ■ ECG monitoring during administration recommended. Monitor BP. At the time of conversion to normal sinus rhythm, PVCs, PACs, sinus bradycardia, sinus tachycardia, skipped beats, and varying degrees of AV nodal block are seen on the ECG in many patients. Usually last only a few seconds and resolve without intervention. ■ Less likely to precipitate hypotension if arrhythmia does not terminate.

Pharmacologic stress testing: ECG monitoring during administration recommended. Monitor HR and BP at regular intervals during infusion. ■ Obtain images when infusion complete and redistribution images 3 to 4 hours later.

Maternal/Child: Category C: use in pregnancy only if clearly needed. Some references recommend avoiding early pregnancy. ■ Safety for use in pediatric patients not established, but has been used for conversion of PSVT in neonates, infants, children, and adolescents. Safety for use in pharmacologic stress testing in patients under 18 years not established.

Elderly: Response similar to that seen in younger patients; however, greater sensitivity of some older patients cannot be ruled out. May have diminished cardiac function, nodal dysfunction, concomitant disease, or drug therapy that may alter hemodynamic function and produce severe bradycardia or AV block.

DRUG/LAB INTERACTIONS

Effects antagonized by methylxanthines (e.g., caffeine, theophylline); larger doses may be required or adenosine may not be effective. ■ Potentiated by dipyridamole (Persantine); smaller doses of adenosine may be indicated. ■ Cardiovascular effects increased by nicotine; lower doses of adenosine may be indicated. ■ May produce a higher degree of heart block with carbamazepine (Tegretol). ■ Before using Adenoscan for pharmacologic stress testing, avoid, or withhold for at least 5 half-lives, adenosine antagonists (e.g., methylxanthines) and/or potentiators (e.g., dipyridamole, papaverine). ■ See Usual Dose.

SIDE EFFECTS

Generally predictable, short lived, and easily tolerated. Most will appear immediately and last less than 1 minute. Chest pressure, dizziness, dyspnea and/or shortness of breath, facial flushing, headache, lightheadedness, nausea, numbness, PACs, PVCs, sinus bradycardia, sinus tachycardia, skipped beats, varying degrees of AV nodal block. Less than 1% of patients complain of apprehension, blurred vision, burning, chest pain, head pressure, heavy arms, hyperventilation, hypotension, metallic taste, neck and back pain, palpitations, pressure in groin, sweating, tight throat, and tingling in arms.

Major: Arrhythmias (persistent), bronchospasm (severe), myocardial infarction, pulmonary edema, third-degree AV block. Asystole with fatal outcome has been reported.

ANTIDOTE

Notify physician of any side effect that lasts more than 1 minute. If a side effect persists, decrease rate of infusion (pharmacologic stress testing). With either use, for progression to a major side effect discontinue adenosine. Treat symptomatically if indicated. Bradycardia may be refractory to atropine. Short half-life generally precludes overdose problems, but aminophylline 50 to 125 mg as a slow infusion is a competitive antagonist. Resuscitate as necessary.

ALATROFLOXACIN MESYLATE

(ah-lat-troh-floks′ah-sin mes′uh-lat)

Trovan IV

Antibacterial
Fluoroquinolone

pH 3.5 to 4.3

USUAL DOSE

200 to 300 mg once every 24 hours. Dose and duration of treatment are based on degree of infection and specific diagnosis based on the chart below. Dose and serum levels similar by oral or IV route: no dose adjustment necessary. Transfer to oral dose as soon as practical. Oral dose form is trovafloxacin (Trovan).

Guidelines for Alatrofloxacin Dosing		
Infection/Location and Type	**Daily Unit Dose and Route of Administration**	**Total Duration**
Nosocomial pneumonia*	300 mg IV† followed by 200 mg oral	10-14 days
Community-acquired pneumonia	200 mg oral or 200 mg IV followed by 200 mg oral	7-14 days
Complicated intraabdominal infections, including postsurgical infections	300 mg IV† followed by 200 mg oral	7-14 days
Gynecologic and pelvic infections	300 mg IV† followed by 200 mg oral	7-14 days
Skin and skin structure infections, complicated, including diabetic foot infections	200 mg oral or 200 mg IV followed by 200 mg oral	10-14 days

*If *Pseudomonas aeruginosa* is a documented or presumptive pathogen, combination therapy with either an aminoglycoside or aztreonam may be clinically indicated.
†Reduce 300-mg IV dose to 200 mg as soon as clinically indicated.

DOSE ADJUSTMENTS

No dose reduction required in impaired renal function, severe renal deficiency (CrCl less than 20 ml/min), hemodialysis, or in the elderly. ■ Half-life is prolonged in impaired hepatic function and dose reduction is recommended in patients with mild to moderate cirrhosis based on the following chart. No data available for patients with severe cirrhosis.

Alatrofloxacin Guidelines for Dosing in Patients With Impaired Hepatic Function	
Indicated Dose (Normal Hepatic Function)	**Adjusted Dose (Chronic Hepatic Disease)**
300 mg IV	200 mg IV
200 mg IV or oral	100 mg IV or oral

DILUTION

Available in single-use vials. Withdraw desired dose (5 mg/ml) from vial. Each 100 mg must be further diluted with a minimum of 30 ml D5W, ½NS, D5/½NS, D5/¼NS, D5LR. Desired concentration is 1 to 2 mg/ml (see chart below). No preservatives; enter vial only once.

Guidelines for Dilution of Alatrofloxacin				
Dosage Strength (mg)	Volume to Withdraw (ml)	Diluent Volume (ml)	Total Volume (ml)	Infusion Concentration (mg/ml)
100 mg	20	30	50	2
100 mg	20	80	100	1
200 mg	40	60	100	2
200 mg	40	160	200	1
300 mg	60	90	150	2
300 mg	60	240	300	1

Storage: Vials stable until expiration date stored at 15° to 30° C (59° to 86° F). Protect from light. Do not freeze. Concentrations of diluted solutions between 0.5 and 2 mg/ml are stable in glass or PVC plastic containers for up to 7 days if refrigerated and for up to 3 days at CRT. Discard any unused portion of vial or diluted solution.

INCOMPATIBLE WITH

Do not dilute with NS or LR alone or in combination with other diluents; a precipitate may form. Do not administer in the same IV or through the same tubing as any solution containing multivalent cations (e.g., calcium, magnesium). Manufacturer recommends that alatrofloxacin be administered separately. Flush line with a compatible solution before and after administration. NS may be used for flushing the IV line.

COMPATIBLE WITH (Underline Indicates Conflicting Compatibility Information)

Consult pharmacist; specific conditions may apply; see Compatibilities, p. xvi.

Y-site: Amikacin (Amikin), cyclosporine (Sandimmune), dopamine (Intropin), droperidol (Inapsine), fentanyl (Sublimaze), gentamicin (Garamycin), hetastarch in electrolytes (Hextend), ketorolac (Toradol), lorazepam (Ativan), LR, <u>midazolam (Versed)</u>, nitroglycerin IV (Nitro-Bid IV), NS, ondansetron (Zofran), potassium chloride (KCl), propofol (Diprivan), sodium bicarbonate, tobramycin (Nebcin), vancomycin (Vancocin).

RATE OF ADMINISTRATION

A single dose must be equally distributed over 60 minutes as an infusion. Severe or life-threatening hypotension has occurred with recommended rate and with too-rapid infusion. May be given through a Y-tube or three-way stopcock of infusion set. Temporarily discontinue other solutions infusing at the same site and flush tubing with compatible solutions before and after alatrofloxacin. NS may be used to flush the IV line.

ACTIONS

A fourth-generation fluoroquinolone antibacterial agent. Has a unique spectrum of activity to a wide range of organisms including gram-positive, gram-negative, aerobic, anaerobic, and atypical microorganisms. Bactericidal through inhibition of DNA gyrase (an essential enzyme involved in synthesis, repair, recombination, and transposition of bacterial DNA) and topoisomerase IV (an enzyme key to the partitioning of DNA during bacterial cell division). Mechanism of fluoroquinolones differs from that of aminoglycosides, penicillins, cephalosporins, macrolides, and tetracyclines, and fluoroquinolones may be active against pathogens resistant to these antibiotics. There is no cross-resistance between fluoroquinolones and these other antibiotics. Alatrofloxacin is rapidly converted to trovafloxacin. Widely distributed into body tissues in concentrations higher than in plasma within 5 to 10 minutes of completion of a 1-hour infusion. Half-life is approximately 11 hours. Steady-state concentrations are achieved by the third daily dose. Metabolized by conjugation in the liver (effect of cytochrome P_{450} oxidative metabolism is minimal). No significant age or gender differences. Primarily excreted in bile through feces with some excretion in urine. Crosses the placental barrier. Secreted in breast milk.

INDICATIONS AND USES

Treatment of serious, life-threatening, or limb-threatening infections caused by susceptible strains of specific organisms (see literature for complete list). Used IV for respiratory tract infections (e.g., nosocomial or community-acquired pneumonia); complicated intraabdominal infections including postsurgical infections, gynecologic and pelvic infections (e.g., endomyometritis, parametritis, septic abortion, postpartum infections); complicated skin and skin structure infections, including diabetic foot infections.

CONTRAINDICATIONS

History of hypersensitivity to alatrofloxacin, trovafloxacin, any components of these products, or any other quinolone antimicrobial agents (e.g., ciprofloxacin [Cipro], levofloxacin [Levaquin], norfloxacin [Noroxin], ofloxacin [Floxin IV]). Not recommended for use when safer, alternative antimicrobial therapy would be effective.

PRECAUTIONS

For IV use only. ■ Trofloxacin and alatrofloxacin have been associated with serious liver injury (e.g., liver enzyme abnormalities, symptomatic hepatitis, jaundice, liver failure, and rare reports of acute hepatic necrosis with eosinophilic infiltration) leading to liver transplantation and/or death. Injury has occurred with both short- and long-term exposure and reexposure. Therapy exceeding 2 weeks has been associated with a significantly increased risk of liver injury. Use of these agents should be reserved for patients with serious, life-threatening or limb-threatening infections who receive their initial therapy in an inpatient setting with adequate laboratory and treatment facilities. These agents should not be used when safer, alternative antimicrobial therapy will be effective. ■ Culture and sensitivity studies indicated to determine susceptibility of the causative organism to alatrofloxacin. ■ Prolonged use may cause superinfection because of overgrowth of nonsusceptible organisms. ■ Use with caution in patients with known CNS disorders that predispose to seizures or alter seizure threshold (e.g., epilepsy, severe cerebral arteriosclerosis, concomitant drug therapy). Convulsions, toxic psychosis, increased intracranial pressure, and CNS stimulation (confusion, depression, hallucinations, insomnia, lightheadedness, nightmares, paranoia, restlessness, tremor) have been reported with quinolones. ■ Use caution in patients with impaired liver function; see Dose Adjustments and Side Effects. Safety and effectiveness in patients with severe cirrhosis (Child-Pugh class C) have not been studied. ■ Cross-resistance may occur with other fluoroquinolones, but some microorganisms resistant to other fluoroquinolones may be susceptible to alatrofloxacin. ■ Pseudomembranous colitis has been reported. May range from mild to life-threatening. Consider in patients that present with diarrhea during or after treatment with alatrofloxacin. ■ Ruptures of shoulder, hand, and/or Achilles tendons that required surgical repair or resulted in prolonged disability have been reported in patients receiving quinolones. ■ Prolongation of the QT interval on the ECG and infrequent cases of arrhythmia (including torsades de pointes) have been reported with the use of fluoroquinolones. The risk of arrhythmia may be reduced by avoiding their use in the presence of hypokalemia, significant bradycardia, cardiomyopathy, or concurrent treatment with class IA antiarrhythmic agents (e.g., quinidine, procainamide [Pronestyl]) or with class III antiarrhythmic agents (e.g., amiodarone [Cordarone], sotalol [Betapace]). ■ Not effective in the treatment of syphilis—antimicrobial treatment may mask symptoms; all patients with gonorrhea should have a serologic test for syphilis at the time of diagnosis. ■ Safety and effectiveness for the treatment of osteomyelitis have not been studied. ■ See Antidote.

Monitor: Hypersensitivity reactions, including anaphylaxis with the first or succeeding doses, have been reported in patients receiving quinolones, even in those without known hypersensitivity. Emergency equipment must always be available. ■ Obtain baseline CBC with differential and platelets and liver function tests (e.g., ALT, AST, alkaline phosphatase, bilirubin). ■ Monitor vital signs. ■ Life-threatening hypotension has been reported. Has occurred when given too rapidly and when given at the recommended rate. ■ Periodic monitoring of organ systems, including hematopoietic, hepatic, and renal, is recommended. ■ Monitor liver function tests in patients who develop S/S consistent with hepatic dysfunction (e.g., abdominal pain, anorexia, dark urine, fatigue, jaundice, pale stool, vomiting). ■ Monitor for S/S of pancreatitis (e.g., abdominal pain, increased serum amylase, nausea and/or vomiting). ■ Maintain adequate hydration to prevent concentrated urine throughout treatment. Other quinolones have formed crystals. ■ Monitor infusion site for inflammation and/or extravasation. ■ See Precautions, Drug/Lab Interactions, and Antidote.

Patient Education: Promptly report skin rash, difficult breathing or swallowing, swelling (e.g., lips, tongue, face), or any other hypersensitivity reaction. ■ Promptly report diarrhea; consult physician before taking any antidiarrhea medication (e.g., Imodium, Kaopectate, Pepto-Bismol). ■ Report any history of convulsions. ■ Promptly report abdominal pain, anorexia, dark urine, fatigue, jaundice, nausea, pale stool, or vomiting. ■ Promptly report skin eruptions. ■ Dizziness or lightheadedness may interfere with ambulation and motor coordination; request assistance for ambulation. Use caution in tasks that require alertness. ■ Drink fluids liberally. ■ Has low potential for photosensitivity, but it may occur; best to avoid excessive sunlight or artificial ultraviolet light. ■ Report tendon pain or inflammation promptly. ■ Additional instruction required with transfer to oral trovafloxacin. ■ See Precautions, Monitor, Drug/Lab Interactions, and Antidote.

Maternal/Child: Category C: safety for use in pregnancy not established; benefits must outweigh risks. Has caused skeletal malformations in rat fetuses. ■ Discontinue breast-feeding. ■ Safety for use in children and adolescents under 18 years of age not established. Quinolones have caused arthropathy and osteochondrosis in juvenile animals.

Elderly: No age-related differences noted.

DRUG/LAB INTERACTIONS

Concomitant administration with cimetidine may reduce alatrofloxacin renal clearance, but dose adjustment is not required. ■ Interactions with theophylline that occur with other quinolones have not been noted, but monitoring of theophylline levels may be indicated with concomitant use. ■ May enhance effects of warfarin (Coumadin). Monitor PT or INR periodically. ■ No dose adjustment required for either drug when alatrofloxacin is administered concomitantly with cyclosporine or digoxin. ■ Alatrofloxacin-induced hypotension may be potentiated by anesthetic agents. ■ Risk of CNS stimulation and seizures may be increased with concurrent use of NSAIDs (e.g., ibuprofen [Advil, Motrin], naproxen [Aleve, Naprosyn]). ■ See literature for additional drug/drug interactions on transfer to oral trovafloxacin. ■ See Precautions.

SIDE EFFECTS

Abdominal pain, diarrhea, dizziness, headache, increased liver function tests (e.g., ALT, AST, alkaline phosphatase, bilirubin), lightheadedness, nausea, pain at injection site, pruritus, rash, vaginitis, and vomiting have occurred in more than 1% of patients. Capable of numerous other reactions (e.g., photosensitivity) in less than 1% of patients.

Major: Allergic reactions (e.g., anaphylaxis, cardiovascular collapse, death, dyspnea, edema [facial, laryngeal, or pharyngeal], hypotension, shock); CNS stimulation (e.g., anxiety, confusion, depression, hallucinations, insomnia, restlessness, nightmares, paranoia, tremor), increased intracranial pressure, and toxic psychoses; hematopoietic changes (e.g., agranulocytosis, aplastic anemia, pancytopenia); hepatic dysfunction (e.g., abdominal pain, anorexia, dark urine; fatigue, pale stool, jaundice, vomiting); fever; rash, skin eruptions, and/or severe dermatologic reactions (e.g., toxic epidermal necrolysis, Stevens-Johnson syndrome). Serious hepatic dysfunction leading to liver transplantation and/or death; and symptomatic pancreatitis (e.g., abdominal pain, increased serum amylase, nausea and/or vomiting) have been reported. See Precautions. Pseudomembranous colitis and pain, inflammation, and ruptures of the shoulder, hand, and Achilles tendon have been reported in patients receiving quinolones.

ANTIDOTE

Keep physician informed of all side effects. Most minor side effects will be treated symptomatically or will resolve with continued dosing (e.g., dizziness, lightheadedness); monitor closely. Discontinue alatrofloxacin at the first sign of any major side effect or phototoxicity. Treat allergic reactions as indicated with epinephrine, airway management, oxygen, IV fluids, antihistamines (e.g., diphenhydramine [Benadryl]), corticosteroids (e.g., Solu-Cortef), and pressor amines (e.g., dopamine [Intropin]). Treat CNS symptoms as indicated; may require diazepam (Valium) for seizures. Oral vancomycin (Vancocin) or metronidazole (Flagyl) is the treatment of choice for antibiotic-related pseudomembranous colitis. Adequate hydration and supplementation of electrolytes and proteins usally indicated. Complete rest is indicated for an affected tendon until treatment is available. Maintain hydration in overdose. No specific antidote; not removed by hemodialysis. Maintain patient until drug is excreted and symptoms subside.

ALBUMIN (HUMAN)

(al-byoo′min)

Plasma volume expander (plasma protein fraction)

Albumarc, Albuminar-5 and -25, Albunex 5%, Albutein 5% & 25%, Buminate 5% & 25%, Normal Serum Albumin, Plasbumin-5, -20, and -25

pH 6.4 to 7.4

USUAL DOSE

Variable, depending on patient condition (e.g., presence of hemorrhage, hypovolemia, or shock, pulse, BP, hemoglobin and hematocrit, and amount of pulmonary or venous congestion present). Fluid and protein requirements and underlying condition determine the concentration of albumin used. 5% is usually indicated in hypovolemic patients, and 25% is appropriate when fluid and sodium intake should be minimized (e.g., cerebral edema, hypoproteinemia, pediatric patients). The initial dose is usually 12.5 to 25 Gm. Amount of 5% given may be increased to 0.5 Gm/lb of body weight (10 ml/lb) with careful monitoring of the patient. Available as 5% solution (5 Gm/100 ml) in 50-ml, 250-ml, 500-ml, and 1,000-ml vials; 20% solution in 100-ml vials; or 25% solution (25 Gm/100 ml) in 20-ml, 50-ml, and 100-ml vials. The maximum dose is 6 Gm/kg/24 hr or 250 Gm in 48 hours (250 Gm is equal to 5 liters of 5% or 1 liter of 25%). In the absence of active hemorrhage, the total dose usually does not exceed the normal circulating mass of albumin (e.g., 2 Gm/kg of body weight).

Hypoproteinemia (hypoalbuminemia): 50 to 75 Gm as a 25% solution. Repeat doses may be required in patients who continue to lose albumin.

Hypovolemia: 25 Gm as a 5% or 25% solution. May be repeated in 15 to 30 minutes if response inadequate. If 25% solution is used, additional fluids may be needed.

Burns: Electrolyte replacement and crystalloids (e.g., IV fluids) to maintain plasma volume are required in the first 24 hours. Then begin with 25 Gm and adjust as necessary to maintain albumin level from 2 to 3 Gm/dl.

Acute nephrosis or acute nephrotic syndrome: 25 Gm of a 25% solution with an appropriate diuretic daily for 7 to 10 days.

Hemodialysis: 25 Gm of a 25% solution.

Red blood cell resuspension: 20 to 25 Gm of a 25% solution/liter of RBCs.

Cardiopulmonary bypass: Achieve a plasma albumin of 2.5 Gm/dl and hematocrit concentration of 20% with either a 5% or 25% solution. Use crystalloids (IV fluids) as a pump prime.

PEDIATRIC DOSE

0.5 to 1 Gm/kg/dose. 25% solution is usually used in infants and children; ***do not use in preterm infants.*** Maximum dose 6 Gm/kg/24 hr or 250 Gm/48 hr.

Hypoproteinemia (hypoalbuminemia): 1 Gm/kg/dose.

Hypovolemia: 0.5 to 1 Gm/kg/dose. May be repeated in 15 to 30 minutes if response inadequate.

Hemolytic disease of the newborn: 1 Gm/kg (4 ml/kg) of 25% albumin. One source recommends giving 1 hour before exchange transfusion. Another recommends 1 to 2 hours before blood transfusion or with transfusion (exchange 50 ml of albumin 25% for 50 ml plasma). ***Do not use in preterm infants.***

Burns: See Usual Dose.

DILUTION

May be given undiluted or further diluted with NS, D5W, or D10W for infusion. NS is the preferred diluent. When sodium restriction is required, D5W may be substituted. The use of SW as a diluent is not recommended. Life-threatening hemolysis and acute renal failure can result if a sufficient volume of SW is used as a diluent. The 5% product is isotonic and osmotically approximates human plasma. One volume of 25% to four volumes of diluent is isotonic. Use only clear solutions.

Storage: Store at CRT. Use within 4 hours after opening. Discard unused portions.

INCOMPATIBLE WITH

Do not use SW as a diluent; see Dilution. Manufacturers state, "Do not mix with protein hydrolysates, amino acid mixtures, or solutions containing alcohol."

COMPATIBLE WITH

Consult pharmacist; specific conditions may apply; see Compatibilities, p. xvi.

Solution: Manufacturers state, "May be administered in conjunction with or combined with other parenterals such as whole blood, plasma, glucose, saline, or sodium lactate." Another adds, "Usual carbohydrate or electrolyte solutions."

Additive: Whole blood, plasma.

Y-site: Diltiazem (Cardizem), lorazepam (Ativan), packed RBCs, plasma, whole blood.

RATE OF ADMINISTRATION

Variable, depending on indication, present blood volume, patient response, and concentration of solution. Any rate greater than 10 ml/min may cause circulatory overload and pulmonary edema. Averages are:

Normal blood volume: 5%, 5 to 10 ml/min; 25%, 2 to 3 ml/min.

Deficient blood volume (hypovolemia): A single dose as rapidly as tolerated. Repeat dose as rapidly as tolerated if indicated. As volume approaches normal, slow 5% to 2 to 4 ml/min and 25% to 1 ml/min to prevent circulatory overload and pulmonary edema.

Hypoproteinemia: 2 to 3 ml/min in adults; a single dose over 30 to 120 minutes in children.

Infants and children: For uses other than hypovolemia and hypoproteinemia, the rate of administration should be about one fourth to one half the adult rate.

ACTIONS

A sterile natural plasma protein substance prepared by a specific process, which makes it free from the danger of serum hepatitis. A blood volume expander that accounts for 70% to 80% of the colloid oncotic pressure of plasma. Expands blood volume proportionately to amount of circulating blood, improves cardiac output, prevents marked hemoconcentration, aids in reduction of edema, and raises serum protein levels. Low sodium content helps to maintain electrolyte balance and should promote diuresis in presence of edema (contains 130 to 160 mEq sodium/L). Also acts as a transport protein that binds both endogenous and exogenous substances, including bilirubin and certain drugs.

INDICATIONS AND USES

Hypovolemia (with or without shock [actual or impending], with or without hemorrhage); 5% if hypovolemic, 25% if adequate hydration or edema is present. ■ Hypoalbuminemia from inadequate production (e.g., burns, congenital analbuminemia, endocrine disorders, infection, liver disease, major injury, malignancy, malnutrition). ■ Hypoalbuminemia from excessive catabolism (e.g., burns, major injury, nephrosis, pancreatitis, pemphigus [chronic relapsing skin disease], thyrotoxicosis). ■ Hypoalbuminemia from loss from the body (e.g., hemorrhage, burn exudates, excessive renal excretion, exfoliative dermatoses, exudative enteropathy [e.g., inflammatory bowel disease]). ■ Hypoalbuminemia from redistribution within the body (e.g., cirrhosis with ascites, inflammatory conditions, major surgery). ■ Hypoalbuminemia secondary to pulmonary edema in adult respiratory distress syndrome (ARDS) (25%). ■ Raising plasma oncotic pressure to treat edema of nephrosis (25%). ■ Cardiopulmonary bypass surgery (25%). ■ Hemolytic disease of the newborn (bilirubin binding activity) as adjunct to exchange transfusion (25%). ■ Provide adequate volume and prevent hypoproteinemia as an adjunct to RBC resuspension.

CONTRAINDICATIONS

Anemia (severe), cardiac failure, history of allergic reaction to albumin, pulmonary edema.

PRECAUTIONS

Whole blood or packed cells probably indicated if more than 1,000 ml 5% albumin required in hemorrhage; are adjunctive to use of large amounts of serum albumin to prevent anemia. Is not a substitute for whole blood in situations where both the oxygen-carrying capacity and plasma volume expansion provided by whole blood are required. ■ May be given regardless of patient blood group. ■ Use caution in hypertension, low cardiac reserve, hepatic or renal failure, or lack of albumin deficiency. ■ Use caution in patients with normal or increased intravascular volume; however, patients with hypoproteinemia may have normal blood volume. Use caution in patients with burns, hypoproteinemia, or hypovolemia; a recent FDA-issued Dear Doctor letter identified concerns of an excess mortality rate. ■ 25 Gm of albumin is the osmotic equivalent of 2 units of fresh-frozen plasma. 25 Gm of albumin provides as much plasma protein as 500 ml of plasma or 2 units of whole blood. ■ Albumin is not a source of nutrition.

Monitor: Monitor BP. ■ Hemoglobin, hematocrit, electrolyte, and serum protein evaluations are mandatory during therapy. Alkaline phosphatase may be elevated. ■ Hyponatremia may result from administration of large volumes of albumin diluted in D5W; additional monitoring of electrolytes may be required. ■ Observe patient carefully for increased bleeding resulting from more normal BP, circulatory embarrassment, pulmonary edema, or lack of diuresis. Central venous pressure readings are most helpful. ■ Maintain hydration with additional fluids, especially in dehydrated patients. ■ Normal plasma albumin is 3.5 to 6 Gm/100 ml.

Maternal/Child: Category C: safety for use during pregnancy not established. ■ Do not use 25% solution in preterm infants.

Elderly: Monitor fluid intake carefully; more susceptible to circulatory overload and pulmonary edema. ■ Plasma albumin levels may be more volatile.

SIDE EFFECTS

Fever, nausea, salivation, vomiting.

Major: Circulatory failure, dyspnea, elevated central venous pressure, precipitous hypotension, pulmonary edema.

ANTIDOTE

Notify the physician of all side effects. Minor side effects are generally tolerated and treated symptomatically. For major side effects, discontinue albumin and treat symptomatically. Resuscitate as necessary.

ALDESLEUKIN

(al-dess-loo'ken)

Antineoplastic
Immunomodulator
Biologic response modifier
Recombinant interleukin-2

Interleukin-2 Recombinant, Proleukin

pH 7.2 to 7.8

USUAL DOSE

Patient selection restricted. Prescreening and baseline studies required; see Precautions/Monitor.

Standard high-dose regimen: ***Intermittent IV:*** 600,000 IU/kg (0.037 mg/kg) every 8 hours for 14 doses. After 9 days of rest, repeat for up to 14 more doses; this constitutes one course (two 5-day [14 or fewer doses] treatment cycles separated by a rest period of 9 days). Treat with 28 doses or until dose-limiting toxicity requiring ICU-level support occurs.

Low-dose regimen (unlabeled): ***Intermittent IV:*** 72,000 IU/kg every 8 hours. Cycles same as standard high-dose regimen. Low-dose regimens are especially useful in patients at greater risk with a higher dose.

In all situations, evaluate for response 4 weeks after course completion and again before scheduling start of the next course. Additional courses are considered if there is some tumor shrinkage following the previous course, a CT scan rules out disease progression, and retreatment is not contraindicated. At least 7 weeks from hospital discharge should elapse before a second course is administered.

Sometimes given in combination with other agents; see Indications.

Unlabeled protocols: Other protocols have been used (see below). These various protocols expressed doses of aldesleukin in Cetus, Roche, or international units. Aldesleukin is available only in international units, 1 Cetus unit = 6 IU, 1 Roche unit = 3 IU. Results from studies include stable disease or disease regression with some decreased toxicity, but efficacy not established.

Continuous IV (unlabeled): 18,000,000 IU/M^2/day as a continuous infusion. Each daily dose is given over 24 hours (interrupted as indicated by patient symptoms) for two 5-day cycles with 5 to 8 days of rest before the second cycle. Another study administered the daily dose for 4 days followed by 3 days off. This cycle is repeated for 4 weeks followed by 2 weeks off. Based on patient tolerance, the entire sequence is usually repeated until some response occurs. Another low-dose regimen given on an outpatient basis uses 18,000,000 IU given over 6 to 8 hours, Monday through Friday, 4 weeks on and 2 weeks off. Beginning with the second cycle, doses on day 1 and 2 are reduced to 9,000,000 IU. Other studies are using SC injection.

DOSE ADJUSTMENTS

Doses are frequently withheld for toxicity. Doses are actually withheld, not reduced in amount. Median number of doses actually administered in a first course is 20. Continuous infusions can be interrupted as indicated by patient symptoms. ■ Hold doses and restart based on the following chart:

Guidelines for Holding Doses of Aldesleukin	
Hold Dose for	**May Give Next Dose if**
CARDIOVASCULAR	
Atrial fibrillation, supraventricular tachycardia, bradycardia that requires treatment or is recurrent or persistent.	Patient is asymptomatic with full recovery to normal sinus rhythm.
Systolic BP <90 mm Hg with increasing requirements for pressors.	Systolic BP ≥90 mm Hg and stable or improving requirements for pressors.
Any ECG change consistent with MI or ischemia with or without chest pain; suspicion of cardiac ischemia or CHF.	Patient is asymptomatic, MI has been ruled out, clinical suspicion of angina is low, there is no incidence of ventricular hypokinesia.
PULMONARY	
O_2 saturation <94% on room air or <90% with 2 L O_2 by nasal prongs.	O_2 saturation >94% on room air or >90% with 2 L O_2 by nasal prongs.
CENTRAL NERVOUS SYSTEM	
Mental status changes (e.g., agitation, confusion, lethargy, somnolence). May result in coma.	Mental status changes completely resolved.
BODY AS A WHOLE	
Sepsis syndrome; patient is clinically unstable.	Sepsis syndrome has resolved, patient is clinically stable, infection is under treatment.
UROGENITAL	
SrCr >4.5 mg/dl or a SrCr of ≥4 mg/dl in presence of severe volume overload, acidosis, or hyperkalemia.	SrCr <4 mg/dl, and fluid and electrolyte status is stable.
Persistent oliguria, urine output of <10 ml/hr for 16 to 24 hr with rising SrCr.	Urine output >10 ml/hr with a decrease of SrCr >1.5 mg/dl or normalization of SrCr.
DIGESTIVE	
Signs of hepatic failure including encephalopathy, increasing ascites, liver pain, hypoglycemia.	Discontinue for remainder of current course. May consider a new course of treatment in 7 weeks if all signs of hepatic failure have resolved.
Stool guaiac repeatedly >3 to 4^+.	Stool guaiac negative.
SKIN	
Bullous dermatitis or marked worsening of preexisting skin condition (avoid topical steroid therapy).	Resolution of all signs of bullous dermatitis.

■ After withholding a dose, no dose should be given until patient is globally assessed and specific criteria for restarting aldesleukin are met.

DILUTION

Each 22,000,000 IU vial (1.3 mg) must be reconstituted with 1.2 ml of preservative-free SW (18,000,000 IU/ml [1.1 mg (1100 mcg)/ml]). Sterile technique imperative. Direct diluent to side of vial and gently swirl to avoid excess foaming. Do not shake. Plastic infusion containers are preferred over glass. Do not use any filters for dilution or administration. Do not use any other diluent or infusion solution; may cause increased aggregation. Bring to room temperature before administration. Must be further diluted in D5W and given as an intermittent or continuous (investigational) IV. Desired concentration is 30 to 70 mcg/ml. The following chart provides an overview of upper and lower limits of aldesleukin content within the IV diluent to remain within 30 to 70 mcg/ml concentration.

Guidelines for Dilution to Achieve Desired Concentrations of Aldesleukin		
Volume of IV Diluent (D5W)	Minimum Amount of Aldesleukin to Maintain At or More Than 30 mcg/ml	Maximum Amount of Aldesleukin to Maintain At or Less Than 70 mcg/ml
*50 ml	1.5 mg (24.3 MIU)	3.5 mg (57 MIU)
100 ml	3 mg (49 MIU)	7 mg (114 MIU)
150 ml	4.5 mg (73 MIU)	10.5 mg (172 MIU)
200 ml	6 mg (97 MIU)	14 mg (229 MIU)
250 ml	7.5 mg (122 MIU)	17.5 mg (286 MIU)

*Recommended volume of IV diluent per package insert.

In specific concentrations albumin must be added to improve stability and maintain aldesleukin in an "aggregated state." To achieve a concentration of 0.1% add 1 ml of 5% (0.2 ml of 25%) albumin to each 50 ml of diluent (D5W). Albumin must be added before adding the reconstituted dose of aldesleukin. See chart below for concentrations requiring albumin at room temperature and body temperature administration.

Final Concentration of Aldesleukin/Albumin Requirements				
Route of Aldesleukin Administration	10-30 mcg/ml	30-70 mcg/ml	70-100 mcg/ml	Greater Than 100 mcg/ml
Intermittent short IV infusion and continuous infusion at *room temperature* (15° to 30° C; 59° to 89° F)	Add albumin to a final concentration of 0.1%	Not necessary to add albumin	**Do not use aldesleukin at this concentration due to poor stability**	Not necessary to add albumin
Continuous infusion at *body temperature* (≥32° C [89° F]) (e.g., CADD Pump)	Add albumin to a final concentration of 0.1%	Add albumin to a final concentration of 0.1%	**Do not use aldesleukin at this concentration due to poor stability**	Not necessary to add albumin

Manufacturer provides a worksheet to guide dilution for continuous IV infusion with a programmed infusion pump; see Storage.

Storage: Store in refrigerator before and after reconstitution and dilution. Do not freeze. No stability problems will occur at CRT for 48 hours after dilution but has no preservatives. Do not use beyond expiration date on vial. Stable for up to 6 days in a programmed infusion pump in a concentration of 100 to 500 mcg/ml without the addition of albumin or in a concentration from 1 to 70 mcg/ml with the addition of albumin. Infusion pump has body temperature conditions.

INCOMPATIBLE WITH

Manufacturer recommends not mixing with other drugs in the same container. Bacteriostatic water for injection (BWFI) or NS will increase aggregation.

COMPATIBLE WITH

Consult pharmacist; specific conditions may apply; see Compatibilities, p. xvi.

Y-site: Amikacin (Amikin), amphotericin B (Fungizone), calcium gluconate, diphenhydramine (Benadryl), dopamine (Intropin), fat emulsion IV (Intralipid), fluconazole (Diflucan), foscarnet (Foscavir), gentamicin (Garamycin), heparin, magnesium sulfate, metoclopramide (Reglan), morphine, ondansetron (Zofran), piperacillin (Pipracil), potassium chloride (KCl), ranitidine (Zantac), sulfamethoxazole-trimethoprim (Bactrim), ticarcillin (Ticar), tobramycin (Nebcin).

RATE OF ADMINISTRATION

Intermittent IV: A single dose as an intermittent infusion over 15 minutes. Flush main line IV with D5W before and after each use. Manufacturer recommends that any keep-open IV in place for intermittent administration be D5W.

Continuous IV (unlabeled): A single dose equally distributed over 24 hours. Only compatible with D5W. May be administered through a programmed infusion pump. The Pharmacia Deltec CADD system has been used in clinical studies. Use of a central venous catheter is appropriate. All recommendations under Dilution (e.g., concentration and addition of albumin) are indicated.

ACTIONS

A genetically engineered recombinant protein that possesses the biologic activity of naturally occurring interleukin-2. It boosts immune system function by increasing production of immune system cells (e.g., T lymphocytes), inducing interferon-gamma activity, and enhancing the activity of other lymphokines. Lymphocytes exposed to interleukin-2 become capable of killing cancer cells and are called lymphokine activitated killer (LAK) cells. Clinically significant numbers of lymphokines become available as contrasted to a smaller quantity generated naturally. It can result in an immune response–related destruction of cancer cells and the reduction or elimination of tumor mass. 30% of a dose initally distributes to plasma and then to extravascular, extracellular spaces; 70% of a dose distributes rapidly into the liver, kidney, and lung. Half-life is from 13 to 85 minutes (distribution to elimination). Metabolized to amino acids in proximal convoluted tubules of the kidney. No active drug is found in urine. May cross blood-brain barrier. Not known if it crosses placental barrier or is secreted in breast milk.

INDICATIONS AND USES

Prescreening mandatory. Eligibility requirements for treatment are specific and directly impact response rate and toxicity (asymptomatic preferred; symptomatic and fully ambulatory may be considered). ■ Treatment of metastatic renal cell carcinoma in adults. May be used as a single agent, in combination with interferon-alfa, or in combination with interferon-alfa and fluorouracil. Response rate is about 15% but may last 2 years; may be complete or partial. ■ Treatment of adults with metastatic melanoma. May be used as a single agent, in combination with interferon-alfa, in combination with chemotherapy, or in combination with interferon-alfa and chemotherapy. Several chemotherapy combinations have been used (Dartmouth regimen [carmustine, dacarbazine, cisplatin, and tamoxifen]; CVD regimen [cisplatin, vinblastine, and dacarbazine]). Response rate is about 16%; median duration of complete or partial response was 9 months. Granted orphan designation for treatment of acute myelogenous leukemia and non-Hodgkin's lymphoma.

Unlabeled uses: Kaposi's sarcoma in combination with zidovudine. ■ Colorectal cancer. ■ Non-Hodgkin's lymphoma. ■ Lung cancer. ■ Ovarian cancer.

CONTRAINDICATIONS

Abnormal thallium stress test or pulmonary function tests. ■ Known hypersensitivity to interleukin-2 or any component of aldesleukin. ■ Patients with organ allografts. ■ Exclude from treatment any patient with significant cardiac, pulmonary, renal, hepatic, or CNS impairment; any patient requiring treatment with steroidal agents; and any patient at higher risk for cardiovascular adverse events during periods of hypotension and fluid shifts.

Retreatment is permanently contraindicated in patients who experienced specific toxicities in a previous course of therapy (see following chart).

Contraindications for Retreatment With Aldesleukin	
Organ System	**Symptom**
Cardiovascular	Sustained ventricular tachycardia ≥5 beats. Cardiac rhythm disturbances not controlled or unresponsive to management. Chest pain with ECG changes consistent with angina or myocardial infarction. Pericardial tamponade.
Pulmonary	Intubation required more than 72 hours.
Renal	Renal dysfunction requiring dialysis for more than 72 hours.
Central nervous system	Coma or toxic psychosis lasting more than 48 hours. Repetitive or difficult-to-control seizures.
Gastrointestinal	Bowel ischemia or perforation. Bleeding requiring surgery.

PRECAUTIONS

Administered in the hospital under the supervision of a qualified physician (usually a medical oncologist and/or immunologist). Intensive care facilities and specialists in cardiopulmonary and/or intensive care medicine must be available. ■ Capillary leak syndrome (CLS [extravasation of plasma proteins and fluid into the extravascular space and loss of vascular tone]) can begin immediately after aldesleukin treatment starts and results in hypotension and reduced organ perfusion that can be severe enough to result in death. ■ Therapy should be restricted to patients with normal cardiac, pulmonary, renal (SrCr less than or equal to 1.5 mg/dl), hepatic, and CNS functions as defined by appropriate tests. Patients who have had a nephrectomy are eligible for treatment if SrCr is less than 1.5 mg/dl (85% of patients in one study). ■ Use extreme caution in patients with normal thallium stress tests and pulmonary function tests who have a history of prior cardiac or pulmonary disease. ■ May exacerbate disease symptoms in clinically unrecognized or untreated CNS metastases. Thoroughly evaluate and treat CNS metastases before aldesleukin therapy. Should be neurologically stable and have a negative CT scan. ■ Use extreme caution in patients with a history of seizures (may cause seizures), patients with fixed requirements for large volumes of fluid (e.g., hypercalcemia), those with autoimmune disorders (e.g., Crohn's disease, ulcerative colitis, psoriasis), previous cytotoxic drug therapy or radiation therapy, and patients sensitive to *Escherichia coli*–derived proteins. ■ May cause autoimmune disease and inflammatory disorders or exacerbate preexisting conditions (e.g., Crohn's disease, scleroderma, inflammatory arthritis, oculobulbar myasthenia gravis, glomerulonephritis, cholecystitis, cerebral vasculitis, Stevens-Johnson syndrome, bullous pemphigoid). ■ Associated with impaired neutrophil function and an increased risk of disseminated infection, including sepsis and bacterial endocarditis. Preexisting bacterial infections should be adequately treated before beginning therapy. ■ Induces significant hypotension; discontinue antihypertensives during treatment. ■ May impair thyroid function; changes may suggest autoimmunity; thyroid replacement therapy has been required in a few patients. ■ May cause hyperglycemia and/or diabetes mellitus. ■ See Drug/Lab Interactions.

Monitor: A central venous catheter (double or triple lumen) is frequently ordered on admission (required for continuous infusion). A minimum of two IV lines is usually required (one for the aldesleukin and its keep-open IV and one for other needed fluids and medications). One line could suffice if absolutely necessary since aldesleukin would be discontinued when colloids are administered. Flushing of line with D5W before and after aldesleukin is imperative. Ability to record CVP and draw blood samples should be available. ■ Admission chest x-ray, ECG, SMA-20, CBC with differential and platelet count, T_3, T_4, PT, PTT, urinalysis, and body weight should be obtained. Adequate pulmonary function, normal arterial blood gases, and normal ejection fraction and unimpaired wall motion (confirmed by thallium stress test and/or a stress echocardiogram) should be documented. ■ Continuous cardiac monitoring is indicated (required with BP below 90 mm Hg or any cardiac irregularity). ■ Monitoring and flexibility in management of fluid and organ perfusion status is imperative. Requires constant management and balancing of effects of fluid shifts to prevent the consequences of hypovolemia (e.g., impaired organ function [such as breakdown of blood-brain barrier]) or fluid accumulation (e.g., edema, pulmonary edema, ascites, pulmonary effusion), which may exceed the patient's tolerance. ■ Assess hypovolemia by central venous catheterization and frequent central venous pressure monitoring. Administer colloids (albumin, plasmanate) or crystalloids (IV fluids) as indicated for a BP drop of 20 mm Hg or greater or a CVP reading lower than 3 to 4 mm H_2O. ▪ Neuro checks (note agitation, blurred vision, confusion, depression, irritability, and persistent somnolence). ▪ Vital signs and strict I & O are required every 2 to 4 hours (much more frequently as side effects develop). ▪ Weigh daily. ▪ Blood is drawn twice daily (AM: CBC with differential and platelet count, SMA-20, PT, PTT; PM: SMA-6, electrolytes and creatinine [to check if evening dose can be given; significant changes in creatinine usually do not occur in less than 12 hr]). ▪ Assess thyroid function periodically. ▪ An ECG and cardiac enzymes are indicated for any S/S of chest pain, murmurs, gallops, irregular rhythm, or palpitations. A repeat thallium study is indicated for evidence of cardiac ischemia or CHF; may indicate ventricular hypokinesia due to myocarditis. ▪ Obtain a urinalysis as indicated, and draw a magnesium level for any respiratory problems, arrhythmias, or other electrolyte disturbances. ▪ Assess pulmonary function through examination, vital signs, and pulse oximetry. Arterial blood gases are indicated for any dyspnea or respiratory impairment. ▪ Some routine medications are indicated prophylactically to reduce incidence of side effects and to promote patient comfort. The morning of the first treatment begin acetaminophen 650 mg PO q 4 hr and indomethacin 25 mg q 6 hr (may increase nephrotoxicity) or naprosyn 500 mg q 12 hr PO for fever and arthralgia. Use ranitidine 150 mg PO q 12 hr or cimetidine 300 mg q 6 hr to prevent GI bleeding. Continue administration of these drugs until 12 hours after last dose of aldesleukin. Low-dose dopamine 1 to 5 mcg/kg can help maintain organ perfusion and urine output if given at initial onset of CLS before hypotension occurs. Give prophylactic ciprofloxacin 250 mg PO q 12 hr for patients with central venous lines (may be given IV [200 mg] or can substitute cefazolin, oxacillin, nafcillin, or vancomycin [must be active against *S. aureus*]; begin when line is placed and continue for 5 days after removal). Antiemetics, antidiarrheals, antichill/rigors (meperidine), antihistamines, and moisturizing skin lotions will also be used throughout treatment; see Antidote for specifics. ▪ If fever occurs several days into treatment or recurs after subsiding, assume infection first, then drug. Confusion, depression, or irritability may also suggest infection. Draw cultures; administer appropriate antibiotics. ▪ Patients who have had nephrectomies may be more at risk for increases in serum BUN or creatinine, electrolyte shifts, and reduced urine output. Evaluate fluid, electrolyte, and acid-base status promptly if any of the above occur. Gradual increases without other complications (marked fluid overload, hyperkalemia, acidosis) are frequently tolerated (SrCr must not exceed 4.5 mg/dl). ▪ Maintain pulmonary status as needed with O_2, diuretics (furosemide) and maintain serum bicarbonate above 15 mEq/L. Assess pulmonary status with chest x-rays. ▪ Monitor central and peripheral IV sites to reduce potential for infection. Change peripheral sites every 3 days. ▪ No restrictions on activity; use caution ambulating (orthostatic hypotension). ▪ No restrictions on diet. Encouragement may be required (anorexia and/or mouth sores). ▪ Monitor for thrombocytopenia (platelet count less than 50,000/mm^3). Initiate precautions to prevent excessive bleeding (e.g., inspect IV sites, skin, and mucous membranes; use extreme care during invasive procedures; test urine, emesis, stool, and secretions for occult blood). ▪

Specific preparation required for discharge; refer to literature. ■ Manufacturer supplies excellent brochures for nurses and physicians with detailed guidelines in chart form on all aspects of monitoring, toxicity, and treatment. ■ Complete review and adequate preparation of all aspects of this therapy with the patient and family are imperative. Can reduce psychologic stress of toxicity. ■ Tumor regression has continued for up to 12 months after one or more courses of therapy. ■ See Dose Adjustments, Contraindications, and Antidote.

Patient Education: Many side effects will occur; report any changes you perceive so they can be evaluated and treated if needed (e.g., changes in breathing, chest or other pain, temperature, mood, lightheadedness, fatigue). ■ Request assistance for ambulation and always sit on the side of the bed first. ■ Take only prescribed medications. ■ Avoid alcohol. ■ Use of effective contraceptive measures recommended for fertile men and women. ■ Use 15 SPF sunscreen in sunlight to protect against photosensitivity. ■ See Appendix D, p. 1148, for additional information. ■ Manufacturer supplies a patient education booklet; review thoroughly and discuss with your physician and nurse.

Maternal/Child: Category C: animal studies not conducted; effects unknown. Benefits must outweigh risks. Contraceptive measures required before initial administration and throughout treatment. ■ Discontinue breast-feeding. ■ Safety for use in children under 18 years of age not established; studies show responsiveness and toxicity similar.

Elderly: May not tolerate toxicity; use caution, consider age-related organ impairment.

DRUG/LAB INTERACTIONS

May cause interactions with psychotropic drugs (e.g., analgesics, antiemetics, narcotics, sedatives, tranquilizers) because aldesleukin also affects central nervous function. ■ Concomitant use with cardiotoxic agents (e.g., doxorubicin [Adriamycin]), hepatotoxic agents (e.g., methotrexate, asparaginase), myelotoxic agents (e.g., cytotoxic chemotherapy, radiation therapy), and nephrotoxic agents (e.g., aminoglycosides, indomethacin) may increase toxicity in these organ systems and/or delay excretion of these agents, increasing their toxicity. ■ Effects may be potentiated by drugs that also cause blood dyscrasias (e.g., penicillins, phenothiazines). ■ May cause severe allergic reactions with iodinated contrast media. ■ Glucocorticoids (e.g., dexamethasone [Decadron]) reduce aldesleukin-induced side effects but also reduce its antitumor effectiveness. ■ Aldesleukin-induced hypotension may be potentiated by beta-blockers (e.g., metoprolol, atenolol) and antihypertensive agents (e.g., nitroglycerin IV, nitroprusside sodium). ■ Concurrent use with interferon-alfa may increase incidence of MI, myocarditis, ventricular hypokinesia, and severe rhabdomyolysis. ■ May cause hypersensitivity reactions in patients receiving combination regimens (high-dose aldesleukin and antineoplastics [e.g., dacarbazine, cisplatin, tamoxifen, interferon-alfa]). ■ Aldesleukin may decrease clearance and increase plasma levels of indinavir (Crixivan). ■ Capable of altering numerous lab values; see literature.

SIDE EFFECTS

Frequent, predictable, often severe; are usually clinically manageable and frequently require intensive care management. Begin to occur shortly after therapy begins (chills, fatigue, fever, hypotension, nausea, vomiting). Frequency and severity are dose-related and schedule-dependent. Most are reversible within 2 or 3 days of discontinuation of therapy. Even with intensive management, side effects can progress to death.

Initially anorexia, arthralgia, chills, fatigue, fever, nausea, and vomiting occur. Initial symptoms of capillary leak syndrome are edema, electrolyte abnormalities, hypotension, oliguria, respiratory distress, significant weight gain, tachycardia. Effects of CLS **successively** result in ***hypovolemia,*** which in turn leads to hypotension→ hypoperfusion→ sinus tachycardia→ angina→ myocardial ischemia and infarction→ arrhythmias (supraventricular and ventricular)→ decreased renal perfusion→ prerenal azotemia→ oliguria→ anuria; ***fluid retention/weight gain,*** which in turn leads to rales→ dyspnea→ cough→ tachypnea→ hypoxia→ pleural effusion→ respiratory insufficiency requiring intubation→ diarrhea→ edema of the bowel→ refractory acidosis→ edema→ ascites; and ***breakdown of blood-brain barrier*** (neuropsychiatric toxicity [e.g., agitation, combativeness, confusion, hallucinations, lethargy, psychosis, somnolence]). Abdominal pain and GI bleeding may be related to diarrhea, vomiting, stomatitis, duodenal ulcer formation, bowel ischemia, infarction, or perforation. Cerebral edema and concomitant medications may impact many side effects. Lethargy and/or somnolence may lead to coma. Anemia and thrombocytopenia may occur; coagulation abnormalities (PT, PTT) reflect liver dysfunction. Hemodynamic effects similar to septic shock may be caused by tumor necrosis factor. Erythematous rash and pruritus (can progress to dry desquamation) can occur in almost all patients and are extremely uncomfortable. See Precautions and Drug/Lab Interactions.

ANTIDOTE

Temporarily discontinue aldesleukin and notify physician immediately of arrhythmias or rhythm changes, chest pain, marked changes in HR, positive neuropsychiatric check (agitation, blurred vision, persistent extreme somnolence), systolic BP below 90 mm Hg, apical HR over 120, temperature over 38° C (100.4° F), respirations over 25/min, complaints of dyspnea, decreased breath sounds, increased sputum production, urinary output less than 200 ml/4 hr, CVP reading below 3 to 4 mm H_2O, weight increase over 4 kg or 10% of baseline over 5 days, abnormal blood or urine tests (e.g., serum bicarbonate less than 15 mEq/L, SrCr greater than 4 to 4.5 mg/dl [based on gradual or sudden rise and if accompanied by other complications]), severe diarrhea associated with refractory acidosis, vomiting refractory to treatment, acute changes in GI status. May be restarted based on patient response. Hold any subsequent dose for failure to maintain organic perfusion; see Dose Adjustments. Fever is routinely treated with acetaminophen and indomethacin or naprosyn; increased doses may be needed; administer rectally if nausea and vomiting are present. Suggested treatments include slow IV meperidine (Demerol) 25 to 50 mg for chills and rigidity; diphenoxylate (Lomotil), or loperamide (Imodium) PO for diarrhea (these meds may not help and diarrhea may be dose-limiting); diphenhydramine (Benadryl) 25 mg PO q 6 hr, a soothing skin cream (Eucerin), and oatmeal baths for urticaria and pruritus; temazepam (Restoril) for insomnia; ondansetron (Zofran) or prochlorperazine (Compazine) for nausea. Treat edema with furosemide (Lasix). IV fluids, albumin or plasmanate, and Trendelenburg positioning are used to maintain fluid balance and BP. If organ perfusion and BP are not sustained by dopamine 2 to 5 mcg/kg as a continuous infusion, increase to 6 to 10 mcg/kg or add phenylephrine (1 to 5 mcg/kg/min). Prolonged use of pressors at relatively high doses may cause cardiac arrhythmias. Treat arrhythmias as indicated (usually sinus or supraventricular tachycardia [adenosine, verapamil]). Use O_2 for decreased PaO_2. Use packed RBCs for anemia and to ensure maximum oxygen-carrying capacity. Platelet transfusions are indicated for thrombocytopenia or to reduce risk of GI bleeding. Use of blood modifiers to treat bone marrow toxicity may be indicated (e.g., darbepoetin alfa [Aranesp], epoetin alfa [Epogen, Procrit], filgrastim [Neupogen], pegfilgrastim [Neulasta], sargramostim [Leukine], oprelvekin [Neumega]). Special precautions may be required (e.g., avoid IM injections; test urine, emesis, stool, secretions for occult blood). All treatment is supportive; recovery should begin within a few hours of cessation of aldesleukin. With normalized BP, diuretics (furosemide [Lasix]) can hasten recovery. Low-dose haloperidol (Haldol) may help severe mental status changes.

More rapid onset of dose-limiting toxicities will occur with overdose. **Dexamethasone (Decadron)** is indicated to counteract life-threatening toxicities. May result in loss of therapeutic effect.

ALEFACEPT

(ah-lef′-a-cept)

Immunosuppressant

Amevive

pH 6.9

USUAL DOSE

7.5 mg as an IV bolus once each week for 12 weeks. Baseline CD4+ T-lymphocyte count must be within normal limits (e.g., 600 to 1,500/mm^3 [consult lab, parameters may vary]) before the initial course of therapy begins. A repeat count is required before each dose. Withhold dose if CD4+ T-lymphocyte counts are below 250 cells/mm^3. A second course may be considered after a 12-week waiting period if CD4+ T-lymphocyte counts are within the normal range. Data limited on retreatment with more than 2 cycles. May be given IM; however, the dose is different (larger) and is supplied in a different kit.

PEDIATRIC DOSE

Safety and effectiveness for use in pediatric patients not studied; not indicated for pediatric use.

DOSE ADJUSTMENTS

Withhold dose if CD4+ T-lymphocyte counts are below 250 cells/mm^3. ■ Discontinue alefacept if counts remain below 250 cells/mm^3 for 1 month.

DILUTION

Supplied in a kit containing a single 7.5-mg vial of alefacept, SW for reconstitution, a syringe, a ¾-inch 23-gauge winged infusion set (butterfly needle), and two 23-gauge 1¼-inch needles. Using the first needle, withdraw 0.6 ml of supplied diluent (SW). Reconstitute the 7.5-mg vial by slowly injecting the diluent toward the sidewall of the vial. Do not shake or vigorously agitate; swirl gently to dissolve (should occur within 2 minutes). Some foaming will occur; avoid excessive foaming. Change to the second needle and withdraw 0.5 ml (7.5 mg of alefacept); some foam may remain in the vial. Prepare 2 syringes with 3 ml of NS in each one. Use the first to prime the winged infusion set before inserting it into the vein. Confirm venous access, then attach the syringe with alefacept. **Storage:** Retain kit in carton until use. Store at CRT, protected from light. Do not use beyond expiration date stamped on kit. Use immediately after reconstitution is preferred, but may be refrigerated in the vial for up to 4 hours if necessary. Discard reconstituted solution after 4 hours.

COMPATIBILITY

Manufacturer states, "Do not add other medications to solutions containing alefacept. Do not reconstitute with other diluents. Do not filter reconstituted solution during preparation or administration."

RATE OF ADMINISTRATION

0.5 ml (7.5 mg) as a bolus injection over no more than 5 seconds. Follow with a flush of 3 ml NS. Remove winged infusion set.

ACTIONS

An immunosuppressive protein produced by recombinant DNA technology in a Chinese Hamster Ovary mammalian cell expression system. Selectively targets the T-cells responsible for chronic plaque psoriasis without disrupting normal immune function. Interferes with lymphocyte activation by specifically binding to the lymphocyte antigen, CD2, and inhibiting LFA-3/CD2 interaction, which plays a role in the pathophysiology of chronic plaque psoriasis. Results in a dose-dependent reduction in circulating CD4+ and CD8+ T-lymphocyte counts. May have some minor effect on cells other than T-lymphocytes. Mean half-life is 270 hours. Onset of response usually begins within 60 days after the start of therapy. Maximum response may not occur until several weeks after the 12-week regimen is complete. Median duration of response in studies was 3.5 months.

INDICATIONS AND USES

Treatment of adults with moderate to severe chronic plaque psoriasis who are candidates for systemic therapy or phototherapy (treatment of a disease by exposure to light).

CONTRAINDICATIONS

Known hypersensitivity to alefacept or any of its components (e.g., sucrose). Do not initiate in patients with a CD4+ T-lymphocyte count below normal (e.g., 600 to 1,500/mm^3), patients with a history of systemic malignancy, or patients with a clinically important infection. See Precautions and Side Effects.

PRECAUTIONS

Administer under the supervision of a physician. ■ May increase the risk of malignancies (e.g., basal or squamous cell skin cancers, lymphomas [Hodgkin's or non-Hodgkin's]). Use caution in patients who may be at high risk for malignancy. Discontinue if a malignancy develops. ■ Use caution in patients with chronic infections or a history of recurrent infection. Discontinue if a serious infection develops. ■ Do not use concurrently with other immunosuppressive agents or phototherapy. May cause excessive immunosuppression. Length of time required between alefacept therapy and initiating another immunosuppressive therapy has not been established. ■ Safety and effectiveness of concurrent administration of live or live-attenuated vaccines not studied; some ability to mount immunity may occur. ■ A protein substance; hypersensitivity reactions have been reported; use caution in patients with allergies. ■ Patients may develop low-titer antibodies to alefacept; no correlation with clinical response or side effects observed. ■ Effects in patients with impaired renal or hepatic function have not been studied.

Monitor: Obtain CD4+ T-lymphocyte count before beginning therapy and repeat each week before dosing. Count should be within normal limits before a regimen is initiated; see Usual Dose and Dose Adjustments. ■ Monitor for symptoms of hypersensitivity reactions; urticaria and angioedema have been reported; see Antidote. ■ Monitor for S/S of infection; see Antidote.

Patient Education: Weekly white blood cell counts required before each dose. ■ May increase risk of developing skin cancers or lymphomas. ■ Susceptibility to infection may be increased; report any S/S of infection (e.g., fever, chills, cold symptoms). ■ Female patients should notify their physician immediately if pregnancy is suspected during therapy or within 8 weeks of completing therapy. If a pregnancy occurs, enrolling in the alefacept Pregnancy Registry is encouraged (1-866-263-8483). ■ See Appendix D, p. 1148.

Maternal/Child: Category B: use during pregnancy only if clearly needed. If pregnancy occurs during therapy, assess risks of continued use. No evidence of harm to animal fetuses; see package insert and Patient Education. Crosses placental barrier in monkeys. ■ Discontinue breast-feeding; has potential for serious harm to the infant.

Elderly: Safety and effectiveness similar to younger patients. ■ Incidence of infections and certain malignancies may be higher in the elderly; use caution.

DRUG/LAB INTERACTIONS

Specific drug interaction studies have not been performed. ■ Do not use concurrently with other immunosuppressive agents or phototherapy. May cause excessive immunosuppression; see Precautions. ■ Safety and effectiveness of concurrent administration of live or live-attenuated vaccines not studied.

SIDE EFFECTS

Treatment-limiting side effects include hypersensitivity reactions (e.g., anaphylaxis, angioedema, urticaria), lymphopenia (CD4+ T-lymphocytes below 250 cells/mm^3), malignancies, and/or serious infections requiring hospitalization (e.g., appendicitis, cholecystitis, gastroenteritis, herpes simplex infection, necrotizing cellulitis, peritonsillar abscess, pneumonia, post-operative and burn wound infection, pre-septal cellulitis, toxic shock). Most frequently reported side effects include accidental injury, chills, dizziness, increased cough, injection site inflammation, myalgia, nausea, pharyngitis, and pruritus.

Overdose: Arthralgia, chills, headache, sinusitis.

ANTIDOTE

Notify physician of all side effects. Most will be treated symptomatically. Discontinue alefacept if CD4+ T-lymphocyte counts remain below 250 cells/mm^3 for 1 month. Discontinue immediately if anaphylaxis or other serious allergic reaction occurs, and treat with oxygen, epinephrine, corticosteroids, and/or antihistamines (e.g., diphenhydramine [Benadryl]) as needed. Discontinue if a malignancy or a serious infection occurs and initiate appropriate treatment. Monitor total lymphocyte count and CD4+ T-lymphocyte count closely in overdose. Resuscitate as indicated.

ALEMTUZUMAB

(al-em-tuz'uh-mab)

Campath

Monoclonal Antibody
Antineoplastic

pH 6.8 to 7.4

USUAL DOSE

Premedication, dose escalation to the recommended maintenance dose, and anti-infective prophylaxis are required.

Premedication: Oral diphenhydramine (Benadryl) 50 mg and acetaminophen (Tylenol) 650 mg should be administered 30 minutes before infusion, at dose escalations, and as clinically indicated. In cases where severe infusion-related reactions have occurred, hydrocortisone (e.g., Solu-Cortef) 200 mg may be administered to help prevent or minimize subsequent reactions.

Dose escalation: Initiate at a dose of 3 mg daily. When this dose is tolerated (infusion-related toxicities are Grade 2 or less), the daily dose should be increased to 10 mg. When the 10-mg dose is tolerated, the maintenance dose of 30 mg may be initiated. In most cases, dose escalation to the maintenance dose of 30 mg can be achieved in 3 to 7 days.

Maintenance dose: 30 mg daily administered three times a week on alternate days (i.e., Monday, Wednesday, Friday). Administered for up to 12 weeks. Single doses greater than 30 mg or cumulative weekly doses greater than 90 mg have been associated with an increased incidence of pancytopenia and should ***not*** be administered.

Anti-infective prophylaxis: To minimize the risk of selected opportunistic infections, administer sulfamethoxazole-trimethoprim (Bactrim DS, Septra DS) twice daily three times a week; famciclovir (Famvir) or equivalent 250 mg twice daily should be initiated at the start of alemtuzumab therapy. Continue prophylaxis for 2 months after completion of therapy or until the $CD4^+$ count is equal to or greater than 200 cells/mm^3, whichever occurs later.

PEDIATRIC DOSE

Safety and effectiveness for use in pediatric patients not established.

DOSE ADJUSTMENTS

Recommendations for dose modification for severe neutropenia or thrombocytopenia are listed in the following chart.

Alemtuzumab Dosing Based on Hematologic Toxicity	
Hematologic Toxicity	**Dose Modification and Reinitiation of Therapy**
For first occurrence of ANC <250/mm^3 and/or platelet count ≤25,000/mm^3	Withhold therapy. When ANC ≥500/mm^3 and platelet count ≥50,000/mm^3, resume therapy at same dose. If delay between dosing is ≥7 days, initiate therapy at 3 mg and escalate to 10 mg and then to 30 mg as tolerated.
For second occurrence of ANC <250/mm^3 and/or platelet count ≤25,000/mm^3	Withhold therapy. When ANC ≥500/mm^3 and platelet count ≥50,000/mm^3, resume therapy at **10 mg.** If delay between dosing is ≥7 days, initiate therapy at 3 mg and escalate to **10 mg only.**
For third occurrence of ANC <250/mm^3 and/or platelet count ≤25,000/mm^3	Discontinue therapy permanently.
For a decrease of ANC and/or platelet count to ≤50% of the baseline value in patients initiating therapy with a baseline ANC ≤500/mm^3 and/or a baseline platelet count ≤25,000/mm^3	Withhold therapy. When ANC and/or platelet count return to baseline value(s), resume therapy. If delay between dosing is ≥7 days, initiate therapy at 3 mg and escalate to 10 mg and then to 30 mg as tolerated.

DILUTION

Do not shake ampule before use. Withdraw the necessary amount of alemtuzumab from the ampule into a syringe. Filter with a sterile, low–protein binding, non–fiber releasing 5-micron filter before dilution and inject into 100 ml of NS or D5W. Gently invert the bag to mix solution. Discard any unused drug.

Storage: Store ampules at 2° to 8° C (36° to 46° F). Do not freeze. Protect from direct sunlight. Prepared solution may be stored at CRT or refrigerated. Protect from light and use within 8 hours of dilution.

COMPATIBILITY

Manufacturer states, "Other drug substances should not be added or simultaneously infused through the same intravenous line." No incompatibilities observed with PVC bags, PVC or polyethylene-lined PVC administration sets, or low–protein binding filters.

RATE OF ADMINISTRATION

A single dose as an infusion over 2 hours. ***Do not administer*** as an IV push or bolus.

ACTIONS

A recombinant, DNA-derived, humanized monoclonal antibody (Campath-1H) that binds to the 21-28 kD cell surface glycoprotein, CD52. CD52 is expressed on the surface of both normal and malignant B and T lymphocytes, NK cells, most monocytes, macrophages, a subpopulation of granulocytes, and tissues of the male reproductive system. Alemtuzumab binding has been observed in lymphoid tissues, the mononuclear phagocyte system, and the male reproductive tract. A proportion of bone marrow cells, including some CD34$^+$ cells, also express variable levels of CD52.

The mechanism of action is thought to be an antibody-dependent lysis of leukemic cells following cell surface binding. Average half-life is 12 days. Steady state is reached by approximately week 6 of therapy. The rise in serum alemtuzumab concentration corresponds with the reduction in malignant lymphocytosis.

INDICATIONS AND USES

Treatment of B-cell chronic lymphocytic leukemia (B-CLL) in patients who have been treated with alkylating agents (e.g., cyclophosphamide [Cytoxan]) and who have failed fludarabine (Fludara) therapy. Determination of the effectiveness of alemtuzumab is based on overall response rates.

CONTRAINDICATIONS

Active systemic infections, underlying immunodeficiency (e.g., seropositive for HIV), or known hypersensitivity or anaphylactic reactions to alemtuzumab or to any one of its components.

PRECAUTIONS

Administered under the supervision of a physician experienced in the use of antineoplastic therapy in a facility equipped to monitor the patient and respond to any medical emergency. ■ Serious and, in rare instances, fatal pancytopenia/marrow hypoplasia, autoimmune idiopathic thrombocytopenia, and autoimmune hemolytic anemia have been reported. Have occurred at recommended dose. Do not exceed maximum daily or weekly recommended dose. See Usual Dose, Dose Adjustments, and Antidote. ■ Serious and sometimes fatal bacterial, viral, fungal, and protozoal infections have been reported. Prophylaxis directed against *Pneumocystis carinii* pneumonia and herpes virus infections has been shown to decrease but not eliminate the occurrence of these infections. See Usual Dose. ■ Because of the potential for graft-versus-host disease in severely lymphopenic patients, irradiation of any blood products is recommended. ■ A small percentage of patients have developed antibodies to alemtuzumab. Patients who develop hypersensitivity to alemtuzumab may have allergic or hypersensitivity reactions to other monoclonal antibodies.

Monitor: Obtain a baseline CBC, including differential and platelet count. Monitor weekly or more frequently if worsening anemia, neutropenia, or thrombocytopenia develops. ■ Infusion reactions, including bronchospasm, chills, fever, hypotension, rash, rigors, and/or shortness of breath, may occur. Reactions may be severe. Acute infusion-related reactions were most common during the first week of therapy in clinical studies. Premedicate patient and monitor carefully during infusion. Gradual escalation to the recommended maintenance dose is required at the initiation of therapy and after interruption of therapy for 7 or more days. See Usual Dose. ■ Monitor blood pressure and hypotensive symptoms carefully in patients with ischemic heart disease and in patients taking antihypertensive medications; see Drug/Lab Interactions. ■ Monitor for thrombocytopenia (platelet count less than 50,000/mm^3). Initiate precautions to prevent excessive bleeding (e.g., inspect IV sites, skin, and mucous membranes; use extreme care during invasive procedures; test urine, emesis, stool, and secretions for occult blood). ■ CD4$^+$ counts should be followed after therapy until recovery to equal to or greater than 200 cells/mm^3. See Usual Dose.

Patient Education: Women of childbearing potential and men of reproductive potential should use effective contraceptive methods during treatment and for a minimum of 6 months following therapy. ■ Report any unusual side effects or signs of infection promptly. ■ See Appendix D, p. 1148.

Maternal/Child: Category C: avoid pregnancy. May cause fetal harm. May cross placental barrier and cause fetal B and T lymphocyte depletion. ■ Discontinue breast-feeding during treatment and for at least 3 months following completion of therapy.

Elderly: Differences in safety and efficacy related to age have not been observed to date, but study numbers have been small.

DRUG/LAB INTERACTIONS

No formal drug interaction studies have been performed. ■ An immune response to alemtuzumab may interfere with subsequent diagnostic serum tests that use antibodies. ■ May cause additive effects with bone marrow–depressing agents, radiation therapy, or agents that cause blood dyscrasias (e.g., amphotericin B, antithyroid agents [Methimazole (Tapazole)], azathioprine [Imuran], chloramphenicol, ganciclovir [Cytovene], interferon, plicamycin [Mithracin], zidovudine [AZT]). ■ May intensify effects of antihypertensive medications; see Monitor. ■ Do not administer chloroquine or live virus vaccines to patients receiving antineoplastic agents.

SIDE EFFECTS

Anorexia, arrhythmias, asthenia, autoimmune hemolytic anemia or autoimmune idiopathic thrombocytopenia, constipation, cough, depression, dizziness, dyspepsia, edema, epistaxis, febrile neutropenia, hematologic toxicity (e.g., anemia, marrow hypoplasia, lymphopenia [profound and prolonged], neutropenia, pancytopenia, thrombocytopenia), infections (e.g., pneumonia and several opportunistic infections), infusion-related reactions (e.g., bronchospasm, dyspnea, diarrhea, fatigue, fever, headache, hypertension, hypotension, nausea, pruritus, rash, rigors, urticaria, vomiting), insomnia, malaise, mucositis, myalgias, pain, purpura, rhinitis, somnolence, tremor, and many others.

ANTIDOTE

Notify physician of all side effects. Treatment of most reactions will be supportive. Therapy should be temporarily discontinued during serious infection, serious hematologic toxicity, or other serious toxicity until the infection or adverse event resolves. Discontinue medication permanently for severe reactions, including autoimmune anemia or thrombocytopenia. Infusion reactions may be treated with acetaminophen, antiemetics (e.g., ondansetron [Zofran]), antihistamines (e.g., diphenhydramine), corticosteroids (e.g., hydrocortisone), and meperidine as indicated. Administration of blood products and/or blood modifiers (e.g., darbepoetin [Aransep], epoetin alfa [Epogen, Procrit], filgrastim [Neupogen], pegfilgrastim [Neulasta], sargramostim [Leukine], oprelvekin [Neumega]) may be indicated to treat bone marrow toxicity. Median durations of neutropenia and thrombocytopenia were 28 and 21 days, respectively. Median time to recovery of CD4+ counts to equal to or greater than $200/mm^3$ is 2 months; however, full recovery of CD4+ and CD8+ counts may take more than 12 months. Discontinue alemtuzumab and provide supportive therapy in overdose. Treat allergic reactions with epinephrine, antihistamines, and corticosteroids as needed. Resuscitate as indicated.

ALFENTANIL HYDROCHLORIDE

(al-fen′ta-nil hye-droe-klor′id)

General anesthetic
Narcotic analgesic agonist
Anesthesia adjunct

Alfenta

pH 4 to 6

USUAL DOSE

Adults and children 12 years of age and older: Dose must be individualized and titrated to the desired effect in each patient according to body weight, physical status, underlying pathologic condition, use of other drugs, and type and duration of surgical procedure and anesthesia. Usually used in conjunction with short-acting barbiturates (e.g., thiopental [Pentothal]), neuromuscular blocking agents (e.g., pancuronium [Pavulon], succinylcholine), and an inhalation anesthetic (e.g., nitrous oxide) to maintain balanced anesthesia. Use reduced doses of a neuromuscular blocking agent prophylactically to prevent muscle rigidity or to induce muscle relaxation after rigidity occurs. Full paralyzing doses may be used after loss of consciousness. Use of a benzodiazepine (e.g., diazepam [Valium], midazolam [Versed]) may reduce induction dose requirements, decrease time to loss of consciousness, and diminish patient recall; see Drug/Lab Interactions. See Dose Adjustments.

Alfentanil Dosing Guidelines For Use During General Anesthesia	
SPONTANEOUSLY BREATHING/ASSISTED VENTILATION	
Procedures lasting up to 30 minutes	Induction of analgesia: 8-20 mcg/kg Maintenance of analgesia: 3-5 mcg/kg q 5-20 min or 0.5-1 mcg/kg/min Total dose: 8-40 mcg/kg
ASSISTED OR CONTROLLED VENTILATION	
Incremental injection in procedures lasting longer than 30 minutes (To attenuate response to laryngoscopy and intubation)	Induction of analgesia: 20-50 mcg/kg Maintenance of analgesia: 5-15 mcg/kg q 5-20 min Total dose: Up to 75 mcg/kg
CONTINUOUS INFUSION	
In procedures lasting longer than 30 minutes (To provide attenuation of response to intubation and incision)	Infusion rates are variable and should be titrated to the desired clinical effect. SEE INFUSION DOSAGE GUIDELINES (NEXT PAGE) Induction of analgesia: 50-75 mcg/kg Maintenance of analgesia: 0.5-3 mcg/kg/min (average rate 1-1.5 mcg/kg/min) Total dose: Dependent on duration of procedure

Continued

Alfentanil Dosing Guidelines For Use During General Anesthesia—cont'd	
ANESTHETIC INDUCTION	
Procedures lasting 45 minutes or longer	Induction of anesthesia: 130-245 mcg/kg Maintenance of analgesia: 0.5-1.5 mcg/kg/min or general anesthetic Total dose: Dependent on duration of procedure At these doses, truncal rigidity should be expected and a muscle relaxant should be utilized Administer slowly (over 3 minutes) Concentration of inhalation agents reduced by 30%-50% for initial hour
MONITORED ANESTHESIA CARE (MAC)	
For sedated and responsive, spontaneously breathing patients	Induction of MAC: 3-8 mcg/kg Maintenance of MAC: 3-5 mcg/kg q 5-20 min or 0.25-1 mcg/kg/min Total dose: 3-40 mcg/kg
INFUSION DOSAGE	
Continuous infusion: 0.5-3 mcg/kg/min administered with nitrous oxide/oxygen in patients undergoing general surgery. Following an anesthetic induction dose of alfentanil, infusion rate requirements are reduced by 30%-50% for the first hour of maintenance. Changes in vital signs that indicate a response to surgical stress or lightening of anesthesia may be controlled by increasing the alfentanil to a maximum of 4 mcg/kg/min and/or administration of bolus doses of 7 mcg/kg. If changes are not controlled after three bolus doses given over a 5-minute period, a barbiturate, vasodilator, and/or inhalation agent should be used. Infusion rates should always be adjusted downward in the absence of these signs until there is some response to surgical stimulation. Rather than an increase in infusion rate, 7 mcg/kg bolus doses of alfentanil or a potent inhalation agent should be administered in response to signs of lightening of anesthesia within the last 15 minutes of surgery. Alfentanil infusion should be discontinued at least 10 to 15 minutes before the end of surgery. Discontinue 10 to 15 minutes before end of procedures in general anesthesia. Continue infusion to end of procedure during MAC, then discontinue.	

PEDIATRIC DOSE

Safety for use in children under 12 years of age not established; not recommended. Half-life and duration of action is decreased in children; more frequent supplemental doses may be required; see Maternal/Child. **Anesthesia adjunct (unlabeled):** ***Loading dose:*** 0.03 to 0.05 mg/kg (30 to 50 mcg/kg). Follow with supplemental single doses of 0.01 to 0.015 mg/kg (10 to 15 mcg/kg) or a continuous infusion at a rate of 0.0005 to 0.0015 mg/kg/min (0.5 to 1.5 mcg/kg/min).

DOSE ADJUSTMENTS

Reduce dose of one or both agents when given in combination with other CNS depressants (e.g., barbiturates, inhalation anesthetics, narcotic analgesics, tranquilizers). ■ Calculate dose based on lean body weight in obese patients (more than 20% above ideal body weight). ■ Reduced initial dose required in elderly or debilitated patients (a 40%

Continued

reduction was required in one study); reduced supplemental doses, a slower infusion rate, or longer intervals between doses may be required based on effects of initial dose. ■ Doses appropriate for general population may cause serious respiratory depression in vulnerable patients. ■ Reduced dose may be required in hypothyroidism and in impaired hepatic function. ■ See Drug/Lab Interactions.

DILUTION

IV injection: Small volumes may be given undiluted (usually by the anesthesiologist). Use of tuberculin syringe recommended (1 ml equals 500 mcg). Further dilution with 5 ml of SW or NS to facilitate titration is appropriate.

Infusion: Dilute 20 ml alfentanil with 230 ml NS, D5NS, D5W, or LR to achieve a concentration of 40 mcg/ml. Desired concentration range is 25 to 80 mcg/ml.

Storage: Store ampules at CRT; protect from light and freezing.

COMPATIBLE WITH

Consult pharmacist; specific conditions may apply; see Compatibilities, p. xvi.

Syringe: Atracurium (Tracrium), midazolam (Versed), ondansetron (Zofran).

Y-site: Cisatracurium (Nimbex), etomidate (Amidate), gatifloxacin (Tequin), hetastarch in electrolytes (Hextend), linezolid (Zyvox), propofol (Diprivan), remifentanil (Ultiva).

RATE OF ADMINISTRATION

IV injection: Administer over a minimum of 3 minutes. Rapid administration of lower doses or administration of full anesthetic doses will result in muscle rigidity, apnea, respiratory paralysis, loss of vascular tone, and hypotension. Titrate rate to desired patient response.

Infusion: See Usual Dose.

ACTIONS

An opioid derivative, narcotic analgesic, and descending CNS depressant. Less potent than fentanyl milligram for milligram, but achieves higher plasma concentrations. Produces hypnosis and respiratory depressant actions that outlast its analgesic effect. Onset of action is immediate. Produces analgesic effects in 1 minute. Peak effect (respiratory depression and analgesia) occurs within 1½ to 2 minutes. With induction doses, loss of consciousness occurs within 1 to 2 minutes. Provides dose-related protection against hemodynamic responses to surgical stress. Histamine release rarely occurs. May cause rigidity of chest, pharynx, and abdominal muscles, inhibiting ventilation; see Precautions/Monitor, Side Effects, Antidote. Duration of action is 5 to 10 minutes. Has a terminal half-life of 90 to 111 minutes. Cumulative effects are somewhat less than with fentanyl or sufentanil, but with repeat doses recovery may be prolonged. Recovery should occur within 10 to 15 minutes of end of procedure or 25 to 30 minutes after last incremental dose or discontinuing the infusion. Metabolized in the liver. Excreted as metabolites in urine. Crosses the placental barrier. Secreted in breast milk.

INDICATIONS AND USES

Analgesic adjunct given in incremental doses in the maintenance of anesthesia with barbiturate/nitrous oxide/oxygen. ■ Analgesic administered by continuous infusion with nitrous oxide/oxygen in the maintenance of general anesthesia. ■ Primary anesthetic agent for the induction of anesthesia in patients undergoing general surgery requiring endotracheal intubation and mechanical ventilation. ■ Analgesic component for monitored anesthesia care (MAC) during surgical or diagnostic procedures.

CONTRAINDICATIONS

Known hypersensitivity to alfentanil or known intolerance to other opioid agonists (e.g., fentanyl, sufentanil). Use during labor and delivery not recommended. In general narcotic analgesics are also contraindicated in acute or severe bronchial asthma and if an upper airway obstruction or significant respiratory depression is present.

PRECAUTIONS

For IV use only. ■ Administered by or under the direct observations of the anesthesiologist. Must have responsibility only for anesthesia and continuous observation of the patient during surgery and/or procedure. ■ Staff must be skilled in medical management of critically ill patients, cardiovascular resuscitation, and airway management. ■ Use caution; plasma clearance reduced and recovery time prolonged in the elderly and in patients with impaired liver function (half-life prolonged [up to 5.8 hours]); reduced dose may be indicated. ■ Use caution in patients with pulmonary disease, decreased respiratory reserve, or potentially compromised respiration. May cause rigidity of chest and abdominal muscles, decrease respiratory drive, and increase airway resistance; may require assisted or controlled ventilation. ■ Use caution in patients with head injury or increased intracranial pressure; risk of respiratory depression is increased. ■ Respiratory depression may cause an increased PCO_2, cerebral vasodilation, and increased intracranial pressure. Clinical course of head injury may be obscured. ■ Use caution in patients with bradyarrhythmias. ■ Use caution in patients with hypothyroidism; risk of respiratory depression and prolonged CNS depression is increased. Reduced doses may be indicated. ■ See Drug/Lab Interactions.

Monitor: Oxygen, controlled ventilation equipment, opioid antagonists (e.g., naloxone [Narcan], nalmefene [Revex]), and neuromuscular blocking agents (e.g., pancuronium [Pavulon], succinylcholine) and all emergency drugs and equipment must be immediately available. Can cause rigidity of respiratory muscles; concurrent use of a neuromuscular blocking agent can prevent or reverse muscle rigidity to permit controlled ventilation. ■ Adequate preoperative hydration is recommended to reduce incidence of hypotension. ■ Observe for hypotension, apnea, upper airway obstruction, and/or oxygen desaturation. Monitor vital signs and oxygen saturation continuously. If not unconscious, patient will appear to be asleep and forget to breathe unless commanded to do so. ■ Additional doses of alfentanil can be used to control tachycardia and hypertension during surgery. ■ Prolonged postoperative monitoring may be indicated; respiratory depression, respiratory arrest, bradycardia, asystole, arrhythmias, and hypotension may occur after initial recovery. ■ Keep patient supine; orthostatic hypotension and fainting may occur. ■ Has a short duration of action; pain medication may be required soon after initial recovery. ■ See Precautions and Drug/Lab Interactions.

Patient Education: Avoid alcohol or other CNS depressants (e.g., antihistamines, benzodiazepines [e.g., diazepam (Valium)]). ■ Blurred vision, dizziness, drowsiness, or lightheadedness may occur; request assistance with ambulation. ■ Review all medications for interactions.

Maternal/Child: Category C: safety for use in pregnancy not established; has embryocidal effects in rats and rabbits. ■ Not recommended for use during labor and delivery. ■ Postpone breast-feeding for at least 24 hours after use of alfentanil. ■ Muscle rigidity is more common in neonates than in older children or adults.

Elderly: See Dose Adjustments and Precautions. ■ May markedly decrease pulmonary ventilation. ■ Decreased protein binding, decreased clearance, and possible increased brain sensitivity may make the elderly more sensitive to effects (e.g., respiratory depression, extended recovery time, urinary retention, constipation). ■ Analgesia should be effective with lower doses. ■ Consider age-related organ impairment; elimination half-life is extended, postoperative recovery may be delayed.

DRUG/LAB INTERACTIONS

Use of benzodiazepines (e.g., diazepam [Valium], midazolam [Versed]) may decrease dose of alfentanil required and decrease patient recall, but when given immediately before or in conjunction with high doses of alfentanil, benzodiazepines may produce vasodilation, severe hypotension, and result in delayed recovery. ■ After an anesthetic induction dose of alfentanil, requirements for volatile inhalation anesthetics (e.g., nitrous oxide) and/or alfentanil infusion are reduced by 30% to 50% for the first hour of maintenance. ■ Beta-adrenergic blocking agents (e.g., metoprolol, timolol) may be used preoperatively to decrease hypertensive episodes during surgical procedures, but chronic use (including ophthalmic preparations) may also increase the risk of initial bradycardia. ■ Respiratory depression, CNS depression, hypotensive effects, and duration of action increased with concomitant administration of other CNS depressants (e.g., antidepressants, antihistamines, barbiturates, benzodiazepines, haloperidol, inhalation anesthetics, narcotic analgesics, phenothiazines). Reduced doses of one or both agents usually required. ■ Clearance decreased by cimetidine (Tagamet) and erythromycin; risk of prolonged or delayed respiratory depression may be increased. ■ Respiratory depressant effects are additive with neuromuscular blocking agents (e.g., pancuronium, succinylcholine). ■ Other opioids have caused severe hypertension with MAO inhibitors (e.g., selegiline [Eldepryl]). Use extreme caution; beta-blockers (e.g., propranolol) and vasodilators (e.g., nitroglycerin) should be available. ■ Duration of action may be prolonged with other agents that inhibit hepatic enzymes (e.g., azole antifungals [e.g., itraconazole (Sporanox)], beta-blockers [e.g., metoprolol (Lopressor), propranolol (Inderal), timolol (Novo-Timol)], calcium channel blockers [e.g., diltiazem (Cardizem), verapamil (Isoptin)], fluoroquinolones [e.g., ciprofloxacin (Cipro), levofloxacin (Levaquin)], MAO inhibitors). ■ Monitor closely for S/S of respiratory depression and CNS depression with concurrent use of protease inhibitors (e.g., saquinavir [Invirase], ritonavir [Norvir]). ■ Use of naltrexone (ReVia) would require increased doses of alfentanil; may cause prolonged respiratory depression and/or circulatory collapse. Discontinue naltrexone several days before elective surgery if use of an opioid is necessary. ■ Analgesic effects may be antagonized by opioid agonist/antagonist analgesics; may also cause additive CNS and respiratory depressant effects. ■ Cerebrospinal fluid pressure may be increased. ■ May delay gastric emptying and invalidate diagnostic tests. ■ May interfere with some hepatobiliary imaging. ■ Delay plasma amylase and lipase measurements for at least 24 hours.

SIDE EFFECTS

Average dose: Bradycardia and hypotension may occur shortly after administration. Respiratory depression caused by alfentanil and/or muscle rigidity may progress to apnea. Agitation, allergic reactions (e.g., anaphylaxis, bronchospasm, itching, laryngospasm, urticaria), arrhythmias (e.g., bradycardia, tachycardia), blurred vision, bradypnea, chest wall rigidity, dizziness, euphoria, headache, hypercapnia (increased CO_2), hypertension, hypotension, muscle rigidity (skeletal muscles including abdomen, chest, pharynx, neck, and extremities), myoclonic movements, nausea, postoperative confusion, respiratory sedation, shivering, skeletal muscle movements, sleepiness, vomiting.

Overdose: Bradycardia; circulatory depression; cold, clammy skin; dizziness (severe); drowsiness (severe); hypotension; nervousness or restlessness (severe); pinpoint pupils of eyes; respiratory depression; weakness (severe).

ANTIDOTE

Many side effects are medical emergencies. Manage respiratory depression during surgery via endotracheal intubation and assisted or controlled ventilation; prolonged mechanical ventilation may be required. Treat postoperative respiratory depression with naloxone (Narcan) or nalmefene (Revex); titrate dose carefully to improve respirations without reversing analgesic effects or causing other adverse effects (hypertension and tachycardia may result in left ventricular failure and pulmonary edema, especially in cardiac patients). Treat bradycardia with atropine, or alfentanil-induced bradycardia can be antagonized with the use of a neuromuscular blocking agent with vagolytic activity (e.g., pancuronium). Treat hypotension by placing the patient in a Trendelenburg position, if possible; administer IV fluids and a vasopressor (e.g., norepinephrine [Levophed], dopamine [Intropin]) if indicated. Naloxone or nalmefene may reverse hypotension postoperatively. Muscle rigidity during anesthesia induction or surgery must be controlled with neuromuscular blocking agents and controlled ventilation with oxygen. Use a neuromuscular blocking agent prophylactically to prevent muscle rigidity or to induce muscle relaxation after rigidity occurs. Neuromuscular blocking agents with vagolytic activity (e.g., pancuronium) may decrease risk of alfentanil-induced bradycardia and hypotension, but may increase the risk of hypertension or tachycardia in some patients. In patients with compromised cardiac function and/or those receiving a beta-adrenergic blocking agent preoperatively, a nonvagolytic neuromuscular blocking agent (e.g., succinylcholine) may increase the incidence and severity of bradycardia and hypotension. Respiratory depressant effects of neuromuscular blocking agents are additive with alfentanil. Postoperatively, naloxone or nalmefene may be used in small incremental doses to reverse skeletal muscle rigidity. Resuscitate as necessary.

ALLOPURINOL SODIUM

(al-oh-pure′i-nole so′de-um)

Antigout
Antihyperuricemic
Antineoplastic adjunct

Aloprim, Zyloprim

pH 10.8 to 11.8

USUAL DOSE

IV and oral doses are therapeutically equivalent. Oral dose can replace an IV dose at any time. See Monitor.

Aloprim: 200 to 400 mg/M^2/day as a single infusion or in equally divided doses at 6-, 8-, or 12-hour intervals. Total dose should not exceed 600 mg/day.

Zyloprim: 300 to 600 mg/day as a single infusion or in equally divided doses at 6-, 8-, or 12-hour intervals. Usually given at 8-hour intervals. An alternate dosing regimen is 40 to 150 mg/M^2 every 8 hours. Higher dose range possibly more effective in adults. Total dose should not exceed 800 mg/day.

PEDIATRIC DOSE

Recommended starting dose is 200 mg/M^2/day. An alternate source suggests 10 mg/kg/day with a maximum total dose of 600 mg/day. Usually given in equally divided doses at 6- to 8-hour intervals. Another source says the daily dose may be given at 6-, 8-, or 12-hour intervals or as a single daily infusion. Studies found no significant difference in dose response in pediatric patients. See comments in Usual Dose.

DOSE ADJUSTMENTS

Dialysis patients may require the usual dose of allopurinol. In patients with impaired renal function not on dialysis, reduce dose based on CrCl according to the following chart.

Allopurinol Dosing in Impaired Renal Function

CrCl ml/min	Dose
10-20	200 mg daily
3-10	100 mg daily
<3	100 mg daily at extended intervals

Treat with the lowest effective dose to minimize side effects. ■ Dose with normal renal function may be increased or decreased based on electrolytes and serum uric acid levels. ■ Lower doses and/or extended intervals may be required in the elderly; see Elderly. ■ See Drug/Lab Interactions.

DILUTION

Available as a single-dose vial containing 500 mg of allopurinol. Reconstitute with 25 ml of SW for injection (yields 20 mg/ml). Swirl until completely dissolved. Must be further diluted with NS or D5W. Maximum concentration for administration is 6 mg/ml. 19 ml of additional diluent per 20 mg (1 ml) yields 1 mg/ml, 9 ml of additional diluent yields 2 mg/ml, and 2.3 ml of additional diluent yields 6 mg/ml.

Storage: Store unopened vials at CRT. ***Aloprim:*** Do not refrigerate the reconstituted and/or diluted product; begin infusion within 10 hours of reconstitution. ***Zyloprim:*** Use reconstituted solution within 24 hours.

INCOMPATIBLE WITH

Manufacturer recommends administering sequentially and flushing before and after administration. Manufacturer lists the following drugs as incompatible: amikacin (Amikin), amphotericin B (Amphotec, Fungizone), carmustine (BiCNU), cefotaxime (Claforan), chlorpromazine (Thorazine), cimetidine (Tagamet), clindamycin (Cleocin), cytarabine (ARA-C), dacarbazine (DTIC), daunorubicin (Cerubidine), diphenhydramine (Benadryl), doxorubicin (Adriamycin), doxycycline (Vibramycin), droperidol (Inapsine), floxuridine (FUDR), gentamicin (Garamycin), haloperidol (Haldol), idarubicin (Idamycin), imipenem-cilastatin (Primaxin), mechlorethamine (Mustargen), meperidine (Demerol), methylprednisolone (Solu-Medrol), metoclopramide (Reglan), minocycline (Minocin), nalbuphine (Nubain), ondansetron (Zofran), prochlorperazine (Compazine), promethazine (Phenergan), sodium bicarbonate, streptozocin (Zanosar), tobramycin (Nebcin), vinorelbine (Navelbine). ***Do not use solutions containing sodium bicarbonate.***

COMPATIBLE WITH

Consult pharmacist; specific conditions may apply; see Compatibilities, p. xvi.

Y-site: Acyclovir (Zovirax), aminophylline, aztreonam (Azactam), bleomycin (Blenoxane), bumetanide (Bumex), buprenorphine (Buprenex), butorphanol (Stadol), calcium gluconate, carboplatin (Paraplatin), cefazolin (Kefzol), cefoperazone (Cefobid), cefotetan (Cefotan), ceftazidime (Fortaz), ceftizoxime (Cefizox), ceftriaxone (Rocephin), cefuroxime (Kefurox), cisplatin (Platinol), cyclophosphamide (Cytoxan), dactinomycin (Cosmegen), dexamethasone (Decadron), doxorubicin liposome (Doxil), enalaprilat (Vasotec IV), etoposide (VePesid), famotidine (Pepcid IV), fluconazole (Diflucan), fludarabine (Fludara), fluorouracil (5-FU), furosemide (Lasix), ganciclovir (Cytovene), granisetron (Kytril), heparin, hydrocortisone (Hydrocortone, Solu-Cortef), hydromorphone (Dilaudid), ifosfamide (Ifex), lorazepam (Ativan), mannitol, mesna (Mesnex), methotrexate (Folex), metronidazole (Flagyl IV), mitoxantrone (Novantrone), morphine, piperacillin (Pipracil), plicamycin (Mithracin), potassium chloride (KCl), ranitidine (Zantac), sulfamethoxazole-trimethoprim (Bactrim), teniposide (Vumon), thiotepa (Thioplex), ticarcillin (Ticar), ticarcillin/clavulanate (Timentin), vancomycin (Vancocin), vinblastine (Velban), vincristine (Oncovin), zidovudine (AZT, Retrovir).

RATE OF ADMINISTRATION

Manufacturer's recommendation not available. A maximum dose should take at least ½ to 1 hour or more based on volume with diluent and patient comfort and/or requirements. Include in hydration fluids. See Incompatible With.

ACTIONS

A xanthine oxidase inhibitor. Metabolized to oxypurinol. Acts on purine catabolism without disrupting the biosynthesis of purines. Reduces the production of uric acid by inhibiting the biochemical reactions immediately preceding its formation. Decreases uric acid concentrations in both serum and urine. Prevents or decreases urate deposition, decreasing the occurrence or progression of gout or urate nephropathy. Onset of action is within 10 minutes. Reduction of serum uric acid concentration occurs in 2 to 3 days. Peak concentrations are related to dose. Pharmacokinetic and plasma profiles of allopurinol and oxypurinol, as well as half-lives and systemic clearance, are similar with IV or oral administration. Systemic exposure to oxypurinol is also similar by both routes at each dose level. Cleared by glomerular filtration; some oxypurinol is reabsorbed in the kidney tubules. Secreted in breast milk.

INDICATIONS AND USES

Management of patients with leukemia, lymphoma, and solid tumor malignancies who are receiving cancer therapy that causes elevations of serum and urinary uric acid levels and who cannot tolerate oral therapy. Consider prophylactic use before initiation of and during chemotherapy in patients who are NPO, are nauseated and vomiting, or have malabsorption problems, dysphagia, or GI tract dysfunctions. IV route is used to attain rapid, significant blood levels; accurately dose pediatric patients; and dose patients with questionable compliance. Used prophylactically before the initiation of and during chemotherapy to prevent tumor lysis syndrome (TLS) and its sequela, acute uric acid nephropathy (AUAN).

Unlabeled uses: Preservation of cadaveric kidneys for transplantation.

CONTRAINDICATIONS

Any patient who has had a severe reaction to allopurinol (usually a hypersensitivity reaction).

PRECAUTIONS

For IV infusion only. ▪ A skin rash or other beginning signs of hypersensitivity may be followed by exfoliative, urticarial, and purpuric lesions; Stevens-Johnson syndrome; generalized vasculitis; irreversible hepatotoxicity; and/or rarely death. ▪ Incidence of hypersensitivity reactions may be increased in patients with decreased renal function especially in those receiving concurrent thiazides (e.g., chlorothiazide [Diuril]); use with caution. ▪ See Drug/Lab Interactions.

Monitor: Whenever possible, begin allopurinol therapy 24 to 48 hours before the start of chemotherapy known to cause tumor cell lysis (including adrenocorticosteroids). ▪ Monitor serum uric acid levels and electrolytes before and during therapy. Monitor serum uric acid levels to determine dose and frequency required to maintain uric acid levels within the normal range. ▪ Hydration with 3,000 ml/M^2/day (twice the level of maintenance fluid replacement) is recommended to promote a high volume of urine output (more than 2 L/day in adults) with low urate concentration. ▪ Maintain urine at neutral or slightly alkaline pH. To increase solubility of uric acid, alkalinity of urine may be increased with sodium bicarbonate. ▪ Monitor renal and hepatic systems before and during therapy. ▪ Monitoring of liver function suggested in patients with preexisting liver disease, in patients with increases in liver function tests, and in patients who develop anorexia, pruritus, or weight loss. ▪ Observe for symptoms of TLS (e.g., hyperuricemia, hyperkalemia, hyperphosphatemia, and hypocalcemia). If untreated, may develop AUAN leading to renal failure requiring hemodialysis. ▪ Bone marrow suppression has been reported; monitor CBC periodically.

Patient Education: Report promptly blood in the urine, painful urination, irritation of the eyes, skin rash, or swelling of the lips or mouth. ▪ Major acute toxicities may be allergic or renal. ▪ May cause drowsiness;

use caution in activities that require alertness. Request assistance for ambulation.

Maternal/Child: Category C: potential benefits must justify potential risks to fetus. ■ Use caution if required during breast-feeding.

Elderly: Lower-end initial doses or extended intervals may be appropriate in the elderly based on potential for decreased organ function, concomitant disease, or other drug therapy.

DRUG/LAB INTERACTIONS

May increase toxicity of didanosine (Videx); concurrent use not recommended. ■ Inhibits metabolism and increases effects and toxicity of thiopurines (e.g., azathioprine [Imuran], mercaptopurine [Purinethol]). Reduce dose of thiopurine to one third to one fourth. ■ Uricosuric agents (e.g., sulfinpyrazone [Anturane], probenecid [Benemid], colchicine) may increase elimination of active metabolites of allopurinol; may increase urinary excretions of uric acid. ■ Prolongs half-life of dicumarol; monitor PT or PTT and adjust anticoagulant dose as indicated. ■ Frequency of skin rash increased with ampicillin/amoxicillin. ■ Bone marrow suppression may be increased when given concurrently with cytotoxic agents (e.g., cyclophosphamide [Cytoxan]); risk of bleeding or infection may be increased. ■ May prolong half-life of chlorpropamide (Diabinese). ■ Hypersensitivity reactions may be increased with ACE inhibitors (e.g., enalaprilat) or thiazide diuretics (e.g., chlorothiazide [Diuril]). ■ Concurrent use with cyclosporine (Sandimmune) may increase cyclosporine serum levels. A reduced dose of cyclosporine may be indicated; monitoring of cyclosporine serum levels suggested. ■ Larger doses (more than 600 mg/day) may decrease clearance and increase toxicity of theophyllines (e.g., Aminophyllin).

SIDE EFFECTS

Fewer than 1% of patients have had side effects directly attributable to allopurinol. Most were allergic in nature (nausea and vomiting, rash, and renal failure/insufficiency) and of mild to moderate severity. Xanthine crystalluria has been rarely reported in long-term therapy with oral allopurinol.

ANTIDOTE

Discontinue allopurinol at the first sign of skin rash or any other allergic reaction. Do not restart. Keep physician informed of all side effects. Symptoms of TLS require immediate intervention and correction of electrolyte abnormalities to avoid kidney damage. Treat allergic reactions as indicated; may require epinephrine (Adrenalin), diphenhydramine (Benadryl), corticosteroids (hydrocortisone), and/or oxygen. Allopurinol is dialyzable, but effectiveness of hemodialysis or peritoneal dialysis in an overdose is not known.

ALPHA$_1$-PROTEINASE INHIBITOR (HUMAN)

(al′fah pro′ten-as in-hib′i-ter [hu′man])

Alpha$_1$-antitrypsin replenisher

Alpha$_1$-antitrypsin, Alpha$_1$-PI, Aralast, Prolastin

pH 7.2 to 7.8 (Aralast) ▪ pH 6.6 to 7.4 (Prolastin)

USUAL DOSE

60 mg/kg once a week as an infusion.

Manufacturers of Prolastin recommend immunizing every patient against hepatitis B before administration. If immediate treatment is required, give a single dose of hepatitis B immune globulin (human) 0.06 ml/kg IM at the same time as the initial dose of hepatitis B vaccine.

DILUTION

Bring components to room temperature (diluent [SW] and lyophilized preparation of alpha$_1$-PI). Insert one end of the double-ended transfer needle (shortest end for Prolastin) into the diluent. Invert the bottle of diluent and insert the other end of the transfer needle at a 45-degree angle into the alpha$_1$-PI; diluent will be drawn into the alpha$_1$-PI by a vacuum. Remove the diluent bottle. Allow the reconstituted solution to stand until contents appear to be in solution, then swirl gently to completely dissolve. ***Do not shake or invert vial until ready to withdraw contents.*** May take 5 to 10 minutes.

Aralast will yield 25 ml/0.5 Gm vial or 50 ml/1 Gm vial. **Prolastin** will yield 20 ml/0.5 Gm vial or 40 ml/1 Gm vial. Must be filtered before or during administration. Manufacturers supply either a filter needle to withdraw alpha$_1$-PI from the vial or an in-line filter (to be used for pooling or in IV line). Several vials may be pooled into an empty sterile IV solution container. Must be given within 3 hours of reconstitution.

Storage: Both products must be refrigerated before reconstitution; avoid freezing. Do not use after expiration date on vials. Before reconstitution, ***Aralast*** can be stored at temperatures not to exceed 25° C (77° F) for up to 1 month.

COMPATIBILITY

Manufacturer states, "Should be given alone, without mixing with other agents or diluting solutions."

RATE OF ADMINISTRATION

0.08 ml/kg/min is recommended. If adverse effects occur, a reduced rate or interruption of the infusion may be indicated until symptoms subside; see Side Effects and Antidote.

ACTIONS

A sterile, stable, lyophilized preparation obtained from human plasma. Increases and maintains functional levels of alpha$_1$-PI in the epithelial lining of the lower respiratory tract. Provides adequate antineutrophil elastase activity in the lungs of individuals with alpha$_1$-antitrypsin deficiency. Numerous processes employed during manufacture to eliminate potential for viral transmission from human plasma; see Precautions.

INDICATIONS AND USES

Treatment of congenital alpha$_1$-antitrypsin deficiency, a potentially fatal disease; used for chronic replacement only in individuals with selected types of clinically demonstrated emphysema.

CONTRAINDICATIONS

Individuals with selective IgA deficiencies (IgA level less than 15 mg/dl for **Aralast**) who have known antibody against IgA (anti-IgA antibody). IgA may be present and severe reactions, including anaphylaxis, can occur.

PRECAUTIONS

Confirm diagnosis of congenital alpha$_1$-antitrypsin deficiency with selected clinically demonstrated emphysema. ■ Each unit of plasma tested and found nonreactive to HIV antibody, Creutzfeldt-Jacob disease, hepatitis B surface antigen, and hepatitis C. Transmission of these viruses is still possible. ■ Will increase plasma volume; use caution in patients at risk for circulatory overload. ■ Long-term effects from continued use are not known.

Monitor: Monitor V/S and observe patient continuously throughout infusion. ■ Blood levels of alpha$_1$-PI have been maintained above the functional level of 80 mg/dl with this replacement therapy. Serum levels determined by commercial immunologic assays may not reflect actual functional alpha$_1$-PI levels. ■ Assess lung sounds and rate and quality of respirations before each infusion. ■ Monitor for S/S of an allergic reaction (e.g., dyspnea, flushing, hypotension, rash, tachycardia); emergency equipment, medications, and supplies must be available.

Patient Education: Inform of risks and of safety precautions taken during manufacturing process. ■ Note changes in breathing pattern or sputum production; avoid smoking.

Maternal/Child: Category C: use in pregnancy only when clearly needed. May present risk to fetus; benefits must justify risks. ■ Safety for use during breast-feeding not established, effects unknown. ■ Safety for use in pediatric patients not established.

DRUG/LAB INTERACTIONS

No specific information available.

SIDE EFFECTS

Aralast: Cough, headache, and pharyngitis are most common. Asthma, back pain, bloating, bronchitis, dizziness, pain, peripheral edema, rash, rhinitis, sinusitis, somnolence, and viral infection may occur.

Prolastin: Mild transient leukocytosis several hours after transfusion. Dizziness, fever, or light-headedness may occur.

All formulations: Consider risk potential of contracting AIDS, Creutzfeldt-Jacob disease, hepatitis B, or hepatitis C. Allergic reactions, including anaphylaxis, chills, dyspnea, hypotension, rash, tachycardia have been reported; see Contraindications.

ANTIDOTE

All side effects except potential transmission of viral diseases usually subside spontaneously. Keep the physician informed. If side effects occur, interrupt or discontinue infusion until symptoms subside, then resume at a tolerated rate. Discontinue alpha$_1$-PI and treat anaphylaxis (antihistamines, epinephrine, corticosteroids) as indicated. Resuscitate as necessary.

ALPROSTADIL

(al-pros'ta-dil)

Prostaglandin
(ductus arteriosus patency adjunct)

Prostaglandin E_1, Prostin VR Pediatric

USUAL DOSE

Begin with 0.05 to 0.1 mcg/kg of body weight/min. When therapeutic response is achieved, reduce infusion rate to lowest dose that maintains the response (0.1 mcg to 0.05 to 0.025 to 0.01 mcg/min). If necessary, dose may be increased gradually to a maximum of 0.4 mcg/kg/min. Generally these higher rates do not produce greater effects. May be given through infusion in a large vein or, if necessary, through an umbilical artery catheter placed at the ductal opening.

DILUTION

Each 500 mcg must be further diluted with NS or D5W. Various volumes may be used depending on infusion pump capabilities and desired infusion rate.

Guidelines for Dilution and Rate of Infusion for Desired Dose of Alprostadil

Diluent	Concentration	Desired Dose	Rate of Infusion
250 ml	2 mcg/ml	0.1 mcg/kg/min	0.05 ml/min/kg
25 ml	20 mcg/ml	0.1 mcg/kg/min	0.005 ml/min/kg

Storage: Refrigerate until dilution. Prepare fresh solution for administration every 24 hours.

COMPATIBILITY

Specific information not available; consult pharmacist before use with any other agent as an additive or at Y-site.

RATE OF ADMINISTRATION

See Usual Dose. Infusion pump capable of delivering 0.005, 0.01, 0.02, or 0.05 ml/min/kg required. Use for the shortest time possible at the lowest rate therapeutically effective. Decrease rate of infusion *stat* if a significant fall in arterial pressure occurs.

ACTIONS

A naturally occurring acidic lipid. Smooth muscle of the ductus arteriosus is susceptible to its relaxing effect, which reduces BP and peripheral resistance and increases cardiac output and rate. In newborns it relaxes and may open the ductus. Metabolized by oxidation almost instantly (80% in one pass through the lungs). Remainder excreted as metabolites in the urine.

INDICATIONS AND USES

Temporarily maintain the patency of the ductus arteriosus until corrective or palliative surgery can be performed on infants with pulmonary atresia, pulmonary stenosis, tricuspid atresia, tetralogy of Fallot, interruption of the aortic arch, coarctation of the aorta, or transposition of the great vessels. ▪ Used by intercavernosal injection to treat impotence.

CONTRAINDICATIONS

None known. Not indicated for respiratory distress syndrome (hyaline membrane disease).

PRECAUTIONS

Usually administered by trained personnel in pediatric intensive care facilities. ■ Establish a diagnosis of cyanotic heart disease (restricted pulmonary blood flow). ■ Response is poor in infants with Po_2 values of 40 mm Hg or those more than 4 days old. More effective with lower Po_2. ■ Use caution in neonates with bleeding tendencies; inhibits platelet aggregation.

Monitor: Monitor respiratory status continuously. Ventilatory assistance must be immediately available. May cause apnea (10% to 12% experience), especially in infants under 2 kg. ■ Monitor arterial pressure intermittently by umbilical artery catheter, auscultation, or Doppler transducer. Decrease rate of infusion *stat* if a significant fall in arterial pressure occurs. ■ Measure effectiveness with increase of Po_2 in infants with restricted pulmonary blood flow and increase of BP and blood pH in infants with restricted systemic blood flow.

DRUG/LAB INTERACTIONS

Inhibits platelet aggregation.

SIDE EFFECTS

Cardiac arrest, cerebral bleeding, cortical proliferation of long bones, diarrhea, DIC, hyperextension of the neck, hyperirritability, hypothermia, seizures, sepsis, tachycardia. Many other side effects have occurred in 1% or less of infants receiving alprostadil.

Overdose: Apnea, bradycardia, flushing, hypotension, pyrexia.

ANTIDOTE

Notify physician of all side effects. Discontinue immediately if apnea or bradycardia occurs. Institute emergency measures. If infusion is restarted use extreme caution. Decrease rate if pyrexia, hypotension, or fall in arterial pressure occurs. Flushing is usually caused by incorrect intraarterial catheter placement. Reposition.

ALTEPLASE, RECOMBINANT

(all'te-place)

Thrombolytic agent (recombinant)

Activase, rt-PA, Tissue Plasminogen Activator, tPA ▪ Cathflo Activase

pH 7.3

USUAL DOSE

Selected indications (e.g., acute ischemic stroke, weight under 65 or 67 kg in acute MI) require exact weight-adjusted dosing. To deliver an accurate dose without possibility of overdose, calculate desired dose and withdraw any amount NOT needed from a 50- or 100-mg vial and discard. In all situations follow total dose with at least 30 ml of NS or D5W through the IV tubing to ensure administration of total dose.

ACUTE MYOCARDIAL INFARCTION

Total dose is based on patient weight and should not exceed 100 mg. Concurrent administration of heparin, aspirin, and/or dipyridamole (Persantine) has been consistently used in MI patients receiving alteplase therapy. MI patients in the ***accelerated infusion*** studies received a loading dose of heparin 5,000 units, followed by 1,000 units/hr by continuous infusion for 48 hours. Dose is adjusted to raise aPTT to between 1.5 to 2 times control. Aspirin therapy was usually concurrent (e.g., 160 mg chewable aspirin on admission, followed by 160 to 325 mg/day) or followed with aspirin after 48 hours. 90% of MI patients receiving the 3-hour infusion also received heparin as a continuous infusion with or without a loading dose and either aspirin or dipyridamole; see Precautions and Monitor. The earlier intervention occurs, the better the results. Most effective if administered within 4 to 6 hours of onset of symptoms of acute myocardial infarction.

Accelerated infusion; weight 67 kg or greater: 100 mg titrated over 90 minutes as an IV infusion. Initially give a bolus of 15 mg over 2 minutes. Follow with 50 mg evenly distributed over 30 minutes. Infuse the remaining 35 mg dose evenly distributed over 60 minutes. See comments under Usual Dose.

Accelerated infusion; weight less than 67 kg: See comments in first paragraph of Usual Dose. Initially give a bolus of 15 mg over 2 minutes. Follow with 0.75 mg/kg (not to exceed a 50-mg dose) evenly distributed over 30 minutes. Then infuse 0.5 mg/kg (not to exceed a 35-mg dose) evenly distributed over 60 minutes. See comments under Usual Dose.

3-hour infusion; weight 65 kg or greater: 100 mg titrated over 3 hours as an IV infusion. Initially, give a bolus of 6 to 10 mg over 2 minutes. Follow with 50 to 54 mg (total 60-mg dose) evenly distributed over the first hour. Follow with 20 mg/hr for 2 hours. See comments under Usual Dose.

3-hour infusion; weight less than 65 kg: Calculate total dose using 1.25 mg/kg of body weight. See comments in first paragraph of Usual Dose. Give three fifths of this total calculated dose divided as above into a bolus and first-hour dose. Give one fifth of this total calculated dose/hr for 2 hours. See comments under Usual Dose.

ACUTE ISCHEMIC STROKE

0.9 mg/kg. Do not exceed the maximum dose of 90 mg. See comments in Usual Dose. Give a bolus of 10% of the calculated dose over 1 minute followed by balance of calculated dose (90%) as an infusion evenly distributed over 60 minutes. Treatment must start within 3 hours of onset of symptoms, but after bleeding in the brain has been ruled out (usually by a non-contrast CT scan of the brain). Do not give aspirin, heparin, or warfarin for 24 hours; see Precautions.

PULMONARY EMBOLISM

100 mg titrated over 2 hours as an IV infusion. Diagnosis should be confirmed by objective means (e.g., lung scan, pulmonary angiography). Begin heparin at end of infusion or immediately after it is complete. Thrombin time (TT) or PTT should be twice normal or less.

CENTRAL VENOUS ACCESS DEVICE (CVAD) OCCLUSIONS, CATHFLO ACTIVASE

See Rate of Administration, Precautions, Monitor, and Maternal/Child. **Patient weight 30 kg or greater:** Instill 2 mg in 2 ml into the occluded catheter. **Patient weight 10 to 29 kg:** Instill 110% of the internal lumen volume of the occluded catheter into the occluded catheter. Do not exceed 2 mg in 2 ml. **Patient weight less than 10 kg:** Safety and effectiveness not established.

Attempt to aspirate blood from the catheter after 30 minutes of dwell time. If catheter function has been restored, aspirate 4 to 5 ml of blood to remove Cathflo Activase and residual clot, then gently irrigate the catheter with NS.

If catheter function has not been restored (unable to aspirate blood), allow the first dose to remain in the catheter for 90 additional minutes of dwell time and then attempt to aspirate again (total elapsed time is 120 minutes). If catheter function has been restored, aspirate and irrigate as above. If function has not been restored, a second dose may be instilled and the dwell time and aspiration process repeated.

DILUTION

Myocardial infarction, stroke, and pulmonary embolism: Must be reconstituted with SW without preservatives (provided by manufacturer). Available in 50- and 100-mg vials (1 mg/ml). May be reconstituted with NS, D5W, but this will result in a hypertonic solution. Consider patient's hemodynamic status. Use of filters or filter needles not recommended. Protein adsorption may occur with resulting drug loss. ***50-mg vials:*** Use a large-bore (18-gauge) needle and direct the stream of diluent into the lyophilized cake. A vacuum must be present when the diluent is added to the powder for injection. Do not use if vacuum not present. Slight foaming is expected; let stand for several minutes to dissipate large bubbles. If necessary, may be further diluted to 0.5 mg/ml immediately before administration with an equal volume of NS or D5W. Do not shake. Mix by swirling or slow inversion; avoid agitation during dilution. Dilution with less than the recommended volume to concentrations greater than 1 mg/ml will also result in a hypertonic solution. Dilution beyond 0.5 mg/ml may cause precipitation. Use balance (at least 30 ml) of 250-ml bottle of NS or D5W to clear tubing after infusion and ensure delivery of total dose; NS is preferred.

Connect NS or D5W to metriset and pump tubing. Clamp between solution and metriset. Add alteplase to metriset. Prime tubing with alteplase. Bolus dose can be given when indicated by IV injection through a med port or by IV pump. Administer balance of dose as outlined in Usual Dose section, adjusting pump rate of delivery as required. Complete by flushing tubing with IV solution.

100-mg vial: Diluent and transfer device provided (does not contain a vacuum). Insert one end of transfer device into upright vial of diluent (do not invert diluent vial yet). Hold alteplase vial upside down and push center of vial down onto piercing pin. Now invert vials and allow diluent to flow into alteplase. Small amount (0.5 ml) of diluent will not transfer. Swirl gently to dissolve. Do not shake. Process takes several minutes. An infusion set may be inserted into puncture site created by piercing pin. Hang by plastic capping on bottom of vial. Prime tubing with alteplase and administer as outlined above for 50-mg vials.

Cathflo Activase for CVAD occlusion: Supplied as a sterile lyophilized powder in 2.2-mg vials. Must be reconstituted with 2.2 mg of SW without preservatives. Direct diluent stream into the powder. Allow to stand undisturbed until large bubbles dissipate; may foam slightly. Mix by swirling gently; do not shake. Should be completely dissolved within 3 minutes. Final concentration is 1 mg/ml. If the 2-mg vials are not available, some pharmacies dilute 50 mg of alteplase with 50 ml of SW without preservatives (1 mg/ml). Withdraw 2.2 ml (2.2 mg) to 2- or 5-ml sterile disposable syringes. In studies these were transferred to sterile glass vials and frozen. Defrost and use as needed (22 prepared doses).

Storage: *Systemic alteplase:* Protect from light in cartons. May be stored at CRT or refrigerated before and/or after reconstitution. Manufacturer recommends reconstitution immediately before use. Must be used within 8 hours of reconstitution. Discard unused solution. Stable as a 0.5 mg/ml solution in NS or D5W for 8 hours at CRT.

Cathflo Activase: Refrigerate unopened vials; protect from light during extended storage. Reconstitution immediately before use is recommended, but solution may be used up to 8 hours after reconstitution if refrigerated at 2° to 30° C. Do not use beyond expiration date on vial. Discard unused solution.

INCOMPATIBLE WITH

Bacteriostatic water for injection (BWFI). Manufacturer states, "No other medication should be added to infusion solutions containing alteplase. Do not use other infusion solutions (e.g., SW or other preservative-containing solutions) for further dilution"; see Dilution. One source suggests D5W used for reconstitution or further dilution may cause a precipitate.

COMPATIBLE WITH

Consult pharmacist; specific conditions may apply; see Compatibilities, p. xvi.

Y-site: Lidocaine, metoprolol (Lopressor), and propranolol (Inderal) through Y-site of free-flowing alteplase infusion.

RATE OF ADMINISTRATION

Systemic alteplase: See specific rates for each diagnosis under Usual Dose. In all situations use an infusion pump (preferred) or a metriset with microdrip (60 gtt/ml) and IV tubing without a filter to facilitate accurate administration. Do not use any filters. Distribute final flush over 30 minutes. NS preferred for flushing of IV line.

Cathflo Activase: Avoid excessive pressure or force while attempting to clear catheters; see Usual Dose, Precautions, and Monitor.

ACTIONS

A tissue plasminogen activator and enzyme produced by recombinant DNA. It binds to fibrin in a thrombus and converts plasminogen to plasmin. Plasmin digests fibrin and dissolves the clot. With therapeutic doses, a decrease in circulating fibrinogen makes the patient susceptible to bleeding. Onset of action is prompt, effecting patency of the vessel within 1 to 2 hours in most patients. Prompt opening of arteries increases probability of improved function. Cleared from the plasma by the liver within 5 (50%) to 10 (80%) minutes after the infusion is discontinued. Some effects may linger for 45 minutes to several hours.

INDICATIONS AND USES

Systemic alteplase: Management of acute myocardial infarction in adults for the lysis of thrombi obstructing coronary arteries, the reduction of infarct size, the improvement of ventricular function, and the reduction of the incidence of congestive heart failure. Recent studies suggest alteplase or reteplase are the drugs of choice. ▪ Current AHA recommendations identify thrombolytic agents as Class I therapy in patients younger than 70 years with recent onset of chest pain (within 6 hours) consistent with acute MI and at least 0.1 mV of ST segment elevation in at least two ECG leads. Use in all other patients based on age, accurate diagnosis, and time from onset of chest pain. ▪ Management of acute ischemic stroke in adults to improve neurologic recovery and reduce incidence of disability. ▪ Management of acute massive pulmonary embolism in adults for the lysis of acute pulmonary emboli either obstructing blood flow to a lobe or multiple segments of the lung or accompanied by unstable hemodynamics (e.g., failure to maintain BP).

Cathflo Activase: Restoration of function to CVADs as assessed by the ability to withdraw blood.

Unlabeled uses: ***Systemic alteplase:*** Treatment of unstable angina pectoris and deep vein thrombosis. Has been shown to restore blood flow to frostbitten limbs (0.075 mg/kg/hr for 6 hours). Has been used to clear thrombi in central venous catheters (2 mg bolus into the blocked catheter), in the occlusion of small blood vessels by microthrombi, and in management of peripheral thromboembolism (0.5 to 1 mg/hr intraarterially).

CONTRAINDICATIONS

Acute myocardial infarction/pulmonary embolism: Active internal bleeding, arteriovenous malformation or aneurysm, bleeding diathesis, cerebrovascular accident, intracranial or intraspinal surgery or trauma within 2 months, intracranial neoplasm, severe uncontrolled hypertension.

Acute ischemic stroke: Active internal bleeding. Evidence of intracranial hemorrhage on pretreatment evaluation. Clinical presentation suggestive of subarachnoid hemorrhage (even with normal CT). History of intracranial hemorrhage, intracranial neoplasm, arteriovenous malformation, or aneurysm. History of intracranial surgery, serious head trauma, or previous stroke within 3 months. Known bleeding diathesis (e.g., current use of oral anticoagulants [e.g., warfarin] with PT greater than 15 seconds). Administration of heparin within 48 hours before onset of stroke with an elevated aPTT as presentation (greater than upper limit of normal for laboratory). Platelet count less than 100,000/mm^3. Seizure observed at the same time as the onset of stroke. Uncontrolled hypertension at time of treatment (e.g., systolic above 185 or diastolic above 110) and patient requires aggressive treatment to reduce BP to within these limits.

Cathflo Activase: Known hypersensitivity to alteplase or its components.

PRECAUTIONS

All systemic indications: A 150-mg dose has caused increased intracranial bleeding; do not use. ■ Administered under the direction of a physician knowledgeable in its use and with appropriate emergency drugs and diagnostic and laboratory facilities available. ■ A greater alteration of hemostatic status than with heparin. Strict bed rest indicated to reduce risk of bleeding. Use extreme care with the patient; avoid any excessive or rough handling or pressure (including too-frequent BPs); avoid invasive procedures (e.g., arterial puncture, venipuncture, IM injection). If these procedures are absolutely necessary, use extreme precautionary methods (use radial artery instead of femoral; use small-gauge catheters and needles, and sites that are easily observed and compressible where bleeding can be controlled; avoid handling catheter sites; and use extended pressure application of up to 30 minutes). Minor bleeding occurs often at catheter insertion sites. Avoid use of razors and toothbrushes. ■ Use extreme caution in the following situations: abnormal blood glucose (less than 50 or greater than 400 mg/dl), major surgery or serious trauma (excluding head trauma; see Contraindications) in the previous 14 days, GI or GU bleeding within 21 days, or puncture of noncompressible vessels (e.g., arterial puncture, spinal puncture, thoracentesis) within the previous 10 days; cerebrovascular disease; hypertension (systolic above 180 or diastolic above 110); mitral stenosis with atrial fibrillation (likelihood of left heart thrombus); acute pericarditis; subacute bacterial endocarditis; coagulation disorders, including those secondary to severe hepatic or renal disease; severe liver dysfunction; pregnancy and first 10 days postpartum; hemorrhagic ophthalmic conditions (e.g., diabetic hemorrhagic retinopathy); septic thrombophlebitis; patients on anticoagulants; patients over 75 years of age; any situation where bleeding might be hazardous or difficult to manage because of location. ■ Not antigenic (does not promote antibody formation). Risk of allergic reactions less than with anistreplase or streptokinase. A second course can be administered if reocclusion occurs. May increase risk of severe hemorrhage, especially if effects of first dose have not subsided.

Myocardial infarction: Reperfusion arrhythmias occur frequently (e.g., sinus bradycardia, accelerated idioventricular rhythm, PVCs, ventricular tachycardia); have antiarrhythmic meds available at bedside. ■ Simultaneous therapy with continuous infusion of heparin (with or without a loading dose and aspirin or dipyridamole) is used to reduce the risk of rethrombosis. Increases risk of bleeding; see Usual Dose. ■ Standard treatment for myocardial infarction continues simultaneously with alteplase therapy except if temporarily contraindicated (e.g., arterial blood gases, unless absolutely necessary).

Acute ischemic stroke: Treatment facility must be able to provide evaluation and management of intracranial hemorrhage. ■ Do not use anticoagulants (e.g., heparin, aspirin, coumadin) during the first 24 hours. If any anticoagulant is indicated after 24 hours, consider performing a non-contrast CT scan or other sensitive diagnostic imaging method to rule out any intracranial hemorrhage before starting an anticoagulant. Another source suggested that antiplatelet agents (e.g., ticlopidine [Ticlid], dipyridamole [Persantine]) and anticoagulants should not be used within the first 24 hours. ■ Risks of alteplase therapy in the treatment of acute ischemic stroke may be increased in patients with severe neurologic deficit at presentation (increased risk of intracranial hemorrhage), patients with major early infarct signs on CT scan (e.g., substantial edema, mass effect, or midline shift). ▪ Treatment may begin before coagulation study results are known in patients without recent use of oral anticoagulants or heparin. Discontinue infusion if pretreatment PT greater than 15 seconds or an elevated aPTT is identified. ▪ Benefits of therapy have not been studied in patients treated with alteplase more than 3 hours after the onset of symptoms; use is not recommended. Risk of intracranial hemorrhage increased; may cause cerebral edema with fatal brain herniation. ▪ Safety and efficacy in patients with minor neurologic deficit or rapidly improving symptoms before treatment is begun has not been studied; caution is recommended.

Pulmonary emboli: Begin heparin at end of infusion or immediately after it is complete. Thrombin time (TT) or PTT should be twice normal or less.

Cathflo Activase: Consider causes of catheter dysfunction other than thrombus formation (e.g., catheter malposition, mechanical failure, constriction by a suture, lipid deposits or drug precipitates within the catheter lumen). ▪ Do not apply vigorous suction during attempts to determine catheter occlusion; may risk damage to the vascular wall or collapse of soft-walled catheters. Avoid excessive pressure during instillation of Cathflo Activase into the catheter; may cause rupture of the catheter or expulsion of the clot into the circulation. ▪ Use caution with patients who have active internal bleeding, thrombocytopenia, other hemostatic defects (including those secondary to hepatic or renal disease). ▪ Use caution in patients who have conditions for which bleeding constitutes a significant hazard, who would be difficult to manage because of location, who are at high risk for embolic complication (e.g., venous thrombosis in the region of the catheter), or who have had any of the following within 48 hours: surgery, obstetrical delivery, percutaneous biopsy of viscera or deep tissues, or puncture of noncompressible vessels. ▪ Use caution in the presence of known or suspected infection in the catheter; may release a localized infection into the systemic circulation. ▪ See Monitor. ▪ Safety and effectiveness of doses greater than 2 mg has not been established.

Monitor: ***All systemic indications:*** Best to establish a separate IV line for alteplase. ▪ Obtain appropriate clotting studies (e.g., PT, TT, PTT, aPTT, CBC, fibrinogen levels, platelets). ▪ Diagnosis-specific baseline studies (e.g., ECG, CPK in myocardial infarction, non-contrast CT brain scan, and neurologic assessment in acute ischemic stroke, and lung scan or pulmonary angiography in pulmonary embolism) are indicated. ▪ Baseline assessment (patient condition, pain, hematomas, petechiae, or recent wounds) should be completed before administration. ▪ Type and crossmatch may also be ordered. ▪ Start IV if indicated (not previously established, other medications being administered through current IV, to have a line available for additional treatment). ▪ Maintain strict bed rest; monitor the patient carefully and frequently for pain and signs of bleeding; observe catheter sites at least every 15 minutes and apply pressure dressings to any recently invaded site; watch for hematuria, hematemesis, bloody stool, petechiae, hematoma, flank pain, muscle weakness; and do neuro checks every hour (or more frequently if indicated). Continue until normal clotting function returns. ▪ Monitor BP and maintain within appropriate limits with antihypertensives or vasopressors as indicated. ▪ Watch for extravasation; may cause ecchymosis and/or inflammation. Restart IV at another site. Moist compresses may be helpful. ■ See Precautions and Drug/Lab Interactions.

Myocardial infarction: Monitor ECG continuously, and record strips with greatest ST segment elevation initially and every 15 minutes for at least 4 hours. A 12-lead ECG is indicated when therapy is complete.

Acute ischemic stroke: Printed protocol guidelines are available from manufacturer and include the following recommendations. ■ Before the initiation of therapy, determine actual time of onset of stroke. ■ Obtain baseline hematocrit, platelet count, and blood glucose. PT or aPTT is recommended in patients with recent use of oral anticoagulants or heparin. Obtain baseline BP, neurologic exam, and non-contrast CT brain scan. ■ Monitor BP every 15 minutes before beginning therapy; should be below 185/110. If over 185/110, BP may be treated with nitroglycerin paste (can be wiped off if BP drops quickly) and/or one or two 10- or 20-mg doses of labetalol (Normodyne, Trandate) give by IV injection within 1 hour. If these measures do not reduce BP below 185/110 and keep it down, the patient should not be treated with alteplase. ■ During and after treatment, monitor BP every 15 minutes for 2 hours, every 30 minutes for 6 hours, then every 1 hour for 18 hours. Avoid hypotension; may decrease perfusion of alteplase; a diastolic BP around 100 helps to maintain sufficient mean arterial pressure to reperfuse stroke area. ***See Antidote for protocol to treat hypertension occurring after treatment has been started.*** ■ Hemorrhage in the brain occurs frequently during treatment with alteplase during the first 36 hours; monitor carefully. Acute neurologic deterioration, new headache, acute hypertension, or nausea and vomiting may indicate the occurrence of intracranial hemorrhage. If intracranial hemorrhage is suspected, discontinue alteplase and obtain a non-contrast CT scan. ■ Monitor for S/S of atrial fibrillation and/or acute MI. ■ Studies did not show an increase in mortality and did confirm that more patients had minimal or no disability at 3 months.

Cathflo Activase: Aseptic technique imperative. ■ Avoid force while attempting to clear catheters; may rupture catheter or dislodge clot into the circulation. ■ To prevent air from entering the open catheter and the circulatory system, instruct the patient to exhale and hold his/her breath any time the catheter is not connected to the IV tubing or a syringe. ■ See Precautions.

Patient Education: Compliance with all measures to minimize bleeding (e.g., strict bed rest) is very important. ■ Avoid use of razors, toothbrushes, and other sharp items. Use caution while moving to avoid excessive bumping. ■ Report all episodes of bleeding and apply local pressure if indicated. Expect oozing from IV sites.

Maternal/Child: ***Systemic alteplase:*** Category C: safety for use in pregnancy, breast-feeding, and children not established.

Cathflo Activase: Category C: use during pregnancy only if benefits justify potential risk to the fetus. ■ Use caution during breast-feeding. ■ Not studied in patients younger than 2 years of age or weighing less than 10 kg. 11% of study participants were between 2 and 16 years of age. No drug-related adverse events were observed in this patient population.

Elderly: ***Systemic alteplase:*** See Indications and Precautions. ■ May have poorer prognosis following acute MI and pre-existing conditions that may increase risk of intracranial bleeding. Select patients carefully to maximize benefits.

Cathflo Activase: No incidents of intracranial hemorrhage, embolic events, or major bleeding events were observed during studies. ▪ Use caution in the elderly with conditions known to increase the risk of bleeding; see Precautions.

DRUG/LAB INTERACTIONS

Risk of bleeding may be increased by any medicine that affects blood clotting including anticoagulants (e.g., heparin, lepirudin [Refludan], warfarin [Coumadin]); Glycoprotein GPIIb/IIIa receptor antagonists (e.g., abciximab [ReoPro], eptifibatide [Integrilin], tirofiban [Aggrastat]); any medication that may cause hypoprothrombinemia, thrombocytopenia, or GI ulceration or bleeding (e.g., selected antibiotics such as cefamandole [Mandol], cefoperazone [Cefobid], cefotetan [Cefotan], ticarcillin [Ticar], aspirin, NSAIDs [e.g., ibuprofen (Advil, Motrin), naproxen (Aleve, Naprosyn), phenylbutazone (Butazolidin)]); and/or any other medication that inhibits platelet aggregation (e.g., clopidogrel [Plavix], dipyridamole [Persantine], plicamycin [Mithracin], sulfinpyrazone [Anturane], ticlopidine [Ticlid], valproic acid [Depacon]). Concurrent use not recommended with the exception of heparin and aspirin (in AMI) to reduce the risk of rethrombosis. If concurrent or subsequent use indicated (e.g., management of acute coronary syndrome, percutaneous coronary intervention) monitor PT and aPTT closely. ▪ Concurrent use with nitroglycerin decreases plasma concentrations of alteplase, impairing the thrombolytic effect. ▪ Coagulation tests will be unreliable; specific procedures can be used; notify the lab of alteplase use.

SIDE EFFECTS

Systemic alteplase: Bleeding is most common: internal (GI tract, GU tract, retroperitoneal, or intracranial sites), epistaxis, gingival, and superficial or surface bleeding (venous cutdowns, arterial punctures, sites of recent surgical intervention). Mild allergic reactions (urticaria) have occurred. Fever, hypotension, nausea and vomiting, reperfusion arrhythmias, and stroke have occurred. Cholesterol embolization syndrome (e.g., acute renal failure, bowel infarction, cerebral infarction, gangrenous digits, hypertension, livedo reticularis, myocardial infarction, pancreatitis, purple toe, retinal artery occlusion, rhabdomyolysis, spinal cord infarction) can occur with thrombolytics but has been reported rarely.

Cathflo Activase: Gastrointestinal bleeding, sepsis, and venous thrombosis have occurred. There were no reports of intracranial hemorrhage or pulmonary emboli during clinical trials.

ANTIDOTE

Systemic alteplase: Notify physician of all side effects. Note even the most minute bleeding tendency. Oozing at IV sites is expected. Control minor bleeding by local pressure. For severe bleeding in a critical location or suspected intracranial bleeding, discontinue alteplase and any heparin therapy immediately. Obtain PT, aPTT, platelet count, and fibrinogen. Draw blood for type and cross-match. Platelets and cryoprecipitate are most commonly used but whole blood, packed RBCs, fresh-frozen plasma, desmopressin, tranexamic acid (Cyklokapron) and aminocaproic acid (Amicar) may be indicated. Topical preparations of aminocaproic acid may stop minor bleeding. Consider protamine if heparin has been used. Treat bradycardia with atropine, reperfusion arrhythmias with lidocaine or procainamide; VT or VF may require cardioversion. If hypotension occurs, reduce rate promptly. If not resolved, vasopressors (e.g., dopamine

[Intropin]), Trendelenburg position, and suitable plasma expanders (e.g., albumin, plasma protein fraction [plasmanate], or hetastarch) may be indicated. Do not use Dextran. ■ ***Protocol for treatment of hypertension occurring during treatment for acute ischemic stroke:*** Monitor BP every 15 minutes; observe for hypertension/hypotension. If diastolic BP is greater than 140 mm Hg, start an IV infusion of nitroprusside sodium (0.5 to 10 mcg/kg/min). If systolic BP greater than 230 mm Hg and/or diastolic BP is 121 to 140 mm Hg, give labetalol 20 mg IV over 1 to 2 minutes. This dose may be repeated and/or doubled every 10 minutes, up to 150 mg. Alternatively, following the first bolus of labetalol, an IV infusion of labetalol 2 to 8 mg/min may be initiated and continued until the desired BP is reached. If satisfactory response is not obtained, use nitroprusside sodium. If systolic BP is 180 to 230 mm Hg and/or diastolic BP is 105 to 120 mm Hg on two readings 5 to 10 minutes apart, give labetalol 10 mg IV over 1 to 2 minutes. The dose may be repeated or doubled every 10 to 20 minutes, up to 150 mg. Alternatively, following the first bolus of labetalol, an IV infusion of labetalol 2 to 8 mg/min may be initiated and continued until the desired BP is reached. Treat minor allergic reactions symptomatically. Discontinue drug and treat anaphylaxis as indicated; resuscitate as necessary.

Cathflo Activase: Discontinue Cathflo Activase and withdraw it from the catheter if serious bleeding in a critical location (e.g., intracranial, gastrointestinal, retroperitoneal, pericardial) occurs. Discontinue drug and treat anaphylaxis as indicated; resuscitate as necessary. In the event of accidental administration of a 2-mg dose directly into the systemic circulation, the concentration of circulating levels of alteplase would be expected to return to exogenous levels of 5 to 10 ng/ml within 30 minutes.

AMIFOSTINE

(a-mi-foss′teen)

Antidote
Antineoplastic adjunct
Cytoprotective agent

Ethyol

USUAL DOSE

PROPHYLACTIC REDUCTION OF CISPLATIN-INDUCED NEPHROTOXICITY, PROPHYLACTIC REDUCTION OF CISPLATIN INDUCED–NEUROTOXICITY (UNLABELED), AND PROPHYLACTIC REDUCTION OF ANTINEOPLASTIC AGENT BONE MARROW TOXICITY (UNLABELED)

Must be administered in conjunction with cisplatin. Adequate hydration and premedication required before administration; see Premedication below and see Monitor.

Premedication: Premedication to prevent severe nausea and vomiting is recommended before each dose. Usual regimen includes dexamethasone 20 mg IV and a serotonin $5HT_3$ receptor antagonist (e.g., ondansetron [Zofran], granisetron [Kytril]) given before and in conjunction with amifostine infusion.

Amifostine: 910 mg/M^2. Cisplatin dose must be given within 30 minutes of starting the amifostine infusion, but only after the full dose of amifostine is administered.

REDUCTION OF MODERATE TO SEVERE XEROSTOMIA FROM RADIATION OF THE HEAD AND NECK

Premedication: Premedication to prevent nausea and vomiting is recommended before each dose. Oral $5HT_3$ receptor antagonists alone or in combination with other antiemetics are recommended. Adequate hydration required; see Monitor.

Amifostine: 200 mg/M^2 once daily as a 3-minute infusion, starting 15 to 30 minutes before standard fraction radiation therapy.

PEDIATRIC DOSE

Safety for use in children not established; see Maternal/Child.

DOSE ADJUSTMENTS

Dosing should be cautious in the elderly. Consider potential for decreased organ function and concomitant disease or drug therapy.

Reduction of cumulative renal toxicity with chemotherapy: Temporarily discontinue the infusion if the systolic BP decreases significantly from the baseline value. See chart below.

Infusion may be restarted to deliver the full dose if the BP returns to normal within 5 minutes and the patient is asymptomatic. If the BP does not return to baseline within 5 minutes and/or the patient is symptomatic (e.g., bradycardia, fainting, unconscious), the full dose cannot be delivered and subsequent doses should be reduced to 740 mg/M^2.

Reduction of moderate to severe xerostomia from radiation of the head and neck: Temporarily discontinue the infusion if the systolic BP decreases significantly from the baseline value. See chart below. Hypotension not as likely with this 200 mg/M^2 dose. Infusion may be restarted to deliver the full dose if the BP returns to normal within 5 minutes and the patient is asymptomatic. If the BP does not return to baseline within 5 minutes and/or the patient is symptomatic (e.g., bradycardia, fainting, unconscious), the full dose cannot be delivered.

Guideline for Interrupting Amifostine Infusion due to Decrease in Systolic Blood Pressure

	Baseline Systolic Blood Pressure (mm Hg)				
	<100	100-119	120-139	140-179	≥180
Decrease in systolic blood pressure during infusion of amifostine (mm Hg)	20	25	30	40	50

DILUTION

Each 500-mg vial should be reconstituted with 9.7 ml of NS (50 mg/ml). May be further diluted with NS to concentrations from 5 to 40 mg/ml. An additional 2.5 ml of NS will yield 40 mg/ml; 90 ml NS will yield 5 mg/ml.

Storage: Store at CRT before reconstitution. Reconstituted or diluted solution prepared in PVC infusion bags is stable for 5 hours at room temperature or 24 hours if refrigerated.

INCOMPATIBLE WITH

Use of any additive, diluent, or solution other than NS is not recommended by manufacturer.

COMPATIBLE WITH

Consult pharmacist; specific conditions may apply; see Compatibilities, p. xvi.

Y-site: Amikacin (Amikin), aminophylline, ampicillin, ampicillin/sulbactam (Unasyn), aztreonam (Azactam), bleomycin (Blenoxane), bumetanide (Bumex), buprenorphine (Buprenex), butorphanol (Stadol), calcium gluconate, carboplatin (Paraplatin), carmustine (BiCNU), cefazolin (Kefzol), cefotaxime (Claforan), cefotetan (Cefotan), cefoxitin (Mefoxin), ceftazidime (Fortaz), ceftizoxime (Cefizox), ceftriaxone (Rocephin), cefuroxime (Zinacef), cimetidine (Tagamet), ciprofloxacin (Cipro IV), clindamycin (Cleocin), cyclophosphamide (Cytoxan), cytarabine (ARA-C), dacarbazine (DTIC), dactinomycin (Cosmegen), daunorubicin (Cerubidine), dexamethasone (Decadron), diphenhydramine (Benadryl), dobutamine (Dobutrex), docetaxel (Taxotere), dopamine (Intropin), doxorubicin (Adriamycin), doxycycline (Vibramycin), droperidol (Inapsine), enalaprilat (Vasotec IV), etoposide (VePesid), famotidine (Pepcid IV), fluconazole (Diflucan), fludarabine (Fludara), fluorouracil (5-FU), furosemide (Lasix), gemcitabine (Gemzar), gentamicin (Garamycin), granisetron (Kytril), haloperidol (Haldol), heparin, hydrocortisone (Hydrocortone, Solu-Cortef), hydromorphone (Dilaudid), idarubicin (Idamycin), ifosfamide (Ifex), imipenem-cilastatin (Primaxin), leucovorin calcium, lorazepam (Ativan), magnesium sulfate, mannitol (Osmitrol), mechlorethamine (nitrogen mustard), meperidine (Demerol), mesna (Mesnex), methotrexate (Folex), methylprednisolone (Solu-Medrol), metoclopramide (Reglan), metronidazole (Flagyl IV), mitomycin (Mutamycin), mitoxantrone (Novantrone), morphine, nalbuphine (Nubain), ondansetron (Zofran), piperacillin (Pipracil), plicamycin (Mithracin), potassium chloride (KCl), promethazine (Phenergan), ranitidine (Zantac), sodium bicarbonate, streptozocin (Zanosar), sulfamethoxazole-trimethoprim (Bactrim), teniposide (Vumon), thiotepa (Thioplex), ticarcillin (Ticar), ticarcillin/clavulanate (Timentin), tobramycin (Nebcin), trimetrexate (Neutrexin), vancomycin (Lyphocin), vinblastine (Velban), vincristine (Oncovin), zidovudine (AZT, Retrovir).

RATE OF ADMINISTRATION

Reduction of cumulative renal toxicity with chemotherapy: A single dose evenly distributed over 15 minutes. Complete amifostine dose but begin cisplatin within 30 minutes after beginning amifostine. Amifostine must be given over 15 minutes; longer infusion times increase the risk of side effects, especially hypotension. Shorter infusion times have not been studied.

Reduction of moderate to severe xerostomia from radiation of the head and neck: A single dose evenly distributed over 3 minutes. Begin infusion 15 to 30 minutes before standard fraction radiation therapy.

ACTIONS

A cytoprotective agent. Rapidly metabolized by alkaline phosphatase in tissues to an active metabolite that can reduce the nephrotoxic effects of cisplatin and the toxic effects of radiation on normal oral tissues. This protective metabolite occurs in greater amounts in normal tissues versus tumor tissues and is available to bind to and detoxify reactive metabolites of cisplatin and/or radiation. It reduces the incidence of cisplatin toxicity including nephrotoxicity but does not cause other toxic reactions. Its protective metabolite can also scavenge reactive oxygen species generated by exposure to either cisplatin or radiation. May adversely affect antitumor effects of cisplatin. Rapidly cleared from plasma with an elimination half-life of 8 minutes. Pretreatment with antiemetics does not alter its actions. Measurable levels of the metabolite have been found in bone marrow; minimal excretion in urine.

INDICATIONS AND USES

Reduce the cumulative renal toxicity associated with repeated administration of cisplatin in patients with advanced ovarian cancer or non–small cell lung cancer. May allow higher cumulative doses of cisplatin and cyclophosphamide, improved response rates and duration. ■ Reduce the incidence of moderate to severe xerostomia (dryness of the mouth from salivary gland dysfunction) in patients undergoing postoperative radiation treatment for head and neck cancer, where the "radiation port" includes a substantial portion of the parotid glands (more than 75%).

Unlabeled uses: Reduce acute and cumulative hematologic toxicity associated with various chemotherapy regimens (e.g., cisplatin, cyclophosphamide, carboplatin; see literature). ■ Decrease frequency or severity of cisplatin-induced neurotoxicity and ototoxicity. ■ Reduce cumulative nephrotoxicity associated with repeated administration of antineoplastic agents in patients with advanced solid tumors of non–germ cell origin. ■ Reduce the damaging effects of paclitaxel on lung fibroblasts.

CONTRAINDICATIONS

Known sensitivity to aminothiol compounds or mannitol. ■ Not recommended for patients receiving chemotherapy for malignancies that are potentially curable; may interfere with effectiveness of chemotherapy regimen and reduce incidence of cure. ■ Not recommended for patients who are hypotensive, dehydrated, or for those receiving antihypertensive therapy that cannot be stopped for 24 hours before amifostine is administered. ■ Not recommended for patients receiving definitive radiotherapy. Tumor-protective effect in this setting has not been ruled out.

PRECAUTIONS

Use caution in the elderly and in patients with preexisting cardiovascular or cerebrovascular conditions (e.g., arrhythmias, congestive heart failure, history of stroke, history of ischemic heart disease). ■ Hypotension and nausea and vomiting can be severe; use caution in any situation where these side effects may have serious consequences. ■ Discontinue antihypertensive therapy 24 hours before administering amifostine. ■ Facilities for monitoring the patient and responding to any medical emergency must be available.

Monitor: ***All indications:*** Adequate hydration required before administration of amifostine. ■ Monitor fluid balance carefully, especially in conjunction with highly emetogenic chemotherapy (e.g., cisplatin). ■ See Usual Dose for premedication requirements. Additional antiemetics may be required to offset nausea and vomiting of chemotherapy drugs. ■ Keep patient in supine position during and immediately after the infusion. ■ Allergic reactions may occur during or after infusion; monitor closely. ■ Monitor serum calcium. Risk of hypocalcemia increased in some patients (e.g., nephrotic syndrome or patients receiving multiple doses). Calcium supplements may be required. ■ See Dose Adjustments, Rate of Administration, and Antidote.

Reduction of cumulative renal toxicity with chemotherapy: Discontinue antihypertensive therapy if indicated; see Contraindications, Precautions, Drug/Lab Interactions. ■ Obtain baseline BP and monitor at least every 5 minutes during and immediately after the infusion. ■ Hypertension may be exacerbated by several causes (e.g., interruption of antihypertensive therapy, IV hydration). Monitor BP closely. ■ Hypotension can occur at any time but is more frequent toward the end of the infusion, and recovery usually begins within 5 to 6 minutes after infusion is discontinued.

Reduction of xerostomia from radiation: Monitor BP before and immediately after the infusion and as indicated by results.

Patient Education: Void before administration. ■ May produce significant hypotension. Effects may be additive with medications currently being taken. Review all medications (prescription and nonprescription) with nurse and/or physician. ■ Must remain in supine position until BP stabilized, then request assistance for ambulation. ■ Report feelings of faintness or nausea promptly.

Maternal/Child: Category C: use only if potential benefits justify risk to fetus; embryotoxic in rabbits at doses lower than required for humans. ■ Discontinue breast-feeding. ■ Safety for use in children not established; experience is limited. In clinical trials, a few children received single doses up to 2,700 mg/M^2 with no unexpected effects.

Elderly: Response similar to younger adults; however, dosing should be cautious; see Dose Adjustments. ■ Monitor fluid balance closely; avoid dehydration. ■ Hypotension may be sudden and severe; monitor closely. ■ See Contraindications and Precautions.

DRUG/LAB INTERACTIONS

Antihypertensive therapy (e.g., ACE inhibitors [e.g., enalaprilat], calcium channel blocking agents [e.g., nicardipine, verapamil], diuretics [e.g., furosemide, torsemide], nitroglycerin, nitroprusside sodium) should be discontinued 24 hours before amifostine administration; see Contraindications. ■ Use extreme caution in any patient receiving medications with hypotensive effects (antidepressants, benzodiazepines, beta-adrenergic blocking agents [e.g., atenolol, esmolol, metoprolol, propranolol], bretylium, lidocaine, magnesium, narcotics, nitrates, paclitaxel, procainamide); will cause additive hypotension.

SIDE EFFECTS

Hypotension and severe nausea and vomiting occur frequently. Hypotension may be associated with apnea, arrhythmias (e.g., atrial fibrillation/flutter, bradycardia, tachycardia), chest pain, dyspnea, hypoxia, myocardial ischemia, and rarely renal failure, respiratory and cardiac arrest, seizures, and unconsciousness. Dehydration, dizziness, feelings of cold or warmth, flushing, hiccups, hypocalcemia, loss of consciousness, somnolence, and/or transient hypertension or exacerbation of preexisting hypertension may occur. Hypersensitivity reactions (e.g., anaphylaxis [rare], arrhythmias, chest tightness, chills, dyspnea, fever, hypoxia, laryngeal edema, mild allergic reactions [sneezing], skin reactions such as erythema multiforme, rash, Stevens-Johnson syndrome [rare], toxic epidermal necrolysis, and urticaria) have been reported.

Overdose: Hypotension is the most likely symptom. Anxiety and reversible urinary retention have occurred at higher doses. Up to 3 doses have been given within 24 hours without unexpected side effects.

ANTIDOTE

Keep physician informed of side effects. Treatment of nausea and vomiting is imperative to encourage patients to continue treatment with full doses of chemotherapeutic agents. Hypotension may be dose-limiting. If the systolic BP decreases significantly (see Dose Adjustments chart), temporarily discontinue the amifostine still infusing, place the patient in Trendelenburg position, and administer an infusion of NS at a separate site. Vasopressors (e.g., dopamine [Intropin], norepinephrine [Levophed]) may be required. If indicated, restart infusion if BP returns to baseline within 5 minutes and patient is asymptomatic. Discontinue amifostine immediately and permanently if an acute allergic reaction occurs. Treat anaphylaxis and resuscitate as necessary.

AMIKACIN SULFATE

(am-i-kay′sin sul′fat)

Amikin

Antibacterial (aminoglycoside)

pH 3.5 to 5.5

USUAL DOSE

Up to 15 mg/kg of body weight/24 hr equally divided into 2 or 3 doses at equally divided intervals (5 mg/kg every 8 hours or 7.5 mg/kg every 12 hours). Dosage based on ideal weight of lean body mass. Do not exceed a total adult dose of 15 mg/kg/24 hr in an average weight patient or 1.5 Gm in heavier patients by all routes in 24 hours.

Recent studies suggest that a single daily dose of 15 to 20 mg/kg (instead of divided into 2 or 3 doses) may provide higher peak levels and enhance drug effectiveness while actually reducing or having no adverse effects on risk of toxicity. Various procedures for monitoring blood levels are in use. Some health facilities are monitoring with trough levels; others may draw levels at predetermined times and plot the concentration on nomograms. Depending on the protocol in place, doses or intervals may be adjusted. See Precautions.

***Mycobacterium avium* complex:** 15 mg/kg/24 hr in equally divided doses every 8 to 12 hours (5 mg/kg every 8 hours or 7.5 mg/kg every 12 hours). Part of a 3- to 5-agent regimen.

PEDIATRIC DOSE

15 to 22.5 mg/kg/24 hr equally divided into 2 or 3 doses and given every 8 to 12 hours (5 to 7.5 mg/kg every 8 hours or 7.5 to 11.25 mg/kg every 12 hours). Do not exceed 1.5 Gm/24 hr. A single daily dose is also being used in children. See comments under Usual Dose.

NEWBORN DOSE

10 mg/kg of body weight as a loading dose, then 7.5 mg/kg/dose. Intervals of 7.5 mg/kg dose adjusted based on age as follows:

Under 28 weeks' gestation and less than 7 days of age: give every 24 hours.

Under 28 weeks' gestation and over 7 days or 28 to 34 weeks' gestation and under 7 days of age: give every 18 hours.

28 to 34 weeks' gestation and over 7 days of age or over 34 weeks' gestation and under 7 days of age: give every 12 hours.

Over 34 weeks' gestation and over 7 days of age: give every 8 hours.

DOSE ADJUSTMENTS

Reduce daily dose commensurate with amount of renal impairment and/or increase intervals between injections. ■ Reduced dose or extended intervals may be required in the elderly. ■ See Drug/Lab Interactions.

DILUTION

Each 500 mg or fraction thereof is diluted with 100 to 200 ml D5W, D5NS, or NS. Amount of diluent may be decreased proportionately with dosage for children and infants. Available for pediatric injection as 50 mg/ml.

Storage: Diluted solution stable at room temperature for 24 hours.

INCOMPATIBLE WITH

Do not physically premix with other drugs; administer separately as recommended by manufacturer. Inactivated in solution with beta-lactam antibiotics (e.g., cephalosporins, penicillins) and vancomycin. Do not mix in the same solution. Appropriate spacing required because of physical incompatibilities. See Drug/Lab Interactions.

COMPATIBLE WITH

Consult pharmacist; specific conditions may apply; see Compatibilities, p. xvi.

Solution: Manufacturer lists D5W, D5/¼NS, D5/½NS, NS, LR, D5 in Normosol M (Plasma-Lyte 56 in D5W), D5 in Normosol R (Plasma-Lyte 148 in D5W). Other sources list additional solutions.

Y-site: Acyclovir (Zovirax), alatrofloxacin (Trovan IV), aldesleukin (Proleukin, IL-2), amifostine (Ethyol), amiodarone (Cordarone), aztreonam (Azactam), cisatracurium (Nimbex), cyclophosphamide (Cytoxan), dexamethasone (Decadron), diltiazem (Cardizem), docetaxel (Taxotere), enalaprilat (Vasotec IV), esmolol (Brevibloc), etoposide phosphate (Etopophos), filgrastim (Neupogen), fluconazole (Diflucan), fludarabine (Fludara), foscarnet (Foscavir), furosemide (Lasix), gatifloxacin (Tequin), gemcitabine (Gemzar), granisetron (Kytril), hetastarch in electrolytes (Hextend), idarubicin (Idamycin), labetalol (Normodyne), levofloxacin (Levaquin), linezolid (Zyvox), lorazepam (Ativan), magnesium sulfate, melphalan (Alkeran), midazolam (Versed), morphine, ondansetron (Zofran), paclitaxel (Taxol), perphenazine (Trilafon), remifentanil (Ultiva), sargramostim (Leukine), teniposide (Vumon), thiotepa (Thioplex), vinorelbine (Navelbine), warfarin (Coumadin), zidovudine (AZT, Retrovir).

RATE OF ADMINISTRATION

A single dose over at least 30 to 60 minutes. Infants should receive a 1- to 2-hour infusion.

ACTIONS

An aminoglycoside antibiotic with neuromuscular blocking action. Bactericidal against many gram-negative organisms resistant to other antibiotics including other aminoglycosides such as gentamicin (Garamycin), kanamycin (Kantrex), and tobramycin (Nebcin). Well distributed through all body fluids. Usual half-life is 2 to 3 hours. Half-life is prolonged in infants, postpartum females, fever, liver disease and ascites, spinal cord injury, cystic fibrosis, and the elderly; shorter in severe burns. Crosses the placental barrier. Excreted in the kidneys. Cross-allergenicity does occur between aminoglycosides.

INDICATIONS AND USES

Short-term treatment of serious infections caused by susceptible organisms (e.g., gram-negative bacteria) generally resistant to alternate drugs that have less potential toxicity. ▪ Effective in infections of the respiratory and urinary tracts, CNS (including meningitis), skin and soft tissue, intraabdominal (including peritonitis), bacterial septicemia (including neonatal sepsis), burns, and postoperative infections. ▪ Considered initial therapy in suspected gram-negative infections after culture and sensitivity is drawn. ▪ Penicillins may be required concomitantly in neonatal sepsis to treat possible infections from gram-positive organisms.

Unlabeled uses: Treatment of *Mycobacterium avium* complex, a common infection in AIDS (part of a multiple [3 to 5] drug regimen).

CONTRAINDICATIONS

Known amikacin or aminoglycoside sensitivity. Sulfite sensitivity may be a contraindication.

PRECAUTIONS

Sensitivity studies indicated to determine susceptibility of causative organism to amikacin. ■ Response should occur in 24 to 48 hours. Use extreme caution if therapy is required over 7 to 10 days. ■ Superinfection may occur from overgrowth of nonsusceptible organisms. ■ May contain sulfites; use caution in patients with asthma. ■ Single daily dosing has been used effectively in abdominal, pelvic inflammatory, and GU infections in patients with normal renal function. Not recommended in bacteremia caused by *Pseudomonas aeruginosa*, endocarditis, meningitis, during pregnancy or in patients less than 6 weeks postpartum. Limited data available for use in all other situations (e.g., burns, cystic fibrosis, elderly, pediatrics, renal impairment). ■ Risk of neurotoxicity (e.g., auditory and vestibular ototoxicity) increased in patients with pre-existing renal damage or in normal renal function with prolonged use. Partial or total irreversible deafness may continue to develop after amikacin discontinued. ■ Pseudomembranous colitis has been reported. May range from mild to life-threatening. Consider in patients that present with diarrhea during or after treatment with amikacin.

Monitor: Maintain good hydration. ■ Narrow range between toxic and therapeutic levels. Periodically monitor peak and trough concentrations to avoid peak serum concentrations above 30 mcg/ml and trough concentrations above 5 to 10 mcg/ml. ■ Monitor urine protein, presence of cells and casts, and decreased specific gravity. Watch for decreased urine output, rising BUN and SrCr, and declining CrCl levels. Dose adjustment may be necessary. ■ Closely monitor patients with impaired renal function for nephrotoxicity and neurotoxicity (e.g., auditory and vestibular ototoxicity); nephrotoxicity may be reversible. ■ Routine serum levels and hearing evaluations are recommended. ■ Monitor serum calcium, magnesium, and sodium; levels may decline. ■ In extended treatment, monitor serum levels, electrolytes, and renal, auditory, and vestibular functions frequently. ■ See Drug/Lab Interactions.

Patient Education: Report promptly any changes in balance, hearing loss, weakness, or dizziness. ■ Consider birth control options.

Maternal/Child: Category D: avoid pregnancy. Potential hazard to fetus. ■ Safety for use during breast-feeding not established; use extreme caution. ■ Peak concentrations are generally lower in infants and young children. ■ Use extreme caution in premature infants and neonates; immature kidney function will result in prolonged half-life.

Elderly: Consider less toxic alternatives. ■ Longer intervals between doses may be more important than smaller doses. ■ Monitor renal function and drug levels carefully. Measurement of CrCl more useful than BUN or SrCr to assess renal function. ■ Half-life prolonged.

DRUG/LAB INTERACTIONS

Synergistic when used in combination with beta-lactam antibiotics (e.g., cephalosporins, penicillins) and vancomycin. Synergism may be inconsistent; see Incompatible With. ■ Concurrent use topically or systemically with any other ototoxic or nephrotoxic agents should be avoided. May have dangerous additive effects with anesthetics (e.g., enflurane), other neuromuscular blocking antibiotics (e.g., kanamycin), diuretics (e.g., furosemide [Lasix]), beta-lactam antibiotics (e.g., cephalosporins), vancomycin, and many others. ■ Neuromuscular blocking muscle relaxants (e.g., doxacurium [Nuromax], succinylcholine) are potentiated by aminoglycosides. *Apnea can occur.* ■ Aminoglycosides are potentiated by anticholinesterases (e.g., edrophonium), antineoplastics (e.g., nitrogen mustard, cisplatin). ■ May be antagonized by bacteriostatic antibiotics (e.g., chloramphenicol, erythromycin, and tetracyclines); bacterial action may be affected.

SIDE EFFECTS

Occur more frequently with impaired renal function, higher doses, prolonged administration, in dehydrated or elderly patients, and in patients receiving other ototoxic or nephrotoxic drugs. Fever, headache, hypotension, nausea, paresthesias, seizures, skin rash, tremor, vomiting.

Major: Albuminuria, anemia, arthralgia, azotemia, eosinophilia, loss of balance, neuromuscular blockade, oliguria, ototoxicity, pseudomembranous colitis, RBCs and WBCs or casts in urine, respiratory depression or arrest, rising SrCr.

ANTIDOTE

Notify physician of all side effects. If minor side effects persist or any major symptom appears, discontinue drug and notify physician. Treatment is symptomatic, or a reduction in dose may be required. In overdose hemodialysis may be indicated. Monitor fluid balance, CrCl, and plasma levels carefully. Complexation with ticarcillin may be as effective as hemodialysis. Consider exchange transfusion in the newborn. Calcium salts or neostigmine may reverse neuromuscular blockade. Resuscitate as necessary.

AMINOCAPROIC ACID

(a-mee-noe-ka-proe′ik as′id)

Antifibrinolytic
Antihemorrhagic

Amicar

pH 6.8

USUAL DOSE

5 Gm initially. Follow with 1 to 1.25 Gm/hr for 6 to 8 hours. Maximum dose is 30 Gm/24 hr.

Prevent recurrence of subarachnoid hemorrhage: 36 Gm/24 hr equally divided into 6 doses.

Reduce need for platelet transfusion in management of amegakaryocytic thrombocytopenia: 8 to 24 Gm/24 hr for 3 days to 13 months.

PEDIATRIC DOSE

100 mg/kg of body weight or 3 Gm/M^2 during the first hour. Follow with a continuous infusion of 33.3 mg/kg/hr or 1 Gm/M^2/hr. Do not exceed 18 Gm/M^2/24 hr; see Maternal/Child.

DOSE ADJUSTMENTS

May be required with impaired renal or hepatic function.

DILUTION

1 Gm equals 4 ml of prepared solution. Further dilute with compatible infusion solutions (NS, D5NS, D5W, DW [SW for injection], or Ringer's solution). Do not use DW in patients with subarachnoid hemorrhage.

Up to 50 ml of diluent may be used for each 1 Gm.

Storage: Before use store at CRT.

COMPATIBILITY

Specific information not available. Consider specific use; consult pharmacist.

RATE OF ADMINISTRATION

5 Gm or fraction thereof over first hour in 250 ml of solution; then administer each succeeding 1 Gm over 1 hour in 50 to 100 ml of solution. Use of an infusion pump for accurate dose recommended. Rapid administration or insufficient dilution may cause hypotension, bradycardia, and/or arrhythmia.

ACTIONS

A monaminocarboxylic acid with the specific action of inhibiting plasminogen activator substances; to a lesser degree inhibits plasmin activity. Increases fibrinogen activity in clot formation by inhibiting the enzyme required for destruction of formed fibrin. Onset of action is prompt, but will last less than 3 hours. Readily excreted in the urine. Easily penetrates RBCs and tissue cells after prolonged administration.

INDICATIONS AND USES

Hemorrhage caused by overactivity of the fibrinolytic system. ■ Systemic hyperfibrinolysis (pathologic), which may result from heart surgery, portacaval shunt, prostatectomy, nephrectomy, aplastic anemia, abruptio placentae, hepatic cirrhosis, or carcinoma of the prostate, lung, stomach, and cervix. ■ Urinary fibrinolysis (normal physiologic phenomenon), which may result from severe trauma, anoxia, shock, surgery of the genitourinary system, or carcinoma of the genitourinary system. ■ Prophylaxis and treatment of postsurgical hemorrhage. ■ Intraoperative and postoperative treatment of hemorrhage in patients with clotting defects other than hemophilia. ■ Prophylaxis and treatment of hemophiliacs during surgery or dental surgery. ■ Treat severe hemorrhage caused by thrombolytic agents (e.g., alteplase [tPA], streptokinase).

Unlabeled uses: Prevent recurrence of subarachnoid hemorrhage. ■ Reduce need for platelet transfusions in management of amegakaryocytic thrombocytopenia.

CONTRAINDICATIONS

Disseminated intravascular coagulation, evidence of thrombosis, first and second trimester of pregnancy.

PRECAUTIONS

Use only in conjunction with general and specific tests to determine the amount of fibrinolysis present. ■ Use extreme care in cardiac, hepatic, or renal diseases. Endocardial hemorrhage, myocardial fat degeneration, teratogenicity, and kidney stones have resulted in animals. ■ Whole blood transfusions may be given if necessary.

Monitor: Vital signs, intake and output, any signs of bleeding, and neurologic assessment should be monitored based on patient condition. ■ Observe for thromboembolic complications (e.g., chest pain, dyspnea, edema, hemoptysis, leg pain, or positive Homans' sign). ■ Monitor lab evaluations as appropriate for diagnosis (e.g., platelet count, clotting factors, CPK, AST [SGOT]).

Patient Education: Move slowly with help to avoid orthostatic hypotension.

Maternal/Child: Category C: safety for use in pregnancy and breast-feeding not established. See Contraindications. ■ Safety for use in children not established but is used.

Elderly: Consider age-related impaired organ function; reduced dose may be indicated.

DRUG/LAB INTERACTIONS

Potential for thrombus formation increased with concurrent use of estrogens. ■ Frequently used with clotting factor complexes (e.g., factor IX complex, antiinhibitor coagulant complex) but risk of thrombus formation may be increased. Delay administration for 8 or more hours after clotting factor complexes. ■ May elevate serum potassium, especially with impaired renal function; reduced dose may be indicated.

SIDE EFFECTS

Cramps, diarrhea, dizziness, grand mal seizure, headache, malaise, nausea, skin rash, stuffy nose, tearing, thrombophlebitis, tinnitus.

ANTIDOTE

Treat side effects symptomatically. Discontinue use of drug with any suspicion of thrombophlebitis, thromboembolic complications, or if CPK is elevated (myopathy). May be removed by hemodialysis or peritoneal dialysis.

AMINOPHYLLINE

(am-in-off'i-lin)

Bronchodilator
Respiratory stimulant

(79% Theophylline), Theophylline Ethylenediamine

pH 8.6 to 9

USUAL DOSE

To obtain maximum benefit with minimal risk of adverse effects, dosing must be individualized based on serum theophylline concentration and patient response. Monitor frequently to avoid toxicity. Only aminophylline premixed in solution or aminophylline containing 20 mg of theophylline for each 25 mg of aminophylline is intended for IV use (approximately 79% theophylline). All doses are based on lean body weight; theophylline does not distribute into fatty tissue. ***All doses listed are milligrams of aminophylline to be administered.***

BRONCHODILATION IN ACUTE ASTHMA OR BRONCHOSPASM

With an average mean volume of distribution of 0.5 L/kg (range is 0.3 to 0.7 L/kg), each mg/kg of theophylline given over 30 minutes should result in an average 2 mcg/ml increase in serum theophylline concentration.

Adults, children, infants and neonates who *HAVE NOT* received a theophylline preparation in the previous 24 hours: An ***initial loading dose*** of 5 to 6 mg/kg of lean body weight (5.7 mg of aminophylline is equal to 4.6 mg/kg of theophylline) should produce a serum concentration of 10 mcg/ml (range 6 to 16 mcg/ml). Measure serum theophylline concentration in 30 minutes to determine if additional loading doses are indicated. Once a serum concentration of 10 to 15 mcg/ml is obtained with loading dose(s), it should be maintained with a continuous infusion. Rate of infusion is based on the pharmacokinetic parameters (e.g., volume of distribution, clearance, concomitant disease states) of the specific patient population and should achieve a target serum concentration of 10 mcg/ml. See Dose Adjustments and Monitor for recommendations of serum theophylline testing after an infusion is started.

Adults, children, infants and neonates who *HAVE* received a theophylline preparation in the previous 24 hours: ***A serum theophylline concentration must be obtained before considering any loading dose.*** Calculate the appropriate loading dose with the following formula.

$$D = (\text{Desired } C - \text{Measured } C) \times (V)$$

D is the loading dose, C is the serum theophylline concentration, and V is the volume of distribution (0.5 L/kg). Desired serum concentration in this situation should be conservative (e.g., 10 mcg/ml) to allow for variability in the volume of distribution; carefully evaluating the patient condition and risk versus benefit. It is not recommended by the manufacturer, but another source suggests that a smaller loading dose may be considered if it is not immediately possible to obtain a theophylline serum concentration. Carefully evaluate the patient's condition and risk versus benefit. The potential for theophylline toxicity must be ruled out. For example, if significant respiratory distress is present, a smaller loading dose of 2.5 mg/kg should increase the theophylline level by approximately 5 mcg/ml. In the absence of toxicity, this increase is unlikely to cause significant side effects and may improve the clinical picture. In all situations, measure serum theophylline concentration in 30 minutes to determine if additional loading doses are indicated. Once a serum concentration of 10 to 15 mcg/ml is obtained with or without loading dose(s), it should be maintained with a continuous infusion. Rate of infusion is based on the pharmacokinetic parameters (e.g., volume of distribution, clearance, concomitant disease states) of the specific patient population and should achieve a target serum concentration of 10 mcg/ml. See Dose Adjustments and Monitor for recommendations of serum theophylline testing after an infusion is started.

Maintenance infusion: Desired theophylline serum concentration is 10 mcg/ml. Most maintenance doses can be reduced within the first 12 hours based on serum theophylline levels and depending on patient condition and response; see Dose Adjustments. Because of a large interpatient variability in theophylline clearance, each patient may differ from the mean value used to calculate these infusion rates. Another serum concentration is recommended one expected half-life after starting the continuous infusion; see Dose Adjustments.

Aminophylline Infusion Rates Following an Appropriate Loading Dose

Patient Population	Aminophylline Infusion Rate in mg/kg/hr[a] (Actual theophylline administered in mg/kg/hr is in parentheses)
Neonates up to 24 days of age	1.25 mg/kg ***every 12 hours*** (1 mg/kg ***every 12 hours***)[b]
Neonates over 24 days of age	1.875 mg/kg ***every 12 hours*** (1.5 mg/kg ***every 12 hours***)[b]
Infants 6 to 52 weeks of age	mg/kg/hr = 0.01 × age in weeks + 0.21[c](0.008 × age in weeks + 0.21)
Children 1 to 9 years	1 mg/kg/hr (0.8 mg/kg/hr)
Children 9 to 12 years	0.875 mg/kg/hr (0.7 mg/kg/hr)
Adolescent smokers 12 to 16 years	0.875 mg/kg/hr (0.7 mg/kg/hr)
Adolescent nonsmokers 12 to 16 years	0.625 mg/kg/hr (0.5 mg/kg/hr)[d]
Adults (healthy nonsmokers 16 to 60 years	0.5 mg/kg/hr (0.4 mg/kg/hr)[d]
Elderly over 60 years	0.375 mg/kg/hr (0.3 mg/kg/hr)[e]
Cardiac decompensation, cor pulmonale, liver dysfunction, sepsis with multi-organ failure, or shock	0.25 mg/kg/hr (0.2 mg/kg/hr)[e]

[a]Lower initial dose may be required for patients receiving other drugs that decrease theophylline clearance (e.g., cimetidine [Tagamet]).
[b] To achieve a target concentration of 7.5 mcg/ml for neonatal apnea.
[c] The 0.21 factor was not adjusted from the theophylline formula because it may not have the same proportional value. See package insert or contact Abbott if additional information desired.
[d] Not to exceed 900 mg/day unless serum levels indicate need for a larger dose.
[e] Not to exceed 400 mg/day or 21 mg/hr (17 mg/hr as theophylline) unless serum levels indicate need for a larger dose.

Continued

REVERSE ADENOSINE-MEDIATED EFFECTS OF DIPYRIDAMOLE IN ADULTS (UNLABELED)
50 to 100 mg over 30 to 60 seconds. Do not exceed a rate of 50 mg/30 sec. Maximum dose is 250 mg.

NEONATAL DOSE

Apnea and bradycardia of prematurity (unlabeled): ***Loading dose:*** 5 to 6 mg/kg given over 20 to 30 minutes. See all criteria under Usual Dose.
Maintenance dose: See Maintenance Infusion under Usual Dose. Manufacturer recommends keeping serum theophylline level at 7.5 mcg/ml. Another source recommends 1 to 2 mg/kg/dose every 6 to 8 hours.

DOSE ADJUSTMENTS

To determine if the concentration is accumulating or declining from the post–loading dose level, a serum concentration is recommended one expected half-life after starting the continuous infusion; see chart below or see literature for a complete summary. If the level is declining (higher than average clearance) consider an additional loading dose or increasing the infusion rate. If the level is increasing, assume accumulation and decrease the infusion rate before the level exceeds 20 mcg/ml.

Theophylline Half-Life (Approximate)	
Age	**Half-Life Mean (Range) in Hours**
Premature neonates, see Maternal/Child	
3 to 15 days	30 (17 to 43)
25 to 57 days	20 (9.4 to 30.6)
Term infants, see Maternal/Child	
1 to 2 days	25.7 (25 to 26.5)
3 to 30 weeks	11 (6 to 29)
Children	
1 to 4 years	3.4 (1.2 to 5.6)
4 to 12 years	Not reported in studies
13 to 15 years	Not reported in studies
6 to 17 years	3.7 (1.5 to 5.9)
Adults (16 to 60 years) and healthy nonsmoking asthmatics	8.7 (6.1 to 12.8)
Elderly (over 60 years); nonsmokers with normal cardiac, liver, and renal function	9.8 (1.6 to 18)

There are huge variances in patients with concurrent illness or altered physiologic states (e.g., acute pulmonary edema, COPD, cystic fibrosis, fever with acute viral respiratory illness in children [9 to 15 years], liver disease, pregnancy, sepsis with multi-organ failure, thyroid disease); see package insert. ■ In patients with cor pulmonale, cardiac decompensation, liver dysfunction, or in those taking drugs that markedly reduce theophylline clearance (e.g., cimetidine [Tagamet]), the initial aminophylline infusion rate should not exceed 21 mg/hr (17 mg/hr as theophylline) unless serum concentrations can be monitored every 24 hours. Up to 5 days may be required before steady state is reached in these patients; see Drug Interactions. ■ To decrease the risk of side effects associated with unexpected large increases in serum theophylline concentration, dose adjustment recommendations should be considered as the upper limit.

Final Dose Adjustment Guided by Serum Theophylline Concentration[a]	
Peak Serum Concentration	**Dose Adjustment**
Less than 9.9 mcg/ml	If symptoms are not controlled and current dose is tolerated, increase infusion rate about 25%. Recheck serum concentration after 12 hours in children and 24 hours in adults for further dose adjustment.
10 to 14.9 mcg/ml	If symptoms are controlled and current dose is tolerated, maintain infusion rate and recheck serum concentration at 24-hour intervals. If symptoms are not controlled and current dose is tolerated, consider adding additional medication(s) to treatment regimen.
15 to 19.9 mcg/ml	Consider 10% decrease in infusion rate to provide greater margin of safety, even if current dose is tolerated.[b]
20 to 24.9 mcg/ml	Decrease infusion rate by 25%, even if no side effects are present. Recheck serum concentration after 12 hours in children and 24 hours in adults to guide further dose adjustment.
25 to 30 mcg/ml	Stop infusion for 12 hours in children and 24 hours in adults and decrease subsequent infusion rate at least 25% even if no side effects are present. Recheck serum concentration after 12 hours in children and 24 hours in adults to guide further dose adjustment. If symptomatic, stop infusion and consider need for overdose treatment; see Antidote.
Over 30 mcg/ml	Stop the infusion and treat overdose as indicated; see Antidote. If aminophylline is subsequently resumed, decrease infusion rate by at least 50% and recheck serum concentration after 12 hours in children and 24 hours in adults to guide further dose adjustment.

[a]Dose increases should not be made in patients with an acute exacerbation of symptoms unless the steady-state serum theophylline concentration is less than 10 mcg/ml.
[b]Dose reduction and/or serum theophylline concentration measurement is indicated whenever side effects are present, physiologic abnormalities that can reduce theophylline clearance occur (e.g., sustained fever), or a drug that interacts with theophylline is added or discontinued; see Precautions and Drug/Lab Interactions.

DILUTION

Check vial carefully; must state, "For IV use." Warm to room temperature. Only the 25 mg/ml solution may be given by IV injection undiluted, but further dilution for infusion in at least 100 to 200 ml of D5W is preferred. NS or dextrose in saline solutions may be used. Available prediluted. Crystals will form if solution pH falls below 8.

Storage: Usually stored between 15° and 30° C (59° and 86° F). Protect from light and freezing.

INCOMPATIBLE WITH

Manufacturer states, "Should not be mixed in a syringe with other drugs but should be added separately to the IV solution," and recommends discontinuing other solutions infusing at the same site if there is a potential problem with admixture incompatibility. Manufacturer recommends avoiding admixtures with alkali labile drugs (e.g., epinephrine, norepinephrine [Levophed], isoproterenol [Isuprel], penicillin G potassium). Precipitation in acidic media may occur with the undiluted solution but not to dilute solutions in IV infusions.

COMPATIBLE WITH **(Underline Indicates Conflicting Compatibility Information)**

Consult pharmacist; specific conditions may apply; see Compatibilities, p. xvi.

Additive: ***See Incompatible With.*** Amikacin (Amikin), ascorbic acid (Cenolate), bretylium (Bretylate), calcium gluconate, chloramphenicol (Chloromycetin), cimetidine (Tagamet), dexamethasone (Decadron), dimenhydrinate (Dinate), diphenhydramine (Benadryl), dopamine (Intropin), erythromycin lactobionate (Erythrocin), esmolol (Brevibloc), flumazenil (Romazicon), furosemide (Lasix), heparin, hydrocortisone sodium succinate (Solu-Cortef), lidocaine, meropenem (Merrem IV), methyldopate (Aldomet), methylprednisolone (Solu-Medrol), nafcillin (Nafcil), nitroglycerin (Nitro-Bid IV), pentobarbital (Nembutal), phenobarbital (Luminal), potassium chloride (KCl), ranitidine (Zantac), sodium bicarbonate, vancomycin (Vancocin), verapamil (Isoptin).

Syringe: ***Not recommended by manufacturer.*** Heparin, metoclopramide (Reglan), pentobarbital (Nembutal), thiopental (Pentothal).

Y-site: Allopurinol (Aloprim, Zyloprim), amifostine (Ethyol), amphotericin B cholesteryl (Amphotec), aztreonam (Azactam), ceftazidime (Fortaz), cimetidine (Tagamet), cisatracurium (Nimbex), cladribine (Leustatin), diltiazem (Cardizem), docetaxel (Taxotere), doxorubicin liposome (Doxil), enalaprilat (Vasotec IV), esmolol (Brevibloc), etoposide phosphate (Etopophos), famotidine (Pepcid IV), filgrastim (Neupogen), fluconazole (Diflucan), fludarabine (Fludara), foscarnet (Foscavir), gatifloxacin (Tequin), gemcitabine (Gemzar), granisetron (Kytril), hetastarch in electrolytes (Hextend), inamrinone (Inocor), labetalol (Normodyne), levofloxacin (Levaquin), linezolid (Zyvox), melphalan (Alkeran), meropenem (Merrem IV), morphine, paclitaxel (Taxol), pancuronium (Pavulon), piperacillin/tazobactam (Zosyn), potassium chloride (KCl), propofol (Diprivan), ranitidine (Zantac), remifentanil (Ultiva), sargramostim (Leukine), tacrolimus (Prograf), teniposide (Vumon), thiotepa (Thioplex), vecuronium (Norcuron).

RATE OF ADMINISTRATION

A single dose over a minimum of 20 to 30 minutes. Most references suggest a minimum of 30 minutes. Do not exceed an average rate of 1 ml or 25 mg/min when giving by IV injection or as an infusion. Rapid administration may cause cardiac arrhythmias. Discontinue primary infusion if theophylline administered by piggyback or additive tubing and a possible incompatibility problem exists.

Reverse adenosine-mediated effects of dipyridamole: See Usual Dose.

ACTIONS

An alkaloid xanthine derivative. It relaxes smooth muscle in the airways (bronchodilation) and suppresses the response of the airways to stimuli (non-bronchodilator prophylactic effects). Cardiac output, urinary output, and sodium excretion are increased. Skeletal and cardiac muscles are stimulated, as is the CNS to a lesser degree. There is peripheral vasodilation. It decreases pulmonary artery pressure and lowers the threshold of the respiratory center to CO_2. Well distributed throughout the body. In adults and children over 1 year of age, 90% of a dose is metabolized in the liver. Because of a large interpatient variability in theophylline clearance, half-life varies extensively based on age, concurrent illness, or altered physiological state; see Dose Adjustments, Precautions, Maternal/Child, and Elderly. Excreted in a changed form in the urine. Crosses the placental barrier. Secreted in breast milk.

INDICATIONS AND USES

Adjunct to inhaled beta-2 selective agonists (e.g., albuterol) and systemic corticosteroids for the treatment of acute exacerbations of the symptoms and reversible airflow obstruction associated with asthma and other chronic lung diseases (e.g., emphysema, chronic bronchitis).

Unlabeled uses: Apnea and bradycardia of prematurity. ■ Reduce bronchospasm in cystic fibrosis and acute descending respiratory infections. ■ Relieve periodic apnea and increase arterial blood pH in patients with Cheyne-Stokes respirations. ■ Reverse adenosine-mediated effects of dipyridamole (Persantine) (e.g., angina pectoris, bronchospasm, severe hypotension, ventricular arrhythmias).

CONTRAINDICATIONS

Known sensitivity to theophylline or ethylenediamine.

PRECAUTIONS

There is an increase in the volume of distribution of theophylline (primarily due to reduction in plasma protein binding) in premature neonates, patients with hepatic cirrhosis, uncorrected acidemia, the elderly, and women during the third trimester of pregnancy. Toxicity may occur in the therapeutic range. ■ Theophylline clearance may be reduced in neonates (term and premature); children less than 1 year; elderly (over 60 years); infants less than 3 months of age with reduced renal function; patients with acute pulmonary edema, congestive heart failure, cor pulmonale, hypothyroidism, liver disease (e.g., cirrhosis, acute hepatitis), sepsis with multi-organ failure, shock; or in patients with a fever of 102° F or more for 24 hours or more, or lesser temperature elevations for longer periods. Risk of severe toxicity increased in these patient populations; dose reduction and more frequent monitoring may be required. ■ Use with extreme caution in patients with active peptic ulcer disease, cardiac arrhythmias (not including bradyarrhythmias), or seizures; may exacerbate these conditions. ■ Initiate oral therapy as soon as symptoms are adequately improved. Wait 4 to 6 hours after last IV dose or measure serum levels. ■ See Maternal/Child and Drug/Lab Interactions.

Monitor: Monitor serum levels as directed in Usual Dose and Dose Adjustments to achieve maximum benefit with minimum risk. Each 0.5 mg/kg will increase serum theophylline by 1 mcg/ml. 10 to less than 20 mcg/ml is considered therapeutic. Peak serum level is best measured 20 to 30 minutes after initial loading dose, a half life after the initial infusion, or 12 to 14 hours into continuous infusion. ■ Monitor vital signs, including lung sounds. ■ Monitor for all signs of toxicity; see Side Effects. Serious toxicity may not be preceded by less severe side effects. ■ Serum theophylline measurements are indicated before making a dose increase; whenever signs or symptoms of toxicity are present; whenever a new illness presents, an existing illness worsens, or a change in treatment regimen is initiated that may alter theophylline clearance (e.g., sustained fever, hepatitis [see Precautions], or drugs that may interact [see Drug/Lab Interactions]); and every 24 hours throughout the infusion. ■ Stop the IV infusion and obtain a serum theophylline concentration immediately in any patient on aminophylline who develops nausea or vomiting (particularly repetitive vomiting) or if any other signs of toxicity occur, even if another cause is suspected. ■ Dose increases should not be made in patients with an acute exacerbation of symptoms unless the steady-state serum theophylline concentration is less than 10 mcg/ml. ■ Patients with a very high initial clearance rate (low steady-state serum theophylline concentrations at above-average doses) are likely to experience large changes in serum concentration in response to dose changes. ■ Maintain hydration. ■ See Precautions, Maternal/Child, Elderly, and Drug/Lab Interactions.

Patient Education: Do not take or discontinue any prescription or over-the-counter medication, including herbal products, without physician's approval. ■ Promptly report S/S of toxicity (e.g., nausea and vomiting).

Maternal/Child: Category C: use in pregnancy only if clearly indicated. ■ Neonates may have therapeutic blood levels and may develop apnea from theophylline withdrawal. ■ Elimination of drug is prolonged in premature infants, neonates, and children up to 1 year. Use with extreme caution in children. Has caused fatal reactions. Elimination reaches maximum values by 1 year of age, remains fairly constant to 9 years of age, and slowly decreases by approximately 50% to adult values at 16 years of age. ■ Children under the age of 1 year, as well as neonates with decreased renal function, require careful attention to dosing and frequent monitoring of serum theophylline concentrations. ■ Secreted in breast milk; some sources recommend discontinuing breast-feeding. If the decision is made to breast-feed, monitor infant for evidence of side effects.

Elderly: Compared to healthy young adults, clearance of theophylline is decreased an average of 30% in healthy elderly. Monitor dosing carefully; frequent serum theophylline concentrations are recommended. See Dose Adjustments, Precautions, and Monitor.

DRUG/LAB INTERACTIONS

Review of patient drug profile by pharmacist imperative at time of initiation of aminophylline and with any change in medication regimen. ■ Do not use one xanthine derivative concurrently with another xanthine derivative, ephedrine, or other sympathomimetic drugs. ■ Xanthines antagonize or potentiate or are themselves antagonized or potentiated by many drug groups. Monitor serum levels as indicated. **Theophylline clearance increased and serum levels decreased** by aminoglutenide, barbiturates, carbamazepine (Tegretol), isoproterenol (Isuprel), hydantoins (e.g., phenytoin [Dilantin]), rifampin (Rifadin), smoking, sulfinpyrazone (Anturane). **Theophylline clearance decreased and serum levels increased** by alcohol, allopurinol, beta-adrenergic blockers (e.g., propranolol [Inderal]), cimetidine (Tagamet), clarithromycin, ciprofloxacin (Cipro IV), disulfiram (Antabuse), erythromycin, estrogen-containing oral contraceptives, fluvoxamine (Luvox), interferon alfa-A, methotrexate (Folex), mexiletine (Mexitil), pentoxifylline (Trental), propafenone (Rythmol), tacrine (Cognex), thiabendazole (Mintezol), ticlopidine (Ticlid), troleandomycin (TAO), verapamil (Isoptin). ■ Inhibits pancuronium (Pavulon); increased doses of pancuronium may be required to achieve neuromuscular blockade. ■ Carbamazepine (Tegretol) and loop diuretics (e.g., furosemide [Lasix]) may increase or decrease serum levels. ▪ Reduces sedative effect of benzodiazepines (e.g., diazepam [Valium], midazolam [Versed]) and of propofol (Diprivan); increased doses of sedatives may be required. To avoid respiratory depression, reduce sedative dose if aminophylline is discontinued or if dose is significantly reduced. ▪ May decrease lithium levels. Dose adjustment and monitoring of lithium levels may be indicated. ▪ Concurrent use with halothane may induce cardiac arrhythmias. ▪ Concurrent use with ketamine may lower aminophylline seizure level. ▪ Concurrent use with ephedrine may increase nausea, nervousness, and insomnia. ▪ May increase lab values for free fatty acids, glucose, HDL, LDL, total cholesterol, uric acid, and urinary free cortisol excretion. ▪ Caffeine and xanthine metabolites in neonates or patients with renal dysfunction may cause readings from some immunoassay techniques to be higher than the actual serum theophylline concentration. ▪ Interferes with dipyridamole-assisted MI perfusion studies.

SIDE EFFECTS

Headache, insomnia, nausea, vomiting most common when peak serum concentrations are less than 20 mcg/ml. Rarely a severe allergic reaction of the skin (e.g., exfoliative dermatitis) may occur. Toxicity resulting in death may occur suddenly at levels less than 20 mcg/ml, especially in certain populations (see Precautions); may occur more frequently with serum levels above 20 mcg/ml. Anxiety, cardiac arrest, arrhythmias (e.g., atrial fibrillation, ventricular fibrillation), convulsions, delirium, dizziness, flushing, hyperpyrexia, intractable seizures, nausea, peripheral vascular collapse, persistent vomiting, restlessness, temporary hypotension.

Overdose: ***Acute:*** Acid/base disturbances, arrhythmias (e.g., sinus tachycardia), hyperglycemia, hypokalemia, seizures (usually with serum concentrations over 100 mcg/ml), vomiting, and death have occurred.

Chronic: All of the above plus various arrhythmias, seizures (with serum concentration greater than 30 mcg/ml), and death.

ANTIDOTE

With onset of any side effect, discontinue drug and notify physician. ▪ Stop the IV infusion and obtain a serum theophylline concentration immediately in any patient on aminophylline who develops nausea or vomiting (particularly repetitive vomiting) or if any other signs of toxicity occur, even if another cause is suspected. ▪ For mild symptoms the physician may choose to continue the drug at a decreased dose and rate of administration. All side effects will be treated symptomatically. Maintain adequate ventilation and adequate hydration. Grand mal seizures may not respond to anticonvulsants. Diazepam (Valium) may be most effective. Treat atrial arrhythmias with verapamil, ventricular arrhythmias with lidocaine or procainamide. Use dopamine (Intropin) for hypotension. Do not use stimulants. Resuscitate as necessary.

MANUFACTURER'S SPECIFIC RECOMMENDATIONS FOR ACUTE AND CHRONIC OVERDOSE
Acute overdose (e.g., excessive loading dose or excessive infusion rate for less than 24 hours) or chronic overdose (e.g., excessive infusion rate for more than 24 hours): Serum concentration 20 to 30 mcg/ml: Stop the infusion, monitor the patient, and obtain a serum theophylline concentration in 2 to 4 hours to ensure that the concentration is decreasing.

Continued

Acute overdose with a serum concentration of 30 to 100 mcg/ml or chronic overdose with serum concentrations greater than 30 mcg/ml in patients less than 60 years of age:
Stop the infusion. Administer multiple-dose oral activated charcoal and measures to control emesis. Monitor the patient and obtain serial theophylline concentrations every 2 to 4 hours to determine the effectiveness of therapy and to determine further treatment decisions. Institute extracorporeal removal if emesis, seizures, or cardiac arrhythmias cannot be adequately controlled.

Acute overdose with a serum concentration greater than 100 mcg/ml or chronic overdose with serum concentrations greater than 30 mcg/ml in patients 60 years or older:
Stop the infusion. Consider prophylactic anticonvulsant therapy. Administer multiple-dose oral-activated charcoal and measures to control emesis. Consider extracorporeal removal, even if the patient has not experienced a seizure. Monitor the patient and obtain serial theophylline concentrations every 2 to 4 hours to determine the effectiveness of therapy and to determine further treatment decisions.

Extracorporeal removal:
Weigh risk versus benefits. Charcoal hemoperfusion is the most effective and increases theophylline clearance up to six-fold, but hypotension, hypocalcemia, and platelet consumption and bleeding diatheses may occur. Hemodialysis is about as efficient as multiple-dose oral-activated charcoal and has a lower risk of serious complications. Consider hemodialysis when charcoal hemoperfusion is not feasible and multiple-dose oral-activated charcoal is ineffective because of intractable emesis. Serum theophylline concentrations may rebound 5 to 10 mcg/ml after either treatment is discontinued due to redistribution of theophylline from the tissue compartment. Peritoneal dialysis is ineffective, and exchange transfusions in neonates have been minimally effective.

AMIODARONE HYDROCHLORIDE

Antiarrhythmic

(a-mee′oh-da-rone hye-droe-klor′id)

Cordarone

pH 4.08

USUAL DOSE

Treatment and Prophylaxis of Ventricular Tachycardia (VT) and Ventricular Fibrillation (VF)

1,000 mg over the first 24 hours in 3 distinct segments; two loading infusions and a maintenance infusion. Use of a dedicated central venous catheter preferred.

Rapid loading infusion: 150 mg specifically diluted solution (1.5 mg/ml) over 10 minutes. Follow immediately with the slow loading infusion.

Slow loading infusion: 360 mg specifically diluted solution (1.8 mg/ml) at 1 mg/min over the next 6 hours.

Maintenance infusion: 540 mg of 1.8 mg/ml solution at 0.5 mg/min over 18 hours. Maintenance infusion is usually continued at 0.5 mg/min for 48 to

96 hours or until ventricular arrhythmias are stabilized. May be continued with caution for up to 2 to 3 weeks. Transfer to oral therapy as soon as feasible (guidelines are in package insert).

Treatment of Breakthrough Ventricular Fibrillation (VF) or Hemodynamically Unstable Ventricular Tachycardia (VT)

At any time that breakthrough VF or hemodynamically unstable VT occurs during administration, a supplemental rapid loading infusion (150 mg over 10 minutes) may be repeated. May be specifically diluted 1.5 mg/ml solution or rate of the maintenance infusion (1.8 mg/ml) may be temporarily increased to equal 150 mg (83.33 ml) over 10 minutes. During trials total doses above 1,800 to 2,100 mg (including added doses for breakthrough VF/VT) increased the risk of hypotension.

Cardiac Arrest (unlabeled)

300 mg (6 ml) or 5 mg/kg as a bolus injection. Flush with 10 ml D5W or NS. Should be given through a separate IV line immediately after the first dose of epinephrine (1 mg) and before the fourth electrical countershock. Supplemental doses of 150 mg (3 ml) may be given for recurrent bouts of VT/VF. AHA guidelines recommend considering a repeat dose of 150 mg IV push in 3 to 5 minutes with a maximum cumulative dose of 2.2 Gm IV/24 hr. After return of spontaneous circulation (ROSC), initiate the slow loading infusion and maintenance infusion as above. If effective, discontinue amiodarone and reassess arrhythmia management within 6 to 24 hours.

Supraventricular Arrhythmias (unlabeled)

150 mg over 10 minutes as a loading dose. Follow with an infusion of 360 mg over 6 hours followed by a maintenance infusion of 0.5 mg/min. Other regimens used during studies to convert atrial fibrillation and atrial flutter to sinus rhythm include 5 mg/kg over 3 to 5 minutes; 5 to 7 mg/kg as a 30 minute infusion followed by a continuous infusion to a maximum total dose of 1500 mg/24 hours; an infusion of 2 mg/kg/hr continued for up to 2 hours after conversion to a stable sinus rhythm or a maximum dose of 2400 mg/24 hr.

PEDIATRIC DOSE

Safety for use in pediatric patients (particularly infants and neonates) not established and not recommended; see Contraindications and Maternal/Child.

Treatment of refractory pulseless VT, VF: 5 mg/kg by rapid IV bolus (Recommendation in AHA guidelines).

Treatment of perfusing supraventricular and ventricular arrhythmias: 5 mg/kg as an infusion over 20 to 60 minutes. May repeat to a maximum of 15 mg/kg/24 hr. (Recommendation in AHA guidelines).

DOSE ADJUSTMENTS

Not required in renal or hepatic disease. Another source suggests a reduced dose in hepatic failure. ▪ Dose selection should be cautious in the elderly. Reduced initial doses may be indicated based on the potential for decreased organ function and concomitant disease or drug therapy.

DILUTION

Do not use evacuated glass intravenous bottles. Use only commercially available D5W solutions in polyolefin or glass containers in any prepared solution that will be given over more than 2 hours. PVC containers are suitable only for dilution of the rapid loading dose; see Incompatible With. **Rapid loading infusion:** Dilute 150 mg (3 ml) in 100 ml D5W (1.5 mg/ml).

Slow loading infusion and maintenance infusion: Dilute 900 mg (18 ml) in 500 ml D5W (1.8 mg/ml). Dilutions from 1 to 6 mg/ml have been used for maintenance solutions after the first 24 hours. Concentrations over 2 mg/ml for longer than 1 hour must be administered through a central venous catheter. Higher concentrations (3 to 6 mg/ml) have caused peripheral vein phlebitis.

Cardiac arrest (unlabeled): Loading dose (300 mg or 5 mg/kg) or supplemental boluses (150 mg) may be given undiluted. Has also been diluted in up to 20 ml D5W.

Storage: Store ampules in their carton at CRT. Use solutions diluted in PVC containers within 2 hours; use those diluted in glass or polyolefin containers within 24 hours.

INCOMPATIBLE WITH

Manufacturer recommendations include: Do not use evacuated glass intravenous bottles. Administer through a dedicated IV line (central venous catheter preferred). Absorbs to PVC tubing but loss accounted for in specified dose; follow infusion regimen closely. Leaches out plasticizers, including DEHP, from IV tubing. The degree of leaching increases when the solution is infused at a higher concentration or a slower infusion rate than recommended.

Y-site: Manufacturer lists aminophylline, cefamandole (Mandol), cefazolin (Kefzol), heparin, mezlocillin (Mezlin), and sodium bicarbonate.

COMPATIBLE WITH **(Underline Indicates Conflicting Compatibility Information)**

Consult pharmacist; specific conditions may apply; see Compatibilities, p. xvi.

Additive: Dobutamine (Dobutrex), <u>furosemide (Lasix)</u>, lidocaine, potassium chloride (KCl), procainamide (Pronestyl), <u>quinidine</u>, verapamil (Isoptin).

Y-site: Amikacin (Amikin), bretylium (Bretylate), clindamycin (Cleocin), dobutamine (Dobutrex), dopamine (Intropin), doxycycline (Vibramycin), erythromycin lactobionate (Erythrocin), esmolol (Brevibloc), gentamicin (Garamycin), insulin (regular), isoproterenol (Isuprel), labetalol (Normodyne), lidocaine, metronidazole (Flagyl IV), midazolam (Versed), morphine, nitroglycerin (Nitro-Bid IV), norepinephrine (Levophed), penicillin G potassium, phentolamine (Regitine), phenylephrine (Neo-Synephrine), potassium chloride (KCl), procainamide (Pronestyl), tobramycin (Nebcin), vancomycin (Vancocin).

RATE OF ADMINISTRATION

Volumetric pump required for administration. Surface properties of diluted solution reduce drop size; use of a drop counter infusion set causes underdosing. Use of a 0.2-micron in-line filter is also recommended. Filtering does not affect potency. A central venous catheter is required for concentrations greater than 2 mg/ml. Adhere to prescribed rates; risk of hypotension is increased in the first hours of treatment and with increased rates; may cause secondary renal or hepatic failure; see Precautions. Avoid IV bolus doses in patients with marked cardiomegaly, a continuous infusion is preferred.

Rapid loading infusion or breakthrough treatment of VF/VT: 150 mg over 10 minutes (15 mg/min). Do not exceed a rate of 30 mg/min.

Slow loading infusion: 1 mg/min or 33.3 ml/hr of 1.8 mg/ml solution for 6 hours.

Maintenance infusion: 0.5 mg/min or 16.6 ml/hr of 1.8 mg/ml solution for 18 hours. A continuing maintenance solution should deliver 720 mg/

24 hr at 0.5 mg/min whether the concentration is 1.8 mg/ml or 6 mg/ml. May be continued at this rate for up to 2 to 3 weeks as described in Usual Dose.

Cardiac arrest (unlabeled): Loading or supplemental doses by IV bolus injection. Follow with 10 ml flush of D5W or NS through Y-tube or three-way stopcock. May be given through a free-flowing infusion of D5W. After ROSC, initiate the slow loading and maintenance infusions as above.

ACTIONS

An antiarrhythmic agent possessing several antiarrhythmic effects that result in a decreased number of VT/VF events. It prolongs the duration of action potentials in cardiac fibers, depresses conduction velocity, slows conduction at the AV node, and exhibits some alpha and beta blockade activity. Raises the threshold for VF and may prevent its recurrence. Also has vasodilatory effects that decrease cardiac workload and myocardial oxygen consumption. Uptake by the myocardium is rapid; antiarrhythmic effect is prompt (clinically relevant within hours); however, full effect may take days. Has an exceptionally long half-life. Metabolized in the liver using cytochrome P_{450} enzymes. Primarily excreted in bile. Crosses placental barrier. Secreted in breast milk.

INDICATIONS AND USES

Treatment of acute life-threatening VT/VF and prophylaxis of frequently recurring VF and hemodynamically unstable VT in patients refractory to other therapy (e.g., bretylium, lidocaine, procainamide). Used until ventricular arrhythmias are stabilized; usually 48 to 96 hours, but may be given for longer periods (i.e., up to 3 weeks). ■ Treatment of patients taking oral amiodarone who are unable to take oral medication.

Unlabeled uses: Treatment of sustained monomorphic VT in patients with acute myocardial infarction (AMI) not accompanied by chest pain, pulmonary congestion, or hypotension in patients who have failed to respond to lidocaine and synchronized DC cardioversion (ACC/AHA Committee on management of AMI). ■ Treatment of peri-arrest (including out-of-hospital) broad complex tachycardia refractory to electrical countershock and lidocaine (Chamberlain and European Resuscitation Council). ■ Termination of persistent atrial fibrillation (AF). ■ Treatment of drug-refractory, symptomatic, recurrent AF. ■ Preoperative prophylaxis against AF occurring after heart surgery. ■ Conversion of supraventricular arrhythmias to sinus rhythm in patients following cardiac surgery. ■ Convert AF in patients with CHF.

CONTRAINDICATIONS

Cardiogenic shock, known hypersensitivity to amiodarone or any of its components, marked sinus bradycardia, second- or third-degree AV block unless a functioning pacemaker is available, sinus node dysfunction. See Drug/Lab Interactions. ■ Not recommended for use in neonates or infants. ■ Contraindicated with ritonavir (Norvir).

PRECAUTIONS

Usually administered by or under the direction of the physician specialist with facilities for monitoring the patient and responding to any medical emergency. ■ Correct hypokalemia and hypomagnesemia before use; may exaggerate a prolonged QTc and cause arrhythmias (e.g., torsades de pointes). ■ May cause transient increases in liver enzymes but abnormal baseline hepatic enzymes is not a contraindication to use. ■ May worsen existing arrhythmias or precipitate new ones, primarily torsades de pointes or new-onset VF. ■ May cause visual impairment (e.g., optic neuropathy or optic neuritis); has progressed to permanent blindness. ■ May cause pulmonary toxicity (e.g., ARDS, bronchospasm, hemoptysis, hypoxemia). Usually seen with long-term use, but acute pulmonary hypersensitivity has been reported after short-term IV use. The elderly, patients with preexisting restrictive lung disease, and patients receiving high concentrations of oxygen may be at increased risk; see Side Effects. ■ Adult respiratory distress syndrome (ARDS) has been reported in patients receiving oral amiodarone following surgery. ■ Monitor patients undergoing general anesthesia closely; may increase sensitivity to myocardial depressant and conduction defects of halogenated inhalation anesthetics (hypotension and atropine-resistant bradycardia). ■ Use caution in patients with cardiomyopathy, hepatic failure, left ventricular dysfunction, or thyroid dysfunction. ■ See Incompatible With and Drug/Lab Interactions. ***Cardiac arrest:*** Incidence of hypotension and/or myocardial depression may be less than with procainamide (Pronestyl) or bretylium. ■ Has been used as an alternative agent in patients who have developed torsades de pointes previously with class Ia antiarrhythmic agents (e.g., disopyramide [Norpace], procainamide, quinidine).

Monitor: Continuous ECG and HR monitoring is mandatory to observe for arrhythmias. Watch for QTc prolongation; may cause proarrhythmia (torsades de pointes). ■ Monitor for bradycardia and AV block. A temporary pacemaker should be available. ■ Monitor BP closely to minimize hypotension (occurs frequently with initial rates). ■ Confirm patency of vein. Reduce rate or concentration for pain or redness at injection site. Incidence of phlebitis markedly increased with concentrations above 2.5 mg/ml; central venous administration preferred. ■ Monitor serum electrolytes and acid-base balance, especially in patients with prolonged diarrhea and those receiving diuretics. ■ Monitor liver enzymes (AST, ALT, GGT) for elevations indicating progressive injury. ■ Monitor pulmonary status (e.g., Fio_2, Sao_2, Pao_2, chest x-ray); baseline pulmonary function tests recommended; repeat as indicated. Monitoring of SrCr, BUN, and thyroid function tests may be indicated. ■ Regular ophthalmic exams, including funduscopy and slit lamp exams, are recommended. Prompt ophthalmic exams recommended at first sign of visual impairment. May require discontinuation of amiodarone therapy. ■ Serum amiodarone levels greater than 2.5 mcg/ml have been associated with a higher incidence of side effects. ■ See Precautions and Drug/Lab Interactions.

Patient Education: Report promptly any feelings of faintness, difficulty breathing, or pain or stinging along injection site. ■ Nonhormonal birth control recommended. ■ Avoid excessive sunlight. May cause sunburn for weeks (extended half-life). Protective clothing and dark glasses may be appropriate outdoors.

Maternal/Child: Category D: avoid pregnancy or use only if benefit to mother justifies risk to fetus. Has caused infrequent neonatal congenital goiter/hypothyroidism and hyperthyroidism in addition to other adverse effects. ■ Discontinue breast-feeding. ■ Safety for use during labor and delivery not established. ■ A manufacturer's warning letter has been issued citing potentially fatal or developmental side effects in infants and neonates; see Contraindications. Another source suggests amiodarone may adversely affect male reproductive tract development in infants, neonates, and toddlers. ■ Contains benzyl alcohol, which has been associated with "gasping syndrome" in neonates (sudden onset of gasping respirations, hypotension, bradycardia, and cardiovascular collapse).

Elderly: Differences in response between the elderly and younger patients have not been identified; however, clearance is slower and half-life may be doubled (up to 47 days). See Dose Adjustments. ■ May be at increased risk for pulmonary toxicity; see Precautions.

DRUG/LAB INTERACTIONS

Amiodarone has a long half-life; drug interactions may persist long after it is discontinued.

Contraindicated with ritonavir (Norvir). Should not be given concurrently with ibutilide (Corvert). ■ Risk of cardiotoxicity increased with pimozide (Orap) and sparfloxacin (Zagam); concurrent use not recommended. ■ Concurrent use with other antiarrhythmic agents (e.g., disopyramide [Norpace], mexiletine [Mexitil], procainamide [Pronestyl], quinidine) increases their serum concentrations and may result in additive increases in QT prolongation and serious arrhythmias. One source recommends reducing the dose of previously given antiarrhythmic agents by 30% to 50% several days after starting amiodarone and then gradually withdrawing them altogether. Another suggests reducing the dose of any antiarrhythmic therapy required in addition to amiodarone to one-half the recommended dose. Monitor serum levels if possible. ■ May decrease metabolism and increase serum levels of digoxin. One source recommends reducing digoxin dose by 50% or withdrawing completely when amiodarone therapy is initiated. ■ Use with potassium-depleting diuretics (e.g., chlorothiazide [Diuril], furosemide [Lasix], indapamide [Lozol]) may lead to increased risk of arrhythmias due to hypokalemia. ■ Inhibits metabolism and increases anticoagulant effect (e.g., increased PT and INR) of warfarin (Coumadin). Dose reduction of the anticoagulant and careful monitoring of PT or INR recommended. Effects may persist long after amiodarone discontinued. ■ May decrease metabolism and increase serum levels of cyclosporine (Sandimmune), flecainide (Tambocor), hydantoins (e.g., phenytoin [Dilantin]), lidocaine, methotrexate, procainamide (Pronestyl), quinidine, and theophyllines (Aminophylline). May cause toxicity; monitor serum levels. Reduced doses indicated. ■ May cause bradycardia, decreased cardiac output, and hypotension with fentanyl (Sublimaze). ■ Therapeutic plasma concentrations of flecainide (Tambocor) can be maintained with reduced doses because amiodarone interferes with flecainide metabolism. ■ Amiodarone clearance increased and plasma levels decreased with cholestyramine (Questran), phenytoin (Dilantin), and rifampin (Rifadin). ■ Cimetidine (Tagamet) and indinavir (Crixivan) may decrease clearance and increase plasma levels of amiodarone. ■ May increase risk of bradycardia and hypotension with beta-blockers (e.g., propranolol [Inderal]). ■ May increase risk of AV block and hypotension with calcium channel blockers (e.g., diltiazem [Cardizem], verapamil [Isoptin]). ■ Monitor patients undergoing general anesthesia closely. May increase sensitivity to myocardial depressant and conduction defects of halogenated inhalation anesthetics (hypotension and atropine-resistant bradycardia). ■ Use for longer than 2 weeks may decrease metabolism and increase serum levels of dextromethorphan (Robitussin DM), methotrexate, and phenytoin. ■ See Precautions.

SIDE EFFECTS

Hypotension or pain at the IV site are the most common side effects. Anaphylaxis, anemia (aplastic and/or hemolytic), angioedema, anorexia, arrhythmias (e.g., AV block, bradycardia, new onset VT/VF, torsades de pointes), adult respiratory distress syndrome (ARDS), ataxia, cardiac arrest, cardiogenic shock, congestive heart failure, dizziness, dry eyes, hepatotoxicity (liver function test abnormalities), myopathy, nausea, nephrotoxicity, neutropenia, pancytopenia, paresthesias, peripheral neuropathy, photosensitivity, pulmonary toxicity (including bronchiolitis obliterans organizing pneumonia [may be fatal]), thyroid dysfunction, and visual impairment/loss of vision may occur. In addition to these side effects, overdose or extended use may cause hepatic and/or renal failure secondary to hypotension.

ANTIDOTE

Keep physician informed of all side effects and treat promptly as appropriate; many are life-threatening. Reduce rate and/or concentration for pain at IV site. Monitor hepatic enzymes closely. Reduce rate or discontinue for progressive hepatic injury. Treat hypotension and cardiogenic shock by slowing the infusion rate. Vasopressors (e.g., dopamine [Intropin], norepinephrine [Levophed]), inotropic agents (e.g., digoxin), and volume expansion may be indicated. Slow infusion rate or discontinue if bradycardia and/or AV block occur; may require a temporary pacemaker. If torsades de pointes occurs, stop all cardioactive drugs (e.g., antiarrhythmics, digoxin, antidepressants, phenothiazines) and normalize electrolytes (e.g., potassium, magnesium). Atrial overdrive pacing may be required to stabilize cardiac rhythm. Amiodarone is not dialyzable. Resuscitate as necessary.

AMPHOTERICIN B ▪ AMPHOTERICIN B LIPID-BASED PRODUCTS

(am-foe-ter'i-sin)

Antifungal
Antiprotozoal
(AmBisome)

Fungizone ▪ Abelcet, AmBisome, Amphotec — **pH 5.7 to 8 ▪ 5 to 6**

USUAL DOSE

Each product has different biochemical, pharmacokinetic, and pharmacodynamic properties. They are not interchangeable from dose to dose in a given patient between each other or traditional amphotericin.

ABELCET (AMPHOTERICIN B LIPID COMPLEX INJECTION)

Adults and children: 5 mg/kg/24 hr as an infusion. Repeat daily until clinical response or mycologic cure.

AMPHOTEC (AMPHOTERICIN B CHOLESTERYL SULFATE COMPLEX FOR INJECTION)

Adults and children: 3 to 4 mg/kg/24 hr as an infusion. Pretreatment with antipyretics, antihistamines, or corticosteroids may be indicated; see Precautions and Antidote. On the first day of treatment, begin with a test dose of 10 ml of the final diluted preparation and infuse over 15 to 30 minutes. Observe the patient for the next 30 minutes. If there is no adverse reaction, continue with the calculated dose. May be increased to 6 mg/kg/24 hr if there is no improvement or if the fungal infection progresses. See Indications.

AMBISOME (AMPHOTERICIN B LIPOSOME FOR INJECTION)

Adults, children, and infants over 1 month of age: All doses are by infusion.

Empirical therapy in febrile, neutropenic patients: 3 mg/kg/24 hr.

Systemic fungal infections (e.g., *Aspergillus, Candida, Cryptococcus*): 3 to 5 mg/kg/24 hr.

Treatment of cryptococcal meningitis in HIV-infected patients: 6 mg/kg/24 hr.

Visceral leishmaniasis in immunocompetent patients: 3 mg/kg/24 hr on days 1 through 5. Repeat 3 mg/kg on day 14 and on day 21. A repeat course of therapy may be useful if parasitic clearance is not achieved.

Visceral leishmaniasis in immunocompromised patients: 4 mg/kg/24 hr on days 1 through 5. Repeat 4 mg/kg on days 10, 17, 24, 31, and 38. During clinical studies parasitic clearance was not achieved or relapse within 6 months occurred in 88.2% of patients. Usefulness of repeat courses not determined.

FUNGIZONE/GENERIC (TRADITIONAL AMPHOTERICIN B)

Adults and children: Begin with a test dose of 0.1 mg/kg up to 1 mg maximum dose in 20 to 50 ml D5W. Infuse over 10 to 30 minutes. Determine size of therapeutic dose by intensity of reaction over a 4-hour period. Usual is 0.25 mg/kg of body weight/24 hr gradually increased in 0.125 to 0.25 mg/kg increments to 1 mg/kg/24 hr or a maximum of 50 mg/day (average dose is 0.5 mg/kg) as tolerance permits. Maximum dose for children is 1 mg/kg/day or 30 mg/M^2/day. Up to 1.5 mg/kg/24 hr may be given on alternate-day therapy. Several months of therapy are usually required and recommended for cure. Dosage must be adjusted to each specific patient. In some instances higher doses can be used.

Mannitol 12.5 Gm immediately before and after each dose of Fungizone or generic amphotericin B may reduce nephrotoxic effects. See Precautions for additional suggestions.

DOSE ADJUSTMENTS

ABELCET: Full dose usually required; base on SrCr and overall patient condition.

AMPHOTEC/AMBISOME: No dose adjustments suggested.

FUNGIZONE/GENERIC: Full dose required even in impaired renal function, but reduce dose or discontinue drug if BUN greater than 40 mg/100 ml or SrCr greater than 3 mg/100 ml. Gradual dose increases are essential. Whenever medicine is not given for 7 days or longer, restart treatment at lowest dosage level.

DILUTION

ABELCET: Available in 50-mg (10-ml) and 100-mg (20-ml) vials. The new 50-mg vial facilitates accurate dosing and reduction of waste. Shake vial until all yellow sediment is dissolved. Maintain aseptic technique. Withdraw an exact total daily dose from one or more vials using one or more syringes and 18-gauge needles. Replace needle(s) on syringe(s) with the 5-micron filter(s) supplied with each vial. A new filter must be used for each 400 mg (80 ml) of Abelcet. Empty syringe contents through filter into an infusion of D5W. 4 ml of diluent (D5W) is required for each 1 ml (5 mg) of Abelcet to achieve a final concentration of 1 mg/ml. For ***pediatric*** and/or fluid-restricted patients (e.g., patients with cardiovascular disease) reduce diluent by half (approximate concentration of 2 mg/ml). pH 5.5 to 6. Use only clear solutions and discard unused portion.

AMPHOTEC: Available in 50-mg or 100-mg vials. Reconstitute by rapidly adding 10 ml of SW for each 50 mg of Amphotec (5 mg/ml). Use of a 20-gauge needle is recommended. Shake gently, rotating the vial until all solids have dissolved. May be opalescent or clear. Must be further diluted for infusion with D5W (see chart). Final desired concentration is approximately 0.6 mg/ml (range with recommended amounts of diluent is 0.16 mg/ml to 0.83 mg/ml). Do not filter or use an in-line filter. See Incompatible With and Rate of Administration.

Guidelines for Dilution of Amphotec		
Dose of Amphotec	**Volume of Reconstituted Amphotec**	**Infusion Bag Size for D5W for Injection**
10-35 mg	2-7 ml	50 ml
35-70 mg	7-14 ml	100 ml
70-175 mg	14-35 ml	250 ml
175-350 mg	35-70 ml	500 ml
350-1,000 mg	70-200 ml	1,000 ml

AMBISOME: Reconstitute each 50-mg vial with 12 ml SW (without a bacteriostatic agent) to yield 4 mg/ml. Shake vial vigorously for 30 seconds; forms a yellow translucent suspension. Withdraw an exact total daily dose from one or more vials using one or more 20-ml syringes and needles. Replace needle(s) with the 5-micron filter(s) supplied with each vial. A new filter must be used for each 50-mg vial. Empty syringe contents through filter into an infusion of D5W. Use sufficient diluent to achieve a final concentration of 1 to 2 mg/ml, pH 5 to 6. For ***pediatric patients:*** may be further diluted to concentrations of 0.2 to 0.5 mg/ml for infants and small children to provide adequate volume for infusion.

FUNGIZONE/GENERIC: A 50-mg vial is initially diluted with 10 ml of SW for injection (without a bacteriostatic agent); 5 mg equals 1 ml. Shake well until solution is clear. Further dilute each 1 mg in at least 10 ml of D5W. Dextrose must have a pH above 4.2. Concentration of solution must not be greater than 0.1 mg/ml. Do not use any other diluent. Use a sterile 20-gauge or larger needle at each step of the dilution. Maintain aseptic technique. Larger pore 1-micron filters may be used. Use only fresh solutions without evidence of precipitate or foreign matter. Light sensitive but protection from light not required unless solution exposed over 8 hours. pH 5.7 to 8.

Storage: ABELCET: Before reconstitution, refrigerate vials and protect from light. Do not freeze. Diluted solution is stable 48 hours if refrigerated and an additional 6 hours at room temperature.

AMPHOTEC: Store unopened vials in carton at CRT. Refrigerate reconstituted or diluted solutions; must be used within 24 hours. Do not freeze. Discard unused drug.

AMBISOME: Refrigerate unopened vials. Vials reconstituted with SW may be refrigerated for up to 24 hours. Do not freeze. Infusion of fully diluted solution must begin within 6 hours. Discard unused drug.

FUNGIZONE/GENERIC: Before reconstitution, refrigerate vials and protect from light. Do not freeze. Preserve concentrate in refrigerator up to 7 days or 24 hours at room temperature. Use diluted solution promptly.

COMPATIBLE WITH **(Underline Indicates Conflicting Compatibility Information)**

ALL FORMULATIONS

Consult pharmacist; specific conditions may apply; see Compatibilities, p. xvi. In all situations, use a separate infusion line or flush an existing line before and after administration.

ABELCET

Do not mix with any other diluent, drug, or solution. Use only D5W. Manufacturer states that compatibility with any other diluent has not been established.

AMBISOME/AMPHOTEC/FUNGIZONE/GENERIC

Do not mix with any other diluent, drug, or solution. Use only SW for reconstitution and D5W for dilution for infusion. Use of any other solution or the presence of a bacteriostatic agent (e.g., benzyl alcohol) may cause precipitation.

AMPHOTEC

Y-site: Acyclovir (Zovirax), aminophylline, cefoxitin (Mefoxin), ceftizoxime (Cefizox), clindamycin (Cleocin), dexamethasone (Decadron), fentanyl (Sublimaze), furosemide (Lasix), ganciclovir (Cytovene), granisetron (Kytril), hydrocortisone sodium succinate (Solu-Cortef), ifosfamide (Ifex), lorazepam (Ativan), mannitol, methotrexate (Folex), methylprednisolone (Solu-Medrol), nitroglycerin (Nitro-Bid IV), sulfamethoxazole-trimethoprim (Bactrim), sufentanil (Sufenta), vinblastine (Velban), vincristine (Oncovin), zidovudine (AZT, Retrovir).

FUNGIZONE/GENERIC

Additive: ***Not recommended by manufacturer;*** fluconazole (Diflucan), heparin, hydrocortisone (Hydrocortone, Solu-Cortef).

Syringe: ***Not recommended by manufacturer;*** heparin.

Y-site: Aldesleukin (Interleukin-2), <u>cisatracurium (Nimbex)</u>, diltiazem (Cardizem), <u>remifentanil (Ultiva)</u>, <u>sargramostim (Leukine)</u>, tacrolimus (Prograf), teniposide (Vumon), thiotepa (Thioplex), zidovudine (AZT, Retrovir).

RATE OF ADMINISTRATION

ALL AMPHOTERICINS: Rapid infusion may cause hypotension, hypokalemia, arrhythmia, and shock. Infusion reactions can occur with all amphotericin B formulations. See Precautions, Side Effects, and Antidote. With all formulations, flush existing line with D5W before and after administration or use a separate IV line.

ABELCET: Total daily dose as an infusion at 2.5 mg/kg/hr. Contents of diluted solution must be mixed by shaking at least every 2 hours. Do not use an in-line filter.

AMPHOTEC: See rate for test dose in Usual Dose. Give total daily dose as an infusion at 1 mg/kg/hr. Infusion time may be shortened to a minimum of 2 hours for patients who show no evidence of intolerance or infusion-related reactions. May be extended for acute reactions or if infusion volume is not tolerated. Do not use filters.

AMBISOME: Total daily dose as an infusion over 2 hours. Use of a controlled infusion device is recommended. Infusion time may be shortened to a minimum of 1 hour for patients who show no evidence of intolerance or infusion-related reactions. Infusion time may be extended for patient discomfort or acute reactions or if infusion volume is not tolerated. Do not use any in-line filter less than 1 micron.

FUNGIZONE/GENERIC: Daily dose over 2 to 6 hours by slow IV infusion. Expected reactions usually less severe with slower rate. A minimum 1-micron filter may be used.

ACTIONS

Antifungal antibiotic agents that bind to fungal cell membranes resulting in leakage of cellular contents. May be fungistatic or fungicidal according to body fluid concentration and susceptibility of the fungus. Abelcet is amphotericin B complexed with two phospholipids in a 1:1 drug-to-lipid ratio. Amphotec is amphotericin B complexed with cholesteryl sulfate in a colloidal dispersion in a 1:1 drug-to-lipid ratio. AmBisome is amphotericin B intercalated into a liposomal membrane with several components. Assay tests cannot distinguish lipid-based amphotericin from traditional (Fungizone/generic). Modification of amphotericin to the various lipid-based products alters the drug's functional properties. It allows for increased levels of drug at the site of action (usually areas where the fungi are). Overall effect is increased effectiveness with less toxicity. Not effective against bacteria, rickettsiae, or viruses. Remains in the body at a therapeutic level up to 20 hours after each infusion (Abelcet has the longest elimination half-life [up to 173 hours]). Actual distribution to organs is somewhat selective and may help to decide which product is best to use in a given situation. Route of metabolism not known. Excreted very slowly in the urine.

INDICATIONS AND USES

Because of their high cost, some clinicians suggest that the lipid-based products should be used only in patients refractory to traditional amphotericin, patients with progressing invasive fungal infections, and patients with nephrotoxicity (SrCr greater than 2.5 mg/dl) or at high risk (e.g., transplant patients on cyclosporine or tacrolimus).

ABELCET: Treatment of invasive fungal infections in patients who are refractory to or intolerant of traditional amphotericin B therapy (e.g., aspergillosis, candidiasis, cryptococcosis, cryptococcal meningitis, fusariosis, zygomycosis). Has orphan drug approval for invasive coccidioidomycosis, invasive protothecosis, and invasive sporotrichosis.

AMPHOTEC: Treatment of invasive aspergillosis in patients refractory to or intolerant of traditional amphotericin B or in patients in whom traditional amphotericin treatment has failed.

AMBISOME: Empirical therapy for presumed fungal infection in febrile, neutropenic patients. ▪ Treatment of patients with aspergillosis, candida, and/or cryptococcus infections refractory to traditional amphotericin B or in patients in whom renal impairment or unacceptable toxicity precludes the use of traditional amphotericin B. ▪ Treatment of visceral leishmaniasis. ▪ Treatment of cryptococcal meningitis in HIV-infected patients. ▪ AmBisome is frequently used in BMT patients on cyclosporine.

FUNGIZONE/GENERIC: Treatment of fungal infections that are progressive and potentially fatal, such as aspergillosis, cryptococcosis, blastomycosis, and disseminated forms of candidiasis, coccidioidomycosis, and histoplasmosis, mucormycosis, and sporotrichosis. These infections must be caused by specific organisms. Not recommended for treatment of noninvasive forms of fungal disease in patients with normal neutrophil counts.

Unlabeled uses: Abelcet is used to prevent fungal infections in bone marrow transplant patients (0.1 mg/kg/day). Lipid-based products are used to treat primary amoebic meningoencephalitis caused by *Naegleria fowleri* and for low-dose chemoprophylaxis in immunocompromised patients at risk for aspergillosis.

CONTRAINDICATIONS

All amphotericin formulations: Known sensitivity to amphotericin B or any components of its formulations unless a life-threatening situation is present.

PRECAUTIONS

ALL AMPHOTERICIN FORMULATIONS: Diagnosis should be positively established by culture or histologic study. ▪ Close clinical observation is imperative. Anaphylaxis has occurred; emergency equipment and supplies must be available. ▪ Infusion reactions are common; pretreatment with antipyretics, antihistamines (e.g., diphenhydramine [Benadryl]), and/or selective use of corticosteroids may be indicated. ▪ Use caution in patients receiving leukocyte transfusions; may cause acute pulmonary toxicity. Separate times of administration as much as possible. ▪ Diabetes must be well controlled before treatment with amphotericin is begun. ▪ Nephrotoxicity is the usual dose-limiting factor for use of traditional amphotericin B. Impairment may improve with dose reduction or alternate day therapy, but some residual dysfunction is possible. Lipid-based formulations are associated with less nephrotoxicity. Most studies show equivalent or superior effectiveness compared to traditional amphotericin. Introduction of lipid-based products to patients with increased CrCl and BUN from traditional amphotericin has decreased the CrCl and BUN. ▪ Pseudomembranous colitis has been reported. May range from mild to life-threatening. Consider in patients that present with diarrhea during or after treatment with amphotericin B.

ABELCET: Renal toxicity is dose dependent but has been consistently less nephrotoxic than uncomplexed amphotericin B.

AMPHOTEC/AMBISOME: Incidence of renal toxicity significantly lower than with uncomplexed amphotericin B.

FUNGIZONE/GENERIC: Hospitalization preferred to initiate therapy. ▪ A small amount of heparin added to the infusion may reduce the incidence of thrombophlebitis. ▪ Meperidine (Demerol) or nonsteroidal antiinflammatory agents (e.g., ibuprofen) before administration or hydrocortisone 0.7 mg/kg of body weight added to the infusion may prevent febrile reactions including chills; corticosteroids not recommended for concomitant use in other situations because they exaggerate hypokalemia. ▪ Prophylactic antiemetics and antihistamines are also appropriate.

Monitor: ***All amphotericin formulations:*** Obtain baseline CBC, PT, serum electrolytes, renal (e.g., creatine kinase, BUN, SrCr) and liver function (e.g., ALT, AST) tests. Repeat frequently during therapy; recommended weekly. Monitor creatine kinase and PT as indicated during therapy. ▪ Discontinue or reduce dose until renal function improves if increase in BUN or SrCr is clinically significant (e.g., BUN greater than 40 mg/dl or SrCr greater than 3 mg/dl). Side effects (e.g., hypokalemia, hypomagnesemia, impaired renal function) may be life threatening. ▪ Monitor vital signs and I & O. Record every 30 minutes for up to 4 hours after infusion is complete. ▪ Encourage fluids to maintain hydration.

Patient Education: ***All amphotericin formulations:*** Review all medical conditions and medications before beginning treatment. ▪ Discomfort associated with infusion. ▪ Report difficulty breathing promptly. ▪ Long-term therapy required to effect a cure. ▪ Report diarrhea, fever, increased or decreased urination, loss of appetite, stomach pain, sore throat, and any unusual bleeding or bruising, tiredness, or weakness.

Maternal/Child: ***All amphotericin formulations:*** Category B: has been used successfully during pregnancy but adequate studies not available. Use only if clearly needed. ▪ Safety for use in breast-feeding and children not established. Discontinue nursing. ▪ Fungizone/generic has been used in children. Lipid-based preparations have been used in children without any unexpected side effects. Safety of use of AmBisome in infants under 1 month of age not established.

Elderly: Consider age-related impaired body functions. Lipid-based preparations have been used without unexpected side effects.

DRUG/LAB INTERACTIONS

Drug interaction studies have not been done for lipid-based preparations, but interactions similar to Fungizone/generic are expected. Corticosteroids will increase hypokalemia and may cause arrhythmias. Use with caution only if indicated to control drug reactions or, if necessary, monitor serum electrolytes and cardiac function closely. ▪ Hypokalemic effect may be increased with thiazides, may potentiate digitalis toxicity, and/or may enhance the curariform effect of neuromuscular blocking agents (e.g., doxacurium [Nuromax], rocuronium [Zemuron], succinylcholine); monitor serum potassium levels. ▪ Avoid use or use extreme caution with other nephrotoxic drugs; aminoglycosides (e.g., gentamicin [Garamycin], tobramycin [Nebcin]), selected antibiotics (e.g., vancomycin), antineoplastics (e.g., cisplatin, nitrogen mustard), anesthetics (e.g., methoxyflurane [Penthrane]), antituberculars (e.g., capreomycin [Capestat]), cyclosporine (Sandimmune), diuretics (e.g., furosemide [Lasix], torsemide [Demadex]), pentamidine. Nephrotoxic effects are additive. Frequent monitoring of renal function indicated if any other nephrotoxic drug must be used. ▪ Nephrotoxicity and myelotoxicity are both increased when given concurrently with zidovudine (AZT). ▪ Potentiates nephrotoxicity of cyclosporine; alternate immunosuppressive therapy recommended. ▪ Concurrent use with antineoplastic agents (e.g., methotrexate) or radiation therapy may increase renal toxicity and incidence of bronchospasm and hypotension. ▪ Enhances antifungal effects of flucytosine (Ancobon) and other antiinfectives. May increase toxicity. ▪ Antagonism between amphotericin B and imidazole antifungals (e.g., ketoconazole, miconazole, fluconazole) has been reported. ▪ Acute pulmonary toxicity occurred in patients receiving leukocyte transfusion; separate administration times as much as possible.

SIDE EFFECTS

LIPID-BASED PREPARATIONS: Most side effects similar to Fungizone but occur with less frequency and intensity. Acute reactions, including fever and chills, may occur within 1 to 2 hours of starting the infusion. Infusion-related cardiorespiratory reactions may include dyspnea, hypertension, hyperventilation, hypotension, hypoxia, tachycardia, and vasodilation. More common with initial doses and subside with subsequent doses. Arrhythmia, bronchospasm, and shock can occur. Anaphylaxis and cardiac arrest from overdose have been reported.

FUNGIZONE/GENERIC: Common even at doses below therapeutic; may begin to occur within 15 to 20 minutes: anorexia, chills, convulsions, diarrhea, fever, headache, phlebitis, vomiting. Anaphylactoid reactions, anemia, cardiac disturbances (including fibrillation and arrest), coagulation defects, hypertension, hypokalemia, hypotension, and numerous other side effects occur fairly frequently. Renal function impaired in 80% of patients. May reverse after treatment ends, but some permanent damage likely. Pseudomembranous colitis has been reported.

ANTIDOTE

ALL AMPHOTERICIN FORMULATIONS: Notify the physician of all side effects. Many are reversible if the drug is discontinued. Some will respond to symptomatic treatment. Acute reactions (e.g., fever, chills, hypotension, nausea, and vomiting) usually lessen with subsequent doses. These acute infusion-related reactions can be managed by pretreatment with antipyretics, antihistamines, and/or corticosteroids or reduction of the rate of infusion and prompt treatment with antihistamines and/or corticosteroids and meperidine (Demerol) for chills. If anaphylaxis or serious respiratory distress occurs, discontinue amphotericin and treat as necessary. Give no further infusions. Hemodialysis not effective in overdose. Discontinue if BUN and alkaline phosphatase are abnormal. Dantrolene has been used to prevent (50 mg PO) or treat (50 mg IV) severe, shaking chills.

FUNGIZONE/GENERIC: Administration of Fungizone/generic on alternate days may decrease the incidence of some side effects. Urinary alkalinizers may minimize renal tubular acidosis.

ABELCET, AMPHOTEC: Overdose has caused cardiac arrest. Discontinue drug and treat symptomatically.

AMPICILLIN SODIUM

(am′pi-sill-in so′de-um)

Antibacterial (penicillin)

✦Ampicin, Omnipen-N, Polycillin N, Totacillin-N

pH 8 to 10

USUAL DOSE

Range is from 1 to 12 Gm/24 hr for adults and children weighing 20 kg or more. Larger doses may be indicated based on the seriousness of the infection. Some clinicians suggest a weight of 40 kg to receive adult dose range.

Respiratory tract or skin and skin structure infections: 250 to 500 mg every 6 hours.

GI or GU infections: 500 mg every 6 hours.

Septicemia or bacterial meningitis: 8 to 14 Gm or 150 to 200 mg/kg/24 hr in equally divided doses every 3 to 4 hours (18.75 to 25 mg/kg every 3 hours or 25 to 33.3 mg/kg every 4 hours). Administer IV a minimum of 3 days; then may be given IV or IM.

Treatment of gonorrhea: 500 mg. Repeat in 8 to 12 hours. May repeat 2-dose regimen IV or IM if indicated. Ceftriaxone (Rocephin) IV or IM is most commonly used.

Listeriosis: 50 mg/kg every 6 hours.

Prevention of bacterial endocarditis in dental or respiratory tract surgery or instrumentation: 2 Gm of ampicillin 30 minutes before procedure.

Prevention of bacterial endocarditis in GI, GU, or biliary tract surgery or instrumentation: ***Low to moderate risk:*** A single dose of 2 Gm of ampicillin 30 minutes before procedure. ***Moderate to high risk:*** 2 Gm of ampicillin in conjunction with gentamicin 1.5 mg/kg (up to 80 mg) 30 minutes before procedure. Repeat 1 Gm of ampicillin or give oral amoxicillin 1 Gm in 6 hours.

Prophylaxis in high-risk cesarean section patients: 1 to 2 Gm immediately after clamping cord.

Prophylaxis of neonatal group B *Streptococcal* disease: 2 Gm to the mother during labor. Should be given at least 4 hours before delivery to ensure amniotic fluid concentrations and placental transfer of ampicillin. May repeat 1 to 2 Gm every 4 to 6 hours until delivery. Continue treatment postpartum if active signs of maternal infection develop. Routine use of prophylaxis in neonates born to these mothers is not recommended; risk must be assessed on an individual basis for each infant.

Leptospirosis (unlabeled): 500 mg to 1 Gm every 6 hours.

Typhoid fever (unlabeled): 25 mg/kg every 6 hours.

PEDIATRIC DOSE

Range is from 25 to 400 mg/kg of body weight/24 hours for pediatric patients weighing less than 20 kg. Some clinicians suggest a weight up to 40 kg is appropriate for pediatric use. Do not exceed adult dose or 12 Gm.

Respiratory tract or skin and skin structure infections: 25 to 50 mg/kg/24 hr in equally divided doses every 4 to 6 hours (4.16 to 8.3 mg/kg every 4 hours or 6.25 to 12.5 mg/kg every 6 hours).

GI or GU infections: 50 to 100 mg/kg/24 hr in equally divided doses every 6 hours (12.5 to 25 mg/kg every 6 hours).

Septicemia or bacterial meningitis: 100 to 200 mg/kg/24 hr in equally divided doses every 3 to 4 hours (12.5 to 25 mg/kg every 3 hours or 16.6 to 33.3 mg/kg every 4 hours).

Empiric treatment of bacterial meningitis in infants and children 2 months to 12 years of age: Some clinicians recommend 200 to 400 mg/kg/24 hr in equally divided doses every 4 to 6 hours (33.3 to 66.6 mg/kg every 4 hours to 50 to 100 mg/kg every 6 hours). Given in conjunction with chloramphenicol. Satisfactory response should occur within 48 hours or initiate alternate therapy. Administer any regimen IV a minimum of 3 days, then may be given IV or IM.

Prevention of bacterial endocarditis in dental or respiratory tract surgery or instrumentation: 50 mg/kg of ampicillin 30 minutes before procedure.

Prevention of bacterial endocarditis in GI, GU, or biliary tract surgery or instrumentation: ***Low to moderate risk:*** A single dose of 50 mg/kg 30 minutes before procedure. ***Moderate to high risk:*** 50 mg/kg of ampicillin in conjunction with gentamicin 1.5 mg/kg (up to 80 mg) 30 minutes before procedure. Repeat 25 mg/kg of ampicillin or oral amoxicillin in 6 hours.

NEONATAL DOSE

Age up to 7 days: ***weight less than 2,000 Gm:*** 25 mg/kg every 12 hours. ***2,000 Gm or more:*** 25 mg/kg every 8 hours.

Over 7 days of age: ***weight less than 1,200 Gm:*** 25 mg every 12 hours. ***1,200 to 2,000 Gm:*** 25 mg/kg every 8 hours. ***More than 2,000 Gm:*** 25 mg/kg every 6 hours.

Empiric treatment of bacterial meningitis in neonates and infants less than 2 months of age: 100 to 300 mg/kg/24 hr in equally divided doses (e.g., 33.3 to 100 mg/kg every 8 hours) in conjunction with IM gentamicin. Administer any regimen IV a minimum of 3 days, then may be given IV or IM.

Bacterial meningitis in neonates and infants less than 2 months of age:

Age up to 7 days: ***weight less than 2,000 Gm:*** 50 to 75 mg/kg every 12 hours. ***2,000 Gm or more:*** 50 to 75 mg/kg every 8 hours.

Over 7 days of age: ***weight less than 2,000 Gm:*** 50 mg/kg every 8 hours. ***2,000 Gm or more:*** 50 mg/kg every 6 hours.

DOSE ADJUSTMENTS

Reduce dose by increasing interval to 12 to 16 hours in severe renal impairment (CrCl less than 10 ml/min). Hemodialysis patients should receive a dose after each dialysis.

DILUTION

Each 500 mg or fraction thereof must be reconstituted with at least 5 ml of SW for injection. Use within 1 hour of reconstitution. May be further diluted in 50 ml or more of selected IV solutions. Stable for 8 hours at concentrations up to 30 mg/ml in NS, LR, sodium lactate, or SW. Stable in D5/½NS or 10% invert sugar in water for 4 hours at concentrations up to 2 mg/ml. Stable in D5W for 4 hours at concentrations up to 2 mg/ml but only for 2 hours at concentrations up to 20 mg/ml. Must be administered before stability expires.

INCOMPATIBLE WITH

Inactivated in solution with aminoglycosides (e.g., amikacin [Amikin], gentamicin [Garamycin]). Do not mix in the same solution. Appropriate spacing and/or separate sites required. See Drug/Lab Interactions.

COMPATIBLE WITH (Underline Indicates Conflicting Compatibility Information)

Consult pharmacist; specific conditions may apply; see Compatibilities, p. xvi.

Additive: ***See Incompatible With.*** Aztreonam (Azactam), cefepime (Maxipime), clindamycin (Cleocin), erythromycin lactobionate (Erythrocin), furosemide (Lasix), heparin, hydrocortisone sodium succinate (Solu-Cortef), metronidazole (Flagyl IV), ranitidine (Zantac), verapamil (Isoptin).

Syringe: Chloramphenicol (Chloromycetin), colistimethate (Coly-Mycin M), heparin, lidocaine, selected dyes used in radiology, streptomycin.

Y-site: Acyclovir (Zovirax), amifostine (Ethyol), aztreonam (Azactam), calcium gluconate, cisatracurium (Nimbex), cyclophosphamide (Cytoxan), diltiazem (Cardizem), docetaxel (Taxotere), doxorubicin liposome (Doxil), enalaprilat (Vasotec IV), esmolol (Brevibloc), etoposide phosphate (Etopophos), famotidine (Pepcid IV), filgrastim (Neupogen), fludarabine (Fludara), foscarnet (Foscavir), gatifloxacin (Tequin), gemcitabine (Gemzar), granisetron (Kytril), heparin, hetastarch in electrolytes (Hextend), hetastarch in NS (Hespan), hydromorphone (Dilaudid), insulin (regular), labetalol (Normodyne), levofloxacin (Levaquin), linezolid (Zyvox), magnesium sulfate, melphalan (Alkeran), meperidine (Demerol), morphine, multivitamins (M.V.I.), ofloxacin (Floxin IV), perphenazine (Trilafon), phytonadione (Aquamephyton), potassium chloride (KCl), propofol (Diprivan), remifentanil (Ultiva), tacrolimus (Prograf), teniposide (Vumon), theophylline, thiotepa (Thioplex), vancomycin (Vancocin).

RATE OF ADMINISTRATION

A single dose over 10 to 15 minutes when given by IV injection. In 100 ml or more of solution, administer at prescribed infusion rate but never exceed IV injection rate. Too-rapid injection may cause seizures.

ACTIONS

A semisynthetic penicillin. Bactericidal against many gram-positive and some gram-negative organisms. Appears in all body fluids. Appears in cerebrospinal fluid only if inflammation is present. Crosses the placental barrier. Excreted in urine. Secreted in breast milk.

INDICATIONS AND USES

Highly effective against severe infections caused by gram-positive and some gram-negative organisms (e.g., respiratory tract, skin and skin structure, GI and GU, bacterial meningitis, endocarditis, listeriosis, septicemia). Not effective with penicillinase-producing staphylococci. ■ Prevention of bacterial endocarditis in dental and respiratory tract surgery or instrumentation. ■ Prevention of bacterial endocarditis in GI, GU, or biliary surgery or instrumentation. Used concurrently with gentamicin. ■ Drug of choice during labor for prevention of neonatal group B streptococcal infections.

Unlabeled use: Prophylaxis in high-risk cesarean section patients. Treatment of leptospirosis. Treatment of typhoid fever.

CONTRAINDICATIONS

Known penicillin or cephalosporin sensitivity (not absolute). Infectious mononucleosis because of increased incidence of rash.

PRECAUTIONS

Sensitivity studies indicated to determine susceptibility of the causative organism to ampicillin. ■ Avoid prolonged use of this drug; superinfection caused by overgrowth of nonsusceptible organisms may result. ■ Pseudomembranous colitis has been reported. May range from mild to life-threatening. Consider in patients that present with diarrhea during or after treatment with ampicillin. ■ Side effects increased in some patients; see Side Effects.

Monitor: Watch for early symptoms of allergic reaction, especially in individuals with a history of allergic problems. ■ AST (SGOT) may be increased. Renal, hepatic, and hematopoietic function should be checked during prolonged therapy. ■ Test all patients with syphilis for HIV. ■ Electrolyte imbalance and cardiac irregularities from sodium content are possible. Contains 2.9 mEq sodium/Gm. May aggravate CHF. Observe for hypokalemia. ■ May cause thrombophlebitis; observe carefully and rotate infusion sites.

Patient Education: May require alternate birth control.

Maternal/Child: Category B: use only if clearly needed. ■ May cause diarrhea, candidiasis, or allergic response in nursing infants. ■ Elimination rate markedly reduced in neonates.

Elderly: Consider degree of age-related impaired renal function.

DRUG/LAB INTERACTIONS

Streptomycin potentiates bactericidal activity against enterococci. ■ May be used concurrently with aminoglycosides (e.g., gentamicin [Garamycin]) but these drugs must never be mixed in the same infusion (mutual inactivation). If given concurrently, administer at separate sites. ■ May be antagonized by bacteriostatic antibiotics (e.g., chloramphenicol, erythromycin, and tetracyclines); may interfere with bactericidal action. ■ Concomitant use with beta-adrenergic blockers (e.g., propranolol [Inderal]) may increase risk of anaphylaxis and inhibit treatment. ■ Potentiated by probenecid (Benemid); toxicity may result. ■ Increased risk of bleeding with heparin. ■ May decrease clearance and increase toxicity of methotrexate. ■ Decreases effectiveness of oral contraceptives; breakthrough bleeding or pregnancy could result. ■ Ampicillin-induced skin rash potentiated by allopurinol (Zyloprim). ■ False-positive glucose reaction with Clinitest and Benedict's or Fehling's solution. ■ May cause false values in other lab tests; see literature.

SIDE EFFECTS

Primarily hypersensitivity reactions such as anaphylaxis, exfoliative dermatitis, rashes, and urticaria. May cause pseudomembranous colitis. Hypersensitivity myocarditis can occur (fever, eosinophilia, rash, sinus tachycardia, ST-T changes, and cardiomegaly). Anemia, leukopenia, and thrombocytopenia have been reported. Thrombophlebitis will occur with long-term use. Higher than normal doses may cause neurologic adverse reactions including convulsions, especially with impaired renal function. Incidence of side effects increased in patients with viral infections or those taking allopurinol (Zyloprim).

ANTIDOTE

Notify the physician of any side effect. For severe symptoms, discontinue the drug, treat allergic reaction (antihistamines, epinephrine, corticosteroids), and resuscitate as necessary. Hemodialysis is effective in overdose.

AMPICILLIN SODIUM AND SULBACTAM SODIUM

(am′pi-sill-in so′de-um and sul-back′tam so′de-um)

Antibacterial (penicillin and beta-lactamase inhibitor)

Unasyn

8 to 10

USUAL DOSE

Adults and children weighing 40 kg or more: 1.5 to 3 Gm every 6 hours (1 Gm ampicillin with 0.5 Gm sulbactam to 2 Gm ampicillin with 1 Gm sulbactam). All commercial preparations in the U.S. have a 2:1 ratio of ampicillin to sulbactam (e.g., 1.5 Gm = 1 Gm ampicillin plus 0.5 Gm sulbactam). Do not exceed 4 Gm ***sulbactam***/24 hr. ***All doses in this monograph include ampicillin and sulbactam within the recommended dose.***

PEDIATRIC DOSE

IV use for more than 14 days is not recommended. See comments under Adult Dose.

Skin and skin structure infections in pediatric patients over 1 year of age and less than 40 kg: 300 mg/kg/day (200 mg/kg ampicillin and 100 mg/kg sulbactam) in equally divided doses as an infusion every 6 hours (75 mg/kg every 6 hours).

The American Academy of Pediatrics suggests use in pediatric patients over 1 month of age in the following doses.

Mild to moderate infections: 150 to 225 mg/kg/day (100 to 150 mg/kg of ampicillin and 50 to 75 mg/kg sulbactam) in equally divided doses as an infusion every 6 hours (37.5 to 56.5 mg/kg every 6 hours).

Severe infections: 300 to 450 mg/kg/day (200 to 300 mg/kg of ampicillin and 100 to 150 mg/kg of sulbactam) in equally divided doses as an infusion every 6 hours (75 mg/kg to 112.5 mg/kg every 6 hours).

DOSE ADJUSTMENTS

May be indicated in the elderly. ■ Reduce total daily dose in impaired renal function according to the following chart.

Ampicillin/Sulbactam Dose Guidelines in Impaired Renal Function

Creatinine Clearance (ml/min per 1.73 M^2)	Dose/Frequency
30 or more	Usual recommended dose q 6 to 8 hr
15 to 29	Usual recommended dose q 12 hr
5 to 14	Usual recommended dose q 24 hr
Hemodialysis patients	Usual recommended dose q 24 hr On day of dialysis, give immediately after dialysis

DILUTION

Each 1.5 Gm or fraction thereof must be initially reconstituted with at least 3.2 ml of SW for injection (375 mg/ml). Allow to stand to dissipate foaming. Solution should be clear. Must be further diluted to a final concentration of 3 to 45 mg/ml in one of the following solutions and given by slow IV injection or as an intermittent IV infusion: D5W, D5/½NS, 10% invert sugar in water, LR, ⅙ M sodium lactate solution, or NS. 3 Gm/L equals 3 mg/ml, 3 Gm/125 ml equals 24 mg/ml. Also available in piggyback vials and ADD-Vantage vials for use with ADD-Vantage infusion containers.

Storage: Store at CRT before dilution. Stable in all specifically listed solutions in any dilution for at least 2 hours. Stability in each solution varies (see literature).

INCOMPATIBLE WITH

May be inactivated in solution with aminoglycosides (e.g., amikacin [Amikin], gentamicin [Garamycin]). Do not mix in the same solution. Appropriate spacing and/or separate sites required. See Drug/Lab Interactions.

COMPATIBLE WITH **(Underline Indicates Conflicting Compatibility Information)**

Consult pharmacist; specific conditions may apply; see Compatibilities, p. xvi.

Additive: ***See Incompatible With.*** Aztreonam (Azactam).

Y-site: Amifostine (Ethyol), aztreonam (Azactam), cefepime (Maxipime), cisatracurium (Nimbex), diltiazem (Cardizem), docetaxel (Taxotere), enalaprilat (Vasotec IV), etoposide phosphate (Etopophos), famotidine (Pepcid IV), filgrastim (Neupogen), fluconazole (Diflucan), fludarabine (Fludara), gatifloxacin (Tequin), gemcitabine (Gemzar), granisetron (Kytril), heparin, hetastarch in electrolytes (Hextend), insulin (regular), linezolid (Zyvox), meperidine (Demerol), morphine, paclitaxel (Taxol), remifentanil (Ultiva), tacrolimus (Prograf), teniposide (Vumon), theophylline, thiotepa (Thioplex), vancomycin (Vancocin).

RATE OF ADMINISTRATION

IV injection: A single dose over a minimum of 15 minutes.

Intermittent IV: A single dose over 15 to 30 minutes or longer, depending on amount of solution. Too-rapid injection may cause seizures.

ACTIONS

A semisynthetic penicillin. The addition of sulbactam improves ampicillin's bactericidal activity against beta-lactamase–producing strains resistant to penicillins and cephalosporins. A broad-spectrum antibiotic and beta-lactamase inhibitor effective against selected gram-positive, gram-negative, and anaerobic organisms (see literature). Peak serum levels achieved by end of infusion. Appears in all body fluids. Crosses the placental barrier. Excreted in the urine. Secreted in breast milk.

INDICATIONS AND USES

Treatment of skin and skin structure and intraabdominal, gynecologic, and urinary tract infections due to susceptible strains of specific organisms.

CONTRAINDICATIONS

Known penicillin, cephalosporin, or beta-lactamase inhibitor sensitivity (not absolute); infectious mononucleosis because of increased incidence of rash.

PRECAUTIONS

Studies indicated to determine the causative organism and susceptibility to ampicillin/sulbactam. ■ Avoid prolonged use of this drug; superinfection caused by overgrowth of nonsusceptible organisms may result. ■ Elimination of sulbactam increased in cystic fibrosis patients. ■ Use caution in patients with CHF, a history of bleeding disorders, or GI disease (e.g., colitis). ■ Pseudomembranous colitis has been reported. May range from mild to life-threatening. Consider in patients that present with diarrhea during or after treatment with ampicillin and sulbactam.

Monitor: Watch for early symptoms of allergic reaction, especially in individuals with a history of allergic problems. ■ AST (SGOT) may be increased. Renal, hepatic, and hematopoietic function should be checked during prolonged therapy. ■ Test all patients with syphilis for HIV. ■ May cause thrombophlebitis. Observe carefully and rotate infusion sites. ■ Electrolyte imbalance and cardiac irregularities from sodium content are possible. Contains 5 mEq sodium/1.5 Gm. May aggravate CHF. Observe for hypokalemia.

Patient Education: Report promptly; fever, rash, sore throat, unusual bleeding or bruising, severe stomach cramps, and/or diarrhea, seizures. ■ May require alternate birth control.

Maternal/Child: Category B: studies in rabbits have not shown adverse effects on fertility or in the fetus. Use only if clearly needed. ■ May cause diarrhea, candidiasis, or allergic response in nursing infants. ■ Safety for use in infants and children over 1 year of age has been established for skin and skin structure infections but not for other uses; however, it is in use. Elimination rate markedly reduced in neonates.

Elderly: Consider degree of age-related impaired renal function. ■ See Dose Adjustments.

DRUG/LAB INTERACTIONS

Streptomycin potentiates bactericidal activity against enterococci. ■ Frequently use concomitantly with aminoglycosides (e.g., gentamicin [Garamycin]) but these drugs must never be mixed in the same infusion (mutual inactivation). If given concurrently, administer at separate sites. ■ May be antagonized by bacteriostatic antibiotics (e.g., chloramphenicol, erythromycin, tetracyclines); may interfere with bactericidal action. ■ Concomitant use with beta-adrenergic blockers (e.g., propranolol [Inderal]) may increase risk of anaphylaxis and inhibit treatment. ■ Potentiated by probenecid (Benemid); higher blood levels may be a positive interaction. ■ Increased risk of bleeding with heparin. ■ May decrease clearance and increase toxicity of methotrexate. ■ Decreases effectiveness of oral contraceptives; breakthrough bleeding or pregnancy could result. ■ Ampicillin-induced skin rash potentiated by allopurinol (Zyloprim). ■ False-positive glucose reaction with Clinitest and Benedict's or Fehling's solution. ■ May cause false values in other lab tests; see literature.

SIDE EFFECTS

Full scope of allergic reactions, including anaphylaxis, are possible. Burning, discomfort, and pain at injection site; diarrhea, rash, and thrombophlebitis occur most frequently. Abdominal distention; candidiasis; chest pain; chills; decreased hemoglobin, hematocrit, RBC, WBC, lymphocytes, neutrophils, and platelets; decreased serum albumin and total protein; dysuria; edema; epistaxis; erythema; facial swelling; fatigue; flatulence; glossitis; headache; hypersensitivity myocarditis (fever, eosinophilia, rash, sinus tachycardia, ST-T changes and cardiomegaly); increased alkaline phosphatase, BUN, creatinine, LDH, AST (SGOT), ALT (SGPT); increased basophils, eosinophils, lymphocytes, monocytes, and platelets; itching, malaise, mucosal bleeding, nausea and vomiting, RBCs and hyaline casts in urine, substernal pain, tightness in throat, and urine retention can occur. May cause pseudomembranous colitis. Higher than normal doses may cause neurologic adverse reactions, including convulsions; especially with impaired renal function.

ANTIDOTE

Notify the physician of any side effect. For severe symptoms, discontinue the drug, treat allergic reaction (antihistamines, epinephrine, corticosteroids), and resuscitate as necessary. Hemodialysis may be effective in overdose.

ANTIHEMOPHILIC FACTOR (HUMAN OR RECOMBINANT)

Antihemorrhagic

(an-tee-hee-moe-fill′ik fak′tor)

AHF, Alphanate, Bioclate, Factor VIII, Helixate, Helixate FS, Hemofil M, Hyate: C Porcine AHF, Koate DVI, Kogenate, Kogenate FS, Monarc-M, Monoclate-P, Recombinate, ReFacto

Available factor VIII products and their origins include the following:

Bioclate, Helixate, Kogenate, Recombinate: Recombinant, stabilized in human albumin.

Helixate FS, Kogenate FS, ReFacto: Recombinant, stabilized without human albumin, formulated with sucrose (amount of sucrose should not affect blood glucose concentrations).

Hemofil M, Monarc-M, Monoclate P: From human plasma, immunoaffinity purified (ultrahigh purity).

Alphanate, Humate P (see AHF & von Willebrand Factor Complex), Koate-DVI: From human plasma, intermediate and high purity.

Hyate C: Porcine AHF: Reserved for patients with inhibitors to human factor VIII.

USUAL DOSE

Adults and children: Completely individualized. Based on degree of deficiency, desired antihemophilic factor level, body weight, severity of bleeding, and presence of factor VIII inhibitors. Identify factor VIII deficiency and level assays before administration. One international unit (IU) is approximately equal to the level of factor VIII activity in 1 ml of fresh pooled human plasma. Recombinant products may be substituted for plasma-derived products without disrupting treatment regimen. A plasma antihemophilic factor level of about 30% of normal is needed for effective hemostasis when hemorrhage is present; greater percentages are required for surgical procedures, and only 5% to 10% of normal may be needed to control hemarthrosis. Each preparation suggests a different formula; end results are similar. An example is:

$$\text{AHF/IU required} = \text{body weight (kg)} \times \text{desired factor VIII increase (\% of normal)} \times 0.5$$

$$\text{Expected factor VIII increase (\% of normal)} = \text{AHF/IU/kg dose administered} \times 2$$

Examples of doses are as follows:

Prophylactic management: (e.g., severe factor VIII deficiency with frequent hemorrhages). Raise factor VIII level to 15% of normal. Repeat every 1 to 2 days. Usually requires 250 units daily in patients weighing less than 50 kg, 500 units daily in patients weighing more than 50 kg. Increase dose until bleeding episodes are adequately controlled.

Early hemarthrosis (blood into a joint or its synovial cavity), muscle bleed, or oral bleed: Raise factor VIII level to 20% to 40%. Usually requires 5 to 10 units/kg initially. Repeat infusion every 12 to 24 hours for 1 to 3 days until the bleeding episode as indicated by pain is resolved or healing is achieved. If early hemarthrosis is treated promptly, lowest doses may be adequate.

More extensive hemarthrosis, muscle bleed, or hematoma: Raise factor VIII level to 30% to 60%. Usually requires 10 to 25 units/kg initially. Adjust dose based on circulating AHF levels and repeat infusion every 8 to 24 hours for 3 days or more until pain and disability are resolved.

Life-threatening bleeds (e.g., head injury, throat bleed, severe abdominal pain): Raise factor VIII level to 60% to 100%. Usually requires 40 to 50 units/kg initially. Adjust dose based on circulating AHF levels and repeat infusion every 8 to 24 hours until threat is resolved.

Minor surgery, including tooth extraction: Raise factor VIII level to 60% to 80%. Usually requires 25 to 40 units/kg. A single infusion plus oral antifibrinolytic therapy within 1 hour is sufficient in 70% of patients.

Major surgery: Raise factor VIII level to 80% to 100%. Usually requires 45 to 50 units/kg initially. Repeat infusion every 8 to 24 hours depending on state of healing. Reduce dose as indicated by state of healing. Increase dose if level falls below 30%.

Maintenance doses vary slightly with specific products; see literature.

Hyate: C Porcine AHF: ***Treatment of hemorrhagic episodes:*** In patients with plasma antibody levels less than 50 Bethesda units/ml, the manufacturer suggests an initial dose of 100 to 150 porcine units/kg. Other sources suggest an initial dose of 50 to 150 porcine units/kg. If a patient has plasma antibody levels greater than 50 Bethesda units/ml, further specific testing must be completed to determine if they will benefit from treatment; see literature. ***Prophylaxis of hemorrhagic episodes:*** 20 to 60 porcine units/kg every other day has been used for long-term prophylaxis in the home. Supplement with 40 to 50 porcine units/kg if hemarthrosis develops.

DOSE ADJUSTMENTS

If AHF does not significantly improve the PTT, factor VIII antibodies are probable; may respond to an increased dose, especially if titer is less than 10 Bethesda units/ml. Frequent determinations of circulating AHF levels indicated.

DILUTION

Consult individual product instructions in the package insert; each product has a specific process for dilution. Information may be updated frequently. All preparations provide diluent and usually provide administration equipment, including needles (single- or double-ended), filters or filter needles, syringes, and/or administration sets for each vial. Actual number of AHF units shown on each vial. Use only the diluent provided, and maintain strict aseptic technique. Use a plastic syringe to prevent binding to glass surfaces. Warm to room temperature (25° C) before dilution and maintain throughout administration to avoid precipitation of active ingredients.

Storage: Before reconstitution, store all formulations except Hyate: C Porcine at 2° to 8° C (35° to 46° F). Do not freeze. Most formulations can be stored at CRT not to exceed 25° C (77° F) for 2 months or more before reconstitution; check individual product. Before reconstitution, store ***Hyate: C Porcine AHF*** at –15° to –20° C (5° to –4° F). Maintain at CRT after dilution. Do not use beyond expiration dates on bottles.

COMPATIBILITY

Administration through a separate line without mixing with other IV fluids or medications is recommended. If antihemophilic factor is given as a continuous IV, one source says heparin 1 to 5 units/ml of concentrate may be added to avoid thrombophlebitis.

RATE OF ADMINISTRATION

Reduce rate of infusion or temporarily discontinue if there is a significant increase in pulse rate or S/S of hypersensitivity occur. Rate is based on patient comfort.

Most preparations suggest beginning with a rate of 2 ml/min and increasing gradually up to 10 mg/min if appropriate. Administration of a single dose in 5 to 10 minutes is generally well tolerated. Consult product information. Other sources list the following information:

Monoclate-P: Begin with a rate of 2 ml/min. Do not exceed 4 ml/min.

Alphanate, Bioclate, Hemofil M, Monarc-M, and Recombinate: May be given at a rate not to exceed 10 ml/min.

Helixate, Helixate FS, Kogenate, Kogenate FS, ReFacto: A single dose over 5 to 10 minutes is usually well tolerated.

ACTIONS

AHF is one of nine major factors in the blood that must act in sequence to produce coagulation, or clotting. It is the specific clotting factor deficient in patients with hemophilia A (classic hemophilia) and can temporarily correct the coagulation defect in these patients. Has a half-life of 10 to 18 hours. One IU of AHF increases the plasma concentration of factor VIII by 2%. **Plasma-based AHF:** A lyophilized concentrate of coagulation factor VIII (antihemophilic factor) prepared by various processes (e.g., heat treatment, chemical inactivation, solvent detergent treatment, immunoaffinity chromatography). Obtained from fresh (less than 3 hours old) human plasma cryoprecipitate. Tested and determined free from hepatitis and HIV viruses and containing acceptable ALT (SGPT) concentrations. **Recombinant AHF:** Produced through genetic engineering technology. Purified using monoclonal antibody purification techniques, ion exchange chromatography, and immunoaffinity chromatography. Risk of viral transmission eliminated because it is not derived from human blood. ReFacto is formulated without human serum albumin in the final product. **Porcine AHF:** No evidence of viral transmission; pigs do not harbor hepatitis or HIV.

INDICATIONS AND USES

Control or prevent bleeding episodes and for surgical prophylaxis in patients with hemophilia A. (Congenital factor VIII deficiency of classic hemophilia.) ReFacto is recommended for short-term routine prophylaxis. Alphanate may be useful in patients with an acquired deficiency (not congenital). Porcine products may be used in patients with plasma antibody levels against human antihemophilic factor with inhibitor titers from 10 to 50 Bethesda units. Must be tested for cross-reactivity before administration.

Unlabeled uses: Adjunct in the treatment of disseminated intravascular coagulation (DIC).

CONTRAINDICATIONS

Hypersensitivity to mouse, hamster, or bovine protein (monoclonal-antibody-derived factor VIII). Not effective for bleeding in patients with von Willebrand's disease.

PRECAUTIONS

Should be administered under the direction of the physician specialist. ■ Treatment of choice when volume or RBC replacement is not needed; avoids hypervolemia and hyperproteinemia. ■ Desmopressin is preferred treatment in mild to moderate hemophilia A. ■ Hepatitis B vaccination indicated in all patients with hemophilia; usually done at birth or time of diagnosis. ■ Risk of transmitting hepatitis or HIV is markedly reduced with newer plasma-based products. There are no reported instances of new seroconversions to HIV with currently marketed products. ■ No risk of any viral transmission (hepatitis or HIV) with recombinant products. ■ Intravascular hemolysis can occur when large volumes are given to individuals with blood groups A, B, or AB. Monitor for progressive anemia. ■ Type-specific cryoprecipitate has been used to maintain adequate factor VIII levels and is appropriate in selected cases; carries risk of possible delayed seroconversion after viral infection (HIV, hepatitis A, B, or C). ■ Inhibitor titers above 10 Bethesda units/ml may make hemostatic control with AHF impossible or impractical because of the large dose required. Inhibitor titer may rise after AHF infusion due to an anamnestic (immunologic memory) response to the AHF antigen. Use of an alternate product may be indicated (e.g., factor IX complex concentrates, antihemophilic factor [Porcine], or anti-inhibitor coagulant complex).

Monitor: Identification of factor VIII deficiency with determination of circulating AHF levels should be obtained before administration and during treatment. Adjust dose as indicated. ■ Monitor pulse before and during treatment. ■ Monitor for the development of factor VIII inhibitors. Should be suspected if factor VIII plasma levels are not obtained or if bleeding is not controlled with an appropriate dose. ■ See Precautions.

Patient Education: Prophylactic hepatitis B vaccine recommended. ■ Instruction for self-administration and proper preparation may be appropriate. ■ Report skin rash or any other hypersensitivity reaction promptly. ■ HIV screening every 2 to 3 months; not required with recombinant products.

Maternal/Child: Category C: use only if clearly needed. ■ Safe for use in children of all ages, including newborns.

SIDE EFFECTS

Usually respond to reduced rate of administration. Massive doses may cause acute hemolytic anemia, hyperfibrinogenemia, increased bleeding tendency, or jaundice (rare).

Plasma-based AHF: Allergic reactions (anaphylaxis, backache, chills, erythema, fever, hives, hypotension, nausea, stinging at infusion site, tightness of chest, urticaria, wheezing); clouding or loss of consciousness, flushing, headache, lethargy, paresthesias, somnolence, tachycardia, or vomiting may occur. Consider risk potential of contracting AIDS or hepatitis; risk of withholding treatment outweighs any risk associated with use.

Recombinant products: Burning, erythema, and pruritus at injection site; chest discomfort, chills, cold feet, diarrhea, dizziness, fever, flushing, headache, hypotension (slight), lethargy, nausea, rash, sore throat, or an unusual taste in the mouth occur occasionally.

ANTIDOTE

Most side effects usually subside spontaneously in 15 to 20 minutes and are generally related to the rate of infusion. Keep the physician informed. Slow or discontinue infusion temporarily if pulse rate increases or beginning S/S of hypersensitivity reactions occur. Discontinue immediately and treat allergic reactions (antihistamines, epinephrine, corticosteroids). Resuscitate as necessary.

ANTIHEMOPHILIC FACTOR ■ VON WILLEBRAND FACTOR COMPLEX (HUMAN), DRIED, PASTEURIZED

Antihemorrhagic

(an-tee-hee-moe-fill′ik fak′tor)

Humate-P

USUAL DOSE

Completely individualized. Based on degree of deficiency, desired antihemophilic factor level, body weight, severity of bleeding, and presence of Factor VIII inhibitors. One International unit (IU) of Factor VIII or 1 IU of von Willebrand factor:Ristocetin Cofactor (vWF:RCof) is approximately equal to the level of factor VIII activity or vWF:RCof found in 1 ml of fresh pooled human plasma.

Treatment of hemophilia A (adults): As a general rule, 1 IU of Factor VIII activity per kg body weight will increase the circulating Factor VIII level by approximately 2 IU/dl. Assess adequacy of treatment by clinical effects and monitoring of Factor VIII activity. See Precautions. The following general dosages are recommended for adult patients:

Dosage Recommendations for the Treatment of Hemophilia A*

Hemorrhage Event	Dosage (IU FVIII:C/kg body weight)
Minor • Early joint or muscle bleed • Severe epistaxis	Loading dose 15 IU FVIII:C/kg to achieve FVIII:C plasma level of approximately 30% of normal; one infusion may be sufficient If needed, half of the loading dose may be given once or twice daily for 1-2 days
Moderate • Advanced joint or muscle bleed • Neck, tongue or pharyngeal hematoma without airway compromise • Tooth extraction • Severe abdominal pain	Loading dose 25 IU FVIII:C/kg to achieve FVIII:C plasma level of approximately 50% of normal Followed by 15 IU FVIII:C/kg every 8-12 hours for first 1-2 days to maintain FVIII:C plasma level at 30% of normal Then same dose once or twice a day for up to 7 days or until adequate wound healing
Life-threatening • Major operations • Gastrointestinal bleeding • Neck, tongue or pharyngeal hematoma with potential for airway compromise • Intracranial, intraabdominal or intrathoracic bleeding • Fractures	Initially 40-50 IU FVIII:C/kg Followed by 20-25 IU FVIII:C/kg every 8 hours to maintain FVIII:C plasma level at 80-100% of normal for 7 days Then continue the same dose once or twice a day for another 7 days in order to maintain the FVIII:C level at 30-50% of normal

*In all cases, the dose should be adjusted individually by clinical judgment of the potential for compromise of a vital structure, and by frequent monitoring of factor VIII activity in the patient's plasma.

Treatment of von Willebrand Disease (vWD) (adults and children): As a rule, 40-80 IU vWF:RCof (corresponding to 16 to 32 IU Factor VIII in Humate-P) per kg body weight given every 8 to 12 hours. Repeat doses are administered as needed based on monitoring of appropriate clinical and laboratory measures. Expected levels of vWF:RCof are based on an expected in vivo recovery of 1.5 IU/dl rise per IU/kg vWF:RCof administered. The administration of 1 IU of Factor VIII per kg body weight can be expected to lead to a rise in circulating vWF:RCof of approximately 3.5 to 4 IU/dl. The following general dosages are recommended for adult and pediatric patients:

Dosage Recommendations for Treatment of von Willebrand Disease

Classification	Hemorrhage	Dosage (IU vWF:RCof/kg body weight)
TYPE 1		
Mild *(Where use of desmopressin is known or suspected to be inadequate)* Baseline vWF:RCof activity typically >30% of normal (i.e., >30 IU/dl)	**Major (examples)** • Severe or refractory epistaxis • GI bleeding • CNS trauma • Traumatic hemorrhage	Loading dose 40 to 60 IU/kg Then 40 to 50 IU/kg every 8 to 12 hours for 3 days to keep the nadir level of vWF:RCof >50% of normal (i.e., >50 IU/dl) Then 40 to 50 IU/kg daily for a total of up to 7 days of treatment
Moderate or Severe Baseline vWF:RCof activity typically <30% of normal (i.e., <30 IU/dl)	**Minor (examples)** • Epistaxis • Oral bleeding • Menorrhagia	40 to 50 IU/kg (1 or 2 doses)
	Major (examples) • Severe or refractory epistaxis • GI bleeding • CNS trauma • Hemarthrosis • Traumatic hemorrhage	Loading dose of 50 to 75 IU/kg Then 40 to 60 IU/kg every 8 to 12 hours for 3 days to keep the nadir level of vWF:RCof >50% of normal (i.e., >50 IU/dl) Then 40 to 60 IU/kg daily for a total of up to 7 days of treatment *Factor VIII:C levels should be monitored and maintained according to the guidelines for hemophilia A therapy**
TYPE 2 (ALL VARIANTS) AND TYPE 3		
	Minor (clinical indications above)	40 to 50 IU/kg (1 or 2 doses)
	Major (clinical indications above)	Loading dose of 60 to 80 IU/kg Then 40 to 60 IU/kg every 8 to 12 hours for 3 days to keep the nadir level of vWF:RCof >50% of normal (i.e., >50 IU/dl) Then 40 to 60 IU/kg daily for a total of up to 7 days of treatment *Factor VIII:C levels should be monitored and maintained according to the guidelines for hemophilia A therapy**

*In instances where both FVIII and vWF levels must be monitored.

Continued

PEDIATRIC DOSE

Treatment of hemophilia A: For immediate control of bleeding, follow the general recommendations for dosing and administration for adults. See Usual Dose and Maternal/Child.

DOSE ADJUSTMENTS

Adjust subsequent doses based on FVIII:C plasma level achieved.

DILUTION

Diluent, sterile transfer set for reconstitution and sterile filter spike for withdrawal of solution are provided. International unit activity of Factor VIII and vWF:RCof is stated on the label of each vial. Warm both diluent and Humate-P to room temperature. Using aseptic technique, pierce the double needle of the transfer set into the diluent vial. Uncap and insert the longer needle of the transfer set into the upright Humate-P vial. Diluent will transfer by vacuum. Remove diluent vial and transfer set and discard. Gently rotate vial until completely dissolved. Do not shake. Aseptically attach the filter spike to a plastic disposable syringe. Plastic syringes are used to prevent binding of protein solution to glass surfaces. Insert filter spike into Humate-P vial and inject air. Draw up solution slowly. If using several syringes, leave the filter spike in the vial. Separate the syringe from the spike and attach the syringe to an infusion kit or a suitable injection needle. Discard filter spike. Do not use filter spike for infusion.

Storage: Refrigerate before use. Avoid freezing. May be stored at CRT for up to 6 months. Administer within 3 hours of reconstitution to assure sterility. Discard any unused solution.

COMPATIBILITY

Specific information not available. Administration through a separate line without mixing with other IV fluids or medications is generally recommended for these products.

RATE OF ADMINISTRATION

Inject solution slowly at a maximum rate of 4 ml/min. Use infusion kit or suitable injection needle.

ACTIONS

A purified, sterile, lyophilized concentrate of antihemophilic factor (Factor VIII) and von Willebrand Factor (vWF). Factor VIII is an essential cofactor in the activation of Factor X, leading ultimately to the formation of thrombin and fibrin. It is the specific clotting factor deficient in patients with hemophilia A (classic hemophilia). vWF is important for correcting the coagulation defect in patients with von Willebrand Disease (vWD). It promotes platelet aggregation and platelet adhesion on damaged vascular endothelium and acts as a stabilizing carrier protein for the procoagulant protein Factor VIII. vWF activity is measured with an assay that uses an agglutinating cofactor called Ristocetin (RCof). The vWF:RCof assay provides a quantitative measurement of vWF function by determining how well vWF helps platelets adhere to one another. Reduced vWF:RCof activity indicates a deficiency of vWF. Following administration of Humate-P, there is a rapid increase of plasma Factor VIII activity, followed by a rapid decrease in activity and then a slower rate of decrease in activity. The mean initial half-life in hemophilic patients is 12.2 hours (range: 8.4 to 17.4 hours). In patients with vWD, bleeding time decreases and median half-life of vWF:RCof is 10.3 hours (range: 6.4 to 13.3 hours). Antihemophilic Factor/von Willibrand Factor Complex is obtained from pooled human fresh-frozen plasma. Pasteurized for 10 hours to inactivate infectious agents, including viruses.

INDICATIONS AND USES

Treatment and prevention of bleeding in adult patients with hemophilia A. ▪ Treatment of spontaneous and trauma-induced bleeding episodes in adult and pediatric patients with severe vWD or with mild or moderate vWD where use of desmopressin is known or suspected to be inadequate. ▪ Safety and efficacy of prophylactic dosing to prevent spontaneous bleeding and to prevent excessive bleeding related to surgery have not been established in patients with vWD. ▪ Only antihemophilic factor approved for use in patients with vWD.

CONTRAINDICATIONS

None known when used as indicated.

PRECAUTIONS

For IV use only. ▪ Important to establish that coagulation disorder is caused by Factor VIII or vWF deficiency. Not useful in treatment of other deficiencies. ▪ Manufactured from human plasma. Risk of transmitting infectious agents (e.g., HIV, hepatitis) has been greatly reduced by screening, testing and manufacturing techniques (e.g., pasteurization). However risk of transmission cannot be totally eliminated. ▪ Administration of hepatitis A and hepatitis B vaccines recommended for patients receiving plasma derivatives.

Monitor: Complex contains blood group isoagglutinins (anti-A and anti-B). When very large or frequently repeated doses are needed, as when inhibitors are present or when presurgical and postsurgical care is involved, patients of blood groups A, B and AB should be monitored for signs of intravascular hemolysis and decreasing hematocrit values. Treat as indicated. ▪ Replacement therapy should be monitored by appropriate coagulation tests, especially in cases involving major surgery. Monitor Factor VIII and vWF:RCof as indicated in dosing guidelines.

Patient Education: Prophylactic hepatitis A and hepatitis B vaccines recommended. ▪ Report symptoms of possibly transmitted viral infections immediately. Symptoms may include anorexia, arthralgias, fatigue, jaundice, low grade fever, nausea, or vomiting. ▪ Report rash or any other sign of hypersensitivity reaction promptly.

Maternal/Child: Category C: use only if clearly needed. ▪ Adequate and well-controlled studies with long term evaluation of joint damage have not been done in pediatric patients. Joint damage may result from suboptimal treatment of hemarthroses. ▪ Safety and effectiveness for use in neonates with vWD has not been established. Has been used safely in infants, children, and adolescents with vWD.

DRUG/LAB INTERACTIONS

Specific information not available.

SIDE EFFECTS

Usually well tolerated. Rare cases of allergic reactions, including anaphylaxis, have been reported (symptoms may include chest tightness, edema, fever, pruritus, rash, urticaria). Other reported side effects include chills, paresthesia, phlebitis, and vasodilation. Inhibitors of Factor VIII may occur.

ANTIDOTE

Keep physician informed of all side effects. Discontinue immediately at first sign of allergic reaction. Treat as necessary (antihistamines, epinephrine, corticosteroids). Resuscitate as necessary.

ANTI-INHIBITOR COAGULANT COMPLEX

Antihemorrhagic

(an′ti in-hib′i-tor ko-ag′u-lant kom-pleks)

Autoplex-T, Feiba VH

USUAL DOSE

A unit of **Feiba VH** is expressed as factor VIII inhibitor bypassing activity. **Autoplex-T** is expressed as factor VIII correctional units. They are not equal to each other, but the dose is the same regardless of the product used. Range is 25 to 100 units/kg. Average dose is 75 units. May be repeated in 6 to 12 hours. Do not exceed 200 units/kg/24 hr. Completely individualized; subsequent doses should be adjusted according to patient response. Identification of factor VIII inhibitor levels and PT mandatory before administration.

DILUTION

All preparations provide diluent for IV infusion. Actual number of units shown on each vial. Use only the diluent provided and maintain strict aseptic technique. Bring to room temperature before reconstitution. Gently swirl. Do not shake. May be given through Y-tube or three-way stopcock of infusion set. To avoid hypotension from prekallikrein activator (PKA), give Autoplex-T within 1 hour of dilution and Feiba VH within 3 hours.

Storage: Refrigerate before reconstitution; do not refrigerate after.

COMPATIBILITY

Specific information not available. Administration through a separate line without mixing with other IV fluids or medications is generally recommended for these products. If anti-inhibitor coagulant is given as a continuous IV, one source says heparin 5 to 10 units/ml of concentrate may be added to avoid thrombophlebitis.

RATE OF ADMINISTRATION

If symptoms of too-rapid infusion (headache, flushing, changes in BP or pulse rate) occur, discontinue until symptoms subside. Restart at a lower rate. **Autoplex-T:** Begin at 2 ml/min. If well tolerated, may gradually increase to 10 ml/min. **Feiba VH:** Do not exceed 2 units/kg/min.

ACTIONS

A 1-unit volume of factor VIII correctional activity (quantity of activated prothrombin complex) will correct clotting time to normal (35 seconds) when added to an equal volume of factor VIII deficient or inhibitor plasma. A dried or freeze-dried concentrate prepared from human plasma by a specific process.

INDICATIONS AND USES

Prophylaxis and treatment of hemorrhagic complications in hemophiliacs (hemophilia A) with factor VIII or factor IX inhibitors who are bleeding or will undergo elective or emergency surgery. Most frequently indicated if factor VIII inhibitor levels are above 2 to 10 Bethesda Units or rise to that level following treatment with AHF. ■ Prophylaxis and treatment of hemorrhagic complications in non-hemophiliacs with acquired inhibitors to factor VIII, XI, and XII.

CONTRAINDICATIONS

Disseminated intravascular coagulation (DIC), history of thromboembolism, symptoms (signs) of fibrinolysis, known hypersensitivity.

PRECAUTIONS

Could transmit HIV and hepatitis. ■ Use extreme caution in newborns and patients with liver disease. ■ Anamnestic responses (development of antibodies, reducing effectiveness of the drug) with a rise in factor VIII inhibitor titers have been seen in up to 20% of cases. ■ Risk of thrombotic complications may be increased in surgical patients and in patients receiving higher doses or prolonged administration. ■ See Drug/Lab Interactions.

Monitor: Monitor PT before and after treatment. Only accurate means of treatment evaluation. Must be two thirds of preinfusion value after treatment if patient is to receive any additional doses. ■ Monitor vital signs before, during, and after the infusion. ■ Monitor for S/S of thrombotic complications (e.g., chest pain, cough, respiratory distress; may indicate intravascular coagulation). ■ Monitor for S/S of allergic reaction (e.g., rash, shortness of breath).

Maternal/Child: Category C: use only if clearly needed. ■ Premature infants and neonates may be at increased risk for developing thrombotic complications and may have a higher morbidity or mortality from hepatitis or HIV caused by contaminated products.

DRUG/LAB INTERACTIONS

Not recommended for use with antifibrinolytic products (aminocaproic acid, tranexamic acid). ■ aPTT, WBCT, and other clotting factor tests do not correlate with actual results and may lead to overdose and DIC.

SIDE EFFECTS

Anaphylaxis, bradycardia, chest pain, chills, cough, decreased fibrinogen concentration, decreased platelet count, DIC, fever, flushing, headache, hypertension, hypotension, myocardial infarction, prolonged PTT, prolonged thrombin time, prolonged PT, respiratory distress, tachycardia, thrombosis or thromboembolism, urticaria. Consider risk potential of contracting AIDS or hepatitis.

ANTIDOTE

If side effects occur, discontinue the infusion and notify the physician. May be resumed at a slower rate or an alternate product may be used. Symptoms of DIC (BP and pulse rate changes, respiratory discomfort, chest pain, cough, prolonged clotting tests, cyanosis of hands and feet, persistent bleeding from puncture sites or mucous membranes) require immediate treatment. Treat anaphylaxis (antihistamines, epinephrine, corticosteroids) and resuscitate as necessary.

ANTITHROMBIN III

(an'tee-throm-bin)

AT-III, Thrombate III

Anticoagulant
Antithrombotic

pH 6.5 to 7.5

USUAL DOSE

Loading dose, maintenance dose, and dosing intervals are completely individualized based on confirmed diagnosis (see Precautions), patient weight, clinical condition, degree of deficiency, type of surgery or procedure involved, physician judgment, desired level of antithrombin III (AT-III), and actual plasma levels achieved as verified by appropriate lab tests. One unit/kg should raise the level of AT-III by 1.4%. The desired AT-III level after the first dose should be about 120% of normal (normal is 0.1 to 0.2 Gm/L). AT-III levels must be maintained at normal or at least above 80% of normal for 2 to 8 days depending on individual patient factors. Usually achieved by administration of a maintenance dose once daily. Concomitant administration of heparin usually indicated; see Drug/Lab Interactions.

Calculate the initial loading dose using the following formula (assumes a plasma volume of 40 ml/kg):

$$\text{Dosage units} = \frac{(\text{desired AT-III level [\%]} - \text{baseline AT-III [\%]} \times \text{body weight kg}}{\div 1.4\%}$$

For a 70-kg patient with a baseline AT-III level of 57% the initial dose of Thrombate III would be $(120\% - 57\%) \times 70 \div 1.4 = 3150$ IU. Measurement of plasma levels is suggested preinfusion, 20 minutes postinfusion (peak), 12 hours postinfusion, and preceding next infusion (trough). If recovery differs from the anticipated rise of 1.4% for each IU/kg, modify the formula accordingly. If the above patient has a 20-minute AT-III level of 147%, the increase in AT-III measured for each 1 IU/kg administered is $(147\% - 57\%) \times 70$ kg $\div 3150$ Units $= 2\%$ rise for each IU/kg administered. This in vivo recovery would be used to calculate future doses. A maintenance dose of approximately 60% of the loading dose every 24 hours is the average required to maintain plasma levels between 80% and 120%. Dose and interval based on plasma levels.

DOSE ADJUSTMENTS

See Drug/Lab Interactions.

DILUTION

Diluent, double-ended needles for dilution, and filter needle for aspiration into a syringe are provided. Warm unopened diluent and concentrate to room temperature. Enter diluent bottle first. Enter vacuum concentrate bottle with needle at an angle. Direct diluent from above to sides of vial to gently moisten all contents. Remove diluent bottle and transfer needle; swirl continuously until completely dissolved. Draw into a syringe through the filter needle. Remove filter needle; replace with an administration set (not provided). For larger doses, several bottles may be drawn into one syringe. Use a separate filter needle for each bottle.

Storage: Store in refrigerator before dilution; avoid freezing. Do not refrigerate after reconstitution. Use within 3 hours of reconstitution.

COMPATIBILITY

Administration through a separate line without mixing with other IV fluids or medications is recommended.

RATE OF ADMINISTRATION

Too-rapid injection may cause dyspnea.

A single dose over 10 to 20 minutes.

ACTIONS

Manufactured from human plasma, purified and heat treated through specific processes, AT-III is a plasma-based protein produced by the body to inactivate specific clotting proteins and control clot formation. Identical to heparin cofactor I, a factor in plasma necessary for heparin to exert its anticoagulant effect. It inactivates thrombin and the activated forms of factors IX, X, XI, and XII (all coagulation enzymes except factors VIIa and Factor XIIIa). Increases AT-III levels within 30 minutes and has a half-life of up to 3 days.

INDICATIONS AND USES

Treatment of patients with hereditary AT-III deficiency to prevent thrombosis during surgical or obstetric procedures (replacement therapy) or during acute thrombotic episodes.

CONTRAINDICATIONS

None when used as indicated.

PRECAUTIONS

For IV use only. ■ Confirm diagnosis of hereditary AT-III deficiency based on a clear family history of venous thrombosis as well as decreased plasma AT-III levels and the exclusion of acquired deficiency. Present laboratory tests may not be able to identify all cases of congenital AT-III deficiency. ■ Every unit of plasma used to manufacture AT-III is tested and found nonreactive for HBsAg and negative for antibody to HIV by FDA-approved tests, then heat-treated by a special process. Even with these precautions, individuals who receive multiple infusions may develop viral infection, particularly non-A, non-B hepatitis. HIV infection remains a remote possibility. ■ May reverse heparin resistance.

Monitor: See varying methods for measuring AT-III levels under Usual Dose. Should be measured at least twice daily until the patient is stabilized and peak and trough levels established, then measured daily. All blood work should be drawn immediately before the next infusion of AT-III.

Patient Education: Inform of risks of thrombosis in connection with pregnancy and surgery and the fact that AT-III deficiency is hereditary.

Maternal/Child: Neonatal AT-III levels should be measured immediately after birth if parents are known to have AT-III deficiency (fatal neonatal thromboembolism [e.g., aortic thrombi] has occurred). Treatment of the neonate should be under the direction of a physician knowledgeable about coagulation disorders. Normal full-term and premature infants have lower than adult averages of AT-III plasma levels. ■ Category B: use only if clearly indicated. Fetal abnormalities not noted when administered in the third trimester. ■ Safety for use in children not established.

DRUG/LAB INTERACTIONS

Half-life of AT-III decreases with concurrent heparin treatment. The anticoagulant effect of heparin is enhanced and a reduced dose of heparin is indicated to avoid bleeding.

SIDE EFFECTS

Bowel fullness, chest pain, chest tightness, chills, cramps, dizziness, fever, film over eye, foul taste in mouth, hives, light-headedness, oozing and hematoma formation, and shortness of breath have occurred with Thrombate III. Some patients with acquired AT-III deficiency diagnosed with disseminated intravascular coagulation (DIC) have had diuretic and vasodilatory effects. Rapid infusion may cause dyspnea.

ANTIDOTE

Levels of 150% to 210% found in a few patients have not caused any apparent complications. Observe for bleeding. Reduce rate of infusion immediately for dyspnea. Decrease rate or interrupt infusion as indicated until side effects subside. Keep physician informed of patient's lab values and condition.

ANTI-THYMOCYTE GLOBULIN (RABBIT)

(an-ti thi′mo-sit glob′u-lin)

Immunosuppressant

Thymoglobulin

pH 7 to 7.4

USUAL DOSE

Premedication: To reduce the incidence and intensity of side effects during the infusion of anti-thymocyte globulin; premedication 1 hour before the infusion with corticosteroids (e.g., dexamethasone [Decadron]), acetaminophen (e.g., Tylenol), and/or an antihistamine (e.g., diphenhydramine [Benadryl]) is recommended.

Anti-thymocyte globulin: 1.5 mg/kg of body weight daily for 7 to 14 days. Given as an infusion into a high flow vein. Used in conjunction with maintenance immunosuppression (e.g., tacrolimus [Prograf], mycophenolate [Cell-Cept]); see Drug/Lab Interactions.

PEDIATRIC DOSE

Safety and effectiveness for use in pediatric patients not established; see Maternal/Child.

DOSE ADJUSTMENTS

Reduce dose by one-half if WBC count is between 2,000 and 3,000 cells/mm^3 or if platelet count is between 50,000 and 75,000 cells/mm^3. ▪ Consider withholding dose or stopping anti-thymocyte therapy if WBC count falls below 2,000 cells/mm^3 or platelets fall below 50,000 cells/mm^3.

DILUTION

Calculate the number of vials required (25 mg/vial), 5 ml of SW as diluent per vial is supplied. Drug and diluent must be warmed to room temperature before dilution. Absolute sterile technique required throughout dilution process. For each vial required use a new syringe and needle. Withdraw 5 ml of diluent and inject into lyophilized powder. Rotate vial gently until powder is completely dissolved. Do not shake. Each reconstituted vial contains 25 mg (5 mg/ml). Must be further diluted by transferring into 50 ml of infusion solution (saline or dextrose) for each 25 mg of anti-thymocyte globulin. Total volume is usually between 50 to 500 ml. Invert the infusion bag gently once or twice to mix the solution.

Storage: Refrigerate and protect from light until removed to prepare for reconstitution. Do not freeze. Do not use after expiration date on vial. Use reconstituted vials within 4 hours. Use infusion solutions immediately. Discard unused drug.

COMPATIBILITY

Specific information not available. Administration through a separate line without mixing with other IV fluids or medications is suggested because of specific use and potential for anaphylaxis.

RATE OF ADMINISTRATION

Use of a high flow vein and a 0.22 micron filter recommended. Well-tolerated and less likely to produce side effects (e.g., chills and fever) when administered at the recommended rate and the patient is premedicated.

Initial dose: A total daily dose equally distributed over a minimum of 6 hours.

Subsequent doses: A total daily dose equally distributed over a minimum of 4 hours.

ACTIONS

A purified, pasteurized, gamma immune globulin, obtained by immunization of rabbits with human thymocytes. Mechanism of action not fully understood. May induce immunosuppression by T-cell depletion and immune modulation. Made up of a variety of antibodies that recognize key receptors on T-cells (those cells responsible for attacking and rejecting a foreign substance within the body). Anti-thymocyte globulin antibodies can inactivate and kill these T-cells, thus reversing the rejection process. May prevent organ loss and reduce the need for retransplantation. T-cell depletion is usually observed within a day of initiating thymoglobulin therapy. Half-life averages 2 to 3 days but the drug remains active, targeting the offending immune cells for days to weeks after treatment.

INDICATIONS AND USES

Treatment of kidney transplant acute rejection in conjunction with concomitant immunosuppression.

Unlabeled uses: Compassionate use in the treatment of acute rejection in bone marrow, heart, and liver transplants. Orphan drug status for the treatment of myelodysplastic syndrome (MDS).

CONTRAINDICATIONS

Patients with a known allergy to rabbit proteins, an acute viral illness, or a history of anaphylaxis during rabbit immunoglobulin administration.

PRECAUTIONS

Administered only under the direction of a physician experienced in immunosuppressive therapy and management of renal transplant patients in a facility with adequate laboratory and supportive medical resources. ■ Not considered effective for treating antibody-mediated (humoral) rejections. ■ Prolonged use or overdose in combination with other immunosuppressive agents may cause over-immunosuppression resulting in severe infections and may increase the incidence of lymphoma or post-transplant lymphoproliferative disease (PTLD) or other malignancies. Use of appropriate antiviral, antibacterial, antiprotozoal, and/or antifungal prophylaxis is recommended. In clinical trials viral prophylaxis with ganciclovir infusion was used. ■ In clinical trials, anti-rabbit antibodies developed in 68% of patients. Controlled studies on repeat use of anti-thymocyte globulin in patients with antirabbit antibodies have not been conducted. Use caution if repeat courses are indicated, monitoring of lymphocyte count is recommended to ensure that T-cell depletion is achieved. ■ If anaphylaxis occurs during or after therapy, further administration of anti-thymocyte globulin is contraindicated.

Monitor: Close clinical observation is imperative. Monitor for side effects during and after infusion. Anaphylaxis has occurred; emergency equipment, medications and supplies must be available. ■ Obtain baseline and monitor WBC and platelet counts during therapy. Thrombocytopenia or neutropenia may occur and are reversible following dose adjustment; see Dose Adjustments. ■ Monitoring of the lymphocyte count (i.e., total lymphocyte count and T-cell counts [absolute and/or subset]) may help assess the degree of T-cell depletion. ■ Monitor carefully for signs of infection. ■ Prophylactic antibiotics may be indicated pending results of C/S in a febrile neutropenic patient. ■ See Precautions and Drug/Lab Interactions.

Patient Education: Imperative that all medications (especially immunosuppressants) be reviewed with physician. ■ Report any previous allergic/anaphylactic reaction. ■ Report acute viral infections immediately. ■ Promptly report chest pain, irregular or rapid heartbeat, shortness of breath, swelling of the face or throat, or wheezing during infusion of medication. ■ See Appendix D, p. 1148. ■ May be associated with an increased risk of malignancy.

Maternal/Child: Category C: safety for use during pregnancy, breast-feeding, and in children not established. Use only if clearly needed. ■ Has been used in children in limited European studies and in the United States for compassionate use. Response similar to adults.

Elderly: Specific information not available.

DRUG/LAB INTERACTIONS

Concurrent use with immunosuppressants (e.g., azathioprine [Imuran], cyclosporine [Sandimmune], mycophenolate [Cell-Cept], tacrolimus [Prograf]) may potentiate the immunosuppressive action of these agents, many transplant centers decrease maintenance immunosuppression therapy during the period of antibody therapy. ■ May stimulate the production of antibodies which crossreact with rabbit immune globulins. ■ May interfere with rabbit antibody-base immunoassays and with cross-match or panel-reactive antibody cytotoxicity assays.

SIDE EFFECTS

Are dose-limiting. Abdominal pain, asthenia, diarrhea, dizziness, dyspnea, fever, headache, hyperkalemia, hypertension, infection, infusion reaction (e.g., chills and fever), leukopenia, malaise, nausea, pain, peripheral edema, tachycardia, and thrombocytopenia were reported frequently. Anaphylaxis has been reported.

Overdose: Leukopenia or thrombocytopenia.

ANTIDOTE

Notify physician of all side effects. Most can be managed symptomatically. Manage leukopenia or thrombocytopenia during therapy or in overdose with dose reduction. Infusion reactions are managed with premedication and reduction in the rate of infusion. Treat infections aggressively; see Precautions. May require discontinuation of therapy. Discontinue infusion and/or therapy immediately if anaphylaxis occurs. Treat anaphylaxis immediately with epinephrine (Adrenalin), diphenhydramine (Benadryl), oxygen, vasopressors (e.g., dopamine [Intropin]), corticosteroids, IV fluids, and ventilation equipment as indicated. Resuscitate as necessary.

ANTIVENIN *(CROTALIDAE)* POLYVALENT

Antivenin

(an-ti-ven′in kro-tal′id-ay pol-e-va′lent)

USUAL DOSE

Testing for sensitivity to horse serum required before use. See Precautions/Monitor for additional pretreatment requirements. Dosage based on severity of envenomation when patient is initially assessed.

No envenomation: None.

Minimal envenomation: 2 to 4 vials (20 to 40 ml).

Moderate envenomation: 5 to 9 vials (50 to 90 ml).

Severe envenomation: 10 to 15 vials (100 to 150 ml).

Additional antivenin need based on clinical response and progression of symptoms. If condition deteriorates, give 1 to 5 additional vials (10 to 50 ml). Most effective within 4 hours of the bite; less effective after 8 hours. In the presence of envenomation, give even after 24 hours have elapsed.

PEDIATRIC DOSE

Not based on weight. Small children bitten by large snakes may require larger doses of antivenin.

DILUTION

Each single vial must be diluted with 10 ml SW for injection. ***Do not use supplied diluent; do not use bacteriostatic water for injection (BWFI).*** Must be further diluted with NS or D5W to a 1:1 to 1:10 solution (1 ml antivenin to 10 ml infusion solution preferred unless patient's condition limits fluid intake). Avoid foaming by gently swirling mix thoroughly.

Storage: Store vials at CRT; do not freeze. Use reconstituted solution within 48 hours and diluted solutions within 12 hours.

COMPATIBILITY

Specific information not available. Administration through a separate line without mixing with other IV fluids or medications is suggested because of specific use and potential for anaphylaxis.

RATE OF ADMINISTRATION

Infuse 5 to 10 ml over a minimum of 3 to 5 minutes. If no adverse reaction occurs, give remaining initial dose at maximum rate of administration based on severity of envenomation and fluid tolerance appropriate for this patient's body weight and condition.

ACTIONS

Prepared from the blood serum of horses immunized against the venom of crotalids (pit vipers) found in North, Central, and South America. Will neutralize the venom of rattlesnakes, copperheads, and cottonmouth moccasins. (See literature for specific species.)

INDICATIONS AND USES

Treatment of patients with symptoms of envenomation sustained from the bite of a rattlesnake, copperhead, cottonmouth moccasin, or other specific pit viper species of snake.

CONTRAINDICATIONS

Hypersensitivity to horse serum unless only treatment available for life-threatening situation. Several techniques, including preload of antihistamines and/or desensitization, may be considered (see literature).

PRECAUTIONS

Read drug literature supplied with antivenin completely before use. Essential to evaluate symptoms and individual status of each patient. ■ IV route preferred; mandatory if shock is present. ■ Determine patient response to any previous injections of serum of any type and history of any allergic-type reactions. ■ Hospitalize patient. ■ Test every patient without exception for sensitivity to horse serum (1-ml vial of 1:10 dilution horse serum supplied). Skin test recommended. ■ Manufacturer in the process of phasing product out of production.

Skin test: Inject 0.02 to 0.03 ml of 1:10 horse serum intradermally. In patients with a history of allergies use a 1:100 solution. A similar injection of NS can be used as a control. Compare in 5 to 30 minutes. An urticarial wheal surrounded by a zone of erythema is a positive reaction.

■ A systemic reaction may occur even when both sensitivity tests are negative. ■ Tetanus prophylaxis is indicated. ■ Corticosteroids are the drugs of choice if antivenin is not available until 24 hours after the snake bite but are not recommended for concomitant administration unless required to treat an allergic reaction. ■ Consider use of broad-spectrum antibiotic. ■ Check with poison control center; many authorities do not recommend packing the bitten extremity in ice.

Monitor: Before antivenin is administered draw adequate blood for baseline studies (type and cross-match, CBC, hematocrit, platelet count, PT, clot retraction, bleeding and coagulation times, BUN, electrolytes, and bilirubin). ■ Monitor all vital signs at frequent intervals. ■ Have urine specimens tested frequently for microscopic erythrocytes. ■ In most cases, the sooner a sensitivity reaction occurs, the greater the sensitivity. Observe patient continuously. ■ Initiate two IV lines as soon as possible; one to be used for supportive therapy, the other for antivenin and electrolytes. ■ Keep emergency equipment available at all times, including oxygen, epinephrine, antihistamines (e.g., diphenhydramine [Benadryl]), vasopressors (e.g., dopamine [Intropin]), corticosteroids, and ventilation equipment. ■ Use of a broad-spectrum antibiotic is recommended if local tissue damage is evident.

Patient Education: Contact physician immediately for any S/S of a delayed allergic reaction (e.g., rash, pruritus, urticaria) after hospital discharge.

Maternal/Child: Category C: use during pregnancy only if clearly needed. ■ Safety for use during breast-feeding not established; no documented problems.

DRUG/LAB INTERACTIONS

Concomitant use of antihistamines may interfere with sensitivity tests.

SIDE EFFECTS

Acute anaphylaxis with urticaria, respiratory distress, and vascular collapse. Serum sickness may occur. Usually appears in 7 to 12 days. Local pain, local erythema, and urticaria without systemic reaction can occur.

ANTIDOTE

Discontinue the drug and notify the physician of all side effects. Treat anaphylaxis immediately. Epinephrine (Adrenalin) and diphenhydramine (Benadryl), oxygen, vasopressors (dopamine), corticosteroids, H_2 antagonists (cimetidine), and ventilation equipment must always be available. Corticosteroids (e.g., hydrocortisone sodium succinate [Solu-Cortef]) are indicated to treat serious delayed reactions. Resuscitate as necessary.

ANTIVENIN CROTALIDAE POLYVALENT IMMUNE FAB (OVINE)

Antivenin

(an-ti-ven′in kro-tal′id-ay pol-e-va′lent i-mun′fab)

CroFab

USUAL DOSE

Contact Poison Control Center for individual treatment advice.

Premedication: Premedication may be indicated for patients with allergies. Obtain blood work before administration; see Contraindications, Precautions, and Monitor. Initiate as soon as possible after crotalid snakebite in patients who develop signs of progressive envenomation (e.g., worsening local injury, coagulation abnormality, or systemic signs of envenomation); see Monitor. Has been effective when given within 6 hours of snakebite.

Initial dose: Skin testing for sensitivity to serum is not required. 4 to 6 vials is the recommended intitial dose based on clinical experience. Adjust based on severity of envenomation when patient is initially assessed. Observe for up to 1 hour after initial dose administered. Desired outcome is complete control of the envenomation (i.e., complete arrest of local manifestations, and return of coagulation tests and systemic signs to normal).

Repeat doses: If control of symptoms is not accomplished by the initial dose, give an additional dose of 4 to 6 vials. This dose may be repeated until initial control of the envenomation syndrome has been achieved. After initial control has been established, give additional 2-vial doses every 6 hours for up to 18 hours (3 doses). Optimal dosing following the 18-hour scheduled dose has not been determined. Additional 2-vial doses may be given as directed by the treating physician, based on the patient's clinical response. Up to 18 vials have been given without any observed direct toxic effect. Scheduled dosing/rather than PRN dosing may provide better control of envenomation symptoms caused by the continued leaking of venom from depot sites.

PEDIATRIC DOSE

Absolute venom dose following snakebite is expected to be the same in children and adults, no dose adjustment for age is required.

DOSE ADJUSTMENTS

No dose adjustments recommended.

DILUTION

Reconstitute each vial with 10 ml SW. Mix by continuous gentle swirling. Further dilute the contents of the reconstituted vial(s) in 250 ml NS and mix by gently swirling.

Storage: Refrigerate unopened vials, do not freeze. Reconstituted vials and diluted solution must be used within 4 hours.

COMPATIBILITY

Specific information not available. Administration through a separate line without mixing with other IV fluids or medications is suggested because of specific use and potential for anaphylaxis.

RATE OF ADMINISTRATION

Infuse at a rate of 25 to 50 ml/hr over the first 10 minutes. Carefully observe for allergic reactions. If no adverse reaction occurs, increase rate to administer 250 ml equally distributed over 1 hour. Reduce rate of administration if infusion-related reactions occur (e.g., fever, low back pain, nausea, wheezing), and monitor closely.

ACTIONS

A venom-specific Fab fragment of immunoglobulin G (IgG) obtained from the blood of healthy sheep flocks immunized with one of four snake venoms; see Indications for specific venoms. To obtain the final product, the four different monospecific antivenins are mixed. Works by binding and neutralizing venom toxins, facilitating their redistribution away from target tissues and their elimination from the body. Half-life is estimated to be 12 to 23 hours.

INDICATIONS AND USES

Management of patients with minimal or moderate North American rattlesnake envenomation *(Crotalus atrox* [Western Diamondback rattlesnake], *Crotalus adamanteus* [Eastern Diamondback rattlesnake], *Crotalus scutulatus* [Mohave rattlesnake], and *Agkistrodon piscivorus* [Cottonmouth or Water Moccasin]). Early use (within 6 hours) is advised to prevent clinical deterioration and the occurrence of systemic coagulation abnormalities. ■ No clinical data is available supporting effectiveness in patients presenting with severe envenomation.

Unlabeled uses: May possess antigenic cross-reactivity against the venoms of some Middle Eastern and North African snakes, no clinical data available.

CONTRAINDICATIONS

Known history of hypersensitivity to sheep, papaya, or papain unless benefits outweigh risks and appropriate management for anaphylactic reactions is readily available.

PRECAUTIONS

Usually administered in the hospital by or under the direction of the physician specialist with adequate diagnostic and treatment facilities readily available. ■ Patients with allergies to dust mites, latex, papain, chymopapain, other papaya extracts, the pineapple enzyme bromelain, or sheep protein may be at risk for an allergic reaction to this antivenin; see Contraindications, use caution. ■ Contains 0.11 mg of mercury per vial (ethyl mercury from thimerosal). Exposure from 18 vial dose is 1.9 mg of mercury. Definitive data not available, literature suggests that information related to methyl mercury toxicities may be applicable. ■ Recurrent coagulation abnormalities (e.g., decreased fibrinogen, decreased platelets, and elevated PT) defined as the return of a coagulation abnormality after it has been successfully treated with antivenin, were observed in patients who experienced coagulation abnormalities during their initial hospitalization and occurred in approximately one-half of patients studied. Crotalidae immune fab has a shorter persistence in the blood than crotalid venoms that can leak from depot sites over a prolonged period of time; repeat dosing to prevent or treat such recurrence may be necessary. Optimal dosing to prevent recurrent coagulopathy has not been determined. ■ Use caution if a repeat course of treatment is required for a subsequent envenomation episode, crotalidae immune fab is a foreign protein and antibodies may develop producing sensitivity.

Monitor: Before antivenin is administered, draw adequate blood for baseline studies (e.g., type and cross-match, CBC, hematocrit, platelet count, PT, clot retraction, bleeding and coagulation times, BUN, electrolytes, and bilirubin). ■ Severity of envenomation is based on six body categories: cardiovascular, gastrointestinal, hematological, local wound (e.g., pain, swelling and ecchymosis), nervous system, and pulmonary effects. Specific parameters of minimal, moderate, and severe envenomation are outlined in the following chart.

Definition of Minimal, Moderate, and Severe Envenomation Used in Clinical Studies of Crotalidae Polyvalent Immune Fab

Envenomation Category	Definition
Minimal	*Swelling, pain, and ecchymosis,* limited to the immediate bite site. *Systemic signs and symptoms* absent. *Coagulation parameters* normal with no clinical evidence of bleeding.
Moderate	*Swelling, pain, and ecchymosis,* involving less than a full extremity or, if bite was sustained on the trunk, head or neck, extending less than 50 cm. *Systemic signs and symptoms,* may be present but not life-threatening, including but not limited to nausea, vomiting, oral paresthesia or unusual tastes, mild hypotension (systolic BP less than 90 mm Hg), mild tachycardia (HR less than 150), and tachypnea. *Coagulation parameters* may be abnormal, but no clinical evidence of bleeding present. Minor hematuria, gum bleeding and nose-bleeds are allowed if they are not considered severe in the investigator's judgment.
Severe	*Swelling, pain, and ecchymosis,* involving more than an entire extremity or threatening the airway. *Systemic signs and symptoms,* are markedly abnormal, including severe alteration of mental status, severe hypotension, severe tachycardia, tachypnea, or respiratory insufficiency. *Coagulation parameters,* are abnormal, with serious bleeding or severe threat of bleeding.

■ Anaphylactic and anaphylactoid reactions, delayed allergic reactions (late serum reaction or serum sickness), and a possible febrile response to immune complexes formed by animal antibodies and neutralized venom components may occur. Observe all patients continuously for signs and symptoms of an acute allergic reaction (e.g., angioedema, bronchospasm with wheezing or cough, erythema, hypotension, pruritus, stridor, tachycardia, urticaria). ■ Monitor all vital signs at frequent intervals. Observe for signs of shock; treat with IV fluids, blood products, plasma expanders, vasopressors (e.g., dopamine [Intropin]) as indicated. ■ Keep emergency equipment available at all times, including oxygen, epinephrine, antihistamines (e.g., IV diphenhydramine [Benadryl]), corticosteroids, albuterol, vasopressors (e.g., dopamine [Intropin]), and ventilation equipment. ■ Initiate two IV lines as soon as possible; one to be used for supportive therapy, the other for antivenin and electrolytes. ■ A decrease in platelets not responsive to whole blood transfusion can occur with rattlesnake bites, platelet count should approach normal limits within 1 hour of administering crotalidae immune fab. ■ Follow-up monitoring is required for S/S of delayed allergic reactions or serum sickness (e.g., arthralgia, fever, myalgia, rash). ■ Test urine specimens for microscopic erythrocytes. ■ If coagulation abnormalities occur, consider other disease processes associated with coagulation disorders (e.g., cancer, collagen disease, CHF, diarrhea, elevated temperature, hepatic disorder, hyperthyroidism, poor nutritional state, steatorrhea, vitamin K deficiency). ■ Monitor patients who experience coagulopathy due to snakebite during hospitalization for initial treatment for several weeks after discharge. Recurrent coagulopathy may persist for 2 weeks or more. Assess the need for retreatment and/or use of anticoagulant or antiplatelet agents. ■ Supportive measures to treat other manifestations of the snakebite (e.g., hypotension, pain, swelling, wound infection) should be implemented.

Patient Education: Immediately report any S/S of delayed allergic reactions or serum sickness (e.g., pruritus, rash, or urticaria occurring after discharge). ■ Promptly report unusual bruising or bleeding (e.g., nosebleeds, excessive bleeding after tooth brushing or superficial injuries, blood in stools or urine, excessive menstrual bleeding, petechiae). May occur for up to 1 week or longer and indicate need for additional treatment.

Maternal/Child: Category C: use during pregnancy only if clearly needed. ■ Use caution, safety for use during breast-feeding not established. ■ Exposure to mercury has been associated with neurological and renal toxicities. Developing fetuses and very young children are most susceptible and are at greater risk.

Elderly: No specific studies on elderly patients.

DRUG/LAB INTERACTIONS

Studies have not been conducted.

SIDE EFFECTS

Pruritus, rash, and urticaria are frequent side effects. Allergic reactions including anaphylaxis, anorexia, back pain, cellulitis, chest pain, chills, circumoral paresthesia, cough, delayed allergic reactions (late serum reaction or serum sickness), ecchymosis, febrile response to immune complexes formed by animal antibodies and neutralized venom components, general paresthesia, hypotension, increased sputum, myalgia, nausea, nervousness, recurrent coagulopathy, and wound infection have occurred.

ANTIDOTE

Keep physician informed of all side effects and extent or progression of envenomation. Reduce the rate of administration if infusion-related reactions occur (e.g., fever, low back pain, nausea, wheezing). Monitor closely and discontinue antivenin if symptoms worsen or an allergic reaction occurs. Treat allergic reactions and/or anaphylaxis immediately with oxygen, epinephrine, antihistamines (e.g., IV diphenhydramine [Benadryl]), corticosteroids, albuterol, vasopressors (e.g., dopamine [Intropin]), and ventilation equipment as indicated. Recurrent coagulopathy may require re-hospitalization and additional antivenin administration. Resuscitate as necessary.

ANTIVENIN *(LATRODECTUS MACTANS)* — Antivenin

(lat′ro-dek′tus mac′tans)

Black Widow Spider Species Antivenin

USUAL DOSE

Testing for sensitivity to horse serum required before use. See Precautions for additional pretreatment requirements.

Entire contents of 1 vial of antivenin (2.5 ml) is recommended for adults and children. One vial is usually enough, but a second dose may be necessary in rare instances. Best results obtained if administered within 4 hours of envenomation.

PEDIATRIC DOSE

Same as adult dose.

DILUTION

Each single dose (6,000 antivenin units) must be initially diluted with 2.5 ml SW for injection (supplied). Keep needle in rubber stopper of antivenin and shake vial to dissolve contents completely. Must be further diluted in 10 to 50 ml NS for IV injection.

Storage: Refrigerate unopened vials; do not freeze. Refrigerate reconstituted and/or diluted solution; discard in 6 hours.

COMPATIBILITY

Specific information not available. Administration through a separate line without mixing with other IV fluids or medications is suggested because of specific use and potential for anaphylaxis.

RATE OF ADMINISTRATION

A single dose over a minimum of 15 minutes.

ACTIONS

Prepared from the blood serum of horses immunized against the venom of the black widow spider. One unit will neutralize one average mouse-lethal dose of black widow spider venom when both are injected simultaneously under lab conditions.

INDICATIONS AND USES

Treatment of patients with symptoms resulting from bites of black widow spiders *(Latrodectus mactans)* and similar spiders.

CONTRAINDICATIONS

Hypersensitivity to horse serum unless only treatment available for a life-threatening situation. Several techniques including preload of antihistamine and/or desensitization may be considered (see literature).

PRECAUTIONS

Read drug literature supplied with antivenin completely before use. Essential to evaluate symptoms and individual status of each patient. ■ Determine patient response to any previous injections of serum of any type and history of any allergic-type reactions. ■ Hospitalize patient if possible. ■ Muscle relaxants may be the initial treatment of choice in healthy individuals between 16 and 60. Antivenin use may be deferred while patient is observed. ■ Test every patient without exception for sensitivity to horse serum (1-ml vial of 1:10 dilution horse serum supplied). Conjunctival test and skin test recommended for maximum safety. Usually begin with the conjunctival test.

Conjunctival test: Instill 1 drop 1:10 horse serum into conjunctival sac for adults (1 drop 1:100 dilution for children). Itching, redness, burning, and/or lacrimation within 10 minutes is a positive reaction. A drop of NS in the opposite eye is used as a control and should be asymptomatic. Reverse adverse effects of positive reaction with 1 drop epinephrine ophthalmic solution.

Skin test: Inject not more than 0.02 ml of 1:10 horse serum intradermally. In patients with a history of allergies use a 1:100 solution. A similar injection of NS can be used as a control. Compare in 10 minutes. An urticarial wheal surrounded by a zone of erythema is a positive reaction.

■ A systemic reaction may occur even when both sensitivity tests are negative. ■ May be given IM. IV preferred in severe cases, if patient is in shock, or in children under 12 years of age.

Monitor: Supportive therapy is indicated. 10 ml of 10% calcium gluconate IV may control muscle pain. Morphine may be needed. Barbiturates or diazepam may be used for restlessness. Prolonged warm baths are helpful; corticosteroids have been used. ■ Observe patient constantly for respiratory paralysis. Can occur from toxin alone, and narcotics and sedatives may precipitate respiratory depression. ■ Observe for serum sickness for 8 to 12 days.

Patient Education: Contact physician immediately for any S/S of a delayed allergic reaction (e.g., rash, pruritus, urticaria) after hospital discharge.

Maternal/Child: Category C: use only if clearly needed. ■ Safety for use in breast-feeding not established. ■ Safety for use in children not established, but there have been no adverse effects when used.

DRUG/LAB INTERACTIONS

Concomitant use of antihistamines may interfere with sensitivity tests. Narcotics and sedatives may precipitate respiratory depression.

SIDE EFFECTS

Acute anaphylaxis with urticaria, respiratory distress, and vascular collapse. Serum sickness may occur. Usually appears in 7 to 12 days. Local pain, local erythema, and urticaria without systemic reaction can occur.

ANTIDOTE

Discontinue the drug and notify the physician of all side effects. Treat anaphylaxis immediately. Epinephrine (Adrenalin), diphenhydramine (Benadryl), oxygen, vasopressors (dopamine), corticosteroids, H_2 antagonists (cimetidine), and ventilation equipment must always be available. Resuscitate as necessary.

ANTIVENIN *(MICRURUS FULVIUS)* — Antivenin
(an-ti-ven′in mi-kroo′rus ful′vi-us)

North American Coral Snake Antivenin — pH 6.5 to 7.5

USUAL DOSE
Testing for sensitivity to horse serum required before use. See Precautions for additional pretreatment requirements.

Entire contents of 3 to 5 vials (30 to 50 ml) is recommended depending on the nature and severity of envenomation. Up to 10 vials may be required if the snake's entire venom load was delivered by the bite. Best results obtained if administered within 4 hours of envenomation.

PEDIATRIC DOSE
Same as adult dose; not adjusted by weight of patient.

DILUTION
Each single vial must be diluted with 10 ml SW for injection. ***Do not use supplied diluent; do not use bacteriostatic water for injection (BWFI).*** Start an IV infusion of 250 to 500 ml NS. May be administered through the tubing of the free-flowing IV or added to the infusion solution after initial 2 ml given without adverse reaction.

Storage: Store vials at CRT; do not freeze. Use reconstituted solution within 48 hours and diluted solution within 12 hours.

COMPATIBILITY
Specific information not available. Administration through a separate line without mixing with other IV fluids or medications is suggested because of specific use and potential for anaphylaxis.

RATE OF ADMINISTRATION
Inject the first 1 to 2 ml over a minimum of 3 to 5 minutes. If no adverse reaction, give remaining initial dose at maximum rate of administration based on severity of envenomation and fluid tolerance appropriate for patient's body weight and condition (e.g., 250 to 500 ml over 30 minutes in a healthy adult, 100 ml in small children followed by 4 ml/min).

ACTIONS
Prepared from the blood serum of horses immunized against the venom of specific coral snakes. Will neutralize the venom of *M. fulvius fulvius* (eastern coral snake) and *M. fulvius tenere* (Texas coral snake). Response should be rapid and dramatic.

INDICATIONS AND USES
Treatment of patients with symptoms resulting from the venom of *M. fulvius fulvius* (eastern coral snake) and *M. fulvius tenere* (Texas coral snake). ■ Not effective for *M. euryxanthus* (Arizona or Sonoran coral snake).

CONTRAINDICATIONS
Hypersensitivity to horse serum unless only treatment available for a life-threatening situation. Several techniques including preload of antihistamines and/or desensitization may be considered (see literature).

PRECAUTIONS
Read drug literature supplied with antivenin completely before use. Essential to evaluate symptoms and individual status of each patient. ■ Determine patient response to any previous injections of serum of any type

and history of any allergic type reactions. ■ Immobilize victim. At a minimum, splint bitten extremity. Hospitalize patient if possible. ■ Test every patient without exception for sensitivity to horse serum (1 ml vial of 1:10 dilution horse serum supplied). Skin test recommended.

Skin test: Inject 0.02 to 0.03 ml of a 1:10 dilution of horse serum in NS. In patients with a history of allergies use a 1:100 dilution. A similar injection of NS can be used as a control. Compare sites in 5 to 30 minutes. An urticarial wheal surrounded by a zone of erythema is a positive reaction.

■ A systemic reaction may occur even when both sensitivity tests are negative. ■ Tetanus prophylaxis indicated.

Monitor: Observe patient constantly. Additional antivenin may be needed. Paralysis can occur within 2 to 2½ hours. Death from respiratory paralysis has occurred within 4 hours. Local tissue reaction does not reflect the amount of envenomation. Observe signs and symptoms to assess amount of toxin injected. Symptoms may begin in 1 hour or be delayed up to 18 hours. ■ Supportive therapy is indicated. Monitoring of electrolytes and continuous bladder drainage (hemoglobinuria) are recommended. Respiratory depressants (e.g., narcotics, sedatives) are contraindicated or used with extreme caution. Keep equipment for artificial ventilation immediately available.

Patient Education: Contact physician immediately for any S/S of a delayed allergic reaction (e.g., rash, pruritus, urticaria) after hospital discharge.

Maternal/Child: Category C: use only if clearly needed. ■ Safety for use during breast-feeding not established; problems not documented.

DRUG/LAB INTERACTIONS

Concomitant use of antihistamines may interfere with sensitivity tests. ■ Narcotics and sedatives may precipitate respiratory depression.

SIDE EFFECTS

Acute anaphylaxis with urticaria, respiratory distress, and vascular collapse. Serum sickness may occur. Usually appears in 7 to 12 days. Local pain, local erythema, and urticaria without systemic reaction can occur.

ANTIDOTE

Discontinue the drug and notify the physician of all side effects. Treat anaphylaxis immediately. Epinephrine (Adrenalin) and diphenhydramine (Benadryl), oxygen, vasopressors (dopamine), H_2 antagonists (cimetidine), and ventilation equipment must always be available. Resuscitate as necessary.

APROTININ INJECTION

(ap′ro-tin′in in-jek′shun)

Antifibrinolytic
Antihemorrhagic

Trasylol

pH 4.5 to 6.5

USUAL DOSE

Administered in one of two dose regimens, Regimen A or Regimen B. Regimen A is most commonly used for high-risk patients. According to the manufacturer's medical information service, Regimen B provides adequate inhibition of plasmin activity while Regimen A promotes more kallikrein inhibiting and anti-inflammatory potential. Both regimens consist of a test dose, a loading dose, a constant infusion dose, and a dose to be added while recirculating the priming fluid of the cardiopulmonary bypass circuit ("pump prime" dose). IV doses must be given through a central venous line with the patient in a supine position. Do not administer any other drug using the same line. Total cumulative doses of more than 7 million kallikrein inhibitor units (KIU) have not been studied in controlled trials. Requires concurrent use of heparin (heparin dose-response required before administration of aprotinin; see below). To avoid physical incompatibility of aprotinin and heparin when adding to the pump prime solution, each agent must be added ***during recirculation*** of the pump prime to ensure adequate dilution before admixture with the other component. See Precautions/Monitor.

HEPARIN

May be administered by a titration regimen or a fixed regimen. See comments under Usual Dose.

Heparin titration regimen: Before administration of aprotinin, obtain a heparin dose response assessed by protamine titration to determine the heparin loading dose. Obtain heparin levels by protamine titration during bypass. Heparin levels during bypass should not be allowed to drop below 2.7 units/ml (2 mg/kg) or below the level indicated by heparin dose-response testing performed before aprotinin administration.

Heparin fixed regimen: A standard loading dose of heparin, administered before cannulation of the heart, and the quantity of heparin added to the prime volume of the cardiopulmonary bypass (CPB) circuit should total at least 350 units/kg. Additional heparin should be administered in a fixed-dose regimen based on patient weight and duration of CPB.

REGIMEN A

Test dose: 1 ml (1.4 mg or 10,000 KIU). Must be given IV at least 10 minutes before the loading dose.

Loading dose: 200 ml (280 mg or 2 million KIU). Given slowly IV over 20 to 30 minutes, after induction of anesthesia but before sternotomy. When complete, follow with a constant infusion of 50 ml/hr (70 mg/hr or 500,000 KIU/hr). Continue until the surgery is complete and the patient leaves the operating room.

"Pump prime dose": 200 ml (280 mg or 2 million KIU). Add to recirculating priming fluid of the cardiopulmonary bypass (CPB) circuit by replacing an aliquot of priming fluid before instituting cardiopulmonary bypass.

REGIMEN B

Test dose: See Regimen A. The ***loading dose*** and ***"pump prime dose"*** for Regimen B are exactly one-half of Regimen A doses. Experience with this lower-dose regimen is limited, but the manufacturer states that in low-risk primary or repeat CABG patients, differences between Regimen A (high-dose) and Regimen B (low-dose) in effectiveness and safety are not statistically significant.

DOSE ADJUSTMENTS

Not required with age or impaired renal function; changes in pharmacokinetics of aprotinin are not great enough. ■ No information available for patients with pre-existing hepatic disease; see Side Effects.

DILUTION

Supplied as a solution. Each 1 ml contains 1.4 mg or 10,000 KIU. May be used without further dilution.

Storage: Store at CRT. Protect from freezing.

COMPATIBILITY

Administered through a central venous line. Manufacturer states, "Do not administer any other drug using the same line." See note regarding heparin in Usual Dose.

RATE OF ADMINISTRATION

Test dose: A single dose over 1 minute.

Loading dose: A single dose over 20 to 30 minutes. Follow with an infusion at 50 ml/hr. Too-rapid administration can cause a transient fall in BP.

ACTIONS

A natural proteinase inhibitor obtained from bovine lung. It modulates the systemic inflammatory response (SIR) associated with cardiopulmonary bypass (CPB) surgery. SIR results in the interrelated activation of the hemostatic, fibrinolytic, cellular, and humoral inflammatory systems. Through its inhibition of multiple mediators (e.g., kallikrein, plasmin), aprotinin results in the attenuation of inflammatory responses, fibrinolysis, and thrombin generation. The net effect is inhibition of both fibrinolysis and turnover of coagulation factors (common results of CPB) and decrease in bleeding. Significantly reduces the donor blood transfusion requirement and decreases mediastinal reexploration for bleeding. Rapidly distributed into the total extracellular space with a rapid initial decrease in plasma concentration. Plasma half-life is 150 minutes. Terminal elimination half-life is about 10 hours. Accumulated in the kidney, and slowly degraded by lysosomal enzymes. Some excretion in urine.

INDICATIONS AND USES

Prophylactic use to reduce perioperative blood loss and the need for blood transfusion in both high-risk and low-risk patients undergoing primary or repeat coronary artery bypass graft surgery (CABG).

CONTRAINDICATIONS

Hypersensitivity to aprotinin.

PRECAUTIONS

Should be used under the direction of a physician specialist and an anesthesiologist. Do not administer to a patient who experiences any allergic reaction to aprotinin. ■ Risk of anaphylaxis (even with test dose) is increased in patients who have received aprotinin or aprotinin-containing products (e.g., fibrin sealants such as Tiseel by Baxter) in the past (especially within the previous 6 months). Emergency equipment and drugs must be immediately available. Do not administer the test dose or loading dose until the conditions for rapid cannulation (if necessary) are present. Delay addition of aprotinin into the pump prime solution until after the loading dose has been safely administered. Consider prophylactic administration of H_1 and H_2 blockers before the test dose; see Monitor. ■ Use caution in patients with a history of allergic reactions. ■ May cause increased renal failure and mortality in patients undergoing deep hypothermic circulatory arrest during surgery of the aortic arch. ■ Use caution in patients with impaired liver function.

Monitor: Primary patient monitoring under the direction of the anesthesiologist. ■ Premedication with diphenhydramine (Benadryl) and H_2 blockers (e.g., ranitidine [Zantac]) is recommended 15 minutes before the loading dose in any patient who has received aprotinin previously. ▪ In prolonged extracorporeal circulation, patients may require additional heparin, even in the presence of activated clotting time (ACT) levels that appear to represent adequate anticoagulation. Maintain a minimal celite-ACT of greater than 750 seconds or a kaolin-ACT of greater than 480 seconds, independent of the effects of hemodilution and hypothermia. Administer heparin either in a fixed-dose regimen based on patient weight and duration of CPB or on the basis of heparin levels measured by a method not affected by aprotinin (e.g., protamine titration); see Usual Dose. ▪ See Precautions and Antidote.

Patient Education: Explain risk of allergic reaction.

Maternal/Child: Category B: use only if clearly needed. ▪ Safety and effectiveness in children not established.

Elderly: Dose adjustment not required. No difference in safety and effectiveness noted between the elderly and younger patients.

DRUG/LAB INTERACTIONS

Had antifibrinolytic activity, may inhibit the effects of fibrinolytic agents (e.g., heparin, alteplase [tPA], anistreplase [Eminase]). ▪ May block the acute hypotensive effect of captopril (Capoten). ▪ Prolongs the ACT in the presence of heparin but is not a heparin-sparing agent; see Monitor.

SIDE EFFECTS

Hypersensitivity reactions including anaphylaxis can occur at any time even if the test dose is negative; risk increased with repeated administration. Elevated PTT and ACT are expected for several hours after surgery. Elevated ALT (SGOT) is more frequent with repeated administration. Increased SrCr (reversible renal dysfunction), serum creatine kinase, and serum glucose may occur. There may be an increased incidence of myocardial infarction and of saphenous vein graft closure. Many reported side effects are not attributable to aprotinin but are common in open-heart surgery (e.g., apnea, arrhythmias, asthma, cardiac arrest, confusion, congestive heart failure, dyspnea, fever, hypotension, kidney failure, myocardial infarction, pneumonia, sepsis, shock).

ANTIDOTE

Discontinue aprotinin and treat anaphylaxis immediately (epinephrine [Adrenalin], corticosteroids, diphenhydramine [Benadryl], ranitidine [Zantac], airway management, oxygen). Keep physician informed. To reverse heparin activity, the amount of protamine administered should be based on the actual amount of heparin given and not on the ACT values. Give protamine by very slow IV injection over a 10-minute period in doses not to exceed 50 mg; too-rapid injection of protamine can cause bradycardia, severe hypotension, and anaphylaxis. Treat all side effects (e.g., arrhythmias) appropriately and resuscitate as necessary.

ARGATROBAN

(are-ga-troe'ban)

Acova

Anticoagulant

pH 3.2 to 7.5

USUAL DOSE

Discontinue all parenteral anticoagulants (e.g., heparin) and obtain baseline blood tests including an aPTT (prophylaxis or treatment) and ACT (PCI) before administration of argatroban; see Monitor.

Prophylaxis or treatment of thrombosis in patients with or at risk for heparin-induced thrombocytopenia (HIT/HITTS): Begin ***argatroban*** with an initial dose of 2 mcg/kg/min as a continuous infusion. Steady-state levels usually obtained within 1 to 3 hours. Check the aPTT in 2 hours. Adjust the mcg/kg/min dose (not to exceed 10 mcg/kg/min) as clinically indicated until the steady-state aPTT is 1.5 to 3 times the initial baseline value (not to exceed 100 seconds).

Anticoagulant in patients with or at risk for HIT/HITTS undergoing percutaneous coronary interventions (PCI): ***Aspirin*** 325 mg 2 to 24 hours before planned PCI was administered in studies. After venous or arterial sheaths are in place, begin ***argatroban*** with an initial infusion of 25 mcg/kg/min via a large-bore IV line. Next, administer a bolus of 350 mcg/kg over 3 to 5 minutes. 5 to 10 minutes after completion of the bolus dose, check the ACT. The PCI may proceed if the ACT is greater than 300 seconds but less than 450 seconds. If the ACT is less than 300 seconds, give an additional IV bolus of 150 mcg/kg, increase the infusion rate to 30 mcg/kg/min, and check the ACT in 5 to 10 minutes. If the ACT is greater than 450 seconds, decrease the infusion rate to 15 mcg/kg/min and recheck the ACT in 5 to 10 minutes. When a therapeutic ACT has been achieved (between 300 and 450 seconds), the infusion dose in effect at the time the therapeutic ACT is achieved should be continued for the duration of the procedure. For situations outside these parameters, see Dose Adjustment. If anticoagulation is required after PCI, continue the argatroban, but lower the infusion rate to between 2.5 and 5 mcg/kg/min. Draw an aPTT in 2 hours and adjust the infusion rate as clinically indicated (not to exceed 10 mcg/kg/min) to reach an aPTT between 1.5 and 3 times baseline value (not to exceed 100 seconds); see All situations in Monitor if transfer to oral anticoagulation is indicated.

PEDIATRIC DOSE

Safety and effectiveness for use in children under 18 years of age not established.

DOSE ADJUSTMENTS

Prophylaxis or treatment of thrombosis in patients with or at risk for heparin-induced thrombocytopenia (HIT/HITTS): Reduce initial dose to 0.5 mcg/kg/min in patients with moderate hepatic impairment. There is a four-fold decrease in argatroban clearance in these patients, titrate dose carefully and monitor aPTT closely.

Anticoagulant in patients with or at risk for HIT/HITTS undergoing percutaneous coronary interventions (PCI): In case of dissection, impending abrupt closure, thrombus formation during the procedure, or inability to achieve or maintain an ACT over 300 seconds, additional bolus doses of 150 mcg/kg may be given and the infusion rate increased to 40 mcg/kg/min. Check the ACT after each additional bolus or change in rate of infusion. ■ See Precautions for patients with clinically significant liver disease.

All situations: No dose adjustment indicated in patients with impaired renal function, or based on age or gender.

DILUTION

Each 250 mg vial must be diluted in 250 ml of NS, D5W, or LR to a concentration of 1 mg/ml. Mix by repeated inversion of the diluent bag for a minimum of 1 minute. Solution may initially be briefly hazy.

Storage: Store vials in carton at CRT, protected from light and freezing. Diluted solution stable at CRT for 24 hours if protected from direct sunlight. Stable for 48 hours if refrigerated and in the dark.

COMPATIBILITY

Specific information not available. Manufacturer states, "Should not be mixed with other drugs prior to dilution in a suitable IV fluid." Consider specific use and dose adjustment requirements.

RATE OF ADMINISTRATION

Prophylaxis or treatment of thrombosis in patients with or at risk for heparin-induced thrombocytopenia (HIT/HITTS):

Argatroban Infusion Rates for 2 mcg/kg/min Dose (1 mg/ml Final Concentration)	
Body Weight (kg)	**Infusion Rate (ml/hr)**
50	6
60	7
70	8
80	10
90	11
100	12
110	13
120	14
130	16
140	17

Anticoagulant in patients with or at risk for HIT/HITTS undergoing percutaneous coronary interventions (PCI): See Usual Dose and/or Dose Adjustments for specific rates and criteria.

ACTIONS

An anticoagulant that is a highly selective synthetic direct thrombin inhibitor derived from L-arginine. It reversibly binds to the thrombin active site and exerts its anticoagulant effects by inhibiting thrombin-catalyzed or induced reactions, including fibrin formation; activation of coagulation factors V, VIII, and XIII; protein C; and platelet aggregation. Highly selective for thrombin with little or no effect on related serine proteases (trypsin, factor Xa, plasmin, and kallikrein). Inhibits both free and clot-bound thrombin. Does not require the co-factor antithrombin III for antithrombic activity, and does not interact with heparin-induced antibodies. Produces a dose-dependent increase in aPTT. Anticoagulant effects are immediate. Steady-state levels of both drug and anticoagulant effect are usually attained within 1 to 3 hours and are maintained until the infusion is discontinued or the dose adjusted. Distribution is primarily in the extracellular fluid. Metabolized in the liver. Half-life range is 39 to 51 minutes. Excreted primarily in feces with some excretion in urine.

INDICATIONS AND USES

An anticoagulant for prophylaxis or treatment of thrombosis in patients with heparin-induced thrombocytopenia (HIT). ■ An anticoagulant in patients with or at risk for heparin-induced thrombocytopenia undergoing percutaneous coronary intervention (PCI). May be used in combination with aspirin.

Unlabeled uses: An alternative to heparin during hemodialysis.

CONTRAINDICATIONS

Hypersensitivity to argatroban or any of its components and patients with overt major bleeding.

PRECAUTIONS

All situations: Use with extreme caution in disease states and other circumstances in which there is an increased danger of hemorrhage, including severe hypertension; immediately following lumbar puncture; spinal anesthesia; major surgery, especially involving the brain, spinal cord, or eye; hematologic conditions associated with increased bleeding tendencies such as congenital or acquired bleeding disorders and gastrointestinal lesions such as ulcerations. ■ Concomitant therapy with thrombolytic agents (e.g., alteplase [tPA], reteplase [Retavase], streptokinase) may increase the risk of bleeding, including life-threatening intracranial bleeding; see Drug/Lab Interactions. ■ Safety and effectiveness of argatroban for cardiac indications other than PCI in patients with HIT not established.
Prophylaxis or treatment of thrombosis: Use caution in patients with hepatic disease, argatroban clearance is decreased four-fold and elimination half-life is increased. Full reversal of anticoagulant effect may require longer than 4 hours. See Dose Adjustments.
PCI: Avoid use of high dose of argatroban in PCI patients with clinically significant hepatic disease or AST/ALT levels greater than 3 times the upper limit of normal. These patients were not included in clinical trials.
Monitor: ***All situations:*** Obtain baseline and monitor platelet count, hemoglobin, hematocrit, and occult blood in stool in addition to required aPTT or ACT; see Usual Dose and specific parameters below. ■ Other coagulation tests (e.g., PT, INR, and TT) are affected by argatroban but therapeutic ranges for these tests have not been identified. ■ Observe carefully for symptoms of a hemorrhagic event (e.g., unexplained fall in hematocrit, fall in BP, or any other unexplained symptom). ■ Recovery of platelet count usually occurs by day 3. ■ HIT is a serious, immune-mediated complication of heparin therapy that may result in subsequent venous and arterial thrombosis. Initial treatment of HIT is to discontinue all heparin, but patients still require anticoagulation for prevention and treatment of thromboembolic events. ■ Initiate oral anticoagulation with warfarin (Coumadin) when appropriate. Do not use a loading dose of warfarin, use the expected daily dose. Monitor INR daily. Concurrent use with warfarin results in prolongation of the PT and INR beyond that produced by warfarin alone. With doses of argatroban up to 2 mcg/kg/min, argatroban

can be discontinued when the INR is greater than 4 on combined therapy. After argatroban is discontinued, repeat the INR in 4 to 6 hours. If the INR is below the desired therapeutic range, resume the infusion of argatroban and repeat the procedure daily until the desired therapeutic range on warfarin alone is reached. See Drug/Lab Interactions. With doses of argatroban more than 2 mcg/kg/min the INR relationship is less predictable. Reduction of dose to 2 mcg/kg/min is recommended.

Prophylaxis or treatment of thrombosis: Obtain a baseline aPTT before treatment begins. Repeat aPTT in 2 hours and as indicated to achieve desired target aPTT of 1.5 to 3 times baseline. ■ No enhancement of aPTT response was observed in subjects receiving repeated administration of argatroban. Repeated administration has been tolerated with no loss of anticoagulant activity and no evidence of neutralizing antibodies. No change in dose is required.

PCI: Obtain a baseline ACT before dosing; repeat ACT 5 to 10 minutes after bolus dosing, after a change in the infusion rate, and at the end of the PCI procedure. Draw additional ACTs every 20 to 30 minutes during a prolonged procedure. ■ Follow standard procedures for maintenance and care of venous or arterial sheaths. Remove sheaths no sooner than 2 hours after discontinuing argatroban and when the ACT has decreased to less than 160 seconds. ■ See Dose Adjustments if anticoagulation is required after PCI.

Patient Education: Report all episodes of bleeding. ■ Report tarry stools. ■ Compliance with all measures to minimize bleeding is very important (e.g., avoid use of razors, toothbrushes, other sharp items). ■ Use caution while moving to avoid excess bumping.

Maternal/Child: Category B: use during pregnancy only if clearly needed. ■ Discontinue breast-feeding.

Elderly: Response similar to that in younger patients. See Dose Adjustments for the elderly with impaired liver function.

DRUG/LAB INTERACTIONS

If argatroban is to be initiated after cessation of heparin therapy, allow sufficient time for heparin's effect on the aPTT to decrease. ■ Risk of bleeding may be increased by any medicine that affects blood clotting, including anticoagulants (e.g., heparin, lepirudin [Refludan], warfarin [Coumadin]); glycoprotein GPIIb/IIIa receptor antagonists (e.g., abciximab [ReoPro], eptifibatide [Integrilin], tirofiban [Aggrastat]); any medication that may cause hypoprothrombinemia, thrombocytopenia, or GI ulceration or bleeding (e.g., selected antibiotics such as cefamandole [Mandol], cefoperazone [Cefobid], cefotetan [Cefotan], ticarcillin [Ticar], aspirin, NSAIDs [e.g., ibuprofen (Advil, Motrin), naproxen (Aleve, Naprosyn), phenylbutazone (Butazolidin)]); and/or any other medication that inhibits platelet aggregation (e.g., clopidogrel [Plavix], dipyridamole [Persantine], plicamycin [Mithracin], sulfinpyrazone [Anturane], ticlopidine [Ticlid], valproic acid [Depacon]). If concurrent or subsequent use is indicated monitor aPTT and PT closely. ■ In clinical testing was not found to interact with digoxin or erythromycin (a potent inhibitor of CYP3A4/5). ■ Concurrent use with warfarin results in prolongation of the PT and INR beyond that produced by warfarin alone; see Monitor. The combination causes no further reduction in vitamin K dependent factor Xa than that seen with warfarin alone. Relationship between INR obtained on combined therapy and INR obtained on warfarin alone is dependent on both the dose of argatroban and the thromboplastin reagent used.

SIDE EFFECTS

All situations: Bleeding is the most frequent adverse event. Allergic reactions (e.g., coughing, dyspnea, hypotension, rash) have been reported, most frequently in patients who also received streptokinase or contrast media.

Prophylaxis or treatment of thrombosis: During clinical trials, intracranial bleeding occurred only in patients with AMI receiving argatroban concurrently with thrombolytic therapy with streptokinase. Other bleeding included a decreased hemoglobin and hematocrit, GI bleeding, GU bleeding, hematuria, hemoptysis, limb and below-knee amputation stump, multisystem hemorrhage and DIC, venous access. Abdominal pain, abnormal renal function, arrhythmias (e.g., atrial fibrillation, ventricular tachycardia), cardiac arrest, cerebrovascular disorder, coughing, diarrhea, fever, hypotension, nausea, pain, pneumonia, sepsis, URI, and vomiting have occurred.

PCI: Retroperitoneal and GI bleeding occurred in a few patients. Other minor bleeding included coronary arteries, a decreased hemoglobin and hematocrit; GI bleeding; GU bleeding; hematuria; groin, hemoptysis, and access site (venous or arterial). Abdominal pain, back pain, bradycardia, chest pain, fever, headache, hypotension. MI and other serious coronary events, nausea, and vomiting have occurred.

Overdose: Symptoms of acute toxicity in animals included clonic convulsions, coma, loss of righting reflex, paralysis of hind limbs, and tremors.

ANTIDOTE

No specific antidote is available. Obtain aPTT, ACT, and/or other coagulation tests. Overdose with or without bleeding may be controlled by discontinuing argatroban or by decreasing the infusion dose; aPTT should return to baseline within 2 to 4 hours after discontinuation. Reversal may take longer in patients with hepatic impairment. If life-threatening bleeding develops and excessive plasma levels of argatroban are suspected, immediately stop argatroban infusion. Determine aPTT and hemoglobin and prepare for blood transfusion as appropriate. Follow current guidelines for treatment of shock as indicated (fluid, vasopressors [e.g., dopamine], Trendelenburg position, plasma expanders [e.g., albumin, hetastarch]).

ARSENIC TRIOXIDE

Antineoplastic

(ahr′se-nik tri-ox′id)

Trisenox

pH 7 to 9

USUAL DOSE

12 lead ECG, serum electrolytes (calcium, magnesium, and potassium), and serum creatinine required before beginning therapy; see Monitor.

Induction schedule: 0.15 mg/kg of body weight daily as an infusion until bone marrow remission. Total induction dose should not exceed 60 doses.

Consolidation schedule: Begin 3 to 6 weeks after completion of induction therapy. 0.15 mg/kg daily for 25 doses over a period of up to 5 weeks.

PEDIATRIC DOSE

Children from 5 to 16 years of age: See Usual Dose. See Maternal/Child.

DILUTION

Specific techniques required; see Precautions. Ampule contains 10 mg/10 ml (1 mg/ml). Dilute each daily dose with 100 to 250 ml D5W or NS immediately after withdrawal from the ampule and give as an infusion. **Storage:** Store ampules at CRT. Do not freeze. Do not use beyond expiration date. Discard unused portions of each ampule, contains no preservatives. Diluted solutions are stable for 24 hours at CRT and 48 hours if refrigerated.

COMPATIBILITY

Manufacturer states, "Do not mix arsenic trioxide with other medications."

RATE OF ADMINISTRATION

A single daily dose as an infusion over 1 to 2 hours. May be extended up to 4 hours if acute vasomotor reactions are observed (e.g., flushing, hypertension, hypotension, pallor). May be given through a peripheral vein, a central venous catheter is not required.

ACTIONS

An antineoplastic agent. Mechanism of action not understood. May cause morphologic changes and DNA fragmentation in selected promyelocytic leukemia cells and damage or degrade selected fusion proteins. In clinical trials, medial time to bone marrow remission was 44 days and to onset of complete remission (absence of visible leukemic cells in bone marrow and peripheral recovery of platelets and WBC with a confirmatory bone marrow about 30 days later) was 53 days. Responses were seen in all age groups ranging from 6 to 72 years. Metabolized in the liver (not by the cytochrome P_{450} family of isoenzymes). Arsenic is stored mainly in liver, kidney, heart, lung, hair, and nails. Excreted in urine. Crosses the placental barrier. Secreted in breast milk.

INDICATIONS AND USES

Induction of remission and consolidation in patients with acute promyelocytic leukemia (APL) who are refractory to, or have relapsed from, retinoid and anthracycline chemotherapy, and whose APL is characterized by the presence of the t(15;17) translocation or PML/RAR-alpha gene expression. ■ Orphan drug approval for treatment of chronic myeloid leukemia (CML) and acute myelocytic leukemia (AML).

Unlabeled uses: As a single agent or in combination with imatinib (Gleevec) to treat patients with CML in chronic, accelerated, and blast crisis.

CONTRAINDICATIONS

Known hypersensitivity to arsenic.

PRECAUTIONS

Follow guidelines for handling cytotoxic agents. See Appendix A, p. 1142. ■ Administered by or under the direction of a physician experienced in the management of patients with acute leukemia, with facilities for monitoring the patient and responding to any medical emergency. ■ Symptoms similar to those associated with retinoic-acid-Acute Promyelocytic Leukemia (RA-APL) or APL differentiation syndrome (dyspnea, fever, pleural or pericardial effusions, pulmonary infiltrates, and weight gain with or without leukocytosis) have been reported in some patients treated with arsenic trioxide and can be fatal. See Monitor and Antidote. ■ May cause QT interval prolongation and complete atrioventricular block. QT prolongation can lead to torsade de pointes, which can be fatal. Risk of torsade de pointes is increased by extent of QT prolongation, concomitant administration of QT prolonging drugs, a history of torsade de pointes, pre-existing QT interval prolongation, congestive heart failure, administration of potassium-wasting diuretics, or other conditions that result in hypokalemia or hypomagnesemia; see Drug/Lab Interactions. QT prolongation was observed between 1 and 5 weeks after infusion and returned toward baseline by the end of 8 weeks after infusions were complete. ■ Has been associated with the development of hyperleukocytosis. WBC counts during induction were higher than during consolidation. Treatment with additional chemotherapy was not required. ■ Use caution in patients with impaired renal function, no dose adjustment recommended, but monitoring of serum creatinine may be indicated; renal excretion is the main route of elimination. ■ Not studied in patients with impaired hepatic function. ■ Thrombocytopenia with disseminated intravascular coagulation (DIC) and bleeding may occur in patients with acute promyelocytic leukemia. Arsenic trioxide may improve symptoms.

Monitor: ***Before initiating therapy:*** Obtain baseline 12 lead ECG, CBC with differential, platelet count, hemoglobin, hematocrit, coagulation profile (e.g., PT), serum electrolytes (e.g., calcium, magnesium, and potassium), and serum creatinine. Correct pre-existing electrolyte abnormalities and if possible, discontinue drugs that are known to prolong the QT interval; see Drug/Lab Interactions. If the QT interval is greater than 500 msec, corrective measures should be completed and the QT interval reassessed with serial ECGs before starting arsenic trioxide. ***During therapy:*** Monitor electrolytes, CBC including differential, platelet count, hemoglobin, hematocrit, and coagulation profile (e.g., PT) at least twice weekly during induction and weekly during consolidation. May be indicated more frequently. Keep potassium concentrations above 4 mEq/dl and magnesium concentrations above 1.8 mg/dl. ■ Monitor ECG weekly and more frequently in unstable patients. No data on the effect of arsenic trioxide on the QT interval during the infusion. If the QT interval is greater than 500 msec at any time during therapy, reassess the patient, correct concomitant risk factors, and consider risk/benefit of continuing versus suspending arsenic trioxide. If syncope, rapid or irregular heartbeat develops, the patient should be hospitalized for ECG monitoring, and monitoring of serum electrolytes. Temporarily discontinue arsenic trioxide. Do not resume therapy until the QT interval is less than 460 msec, electrolyte abnormalities are corrected, and the syncope and irregular heartbeat cease. ■ Monitor for thrombocytopenia (platelet count less than 50,000/mm^3). Initiate precautions to prevent excessive bleeding (e.g., inspect IV sites, skin, and mucous membranes; use extreme care during invasive procedures; test urine, emesis, stool, and secretions for occult blood). ■ Monitor for signs of APL differentiation syndrome (i.e., abnormal chest auscultatory findings or radiographic abnormalities, dyspnea, weight gain, and unexplained fever). If symptoms occur, irrespective of the leukocyte count, begin immediate treatment with high-dose steroids (e.g., dexamethasone 10 mg IV BID); continue for at least 3 days or longer until S/S resolve. Termination of arsenic trioxide treatment is not usually required.

Patient Education: Avoid pregnancy, may cause fetal harm. Nonhormonal birth control recommended. Notify physician immediately if a pregnancy is suspected. ■ Report dizziness, dyspnea, fainting, fever, rapid or irregular heartbeat, and weight gain immediately. ■ Review all prescription and nonprescription drugs with your physician. ■ See Appendix D, p. 1148.

Maternal/Child: Category D: avoid pregnancy. May cause fetal harm. Effective birth control required. ■ Discontinue breast-feeding. ■ Limited clinical data for pediatric use. Five patients ranging in age from 5 to 16 years were included in clinical studies, 3 achieved a complete response. ■ Safety and effectiveness for children under 5 years of age not established.

Elderly: Response similar to that in younger patients. ■ Monitor renal function closely.

DRUG/LAB INTERACTIONS

Concurrent use with other drugs that prolong the QT interval, including antiarrhythmics (e.g., amiodarone [Cordarone], disopyramide [Norpace], ibutilide [Corvert], mexiletine [Mexitil], procainamide [Pronestyl], quinidine), antihistamines, azole antifungals (e.g., itraconazole [Sporanox]), fluoroquinolones (e.g., levofloxacin [Levaquin]), phenothiazines (e.g., thioridazine [Mellaril]), and tricyclic antidepressants (e.g., amitriptyline [Elavil]) may cause torsade de pointes and could be fatal. ■ Concurrent use with drugs that may cause hypokalemia or other electrolyte abnormalities (e.g., amphotericin B, diuretics [e.g., furosemide (Lasix)]) may increase the risk of hypokalemia and cardiac arrhythmias.

SIDE EFFECTS

Abdominal pain, anemia, chest pain, cough, diarrhea, dizziness, dyspnea, edema, fatigue, headache, hyperglycemia, hyperkalemia, hypertension, hypokalemia, hypomagnesemia, hypotension, hypoxia, itching, leukocytosis, nausea, neutropenia (may be febrile), palpitations, pleural effusion, rash, thrombocytopenia, URI, and vomiting. Numerous other side effects have been reported (see literature).

Major: Adverse events rated grade 3 or 4 on the NCI Common Toxicity Criteria were common. APL differentiation syndrome, atrial arrhythmias, hyperglycemia, hyperleukocytosis, QT interval 500 msec or more (with or without torsade de pointes) also occurred.

Overdose: Acute arsenic toxicity (e.g., confusion, convulsions, and muscle weakness).

ANTIDOTE

Keep physician informed of all side effects. Those classified as average will usually be treated symptomatically. Major side effects may be fatal and require aggressive treatment as well as temporarily withholding or discontinuing arsenic trioxide. In all situations, monitor electrolytes; maintain potassium and magnesium within prescribed limits. Treat APL differentiation syndrome immediately with high-dose steroids (dexamethasone [Decadron] 10 mg IV BID) for at least 3 days or until signs and symptoms resolve (interruption of arsenic trioxide therapy not consistently required). Temporarily discontinue arsenic trioxide for QT prolongation 500 msec or more; see Monitor for recommendations and treat any serious or symptomatic arrhythmia (e.g., conduction abnormalities, VT, torsade de pointes) promptly. Discontinue therapy and treat acute arsenic intoxication with dimercaprol (BAL) 3 mg/kg IM every 4 hours until immediate life-threatening toxicity subsides. Then treat with penicillamine 250 mg PO up to four times a day (approximately 1 Gm/day). Hyperleukocytosis was not treated with additional chemotherapy during clinical trials.

ASCORBIC ACID

(a-skor′bic as′id)

Nutritional supplement (vitamin)

Cenolate, ✤Redoxon, Sodium Ascorbate, Vitamin C

pH 5.5 to 7

USUAL DOSE

Up to 6 Gm/24 hr has been given without toxicity.

Nutritional protection: 70 to 150 mg daily. 100 to 200 mg daily may be required during chronic dialysis.

Prevention or treatment of scurvy: 100 to 250 mg 1 to 3 times daily. Give for a minimum of several days; up to 2 to 3 weeks may be indicated.

Enhance wound healing: 300 to 500 mg daily for 7 to 10 days.

Burns: 1 to 2 Gm daily.

PEDIATRIC DOSE

Nutritional protection: 30 mg daily. ***Premature infants*** may require 75 to 100 mg daily.

Prevention or treatment of scurvy: 100 to 300 mg/24 hr. Give in divided doses. Give for a minimum of several days; up to 2 to 3 weeks may be indicated.

DILUTION

May be given undiluted or may be administered diluted in IV infusion solutions. Soluble in the more commonly used solutions, such as D5W, D5NS, NS, LR, Ringer's injection, or sodium lactate injection. Slight coloration does not affect the medication.

Storage: Protect from freezing and from light.

COMPATIBLE WITH **(Underline Indicates Conflicting Compatibility Information)**

Consult pharmacist; specific conditions may apply; see Compatibilities, p. xvi.

Additive: Amikacin (Amikin), aminophylline, calcium chloride, calcium gluconate, chloramphenicol (Chloromycetin), chlorpromazine (Thorazine), colistimethate (Coly-Mycin M), diphenhydramine (Benadryl), erythromycin lactobionate (Erythrocin), heparin, hydrocortisone sodium succinate (Solu-Cortef), kanamycin (Kantrex), methyldopate (Aldomet), penicillin G potassium, prochlorperazine (Compazine), promethazine (Phenergan), verapamil (Isoptin).

Syringe: Metoclopramide (Reglan).

Y-site: Warfarin (Coumadin).

RATE OF ADMINISTRATION

IV injection: 100 mg or fraction thereof over 1 minute.

Infusion: Administer at ordered rate for standard infusion (e.g., over 4 to 8 hours).

ACTIONS

This water-soluble vitamin is necessary for the formation of collagen in all fibrous tissue, carbohydrate metabolism, connective tissue repair, maintenance of intracellular stability of blood vessels, and many other body functions. Not stored in the body. Daily requirements must be met. Completely utilized; excess is excreted unchanged in the urine. Crosses placental barrier. Secreted in breast milk.

INDICATIONS AND USES

Prevention and treatment of vitamin C deficiency, which may lead to scurvy. ■ Give pre-op and post-op to enhance wound healing. ■ Prolonged IV therapy. ■ Increased vitamin requirements or replacement therapy in severe burns, extensive injuries, and severe infections. ■ Prematurity. ■ Deficient intestinal absorption of water-soluble vitamins. ■ Prolonged or wasting diseases. ■ Hemovascular disorders and delayed fracture and wound healing require increased intake.

CONTRAINDICATIONS

There are no absolute contraindications.

PRECAUTIONS

Vitamin C is better absorbed and utilized by IM injection. ■ Use caution in cardiac patients. Sodium or calcium content may antagonize other drugs or overall condition. ■ Use caution in diabetics and patients prone to recurrent renal calculi or undergoing stool occult blood tests. May contain sulfites; use caution in allergic individuals.

Monitor: Increased urinary excretion is diagnostic for vitamin C saturation. ■ Continue curative doses until clinical symptoms subside or urinary saturation occurs.

Maternal/Child: Use caution in pregnancy; high dose may adversely affect fetus.

DRUG/LAB INTERACTIONS

Potentiates oral contraceptives, ferrous iron absorption, salicylates, and sulfonamides. ■ May antagonize anticoagulants. ■ 2 Gm/day will lower urine pH and will cause reabsorption of acidic drugs and crystallization with sulfonamides. ■ May inhibit phenothiazines. ■ Plasma levels decreased by smoking cigarettes; increased doses of ascorbic acid may be required. ■ May cause false-negative occult blood in stool. ■ May cause false-positive or false-negative in urine glucose tests. ■ Can alter numerous test results; must be individually evaluated.

SIDE EFFECTS

Occur only with too-rapid injection: temporary dizziness or faintness. Diarrhea or renal calculi may occur with large doses.

ANTIDOTE

Discontinue administration temporarily. Resume administration at a decreased rate. If side effects persist, discontinue drug and notify the physician.

ASPARAGINASE

(a-spare′a-gi-nase)

Elspar, ✤Kidrolase

Antineoplastic (enzyme)

pH 7.4

USUAL DOSE

Skin test: Required before initial dose and whenever 7 days or more elapse between doses. See Dilution for preparation. Give 2 IU intradermally and observe for 1 hour for the appearance of a wheal or erythema.

Intermittent IV: Very specific amount to be given on a specific day or days in a specific regimen of other chemotherapeutic agents, i.e., 1,000 IU/kg of body weight/day for 10 successive days beginning on day 22 of regimen with specific prednisone and vincristine doses. When used as a single agent (rare), the usual dose for adults and children is 200 IU/kg/day for 28 days.

Desensitization process for administration: Extensive process. See drug literature.

DILUTION

Specific techniques required; see Precautions. Initially reconstitute each 10-ml vial (10,000 IU) with 4 ml of SW for Kidrolase and 5 ml of SW or NS for Elspar. Both result in 2,000 IU/ml.

Skin test: Withdraw 0.1 ml from the above solution and further dilute with 9.9 ml NS (20 IU/ml). 0.1 ml of this solution equals 2 IU.

Intermittent IV: Use 2,000 IU/ml solution. Should be further diluted with 50 to 100 ml of D5W or NS and administered as an infusion through Y-tube or three-way stopcock of a free-flowing infusion of D5W or NS. Use only clear solutions. May contain fiberlike particles; use of 5-micron filter recommended.

Storage: Refrigerate before and after dilution. Discard Elspar after 8 hours. Reconstituted Kidrolase may be refrigerated up to 14 days. Discard any solution that is cloudy.

COMPATIBLE WITH

Consult pharmacist; specific conditions may apply; see Compatibilities, p. xvi.

Y-site: Methotrexate (Folex), sodium bicarbonate.

RATE OF ADMINISTRATION

Intermittent IV: Each dose evenly distributed over at least 30 minutes.

ACTIONS

An enzyme derived from *Escherichia coli* that rapidly depletes asparagine from cells. Some malignant cells have a metabolic defect that makes them dependent on exogenous asparagine for survival, but they are unable to synthesize asparagine as normal cells do. Undergoes metabolic degradation. Range of plasma half-life is 8 to 30 hours. Trace amounts excreted in urine.

INDICATIONS AND USES

Induces remissions in acute lymphocytic leukemia. Primarily used in specific combinations with other chemotherapeutic agents. ■ May be useful in other leukemias and non-Hodgkin's lymphoma.

CONTRAINDICATIONS

Hypersensitivity to asparaginase, pancreatitis, or history of pancreatitis.

PRECAUTIONS

Follow guidelines for handling cytotoxic agents. See Appendix A, p. 1142. ■ A lethal drug; administered by or under the direction of the physician specialist. ■ Rarely used as a single agent; not recommended for maintenance therapy. ■ Impairs liver function; may increase toxicity of other drugs.

Monitor: Toxicity and short-term effectiveness limit use. More toxic in adults than in children. ■ Avoid giving at night. ■ Observe patient carefully during and after infusion. Monitor BP every 15 minutes for at least 1 hour. ■ Appropriate treatment for anaphylaxis must always be available. Risk increased if patient has received asparaginase before. ■ Allopurinol, increased fluid intake, and alkalinization of the urine may be required to reduce uric acid levels. ■ Frequent blood cell counts, bone marrow evaluation, serum amylase, blood sugar, and evaluation of liver and kidney function are necessary. ■ Nausea and vomiting can be severe. Prophylactic administration of antiemetics recommended to increase patient comfort. ■ Predisposition to infection probable. Prophylactic antibiotics may be indicated pending results of C/S in a febrile neutropenic patient. ■ Monitor for thrombocytopenia (platelet count less than 50,000/mm^3). Initiate precautions to prevent excessive bleeding (e.g., inspect IV sites, skin, and mucous membranes; use extreme care during invasive procedures; test urine, emesis, stool, and secretions for occult blood).

Patient Education: Report all symptoms promptly; verbalize all questions. ■ Assess birth control requirements. Nonhormonal contraception advised. ■ See Appendix D, p. 1148.

Maternal/Child: Category C: will have teratogenic effects on the fetus. Evaluate benefit versus risk for anyone who is pregnant or may become pregnant. ■ Discontinue breast-feeding.

Elderly: Toxicity may be more severe. ■ Consider age-related organ impairment.

DRUG/LAB INTERACTIONS

Toxicity of all agents may be increased if asparaginase is given before or concurrently with vincristine and prednisone. May be less pronounced if asparaginase is given 12 to 24 hours after vincristine and prednisone. ■ Blocks the effects of methotrexate for as long as asparagine concentrations are suppressed. Some suggest administering asparaginase 24 hours after methotrexate; others suggest these agents should not be used together while asparagine concentrations are suppressed. ■ May interfere with thyroid function test interpretation. ■ Do not administer any live vaccine to patients receiving antineoplastic drugs. ■ See Precautions.

SIDE EFFECTS

Occur frequently (usually within 30 minutes), even with the initial dose, and may cause death. Allergic reactions including anaphylaxis (even if skin test negative and/or allergic symptoms have not occurred with previous doses), agitation, azotemia, bleeding, bone marrow depression, coma, confusion, depression, fatigue, hallucinations, hyperglycemia, hyperthermia (fatal), pulmonary embolism or thrombosis from hypofibrinogenemia and depression of other clotting factors, nausea and vomiting, fulminating pancreatitis (fatal).

ANTIDOTE

Notify physician of all side effects. Asparaginase may have to be discontinued until recovery or permanently discontinued. Symptomatic and supportive treatment is indicated. Treat anaphylaxis with epinephrine, corticosteroids, oxygen, and antihistamines. There is no specific antidote.

ATENOLOL

(a-ten'oh-lol)

Beta-adrenergic blocking agent

Tenormin

pH 5.5 to 6.5

USUAL DOSE

5 mg. Initiate as soon as the patient's hemodynamic condition has stabilized and eligibility has been established. If initial dose is well tolerated, repeat in 10 minutes. If full IV dose is well tolerated, give 50 mg PO 10 minutes after last bolus. Repeat in 12 hours. Follow with an oral maintenance dose of 100 mg daily or 50 mg twice a day for 6 to 9 days or until discharged from hospital. Discontinue if bradycardia, hypotension requiring treatment, or other untoward effects occur (e.g., bronchospasm, cardiac arrest, cardiac failure, cardiogenic shock, first-degree heart block, reinfarction). Best results achieved if administered within 2 to 4 hours of symptom onset or thrombolytic therapy.

Used concurrently with digitalis, alpha-adrenergic blockers (e.g., phentolamine [Regitine]), vasodilators (e.g., nitroglycerin), and clot-dissolving drugs (e.g., alteplase recombinant [tPA]), as indicated.

Unstable angina (unlabeled): 5 mg IV over 5 minutes for up to 3 doses. Follow with 25 to 100 mg/day PO.

DOSE ADJUSTMENTS

Use with caution and reduce dose by one half in patients with asthma or other bronchospastic disease. Isoproterenol (Isuprel) should be available. ■ Reduced dose may be indicated in patients already taking a beta blocker (e.g., propranolol [Inderal]). Titrate by clinical observations. ■ Dosing should be cautious in the elderly. Consider potential for decreased cardiac, hepatic, and renal function; concomitant disease; or other drug therapy. ■ Reduce oral follow-up dose to 50 mg daily in patients with a CrCl of 15 to 35 ml/min/1.73 M^2 and to 50 mg every other day with a CrCl less than 15 ml/min/1.73 M^2.

DILUTION

May be given undiluted by IV injection or diluted in 10 to 50 ml NS or dextrose solutions in water or saline and given as an infusion.

Storage: Stable for 48 hours after dilution.

COMPATIBLE WITH

Consult pharmacist; specific conditions may apply; see Compatibilities, p. xvi.

Y-site: Meperidine (Demerol), meropenem (Merrem IV), morphine.

RATE OF ADMINISTRATION

Distribute a single dose evenly over 5 minutes. Monitor ECG, HR, and BP and discontinue atenolol if adverse symptoms occur (bradycardia less than 45 beats/min, heart block greater than first degree, systolic BP less than 90 mm Hg, or moderate to severe cardiac failure).

ACTIONS

Atenolol is a cardioselective ($beta_1$-) adrenergic blocking agent. Its mechanism of action in patients with suspected or definite myocardial infarction is not known. Reduces HR, cardiac output, BP, and myocardial oxygen consumption. Promotes redistribution of blood flow from adequately supplied areas of the heart to ischemic areas. May also reduce chest pain. It reduces the incidence of recurrent myocardial infarctions (MI) and reduces the size of the infarct and the incidence of fatal arrhythmias. Inhibits isoproterenol-induced tachycardia and reduces reflex orthostatic tachycardia. Well distributed throughout the body. Peak plasma levels are reached within 5 minutes and decline rapidly over approximately 7 hours. Undergoes little or no metabolism by the liver. Excreted in urine. Crosses the placental barrier. Secreted in breast milk.

INDICATIONS AND USES

An additional treatment to standard Coronary Care therapy. Reduces cardiac mortality, recurrent MI, and incidence of ventricular fibrillation in hemodynamically stable individuals with suspected or definite MI. ■ Reduces incidence of ventricular fibrillation in post-MI patients who do not receive thrombolytic agents. ■ Used within 2 to 4 hours of thrombolytic agents, may reduce rate of nonfatal reinfarction and recurrent ischemia; used within 2 hours of symptom onset, may reduce mortality and recurrent MI. ■ Oral form also used to treat hypertension and angina pectoris.

Unlabeled uses: Treatment of unstable angina.

CONTRAINDICATIONS

Cardiogenic shock, heart block greater than first degree, overt cardiac failure, and sinus bradycardia. History of hypersensitivity to atenolol or its components. Not recommended for use in patients with untreated pheochromocytoma.

PRECAUTIONS

Usually administered in an intensive care setting under the direction of the physician specialist with facilities for monitoring the patient and responding to any medical emergency. ■ Use caution in the presence of heart failure. ■ Use caution in heart failure controlled by digitalis; both drugs slow AV conduction. ■ Use caution in any patient with lung disease and/or bronchospasm. Use suggested only in those patients who do not respond to or cannot tolerate other antihypertensive treatment. ■ May mask tachycardia occurring with hypoglycemia in diabetes and tachycardia of hyperthyroidism. Abrupt withdrawal in patients with thyroid disease may precipitate a thyroid storm. ■ Discontinuation of beta-blockers before OR is controversial (beta blockade interferes with cardiac response to reflex stimuli and can cause severe hypotension and difficulty starting or maintaining a heartbeat during surgery); however, some authorities recommend administering throughout the perioperative period. May cause arrhythmia, angina, MI, or death if stopped abruptly. ■ If withdrawal of atenolol is planned, reduce oral dose gradually over approximately 2 weeks to avoid rebound angina, MI, or ventricular arrhythmias.

Monitor: Continuous ECG, HR, and BP monitoring are mandatory during administration of IV atenolol. ■ See Precautions, Drug/Lab Interactions, and Antidote.

Patient Education: Report any breathing difficulty promptly. ■ Avoid pregnancy if oral atenolol is prescribed. Nonhormonal birth control recommended.

Maternal/Child: Category D: avoid use during pregnancy; may cause fetal harm. ■ Use with caution during breast-feeding; clinically significant bradycardia has been reported in breast-feeding infants. ■ Safety for use in children not established. ■ Premature infants or infants with impaired renal function are at increased risk for adverse effects.

Elderly: Response similar to younger adults; however, dosing should be cautious; see Dose Adjustments. ■ Reduced benefit noted in elderly patients with suspected acute MI and a systolic BP less than 120 mm Hg. ■ Serum levels increased and half-life markedly extended in the elderly; monitor renal function. ■ Monitor BP.

DRUG/LAB INTERACTIONS

Synergistic with digitalis; both drugs slow AV conduction; see Precautions. ■ Beta-adrenergic blocking agents may be inhibited by NSAIDs (e.g., ibuprofen [Advil, Motrin], naproxen [Aleve, Naprosyn]), sympathomimetics (e.g., epinephrine, norepinephrine, isoproterenol [Isuprel], dopamine [Intropin], dobutamine [Dobutrex]), and ritodrine. ■ May potentiate catecholamine-depleting drugs (e.g., reserpine), lidocaine, prazosin (Minipress), disopyramide (Norpace), and verapamil (Isoptin). ■ Use with calcium channel blockers (e.g., diltiazem [Cardizem], verapamil [Isoptin]) may potentiate both drugs and result in severe depression of myocardium and AV conduction and severe hypotension. ■ May cause severe hypotension and/or bradycardia with catecholamine-depleting drugs (e.g., reserpine); observe patient closely. ■ Use with clonidine may precipitate acute hypertension. May aggravate rebound hypertension if clonidine stopped abruptly; discontinue atenolol several days before gradual withdrawal of clonidine. ■ Some authorities recommend that beta-adrenergic blockers be discontinued 48 hours before major surgery (beta blockage interferes with cardiac response to reflex stimuli). If continued, use caution administering general anesthetics that depress the myocardium (e.g., cyclopropane, trichloroethylene). ■ May be potentiated by atropine.

SIDE EFFECTS

Bradycardia and hypotension are most common. Other side effects include AV conduction delays, bradyarrhythmias, bronchospasm, cardiac arrest, cardiac failure, cardiac reinfarction, cold extremities, depression, diarrhea, dizziness, dreaming, drowsiness, dyspnea, fatigue, heart block, hypoglycemia, hypotension, leg pain, lethargy, light-headedness, nausea, postural hypotension, pulmonary emboli, respiratory distress (severe), supraventricular tachycardia, ventricular tachycardia, vertigo, wheezing. Death has been reported.

Overdose: Bradycardia, bronchospasm, CHF, hypoglycemia, hypotension, lethargy, respiratory distress (severe), sinus pause, wheezing.

ANTIDOTE

For any side effect, discontinue the drug and notify the physician immediately. Physician may elect to continue atenolol at a reduced dose. Patients with MI may be more hemodynamically unstable; treat with caution. Bradycardia and hypotension may respond spontaneously after atenolol discontinued. If indicated, use atropine for bradycardia; use isoproterenol with caution if atropine is not effective. Glucagon, 5 to 10 mg IV, may be effective if atropine and isoproterenol are not (unlabeled use). Transvenous cardiac pacing may be needed. Treatment of heart block may require isoproterenol or a transverse cardiac pacemaker. Treat hypotension with IV fluids if indicated or vasopressors (e.g., dopamine [Intropin], norepinephrine [levarterenol]). Treat cause of hypotension (e.g., bradycardia) and monitor BP continuously. Use all vasopressors with extreme caution; severe hypotension can result. Use digitalis and diuretics at first signs of cardiac failure; glucagon has been reported to be useful. If symptoms continue after adequate treatment, discontinue atenolol. Use a $beta_2$ stimulant (e.g., aminophylline, isoproterenol, or terbutaline [Brethine]) with extreme care for bronchospasm. Use IV glucose for hypoglycemia. Treat other side effects symptomatically and resuscitate as necessary. Hemodialysis is effective in overdose.

ATRACURIUM BESYLATE

(a-tra-kyoor′ee-um bes′uh-lat)

Neuromuscular blocking agent (nondepolarizing)
Anesthesia adjunct

Atracurium besylate PF, Tracrium

pH 3.25 to 3.65

USUAL DOSE

Adjunct to general anesthesia for adults and children over 2 years of age: Must be individualized, depending on previous drugs administered and degree and length of muscle relaxation required. 0.4 to 0.5 mg/kg of body weight initially as an IV bolus. Must be used with adequate anesthesia and/or sedation and after unconsciousness induced. Determine need for maintenance dose based on beginning symptoms of neuromuscular blockade reversal determined by a peripheral nerve stimulator. To maintain muscle relaxation a maintenance dose may be given as a bolus injection of 0.08 to 0.10 mg/kg and is required in approximately 25 to 40 minutes and every 15 to 25 minutes. May alternately be given as a continuous IV infusion of 2 to 15 mcg/kg/min. Repeated doses have no cumulative effect if recovery is allowed to begin before administration.

Adjunct to general anesthesia for infants and children 1 month to 2 years of age: 0.3 to 0.4 mg/kg for infants and children under halothane anesthesia. See Usual Dose for maintenance dose; may be required on a more frequent basis.

Support of intubated, mechanically ventilated, or respiratory-controlled adult ICU patients (unlabeled): An initial infusion rate of 11 to 13 mcg/kg/min (range 4.5 to 29.5) provides adequate neuromuscular blockade. Published reports describe a wide interpatient variability in dosing requirements for maintenance ranging from 2.3 to 23 mcg/kg/min (0.14 to 1.38 mg/kg/hr) in adult ICU patients. Occasional adult patients have needed very high infusion rates (greater than 60 mcg/kg/min). In ***pediatric*** ICU patients maintenance doses ranged from 10 to 30 mcg/kg/min (0.6 to 1.8 mg/kg/hr). A specific initial dose for pediatric patients has not yet been defined.

DOSE ADJUSTMENTS

Reduce dose by one third (0.25 to 0.35 mg/kg) if isoflurane or enflurane are used as general anesthetics. ■ Reduce dose to 0.3 to 0.4 mg/kg if using halothane anesthetic, in patients with a history of cardiovascular disease, or a history suggesting greater risk of histamine release (allergies), or following succinylcholine administration. Succinylcholine must show signs of wearing off before atracurium is given. Use caution. ■ Reduce maintenance dose by one half where hypothermia is induced (e.g., cardiac bypass). ■ See Drug/Lab Interactions.

DILUTION

Initial IV bolus may be given undiluted. Maintenance dose for anesthesia and mechanical ventilation support must be further diluted in NS, D5W, or D5NS and given as a continuous infusion titrated to symptoms of neuromuscular blockade reversal. 20 mg (2 ml) diluted in 98 ml yields 200 mcg/ml (0.2 mg/ml). 50 mg (5 ml) diluted in 95 ml yields 500 mcg/ml (0.5 mg/ml).

Storage: Refrigerate. Diluted solution stable for 24 hours refrigerated or at room temperature.

COMPATIBLE WITH

Consult pharmacist; specific conditions may apply; see Compatibilities, p. xvi.

Additive: Bretylium (Bretylate), cimetidine (Tagamet), dobutamine (Dobutrex), dopamine (Intropin), esmolol (Brevibloc), gentamicin (Garamycin), isoproterenol (Isuprel), lidocaine, morphine, potassium chloride (KCl), procainamide (Pronestyl), vancomycin (Vancocin).

Syringe: Alfentanil (Alfenta), fentanyl (Sublimaze), midazolam (Versed), sufentanil (Sufenta).

Y-site: Cefazolin (Kefzol), cefuroxime (Zinacef), cimetidine, (Tagamet), dexmedetomidine (Precedex), dobutamine (Dobutrex), dopamine (Intropin), epinephrine (Adrenalin), esmolol (Brevibloc), etomidate (Amidate), fentanyl (Sublimaze), gentamicin (Garamycin), heparin, hetastarch in electrolytes (Hextend), hydrocortisone sodium succinate (Solu-Cortef), isoproterenol (Isuprel), lorazepam (Ativan), midazolam (Versed), milrinone (Primacor), morphine, nitroglycerin (Nitro-Bid IV), nitroprusside sodium, ranitidine (Zantac), sulfamethoxazole-trimethoprim (Bactrim), vancomycin (Vancocin).

RATE OF ADMINISTRATION

In adults or children, adjust infusion rate according to clinical assessment of the patient's response. Use of a peripheral nerve stimulator is recommended.

Adjunct to general anesthesia: Initial IV bolus over 30 to 60 seconds.

Maintenance dose: In the 200 mcg/ml dilution, 5 mcg/kg/min will be delivered by a rate of 0.025 ml/kg/min or 1.75 ml/min for a 70-kg patient. Adjust rate to specific dose desired. Drug literature has additional rate calculations.

Mechanical ventilation support in ICU: See Usual Dose for specific rates and criteria.

ACTIONS

A nondepolarizing skeletal muscle relaxant with duration of blockade one third to one half that of tubocurarine chloride (curare). A less potent histamine releaser than tubocurarine or metocurine. Causes paralysis by interfering with neural transmission at the myoneural junction. Onset of action is dose dependent. Produces maximum neuromuscular blockade within 3 to 5 minutes and lasts about 25 minutes. When infusion is discontinued, some recovery occurs within 30 minutes. Recovery to 75% averages 60 minutes (range 32 to 108 minutes). It may be several hours before complete recovery occurs. Excreted as metabolites in bile and urine. Crosses the placental barrier.

INDICATIONS AND USES

Adjunctive to general anesthesia to facilitate endotracheal intubation and to relax skeletal muscles during surgery or mechanical ventilation.

Unlabeled uses: Support of intubated, mechanically ventilated, or respiratory-controlled patients in ICU.

CONTRAINDICATIONS

Known hypersensitivity to atracurium.

PRECAUTIONS

For IV use only. ■ Administered by or under the observation of the anesthesiologist. ■ Use extreme caution in patients with significant cardiovascular disease or a history of allergies or allergic reaction. ■ Myasthenia gravis and other neuromuscular diseases increase sensitivity to drug. Can cause critical reactions. ■ Respiratory depression with propofol (Diprivan) or morphine may be preferred in some patients requiring mechanical ventilation. ■ Bradycardia is fairly common since atracurium will not counteract the bradycardia produced by many anesthetic agents or vagal stimulation. ■ Acid-base and/or electrolyte imbalance, debilitation, hypoxic episodes, and/or the use of other drugs (e.g., broad-spectrum antibiotics, narcotics, steroids) may prolong the effects of atracurium.

Monitor: This drug produces apnea. Controlled artificial ventilation with oxygen must be continuous and under direct observation at all times. Maintain a patent airway. ■ Use a peripheral nerve stimulator to monitor response to atracurium and avoid overdose. ■ Patient may be conscious and completely unable to communicate by any means. Has no analgesic or sedative properties. ■ Action potentiated by hypokalemia and some carcinomas. ■ Action is altered by dehydration, electrolyte imbalance, body temperature, and acid-base imbalance. ***Mechanical ventilation support in ICU:*** Physical therapy is recommended to prevent muscular weakness, atrophy, and joint contracture. Muscular weakness may be first noticed during attempts to wean patient from the ventilator.

Maternal/Child: Category C: use in pregnancy only if use justifies potential risk to fetus. Has been used during cesarean section; monitor infant carefully. ■ Use caution during breast-feeding. ■ Safety for use in infants under 1 month of age not established. ■ Contains benzyl alcohol; may cause "gasping syndrome" in premature infants.

Elderly: No adjustments identified.

DRUG/LAB INTERACTIONS

Potentiated by general anesthetics (e.g., enflurane, isoflurane, halothane), many antibiotics (e.g., lincosamides [clindamycin (Cleocin)], aminoglycosides [kanamycin (Kantrex), gentamicin (Garamycin)], polypeptides [bacitracin, colistimethate]), corticosteroids, diuretics, diazepam (Valium) and other muscle relaxants, magnesium sulfate, meperidine, morphine, procainamide (Pronestyl), quinidine, succinylcholine, verapamil, and others. May need to reduce dose of atracurium; use with caution. ■ Duration of neuromuscular block may be shorter and dose requirements may be higher during maintenance infusion in patients stabilized on carbamazepine (Tegretol) and phenytoin (Dilantin). ■ Antagonized by acetylcholine, anticholinesterases, azathioprine, and theophylline. ■ Succinylcholine must show signs of wearing off before atracurium is given. Use caution.

SIDE EFFECTS

Prolonged action resulting in respiratory insufficiency or apnea. Airway closure caused by relaxation of epiglottis, pharynx, and tongue muscles. Hypersensitivity reactions including anaphylaxis are possible. Bradycardia, bronchospasm, dyspnea, flushing, histamine release, hypotension, laryngospasm, reaction at injection site, shock, and tachycardia may occur. Rare reports of seizures with use of atracurium in ICU could be caused by other conditions or medications. Malignant hyperthermia is rare but may occur.

ANTIDOTE

All side effects are medical emergencies. Treat symptomatically. Controlled artificial ventilation must be continuous. Pyridostigmine (Mestinon) or neostigmine (Prostigmin) given with atropine will probably reverse the muscle relaxation. Not effective in all situations; may aggravate severe overdosage. Resuscitate as necessary.

ATROPINE SULFATE

(a'troe-peen sul'fat)

Anticholinergic
Antiarrhythmic
Antidote

pH 3.5 to 6.5

USUAL DOSE

Bradyarrhythmias: 0.4- to 1-mg bolus repeated every 3 to 5 minutes up to a total dose of 2 mg can be used to achieve a desired pulse rate above 60. AHA guidelines recommend 0.5 to 1 mg every 3 to 5 minutes as needed, the ***total dose not to exceed 0.04 mg/kg.*** The use of shorter dosing intervals (3 minutes) and higher maximum dose range (0.04 mg/kg) is suggested in severe clinical conditions. Subsequent doses of 0.5 to 1 mg may be given at 4- to 6-hour intervals. Doses under 0.5 mg may cause paradoxical slowing of HR.

Smooth muscle relaxation and suppression of secretions: 0.4 to 0.6 mg every 4 to 6 hours.

During surgery: Above doses appropriate except during cyclopropane anesthesia. Start with 0.4 mg or less. Administer very slowly to avoid ventricular arrhythmias; see Drug/Lab Interactions.

Cardiac asystole or pulseless electrical activity: 1-mg bolus recommended in asystole with specific protocol. May be repeated in 3 to 5 minutes if asystole persists. Usual total dose does not exceed 2 to 2.5 mg within 2½ hours, but 0.04 mg/kg may be given only in cardiac asystole. AHA guidelines recommend a maximum dose of 0.03 to 0.04 mg/kg. Use caution; a total dose of 3 mg causes full vagal blockade.

Antidote to reverse muscarinic effects of anticholinesterase agents: 0.6 to 1.2 mg for each 0.5 to 2.5 mg of neostigmine or 10 to 20 mg of pyridostigmine administered. Administer in a separate syringe, concurrently or a few minutes before the anticholinesterase agent. If bradycardia is present, bring pulse up to 80 by giving IV atropine first. See neostigmine, pyridostigmine, or physostigmine monographs.

Antidote for acute poisoning from exposure to anticholinesterase compounds (e.g., organophosphate pesticides, nerve gases, and mushroom poisoning): 1 to 2 mg may be given in a single dose and repeated every 5 to 60 minutes. In severe poisoning 2 to 6 mg may be given and repeated at 5- to 60-minute intervals until muscarinic signs and symptoms subside and repeated if they appear. Up to 50 mg may be required in the first 24 hours. Use oral atropine for maintenance; withdraw gradually to avoid recurrence of symptoms (e.g., pulmonary edema). A cholinase reactivator (e.g., pralidoxime) is administered concomitantly except in carbamate exposure.

PEDIATRIC DOSE

Fatal dose of atropine in children may be as low as 10 mg.

Bradyarrhythmias: 0.01 to 0.03 mg/kg of body weight can be used to achieve a pulse rate above 80 in a distressed infant under 6 months or above 60 in a child. Minimum dose is 0.1 mg. Maximum single dose is 0.5 mg in a child, 1 mg for an adolescent. May be repeated in 5-minute intervals times 2. AHA guidelines recommend 0.02 mg/kg. Double to 0.04 mg/kg if a second dose is required. Maximum total dose for a child is 1 mg, for an adolescent 2 mg. When used for bradycardia or asystole in infants and small children, vagolytic doses are required. Smaller doses may cause paradoxical bradycardia.

Smooth muscle relaxation and suppression of secretions: 0.01 mg/kg. Minimum dose is 0.1 mg in the newborn; up to 0.4 mg for a 12-year-old. Usually given SC. May repeat every 4 to 6 hours.

Bronchospasm: 0.05 mg/kg in 2.5 ml NS every 6 to 8 hours. Minimum dose 0.25 mg; maximum dose is 1 mg.

Antidote to reverse muscarinic effects of anticholinesterase agents: 0.02 mg/kg of atropine concomitantly with 0.04 mg/kg of neostigmine. See Usual Dose for additional information.

Antidote for acute poisoning from exposure to anticholinesterase compounds (e.g., organophosphate compounds, nerve gases, mushroom poisoning): 0.05 mg/kg; repeat every 10 to 30 minutes until muscarinic signs and symptoms subside, and repeat if they reappear. See Usual Dose for additional information.

DOSE ADJUSTMENTS

Reduced dose may be indicated in the elderly. ■ See Drug/Lab Interactions and Pediatric Dose.

DILUTION

May be given undiluted, but may prefer to dilute desired dose in at least 10 ml of SW for injection. Do not add to IV solutions. Inject through Y-tube or three-way stopcock of infusion set. Also available in combination with edrophonium (Enlon-Plus) to reverse cholinesterase toxicity caused by reversal of nondepolarizing muscle relaxants.

COMPATIBLE WITH (Underline Indicates Conflicting Compatibility Information)

Consult pharmacist; specific conditions may apply; see Compatibilities, p. xvi.

Additive: Buprenorphine (Buprenex), butorphanol (Stadol), dobutamine (Dobutrex), furosemide (Lasix), meropenem (Merrem IV), verapamil (Isoptin).

Syringe: Butorphanol (Stadol), chlorpromazine (Thorazine), cimetidine (Tagamet), dimenhydrinate (Dinate), diphenhydramine (Benadryl), droperidol (Inapsine), fentanyl (Sublimaze), glycopyrrolate, heparin, hydromorphone (Dilaudid), meperidine (Demerol), metoclopramide (Reglan), midazolam (Versed), milrinone (Primacor), morphine, nalbuphine (Nubain), ondansetron (Zofran), pentazocine (Talwin), <u>pentobarbital (Nembutal)</u>, perphenazine (Trilafon), prochlorperazine (Compazine), promethazine (Phenergan), ranitidine (Zantac), scopolamine, sufentanil (Sufenta).

Y-site: Dexmedetomidine (Precedex), etomidate (Amidate), famotidine (Pepcid IV), fentanyl (Sublimaze), heparin, hydrocortisone sodium succinate (Solu-Cortef), hydromorphone (Dilaudid), inamrinone (Inocor), meropenem (Merrem IV), morphine, nafcillin (Nafcil), potassium chloride (KCl), <u>propofol (Diprivan)</u>, sufentanil (Sufenta).

RATE OF ADMINISTRATION

1 mg or fraction thereof over 1 minute.

ACTIONS

Atropine is an anticholinergic drug and a potent belladonna alkaloid. It produces local, central, and peripheral effects on the body. The main therapeutic uses of atropine are peripheral, affecting smooth muscle, cardiac muscle, and gland cells. Reverses cholinergic-mediated decreases in HR, systemic vascular resistance, and BP. This drug can interfere with vagal stimuli. It is widely distributed in all body fluids. Metabolized by the liver and excreted in urine and bile. Crosses placental barrier. Secreted in breast milk.

INDICATIONS AND USES

Treatment of symptomatic sinus bradycardia, syncope from Stokes-Adams syndrome, and high-degree atrioventricular block with profound bradycardia. ■ AHA guidelines recommend as the primary drug to treat symptomatic sinus bradycardia and as the second drug (after) epinephrine for asystole or pulseless electrical activity. ■ Suppression of salivary, gastric, pancreatic, and respiratory secretions. ■ To relieve pylorospasm, hypertonicity of the small intestine, and hypermotility of the colon. ■ To relieve biliary and ureteral colic. ■ Antidote to reverse cholinesterase toxicity (muscarinic effects) caused by reversal of nondepolarizing muscle relaxants by neostigmine, physostigmine, and pyridostigmine. ■ Antidote for specific poisons such as organophosphorus insecticides, nerve gases, and mushroom poisoning *(Amanita muscaria).* ■ Temporary, reversible muscarinic blockade when excessive (or sometimes normal) muscarinic effects are judged to be life threatening or are producing severe symptoms. ■ Used in combination with many other drugs to produce a desired effect (e.g., edrophonium [Enlon, Enlon-Plus]).

CONTRAINDICATIONS

Hypersensitivity to atropine, acute glaucoma, acute hemorrhage with unstable cardiovascular status, asthma, hepatic disease, intestinal atony of the elderly or debilitated, myasthenia gravis, myocardial ischemia, obstructive disease of the GI or GU tracts, paralytic ileus, pyloric stenosis, renal disease, severe ulcerative colitis, tachycardia, toxic megacolon.

PRECAUTIONS

Use caution in prostatic hypertrophy, chronic lung disease, infants and small children, the elderly and debilitated, in urinary retention, during cyclopropane anesthesia, and in myocardial ischemia or infarction. ■ Increases myocardial oxygen demand and can trigger tachyarrhythmias. ■ Doses less than 0.5 mg may further slow HR. ■ May be given endotracheally. ■ Considered possibly harmful in AV block at the His-Purkinje level or with newly appearing wide QRS complexes.

Monitor: Vital signs and/or ECG based on specific situation.

Patient Education: Use caution if task requires alertness; may cause blurred vision, dizziness, or drowsiness. ■ Report eye pain, flushing, or skin rash promptly. ■ Report dry mouth, difficulty urinating, constipation, or increased light sensitivity.

Maternal/Child: Category C: safety for use in pregnancy, breast-feeding, and children not established. ■ Toxicity to nursing infants probable.

Elderly: May produce excitement, agitation, confusion, or drowsiness. ■ May precipitate undiagnosed glaucoma. ■ Potential for constipation and urinary retention increased. ■ Has potential to increase memory impairment. ■ See Dose Adjustments and Precautions.

DRUG/LAB INTERACTIONS

Potentiated by other drugs with anticholinergic activity (e.g., amantadine, [Symmetrel], glycopyrrolate, phenothiazines [e.g., prochlorperazine (Compazine)], tricyclic antidepressants [e.g., amitriptyline (Elavil)]). Reduce dose of atropine. ■ Antipsychotic effects of phenothiazines (e.g., prochlorperazine [Compazine]) may be decreased. ■ Concurrent use with cyclopropane anesthesia may cause ventricular arrhythmias; use of glycopyrrolate in increments of 0.1 mg or less is preferred. ■ Potentiates effects of many oral drugs by delaying gastric emptying and increasing rate of absorption (e.g., atenolol, digoxin, nitrofurantoin, thiazide diuretics). ■ Antagonistic to many drugs (e.g., edrophonium [Tensilon], pyridostigmine [Mestinon]).

SIDE EFFECTS

Anhidrosis, anticholinergic psychosis, blurred vision, bradycardia (temporary), constipation, dilation of the pupils, dryness of the mouth, flushing, gastroesophageal reflux, heat prostration from decreased sweating, nausea, paralytic ileus, postural hypotension, tachyarrhythmias, urinary hesitancy and retention (especially in males), and vomiting may occur.

Overdose: Coma, death, delirium, elevated BP, fever, paralytic ileus, rash, respiratory failure, stupor, tachycardia.

ANTIDOTE

Discontinue if side effects increase or are severe. Notify physician. Use standard treatments to manage cardiac arrhythmias. Physostigmine salicylate (Antilirium) reverses most cardiovascular and CNS effects; however, it may cause profound bradycardia, seizures, or asystole. Administer pilocarpine, 10 mg (SC), until the mouth is moist. Sustain physiologic functions at a normal level. Use diazepam (Valium), phenobarbital (Luminal), or chloral hydrate to relieve excitement. Neostigmine methylsulfate (Prostigmin) is an alternate antidote.

AZATHIOPRINE SODIUM

Immunosuppressant

(ay-za-thye′oh-preen so′de-um)

Imuran **pH 9.6**

USUAL DOSE

3 to 5 mg/kg of body weight/24 hr. Begin treatment within 24 hours of renal homotransplantation. In some cases, doses are given 1 to 3 days prior to transplantation. Maintenance dose is 1 to 3 mg/kg/24 hr. Individualized adjustment is imperative and may be required on a daily basis. Do not increase to toxic levels because of threatened rejection. Oral and IV doses are therapeutically equivalent; transfer to oral therapy as soon as practical.

DOSE ADJUSTMENTS

Reduce dose in impaired kidney function (especially immediately after transplant or with cadaveric kidneys) and in persistent negative nitrogen balance. ■ See Drug/Lab Interactions and Precautions/Monitor.

DILUTION

Specific techniques suggested; see Precautions. Each 100 mg should be initially reconstituted with 10 ml of SW. Swirl the vial gently until completely in solution. May be further diluted in a minimum of 50 ml of NS, D5W, or D5NS and given as an infusion. See Compatibility. Use within 24 hours.

COMPATIBILITY

Specific information not available. Listed as incompatible with preservatives (e.g., methylparaben, phenol, propylparaben). Administer separately. Converts to 6-mercaptopurine in alkaline solutions and sulfhydryl compounds (e.g., cysteine). Flush IV line with a compatible IV fluid before and after administration.

RATE OF ADMINISTRATION

A single dose properly diluted over 30 to 60 minutes. Actual range may be 5 minutes to 8 hours.

ACTIONS

An immunosuppressive drug. It is a derivative of the antineoplastic preparation mercaptopurine. Maximum response occurs if administered when antibody response begins. Has a selective action but achieves good response in many situations. Metabolized readily with small amounts excreted in the urine.

INDICATIONS AND USES

Adjunct to prevent rejection in renal homotransplantation. ■ Used PO to treat rheumatoid arthritis; see package insert.

CONTRAINDICATIONS

Anuria, known hypersensitivity, severe rejection.

PRECAUTIONS

■ Follow guidelines for handling cytotoxic agents (see Appendix A, p. 1142). ■ Usually administered in the hospital by or under the direction of a physician experienced in immunosuppressive therapy and management of organ transplant patients. ■ Adequate laboratory and supportive medical resources must be available. ■ May increase possibility of malignant tumor growth; patients previously treated with alkylating agents (e.g., cyclophosphamide [Cytoxan]) may be at increased risk. ■ Use caution with other myelosuppressive drugs or radiation therapy. ■ Toxic hepatitis or biliary status may necessitate discontinuing drug. ■ Rapid bone marrow suppression progressing to severe, life-threatening myelotoxicity may occur in patients with inherited low or absent thiopurine methyltransferase (TPMT). Genotyping or phenotyping may help identify these patients. **Monitor:** Monitor platelet count, RBC, WBC, and BUN frequently. Drug should be withdrawn or dose reduced at first sign of abnormally large fall in the leukocyte count or other evidence of persistent bone marrow depression. ■ Observe constantly for signs of infection. Prophylactic antibiotics may be indicated pending results of C/S in a febrile neutropenic patient. **Patient Education:** Avoid pregnancy; nonhormonal birth control recommended. ■ Promptly report unusual bruising or bleeding and/or S/S of infection. ■ Obtain all lab work as directed. ■ See Appendix D, p. 1148. **Maternal/Child:** Category D: avoid pregnancy. Can cause fetal harm. ■ Discontinue breast-feeding. ■ Safety and effectiveness for use in children not established.

DRUG/LAB INTERACTIONS

Potentiated by allopurinol (Zyloprim). Reduce dose to one third or one fourth of usual. ■ Inhibits anticoagulant effects of warfarin (Coumadin). ■ Concurrent use with bone marrow depressants, radiation therapy, other immunosuppressants (e.g., cyclosporine [Sandimmune]) or other drugs that may cause blood dyscrasias (e.g., sulfamethoxazole/trimethoprim [Bactrim]) may increase toxicity. ■ Concurrent use with ACE inhibitors (e.g., captopril [Capoten]) may induce anemia and severe leukopenia. ■ Plasma levels of the metabolite 6-MP may be increased by methotrexate. ■ Antibody response to vaccines may be suppressed. Do not use live vaccines in patients receiving azathioprine.

SIDE EFFECTS

Leukopenia and/or thrombocytopenia are dose-dependent and dose limiting. Other side effects include alopecia, anemia, anorexia, arthralgia, bleeding, diarrhea, elevated liver enzymes (e.g., ALT, LDH), fever, hypotension, jaundice, malaise, myalgias, nausea, oral lesions, pancreatitis, skin rash, vomiting. A GI hypersensitivity reaction (e.g., severe nausea and vomiting) has been reported.

ANTIDOTE

Notify the physician of all side effects. Most can be treated symptomatically and may reverse when the drug is discontinued. Reactions can occur within hours of a rechallenge. Drug may be decreased or discontinued or other immunosuppressive agents utilized. Hematopoietic depression may require temporary or permanent discontinuation of treatment and may be indicated even if rejection of graft may occur.

AZITHROMYCIN

(ay-zi-thro-mye′sin)

Antibacterial (azalide/macrolide)

Zithromax

USUAL DOSE

Community-acquired pneumonia: 500 mg as a single daily dose for a minimum of 2 days. Follow with 500 mg of oral azithromycin as a single daily dose. Total course of therapy (IV + oral) should be 7 to 10 days. **Pelvic inflammatory disease:** 500 mg as a single daily dose for 1 to 2 days. Follow with 250 mg of oral azithromycin as a single daily dose. Total course of therapy (IV + oral) should be 7 days. If anaerobic microorganisms are also suspected, concurrent administration of an antibacterial agent with anaerobic activity is recommended (e.g., metronidazole [Flagyl]).

PEDIATRIC DOSE

Safety and effectiveness for children under 16 years of age not established. See Maternal/Child.

DOSE ADJUSTMENTS

Reduced dose may be required in impaired liver or renal function; see Precautions. ■ See Drug/Lab Interactions.

DILUTION

Each 500-mg vial must be reconstituted with 4.8 ml SW. Shake well to ensure dilution (100 mg/ml). Further dilute each 500 mg of reconstituted solution with 250 to 500 ml of one of the following solutions: D5W, NS, ½NS, D5/⅓NS, D5/½NS, D5/½NS with 20 mEq KCl, LR, D5LR, D5/Normosol M, D5/Normosol R. 500 ml diluent yields 1 mg/ml, 250 ml yields 2 mg/ml. Concentrations greater than 2 mg/ml have caused local IV site reactions and should be avoided.

Storage: Reconstituted or diluted solution stable at CRT for 24 hours. Diluted solution stable for up 7 days if refrigerated.

COMPATIBILITY

Manufacturer states, "Other IV substances, additives, or medications should not be added to azithromycin, or infused simultaneously through the same IV line." Flush IV line with a compatible IV fluid before and after administration.

RATE OF ADMINISTRATION

Do not give by IV bolus; must be infused over at least 1 hour.

1 mg/ml dilution: A single dose equally distributed over a minimum of 1 hour; over 3 hours is preferred.

2 mg/ml dilution: A single dose equally distributed over at least 1 hour.

ACTIONS

An azalide (subclass of macrolide) antibiotic. Bactericidal and bacteriostatic to selected organisms, including aerobic gram-positive and gram-negative organisms, *Chlamydia*, and *Mycoplasma pneumoniae*. It is derived from erythromycin but is chemically different. Interferes with microbial protein synthesis by binding a ribosomal subunit of a susceptible microorganism. Concentration in phagocytes and fibroblasts may contribute to distribution in inflamed tissues. Activity not affected by beta-lactamase production. Compared to oral dosing, IV route plasma concentrations are consistently higher throughout a 24-hour interval. Trough levels increase with successive doses. Has a long tissue half-life permitting once-a-day dosing. Metabolized in the liver. Primarily excreted as unchanged drug in bile. Up to 14% excreted in urine within 24 hours.

INDICATIONS AND USES

Treatment of community-acquired pneumonia and pelvic inflammatory disease caused by specific organisms (e.g., *Staphylococcus aureus*, *Streptococcus pneumoniae*, *Haemophilus influenzae*, *Neisseria gonorrhoeae*, *Chlamydia trachomatis*. See product insert for complete list). Many other indications for oral use.

CONTRAINDICATIONS

Hypersensitivity to azithromycin, erythromycin, or any macrolide antibiotic.

PRECAUTIONS

For IV use only. ■ Specific sensitivity studies are indicated to determine susceptibility of the causative organism to azithromycin. ■ Has demonstrated cross-resistance with erythromycin-resistant gram-positive organisms. Most strains of *Enterococcus faecalis* and methicillin-resistant staphylococci are resistant to azithromycin. ■ Use extreme caution; allergic symptoms have recurred even after azithromycin was discontinued and allergic symptoms treated. Anaphylaxis resulting in fatalities has been reported rarely. ■ Principally eliminated in the liver; use caution in patients with impaired hepatic function. ■ Use caution in patients with impaired renal function; no data available on effects of IV azithromycin. ■ Use caution in patients with prolonged QT intervals; other macrolide antibiotics have caused ventricular arrhythmias, including ventricular tachycardia and torsades de pointes. ■ Timing of transfer to oral therapy should be based on clinical response. ■ Avoid prolonged use; superinfection caused by overgrowth of nonsusceptible organisms may result. ■ Pseudomembranous colitis has been reported. May range from mild to life-threatening. Consider in patients that present with diarrhea during or after treatment with azithromycin. ■ May cause photosensitivity.

Monitor: Monitor vital signs. ■ Observe closely for signs of allergic reaction. ■ Monitoring of liver function may be indicated. ■ Monitor infusion site for inflammation and/or extravasation. ■ Contains 4.96 mEq of sodium/vial. Observe for electrolyte imbalance and cardiac irregularities. May aggravate CHF. ■ See Drug/Lab Interactions and Antidote.

Patient Education: Discontinue azithromycin and report any signs of an allergic reaction immediately (difficulty breathing, itching, rash, swelling). ■ Oral azithromycin should be taken 1 hour before or 2 hours after a meal; should not be taken with food. ■ Do not take antacids containing aluminum or magnesium simultaneously with oral azithromycin.

Maternal/Child: Category B: safety for use during pregnancy and breast-feeding not established; use with caution and only if clearly needed. ■ Has been administered to pediatric patients age 6 months to 16 years by the oral route. The most common side effects in this age-group included abdominal pain, diarrhea, headache, nausea, rash, and vomiting.

Elderly: Response similar to that seen in younger adults. ■ Consider age-related organ impairment.

DRUG/LAB INTERACTIONS

Other macrolide antibiotics cause interactions when given concomitantly with the following drugs; azithromycin has not been studied. May increase serum concentrations of theophylline; monitoring of theophylline levels indicated. ■ May increase anticoagulant effects of warfarin (Coumadin); monitoring of PT indicated. ■ May increase digoxin levels; monitoring of digoxin levels indicated. ■ May cause acute ergot toxicity (severe peripheral vasospasm and dysesthesia) with ergotamine or dihydroergotamine. ■ May inhibit metabolism and increase serum levels and effects of triazolam (Halcion) and drugs metabolized by the cytochrome P_{450} system (e.g., carbamazepine [Tegretol], cimetidine [Tagamet], cyclosporine [Sandimmune], phenytoin [Dilantin]); reduced doses of these drugs may be indicated.

SIDE EFFECTS

Usually mild to moderate in severity and reversible after azithromycin discontinued. Abdominal pain; anemia; anorexia; arrhythmias; cough; diarrhea; dizziness; dyspnea; facial edema; fatigue; fungal infections; hypotension; increase in AST (SGOT), ALT (SGPT), and/or alkaline phosphatase levels; injection site pain or local inflammation; leukopenia; malaise; nausea; oral candidiasis; pancreatitis; pharyngitis; pleural effusion; rashes; rhinitis; stomatitis; vaginitis; vomiting. Serious abnormal liver function, including hepatitis and cholestatic jaundice, rare cases of hepatic and cholestatic jaundice, rare cases of hepatic necrosis and hepatic failure (some resulting in death) have occurred. Acute interstitial nephritis (fever, joint pain, skin rash) is rare but may cause acute renal failure. Allergic reactions (e.g., angioedema, anaphylaxis, and dermatologic reactions including Stevens-Johnson syndrome and toxic epidermal necrolysis) have been reported rarely and may be fatal; see Precautions. Pseudomembranous colitis has been reported.

ANTIDOTE

Notify physician of any side effects. Discontinue azithromycin for allergic reaction. Treat allergic reaction as indicated and resuscitate as necessary. Additional allergic symptoms have recurred after azithromycin has been discontinued and initial allergic treatment completed. Prolonged observation is required. Mild cases of colitis may respond to discontinuation of azithromycin. Fluids, electrolytes, and protein supplements may be indicated. Oral vancomycin (Vancocin) or metronidazole (Flagyl) is the treatment of choice for antibiotic-related pseudomembranous colitis.

AZTREONAM

(az-tree′oo-nam)

Azactam

Antibacterial (monobactam)

pH 4.5 to 7.5

USUAL DOSE

Urinary tract infection: 500 mg to 1 Gm every 8 or 12 hours.

Moderately severe systemic infections: 1 or 2 Gm every 8 to 12 hours.

Severe systemic, or life-threatening infections: 2 Gm every 6 or 8 hours. Use the full suggested dose. Do not exceed 8 Gm/24 hr.

Normal renal function required. Continue for at least 2 days after all symptoms of infection subside. Can produce therapeutic serum levels given intraperitoneally in dialysis fluid.

PEDIATRIC DOSE

Mild to moderate infections: 30 mg/kg every 8 hours.

Moderate to severe infections: 30 mg/kg every 6 or 8 hours. Maximum recommended dose is 120 mg/kg/24 hr.

Cystic fibrosis: 50 mg/kg every 6 to 8 hours. Maximum dose is 8 Gm/24 hr.

NEONATAL DOSE

30 mg/kg/dose. Interval between doses based on age and weight as follows:

Less than 1,200 Gm and 0 to 4 weeks of age or less than 2,000 Gm and 0 to 7 days of age: Give every 12 hours.

1,200 to 2,000 Gm and over 7 days of age or more than 2,000 Gm and 0 to 7 days of age: Give every 8 hours.

More than 2,000 Gm and over 7 days of age: Give every 6 hours.

DOSE ADJUSTMENTS

Prolonged serum levels may occur in patients with renal insufficiency. After an initial loading dose of 1 or 2 Gm, reduce succeeding doses by 50% in patients with CrCl between 10 and 30 ml/min/1.73 M^2. ■ After an initial loading dose of 500 mg, 1 Gm, or 2 Gm, reduce succeeding doses by 75% in patients with CrCl less than 10 ml/min/1.73 M^2 or in patients supported by dialysis. In addition 12.5% of the maintenance dose may be given after a dialysis session in serious or life-threatening situations. ■ Reduce dose in the elderly based on CrCl.

DILUTION

Usually light yellow, may become slightly pink on standing; does not affect potency.

IV injection: Reconstitute a single dose with 6 to 10 ml of SW for injection. Shake immediately and vigorously. Use immediately and discard any unused solution.

Intermittent IV: Initially reconstitute each single dose with a minimum of 3 ml of SW for injection. Shake immediately and vigorously. Must be further diluted in at least 50 ml of D5W, NS, or other compatible infusion solutions for each 1 Gm of aztreonam (see chart on inside back cover or literature). Concentration should not exceed 20 mg/ml. Available in vials and premixed Galaxy infusion bags.

Storage: Stable for 48 hours at room temperature or up to 7 days if refrigerated. When specific diluents are used, may be frozen for up to 3 months. Thaw at room temperature (see literature); do not refreeze.

INCOMPATIBLE WITH

Manufacturer lists metronidazole (Flagyl IV), nafcillin (Nafcil).

COMPATIBLE WITH **(Underline Indicates Conflicting Compatibility Information)**

Consult pharmacist; specific conditions may apply; see Compatibilities, p. xvi.

Manufacturer lists ampicillin, cefazolin (Kefzol), clindamycin (Cleocin), gentamicin (Garamycin), and tobramycin (Nebcin) diluted in specific concentrations and in specific solutions and states "other admixtures are not recommended."

Other sources list the following:

Additive: Ampicillin/sulbactam (Unasyn), cefoxitin (Mefoxin), ciprofloxacin (Cipro IV), linezolid (Zyvox), vancomycin (Vancocin).

Syringe: Clindamycin (Cleocin).

Y-site: Allopurinol (Aloprim, Zyloprim), amifostine (Ethyol), amikacin (Amikin), aminophylline, ampicillin, ampicillin/sulbactam (Unasyn), bleomycin (Blenoxane), bumetanide (Bumex), buprenorphine (Buprenex), butorphanol (Stadol), calcium gluconate, carboplatin (Paraplatin), carmustine (BiCNU), cefazolin (Kefzol), cefepime (Maxipime), cefoperazone (Cefobid), cefotaxime (Claforan), cefotetan (Cefotan), cefoxitin (Mefoxin), ceftazidime (Fortaz), ceftizoxime (Cefizox), ceftriaxone (Rocephin), cefuroxime (Zinacef), cimetidine (Tagamet), ciprofloxacin (Cipro IV), cisatracurium (Nimbex), cisplatin (Platinol), clindamycin (Cleocin), cyclophosphamide (Cytoxan), cytarabine (ARA-C), dacarbazine (DTIC), dactinomycin (Cosmegen), dexamethasone (Decadron), diltiazem (Cardizem), diphenhydramine (Benadryl), dobutamine (Dobutrex), docetaxel (Taxotere), dopamine (Intropin), doxorubicin (Adriamycin), doxorubicin liposome (Doxil), doxycycline (Vibramycin), droperidol (Inapsine), enalaprilat (Vasotec IV), etoposide (VePesid, Etopophos), famotidine (Pepcid IV), filgrastim (Neupogen), fluconazole (Diflucan), fludarabine (Fludara), fluorouracil (5-FU), foscarnet (Foscavir), furosemide (Lasix), gatifloxacin (Tequin), gemcitabine (Gemzar), gentamicin (Garamycin), granisetron (Kytril), haloperidol (Haldol), heparin, hydrocortisone (Hydrocortone, Solu-Cortef), hydromorphone (Dilaudid), idarubicin (Idamycin), ifosfamide (Ifex), imipenem-cilastatin (Primaxin), insulin (regular), leucovorin calcium, linezolid (Zyvox), magnesium sulfate, mannitol, mechlorethamine (nitrogen mustard), melphalan (Alkeran), meperidine (Demerol), mesna (Mesnex), methotrexate (Folex), methylprednisolone (Solu-Medrol), metoclopramide (Reglan), minocycline (Minocin), morphine, nalbuphine (Nubain), ondansetron (Zofran), piperacillin (Pipracil), piperacillin/tazobactam (Zosyn), plicamycin (Mithracin), potassium chloride (KCl), promethazine (Phenergan), propofol (Diprivan), ranitidine (Zantac), remifentanil (Ultiva), sargramostim (Leukine), sodium bicarbonate, sulfamethoxazole-trimethoprim (Bactrim), teniposide (Vumon), theophylline, thiotepa (Thioplex), ticarcillin (Ticar), ticarcillin/clavulanate (Timentin), tobramycin, vancomycin (Vancocin), vinblastine (Velban), vincristine (Oncovin), vinorelbine (Navelbine), zidovudine (AZT, Retrovir).

RATE OF ADMINISTRATION

IV injection: A single dose equally distributed over 3 to 5 minutes.

Intermittent IV: A single dose over 20 to 60 minutes. May be given through Y-tube or three-way stopcock of infusion set. Do not infuse simultaneously with other drugs or solutions except in proven compatibility. Flush common IV tubing before and after administration.

ACTIONS

A synthetic monobactam antibiotic. Bactericidal through inhibition of bacterial cell wall synthesis to a wide spectrum of specific gram-negative aerobic organisms including *Pseudomonas aeruginosa*. Effective against many otherwise resistant organisms. Therapeutic levels widely distributed into many body fluids and tissues. Serum half-life averages 1.7 hours; range is 1.5 to 2 hours. Primarily excreted in the urine with some excretion through feces. Crosses placental barrier. Secreted in breast milk.

INDICATIONS AND USES

Treatment of serious lower respiratory tract, urinary tract, skin and skin structure, gynecologic, and intraabdominal infections and bacterial septicemia. Most effective against specific gram-negative organisms (see literature). ■ Adjunctive therapy to surgery for the management of infections.

CONTRAINDICATIONS

Known hypersensitivity to aztreonam.

PRECAUTIONS

Specific studies are indicated to identify the causative organism and susceptibility to aztreonam. ■ Before C/S data are available, antimicrobial therapy with agents to cover gram-positive and/or anaerobic microorganisms may be indicated. ■ Avoid prolonged use of drug; superinfection caused by overgrowth of nonsusceptible organisms may result. ■ Pseudomembranous colitis has been reported. May range from mild to life-threatening. Consider in patients that present with diarrhea during or after treatment with aztreonam. ■ Epidermal necrolysis has been reported rarely in patients receiving aztreonam who have undergone BMT and have other risk factors (e.g., graft-versus-host disease, radiation therapy, sepsis).

Monitor: Watch for early symptoms of allergic reaction. Use caution in patients with known sensitivity to penicillins, cephalosporins, or carbapenems. ■ Monitor renal and hepatic function, especially in the elderly. ■ May cause thrombophlebitis. Use small needles, large veins, and rotate infusion sites.

Maternal/Child: Category B: use in pregnancy and breast-feeding only if clearly needed. ■ Consider discontinuation of breast-feeding. ■ Safety for use in infants and children not established.

Elderly: Response is similar to that seen in younger patients; however, clearance is decreased and half-life is prolonged. Reduced doses may be indicated based on potential for decreased organ function and concomitant disease or drug therapy. Monitor renal function; see Dose Adjustments.

DRUG/LAB INTERACTIONS

Adverse interaction may occur with beta-lactamase–inducing antibiotics (e.g., cefoxitin, imipenem); do not use concurrently. ■ May be used concomitantly with aminoglycosides in severe infections. Nephrotoxicity and ototoxicity can be markedly increased when both drugs are utilized. ■ Probenecid and furosemide do increase blood levels; not clinically significant. ■ Bactericidal activity of aztreonam may be antagonized by chloramphenicol (Chloromycetin). ■ See Side Effects.

SIDE EFFECTS

Full scope of allergic reactions including anaphylaxis. Burning, discomfort, and pain at injection site; diarrhea; nausea and vomiting; pseudomembranous colitis; and rash occur most frequently. Abdominal cramps; altered taste; confusion; diaphoresis; diplopia; dizziness; dyspnea; elevated alkaline phosphatase, AST (SGOT), ALT (SGPT), and SrCr; eosinophilia;

erythema multiforme; exfoliative dermatitis; fever; halitosis; headache; hematologic changes; hepatitis; hypotension; insomnia; jaundice; mouth ulcer; nasal congestion; numb tongue; paresthesia; petechiae; positive Coombs' test; prolonged PT and PTT; pruritus; purpura; transient ECG changes (ventricular bigeminy and PVCs); seizures; sneezing; tinnitus; urticaria; vaginitis; vertigo can occur.

ANTIDOTE

Notify physician of any side effects. Discontinue the drug if indicated. Treat allergic reaction as indicated and resuscitate as necessary. Mild causes of colitis may respond to discontinuation of drug. Oral vancomycin (Vancocin) or metronidazole (Flagyl) is the treatment of choice for antibiotic-related pseudomembranous colitis. Hemodialysis or peritoneal dialysis may be useful in overdose.

BASILIXIMAB

(bas-ih-liks'ih-mab)

Recombinant monoclonal antibody
Immunosuppressant

Simulect

USUAL DOSE

Basiliximab should only be administered once it has been determined that the patient will receive the graft and concomitant immunosuppression. Patients who have received a previous course of basiliximab should only be re-exposed to a subsequent course of therapy with extreme caution. Used concurrently with cyclosporine (Sandimmune) and corticosteroids.
Organ rejection prophylaxis in renal transplant: 2 doses of 20 mg each as an infusion. Administer the first dose within 2 hours before transplantation. Give the second dose 4 days after transplantation. Withhold the second dose if complications such as severe hypersensitivity reactions to basiliximab or graft loss occurs.

PEDIATRIC DOSE

Less than 35 kg: 2 doses of 10 mg each (discard remaining product after each dose).
35 kg or more: 2 doses of 20 mg each.

In all pediatric patients, administer the first dose within 2 hours before transplantation. Give the second dose 4 days after transplantation. See Actions and Maternal/Child. Withhold second dose if complications occur (e.g., hypersensitivity reactions or graft loss).

DOSE ADJUSTMENTS

No dose adjustments indicated.

DILUTION

Reconstitute each single dose with 5 ml of SW. Shake gently to dissolve powder. After reconstitutions may be given as an IV injection or may be further diluted to 50 ml with NS or D5W. When mixing, gently invert to avoid foaming; do not shake.
Storage: Store unopened vials in the refrigerator (2° to 8° C [36° to 46° F]). Should be used within 4 hours of reconstitution. If necessary, may be refrigerated for up to 24 hours. Discard prepared solution after 24 hours.

COMPATIBILITY

Manufacturer states, "Other drug substances should not be added or infused simultaneously through the same IV line." No incompatibilities observed with polyvinyl chloride bags and administration sets.

RATE OF ADMINISTRATION

May be given through a peripheral or central vein.

IV injection: May be given as a bolus injection over 30 to 60 seconds. Incidence of N/V and local reaction including pain increased.

Infusion: A single dose properly diluted over 20 to 30 minutes.

ACTIONS

A chimeric (murine/human) monoclonal antibody produced by recombinant DNA technology. Functions as an immunosuppressant. Specifically binds to and blocks the interleukin-2 receptor alpha chain (IL-2Rα, also known as CD25 antigen), thereby inhibiting IL-2 driven proliferation of activated T cells which play a key role in organ rejection. Reduces/minimizes acute rejection. IL-2Rα is expressed selectively on activated, but not resting, T cells. This selectivity prevents the profound generalized immunosuppression seen with other immunosuppressants used in organ transplantation and may decrease the risk of infection and development of lymphoproliferative disorders. Two 20-mg doses block the receptor for 4 to 6 weeks posttransplantation, the critical risk period for acute organ rejection. Has reduced the incidence of biopsy-confirmed acute rejections while minimizing side effects seen with other immunosuppressants. Clinical benefit demonstrated in a broad range of patients, regardless of age, gender, race, donor type, or history of diabetes mellitus as long as serum levels exceed 0.2 mg/ml (by ELISA). Mean half-life is 4 to 10.4 days. Half-life is increased (5.2 to 17.8 days) and distribution volume and clearance are decreased by about 50% in children 2 to 11 years of age. Crosses the placental barrier. May be secreted in breast milk.

INDICATIONS AND USES

Prophylaxis of acute organ rejection in patients receiving renal transplants. Used as part of an immunosuppresive regimen that includes cyclosporine and corticosteroids. Dosing regimen may also include either azathioprine (Imuran) or mycophenolate mofetil (CellCept).

CONTRAINDICATIONS

Known hypersensitivity to basiliximab or any of its components (composite of human and murine antibodies).

PRECAUTIONS

Usually administered by or under the direction of a physician experienced in immunosuppressive therapy and management of organ transplant patients. Adequate laboratory and supportive medical resources must be available. ■ Severe acute (onset within 24 hours) hypersensitivity reactions including anaphylaxis have been reported both with initial exposure and/or following re-exposure after several months. Emergency equipment and drugs for the treatment of severe hypersensitivity reactions must be readily available. Withhold the second dose of basiliximab if a hypersensitivity reaction occurs. ■ Re-administration after an initial course of therapy has not been studied in humans, but other monoclonal antibodies have precipitated anaphylactoid reactions. ■ Potential for causing lymphoproliferative disorders, CMV, and other opportunistic infections is unknown. ■ Use with caution in patients with infections or malignancies. ■ It is not known whether basiliximab use will have a long-term effect on the ability of the immune system to respond to antigens first encountered during induced immunosuppression. ■ Low titers of anti-idiotype antibodies and human antimurine antibodies (HAMA) to basiliximab have been detected in some patients during treatment; no adverse effects have been noted.

Monitor: Obtain baseline CBC with differential and platelets and baseline renal and liver tests if not already completed for other immunosuppressant agents. ■ Monitor vital signs. ■ Observe closely for signs of infection (fever, sore throat, tiredness) or unusual bleeding or bruising. ■ Prophylactic antibiotics may be indicated pending results of C/S in a febrile immunosuppressed patient. ■ Symptoms of cytokine release syndrome (e.g., chills, fever, dyspnea, and malaise) have not been reported but may occur; observe carefully. ■ See Drug/Lab Interactions.

Patient Education: Report difficulty in breathing or swallowing, rapid heartbeat, rash, or itching immediately. ■ Report swelling of lower extremities and weakness. ■ Avoid pregnancy; non-hormonal birth control preferred. Women with childbearing potential should use effective contraception before beginning basiliximab therapy, during therapy, and for 2 months after completion. ■ See Appendix D, p. 1148.

Maternal/Child: Category B: use during pregnancy only if benefits justify the potential risk to the fetus. Avoid pregnancy; effective contraception required; see Patient Education. ■ Discontinue breast-feeding. ■ Has been used in children from 2 to 15 years of age. No adequate or well-controlled studies completed. See differences in Actions. Most frequent side effects were fever and urinary infections.

Elderly: Age-related dosing not required. Adverse events similar to younger adults. Use caution when giving immunosuppressive drugs to the elderly.

DRUG/LAB INTERACTIONS

Has been administered concurrently with antilymphocyte globulin (ALG), antithymocyte globulin (ATG), azathioprine (Imuran), corticosteroids, cyclosporine, muromonab CD3 (Orthoclone), and mycophenolate mofetil (CellCept); no additional adverse reactions noted. ■ May increase or decrease numerous lab values, including serum calcium and potassium and fasting blood glucose.

SIDE EFFECTS

Basiliximab did not appear to alter the pattern, frequency, or severity of known side effects associated with the use of immunosuppressive drugs. Abdominal pain, anemia, constipation, diarrhea, edema, fever, headache, hyperkalemia, hypersensitivity reactions (including anaphylaxis, bronchospasm, capillary leak syndrome, cardiac failure, cytokine release syndrome, dyspnea, hypotension, pruritus, pulmonary edema, rash, respiratory failure, sneezing, tachycardia, urticaria, wheezing), hypokalemia, hypertension, insomnia, nausea, pain, peripheral edema, upper respiratory infections, urinary tract infections. Incidence of N/V and local reaction including pain increased with bolus injection. Severe hypersensitivity reactions (including anaphylaxis), capillary leak syndrome, and cytokine release syndrome have been reported. Incidence of infections, lymphomas, or other malignancies similar to placebo groups in studies.

ANTIDOTE

Notify physician of all side effects. Most will be treated symptomatically. Basiliximab may be discontinued or alternate immunosuppressive agents substituted. Discontinue immediately if anaphylaxis occurs, and treat with oxygen, epinephrine, corticosteroids, and/or antihistamines (e.g., diphenhydramine [Benadryl]). Resuscitate as necessary.

BIVALIRUDIN

(bye-va-leer′u-din)

Anticoagulant

Angiomax

pH 5 to 6

USUAL DOSE

Obtain baseline blood tests before administration; see Monitor and Drug/Lab Interactions. Initiate just prior to percutaneous coronary intervention (PCI). Given in combination with aspirin.

Aspirin: 300 to 325 mg before PCI and daily thereafter.

Bivalirudin: Begin with an IV bolus dose of 1 mg/kg. Follow with an infusion at 2.5 mg/kg/hr for 4 hours. If indicated an additional infusion at 0.2 mg/kg/hr may be continued for up to 20 hours. See Dosing table in Rate of Administration.

A recent study suggests an alternate dosing regimen for patients undergoing PCI (not limited to those with unstable angina [unlabeled]). The primary purpose of this study was to demonstrate that during PCI, bivalirudin with provisional (used when indicated) glycoprotein IIb/IIIa blockade was as effective as heparin with planned glycoprotein IIb/IIIa blockade and was associated with less bleeding. This regimen is currently being reviewed by the FDA and includes:

Aspirin: 300 to 325 mg before PCI and daily thereafter.

Thienopyridines: Clopidogrel (Plavix) 300 mg 2 to 12 hours before PCI and 75 mg daily thereafter for 30 days.

Bivalirudin: Begin with an IV bolus dose of 0.75 mg/kg. Follow with an infusion at 1.75 mg/kg/hr for the duration of PCI.

Glycoprotein IIb/IIIa antagonist: Administration was provisional. Suggested indications for provisional use included, but were not limited to, abrupt or side-branch closure, obstructive dissection, new or suspected thrombus, impaired or slow coronary flow, distal embolization, persistent residual stenosis, unplanned stent placement, prolonged ischemia, or other clinical instability. Abciximab (ReoPro) or eptifibatide (Integrilin) were used during the study. 7.2% of patients in the study required provisional use.

DOSE ADJUSTMENTS

Reduce dose in impaired renal function as indicated in the following chart.

Guidelines for Bivalirudin Dose Adjustments in Impaired Renal Function*			
Renal Function (GFR, ml/min)	Clearance (ml/min/kg)	Half-life (minutes)	% Reduction in Infusion Dose
Normal renal function (≥90 ml/min)	3.4	25	0
Mild renal impairment (60-90 ml/min)	3.4	22	0
Moderate renal impairment (30-59 ml/min)	2.7	34	20
Severe renal impairment (10-29 ml/min)	2.8	57	60
Dialysis-dependent patients (off dialysis)	1.0	3.5 hours	90

*The ACT should be monitored in renally-impaired patients

DILUTION

Bolus and initial infusion: Reconstitute each 250 mg vial with 5 ml SW. Gently swirl to dissolve. Each 250 mg vial must be further diluted in 50 ml of D5W or NS to yield a final concentration of 5 mg/ml (e.g., 1 vial in 50 ml, 2 vials in 100 ml, and 5 vials in 250 ml).

Low rate or subsequent infusion: After reconstitution as above, the 250 mg vial should be further diluted in 500 ml of D5W or NS to yield a final concentration of 0.5 mg/ml.

Storage: Refrigerate unopened vials. Do not freeze reconstituted or diluted solution. Reconstituted solution stable for 24 hours refrigerated. Concentrations between 0.5 mg/ml and 5 mg/ml are stable at CRT for up to 24 hours. Discard unused portion of reconstituted solution.

INCOMPATIBLE WITH

Manufacturer states, "No other medications should be mixed with bivalirudin before or during administration," and lists alteplase (Activase, tPA), amiodarone (Cordarone), amphotericin B (Fungizone), chlorpromazine (Thorazine), diazepam (Valium), prochlorperazine (Compazine), reteplase (Retavase, rPA), streptokinase, and vancomycin (Vancocin) as incompatible through the same IV line (Y-site or piggyback). No incompatibilities observed with glass bottles or polyvinyl chloride bags and administration sets.

RATE OF ADMINISTRATION

The following chart details by patient weight in kilograms, the amount of the bolus dose, the rate in ml/hr of the initial infusion, and the rate in ml/hr of the subsequent infusion.

Bivalirudin Dosing Guidelines			
Using 5 mg/ml Concentration			Using 0.5 mg/ml Concentration
Weight (kg)	Bolus (1 mg/kg) (ml)	Initial 4-hour Infusion (2.5 mg/kg/hr) (ml/hr)	Subsequent Low-rate Infusion (0.2 mg/kg/hr) (ml/hr)
43-47	9	22.5	18
48-52	10	25	20
53-57	11	27.5	22
58-62	12	30	24
63-67	13	32.5	26
68-72	14	35	28
73-77	15	37.5	30
78-82	16	40	32
83-87	17	42.5	34
88-92	18	45	36
93-97	19	47.5	38
98-102	20	50	40
103-107	21	52.5	42
108-112	22	55	44
113-117	23	57.5	46
118-122	24	60	48
123-127	25	62.5	50
128-132	26	65	52
133-137	27	67.5	54
138-142	28	70	56
143-147	29	72.5	58
148-152	30	75	60

ACTIONS

An anticoagulant that is a specific and reversible direct thrombin inhibitor. It directly inhibits thrombin by specifically binding both to the catalytic site and to the anion-binding exosite of circulating and clot-bound thrombin. Inhibits both free and clot-bound thrombin without requiring endogenous cofactors (i.e., mode of action is independent of antithrombin III and is not inhibited by components of the platelet release reaction [e.g., platelet factor 4]). Produces a dose-dependent increase in aPTT, PT, TT, and ACT. Anticoagulant effect is immediate. Steady-state concentrations of 12.3 ± 1.7 mcg/ml is achieved following the bolus dose and 4-hour infusion. Cleared from plasma by a combination of renal mechanisms and proteolytic cleavage. The binding of bivalirudin to thrombin is reversible resulting in recovery of thrombin active site functions. Half-life averages 25 minutes. 20% of unchanged drug excreted in urine.

INDICATIONS AND USES

An anticoagulant for use in patients with unstable angina undergoing PCI. (Used in place of heparin.) Used concurrently with aspirin.

Unlabeled uses: As an anticoagulant for use in patients undergoing PCI (not limited to those with unstable angina). Used in combination with aspirin and thienopyridines (clopidogrel [Plavix]) and may be used in combination with glycoprotein IIb/IIIa antagonists (e.g., abciximab [ReoPro], eptifibatide [Integrilin]) as medically indicated. Used in place of glycoprotein IIb/IIIa antagonists in combination with heparin. ▪ Has been used in place of heparin in cardiac catheterization, AMI, and unstable angina; safety and effectiveness not established. ▪ Treatment of heparin-associated thrombocytopenia. ▪ Limited information available for treatment of patients with heparin-induced thrombocytopenia/heparin-induced thrombocytopenia-thrombosis syndrome (HIT/HITTS). ▪ Has been given SC in orthopedic surgeries.

CONTRAINDICATIONS

Hypersensitivity to bivalirudin or its components; active major bleeding.

PRECAUTIONS

For IV or SC use only. Do not administer IM. ▪ Most bleeding associated with the use of bivalirudin in PCI occurs at the site of arterial puncture, however, hemorrhage can occur at any site. Consider a hemorrhagic event if there is an unexplained fall in BP or hematocrit or other unexplained symptom and discontinue bivalirudin. ▪ Use with caution in disease states and other circumstances in which there is an increased danger of hemorrhage including severe hypertension; immediately following lumbar puncture; spinal anesthesia; major surgery, especially involving the brain, spinal cord, or eye; hematologic conditions associated with increased bleeding tendencies such as congenital or acquired bleeding disorders and gastrointestinal lesions such as ulcerations. ▪ Safety for use with platelet inhibitors other than aspirin (e.g., glycoprotein IIb/IIIa inhibitors such as abciximab [ReoPro], eptifibatide [Integrilin], tirofiban [Aggrastat]) has not been established; see Drug/Lab Interactions. ▪ Safety for use in combination with thrombolytic agents (e.g., alteplase [tPA], reteplase [Retavase], streptokinase) has not been established; see Drug/Lab Interactions. ▪ Safety for use in patients with unstable angina who are not undergoing PCI or in patients with other acute coronary syndromes has not been established. ▪ Half-life extended in patients with impaired renal function; see Dose Adjustments. ▪ Limited data regarding reexposure to bivalirudin; positive antibodies developed in 2 patients and neither developed clinical evidence of an allergic reaction.

Monitor: Discontinue low molecular weight heparin at least 8 hours prior to the procedure and administration of bivalirudin. ▪ Before therapy obtain platelet count, hemoglobin or hematocrit, SrCr, ACT, aPTT, TT, and PT. ▪ Dose is not titrated to ACT; however the ACT was checked at 5 minutes and again in 45 minutes during original clinical studies. An additional bolus of heparin was given if the ACT was less than 350 seconds. ▪ In the most recent studies (unlabeled use), the ACT was checked at 5 minutes after a bolus dose. An additional bivalirudin dose (0.3 mg/kg) was given if the ACT was less than 225 seconds. ▪ Also in the most recent studies (unlabeled), unless a closure device was used, vascular access sheaths were removed following the procedure once the ACT was 175 seconds or less or the aPTT was 50 seconds or less. ■ Monitor anticoagulation status in patients with impaired renal function receiving reduced doses. ■ Observe carefully for symptoms of a hemorrhagic event (e.g., unexplained fall in hematocrit, fall in BP, or any other unexplained symptom).

Patient Education: Report all episodes of bleeding. ■ Report tarry stools. ■ Compliance with all measures to minimize bleeding is very important (e.g., avoid use of razors, toothbrushes, other sharp items). ■ Use caution while moving to avoid excess bumping.

Maternal/Child: Category B: safety for use during pregnancy not established. May have adverse effects on the fetus and the potential for maternal bleeding is increased, particularly during the third trimester. Use only if clearly needed. ■ Not known if bivalirudin is secreted in human milk, use caution if required during breast-feeding. ■ Safety and effectiveness for use in children have not been established.

Elderly: Response similar to younger adults. ■ See Dose Adjustments for the elderly with impaired renal function. ■ Puncture site hemorrhage and hematoma were observed more frequently in patients over 65 years of age.

DRUG/LAB INTERACTIONS

Discontinue low molecular weight heparin at least 8 hours prior to the procedure and administration of bivalirudin. ■ Risk of bleeding may be increased by any medicine that affects blood clotting including anticoagulants (e.g., heparin, lepirudin [Refludan], warfarin [Coumadin]); glycoprotein GPIIb/IIIa receptor antagonists (e.g., abciximab [ReoPro], eptifibatide [Integrilin], tirofiban [Aggrastat]); any medication that may cause hypoprothrombinemia, thrombocytopenia, or GI ulceration or bleeding (e.g., selected antibiotics such as cefamandole [Mandol], cefoperazone [Cefobid], cefotetan [Cefotan], ticarcillin [Ticar], aspirin, NSAIDs [e.g., ibuprofen (Advil, Motrin), naproxen (Aleve, Naprosyn), phenylbutazone (Butazolidin)]); and/or any other medication that inhibits platelet aggregation (e.g., clopidogrel [Plavix], dipyridamole [Persantine], plicamycin [Mithracin], sulfinpyrazone [Anturane], ticlopidine [Ticlid], valproic acid [Depacon]). If concurrent or subsequent use is indicated monitor closely.

SIDE EFFECTS

Bleeding is the most frequent adverse event; incidence in clinical studies was less than with heparin. Abdominal pain, anxiety, back pain, bradycardia, dyspepsia, fever, headache, hypertension, hypotension, injection site pain, insomnia, nausea, nervousness, pain, pelvic pain, and urinary retention have occurred.

ANTIDOTE

No specific antidote is available. Overdose with or without bleeding may be controlled by discontinuing bivalirudin. Discontinuation leads to a gradual reduction in anticoagulant effects due to metabolism of the drug depending on dose/overdose and concentration achieved. ACT or aPTT should return to normal within 1 to 4 hours after discontinuation. Reversal may take longer in patients with renal impairment. If life-threatening bleeding develops and excessive plasma levels of bivalirudin are suspected, immediately stop infusion. Determine aPTT, ACT, and hemoglobin and prepare for blood transfusion as appropriate. Follow current guidelines for treatment of shock as indicated (fluid, vasopressors [e.g., dopamine], Trendelenburg position, plasma expanders [e.g., albumin, hetastarch]). Bivalirudin is removed by hemodialysis.

BLEOMYCIN SULFATE

(blee-oh-mye'sin sul'fat)

Blenoxane

Antineoplastic (antibiotic)

pH 4.5 to 6

USUAL DOSE

0.25 to 0.5 unit/kg of body weight/24 hr (10 to 20 units/M^2), once or twice weekly (1 unit equals 1 mg). The first two doses in lymphoma patients should not exceed 2 units in order to rule out hypersensitivity.

Hodgkin's disease: Dosage as above. After a 50% response, a maintenance dose of 1 unit daily or 5 units weekly is recommended.

DOSE ADJUSTMENTS

Unit/kg dose based on average weight in presence of edema or ascites. ■ Reduce dose in impaired renal function. Based on CrCl; see literature.

DILUTION

Specific techniques required; see Precautions. Each 15 units or fraction thereof must be reconstituted with 5 ml or more of NS to achieve concentrations not greater than 3 units (mg)/ml. For IV injection, further dilution is not necessary, but has been further diluted in 50 ml NS and given as an intermittent infusion. Has also been further diluted in larger amounts of NS and given as a continuous infusion (15 to 20 units/M^2/day) over 3 to 7 days. May be given through Y-tube or three-way stopcock of a free-flowing IV.

Storage: Refrigerate powder. Diluted solution stable at room temperature for 24 hours.

COMPATIBLE WITH **(Underline Indicates Conflicting Compatibility Information)**

Consult pharmacist; specific conditions may apply; see Compatibilities, p. xvi.

Additive: Amikacin (Amikin), cyclophosphamide (Cytoxan), dexamethazsone (Decadron), diphenhydramine (Benadryl), doxorubicin (Adriamycin), fluorouracil (5-FU), gentamicin (Garamycin), heparin, hydrocortisone sodium phosphate (Hydrocortone), mesna (Mesnex), phenytoin (Dilantin), streptomycin, tobramycin (Nebcin), vinblastine (Velban), vincristine (Oncovin).

Syringe: Cisplatin (Platinol), cyclophosphamide (Cytoxan), doxorubicin (Adriamycin), droperidol (Inapsine), fluorouracil (5-FU), furosemide (Lasix), heparin, leucovorin calcium, methotrexate (Folex), metoclopramide (Reglan), mitomycin (Mutamycin), vinblastine (Velban), vincristine (Oncovin).

Y-site: Allopurinol (Aloprim, Zyloprim), amifostine (Ethyol), aztreonam (Azactam), cefepime (Maxipime), cisplatin (Platinol), cyclophosphamide (Cytoxan), doxorubicin (Adriamycin), doxorubicin liposome (Doxil), droperidol (Inapsine), etoposide phosphate (Etopophos), filgrastim (Neupogen), fludarabine (Fludara), fluorouracil (5-FU), gemcitabine (Gemzar), granisetron (Kytril), heparin, leucovorin calcium, melphalan (Alkeran), mesna (Mesnex), methotrexate (Folex), metoclopramide (Reglan), mitomycin (Mutamycin), ondansetron (Zofran), paclitaxel (Taxol), piperacillin/tazobactam (Zosyn), sargramostim (Leukine), teniposide (Vumon), thiotepa (Thioplex), vinblastine (Velban), vincristine (Oncovin), vinorelbine (Navelbine).

RATE OF ADMINISTRATION

IV injection: Each 15 to 30 unit dose over 10 minutes.

Intermittent infusion: A single dose over 15 minutes or longer.

Continuous IV: A daily dose equally distributed over 24 hours. Repeated each day for 3 to 7 days.

ACTIONS

An antibiotic antineoplastic agent, cell cycle phase-specific, that seems to act by splitting and fragmentation of double-stranded DNA, leading to chromosomal damage. It localizes in tumors. Improvement usually noted within 2 weeks. Well distributed in skin, lungs, kidneys, peritoneum, and lymphatics. About 60% to 70% excreted in urine.

INDICATIONS AND USES

Testicular carcinoma; may induce complete remission with vinblastine and cisplatin. ▪ Palliative treatment, adjunct to surgery or radiation, in patients not responsive to other chemotherapeutic agents or those with squamous cell carcinoma of the skin, head, esophagus, neck, or GU tract, including the cervix, vulva, scrotum, and penis; in Hodgkin's disease and other lymphomas. ▪ Orphan drug approval for treatment of pancreatic cancer. ▪ Injected into pleural cavity to treat malignant pleural effusion.

CONTRAINDICATIONS

Known hypersensitivity to bleomycin, elderly patients with pulmonary disease.

PRECAUTIONS

Follow guidelines for handling cytotoxic agents. See Appendix A, p. 1142. ▪ Administered by or under the direction of the physician specialist. ▪ May be used with other antineoplastic drugs to achieve tumor remission. ▪ May cause severe anaphylaxis with lymphomas; use a test dose.

Monitor: Obtain a baseline chest x-ray, and recheck every 1 to 2 weeks to detect pulmonary changes. ▪ Monitor renal, hepatic, and central nervous systems and skin for symptoms of toxicity. ▪ Determine patency of vein; avoid extravasation. ▪ Pulmonary toxicity increases markedly with advancing age, larger doses, or in smokers; may occur at lower doses when bleomycin is used in combination with other antineoplastic agents. To identify subclinical pulmonary toxicity, monitor pulmonary diffusion capacity for carbon monoxide monthly. Should remain 30% to 35% above pretreatment value. Most toxic when total cumulative dose exceeds 350 to 450 units. Some references suggest that the total lifetime dose should never exceed 400 units, and that many physicians limit the total lifetime dose to 300 units. ▪ Maintain adequate hydration. ▪ Prophylactic antiemetics may reduce nausea and vomiting and increase patient comfort. ▪ Observe closely for all signs of infection. Prophylactic antibiotics may be indicated pending results of C/S in a febrile neutropenic patient. ▪ Acetaminophen, diphenhydramine (Benadryl), and steroids (e.g., hydrocortisone) may be used prophylactically to reduce incidence of fever and anaphylaxis.

Patient Education: Use nonhormonal contraception. ▪ Report any possible side effects promptly. ▪ Report stinging or burning at IV site promptly. ▪ See Appendix D, p. 1148. ▪ Pulmonary toxicity more likely in smokers.

Maternal/Child: Avoid pregnancy. ▪ Not recommended during breast-feeding.

Elderly: Response similar to that seen in younger adults; however, pulmonary toxicity is more common in patients older than 70 years of age. ▪ Consider age-related renal impairment.

DRUG/LAB INTERACTIONS

See Precautions. ■ Vascular toxicities (e.g., myocardial infarction, CVA, thrombotic microangiopathy, cerebral arteritis) or Raynaud's phenomenon have occurred rarely when bleomycin is used in combination with other antineoplastic agents. ■ May decrease GI absorption of digoxin and hydantoins (e.g., phenytoin). ■ Do not administer live vaccines to patients receiving antineoplastic drugs. ■ Causes sensitization of lung tissue to O_2; increases risk of pulmonary toxicity with O_2 and general anesthetics. ■ Cisplatin may inhibit renal elimination and increase toxicity. ■ Effects of bleomycin significantly enhanced if vinblastine is administered 6 to 8 hours before bleomycin.

SIDE EFFECTS

Alopecia, anorexia, chills, dyspnea, fever, hypotension, malaise, nausea, phlebitis (infrequent), rales, scleroderma-like skin changes, tenderness of the skin, tumor site pain, vomiting, weight loss.

Major: Anaphylaxis (up to 6 hours after test dose), chest pain (acute with sudden onset suggestive of pleuropericarditis), pneumonitis, pulmonary fibrosis, skin toxicity (including nodules on hands, desquamation of skin, hyperpigmentation, and gangrene).

ANTIDOTE

Notify the physician of all side effects. Minor side effects will be treated symptomatically. Discontinue the drug immediately and notify the physician of any symptom of major side effects. Provide immediate treatment (epinephrine [Adrenalin] and diphenhydramine [Benadryl] for anaphylaxis, antibiotics and steroids for pneumonitis) or supportive therapy as indicated.

BRETYLIUM TOSYLATE

(bre-til'ee-um to'suh-late)

Antiarrhythmic

✤Bretylate, Bretylium Tosylate PF

pH 4.5 to 7

USUAL DOSE

Life-threatening ventricular arrhythmias: 5 mg/kg of body weight. Defibrillate. If ventricular arrhythmia persists, increase to 10 mg/kg and repeat every 5 to 30 minutes as necessary. Maximum total dose is 35 mg/kg.

Other ventricular arrhythmias: 5 to 10 mg/kg by IV infusion. Repeat in 1 to 2 hours if arrhythmia persists.

Maintenance dose: 5 to 10 mg/kg by intermittent infusion every 6 hours or a continuous infusion at 1 to 2 mg/min. Replace with oral antiarrhythmic therapy as soon as practical, usually within 24 hours. Reduce dose under ECG monitoring.

PEDIATRIC DOSE

Same as adult doses except total dose should not exceed 30 mg/kg. See Maternal/Child.

DOSE ADJUSTMENTS

May be required in impaired renal function. ■ Reduced doses may be indicated in the elderly based on potential for decreased organ function and concomitant disease or drug therapy.

DILUTION

May be given undiluted in ventricular fibrillation. For other ventricular arrhythmias each dose must be diluted with 50 ml or more of D5W or NS to be given as an intermittent infusion. Larger amounts may be further diluted in any amount of the above solutions and given as a continuous infusion (1 Gm in 1,000 ml equals 1 mg/ml). 1 Gm in 250 ml (4 mg/ml) may be used to deliver bolus doses. Available premixed as 2 mg/ml and 4 mg/ml in 250 ml D5W.

COMPATIBLE WITH

(Underline Indicates Conflicting Compatibility Information)

Consult pharmacist; specific conditions may apply; see Compatibilities, p. xvi.

Solution: D5W, D5/½NS, D5NS, D5LR, NS, 5% sodium bicarbonate, 20% mannitol, ⅙ M sodium lactate, LR, calcium chloride (54.4 mEq/L) in D5W, potassium chloride (40 mEq/L) in D5W.

Additive: Aminophylline, atracurium (Tracrium), calcium chloride, calcium gluconate, digoxin (Lanoxin), <u>dobutamine (Dobutrex)</u>, dopamine (Intropin), esmolol (Brevibloc), insulin (regular), lidocaine, <u>nitroglycerin (Nitro-Bid IV)</u>, potassium chloride (KCl), <u>procainamide (Pronestyl)</u>, quinidine, verapamil (Isoptin).

Y-site: Amiodarone (Cordarone), cisatracurium (Nimbex), diltiazem (Cardizem), dobutamine (Dobutrex), famotidine (Pepcid IV), gatifloxacin (Tequin), inamrinone (Inocor), isoproterenol (Isuprel), linezolid (Zyvox), ranitidine (Zantac), remifentanil (Ultiva).

RATE OF ADMINISTRATION

Life-threatening ventricular arrhythmias: A single dose over 1 minute.

Intermittent infusion: A single dose over a minimum of 8 to 10 minutes. More rapid infusion may cause nausea and vomiting in all patients and orthostatic hypotension in the elderly.

Continuous infusion: 1 to 2 mg diluted solution/min. Use an infusion pump or microdrip (60 gtt/ml). Adjust as indicated by progress in patient's condition.

ACTIONS

A quaternary ammonium compound with antiarrhythmic effects. It increases the ventricular fibrillation threshold, suppresses ventricular arrhythmias and aberrant impulses, and increases the refractory period without increasing HR. Probably effective through its adrenergic blocking action. Antifibrillatory effects occur within minutes; suppression of ventricular tachycardia and other ventricular arrhythmias develop over 15 to 20 minutes. Suppression of premature beats requires constant plasma levels. Half-life ranges from 4 to 17 hours. Excreted in the urine.

INDICATIONS AND USES

Prophylaxis and treatment of ventricular fibrillation and treatment of life-threatening ventricular arrhythmias. Not a first-line antiarrhythmic agent. Recommended when defibrillation, epinephrine, and lidocaine have failed to convert VF, when VF has recurred despite epinephrine and lidocaine, when lidocaine and procainamide have not controlled VT associated with a pulse, or when lidocaine and adenosine have not controlled wide-complex tachycardias.

CONTRAINDICATIONS

None when used as indicated.

PRECAUTIONS

May cause severe hypotension if fixed cardiac output present (aortic stenosis, pulmonary hypertension). ■ May cause transient hypertension and increased frequency of arrhythmias. ■ Use caution if renal function is impaired.

Monitor: Monitor the patient's ECG and BP continuously. ■ Keep patient in supine position; postural hypotension is almost always present. Tolerance to hypotensive effect may develop after several days. ■ Correct dehydration or hypovolemia. ■ Observe for increased anginal pain in susceptible patients.

Maternal/Child: Used during pregnancy or in children only in life-threatening situations. ■ Safety and effectiveness for use in children not established.

Elderly: Reduced doses may be indicated; see Dose Adjustments. Monitoring of renal function suggested. ■ Risk of orthostatic hypotension increases with a rapid rate of infusion.

DRUG/LAB INTERACTIONS

May aggravate digitalis toxicity; use with caution if patient receiving digitalis; avoid simultaneous initiation of therapy. ■ Will potentiate catecholamines (e.g., dopamine [Intropin]); use diluted solution and monitor BP closely. ■ Risk of cardiotoxicity increased with pimozide (Orap) and sparfloxacin (Zagam); concurrent use not recommended.

SIDE EFFECTS

Anginal attacks, bradycardia, dizziness, hypotension and postural hypotension, increased frequency of PVCs, initial increase in arrhythmias, light-headedness, nausea and vomiting, substernal pressure, syncope, transitory hypertension, vertigo.

ANTIDOTE

Notify the physician of all side effects. Nausea and vomiting may subside with reduction in rate of administration. Use dopamine or norepinephrine (Levophed) and IV fluids to correct hypotension. Treat hypertension with a short-acting antihypertensive agent (e.g., nitroprusside sodium). Resuscitate as necessary.

BUMETANIDE

(byoo-met′a-nide)

Diuretic (loop)

Bumex

pH 6.8 to 7.8

USUAL DOSE

0.5 to 1 mg. May be repeated at 2- to 3-hour intervals. Do not exceed 10 mg/24 hr. Can be used for patients allergic to furosemide. 1:40 mg ratio (bumetanide to furosemide) is used to determine dose.

PEDIATRIC DOSE

Safety for use in pediatric patients not established; see Maternal/Child.

DOSE ADJUSTMENTS

Start at lower end of dosing range in the elderly. Consider decreased cardiac, hepatic, or renal function; concomitant disease; and other drug therapy.

DILUTION

May be given undiluted. Not usually added to IV solutions but compatible with D5W, NS, and LR. Usually given through Y-tube or three-way stopcock of infusion set. Use only freshly prepared solutions for infusion. Discard after 24 hours.

INCOMPATIBLE WITH

May precipitate with milrinone (Primacor) infusions.

COMPATIBLE WITH (Underline Indicates Conflicting Compatibility Information)

Consult pharmacist; specific conditions may apply; see Compatibilities, p. xvi.

Additive: Furosemide (Lasix).

Syringe: Doxapram (Dopram).

Y-site: Allopurinol (Aloprim, Zyloprim), amifostine (Ethyol), aztreonam (Azactam), cefepime (Maxipime), cisatracurium (Nimbex), cladribine (Leustatin), diltiazem (Cardizem), docetaxel (Taxotere), etoposide phosphate (Etopophos), filgrastim (Neupogen), gemcitabine (Gemzar), granisetron (Kytril), hetastarch in electrolytes (Hextend), lorazepam (Ativan), melphalan (Alkeran), meperidine (Demerol), <u>milrinone (Primacor)</u>, morphine, piperacillin/tazobactam (Zosyn), propofol (Diprivan), remifentanil (Ultiva), teniposide (Vumon), thiotepa (Thioplex), vinorelbine (Navelbine).

RATE OF ADMINISTRATION

A single dose by IV injection over 1 to 2 minutes. Give infusion at prescribed rate.

ACTIONS

A sulfonamide diuretic, antihypertensive, and antihypercalcemic agent related to the thiazides. A loop diuretic agent. Extremely potent. Onset of action is within minutes and duration of action may last 4 to 6 hours. Apparently acts on the proximal and distal ends of the tubule and the ascending limb of the loop of Henle to excrete water, sodium, chloride, and potassium. Will produce diuresis in alkalosis or acidosis. Rapidly distributed, it is excreted primarily in the urine.

INDICATIONS AND USES

Edema associated with congestive heart failure, cirrhosis of the liver with ascites, renal diseases including nephrotic syndrome. ▪ Acute pulmonary edema. ▪ Edema unresponsive to other diuretic agents. ▪ Diuresis in patients allergic to furosemide. ▪ Adjunct in combination with other antihypertensive agents in the treatment of hypertensive crisis.

Unlabeled uses: Treatment of hypercalcemia.

CONTRAINDICATIONS

Anuria, known hypersensitivity to bumetanide. Use caution in patients with hepatic coma or in states of severe electrolyte depletion. Do not use until condition is improved or corrected.

PRECAUTIONS

May be used concurrently with aldosterone antagonists (e.g., spironolactone [Aldactone]) for more effective diuresis and to prevent excessive potassium loss. ▪ May increase blood glucose; has precipitated diabetes mellitus. ▪ May lower serum calcium level, causing tetany. ▪ In rare instances may precipitate an acute attack of gout. ▪ Risk of ototoxicity increased with higher doses, rapid injection, decreased renal function, or concurrent use with other ototoxic drugs; see Drug/Lab Interactions. ▪ Patients allergic to sulfonamides may have an allergic reaction to bumetanide.

Monitor: May precipitate excessive diuresis with water and electrolyte depletion. Routine checks on electrolyte panel, CO_2, serum glucose, uric acid, and BUN are necessary during therapy. Potassium chloride replacement may be required.

Patient Education: Hypotension may cause dizziness; move slowly, and request assistance to sit on edge of bed or ambulate. ▪ May decrease potassium levels and require a supplement.

Maternal/Child: Category C: use in pregnancy only if clearly needed. ▪ Consider discontinuing breast-feeding. ▪ Has been used in infants age 4 days to 6 months at doses ranging from 0.005 mg/kg to 0.1 mg/kg. Maximal diuretic effect seen at doses of 0.035 to 0.04 mg/kg. Elimination half-life decreases during the first month of life from approximately 6 hours at birth to 2.4 hours at 1 month.

Elderly: Response similar to that seen in younger patients; however, dose selection should be cautious; see Dose Adjustments. Consider increased sensitivity to hypotensive and electrolyte effects and increased risk of circulatory collapse or thromboembolic episodes. ▪ Monitoring of renal function suggested.

DRUG/LAB INTERACTIONS

Causes excessive potassium depletion with corticosteroids, thiazide diuretics (e.g., hydrochlorothiazide [Hydrodiuril]), amphotericin B (all formulations). ▪ Potentiates antihypertensive drugs (e.g., nitroglycerin, nitroprusside sodium); reduced dose of the antihypertensive agent or both drugs may be indicated. ■ May cause transient or permanent deafness with doses exceeding the usual or when given in conjunction with other ototoxic drugs (e.g., aminoglycosides [e.g., gentamicin], cisplatin). ■ Amphotericin B (all formulations) may increase potential for ototoxicity and nephrotoxicity, avoid concurrent use. ■ Nephrotoxicity increased by other nephrotoxic agents (e.g., acyclovir [Zovirax], aminoglycocides, ciprofloxacin [Cipro IV], cyclosporine [Sandimmune], vancomycin [Vancocin]); avoid concurrent use. ■ May increase activity of anticoagulants (e.g., warfarin [Coumadin], heparin, streptokinase); monitor PT. ■ May increase serum levels of lithium (may cause toxicity). ■ May cause cardiac arrhythmias with amiodarone (Cordarone) or digitalis (potassium depletion). ■ Risk of cardiotoxicity increased with pimozide (Orap) and sparfloxacin (Zagam); concurrent use not recommended. ■ May enhance or inhibit actions of nondepolarizing muscle relaxants (e.g., mivacurium [Mivacron]) or theophyllines. ■ May cause hyperglycemia with insulin or sulfonylureas (e.g., tolbutamide) by decreasing glucose tolerance. ■ Effects may be inhibited by ACE inhibitors (e.g., captopril [Capoten]), NSAIDs (e.g., ibuprofen [Motrin]), probenecid, or in patients with cirrhosis and ascites on salicylates. ■ May cause profound diuresis and serious electrolyte abnormalities with thiazide diuretics (e.g., chlorothiazide [Diuril]) because of synergistic effects. ■ Do not use concomitantly with ethacrynic acid (Edecrin); risk of ototoxicity markedly increased. ■ Smoking may increase secretion of ADH-decreasing diuretic effects and cardiac output. ■ See Precautions.

SIDE EFFECTS

Usually occur in prolonged therapy, seriously ill patients, or following large doses.

Abdominal pain, arthritic pain, azotemia, dizziness, ECG changes, elevated SrCr, encephalopathy, headache, hyperglycemia, hyperuricemia, hypochloremia, hyponatremia, hypotension, impaired hearing, muscle cramps, nausea, pruritus, rash.

Major: Anaphylactic shock, blood volume reduction, circulatory collapse, dehydration, excessive diuresis, hypokalemia, metabolic acidosis, thrombocytopenia, vascular thrombosis, and embolism.

ANTIDOTE

If minor side effects are noted, discontinue the drug and notify the physician, who may treat the side effects symptomatically and continue the drug. If side effects are progressive or any major side effect occurs, discontinue the drug immediately and notify the physician. Treatment of major side effects is symptomatic and aggressive and includes fluid and electrolyte replacement. Resuscitate as necessary.

BUPRENORPHINE HYDROCHLORIDE

(byoo-pre-nor′feen hye-droe-klor′id)

Narcotic analgesic (agonist-antagonist)
Anesthesia adjunct

Buprenex

pH 3.5 to 5.5

USUAL DOSE

Pain control: 0.3 mg (1 ml). Repeat every 6 hours as necessary. May be repeated in 30 to 60 minutes, if indicated. These dose recommendations have been lowered because of excessive respiratory depression with doses up to 0.6 mg. 25 to 250 mcg/hr has been given as a continuous infusion to manage postoperative pain.

Reverse fentanyl-induced anesthesia (unlabeled): 0.3 to 0.8 mg 1 to 4 hours after induction of anesthesia and 30 minutes before end of surgery.

PEDIATRIC DOSE

2 to 12 years of age: Pain control: 2 to 6 mcg/kg of body weight every 4 to 8 hours. A repeat dose in 30 to 60 minutes is not recommended. Longer intervals (6 to 8 hours) are suggested and should provide sufficient pain relief. Determine appropriate interval through clinical assessment.

DOSE ADJUSTMENTS

Reduce dose by one half in high-risk patients (e.g., elderly or debilitated, respiratory disease), when other CNS depressants have been given, and in the immediate postoperative period; see Drug/Lab Interactions. ■ Reduced dose may be required in impaired liver function.

DILUTION

IV injection: May be given undiluted.

Infusion: May be further diluted with NS, D5W, D5NS, or LR injection and given as an infusion. 1 mg in 250 ml = 4 mcg/ml, 3 mg in 250 ml = 12 mcg/ml.

Storage: Before use, store at CRT. Avoid freezing and/or prolonged exposure to light.

COMPATIBLE WITH

Consult pharmacist; specific conditions may apply; see Compatibilities, p. xvi.

Syringe: Atropine, diphenhydramine (Benedryl), droperidol (Inapsine), glycopyrrolate, haloperidol (Haldol), heparin, midazolam (Versed), promethazine (Phenergan), scopolamine.

Y-site: Allopurinol (Aloprim, Zyloprim), amifostine (Ethyol), aztreonam (Azactam), cefepime (Maxipime), cisatracurium (Nimbex), cladribine (Leustatin), docetaxel (Taxotere), etoposide phosphate (Etopophos), filgrastim (Neupogen), gatifloxacin (Tequin), gemcitabine (Gemzar), granisetron (Kytril), linezolid (Zyvox), melphalan (Alkeran), piperacillin/tazobactam (Zosyn), propofol (Diprivan), remifentanil (Ultiva), teniposide (Vumon), thiotepa (Thioplex), vinorelbine (Navelbine).

RATE OF ADMINISTRATION

Titrate slowly according to symptom relief and respiratory rate.

IV injection: A single dose over 3 to 5 minutes.

Infusion: See Usual Dose. Use of a metriset (60 gtt/min) or a controlled infusion device recommended.

ACTIONS

A synthetic narcotic agonist-antagonist analgesic. Thirty times as potent as morphine in analgesic effect (0.3 mg equivalent to 10 mg morphine) and has the antagonist effect of naloxone in larger doses. Does produce respiratory depression. Pain relief is effected in 2 to 3 minutes and lasts up to 6 hours. Metabolized in the liver. Primarily excreted through feces. Crosses the placental barrier. Secreted in breast milk.

INDICATIONS AND USES

Relief of moderate to severe pain.

Unlabeled use: Reverse fentanyl-induced anesthesia.

CONTRAINDICATIONS

Children 2 years of age and younger, hypersensitivity to buprenorphine.

PRECAUTIONS

Usually given IM. ■ May precipitate withdrawal symptoms if stopped too quickly after prolonged use or if patient has been on opiates. ■ Use caution in asthma, respiratory depression or difficulty from any source, impaired renal or hepatic function, the elderly or debilitated, myxedema or hypothyroidism, adrenocortical insufficiency, CNS depression or coma, toxic psychoses, prostatic hypertrophy or urethral stricture, acute alcoholism, delirium tremens, or kyphoscoliosis. ■ May elevate cerebrospinal fluid pressure; use caution in head injury, intracranial lesions, and other situations with increased intracranial pressure.

Monitor: Naloxone (Narcan), oxygen, and controlled respiratory equipment must be available. Naloxone is only partially effective in reversing respiratory depression. ■ Observe patient frequently and monitor vital signs. ■ Keep patient supine to minimize side effects; orthostatic hypotension and fainting may occur. Observe closely during ambulation. ■ Pain control usually more effective with routinely administered doses. Determine appropriate interval through clinical assessment.

Patient Education: Avoid use of alcohol or other CNS depressants (e.g., antihistamines, diazepam [Valium]). ■ Use caution performing any task requiring alertness; may cause dizziness, euphoria, and sedation. ■ Request assistance for ambulation. ■ May be habit forming.

Maternal/Child: Category C: safety for use during pregnancy, labor and delivery, or breast-feeding not established. Use only when clearly needed. ■ Not recommended in children under 2 years of age but has been used in children as young as 9 months of age.

Elderly: See Dose Adjustments. ■ May be more sensitive to effects (e.g., respiratory depression, urinary retention, constipation, dizziness). ■ Analgesia should be effective with lower doses. ■ Consider possibility of decreased organ function.

DRUG/LAB INTERACTIONS

Respiratory and CNS effects may be additive with barbiturate anesthetics (e.g., thiopental [Pentothal]); reduced doses of both drugs may be indicated. ■ May cause respiratory depression and cardiovascular collapse with diazepam (Valium); reduced doses of both drugs may be indicated. ■ May decrease analgesic effects of other narcotics; avoid concurrent use. ■ Clearance decreased and serum levels increased by cytochrome P_{450} inhibitors (e.g., azole antifungal agents [e.g., itraconazole (Sporanox)], macrolide antibiotics [e.g., erythromycin], protease inhibitors [e.g., ritonavir (Norvir)]). Monitor with concurrent use; dose adjustment may be indicated. ■ Clearance increased and serum levels decreased by cytochrome P_{450} inducers (e.g., carbamazepine [Tegretol], phenytoin [Dilantin], rifampin [Rifadin]). Use caution; dose adjustments may be indicated.

SIDE EFFECTS

Excessive sedation is a major side effect. Has caused death from respiratory depression. Anaphylaxis, bradycardia, clammy skin, constipation, cyanosis, dizziness, dyspnea, headache, hypertension, hypotension, nausea, pruritus, tachycardia, vertigo, visual disturbances, vomiting.

ANTIDOTE

With increasing severity of any side effect or onset of symptoms of overdose, discontinue the drug and notify the physician. Naloxone hydrochloride (Narcan) will help to reverse respiratory depression, but is not as effective as it is with other narcotics. A patent airway, artificial ventilation, oxygen therapy, and other symptomatic treatment must be instituted promptly. Treat anaphylaxis and resuscitate as necessary.

BUSULFAN

(byoo-sul′fan)

Busulfex

Antineoplastic (alkylating agent)

pH 3.4 to 3.9

USUAL DOSE

Administered in combination with cyclophosphamide as a component of a conditioning regimen prior to bone marrow or peripheral blood progenitor cell replacement support.

Premedication: Premedicate patients with phenytoin (use of other anticonvulsants not recommended) and an antiemetic (e.g., $5HT_3$ antiemetics such as ondansetron [Zofran], granisetron [Kytril]). Continue antiemetic administration on a fixed schedule throughout busulfan therapy. See Monitor, Drug Interactions and Side Effects.

Busulfan: 0.8 mg/kg of ideal body weight (IBW) or actual body weight, whichever is lower, administered through a central venous catheter every 6 hours for 4 days (16 doses). Six hours after the 16th busulfan dose (on BMT day minus 3 [3 days prior to BMT]), begin cyclophosphamide at a dose of 60 mg/kg/day for 2 days. Before and after each infusion, flush the catheter line with 5 ml NS or D5W.

DOSE ADJUSTMENTS

In obese or severely obese patients, dose should be based on an adjusted ideal body weight (AIBW). Calculate as follows:

$$\text{AIBW} = \text{IBW} + 0.25 \times (\text{actual weight} - \text{IBW})$$

■ Busulfan has not been studied in patients with renal or hepatic insufficiency. See Precautions.

DILUTION

Specific techniques required; see Precautions. Supplied in ampules containing 60 mg/10 ml (6 mg/ml). Must be diluted prior to infusion with either NS or D5W. The diluent volume should be 10 times the busulfan volume to ensure a final concentration of approximately 0.5 mg/ml. Remove calculated dose of busulfan from ampule, using a syringe fitted with a needle and a 5-micron Nylon filter (provided). Use of filters other than the specific type included in the package is not recommended. Remove the needle and filter, replace with a new needle and dispense the contents of the syringe into an intravenous bag or syringe that contains the calculated amount of diluent. Always add the busulfan to the diluent rather than the diluent to the busulfan. Mix thoroughly by inverting several times. The dose for a 70-kg patient would be prepared using the following steps:

1. 70 kg × 0.8 mg/kg = 56 mg.
2. 56 mg ÷ 6 mg/ml = 9.3 ml busulfan needed.
3. 9.3 × 10 = 93 ml.
4. Add 9.3 ml of busulfan to 93 ml of NS or D5W.
5. Final concentration = 56 mg ÷ 102.3 ml = 0.54 mg/ml.

Storage: Refrigerate. Busulfan diluted with NS or D5W is stable for 8 hours at room temperature, but infusion must be completed within that time. When diluted with NS and refrigerated, it is stable for 12 hours, but infusion must be completed within that time.

COMPATIBILITY

Do not use polycarbonate syringes. Manufacturer states, "Do not infuse concomitantly with another intravenous solution of unknown compatibility. Flush central venous catheter line before and after administration with at least 5 ml of NS or D5W."

RATE OF ADMINISTRATION

Before and after each infusion, flush the catheter line with 5 ml NS or D5W.

Busulfan: Infuse over 2 hours using an infusion pump.

Cyclophosphamide: Infuse over 1 hour.

ACTIONS

A bifunctional alkylating agent. Cell cycle phase–nonspecific. Interferes with DNA replication, leading to cytotoxicity and cell death. Distributes equally into plasma and CSF. Metabolized in the liver. Excreted partially in the urine, primarily as metabolites.

INDICATIONS AND USES

For use in combination with cyclophosphamide as a conditioning regimen prior to allogeneic hematopoietic progenitor cell transplantation for chronic myelogenous leukemia. ■ Has orphan drug approval as preparative therapy for treatment of malignancies with BMT and treatment of brain cancer.

CONTRAINDICATIONS

Previous hypersensitivity to busulfan or any of its components (polyethylene glycol and dimethylacetamide).

PRECAUTIONS

Follow guidelines for handling cytotoxic agents. See Appendix A, p. 1142. ■ Administered by or under the direction of a physician who is experienced in allogeneic hematopoietic stem cell transplantation, the use of cancer chemotherapeutic drugs, and the management of patients with severe pancytopenia. ■ Adequate diagnostic and treatment facilities must be readily available to manage therapy and any complications that arise. ■ Profound myelosuppression, including granulocytopenia, thrombocytopenia, anemia, or any combination of these will occur. ■ Seizures have been reported. Use caution when administering to patients with a history of seizures or head trauma or patients who are receiving other potentially epileptogenic drugs (e.g., imipenem-cilastatin [Primaxin], meperidine [Demerol]). ■ Anticonvulsant prophylactic therapy should be initiated with phenytoin before busulfan treatment. ■ High busulfan AUC values (greater than 1,500 μM•min) may be associated with an increased risk of developing hepatic veno-occlusive disease (VOD). Patients who have received prior radiation therapy, three or more cycles of chemotherapy, or a prior progenitor cell transplant may be at an increased risk of developing hepatic VOD with the recommended busulfan dose and regimen. ■ Cardiac tamponade has been reported in pediatric patients with thalassemia who received high doses of oral busulfan and cyclophosphamide. No patients treated in the busulfan injection trials experienced cardiac tamponade. ■ Bronchopulmonary dysplasia with pulmonary fibrosis is a rare but serious complication following chronic busulfan therapy. Average onset of symptoms is 4 years after therapy (range: 4 months to 10 years). ■ May cause cellular dysplasia in many organs. Dysplasia may be severe enough to cause difficulty in interpretation of exfoliative cytologic examinations of the lungs, bladder, breast and the uterine cervix.

Monitor: Obtain a baseline and a daily CBC, including differential and platelet count, during treatment and until engraftment is demonstrated. Absolute neutrophil count (ANC) dropped below 0.5×10^9/L at a median of 4 days posttransplant and recovered at a median of 13 days when prophylactic G-CSF was used. Thrombocytopenia (platelets less than 25,000/mm^3 or platelet transfusion required) occurred at a median of 5-6 days. ■ Monitor for signs of local or systemic infection or bleeding. Antibiotic therapy and platelet and RBC support should be used when medically indicated. ■ Monitor for thrombocytopenia (platelet count less than 50,000/mm^3). Initiate precautions to prevent excessive bleeding (e.g., inspect IV sites, skin, and mucous membranes; use extreme care during invasive procedures; test urine, emesis, stool, and secretions for occult blood). ■ Serum transaminases, alkaline phosphatase, and bilirubin should be obtained daily through transplant day 28 to monitor for signs of hepatotoxicity, and the onset of hepatic VOD. Jones' criteria may be used to diagnose VOD (hyperbilirubinemia, and two of the following three findings: painful hepatomegaly, weight gain more than 5%, or ascites). ■ Obtain baseline and periodic uric acid concentrations. ■ Use of anticonvulsants other than phenytoin may result in higher busulfan plasma AUCs and an increased risk of VOD or seizures. When other anticonvulsants are used, plasma busulfan AUC should be monitored; see Drug/Lab Interactions.

Patient Education: Nonhormonal birth control recommended. ■ May be at increased risk of developing a secondary malignancy. ■ See Appendix D, p. 1148.

Maternal/Child: Category D: avoid pregnancy. Can cause fetal harm. Has mutagenic potential. ■ Discontinue breast-feeding. ■ Safety and efficacy in children not established. Clearance has been shown to be higher in children than adults, necessitating the development of alternative dosing regimens for oral busulfan in children. Studies are under way to define the pharmacokinetics of busulfan injection in children. The recommended dose of busulfan injection has not yet been defined.

Elderly: Has been used in a small number of patients over 55 years of age. All achieved myeloablation and engraftment.

DRUG/LAB INTERACTIONS

Itraconazole (Sporanox) decreases busulfan clearance, increasing the AUC and risk of toxicity. ■ Phenytoin increases the clearance of busulfan. Because the pharmacokinetics of busulfan were studied in patients treated with phenytoin, the clearance of busulfan at the recommended dose may be lower and the AUC higher in patients not treated with phenytoin. ■ Acetaminophen (Tylenol) may decrease clearance of busulfan. Avoid administration of acetaminophen 72 hours prior to or with busulfan therapy. ■ Do not administer live virus vaccines to patients receiving antineoplastic drugs. ■ Busulfan has been used with fluconazole (Diflucan), ondansetron (Zofran), and granisetron (Kytril). ■ May cause additive effects with bone-marrow–depressing agents or agents that cause blood dyscrasias (e.g., amphotercin B, antithyroid agents, azathioprine [Imuran], chloramphenicol, ganciclovir [Cytovene], interferon, plicamycin [Mithracin], zidovudine) and radiation therapy. Adjust busulfan dose based on blood cell counts. ■ Risk of uric acid nephropathy increased with sulfinpyrazone (Anturan), allopurinol may be preferred to prevent or treat hyperuricemia. ■ See Precautions.

SIDE EFFECTS

Profound myelosuppression, including granulocytopenia, thrombocytopenia, anemia, or a combination of these, will occur in 100% of patients. ■ Other nonhematologic adverse events occurring in more than 20% of patients include abdominal pain or enlargement, allergic reactions, anorexia, anxiety, asthenia, back pain, chest pain, chills, constipation, cough, creatinine elevation, depression, diarrhea, dizziness, dry mouth, dyspepsia, dyspnea, edema, epistaxis, fever, headache, hyperbilirubinemia, hyperglycemia, hypertension, hypocalcemia, hypokalemia, hypomagnesemia, infection, inflammation or pain at injection site, insomnia, lung disorders, nausea, pain, pruritus, rash, rectal disorder, rhinitis, seizures, SGPT elevation, stomatitis (mucositis), tachycardia, thrombosis, vasodilation (flushing or hot flashes), vomiting. ■ Graft-versus-host disease, hepatic veno-occlusive disease and death have also been reported. ■ Dimethylacetamide (DMA), the solvent used in busulfan formulation, has been associated with adverse reactions such as confusion, hallucinations, hepatotoxicity, lethargy, and somnolence. The relative contribution of DMA to neurologic and hepatic toxicities observed with busulfan is difficult to determine. Numerous other side effects have occurred.

ANTIDOTE

Treat minor side effects symptomatically. In the absence of hematopoietic progenitor cell transplantation, the normal dosage of busulfan injection constitutes an overdose. Monitor hematologic status closely, and institute supportive measures as indicated. Administration of whole blood products (e.g., packed RBCs, platelets, leukocytes) and/or blood modifiers (e.g., darbepoetin alfa [Aranesp], epoetin alfa [Epogen, Procrit], filgrastim [Neupogen], pegfilgrastim [Neulasta], sargramostim [Leukine], oprelvekin [Neumega]) may be indicated to treat bone marrow toxicity. Dialysis and administration of glutathione may be considered in an overdose (busulfan is metabolized by conjugation with glutathione).

BUTORPHANOL TARTRATE

(byoo-tor′fa-nole tahr′trat)

Narcotic analgesic (agonist-antagonist)
Anesthesia adjunct

Stadol, Stadol PF

pH 3 to 5.5

USUAL DOSE

Pain control: 1 mg. Repeat every 3 to 4 hours as necessary. Range is 0.5 to 2 mg.

Preoperative or preanesthetic: 2 mg 30 to 60 minutes before surgery. Individualize dose. Usually given IM.

Labor: 1 to 2 mg at full term in early labor; may be repeated after 4 hours. Use alternate analgesia if delivery is expected to occur within 4 hours.

Adjunct to balanced anesthesia: 2 mg just before induction or 0.5 to 1 mg in increments during anesthesia. Increments may be up to 0.06 mg/kg and should be based on previous sedative, analgesic, and hypnotic drugs. A total dose exceeding 4 mg is seldom required, but the range is from 4 to 12.5 mg (0.06 to 0.18 mg/kg). Administered only under the direction of the anesthesiologist.

PEDIATRIC DOSE

Safety and effectiveness for use in pediatric patients not established; see Maternal/Child.

DOSE ADJUSTMENTS

Reduce dose and/or increase the interval between doses in high-risk patients (e.g., elderly or debilitated, respiratory disease); adjust as indicated by patient response. ■ Reduce dose when other CNS depressants have been given and in the immediate postoperative period. Use the smallest effective dose and extend intervals between doses. ■ Extend intervals to 6 or 8 hours in impaired liver or renal function; adjust as indicated by patient response. ■ See Drug/Lab Interactions.

DILUTION

May be given undiluted. Avoid aerosol spray while preparing a syringe for use. Rinse with cool water following skin contact. Available preservative free.

Storage: Store at CRT. Protect from light and freezing.

COMPATIBLE WITH

(Underline Indicates Conflicting Compatibility Information)

Consult pharmacist; specific conditions may apply; see Compatibilities, p. xvi.

Additive: Atropine sulfate, promethazine (Phenergan).

Syringe: Atropine sulfate, chlorpromazine (Thorazine), cimetidine (Tagamet), diphenhydramine (Benadryl), droperidol (Inapsine), fentanyl (Sublimaze), meperidine (Demerol), metoclopramide (Reglan), <u>midazolam (Versed)</u>, morphine, pentazocine (Talwin), perphenazine (Trilafon), prochlorperazine (Compazine), promethazine (Phenergan), scopolamine.

Y-site: Allopurinol (Aloprim, Zyloprim), amifostine (Ethyol), aztreonam (Azactam), cefepime (Maxipime), cisatracurium (Nimbex), cladribine (Leustatin), docetaxel (Taxotere), doxorubicin liposome (Doxil), enalaprilat (Vasotec IV), esmolol (Brevibloc), etoposide phosphate (Etopophos), filgrastim (Neupogen), fludarabine (Fludara), gatifloxacin (Tequin), gemcitabine (Gemzar), granisetron (Kytril), hetastarch in electrolytes

(Hextend), labetalol (Normodyne), linezolid (Zyvox), melphalan (Alkeran), paclitaxel (Taxol), piperacillin/tazobactam (Zosyn), propofol (Diprivan), remifentanil (Ultiva), sargramostim (Leukine), teniposide (Vumon), thiotepa (Thioplex), vinorelbine (Navelbine).

RATE OF ADMINISTRATION

Each 2 mg or fraction thereof over 3 to 5 minutes. Frequently titrated according to symptom relief and respiratory rate.

ACTIONS

A potent narcotic analgesic with some narcotic agonist-antagonist effects. Exact mechanism of action is unknown. Analgesia similar to morphine is produced. Does produce respiratory depression, but this does not increase markedly with larger doses. Pain relief is effected almost immediately, peaks at 30 minutes, and lasts about 2 to 4 hours. Causes some hemodynamic changes that increase the workload of the heart. Metabolized in the liver. Excreted in urine and feces. Crosses the blood-brain barrier and placental barrier. Secreted in breast milk.

INDICATIONS AND USES

Relief of moderate to severe pain. ■ Preoperative or preanesthetic medication, as a supplement to anesthesia. ■ Relief of pain during early labor.

CONTRAINDICATIONS

Hypersensitivity to butorphanol or its components (some products contain benzethonium chloride).

PRECAUTIONS

Not used for narcotic-dependent patients because of antagonist activity. ■ May increase cardiac workload; use in myocardial infarction, ventricular dysfunction, and coronary insufficiency only if benefits outweigh risks. ■ Use caution in respiratory depression or difficulty from any source, obstructive respiratory conditions, head injury, and impaired liver or kidney function. ■ Prolonged continuous use may result in physical dependence or tolerance. ■ In overdose situations, always consider the possibility of multiple drug ingestion.

Monitor: Naloxone (Narcan), oxygen, and controlled respiratory equipment must be available. Duration of action of butorphanol usually exceeds that of naloxone; repeated dosing may be necessary. ■ Observe patient frequently and monitor vital signs. ■ Keep patient supine to minimize side effects; orthostatic hypotension and fainting may occur. Observe closely during ambulation. ■ Pain control usually more effective with routinely administered doses. Determine appropriate interval through clinical assessment.

Patient Education: Avoid use of alcohol or other CNS depressants (e.g., antihistamines, diazepam [Valium]). ■ Use caution performing any task requiring alertness; may cause dizziness, euphoria, and sedation. ■ Request assistance for ambulation. ■ May be habit forming.

Maternal/Child: Category C: safety for use in pregnant women before 37 weeks' gestation not established; use only if benefit justifies potential risk to fetus. ■ Has been used safely during labor of term infants. Has been associated with transient (10 to 90 minutes) sinusoidal fetal heart rate patterns. Use caution if abnormal fetal heart rate is present; manufacturer states "was not associated with adverse outcomes." Alternative analgesia suggested if delivery is expected to occur within 4 hours. ■ Use caution in breast-feeding; an estimated 4 mcg/L has been found in breast milk;

may be clinically insignificant. ■ Safety and effectiveness not established for children under 18 years.

Elderly: Mean half-life may be extended by 25%, may be more sensitive to effects (e.g., respiratory depression, constipation, dizziness, urinary retention). ■ Analgesia should be effective with lower doses; see Dose Adjustments. ■ Consider decreased organ function, concomitant disease, or other drug therapy.

DRUG/LAB INTERACTIONS

Potentiated by cimetidine (Tagamet), phenothiazines (e.g., chlorpromazine [Thorazine]), droperidol (Inapsine), and CNS depressants such as narcotic analgesics, general anesthetics, alcohol, anticholinergics, antihistamines, barbiturates, benzodiazepines (e.g., diazepam [Valium]), hypnotics, MAO inhibitors, neuromuscular blocking agents (e.g., mivacurium [Mivacron]), psychotropic agents, and sedatives. Reduced doses of both drugs may be indicated; use the smallest effective dose of butorphanol and/or extend intervals between doses. ■ Effects may be altered by other medications that affect hepatic metabolism of drugs (e.g., aminophyline, erythromycin). Reduced doses of butorphanol and/or longer intervals between doses may be indicated. ■ May decrease analgesic effects of other narcotics; avoid concurrent use. ■ Will cause an increase in conjunctival changes with pancuronium (Pavulon).

SIDE EFFECTS

Dizziness, nausea and/or vomiting, and somnolence occur most frequently. Abdominal pain, anorexia, anxiety, asthenia, bronchitis, clammy skin, confusion, constipation, cough, diplopia, dizziness, drug dependence, dry mouth, dyspnea, euphoria, floating feeling, flushing, hallucinations, headache, hypersensitivity reactions (e.g., pruritis), hypotension, insomnia, lethargy, nervousness, palpitations, paresthesia, respiratory depression, sweating, tremor, unusual dreams, vasodilation, vertigo, warmth. May cause increased pulmonary artery pressure, pulmonary wedge pressure, left ventricular end-diastolic pressure, systemic arterial pressure, pulmonary vascular resistance, and cardiac workload.

Overdose: Cardiovascular insufficiency, hypoventilation, coma, and death. May be associated with ingestion of multiple drugs.

ANTIDOTE

With increasing severity of any side effect or onset of symptoms of overdose, discontinue the drug and notify the physician. Most side effects will be treated symptomatically. Treat hypertension with antihypertensives (e.g., nitroglycerin, nitroprusside sodium). Naloxone hydrochloride (Narcan) will reverse respiratory depression. Duration of action of butorphanol usually exceeds that of naloxone; repeated dosing may be necessary. A patent airway, adequate ventilation, oxygen therapy, and other symptomatic treatment must be instituted promptly. Vasodilation may cause hypotension.

CAFFEINE CITRATE

(kaf′een sit′rat)

Cafcit

CNS stimulant
Respiratory stimulant adjunct

pH 4.7

USUAL DOSE

The dose expressed as caffeine base is one half the dose when expressed as caffeine citrate. The recommended loading dose and maintenance dose are listed in the chart below:

Guidelines for Loading and Maintenance Doses of Caffeine Citrate			
	Dose of Cafcit (volume)	Dose Expressed as Caffeine Citrate	Dose Expressed as Caffeine Base
Loading dose	1 ml/kg	20 mg/kg	10 mg/kg
Maintenance dose	0.25 ml/kg	5 mg/kg	2.5 mg/kg

Begin maintenance dose 24 hours after loading dose. Maintenance dose may be given IV or orally. Duration of treatment beyond 10 to 12 days has not been studied. See Precautions.

DOSE ADJUSTMENTS

May adjust maintenance dose using serum concentrations of caffeine. ■ To avoid toxicity in neonates with impaired renal or hepatic function, use with caution and monitor serum concentrations.

DILUTION

Supplied in a vial containing 60 mg/3 ml of caffeine citrate (30 mg/3 ml of caffeine base). Withdraw calculated dose and dilute with sufficient D5W to administer at the recommended rate of administration.

Storage: Store at CRT. Single-use vial. Discard any unused solution. Stable for 24 hours at room temperature when mixed with any of the solutions listed in Compatible With.

COMPATIBLE WITH

Consult pharmacist; specific conditions may apply; see Compatibilities, p. xvi.

Additive: Manufacturer lists amino acid solution 8.5% (Aminosyn 8.5%), calcium gluconate 10%, D5W, dextrose 50%, dopamine 40 mg/ml diluted to 0.6 mg/ml with D5W, fentanyl diluted to 10 mcg/ml with D5W, heparin sodium diluted to 1 unit/ml with D5W, IV fat emulsion 20% (Intralipid 20%).

RATE OF ADMINISTRATION

Use of a syringe pump infuser is recommended.

Loading dose: Infuse over 30 minutes.

Maintenance dose: Infuse over 10 minutes.

ACTIONS

A bronchial smooth muscle relaxant, a CNS and cardiac stimulant, and a diuretic. Structurally related to other methylxanthines (e.g., theophylline and theobromine). Exact mechanism of action in apnea of prematurity is not known. Postulated mechanisms include stimulation of the respiratory center, increased minute ventilation, decreased threshold to hypercapnia, increased response to hypercapnia, increased skeletal muscle tone, decreased diaphragmatic fatigue, increased metabolic rate, increased oxygen consumption, blood vessel dilatation, central vessel vasoconstriction, and smooth muscle relaxation. Readily distributes into the brain. Caffeine levels in the CSF of preterm neonates approximate plasma levels. Metabolized in the liver by the cytochrome P_{450} system. Metabolism and elimination in the preterm neonate are much slower than in adults due to immature hepatic and/or renal function. Mean half-life and fraction excreted unchanged in the urine is inversely related to gestational/postconceptual age. In neonates, the half-life is approximately 3 to 4 days and the fraction excreted unchanged in the urine is approximately 86% (within 6 days). By 9 months of age, the metabolism of caffeine approximates that seen in adults (half-life is 5 hours and amount excreted unchanged is 1%). Interconversion between caffeine and theophylline have been reported in preterm neonates. After theophylline administration, caffeine levels are approximately 25% of theophylline levels. After caffeine administration, 3% to 5% of caffeine administered converts to theophylline.

INDICATIONS AND USES

Short-term treatment of apnea of prematurity in infants more than 28 but less than 33 weeks' gestational age. In one study apnea of prematurity was defined as having at least 6 apnea episodes of more than 20 seconds duration in a 24-hour period with no other identifiable cause of apnea. **Unlabeled uses:** Prevention of postoperative apnea in former preterm infants.

CONTRAINDICATIONS

Hypersensitivity to any of its components.

PRECAUTIONS

Reports in the literature suggest a possible association between the use of methylxanthines and the development of necrotizing enterocolitis. Necrotizing enterocolitis, resulting in death in some cases, has been reported in neonates receiving caffeine citrate. ■ Apnea of prematurity is a diagnosis of exclusion. Other causes of apnea (e.g., CNS disorders, primary lung disease, anemia, sepsis, metabolic disturbances, cardiovascular abnormalities, or obstructive apnea) should be ruled out or properly treated prior to initiating therapy with caffeine citrate. ■ Is a CNS stimulant. Use with caution in infants with seizure disorders. ■ May increase heart rate, left ventricular output, and stroke volume. Use with caution in infants with cardiovascular disease. ■ Duration of treatment of apnea of prematurity in trials has been limited to 10 to 12 days. Safety and efficacy of therapy beyond this time have not been established. ■ Safety and efficacy for use in prophylactic treatment of sudden infant death syndrome (SIDS) or before extubation in mechanically ventilated infants have not been established. ■ Use with caution in infants with impaired renal or hepatic function; see Dose Adjustments and Monitor. ■ Patients sensitive to other xanthines (e.g., aminophylline) may also be sensitive to caffeine.

Monitor: Obtain baseline serum caffeine levels in infants previously treated with theophylline, since preterm infants metabolize theophylline to caffeine; see Actions. Levels should also be obtained in infants born to mothers who ingested caffeine before delivery, as caffeine readily crosses the placenta. Caffeine levels ranged from 8 to 40 mg/L in clinical trials. A therapeutic plasma concentration range has not been determined, but one source suggests 5 to 25 mcg/ml. Serious toxicity has been reported at levels exceeding 50 mg/L. Monitor levels periodically during treatment to avoid toxicity. Monitoring is especially important in infants with impaired renal or hepatic function. ■ Monitor serum glucose periodically. Hypoglycemia and hyperglycemia have been reported.

Patient Education: Caregivers should be instructed to consult physician if infant continues to have apnea events and to not increase the dose of caffeine citrate without consulting a physician. ■ Contact physician at the first sign of lethargy or GI intolerance (e.g., abdominal distention, vomiting, or bloody stools). ■ Dose must be accurately measured, and any unused solution must be discarded.

Maternal/Child: Category C: no controlled studies; benefits should outweigh risks. ■ Half-life is increased in pregnant women. ■ Half-life may be in excess of 100 hours in infants under 6 months of age due to immature liver function.

DRUG/LAB INTERACTIONS

Metabolized by the cytochrome P_{450} system. Lower caffeine doses may be required with coadministration of medications that inhibit the P_{450} system, decreasing the elimination of caffeine (e.g., cimetidine [Tagamet] and ketoconazole [Nizoral]). Higher caffeine doses may be needed with coadministration of medications that induce the P_{450} system, increasing the elimination of caffeine (e.g., phenobarbital and phenytoin). ■ Interconversion between caffeine and theophylline has been reported. Concurrent use of these drugs is not recommended; see Actions.

SIDE EFFECTS

Cardiovascular effects (e.g., tachycardia, increased left ventricular output, and increased stroke volume), CNS stimulation (e.g., irritability, jitteriness, restlessness), GI effects (e.g., feeding intolerance, gastritis, increased gastric aspirate, and necrotizing enterocolitis), hyperglycemia, hypoglycemia, renal effects (e.g., increased urine output, increased CrCl, and increased sodium and calcium excretion).

Overdose: Signs and symptoms of caffeine overdose in the preterm infant may include: elevated BUN, elevated total leukocyte concentration, fever, fine tremor of extremities, hyperglycemia, hypertonia, insomnia, jitteriness, nonpurposeful jaw and lip movements, opisthotonos, seizures, tachypnea, tonic-clonic movements, or vomiting.

ANTIDOTE

Notify the physician of any side effects. Treatment of overdose is primarily symptomatic and supportive. Seizures may be treated with intravenous administration of diazepam (Valium) or a barbiturate such as pentobarbital (Nembutal). Caffeine levels have been shown to decrease after exchange transfusions. Resuscitate as necessary.

CALCITRIOL

(kal-si-trye′ole)

Calcijex

Vitamin D

pH 6.5 to 8

USUAL DOSE

Effectiveness of calcitriol therapy is dependent on adequate daily intake of calcium. The RDA of calcium in adults is 800 mg. Calcium supplementation or proper dietary measures must be initiated and maintained.

Hypocalcemia and/or secondary hyperparathyroidism: Recommended initial dose, depending on the severity of hypocalcemia and/or secondary hyperparathyroidism, is 1 mcg (0.02 mcg/kg) to 2 mcg administered at each hemodialysis treatment (three times weekly, approximately every other day). Initial doses have ranged from 0.5 to 4 mcg three times weekly.

Information supplied by the manufacturer suggests that the relative dosing of paricalcitol to calcitriol is 4:1. When converting a patient from calcitriol to paricalcitol, the initial dose of paricalcitol should be four times greater than the patient's dose of calcitriol.

PEDIATRIC DOSE

Hypocalcemia in end stage renal disease (ESRD) (unlabeled): 0.01 to 0.05 mcg/kg/dose given 3 times a week; see Maternal/Child. See all comments under Usual Dose.

DOSE ADJUSTMENTS

Adjust dosing based on patient response. Begin dosing at lower end of dose range in the elderly; see Elderly. If a satisfactory response is not observed, dose may be increased by 0.5 to 1 mcg at 2- to 4-week intervals. Monitor serum calcium, phosphorus, and calcium × phosphorus product (Ca × P) frequently during any dose adjustment period; see Monitor. ■ Discontinue therapy if elevated calcium level or a Ca × P product of greater than 70 is noted. Reinitiate therapy at a lower dose when parameters normalize. ■ Calcitriol dose may need to be reduced as the parathyroid hormone (PTH) levels decrease in response to therapy. The currently accepted target range for intact parathyroid hormone (iPTH) in chronic renal failure (CRF) patients is no more than 1.5 to 3 times the non-uremic upper limit of normal. Incremental dosing must be individualized and commensurate with PTH, serum calcium, and phosphorus levels. The following chart is a suggested approach to dose titration:

Calcitriol Suggested Dosing Guidelines

PTH Levels	Calcitriol Dose
The same or increasing	Increase
Decreasing by <30%	Increase
Decreasing by >30% but <60%	Maintain
Decreasing by >60%	Decrease
One and one-half to three times the upper limit of normal	Maintain

DILUTION

May be given undiluted. Available in 1- and 2-mcg/ml ampules.

Storage: Store ampules at CRT. Protect from light. Calcitriol may be drawn up into a syringe up to 8 hours prior to administration but must be protected from direct sunlight.

COMPATIBILITY

Specific information not available; consult pharmacist.

RATE OF ADMINISTRATION

Administer as a bolus dose into the venous line at the end of hemodialysis.

ACTIONS

The active form of vitamin D_3 (cholecalciferol). Must be metabolically activated in liver and kidney before it is fully active on its target tissues. In bone, acts with PTH to stimulate resorption of calcium. In kidneys, increases tubular reabsorption of calcium. Stimulates intestinal calcium transport, and directly suppresses synthesis and release of PTH from the parathyroid gland. A vitamin D–resistant state may exist in uremic patients because of the failure of the kidney to adequately convert precursors to the active compound, calcitriol. Plasma half-life is 3 to 6 hours. Duration of action is 3 to 5 days. Eliminated in bile and urine.

INDICATIONS AND USES

Management of hypocalcemia in patients undergoing chronic renal dialysis. Has been shown to significantly reduce elevated PTH levels, which results in improvement in renal osteodystrophy.

Unlabeled uses: Treatment of hypercalcemia in pediatric patients with ESRD.

CONTRAINDICATIONS

Patients with hypercalcemia or evidence of vitamin D toxicity.

PRECAUTIONS

Since calcitriol is the most potent form of vitamin D available, oral vitamin D supplements should be discontinued during treatment. ■ Dietary phosphorus should be restricted and a non–aluminum phosphate–binding compound (e.g., calcium acetate [Phos-Lo], sevelamer [Renagel]) should be administered to control serum phosphorus levels in patients undergoing dialysis. ■ Consider a 2.5-mEq/L calcium dialysate concentration if patient has a history of hypercalcemia and/or is receiving a calcium-based phosphate binder (calcium acetate [Phos-Lo]).

Monitor: Obtain baseline serum calcium, phosphorus, aluminum, albumin, and PTH assays. ■ Serum calcium levels should be corrected for serum albumin using the following equation: Corrected Ca = observed Ca + 0.8 × (normal albumin − observed albumin). For example: If serum calcium is 7 mg/dl and observed albumin is 2.5 Gm/dl, Corrected Ca = $7 + 0.8 \times (4 - 2.5) = 8.2$ mg/dl. All decisions regarding therapy should be based on corrected calcium values. ■ Monitor magnesium, alkaline phosphatase, and 24-hour urinary calcium and phosphorus periodically. ■ Criteria used to determine if calcitriol should be administered include: serum calcium less than 11.5 mg/dl, Ca × P less than 70, serum albumin less than 60 mcg/L (within normal limits), and PTH more than 3 times the upper limit of normal. ■ Serum calcium, phosphorus, and the Ca × P product should be monitored twice weekly during dose titration. Once stable, decrease monitoring to once monthly. See Dose Adjustments. ■ PTH levels, once stable, should be monitored every 3 months.

Adynamic bone lesions may develop if PTH levels are suppressed to abnormal levels. If PTH levels fall below the target range (1.5 to 3 times the upper limit of normal), the calcitriol dose should be reduced. Discontinuation may result in rebound effect. Therefore, gradual titration downward to a new maintenance dose is recommended; see Dose Adjustments. ▪ Overdosage of vitamin D is dangerous. May induce hypercalcemia and/or hypercalciuria. If clinically significant hypercalcemia develops, dose should be reduced or held. Chronic hypercalcemia can lead to generalized vascular calcification, nephrocalcinosis, and other soft-tissue calcification. The serum Ca × P product should not be allowed to exceed 70. Radiographic evaluation of suspect anatomical regions may be useful in early detection of this condition; see Side Effects and Antidote. ▪ Use with caution in patients receiving digitalis. Hypercalcemia may precipitate cardiac arrhythmias; see Drug/Lab Interactions.

Patient Education: Report symptoms of hypercalcemia promptly. Dose adjustment or treatment may be required. Strict adherence to dietary supplementation of calcium and restriction of phosphorus is required to ensure optimal effectiveness of therapy. Phosphate-binding compounds (e.g., calcium acetate [Phos-Lo]) may be needed to control serum phosphorus levels in patients with CRF, but excessive use of aluminum-containing products (e.g., aluminum hydroxide gel [Alternagel]) should be avoided. ▪ Avoid use of unapproved nonprescription medications, including magnesium-containing antacids.

Maternal/Child: Category C: safety for use in pregnancy not established. Benefits must outweigh risks. ▪ Safety for use in breast-feeding not established. A decision should be made whether to discontinue nursing or to discontinue the drug. ▪ Safety and effectiveness have been studied in a small number of pediatric patients, ages 13 to 18 years, with ESRD on hemodialysis. The mean weekly dose ranged from 1 to 1.4 mcg. Use in this study program appeared to be safe and effective. See package insert for study information.

Elderly: Begin dosing at lower end of dose range. Consider age-related organ impairment, concomitant disease, and/or drug therapy; see Dose Adjustments.

DRUG/LAB INTERACTIONS

Specific interaction studies have not been performed. ▪ Digitalis toxicity is potentiated by hypercalcemia. Use caution when calcitriol is prescribed concomitantly with digitalis compounds. ▪ Phosphate or vitamin D-related compounds should not be taken concomitantly with calcitriol. ▪ Magnesium-containing antacids and calcitriol should not be used concomitantly. Hypermagnesemia may result. ▪ May reduce serum alkaline phosphatase levels.

SIDE EFFECTS

Overdose or chronic administration may lead to hypercalcemia, hypercalciuria, and hyperphosphatemia. High intake of calcium and phosphate concomitant with calcitriol therapy may lead to similar abnormalities. Signs and symptoms of vitamin D intoxication associated with hypercalcemia include ***Early:*** bone pain, constipation, dry mouth, headache, metallic taste, muscle pain, nausea, somnolence, vomiting, and weakness. ***Late:*** albuminuria, anorexia, cardiac arrhythmias, conjunctivitis (calcific), decreased libido, ectopic calcification, elevated BUN, elevated SGOT and

SGPT, hypercholesterolemia, hypertension, hyperthermia, nocturia, overt psychosis (rare), pain at injection site, pancreatitis, photophobia, polydipsia, polyuria, pruritus, rhinorrhea, and weight loss.

ANTIDOTE

Notify physician of any side effects. Treatment of patients with clinically significant hypercalcemia (more than 1 mg/dl above the upper limit of normal range) consists of supportive measures, immediate dose reduction or interruption of therapy, initiation of a low-calcium diet, withdrawal of calcium supplements, patient mobilization, attention to fluid and electrolyte imbalances, assessment of electrocardiographic abnormalities (critical in patients receiving digitalis), and hemodialysis or peritoneal dialysis against a calcium-free dialysate, as warranted. Hypercalcemia usually resolves in 2 to 7 days. Monitor serum calcium levels frequently until calcium levels return to within normal limits. May reinitiate calcitriol therapy at a dose 0.5 mcg less than prior dose. See Dose Adjustments.

CALCIUM CHLORIDE

(kal′se-um klor′id)

Electrolyte replenisher
Antihypocalcemic
Cardiotonic
Antihyperkalemic
Antihypermagnesemic

pH 5.5 to 7.5

USUAL DOSE

In a 10% solution, 10 ml (1 Gm) contains 13.6 mEq (272 mg) of calcium; 1 ml (100 mg), 1.36 mEq (27.2 mg). All doses based on a 10% solution.

Hypocalcemic disorders (prophylaxis, treatment, electrolyte replacement, maintenance): 5 to 10 ml (500 mg to 1 Gm) at intervals of 1 to 3 days. Repeat doses may be required and are based on patient response or serum calcium levels. May be given as part of a TPN program.

Magnesium intoxication: 5 ml (500 mg). Observe for signs of recovery before giving any additional calcium.

Hyperkalemia ECG disturbances of cardiac function: 1 to 10 ml (100 mg to 1 Gm); titrate dose by monitoring ECG changes. AHA guidelines recommend 8 to 16 mg/kg (usually 5 to 10 ml of a 10% solution), repeat as needed.

Cardiac resuscitation (see Indications for specific uses): 0.02 to 0.04 ml/kg (2 to 4 mg/kg); repeat at 10-minute intervals as indicated or as measured by serum deficits of calcium. Consider need for calcium (usually gluconate or gluceptate) for every 500 ml of whole blood if arrest occurs in a situation requiring copious blood replacement.

Overdose of calcium channel blockers or beta adrenergic blockers (unlabeled): AHA guidelines recommend 0.08 to 0.16 ml/kg (8 to 16 mg/kg). Average dose range is 5 to 10 ml. May repeat as needed.

Prophylaxis of hypotension of calcium channel blockers (unlabeled): AHA guidelines recommend 0.02 to 0.04 ml/kg (2 to 4 mg/kg). Average dose range is 2 ml given before administration of IV calcium channel blockers (e.g., diltiazem [Cardizem], verapamil [Isoptin]).

PEDIATRIC DOSE

Do not administer into a scalp vein in pediatric patients; see Precautions, Monitor, and Maternal/Child.

Hypocalcemic disorders: 0.027 to 0.05 ml/kg of body weight (2.7 to 5 mg/kg) of a 10% solution. Up to 10 ml (1 Gm)/day may be required. No data from clinical trials is available regarding repeat doses. Sources suggest repeat doses every 4 to 6 hours based on patient response or serum calcium levels.

Cardiac resuscitation (see Indications for specific uses): 0.2 ml of a 10% solution/kg of body weight (20 mg/kg). Repeat as indicated at 10-minute intervals. AHA guidelines recommend consideration of this dose in hypomagnesemia and calcium channel blocker overdose.

DILUTION

May be given undiluted, but preferably diluted with an equal amount of SW or NS for injection to make a 5% solution. Solution should be warmed to body temperature. May be further diluted with most common infusion solutions and given as an intermittent or continuous infusion.

INCOMPATIBLE WITH

Calcium salts not generally mixed with carbonates, phosphates, sulfates, or tartrates. ***Extreme caution and a specific multi-step process are required when calcium and phosphates are combined in parenteral nutrition solutions. Consult pharmacist.***

COMPATIBLE WITH **(Underline Indicates Conflicting Compatibility Information)**

Consult pharmacist; specific conditions may apply; see Compatibilities, p. xvi.

Additive: Amikacin (Amikin), ascorbic acid (Cenolate), bretylium (Bretylate), chloramphenicol (Chloromycetin), <u>dobutamine (Dobutrex)</u>, dopamine (Intropin), hydrocortisone sodium succinate (Solu-Cortef), isoproterenol (Isuprel), lidocaine, norepinephrine (Levophed), penicillin G potassium and sodium, pentobarbital (Nembutal), phenobarbital (Luminal), sodium bicarbonate, verapamil (Isoptin).

Syringe: Milrinone (Primacor).

Y-site: Dobutamine (Dobutrex), epinephrine (Adrenalin), esmolol (Brevibloc), gatifloxacin (Tequin), inamrinone (Inocor), morphine, paclitaxel (Taxol).

RATE OF ADMINISTRATION

0.5 to 1 ml of solution over 1 minute. Administration into a central or deep vein is preferred; see Monitor. Stop or slow infusion rate if patient complains of discomfort. Do not exceed the equivalent of 1 ml calcium chloride/minute by IV injection or infusion. Rapid administration may cause bradycardia; heat waves; local burning sensation; metallic, calcium, or chalky taste; moderate drop in BP; peripheral vasodilation; or a sense of oppression.

ACTIONS

Calcium is a basic element prevalent in the human body. It affects bones, nerves, muscles, glands, cardiac and vascular tone, and normal coagulation of the blood. It is excreted in the urine and feces.

INDICATIONS AND USES

Calcium preparations other than calcium chloride are often preferred except in cardiac resuscitation or calcium channel blocker toxicity. ■

Increase plasma calcium levels in hypocalcemic disorders (e.g., tetany [neonatal, parathyroid deficiency], vitamin D deficiency, alkalosis, conditions associated with intestinal malabsorption). ■ Treat ECG disturbances caused by hyperkalemia. ■ Adjunctive therapy in sensitivity reactions (especially with urticaria), insect bites or stings (relieve muscle cramping), acute symptoms of lead colic, rickets, or osteomalacia. ■ Cardiac resuscitation only to treat hypocalcemia, hyperkalemia, or calcium-channel blocker toxicity (verapamil, diltiazem), or after open heart surgery if epinephrine does not produce effective myocardial contractions. ■ Antidote for cardiac and respiratory depression of magnesium sulfate toxicity.

Unlabeled uses: Treatment of arrhythmias and/or hypotension caused by an overdose of calcium channel blockers (e.g., diltiazem [Cardizem], verapamil [Isoptin] or beta-adrenergic blockers (e.g., atenolol [Tenormin], metoprolol [Lopressor], propranolol [Inderal]). ■ Prevention of hypotension caused by calcium channel blockers.

CONTRAINDICATIONS

Digitalized patients, hypercalcemia, ventricular fibrillation. Not recommended in the treatment of asystole and electromechanical dissociation.

PRECAUTIONS

Three times more potent than calcium gluconate. ■ For IV use only. ■ See Drug/Lab Interactions.

Monitor: Confirm patency of vein; select a large vein and use a small needle to reduce vein irritation. Administration into a central or deep vein is preferred. Necrosis and sloughing will occur with IM or SC injection or extravasation. ■ Keep patient recumbent after injection to prevent postural hypotension. ■ Monitor vital signs carefully. ■ Monitor serum calcium levels as indicated. May cause hyperchloremic acidosis.

Maternal/Child: Category C: safety for use in pregnancy and breast-feeding not established. Use only when clearly needed. ■ Rarely used IV in children. Use of a less irritating salt preferred because of small vein size.

DRUG/LAB INTERACTIONS

Will increase digitalis toxicity and may cause arrhythmias. If necessary, give small amounts very slowly. ■ Potentiated by thiazide diuretics (e.g., chlorothiazide [Diuril]); may cause hypercalcemia or calcium toxicity. ■ May reduce plasma levels of atenolol (Tenormin). ■ Can reduce neuromuscular paralysis and respiratory depression produced by antibiotics such as kanamycin (Kantrex). ■ Antagonizes verapamil; can reverse clinical effects. ■ May cause metabolic alkalosis and inhibit binding of potassium with sodium polystyrene sulfonate.

SIDE EFFECTS

Usual doses will produce a local burning sensation, moderate drop in BP, and peripheral vasodilation. May cause bradycardia, cardiac arrest, heat waves; metallic, calcium, or chalky taste; prolonged state of cardiac contraction, sense of oppression, or tingling sensation, especially with a too-rapid rate of administration.

Overdose: Coma, intractable nausea and vomiting, lethargy, markedly elevated plasma calcium level, weakness, and sudden death.

ANTIDOTE

If side effects occur, further dilution and decrease in the rate of administration may be necessary. If side effects persist, discontinue the drug and notify the physician. IV infusion of sodium chloride (to maintain normovolemia) and furosemide (Lasix) 80 to 100 mg IV every 2 to 4 hours (with caution) is recommended in overdose. Sodium chloride competes with calcium for reabsorption in the renal tubules; furosemide enhances the activity. Together they will reduce hypercalcemia by causing a marked increase in calcium excretion. Monitoring of fluid, electrolytes, and cardiac and respiratory status is imperative. Disodium edetate may be used with extreme caution as a calcium chelating agent if overdose is critical. For extravasation inject affected area with 1% procaine hydrochloride and hyaluronidase to reduce venospasm and dilute calcium. Use a 27- or 25-gauge needle. Warm, moist compresses may be helpful. Resuscitate as necessary.

CALCIUM GLUCONATE
(kal′se-um gloo′ko-nat)

Electrolyte replenisher
Antihypocalcemic
Cardiotonic
Antihyperkalemic
Antihypermagnesemic

pH 6 to 8.2

USUAL DOSE

All doses based on a 10% solution.

Hypocalcemia disorders/maintenance: 5 to 20 ml (2.3 to 9.3 mEq). Repeat as required. Daily dose ranges from 4.65 to 70 mEq. Larger amounts may be given as an intermittent or continuous IV infusion. 10 ml (1 Gm in a 10% solution) contains 4.65 mEq (93 mg) of calcium.

Emergency elevation of serum calcium: 15 to 30.1 ml (7 to 14 mEq). Repeat every 1 to 3 days based on patient response.

Cardiac resuscitation (see Indications for specific uses): 5 to 8 ml (2.3 to 3.6 mEq). Repeat at 10-minute intervals as indicated by clinical condition or serum calcium level.

Hyperkalemia with secondary cardiac toxicity: 4.8 to 30.1 ml (2.25 to 14 mEq). ECG monitoring required; observe results and repeat in 1 to 2 minutes if indicated.

Hypocalcemic tetany: 9.7 to 34.4 ml (4.5 to 16 mEq). Repeat as indicated to control tetany.

Magnesium intoxication: 9.7 to 19.4 ml (4.5 to 9 mEq). Repeat as indicated by patient response; observe for signs of recovery before giving additional calcium.

Exchange transfusion: Approximately 2.9 ml (1.35 mEq) with each 100 ml of citrated blood.

PEDIATRIC DOSE

Do not administer into a scalp vein in pediatric patients; see Precautions/Monitor.

Hypocalcemia disorders/maintenance: 5 ml/kg/day (2.3 mEq/kg/day) or 120 ml/M^2/day (56 mEq/M^2/day) in divided doses.

Emergency elevation of serum calcium: 2.2 to 15 ml (1 to 7 mEq). Repeat every 1 to 3 days based on patient response.

Hypocalcemic tetany: 1.1 to 1.5 ml/kg (0.5 to 0.7 mEq/kg) 3 or 4 times daily until tetany is controlled.

Cardiac resuscitation (see Indications for specific uses): 0.6 to 1 ml/kg of a 10% solution (60 to 100 mg/kg). Repeat if indicated. AHA guidelines recommend consideration of this dose in hypomagnesemia and calcium channel blocker overdose.

NEONATAL DOSE

Do not administer into a scalp vein in neonates; see Precautions/Monitor.

Hypocalcemia disorders/maintenance: Not more than 2 ml (0.93 mEq).

Emergency elevation of serum calcium: Up to 2.2 ml (1 mEq). Repeat every 1 to 3 days based on patient response.

Hypocalcemic tetany: 5.2 ml/kg/24 hr (2.4 mEq/kg/24 hr) in divided doses.

Exchange transfusion: 1 ml (0.45 mEq) with each 100 ml of citrated blood.

DILUTION

May be given undiluted or may be further diluted in up to 1,000 ml of NS for infusion. Solution should be warmed to body temperature. Solution must be clear and free of crystals. Crystals can be dissolved by heating to 80° C (146° F) in a dry heat oven for at least 1 hour. Shake vigorously; cool to room temperature. Discard if crystals persist.

Pediatric and neonatal dilution: Must be further diluted with NS.

INCOMPATIBLE WITH

Calcium salts not generally mixed with carbonates, phosphates, sulfates, or tartrates. ***Extreme caution and a specific multi-step process are required when calcium and phosphates are combined in parenteral nutrition solutions. Consult pharmacist.***

COMPATIBLE WITH (Underline Indicates Conflicting Compatibility Information)

Consult pharmacist; specific conditions may apply; see Compatibilities, p. xvi.

Additive: Amikacin (Amikin), aminophylline, ascorbic acid (Cenolate), bretylium (Bretylate), chloramphenicol (Chloromycetin), dimenhydrinate (Dinate), furosemide (Lasix), heparin, hydrocortisone sodium succinate (Solu-Cortef), lidocaine, magnesium sulfate, norepinephrine (Levophed), penicillin G potassium and sodium, phenobarbital (Luminal), potassium chloride (KCl), <u>prochlorperazine (Compazine)</u>, tobramycin (Nebcin), vancomycin (Vancocin), verapamil (Isoptin).

Y-site: Aldesleukin (Proleukin, IL-2), allopurinol (Aloprim, Zyloprim), amifostine (Ethyol), <u>ampicillin</u>, aztreonam (Azactam), cefazolin (Kefzol), cefepime (Maxipime), ciprofloxacin (Cipro IV), cisatracurium (Nimbex), cladribine (Leustatin), dobutamine (Dobutrex), docetaxel (Taxotere), doxorubicin liposome (Doxil), enalaprilat (Vasotec IV), epinephrine (Adrenalin), etoposide phosphate (Etopophos), famotidine (Pepcid IV), filgrastim (Neupogen), gatifloxacin (Tequin), gemcitabine (Gemzar), granisetron (Kytril), hetastarch in electrolytes (Hextend), labetalol (Normodyne), linezolid (Zyvox), melphalan (Alkeran), <u>meropenem (Merrem IV)</u>, midazolam (Versed), milrinone (Primacor), piperacillin/tazobactam (Zosyn), potassium chloride (KCl), prochlorperazine (Compazine), propofol (Diprivan), remifentanil (Ultiva), sargramostim (Leukine), tacrolimus (Prograf), teniposide (Vumon), thiotepa (Thioplex), vinorelbine (Navelbine).

RATE OF ADMINISTRATION

In all situations stop or slow infusion rate if patient complains of discomfort. Rapid administration may cause vasodilation, decreased BP, cardiac arrhythmias, syncope, and cardiac arrest.

IV injection: Undiluted, each 0.5 ml or fraction thereof over 1 minute. Do not exceed 2 ml/min (200 mg).

Intermittent IV: Do not exceed a rate of 200 mg/min (IV injection rate).

Infusion: Diluted in 1,000 ml of NS, it may be given over 12 to 24 hours. Do not exceed 200 mg/min.

Pediatric and neonatal rate of administration: Slow rate of administration considerably. Observe continuously.

ACTIONS

Calcium is a basic element prevalent in the human body. It affects bones, nerves, glands, cardiac and vascular tone, and normal coagulation of the blood. It crosses the placental barrier and is secreted in breast milk. It is excreted in the urine and feces.

INDICATIONS AND USES

■ Increase plasma calcium levels in hypocalcemic disorders (e.g., tetany [neonatal, parathyroid deficiency], vitamin D deficiency, alkalosis, conditions associated with intestinal malabsorption). ■ Adjunctive therapy in sensitivity reactions (especially with urticaria), insect bites or stings (relieve muscle cramping), acute symptoms of lead colic, rickets, or osteomalacia. ■ Cardiac resuscitation only to treat hypocalcemia, hyperkalemia, or calcium-channel blocker overdose (verapamil, diltiazem). ■ Antidote for cardiac and respiratory depression of magnesium sulfate toxicity. ■ Prevention of hypocalcemia during exchange transfusions. ■ Decrease capillary permeability in allergic conditions, nonthrombocytopenic purpura and exudative dermatoses (e.g., dermatitis herpetiformis). ■ Treat pruritus of eruptions caused by drugs. ■ Treat ECG disturbances caused by hyperkalemia or verapamil-induced hypotension.

Unlabeled uses: Treatment of verapamil overdose, acute hypotension from verapamil, and prevention of initial hypotension when it could be detrimental to a specific patient and verapamil is required.

CONTRAINDICATIONS

IM use in infants and small children. Digitalized patients, hypercalcemia, ventricular fibrillation.

PRECAUTIONS

Has only one third the potency of calcium chloride. ■ For IV use only; IM use permitted in adults only if IV administration cannot be accomplished; see Monitor.

Monitor: Confirm patency of vein; select a large vein and use a small needle to reduce vein irritation. Local necrosis and abscess formation can occur with IM or SC injection or extravasation. ■ Keep patient recumbent after injection to prevent postural hypotension. ■ Monitor vital signs carefully.

Maternal/Child: Category C: safety for use in pregnancy not established; benefits must outweigh risk. ■ See Contraindications.

DRUG/LAB INTERACTIONS

Will increase digitalis toxicity and may cause arrhythmias. If necessary, give small amounts very slowly. ■ Potentiated by thiazide diuretics (e.g., chlorothiazide [Diuril]); may cause hypercalcemia or calcium toxicity. ■ May reduce plasma levels of atenolol (Tenormin). ■ Antagonizes verapamil; can reverse clinical effects. ■ May cause metabolic alkalosis and inhibit binding of potassium with sodium polystyrene sulfonate.

SIDE EFFECTS

Rare when given as recommended: bradycardia, cardiac arrhythmias, cardiac arrest, heat waves, hypotension; metallic, calcium, or chalky taste; sense of oppression, syncope, tingling, and vasodilation can occur with too-rapid rate of administration. Depression of neuromuscular function, flushing, prolonged state of cardiac contraction can occur.

Overdose: Coma, intractable nausea and vomiting, lethargy, markedly elevated plasma calcium level, weakness, and sudden death.

ANTIDOTE

If side effects occur, further dilution and decrease in the rate of administration may be necessary. If side effects persist, discontinue the drug and notify the physician. IV infusion of sodium chloride (to maintain normovolemia) and furosemide (Lasix) 80 to 100 mg IV every 2 to 4 hours (with caution) are recommended in overdose. Sodium chloride competes with calcium for reabsorption in the renal tubules; furosemide enhances the activity. Together they will reduce hypercalcemia by causing a marked increase in calcium excretion. Monitoring of fluid, electrolytes, and cardiac and respiratory status is imperative. Disodium edetate may be used with extreme caution as a calcium chelating agent if overdosage is critical. For extravasation inject affected area with 1% procaine hydrochloride and hyaluronidase to reduce venospasm and dilute calcium. Use a 27- or 25-gauge needle. Warm, moist compresses may be helpful. Resuscitate as necessary.

CAPREOMYCIN

(kap-ree-oh-mye'sin)

Capastat

Antibacterial (antituberculosis)

USUAL DOSE

1 Gm daily, not to exceed 20 mg/kg/day. Give for 60 to 120 days, followed by 1 Gm two or three times weekly. Therapy for tuberculosis should be maintained for 12 to 24 months. Administered in combination with at least one other antituberculosis agent to which the patient's strain of tubercle bacilli is susceptible.

DOSE ADJUSTMENTS

The elderly and patients with reduced renal function should have dosage reduction based on CrCl using the guidelines in the chart below. These dosages are designed to achieve a mean steady-state capreomycin level of 10 mcg/ml. Elevation of BUN above 30 mg/dl or any other evidence of decreasing renal function warrants evaluation of patient. Dose reduction or discontinuation of therapy may be required.

Estimated Dosages to Attain Mean Steady-State Serum Capreomycin Concentration of 10 mcg/ml Based on CrCl

	Dose* (mg/kg) Based on Dosing Intervals		
CrCl (ml/min)	24 hr	48 hr	72 hr
0	1.29	2.58	3.87
10	2.43	4.87	7.30
20	3.58	7.16	10.7
30	4.72	9.45	14.2
40	5.87	11.7	
50	7.01	14.0	
60	8.16		
80	10.4†		
100	12.7†		
110	13.9†		

*Optional dosing intervals are given. Longer intervals are expected to provide greater peaks and lower trough serum levels than shorter intervals.

†See Usual Dose.

DILUTION

Reconstitute each 1-Gm vial with 2 ml of NS or SW. Allow 2 to 3 minutes for complete dissolution. Withdraw calculated dose and further dilute in 100 ml NS.

Storage: Store at CRT before reconstitution. After reconstitution, stable for 24 hours if refrigerated.

COMPATIBILITY

Specific information not available; consult pharmacist.

RATE OF ADMINISTRATION

A single dose as an infusion over 60 minutes. Neuromuscular blockade or respiratory paralysis may occur following rapid intravenous infusion. See Precautions and Side Effects.

ACTIONS

A polypeptide antibiotic isolated from *Streptomyces capreolus.* Active against strains of *Mycobacterium tuberculosis.* Half-life is 3 to 6 hours in patients with normal renal function. Excreted primarily unchanged in urine. Small amounts excreted in bile. Crosses the placenta. Does not penetrate into CSF.

INDICATIONS AND USES

Used concomitantly with other appropriate antituberculosis agents for treatment of pulmonary infections caused by capreomycin-susceptible strains of *M. tuberculosis* when the primary agents (isoniazid, rifampin, ethambutol, aminosalicylic acid, and streptomycin) have been ineffective or cannot be used because of toxicity or the presence of resistant tubercle bacilli.

CONTRAINDICATIONS

Hypersensitivity to capreomycin.

PRECAUTIONS

Usually given IM; IV used in patients with limited muscle mass. ■ Sensitivity studies necessary to determine susceptibility of causative organism to capreomycin. ■ Use with caution in patients with pre-existing auditory impairment, dehydration, or renal insufficiency or when used concomitantly with other potentially ototoxic or nephrotoxic drugs (e.g., aminoglycosides [e.g., amikacin (Amikin), colistin sulfate, gentamicin (Garamycin), polymyxin A, streptomycin, tobramycin (Nebcin)], vancomycin (Vancocin). Must weigh risk of additional cranial nerve VIII (auditory and vestibular) damage or renal injury against benefit of therapy. ■ Renal injury, with tubular necrosis, elevation of BUN or SrCr, and abnormal urinary sediment (casts, RBCs, WBCs), has been reported. Elderly patients, patients with abnormal renal function or dehydration, and patients receiving other nephrotoxic drugs are at increased risk for developing acute tubular necrosis. ■ Elevation of BUN above 30 mg/dl or other evidence of decreasing renal function warrants evaluation of patient. Dose reduction or discontinuation of drug may be necessary; see Dose Adjustments. Clinical significance of abnormal urine sediment and slight increase in BUN or SrCr during long-term therapy is not known. ■ The peripheral neuromuscular blocking action seen with other polypeptide antibiotics (colistin sulfate, polymyxin A sulfate) and aminoglycosides (e.g., kanamycin, neomycin, streptomycin) has been reported with capreomycin. ■ Cross-resistance between capreomycin and kanamycin, neomycin and viomycin has been reported. No cross-resistance has been observed between capreomycin and aminosalicylic acid, cycloserine, ethambutol, ethionamide, isoniazid, and streptomycin.

Monitor: Audiometric measurements and assessment of vestibular function should be performed before initiation of therapy and at regular intervals during treatment. ■ Obtain baseline SrCr, BUN, liver function tests, and electrolytes before initiating therapy. Reduced dosage required for patients with impaired renal function; see Dose Adjustments. Weekly monitoring of renal function and periodic monitoring of electrolytes and liver function tests are recommended.

Patient Education: Compliance with full course of therapy is imperative. Report any side effects promptly.

Maternal/Child: Category C: safety for use during pregnancy and breast-feeding not established. Benefits must outweigh risks. Crosses the placenta. ■ Safety and effectiveness in children not established.

Elderly: May be at increased risk of toxicity because of age-related decrease in renal function; see Dose Adjustments and Precautions.

DRUG/LAB INTERACTIONS

Neuromuscular blockade of non-depolarizing neuromuscular blocking agents (e.g., vecuronium [Norcuron]) may be enhanced with concurrent use of capreomycin because of synergistic effects and may be further enhanced by ether or methoxyflurane anesthesia. ■ Risk of neuromuscular blockade increased when administered concurrently or sequentially with polymyxins or aminoglycosides (e.g., kanamycin, neomycin, streptomycin); see Precautions. ■ Neuromuscular blockade antagonized by neostigmine. ■ Risk of ototoxicity, nephrotoxicity, and respiratory paralysis increased when administered concurrently or sequentially with other potentially ototoxic or nephrotoxic medications (e.g., aminoglycosides [e.g., amikacin (Amikin), gentamicin (Garamycin), streptomycin, tobramycin (Nebcin)], colistin sulfate, polymyxin A, vancomycin [Vancocin]); see Precautions.

SIDE EFFECTS

Abnormal liver function tests, abnormal urine sediment, dizziness, electrolyte disturbances resembling Bartter's syndrome, as well as hypocalcemia, hypokalemia, and hypomagnesemia, elevated BUN or SrCr, eosinophilia, febrile reactions, hypersensitivity, leukocytosis, leukopenia, maculopapular skin rash, pain and induration at injection site, subclinical auditory loss (high-tone acuity), thrombocytopenia, tinnitus, toxic nephritis, urticaria, vertigo.

ANTIDOTE

Protect airway and support ventilation and perfusion. Hydrate patient to maintain urine output of 3 to 5 ml/kg/hr. Monitor fluid balance, electrolytes, renal function, vital signs, and blood gases; treat abnormalities as indicated. Hemodialysis may be useful. Resuscitate as necessary.

CARBOPLATIN

(kar-boe-pla'tin)

Antineoplastic (alkylating agent)

Paraplatin, ✤Paraplatin-AQ

pH 5 to 7

USUAL DOSE

Before giving a dose in a cycle, it is recommended that platelets be above 100,000/mm^3 and neutrophils above 2,000/mm^3; see Dose Adjustments. Recently a new dosing formula (Calvert formula for carboplatin dosing) based on pre-existing renal function and/or desired platelet nadir has been implemented.

$$\text{Total dose (mg)} = (\text{target AUC}) \times (\text{GFR} + 25)$$

Dose is calculated in milligrams, not mg/M^2. The ordering physician determines the target AUC (area under the curve) and supplies the required information on the GFR (glomerular filtration rate) or CrCl, as well as the desired response. The pharmacist calculates the correct dose. See package insert for additional information.

Palliative treatment of recurrent ovarian cancer after prior chemotherapy: ***As a single agent:*** With normal renal function (CrCl greater than 60 ml/min), give 360 mg/M^2 on day 1 every 4 weeks or a dose targeted by Calvert equation to an AUC of 4 to 6 appears to provide an appropriate dose range in these patients.

Treatment of brain tumor (unlabeled): ***As a single agent:*** 560 mg/M^2 every 4 weeks.

Initial treatment of advanced ovarian cancer in combination with cyclophosphamide: Carboplatin 300 mg/M^2 plus cyclophosphamide 600 mg/M^2 on day 1 every 4 weeks for 6 cycles or carboplatin dose targeted by Calvert equation to an AUC of 6 to 7 plus cyclophosphamide 600 mg/M^2 on day 1 every 4 weeks.

Treatment of unresectable non–small-cell lung cancer (NSCLC [unlabeled]): Given in combination with paclitaxel (Taxol). Many dosage regimens are being used. Examples are: paclitaxel 135 to 175 mg/M^2 as either a continuous infusion over 24 hours or an intermittent IV over 3 hours on day 1. Follow on day 2 with carboplatin 300 mg/M^2 or dose targeted by Calvert equation to an AUC of 6. Repeat this cycle every 4 weeks for up to 6 cycles. Another source suggests paclitaxel 135 mg/M^2 as a continuous infusion over 24 hours on day 1 or 175 mg/M^2 IV over 3 hours on day 1. Follow either of these doses with carboplatin dose targeted by Calvert equation to an AUC of 7.5. Repeat cycle every 21 days.

DOSE ADJUSTMENTS

Single agent or combination therapy. Dose adjustment is based on nadir after prior dose according to the following chart.

Carboplatin Dose Based on Bone Marrow Suppression		
Platelets/mm^3	Neutrophils/mm^3	Adjusted Dose (From Prior Course)
>100,000	>2,000	Increase to 125%
50,000-100,000	500-2,000	No adjustment
<50,000	<500	Decrease to 75%

Once the dose has been increased to 125% of the starting dose, no further dose increases are indicated. ■ With impaired renal function (CrCl 16 to 40 ml/min), give 200 mg/M^2; CrCl 40 to 59 ml/min, give 250 mg/M^2. Adjust dose by percentages and criteria as indicated for normal renal function. ■ Bone marrow suppression is more severe in patients who have had prior therapy, especially with cisplatin and when carboplatin is used with other bone marrow–suppressing therapies or radiation, and may be more severe in the elderly. Reduced dose may be indicated. Monitor carefully and manage dose and timing to reduce additive effects.

DILUTION

Specific techniques required; see Precautions. Immediately before use dilute each 10 mg of carboplatin with 1 ml of SW for injection, D5W, or NS (50 mg with 5 ml, 150 mg with 15 ml, 450 mg with 45 ml). All yield 10 mg/ml. Should be further diluted with NS or D5W to 1 to 4 mg/ml (add 10 ml additional diluent to each 10 mg to obtain 1 mg/ml and 2.5 ml to each 10 mg to obtain 4 mg/ml). Do not use needles or IV tubing with aluminum parts to mix or administer; a precipitate will form and decrease potency. Best to mix immediately before use. Discard solution 8 hours after dilution at room temperature, 24 hours if refrigerated.

Storage: Store unopened vials at 15° to 30° C (59° to 86° F). Protect from light.

INCOMPATIBLE WITH

Forms a precipitate if in contact with aluminum (e.g., needles, syringes, catheters).

COMPATIBLE WITH

Consult pharmacist; specific conditions may apply; see Compatibilities, p. xvi.

Additive: Cisplatin (Platinol), etoposide (VePesid), ifosfamide (Ifex), paclitaxel (Taxol).

Y-site: Allopurinol (Aloprim, Zyloprim), amifostine (Ethyol), aztreonam (Azactam), cefepime (Maxipime), cladribine (Leustatin), doxorubicin liposome (Doxil), etoposide phosphate (Etopophos), filgrastim (Neupogen), fludarabine (Fludara), gatifloxacin (Tequin), gemcitabine (Gemzar), granisetron (Kytril), linezolid (Zyvox), melphalan (Alkeran), ondansetron (Zofran), paclitaxel (Taxol), piperacillin/tazobactam (Zosyn), propofol (Diprivan), sargramostim (Leukine), teniposide (Vumon), thiotepa (Thioplex), topotecan (Hycamtin), vinorelbine (Navelbine).

RATE OF ADMINISTRATION

A single dose as an infusion over a minimum of 15 minutes. Extend administration time based on amount of diluent and patient condition.

ACTIONS

An alkylating agent. An improved platinum-based compound similar to cisplatin but with improved therapeutic effects. Better tolerated by patients, carboplatin causes less nausea and vomiting, less neurotoxicity, and less nephrotoxicity than cisplatin. Myelosuppression is generally reversible and manageable with antibiotics and transfusions. Produces interstrand DNA cross-links and is cell cycle nonspecific. Not as heavily protein bound as cisplatin. Majority of carboplatin is excreted in the urine within 24 hours.

INDICATIONS AND USES

Initial treatment of advanced ovarian cancer in combination with other approved chemotherapeutic agents (e.g., cyclophosphamide). ■ Palliative treatment of recurrent ovarian cancer after prior chemotherapy, including patients treated with cisplatin.

Unlabeled uses: In combination with paclitaxel (Taxol) to treat unresectable non–small-cell lung cancer (NSCLC) and fallopian tube and peritoneal cancers of ovarian origin. ■ Treatment of brain tumors. ■ Treatment of breast and bladder cancers, lymphomas (Hodgkin's and non-Hodgkin's), malignant melanoma, small-cell lung cancer, and retinoblastoma; and to replace cisplatin in treatment of endometrial, esophageal, head and neck, lung, and testicular cancers and relapsed and refractory acute leukemia. May be used as a single agent but most effective in protocols.

CONTRAINDICATIONS

Hypersensitivity to cisplatin or other platinum-containing compounds or mannitol; severe bone marrow depression; significant bleeding.

PRECAUTIONS

■ Follow guidelines for handling cytotoxic agents. See Appendix A, p. 1142. ■ Usually administered by or under the direction of the physician specialist. ■ Peripheral neurotoxicity is infrequent but may increase in patients over 65 years of age and in patients previously treated with cisplatin. ■ Risk of allergic reaction increased in patients previously exposed to platinum therapy. Patients sensitive to other platinum compounds (e.g., cisplatin) may be sensitive to carboplatin.

Monitor: BUN and SrCr should be done before each dose. CrCl, WBC, platelet count, and hemoglobin are recommended before each dose and weekly thereafter. Platelet count recommended to be 100,000/mm^3 and neutrophils 2,000/mm^3 before a dose can be repeated; see Dose Adjustments. Anemia is frequent and cumulative. Transfusion is often indicated. ■ Excessive hydration or forced diuresis not required, but maintain adequate hydration and urinary output. ■ Nausea and vomiting are frequently severe but less than with cisplatin; generally last 24 hours. Prophylactic administration of antiemetics is indicated. Various protocols, including metoclopramide (Reglan) and ondansetron (Zofran), dexamethasone (Decadron) and lorazepam (Ativan), droperidol (Inapsine) or haloperidol (Haldol) and dexamethasone, or prochlorperazine (Compazine) are used. ■ Observe for symptoms of allergic reaction during administration; epinephrine, corticosteroids, and antihistamines should be available. ■ Observe closely for symptoms of infection. Prophylactic antibiotics may be indicated pending results of C/S in a febrile neutropenic patient. ■ Monitor for thrombocytopenia (platelet count less than 50,000/mm^3). Initiate precautions to prevent excessive bleeding (e.g., inspect IV sites, skin, and mucous membranes; use extreme care during invasive procedures; test urine, emesis, stool, and secretions for occult blood).

Patient Education: Nonhormonal birth control recommended. Manufacturer provides a patient information booklet. ■ See Appendix D, p. 1148.

Maternal/Child: Category D: avoid pregnancy. ■ Discontinue breastfeeding. ■ Significant hearing loss has been reported in children; occurred with higher-than-recommended doses of carboplatin in combination with other ototoxic agents.

Elderly: Neurotoxicity and myelotoxicity may be more severe. ■ Consider possibility of decreased renal function. ■ See Dose Adjustments and Precautions.

DRUG/LAB INTERACTIONS

Nephrotoxicity and ototoxicity is additive when used with other ototoxic or nephrotoxic agents (e.g., acyclovir [Zovirax], aminoglycosides [e.g., gentamicin (Garamycin)], cisplatin [Platinol-AQ], rifampin [Rifadin], quinidine). Use with caution. ■ Bone marrow toxicity increased with other antineoplastic agents, radiation therapy, and/or other agents that may cause blood dyscrasias (e.g., anticonvulsants [e.g., phenytoin (Dilantin)], cephalosporins, mycophenolate [CellCept], rituximab [Rituxan]). Dose adjustment of either or both drugs may be indicated. ■ Do not administer live virus vaccines to patients receiving antineoplastic drugs. ■ See Dose Adjustments.

SIDE EFFECTS

Allergic reactions, including anaphylaxis, can occur during administration. Alopecia (rare), anemia, anorexia, bleeding, bone marrow suppression (usually reversible), bronchospasm, bruising, changes in taste, constipation, death, decreased urine output, decreased serum electrolytes, dehydration, diarrhea, erythema, fatigue, fever, hemolytic uremic syndrome (rare, cancer associated), hypotension, infection, laboratory test abnormalities (alkaline phosphatase, aspartate aminotransferase [AST], BUN, SrCr, total bilirubin), nausea and vomiting (severe), neutropenia, ototoxicity, peripheral neuropathies, pruritus, rash, thrombocytopenia, urticaria, visual disturbances, weakness.

ANTIDOTE

Notify physician of all side effects. Symptomatic and supportive treatment is indicated. Withhold carboplatin until myelosuppression is reversed. Administration of whole blood products (e.g., packed RBCs, platelets, leukocytes) may be required. Blood modifiers (e.g., darbepoetin alfa [Aranesp], epoetin alfa [Epogen, Procrit], filgrastim [Neupogen], pegfilgrastim [Neulasta], sargramostim [Leukine], oprelvekin [Neumega]) may be indicated to treat bone marrow toxicity. Treat anaphylaxis with epinephrine, corticosteroids, oxygen, and antihistamines. There is no specific antidote.

CARMUSTINE (BCNU)

(kar-mus′teen)

BiCNU

Antineoplastic (alkylating agent/nitrosourea)

pH 5.6 to 6

USUAL DOSE

Initial dose is 150 to 200 mg/M^2. May be given as a single dose, or one half of the calculated dose may be given initially and repeated the next day. Repeat every 6 weeks if bone marrow is sufficiently recovered. Repeat doses adjusted according to hematologic response of previous dose (see Dose Adjustments).

DOSE ADJUSTMENTS

Carmustine Dose Adjustment Based on Bone Marrow Suppression		
Nadir After Prior Dose		Percentage of Prior Dose to be Given
Leukocytes/mm^3	Platelets/mm^3	%
>4000	>100,000	100
3000-3999	75,000-99,999	100
2000-2999	25,000-74,999	70
<2000	<25,000	50

DILUTION

Specific techniques required; see Precautions. Initially dilute 100-mg vial with supplied sterile diluent (3 ml of absolute ethanol). Further dilute with 27 ml of SW for injection. Each ml will contain 3.3 mg carmustine. Withdraw desired dose and further dilute in 100 to 500 ml D5W or NS and give as an infusion. Use of glass containers preferred; loss of potency occurs in PVC containers and IV tubing.

Storage: Protect from light. Store in refrigerator (2° to 8° C [35° to 46° F]) in all forms. Stable 24 hours after reconstitution and up to 48 hours after dilution. Temperatures above 27° C (80° F) will cause liquefaction of the drug powder; discard immediately.

INCOMPATIBLE WITH

Polyvinyl chloride infusion bags; use only glass containers.

COMPATIBLE WITH **(Underline Indicates Conflicting Compatibility Information)**

Consult pharmacist; specific conditions may apply; see Compatibilities, p. xvi.

Additive: Cisplatin (Platinol), dacarbazine (DTIC).

Y-site: Amifostine (Ethyol), aztreonam (Azactam), cefepime (Maxipime), etoposide phosphate (Etopophos), filgrastim (Neupogen), fludarabine (Fludara), gemcitabine (Gemzar), granisetron (Kytril), melphalan (Alkeran), ondansetron (Zofran), piperacillin/tazobactam (Zosyn), sargramostim (Leukine), teniposide (Vumon), thiotepa (Thioplex), vinorelbine (Navelbine).

RATE OF ADMINISTRATION

Each single dose must be given as an infusion over a minimum of 1 hour. Reduce rate for pain or burning at injection site, flushing of the skin, or suffusion of the conjunctiva. Usually given over 1 to 2 hours.

ACTIONS

An alkylating agent of the nitrosourea group with antitumor activity, cell cycle phase nonspecific. Degraded to metabolites within 15 minutes of administration. Effectively crosses the blood-brain barrier; concentration higher in cerebrospinal fluid than in plasma. Excreted in changed form in urine. Small amounts excreted as respiratory CO_2.

INDICATIONS AND USES

Suppress or retard neoplastic growth of brain tumors; multiple myeloma; GI, breast, bronchogenic, and renal carcinomas; meningeal leukemia; Hodgkin's disease; and some non-Hodgkin's lymphomas.

CONTRAINDICATIONS

Hypersensitivity to carmustine, previous chemotherapy, or other causes that result in insufficient circulating platelets, leukocytes, or erythrocytes.

PRECAUTIONS

■ Follow guidelines for handling cytotoxic agents. See Appendix A, p. 1142. Administered by or under the direction of the physician specialist. ■ Often used with other antineoplastic drugs in reduced doses to achieve tumor remission. ■ Pulmonary toxicity associated with a cumulative dose greater than 1,400 mg/M^2. Delayed onset pulmonary fibrosis has occurred up to 15 years after treatment with injectable carmustine in patients who received it in childhood or early adolescence.

Monitor: Determine absolute patency and quality of vein and adequate circulation of extremity. Severe cellulitis may result from extravasation. ■ Delayed toxicity probable in 4 to 6 weeks; wait at least 6 weeks between doses; frequent CBCs including leukocyte and platelet counts indicated. ■ Nausea and vomiting can be severe. Prophylactic administration of antiemetics recommended. ■ Avoid contact of carmustine solution with the skin. ■ Observe for any signs of infection. Prophylactic antibiotics may be indicated pending results of C/S in a febrile neutropenic patient. ■ Maintain hydration. ■ Monitor for thrombocytopenia (platelet count less than 50,000/mm^3). Initiate precautions to prevent excessive bleeding (e.g., inspect IV sites, skin, and mucous membranes; use extreme care during invasive procedures; test urine, emesis, stool, and secretions for occult blood).

Patient Education: Nonhormonal birth control recommended. ■ Report stinging or burning at IV site promptly. ■ See Appendix D, p. 1148.

Maternal/Child: Category D: avoid pregnancy; will produce teratogenic effects in rats; has mutagenic potential. ■ Discontinue breast-feeding.

Elderly: Consider age-related renal impairment; toxicity may be increased.

DRUG/LAB INTERACTIONS

Potentiates or is potentiated by hepatotoxic or nephrotoxic medications and radiation therapy. ■ Potentiated by cimetidine (Tagamet); may cause increased myelosuppression. ■ Inhibits digoxin and phenytoin (Dilantin); may reduce serum levels. ■ May cause corneal and conjunctival epithelial damage with mitomycin. ■ Do not administer vaccine or chloroquine to patients receiving antineoplastic drugs. ■ See Dose Adjustments.

SIDE EFFECTS

Most are dose related and can be reversed. Bone marrow toxicity (especially leukopenia and thrombocytopenia) is most pronounced at 4 to 6 weeks; can be severe and cumulative with repeated dosage. Anemia, elevated liver function test results, flushing of skin and suffusion of conjunctiva from too-rapid infusion rate, hyperpigmentation and burning of skin (from actual contact with solution), nausea and vomiting, pulmonary infiltrates or fibrosis with long-term therapy, renal abnormalities, retinal hemorrhage.

ANTIDOTE

Notify physician of all side effects. Most will decrease in severity with reduced dosage, increased time span between doses, or symptomatic treatment. May reduce therapeutic effectiveness. Bone marrow depression may require withholding carmustine until recovery occurs. Administration of whole blood products (e.g., packed RBCs, platelets, leukocytes) may be required. Blood modifiers (e.g., darbepoetin alfa [Aranesp], epoetin alfa [Epogen, Procrit], filgrastim [Neupogen], pegfilgrastim [Neulasta], sargramostim [Leukine], oprelvekin [Neumega]) may be indicated to treat bone marrow toxicity. There is no specific antidote. Supportive therapy as indicated will help sustain the patient in toxicity. For extravasation, elevate extremity; consider injection of long-acting dexamethasone (Decadron LA) or hyaluronidase (Wydase) throughout extravasated tissue. Use a 27- or 25-gauge needle. Apply warm, moist compresses.

CASPOFUNGIN ACETATE

Antifungal

(kas′poh-fun′-jin as′ah-tat)

Cancidas

pH 6.6

USUAL DOSE

Candidemia and other *Candida* infections: 70 mg as an infusion on day 1. Beginning on day 2, reduce subsequent doses to 50 mg/day. Duration of treatment is based on clinical and microbiologic response. Usually continued for at least 14 days after the last positive culture. Persistently neutropenic patients may require a longer course of therapy pending resolution of the neutropenia.

Esophageal candidiasis: 50 mg daily as an infusion. Suppressive oral therapy following treatment with caspofungin may be considered to decrease the risk of relapse of oropharyngeal candidiasis in patients with HIV infections.

Invasive aspergillosis: 70 mg as an infusion on day 1. Beginning on day 2, reduce subsequent doses to 50 mg/day. Duration of treatment is based on severity of the underlying disease, recovery from immunosuppression, and clinical response.

DOSE ADJUSTMENTS

All diagnoses: Dose adjustment is not indicated based on age, gender, or race. ■ Dose adjustment is not indicated in patients with impaired renal function or in patients with mild impaired hepatic function (Child-Pugh score 5 to 6). ■ In patients receiving concurrent administration of rifampin (Rifadin), increase the daily dose to 70 mg. An increase in the daily dose to 70 mg/day should be considered in patients who are not clinically responding and are taking other inducers and/or mixed inducers/inhibitors of caspofungin clearance, specifically carbamazepine (Tegretol), dexamethasone (Decadron), efavirenz (Sustiva), nevirapine (Viramune), and phenytoin (Dilantin). ■ See Drug/Lab Interactions.

Esophageal candidiasis and/or oropharyngeal candidiasis: In patients with moderate hepatic insufficiency (Child-Pugh score 7 to 9), reduce dose to 35 mg daily.

Invasive aspergillosis: In patients with moderate hepatic insufficiency (Child-Pugh score 7 to 9) after the initial loading dose of 70 mg, reduce subsequent daily doses to 35 mg. ■ Dose may be increased from 50 to 70 mg daily in patients not clinically responding to the 50-mg dose; experience limited. Doses above 70 mg/day have not been studied.

DILUTION

Available in 70-mg and 50-mg vials. Select appropriate dose and allow vial of caspofungin to come to room temperature. Reconstitute selected dose with 10.5 ml of NS, SW, or BWFI. Mix gently to achieve a clear solution, should dissolve completely. The 70-mg vial will yield 7.2 mg/ml, the 50-mg vial will yield 5.2 mg/ml. Withdraw 10 ml of reconstituted solution and add to 250 ml of NS, ½NS, ¼NS, or LR for infusion. If a 70-mg vial is not available, reconstitute two 50-mg vials and withdraw a total of 14 ml to be further diluted in 250 ml NS of the above solutions. When preparing a 35-mg dose, withdraw 7 ml from the reconstituted 50-mg vial and further dilute in 250 ml NS of the above solutions. If medically necessary, the amount of infusion solution for the 50-mg or 35-mg dose may be reduced from 250 ml to 100 ml.

Storage: Refrigerate unopened vials. Reconstituted vials may be kept at CRT for one hour before preparing as an infusion solution. Fully diluted solutions may be stored at CRT for 24 hours or refrigerated for 48 hours.

COMPATIBILITY

Manufacturer states, "Do not mix or co-infuse caspofungin with other medications. Do not use diluents containing dextrose."

RATE OF ADMINISTRATION

A single dose as an infusion evenly distributed over 1 hour.

ACTIONS

An antifungal. An echinocandin or glucan synthesis inhibitor. It attacks the fungal cell wall and inhibits the synthesis of beta (1,3)-D-glucan, an essential component of the cell wall of susceptible filamentous fungi that is not found in human cells. Extensively bound to albumin (97%). After completion of an IV infusion, plasma concentrations decline in several phases, each with its own half-life (e.g., 9 to 11 hours, 40 to 50 hours). Distribution, rather than excretion or biotransformation, is the primary mechanism influencing plasma clearance. Slowly metabolized by hydrolysis and N-acetylation, eventually breaking down to amino acids and their degradates. Excreted in urine and feces.

INDICATIONS AND USES

Treatment of invasive aspergillosis in patients who are refractory to or intolerant of other therapies (i.e., amphotericin B [Fungizone], lipid formulations of amphotericin B [e.g., Abelcet, AmBisome, Amphotec], and/or itraconazole [Sporanox]). Has not been studied for initial therapy for invasive aspergillosis. ■ Treatment of esophageal candidiasis. ■ Treatment of candidemia and the following *Candida* infections: intra-abdominal abscesses, peritonitis, and pleural space infections. Has not been studied in endocarditis, osteomyelitis, and meningitis due to *Candida.*

CONTRAINDICATIONS

Known hypersensitivity to caspofungin or any of its components.

PRECAUTIONS

Concomitant use with cyclosporine is not recommended unless the potential benefit outweighs the risk; see Drug/Lab Interactions. ■ Extended courses of therapy (up to 162 days in selected patients) have been well tolerated, but information on administration for longer than 2 weeks is limited. ■ There is no clinical experience in patients with severe hepatic insufficiency (Child-Pugh score greater than 9). ■ Drug resistance in patients with invasive aspergillosis has not been observed.

Monitor: Most patients have serious underlying medical conditions (e.g., bone marrow transplant, HIV, malignancies) requiring multiple concomitant medications. Obtain baseline studies as required and repeat as indicated. ■ Monitor vital signs. ■ Observe for S/S of allergic reaction. ■ Encourage fluids to maintain hydration. ■ Effects of severe hepatic impairment unknown; monitor liver function tests (e.g., AST, ALT) in patients with pre-existing impaired hepatic function and any time S/S suggestive of liver dysfunction develop (e.g., jaundice, lethargy). ■ See Drug/Lab Interactions.

Patient Education: Review all medical conditions and medications before beginning treatment. ■ Promptly report pain at infusion site and symptoms of histamine reactions (e.g., facial swelling, pruritus, rash, sensation of warmth).

Maternal/Child: Category C: use during pregnancy only if benefits outweigh potential risks to fetus. Has been found to be embryotoxic in rats and rabbits. ■ Has been found in the milk of lactating, drug-treated rats; use caution if required during breast-feeding or discontinue breast-feeding. CDC advises HIV-infected women not to breast-feed. ■ Safety and effectiveness for use in pediatric patients not studied.

Elderly: Response similar to that in younger patients. Dose adjustment is not recommended; however, use caution; may have greater sensitivity to its effects.

DRUG/LAB INTERACTIONS

Concomitant use with cyclosporine (Sandimmune) is not recommended unless benefit outweighs risk. By day 10 of concomitant administration some patients had a transient ALT (SGOT) 2 to 3 times the upper limit of normal, and the AUC of caspofungin had increased by about 35%. ■ Pharmacokinetics of caspofungin are not altered by amphotericin B, itraconazole, mycophenolate (Cell-Cept), or tacrolimus (Prograf). Serum concentrations of tacrolimus may be somewhat decreased with concomitant administration, monitor tacrolimus concentrations and adjust dose as indicated. ■ Inducers and/or mixed inducers/inhibitors of caspofungin clearance (e.g., carbamazepine [Tegretol], dexamethasone [Decadron], efavirenz [Sustiva], nevirapine [Viramune], phenytoin [Dilantin], rifampin [Rifadin]) may significantly increase caspofungin clearance and require an increase in dose; see Dose Adjustments. ■ Although its clearance may be affected by the enzyme inducers previously mentioned, caspofungin is not an inhibitor or inducer of any enzyme in the cytochrome P_{450} (CPY) system. It is not a substrate (a substance on which an enzyme acts) for P-glycoprotein and is a poor substrate for cytochrome P_{450} enzymes. It is not expected to interact with drugs metabolized by this system (e.g., amiodarone [Cordarone], calcium channel blockers [e.g., diltiazem (Cardizem), verapamil (Isoptin)], cimetidine [Tagamet], MAO inhibitors [e.g., selegiline (Eldepryl)]).

SIDE EFFECTS

Incidence difficult to assess because of multiple medical conditions and multiple medications. ARDS, fever, flushing, headache, hypokalemia, increased liver function tests (e.g., alkaline phosphatase, ALT, AST), increased RBCs and protein in urine, injection site reactions, nausea, phlebitis, pulmonary edema, radiographic infiltrates, and vomiting. Allergic responses (e.g., facial swelling, pruritus, rash, sensation of warmth) including one anaphylactic reaction with dyspnea, stridor, and worsening of rash have been reported.

ANTIDOTE

Notify physician of all side effects; most will be treated symptomatically. Discontinue caspofungin and notify physician of abnormal liver function tests progressing to clinical S/S of liver disease. Rash may be the first sign of an exfoliative skin disorder in immunocompromised patients; discontinue caspofungin and notify physician. Not removed by hemodialysis. Treat anaphylaxis as indicated and/or resusitate as necessary.

CEFAMANDOLE NAFATE

(sef-a-man′dole naf′ate)

Mandol

Antibacterial
Cephalosporin

pH 6 to 8

USUAL DOSE

Range is from 500 mg to 2 Gm every 4 to 8 hours. Severe infections may require 1 Gm every 4 to 6 hours. Life-threatening infections may require 2 Gm every 4 hours. Larger doses may also be required with less susceptible organisms. Do not exceed 12 Gm/24 hr. Maximum recommended dose is 1.5 Gm every 6 hours in the elderly (over 75 years of age) even if their SrCr is normal.

Uncomplicated pneumonia, skin and soft tissue infections: 500 mg every 6 hours.

GU infections: 500 mg every 8 hours. Increase to 1 Gm every 8 hours in serious GU infections.

Perioperative prophylaxis: 1 or 2 Gm 30 minutes to 1 hour before incision. Follow with 1 to 2 Gm every 6 hours for 24 to 48 hours. Extend to 72 hours in patients undergoing prosthetic arthroplasty. During ***cesarean section,*** initial dose is given immediately before surgery or just after the cord is clamped.

PEDIATRIC DOSE

Mild to moderate infections, children and infants over 1 month of age: 8.3 to 33.3 mg/kg of body weight every 4 to 8 hours. Do not exceed 150 mg/kg/24 hr or maximum adult dose.

Severe infections, children and infants over 1 month of age: 25 to 50 mg/kg every 4 to 8 hours. Do not exceed 150 mg/kg/24 hr or maximum adult dose.

Perioperative prophylaxis, children and infants over 3 months of age: 12.5 to 25 mg/kg/dose. Give first dose 30 minutes to 1 hour before incision and then every 6 hours for up to 24 to 48 hours.

DOSE ADJUSTMENTS

In impaired renal function, the initial dose should be as above, but all remaining doses should be based on CrCl according to the following chart. ■ See Drug/Lab Interactions.

Cefamandole Recommended Maintenance Schedule in Impaired Renal Function

Creatinine Clearance (ml/min/1.73 M^2)	Less Severe Infections	Life-Threatening Infections (maximum dose)
Normal recommended dosing schedule (CrCl >80)	1-2 Gm q 6 hr	2 Gm q 4 hr
50-80 (mild)	0.75-1.5 Gm q 6 hr	1.5 Gm q 4 hr or 2 Gm q 6 hr
25-50 (moderate)	0.75-1.5 Gm q 8 hr	1.5 Gm q 6 hr or 2 Gm q 8 hr

Continued

Cefamandole Recommended Maintenance Schedule in Impaired Renal Function—cont'd		
Creatinine Clearance (ml/min/1.73 M^2)	**Less Severe Infections**	**Life-Threatening Infections (maximum dose)**
10-25 (severe)	0.5-1 Gm q 8 hr	1 Gm q 6 hr or 1.25 Gm q 8 hr
2-10 (marked)	0.5-0.75 Gm q 12 hr	0.67 Gm q 8 hr or 1 Gm q 12 hr
<2 (none)	0.25-0.5 Gm q 12 hr	0.5 Gm q 8 hr or 0.75 Gm q 12 hr

DILUTION

Forms carbon dioxide after initial dilution; use caution when drawing from vial; do not store in syringe.

IV injection: Each 1 Gm or fraction thereof must be reconstituted with at least 10 ml NS, D5W, D10W, D5NS, D5/½NS, D5/¼NS, sodium lactate, or SW. If using SW as the diluent, increase amount to 20 ml/Gm to avoid a hypotonic solution.

Intermittent infusion: Further dilute in 50 to 100 ml D5W or NS for infusion and give through Y-tube, three-way stopcock, or additive infusion set.

Continuous infusion: May be further diluted in up to 1,000 ml compatible infusion solutions (e.g., D5W, D10W, 2%, 0.45%, or 0.9% NS with or without dextrose, ⅙ M lactate).

Storage: Administer within 24 hours of preparation if unrefrigerated or within 96 hours if refrigerated.

INCOMPATIBLE WITH

Solutions containing calcium or magnesium ions or tromethamine (Tham). Manufacturer recommends temporarily discontinuing other solutions infusing at the same site during intermittent infusion. May be used concomitantly with aminoglycosides (e.g., amikacin [Amikin], gentamicin [Garamycin]), but these drugs must never be mixed in the same infusion (mutual inactivation). If given concurrently, administer at separate sites.

COMPATIBLE WITH

(Underline Indicates Conflicting Compatibility Information)

Consult pharmacist; specific conditions may apply; see Compatibilities, p. xvi.

Additive: Cimetidine (Tagamet), clindamycin (Cleocin), furosemide (Lasix), lidocaine, metronidazole (Flagyl IV), verapamil (Isoptin).

Syringe: Heparin.

Y-site: Acyclovir (Zovirax), cyclophosphamide (Cytoxan), diltiazem (Cardizem), hydromorphone (Dilaudid), magnesium sulfate, meperidine (Demerol), morphine, perphenazine (Trilafon).

RATE OF ADMINISTRATION

See Incompatible With. Each 1 Gm or fraction thereof over 3 to 5 minutes or longer as indicated by amount of solution and condition of the patient. Rate of continuous infusion should be by physician order.

ACTIONS

A semisynthetic, second-generation, broad-spectrum cephalosporin antibiotic that is bactericidal to specific gram-positive, gram-negative, and anaerobic organisms. Peak serum levels achieved by end of infusion. Widely distributed in most tissues, body fluids (CSF minimal), bone, gallbladder, myocardium, and skin and soft tissue. Crosses the placental barrier. Excreted rapidly in the urine. Secreted in breast milk.

INDICATIONS AND USES

Treatment of serious respiratory tract, GU tract, bone, joint, soft tissue, and skin infections; septicemia; and peritonitis. Effective only if the causative organism is susceptible. ■ Perioperative prophylaxis.

CONTRAINDICATIONS

Previous allergic reaction to cephalosporins or related antibiotics (penicillins). Absolute only if reaction was serious.

PRECAUTIONS

Sensitivity studies indicated to determine susceptibility of the causative organism to cefamandole. ■ Continue for at least 2 to 3 days after all symptoms of infection subside. ■ Avoid prolonged use of drug; superinfection caused by overgrowth of nonsusceptible organisms may result. ■ Use caution in patients with impaired renal function; a history of GI disease (especially colitis), bleeding disorders, or allergies; and those receiving an extended course of cephalosporins. ■ Pseudomembranous colitis has been reported. May range from mild to life-threatening. Consider in patients that present with diarrhea during or after treatment with cefamandole.

Monitor: Watch for early symptoms of allergic reaction. ■ Use extreme caution in the penicillin-sensitive patient; incidence of cross-sensitivity may range from 3% to 16%. ■ Observe for electrolyte imbalance and cardiac irregularities. Each gram contains 3.3 mEq of sodium. ■ May cause hypoprothrombinemia (deficiency of prothrombin [Factor II]); 10 mg/week of prophylactic vitamin K may be indicated in elderly, debilitated, or other patients with vitamin K deficiency. Monitor PT. ■ Thrombophlebitis may result from prolonged or high dosage; use small needles, larger veins, and rotate infusion sites. ■ See Drug/Lab Interactions; additional monitoring may be indicated (e.g., renal function, drug serum levels, PT).

Patient Education: Avoid alcohol or alcohol-containing preparations; may cause abdominal cramps, headache, flushing, nausea and vomiting, shortness of breath, sweating, and tachycardia. ■ Report promptly any bleeding or bruising, diarrhea, symptoms of allergy (e.g., difficulty breathing, hives, itching, rash).

Maternal/Child: Category B: safety for use during pregnancy and breastfeeding not established. No problems documented. ■ Safety for use in infants under 1 month of age not established; immature renal function will increase blood levels.

Elderly: No specific problems documented. Consider age-related impaired organ function and nutritional status; reduced dose or extended intervals may be indicated. ■ See Usual Dose.

DRUG/LAB INTERACTIONS

May produce symptoms of acute alcohol intolerance with alcohol (a disulfiram-like reaction [abdominal cramps, headache, flushing, nausea and vomiting, shortness of breath, sweating, tachycardia]). Patient must abstain from alcohol during treatment until at least 72 hours after discontinued. ■ Risk of nephrotoxicity may be increased with aminoglycosides and other nephrotoxic agents (e.g., loop diuretics [e.g., furosemide [Lasix]). ■ Probenecid inhibits excretion and may require reduction in dosage. ■ May be antagonized by bacteriostatic antibiotics (e.g., chloramphenicol, erythromycin, tetracyclines); may interfere with bactericidal action. ■ Bleeding tendency may be increased with any medicine that affects blood clotting (e.g., heparin and oral anticoagulants [warfarin (Coumadin)], thrombolytic agents [e.g., alteplase (tPA)], salicylates, NSAIDs [e.g., ibuprofen (Advil, Motrin), naproxen (Aleve, Naprosyn)], sulfinpyrazone [Anturane]). ■ Large amounts of cephalosporins and/or salicylates may induce hypoprothrombinemia. ■ False-positive reaction for urine glucose except with enzyme-based tests (e.g., Chemstix). ■ May produce false-positive test for proteinuria. ■ See Incompatible With and Side Effects.

SIDE EFFECTS

Allergic reactions including anaphylaxis; anorexia; bleeding episodes; diarrhea; jaundice; leukopenia; local site pain; nausea and vomiting; neutropenia; oral thrush; phlebitis; positive direct Coombs' test; prolonged PT; pseudomembranous colitis; transient elevation of AST (SGOT), ALT (SGPT), BUN, and alkaline phosphatase; proteinuria; seizures (large doses); thrombophlebitis; vaginal itching or discharge. Hypoprothrombinemia (rare) and hemolytic anemia may occur. Serum sickness–like reactions have occurred (e.g., arthralgia, fever, polyarthritis, skin rashes), usually after a second course of therapy. Usually resolve after cephalosporins are discontinued.

ANTIDOTE

Notify physician of any side effects. Discontinue drug if indicated. Treat allergic reaction as indicated and resuscitate as necessary. Hemodialysis or peritoneal dialysis may be useful in overdose. Vitamin K, fresh-frozen plasma, packed red cells, or platelet concentrates may be indicated in abnormal bleeding tendencies confirmed by lab evaluations. If bleeding is due to platelet dysfunction, discontinue and use an alternate antibiotic. Treat antibiotic-related pseudomembranous colitis with oral vancomycin or metronidazole (Flagyl). Antihistamines and corticosteroids may be indicated to manage symptoms of serum sickness.

CEFAZOLIN SODIUM

(sef-a'zoe-lin so'de-um)

Ancef, Kefzol

Antibacterial (cephalosporin)

pH 4.5 to 7

USUAL DOSE

250 mg to 1.5 Gm every 6 to 8 hours. Up to 6 Gm is usual, but 12 Gm in 24 hours has been used, depending on severity of infection. Maximum recommended dose is 500 mg every 8 hours in the elderly (over 75 years of age) even if their SrCr is normal.

Mild infections: 250 to 500 mg every 8 hours.

Moderate to severe infections: 500 mg to 1 Gm every 6 to 8 hours.

Life-threatening infections (e.g., [endocarditis, unlabeled], septicemia): 1 to 1.5 Gm every 6 hours.

Pneumococcal pneumonia: 500 mg every 12 hours.

Uncomplicated GU infections: 1 Gm every 12 hours.

Perioperative prophylaxis: 1 Gm 30 minutes to 1 hour before incision. 0.5 to 1 Gm may be repeated in 2 hours in the OR and every 6 to 8 hours for 24 hours.

Endocarditis prophylaxis (unlabeled): 1 Gm 30 minutes before start of surgery.

PEDIATRIC DOSE

Over 1 month of age: 6.25 to 25 mg/kg of body weight every 6 hours, or 8.3 to 33.3 mg/kg every 8 hours. Do not exceed adult dose.

Endocarditis prophylaxis (unlabeled): 25 mg/kg 30 minutes before start of surgery. Do not exceed 1 Gm.

NEONATAL DOSE

See Maternal/Child.

Less than 7 days of age or over 7 days but under 2,000 Gm: 20 mg/kg every 12 hours.

7 days to 1 month of age and 2,000 Gm or more: 20 mg/kg every 8 hours.

DOSE ADJUSTMENTS

In impaired renal function, the initial dose in adults and children should be as above. Reduce all subsequent doses according to the following charts.

Cefazolin Dose Guidelines in Impaired Renal Function for Adults		
Creatinine Clearance	**Dose**	**Frequency**
>55 ml/min	Full	Normal
35-54 ml/min	Full	q 8 hr or less frequently
11-34 ml/min	≈ Usual dose	q 12 hr
10 ml/min or less	≈ Usual dose	q 18-24 hr

Cefazolin Dose Guidelines in Impaired Renal Function for Pediatric Patients		
Creatinine Clearance	Dose	Frequency
>70 ml/min	Full	Normal
40-70 ml/min	7.5 to 30 mg/kg	q 12 hr
20-40 ml/min	3.1 to 12.5 mg/kg	q 12 hr
5-20 ml/min	2.5 to 10 mg/kg	q 24 hr

DILUTION

Each 1 Gm or fraction thereof must be reconstituted with at least 10 ml of SW for injection. To reduce the incidence of thrombophlebitis, may be further diluted in 50 to 100 ml of D5W, NS, or other compatible infusion solutions (see chart on inside back cover or literature) and given as an intermittent infusion. Available premixed and in ADD-Vantage vials for use with ADD-Vantage infusion containers. May be administered through Y-tube, three-way stopcock, or additive infusion set.

Storage: Before reconstitution, protect from light and store at CRT. Give within 24 hours of preparation, or within 10 days if under refrigeration.

INCOMPATIBLE WITH

May be used concomitantly with aminoglycosides (e.g., amikacin [Amikin], gentamicin [Garamycin]), but these drugs must never be mixed in the same infusion (mutual inactivation). If given concurrently, administer at separate sites.

COMPATIBLE WITH **(Underline Indicates Conflicting Compatibility Information)**

Consult pharmacist; specific conditions may apply; see Compatibilities, p. xvi.

Additive: Aztreonam (Azactam), cimetidine (Tagamet), clindamycin (Cleocin), famotidine (Pepcid IV), fluconazole (Diflucan), linezolid (Zyvox), meperidine (Demerol), metronidazole (Flagyl IV), verapamil (Isoptin).

Syringe: Heparin, hydromorphone (Dilaudid).

Y-site: Acyclovir (Zovirax), allopurinol (Aloprim, Zyloprim), amifostine (Ethyol), amiodarone (Cordarone), atracurium (Tracrium), aztreonam (Azactam), calcium gluconate, cisatracurium (Nimbex), cyclophosphamide (Cytoxan), diltiazem (Cardizem), docetaxel (Taxotere), doxorubicin liposome (Doxil), enalaprilat (Vasotec IV), esmolol (Brevibloc), etoposide phosphate (Etopophos), famotidine (Pepcid IV), filgrastim (Neupogen), fluconazole (Diflucan), fludarabine (Fludara), foscarnet (Foscavir), gatifloxacin (Tequin), gemcitabine (Gemzar), granisetron (Kytril), heparin, hetastarch in electrolytes (Hextend), hetastarch in NS (Hespan), hydromorphone (Dilaudid), insulin (regular), labetalol (Normodyne), lidocaine, linezolid (Zyvox), magnesium sulfate, melphalan (Alkeran), meperidine (Demerol), midazolam (Versed), morphine, multivitamins (M.V.I.), ondansetron (Zofran), pancuronium (Pavulon), perphenazine (Trilafon), propofol (Diprivan), ranitidine (Zantac), remifentanil (Ultiva), sargramostim (Leukine), tacrolimus (Prograf), teniposide (Vumon), theophylline, thiotepa (Thioplex), vancomycin (Vancocin), vecuronium (Norcuron), warfarin (Coumadin).

RATE OF ADMINISTRATION

IV injection: Each 1 Gm or fraction thereof over 3 to 5 minutes. Extend administration time as indicated by amount of solution and condition of patient.

ACTIONS

A semisynthetic, first-generation, broad-spectrum cephalosporin antibiotic that is bactericidal through inhibition of cell wall synthesis to some gram-positive and gram-negative organisms, including staphylococci and streptococci. A number of organisms are resistant to this cephalosporin. Peak serum levels achieved by end of infusion. Widely distributed in most tissues, body fluids (CSF minimal), bone, gallbladder, myocardium, and skin and soft tissue. Crosses the placental barrier. Excreted rapidly in the urine. Secreted in breast milk.

INDICATIONS AND USES

Treatment of serious infections of the bone, joints, skin, soft tissue, respiratory tract, biliary tract, and GU tract; septicemia and endocarditis. Effective only if the causative organism is susceptible. ■ Perioperative prophylaxis. ■ Not recommended for prophylaxis in GU procedures.

Unlabeled uses: Prophylaxis of bacterial endocarditis.

CONTRAINDICATIONS

Previous allergic reaction to cephalosporins or related antibiotics (penicillins). Absolute only if reaction was serious.

PRECAUTIONS

Sensitivity studies indicated to determine susceptibility of the causative organisms to cefazolin. ■ Continue for at least 2 to 3 days after all symptoms of infection subside. ■ Avoid prolonged use of drug; superinfection caused by overgrowth of nonsusceptible organisms may result. ■ Use caution in patients with impaired renal function, allergies, or a history of GI disease (especially colitis). ■ Pseudomembranous colitis has been reported. May range from mild to life-threatening. Consider in patients that present with diarrhea during or after treatment with cefazolin. ■ Continuous IV infusion not recommended; markedly increases incidence of phlebitis; see Monitor.

Monitor: Watch for early symptoms of allergic reaction. ■ Use extreme caution in the penicillin-sensitive patient; incidence of cross-sensitivity may range from 3% to 16%. ■ Observe for electrolyte imbalance and cardiac irregularities. Contains 2.1 mEq sodium per Gm. ■ Thrombophlebitis may result from prolonged or high dosage; use small needles, larger veins, and rotate infusion sites. ■ See Drug/Lab Interactions; additional monitoring may be indicated (e.g., renal function, drug serum levels, PT).

Patient Education: Report promptly any bleeding or bruising, diarrhea, or symptoms of allergy (e.g., difficulty breathing, hives, itching, rash).

Maternal/Child: Category B: safety for use during pregnancy and breastfeeding not established. No problems documented. ■ Safety for use in infants under 1 month of age not established; immature renal function will increase blood levels.

Elderly: No specific problems documented. Consider age-related impaired organ function and nutritional status; reduced dose or extended intervals may be indicated. ■ See Usual Dose.

DRUG/LAB INTERACTIONS

Risk of nephrotoxicity may be increased with aminoglycosides and other nephrotoxic agents (e.g., loop diuretics [e.g., furosemide (Lasix)]). ■ Probenecid inhibits excretion and may require reduced dose. ■ May be antagonized by bacteriostatic antibiotics (e.g., chloramphenicol, erythromycin, tetracyclines); may interfere with bactericidal action. ■ Large amounts of cephalosporins and/or salicylates may induce hypoprothrombinemia (deficiency of prothrombin [Factor II]). The addition of agents that may affect platelet aggregation and/or may have GI ulcerative potential (e.g., NSAIDs [ibuprofen (Advil, Motrin), naproxen (Aleve, Naprosyn)], or sulfinpyrazone [Anturane]) may increase risk of hemorrhage. ■ False-positive reaction for urine glucose except with enzyme-based tests (e.g., Chemstix). ■ See Incompatible With and Side Effects.

SIDE EFFECTS

Allergic reactions including anaphylaxis, anorexia, diarrhea, leukopenia, local site pain, nausea and vomiting, neutropenia, oral thrush, phlebitis, positive direct and indirect Coombs' test, prolonged PT, pseudomembranous colitis, transient elevation of AST (SGOT), ALT (SGPT), BUN, and alkaline phosphatase, seizures (large doses), thrombophlebitis, vaginal itching or discharge. Hypoprothrombinemia (rare) and hemolytic anemia may occur. Serum sickness–like reactions have occurred (e.g., arthralgia, fever, polyarthritis, skin rashes), usually after a second course of therapy. Usually resolve after cephalosporins are discontinued.

ANTIDOTE

Notify the physician of any side effects. Discontinue the drug if indicated. Mild cases of colitis may respond to discontinuation of drug. Treat antibiotic-related pseudomembranous colitis with fluids, electrolytes, protein supplements, and oral vancomycin or metronidazole (Flagyl) as indicated. Antihistamines and corticosteroids may be indicated to manage symptoms of serum sickness. Discontinue cefazolin and treat allergic reaction as indicated (airway, oxygen, IV fluids, antihistamines [e.g., diphenhydramine], corticosteroids [e.g., dexamethasone], epinephrine, pressor-amines [e.g., dopamine]) and resuscitate as necessary. Hemodialysis may be useful in overdose.

CEFEPIME HYDROCHLORIDE

(sef′e-peem hye-droe-klor′id)

Maxipime

Antibacterial (cephalosporin)

pH 4 to 6

USUAL DOSE

Adults and children over 12 years of age: Range is from 0.5 Gm to 2 Gm. Usually given every 12 hours. Dose based on severity of disease and/or specific organism according to the following chart.

Cefepime Dose Guidelines			
Site and Type of Infection	Dose	Frequency	Duration (days)
Mild to Moderate Uncomplicated or complicated urinary tract infections	0.5-1 Gm IV/IM	q 12 hr	7-10
Severe Uncomplicated or complicated urinary tract infections	2 Gm IV	q 12 hr	10
Moderate to Severe Pneumonia	1-2 Gm IV	q 12 hr	10
Moderate to Severe Uncomplicated skin and skin structure infections Septicemia (unlabeled)	2 Gm IV	q 12 hr	10
Empiric Therapy For febrile neutropenic patients	2 Gm IV	q 8 hr	7 or until neutropenia resolves
Complicated Intraabdominal infections	Cefepime 2 Gm IV q 12 hr in combination with metronidazole 500 mg or 7.5 mg/kg q 6 hr, not to exceed 4 Gm/24 hr of metronidazole		7-10

PEDIATRIC DOSE

Children 2 months to 16 years and up to 40 kg: 50 mg/kg every 12 hours for 7 to 10 days. Increase frequency to every 8 hours for empiric monotherapy in febrile neutropenia. Do not exceed adult dose.

DOSE ADJUSTMENTS

In impaired renal function, the initial dose should be as above, but all remaining doses should be reduced based on CrCl according to the following chart (e.g., if the normal dose is 1 Gm every 12 hours with a CrCl greater than 60, the maintenance dose would be reduced to 1 Gm every 24 hours with a CrCl between 30 and 60 ml/min). Dose reductions should be comparable in ***pediatric patients.***

Cefepime Dose Guidelines in Impaired Renal Function				
Creatinine Clearance (ml/min)	Recommended Maintenance Schedule (relative to normal dosing schedule)			
Normal Recommended Dosing Schedule (>60)	**500 mg q 12 hr**	**1 Gm q 12 hr**	**2 Gm q 12 hr**	**2 Gm q 8 hr**
30-60	500 mg q 24 hr	1 Gm q 24 hr	2 Gm q 24 hr	2 Gm q 12 hr
11-29	500 mg q 24 hr	500 mg q 24 hr	1 Gm q 24 hr	2 Gm q 24 hr
≤10	250 mg q 24 hr	250 mg q 24 hr	500 mg q 24 hr	1 Gm q 24 hr

Consult literature for conversion formula if dose is to be based on SrCr. ■ Give a repeat dose equal to the initial dose at the end of each hemodialysis session. ■ Give the usual dose to patients on continuous ambulatory peritoneal dialysis, but increase intervals between each dose to 48 hours. ■ Reduced dose may be required in the elderly based on renal function. ■ Dose adjustment not required in impaired hepatic function.

DILUTION

Available in vials (IM/IV), piggyback, and ADD-Vantage preparations. ***Vials*** may be reconstituted (see following chart) and then further diluted with NS, D5W, D10W, D5NS, D5LR, ⅙ M sodium lactate, Normosol-R, or D5/Normosol M. Concentrations between 1 mg/ml and 40 mg/ml are acceptable. (500 mg reconstituted with 5 ml = 100 mg/ml, further diluted with 95 ml = 5 mg/ml, with 45 ml = 10 mg/ml.)

Piggyback preparations must be diluted with 50 to 100 ml of any of the above compatible solutions.

ADD-Vantage vials must only be diluted with 50 to 100 ml of NS or D5W in ADD-Vantage infusion containers.

Cefepime Dilution Guidelines			
Single-Dose Vials for Intravenous/ Intramuscular Administration	Amount of Diluent to be Added (ml)	Approximate Available Volume (ml)	Approximate Cefepime Concentration (mg/ml)
CEFEPIME VIAL CONTENT			
500 mg (IV)	5	5.6	100
500 mg (IM)	1.3	1.8	280
1 Gm (IV)	10	11.3	100
1 Gm (IM)	2.4	3.6	280
2 Gm (IV)	10	12.5	160

Continued

Cefepime Dilution Guidelines—cont'd			
Single-Dose Vials for Intravenous/ Intramuscular Administration	Amount of Diluent to be Added (ml)	Approximate Available Volume (ml)	Approximate Cefepime Concentration (mg/ml)
PIGGYBACK (100 ml)			
1 Gm bottle	50	50	20
1 Gm bottle	100	100	10
2 Gm bottle	50	50	40
2 Gm bottle	100	100	20
ADD-VANTAGE			
1 Gm vial	50	50	20
1 Gm vial	100	100	10

Storage: Store cefepime in the dry state between 2° to 25° C (36° to 77° F); protect from light. Reconstituted or diluted solutions are stable for 24 hours at CRT and 7 days if refrigerated.

INCOMPATIBLE WITH

Manufacturer recommends temporarily discontinuing other solutions infusing at the same site during intermittent infusion. May be used concomitantly with aminoglycosides (e.g., amikacin [Amikin], gentamicin [Garamycin], tobramycin [Nebcin]), aminophylline, metronidazole (Flagyl IV), and vancomycin (Vancocin), but these drugs must never be mixed in the same infusion (mutual inactivation or other potential interactions). If given concurrently, administer at separate sites.

COMPATIBLE WITH (Underline Indicates Conflicting Compatibility Information)

Consult pharmacist; specific conditions may apply; see Compatibilities, p. xvi.

Additive: Manufacturer lists specific concentrations of amikacin (Amikin), ampicillin, clindamycin (Cleocin), heparin, potassium chloride (KCl), and theophylline. Other sources add metronidazole (Flagyl IV) and vancomycin (Vancocin).

Y-site: Ampicillin/sulbactam (Unasyn), aztreonam (Azactam), bleomycin (Blenoxane), bumetanide (Bumex), buprenorphine (Buprenex), butorphanol (Stadol), calcium gluconate, carboplatin (Paraplatin), carmustine (BiCNU), cyclophosphamide (Cytoxan), cytarabine (ARA-C), dactinomycin (Cosmegen), dexamethasone (Decadron), docetaxel (Taxotere), doxorubicin liposome (Doxil), fluconazole (Diflucan), fludarabine (Fludara), fluorouracil (5-FU), furosemide (Lasix), granisetron (Kytril), hetastarch in electrolytes (Hextend), hydrocortisone (Hydrocortone, Solu-Cortef), hydromorphone (Dilaudid), imipenem-cilastatin (Primaxin), leucovorin calcium, lorazepam (Ativan), melphalan (Alkeran), mesna (Mesnex), methotrexate (Folex), methylprednisolone (Solu-Medrol), metronidazole (Flagyl IV), paclitaxel (Taxol), piperacillin/tazobactam (Zosyn), propofol (Diprivan), ranitidine (Zantac), sargramostim (Leukine), sodium bicarbonate, sulfamethoxazole-trimethoprim (Bactrim), thiotepa (Thioplex), ticarcillin/clavulanate (Timentin), zidovudine (AZT, Retrovir).

RATE OF ADMINISTRATION

May be given through Y-tube or three-way stopcock of infusion set; see Incompatible With.

Intermittent infusion: A single dose equally distributed over 30 minutes.

ACTIONS

A semisynthetic, extended-spectrum, fourth-generation cephalosporin antibiotic. Bactericidal to both gram-positive and gram-negative organisms, including many strains resistant to third-generation cephalosporins and aminoglycosides. Acts by inhibition of bacterial wall synthesis. Has a well-balanced spectrum with good antistaphylococcal activity, enhanced activity against gram-negative organisms, and good antipseudomonal activity. Peak serum levels achieved by end of infusion; half-life is 2.2 hours. Therapeutic levels last for 12 hours, allowing for twice-daily dosing. Well distributed into many body fluids and tissues. Crosses inflamed meninges to enter CSF. Partially metabolized; 85% excreted unchanged in urine. Crosses the placental barrier. Secreted in breast milk.

INDICATIONS AND USES

Treatment of moderate to severe pneumonia caused by susceptible nosocomial pathogens, as well as severe pneumonias complicated by pneumococcal bacteremia. ■ Treatment of uncomplicated and complicated urinary tract infections caused by susceptible organisms, including pyelonephritis and cases associated with concurrent bacteremia. ■ Treatment of uncomplicated skin and skin structure infections caused by susceptible organisms. ■ Empiric monotherapy in the treatment of febrile neutropenic patients. ■ Treatment of complicated intraabdominal infections in adults; used in combination with metronidazole (Flagyl). ■ See literature for list of susceptible organisms.

Unlabeled uses: Treatment of bronchitis and septicemia.

CONTRAINDICATIONS

Patients who have shown immediate hypersensitivity reactions to cefepime, any cephalosporin, cephamycins, penicillamine, penicillins, or other beta-lactam antibiotics.

PRECAUTIONS

Specific sensitivity studies are indicated to determine susceptibility of the causative organism to cefepime. ■ Generally more resistant to hydrolysis by beta-lactamases than third-generation cephalosporins are. ■ IM injection is used only for mild to moderate urinary tract infections. ■ Avoid prolonged use of drug; superinfection caused by overgrowth of nonsusceptible organisms may result. ■ Continue for at least 2 days after all symptoms of infection subside. ■ May decrease prothrombin activity, especially in patients with impaired renal or hepatic function, those in a poor nutritional state, and those receiving extended courses of antimicrobial therapy. ■ Use caution in patients with a history of GI disease (especially colitis). ■ Serious adverse events, including encephalopathy, myoclonus, seizures, and other life-threatening or fatal events have occurred. Patients with impaired renal function may be at greater risk, especially if doses are not properly adjusted; see Dose Adjustments and monitor closely. ■ Use extreme caution in the penicillin-sensitive patient; incidence of cross-sensitivity among beta-lactam antibiotics may be up to 10%. ■ Pseudomembranous colitis has been reported. May range from mild to life-threatening. Consider in patients that present with diarrhea during or after treatment with cefepime. ■ Contains arginine, which may alter glucose metabolism and elevate serum potassium. ■ Higher-end doses may increase incidence and severity of rash and require cefepime to be discontinued. ■ Insufficient data exist for treatment of febrile neutropenia in patients at high risk for severe infection (e.g., history of recent bone marrow transplant, hypotension on presentation, underlying hematologic malignancy, severe or prolonged neutropenia). No data are available for patients with septic shock.

Monitor: Watch for early symptoms of allergic reaction. ■ Obtain baseline CBC with differential and platelets and SrCr. ■ Record vital signs at least 3 times daily. ■ Obtain baseline PT and monitor, especially in at-risk patients (see Precautions); vitamin K may be indicated. ■ Monitoring of serum glucose and electrolytes (e.g., potassium, calcium) may be indicated. ■ May cause thrombophlebitis. ■ Monitor and reevaluate frequently the need for continued antimicrobial treatment in patients whose fever resolves but who remain neutropenic for more than 7 days. ■ Thrombophlebitis may result from prolonged or high dosage; use small needles, larger veins, and rotate infusion sites. ■ See Drug/Lab Interactions.

Patient Education: Promptly report any bleeding or bruising, diarrhea, or symptoms of allergy (e.g., difficulty breathing, hives, itching, rash).

Maternal/Child: Category B: safety for use during pregnancy and breastfeeding not established; use only if clearly needed. ■ A nursing infant consuming 1 quart of breast milk in a day would receive about 0.5 mg of cefepime. ■ Safety and effectiveness not established for infants under 2 months of age. ■ Pharmacokinetics in children and adults are similar. Dose modification similar to adults is indicated in impaired renal function; see Dose Adjustments. ■ Immature renal function of infants and small children will increase blood levels of all cephalosporins.

Elderly: No specific problems documented. Consider age-related impaired organ function and nutritional status; reduced dose or extended intervals may be indicated; see Dose Adjustments. Monitor for hypocalcemia.

DRUG/LAB INTERACTIONS

Risk of nephrotoxicity may be increased with aminoglycosides and other nephrotoxic agents (e.g., loop diuretics [e.g., furosemide (Lasix)]); monitor renal function closely. ■ May cause a false-positive direct Coombs' test. ■ May have a false-positive reaction for urine glucose except with enzyme-based tests (e.g., Clinistix). ■ See Side Effects. ■ While it has not been specifically studied with cefepime, other cephalosporins have the following drug interactions. May be antagonized by bacteriostatic antibiotics (e.g., chloramphenicol, erythromycin, tetracyclines); may interfere with bactericidal action. ■ Large amounts of cephalosporins and/or salicylates may induce hypoprothrombinemia (deficiency of prothrombin [Factor II]). The addition of agents that affect platelet aggregation and/or may have GI ulcerative potential (e.g., NSAIDs [ibuprofen (Advil, Motrin), naproxen (Aleve, Naprosyn)], or sulfinpyrazone [Anturane]) may increase risk of hemorrhage. ■ See Incompatible With.

SIDE EFFECTS

Full scope of allergic reactions (e.g., anaphylaxis, itching, rash, shock, urticaria). Burning, discomfort, pain, or phlebitis at injection site; diarrhea; elevated alkaline phosphatase, AST (SGOT), ALT (SGPT), BUN; fever; headache; nausea and vomiting; oral moniliasis; prolonged PT; pseudomembranous colitis; seizures (large doses or standard doses in renally impaired); vaginitis. Serum sickness–like reactions have occurred (e.g., arthralgia, fever, polyarthritis, skin rashes), usually after a second course of therapy. Usually resolve after cephalosporins are discontinued. Hypoprothrombinemia (rare) and hemolytic anemia may occur.

Overdose: Encephalopathy (disturbances of consciousness, including confusion, hallucinations, stupor, and coma), myoclonus, neuromuscular excitability, seizures.

ANTIDOTE

Notify physician of any side effects. Discontinue cefepime and treat allergic reaction as indicated (airway, oxygen, IV fluids, epinephrine, corticosteroids, pressor amines [e.g., dopamine], antihistamines [e.g., diphenhydramine]). Resuscitate as necessary. Discontinue cefepime if seizures occur and treat with anticonvulsants (e.g., diazepam [Valium]). Mild cases of colitis may respond to discontinuation of cefepime. Oral vancomycin (Vancocin) or metronidazole (Flagyl) is the treatment of choice for antibiotic-related pseudomembranous colitis. Antihistamines and corticosteroids may be indicated to manage symptoms of serum sickness. Hemodialysis may be useful in overdose.

CEFOPERAZONE SODIUM

(sef-oh-per′a-zone so′de-um)

Antibacterial (cephalosporin)

Cefobid

pH 4.5 to 6.5

USUAL DOSE

Moderate infections: 1 to 2 Gm every 12 hours.

Severe infections: 2 to 4 Gm every 8 hours or 3 to 6 Gm every 12 hours. Up to 12 to 16 Gm has been given in 24 hours.

PEDIATRIC DOSE

33.3 to 66.6 mg/kg of body weight every 8 hours or 50 to 100 mg/kg every 12 hours. See Maternal/Child.

DOSE ADJUSTMENTS

With average doses, no dose adjustment is required in impaired renal function. Monitor serum levels with higher doses. ■ Administer a dose following hemodialysis. ■ Reduce total daily dose to 1 to 2 Gm/24 hr if both renal and hepatic function are impaired. ■ Reduce total daily dose to 2 to 4 Gm/24 hr in impaired hepatic function or biliary obstruction. Begin at the low end of the dosing range in the elderly. Consider potential for decreased organ function and concomitant disease or drug therapy. ■ See Drug/Lab Interactions.

DILUTION

Each 1 Gm must be reconstituted with 5 ml SW. Difficult to put into solution. Shake vigorously to ensure solution; then allow to sit and examine for clarity. Should be further diluted with 20 to 40 ml D5W, NS, or other compatible solutions (see chart on inside back cover or literature) to a maximum concentration of 50 mg/ml and given as an intermittent infusion. Available premixed in 50 ml diluent. May be further diluted to 2 to 25 mg/ml and given as a continuous infusion.

Storage: Store unopened vials in carton at CRT. Protect from light. Administer within 24 hours of preparation. Selected solutions may be preserved 5 days with refrigeration.

INCOMPATIBLE WITH

May be used concomitantly with aminoglycosides (e.g., amikacin [Amikin], gentamicin [Garamycin]), but these drugs must never be mixed in the same infusion (mutual inactivation). If given concurrently, administer at separate sites. If administered sequentially, manufacturer recommends administration of cefoperazone before the aminoglycoside using a separate secondary IV tubing and flushing of the primary IV line before and after administration.

COMPATIBLE WITH (Underline Indicates Conflicting Compatibility Information)

Consult pharmacist; specific conditions may apply; see Compatibilities, p. xvi.

Additive: Cimetidine (Tagamet), clindamycin (Cleocin), furosemide (Lasix).

Syringe: Heparin.

Y-site: Acyclovir (Zovirax), allopurinol (Aloprim, Zyloprim), aztreonam (Azactam), cyclophosphamide (Cytoxan), <u>diltiazem (Cardizem)</u>, docetaxel (Taxotere), enalaprilat (Vasotec IV), esmolol (Brevibloc), etoposide phosphate (Etopophos), famotidine (Pepcid IV), fludarabine (Fludara), foscarnet (Foscavir), granisetron (Kytril), hetastarch in electrolytes (Hextend), hydromorphone (Dilaudid), linezolid (Zyvox), magnesium sulfate, melphalan (Alkeran), morphine, propofol (Diprivan), ranitidine (Zantac), <u>remifentanil (Ultiva)</u>, teniposide (Vumon), thiotepa (Thioplex).

RATE OF ADMINISTRATION

See Incompatible With.

Intermittent IV: A single dose over 15 to 30 minutes.

Continuous infusion: 500 to 1,000 ml over 6 to 24 hours, depending on total dose and concentration.

ACTIONS

A broad-spectrum, third-generation cephalosporin antibiotic. Bactericidal to many gram-negative, gram-positive, and anaerobic organisms. Effective against organisms resistant to other second- and third-generation cephalosporins. Peak serum levels achieved by end of infusion. Widely distributed in most tissues, body fluids (including inflamed meninges), bone, gallbladder (high biliary concentrations), myocardium, and skin and soft tissue. Excreted in bile. Crosses placental barrier. Secreted in breast milk.

INDICATIONS AND USES

Treatment of serious respiratory tract, intraabdominal, skin and skin structure, GU infections, and bacterial septicemia. Most effective against specific organisms (see literature).

Unlabeled uses: Treatment of bone and joint infections.

CONTRAINDICATIONS

Previous allergic reaction to cephalosporins or related antibiotics (penicillins). Absolute only if reaction was serious.

PRECAUTIONS

Sensitivity studies indicated to determine susceptibility of the causative organism to cefoperazone. ■ Continue for at least 2 to 3 days after all symptoms of infection subside. ■ Avoid prolonged use of drug; superinfection caused by overgrowth of nonsusceptible organisms may result. ■ Use caution in patients with impaired liver function or biliary obstruction; impaired renal function; a history of GI disease (especially colitis), bleeding disorders, or allergies; and those receiving an extended course of cephalosporins. ■ Pseudomembranous colitis has been reported. May range from mild to life-threatening. Consider in patients that present with diarrhea during or after treatment with cefoperazone.

Monitor: Watch for early symptoms of allergic reaction. ■ Use extreme caution in the penicillin-sensitive patient; incidence of cross-sensitivity may range from 3% to 16%. ■ May cause thrombophlebitis. Use small needles and large veins, and rotate infusion sites. ■ Observe for electrolyte imbalance and cardiac irregularities. Contains 1.5 mEq sodium per Gm. ■ May cause hypoprothrombinemia (deficiency of prothrombin [Factor II]); 10 mg/week of prophylactic vitamin K may be indicated in elderly, debilitated, or other patients with vitamin K deficiency. Monitor PT. ■ See Drug/Lab Interactions; additional monitoring may be indicated (e.g., renal function, drug serum levels, PT).

Patient Education: Avoid alcohol or alcohol-containing preparations; may cause abdominal cramping, flushing, headache, nausea and vomiting, shortness of breath, sweating, and tachycardia. ■ Report promptly any bleeding or bruising, diarrhea, symptoms of allergy (e.g., difficulty breathing, hives, itching, rash).

Maternal/Child: Category B: safety for use during pregnancy and breast-feeding not established. No problems documented. ■ Safety and effectiveness for use in children under 12 years not established.

Elderly: Response similar to younger adults; however, dosing should be cautious; see Dose Adjustments.

DRUG/LAB INTERACTIONS

May produce symptoms of acute alcohol intolerance with alcohol (a disulfiram-like reaction with abdominal cramps, headache, flushing, nausea and vomiting, shortness of breath, sweating, tachycardia). Patient must abstain from alcohol during treatment and until at least 72 hours after discontinuation. ■ Risk of nephrotoxicity may be increased with aminoglycoside and other nephrotoxic agents (e.g., loop diuretics such as furosemide [Lasix]). ■ Is not inhibited by probenecid as other cephalosporins are because of biliary excretion. ■ May be antagonized by bacteriostatic antibiotics (e.g., chloramphenicol, erythromycin, tetracyclines); may interfere with bactericidal action. ■ Bleeding tendency may be increased with any medicine that affects blood clotting (e.g., heparin and oral anticoagulants [warfarin (Coumadin)], thrombolytic agents [e.g., alteplase (tPA)], salicylates, NSAIDs [e.g., ibuprofen (Advil, Motrin), naproxen (Aleve, Naprosyn)], sulfinpyrazone [Anturane]). ■ Large amounts of cephalosporins and/or salicylates may induce hypoprothrombinemia. ■ Positive Coombs' test. ■ False-positive reaction for urine glucose except with enzyme-based tests (e.g., Chemstix). ■ See Incompatible With and Side Effects.

SIDE EFFECTS

Full scope of allergic reactions including anaphylaxis. Abnormal bleeding; decreased hemoglobin or decreased hematocrit; decreased platelet functions; diarrhea, eosinophilia; elevation of AST (SGOT), ALT (SGPT), total bilirubin, alkaline phosphatase, LDH, and BUN (transient); fever; leukopenia; local site pain; positive Coombs' test; prolonged PT; pseudomembranous colitis; seizures (large doses); thrombocytopenia; thrombophlebitis; transient neutropenia; vaginitis; vomiting. Hypoprothrombinemia (rare) and hemolytic anemia may occur. Serum sickness–like reactions have occurred (e.g., arthralgia, fever, polyarthritis, skin rashes), usually after a second course of therapy. Generally resolve after cephalosporins are discontinued.

ANTIDOTE

Notify the physician of any side effects. Discontinue the drug if indicated. Treat allergic reaction as indicated and resuscitate as necessary. Mild cases of colitis may respond to discontinuation of cefoperazone. Oral vancomycin (Vancocin) or metronidazole (Flagyl) is the treatment of choice for antibiotic-related pseudomembranous colitis. Hemodialysis only slightly useful in overdose. Vitamin K, fresh-frozen plasma, packed red cells, or platelet concentrates may be indicated in abnormal bleeding tendencies confirmed by lab evaluations. If bleeding is due to platelet dysfunction, discontinue and use an alternate antibiotic. Antihistamines and corticosteroids may be indicated to manage symptoms of serum sickness.

CEFOTAXIME SODIUM

(sef-oh-taks′eem so′de-um)

Antibacterial (cephalosporin)

Claforan

pH 4.5 to 7.5

USUAL DOSE

Range is 2 to 12 Gm/24 hr. Depends on seriousness of infection. Maximum daily dose is 12 Gm.

Uncomplicated infections: 1 Gm every 12 hours.

Moderate to severe infections: 1 to 2 Gm every 8 hours.

Serious infections and septicemia: 2 Gm every 6 to 8 hours.

Life-threatening infections: 2 Gm every 4 hours.

Higher doses often reduced with positive clinical response.

Disseminated gonococcal infections: 1 Gm every 8 hours (usually given IM).

Gonococcal ophthalmia (penicillinase producing *Neisseria gonorrhoeae* [PPNG]): 500 mg every 6 hours.

Perioperative prophylaxis: 1 Gm 30 to 90 minutes before incision. May be repeated in a lengthy procedure. In ***cesarean section*** give initial dose after cord is clamped, then 1 Gm at 6 and 12 hours postoperatively.

PEDIATRIC DOSE

Maximum daily dose 12 Gm/24 hr. Differentiation between premature and normal gestational age is not necessary.

0 to 1 week of age: 50 mg/kg/dose every 12 hours.

1 to 4 weeks of age: 50 mg/kg/dose every 8 hours. One source increases the interval to every 12 hours in infants weighing less than 1,200 Gm.

1 month to 12 years, weight less than 50 kg: 50 to 180 mg/kg/24 hr equally divided into 4 to 6 doses (8.3 to 30 mg/kg/dose every 4 hours or 12.5 to 45 mg/kg/dose every 6 hours). Use higher-end doses for serious infections, including meningitis.

Weight 50 kg or more: See Usual Dose.

DOSE ADJUSTMENTS

In impaired renal function with a CrCl less than 20 ml/min/1.73 M^2, reduce dose by one half and maintain same dosing interval. ■ See Usual Dose and Drug/Lab Interactions.

DILUTION

Each dose (500 mg, 1 Gm, 2 Gm) must be reconstituted with 10 ml SW, D5W, NS, or other compatible infusion solution (see chart on inside back cover or literature). Available premixed and in ADD-Vantage vials for use with ADD-Vantage infusion containers. May be further diluted with 50 to 100 ml of compatible solutions and given as an intermittent infusion or added to larger volumes and given as a continuous infusion. (1 Gm in 14 ml of SW is isotonic.)

Storage: Store unopened cartons at CRT. Protect from excessive light. Administer diluted solution within 24 hours or within 5 days if refrigerated.

INCOMPATIBLE WITH

May be used concomitantly with aminoglycosides (e.g., amikacin [Amikin], gentamicin [Garamycin]), but these drugs must never be mixed in the same infusion (mutual inactivation). If given concurrently, administer at separate sites. Manufacturer recommends temporarily discontinuing other solutions infusing at the same site during intermittent infusion and states, "Do not add supplementary medications to premixed plastic IV containers."

COMPATIBLE WITH **(Underline Indicates Conflicting Compatibility Information)**

Consult pharmacist; specific conditions may apply; see Compatibilities, p. xvi.

Additive: Clindamycin (Cleocin), metronidazole (Flagyl IV), verapamil (Isoptin).

Syringe: Heparin, ofloxacin (Floxin IV).

Y-site: Acyclovir (Zovirax), amifostine (Ethyol), aztreonam (Azactam), <u>cisatracurium (Nimbex)</u>, cyclophosphamide (Cytoxan), diltiazem (Cardizem), docetaxel (Taxotere), etoposide phosphate (Etopophos), famotidine (Pepcid IV), fludarabine (Fludara), granisetron (Kytril), hetastarch in electrolytes (Hextend), hydromorphone (Dilaudid), levofloxacin (Levaquin), lorazepam (Ativan), magnesium sulfate, melphalan (Alkeran), meperidine (Demerol), midazolam (Versed), morphine, ondansetron (Zofran), perphenazine (Trilafon), propofol (Diprivan), remifentanil (Ultiva), sargramostim (Leukine), teniposide (Vumon), thiotepa (Thioplex), <u>vancomycin (Vancocin)</u>, vinorelbine (Navelbine).

RATE OF ADMINISTRATION

See Incompatible With. Injection and intermittent infusion may be given through Y-tube or three-way stopcock of infusion set.

IV injection: A single dose equally distributed over 3 to 5 minutes.

Intermittent IV: A single dose over 30 minutes.

Continuous infusion: 500 to 1,000 ml over 6 to 24 hours, depending on total dose and concentration.

ACTIONS

A broad-spectrum, third-generation cephalosporin antibiotic. Bactericidal to many gram-negative, gram-positive, and anaerobic organisms. Effective against many otherwise resistant organisms. Peak serum levels achieved within 30 minutes. Distributed into most body tissues and fluids, including inflamed meninges. Some metabolites formed. Excreted in the urine. Crosses placental barrier. Secreted in breast milk.

INDICATIONS AND USES

Treatment of serious lower respiratory tract, urinary tract, skin and skin structure, intraabdominal, bone and joint, CNS, gynecologic infections, and bacteremia/septicemia. Most effective against specific organisms (see literature). ■ Perioperative prophylaxis. ■ Used IM to treat disseminated gonococcal infections.

Unlabeled uses: Treatment of Lyme disease.

CONTRAINDICATIONS

Previous allergic reaction to cephalosporins or related antibiotics (penicillins). Absolute only if reaction was serious.

PRECAUTIONS

Sensitivity studies indicated to determine susceptibility of the causative organism to cefotaxime. ■ Continue for 2 to 3 days after all symptoms of infection subside. ■ Avoid prolonged use of drug; superinfection caused by overgrowth of nonsusceptible organisms may result. ■ Use caution in patients with impaired renal function, allergies, or a history of GI disease (especially colitis). ■ Pseudomembranous colitis has been reported. May range from mild to life-threatening. Consider in patients that present with diarrhea during or after treatment with cefotaxime.

Monitor: Watch for early symptoms of allergic reaction. ■ Use extreme caution in the penicillin-sensitive patient; incidence of cross-sensitivity may range from 3% to 16%. ■ May cause thrombophlebitis. Use small needles and large veins, and rotate infusion sites. ■ Observe for electrolyte imbalance or cardiac irregularities. Contains 2.2 mEq sodium per Gm. ■ See Drug/Lab Interactions; additional monitoring may be indicated (e.g., renal function, drug serum levels, PT).

Patient Education: Report promptly any bleeding or bruising, diarrhea, or symptoms of allergy (e.g., difficulty breathing, hives, itching, rash).

Maternal/Child: Category B: safety for use during pregnancy and breast-feeding not established. No problems documented. ■ Immature renal function of infants and small children will increase blood levels of all cephalosporins.

Elderly: No specific problems documented. Consider age-related impaired organ function and nutritional status; reduced dose or extended intervals may be indicated.

DRUG/LAB INTERACTIONS

Risk of nephrotoxicity may be increased with aminoglycosides and other nephrotoxic agents (e.g., loop diuretics [such as furosemide (Lasix)]). ■ Probenecid inhibits excretion and may require reduced dosage. ■ May be antagonized by bacteriostatic antibiotics (e.g., chloramphenicol, erythromycin, tetracyclines); may interfere with bactericidal action. ■ Large amounts of cephalosporins and/or salicylates may induce hypoprothrombinemia (deficiency of prothrombin [Factor II]). The addition of agents that affect platelet aggregation and/or may have GI ulcerative potential (e.g., NSAIDs [ibuprofen (Advil, Motrin), naproxen (Aleve, Naprosyn)], or sulfinpyrazone [Anturane]) may increase risk of hemorrhage. ■ See Incompatible With and Side Effects.

SIDE EFFECTS

Full scope of allergic reactions including anaphylaxis. Decreased hemoglobin or decreased hematocrit; decreased platelet functions; diarrhea;

dyspnea; elevation of AST (SGOT), ALT (SGPT), total bilirubin, alkaline phosphatase, LDH, and BUN (transient); eosinophilia; fever; leukopenia; local site pain; nausea; oral thrush; positive direct Coombs' test; prolonged PT; pseudomembranous colitis; seizures (large doses); thrombocytopenia; thrombophlebitis; transient neutropenia; vaginitis; vomiting. Cutaneous reactions (e.g., erythema multiforme, Stevens-Johnson syndrome, toxic epidermal necrolysis), hypoprothrombinemia (rare), and hemolytic anemia may occur. Serum sickness–like reactions have occurred (e.g., arthralgia, fever, polyarthritis, skin rashes), usually after a second course of therapy. Generally resolve after cephalosporins are discontinued.

ANTIDOTE

Notify the physician of any side effects. Discontinue the drug if indicated. Mild cases of colitis may respond to discontinuation of cefotaxime. Oral vancomycin (Vancocin) or metronidazole (Flagyl) is the treatment of choice for antibiotic-related pseudomembranous colitis. Antihistamines and corticosteroids may be indicated to manage symptoms of serum sickness. Treat allergic reaction as indicated and resuscitate as necessary. Hemodialysis may be useful in overdose.

CEFOTETAN DISODIUM

(sef′oh-tee-tan dye-so′de-um)

Cefotan

Antibacterial (cephalosporin)

pH 4 to 6.5

USUAL DOSE

Range is 1 to 6 Gm/24 hr for 5 to 10 days. Do not exceed 6 Gm/24 hr.

Urinary tract infections: 500 mg to 2 Gm every 12 hours or 1 to 2 Gm every 12 to 24 hours.

Moderate infections: 1 or 2 Gm every 12 hours.

Moderate infections of skin and skin structure: 2 Gm every 24 hours or 1 Gm every 12 hours. Give 1 or 2 Gm every 12 hours if *Klebsiella pneumoniae* is the causative organism.

Serious infections: 2 Gm every 12 hours.

Life-threatening infections: 3 Gm every 12 hours.

Pelvic inflammatory disease: 2 Gm every 12 hours for 14 days. Transfer to oral therapy at any time it is clinically appropriate, usually 48 hours after clinical improvement.

Perioperative prophylaxis: 1 to 2 Gm IV 30 to 60 minutes before incision except during ***cesarean section.*** Given only after clamping the umbilical cord in cesarean section.

PEDIATRIC DOSE

20 to 40 mg/kg of body weight every 12 hours; see Maternal/Child.

DOSE ADJUSTMENTS

Reduce total daily dose if renal function impaired according to the following chart.

Cefotetan Dose Guidelines in Impaired Renal Function

Creatinine Clearance (ml/min)	Dose/Frequency
>30	Usual recommended dose q 12 hr
10-30	Usual recommended dose q 24 hr or ½ usual recommended dose q 12 hr
<10	Usual recommended dose q 48 hr or ¼ usual recommended dose q 12 hr
Hemodialysis patients	¼ usual adult dose q 24 hr on days between dialysis sessions ½ usual adult dose on the day of dialysis

DILUTION

Available in vials, piggyback, ADD-Vantage vials for use with ADD-Vantage infusion containers, and in Galaxy infusion bags. With all preparations, after dilution shake well and let stand until clear.

IV injection: Reconstitute each 1 Gm with 10 ml of SW for injection (2 Gm with 20 ml).

Intermittent IV: ***Vials:*** A single dose may be further diluted or initially diluted with 50 to 100 ml of D5W or NS.

Piggyback preparations may be diluted with 50 to 100 ml D5W or NS. ***ADD-Vantage preparations*** must be diluted with 50, 100, or 250 ml of NS or D5W in ADD-Vantage infusion containers. Follow manufacturer's instructions.

Storage: Store vials below 22° C (72° F); protect from light. Administer within 24 hours of preparation or within 96 hours if refrigerated. Stable after dilution for 1 week if frozen; thaw at room temperature before use, discard remaining solution; do not refreeze. Slight yellowing does not affect potency.

INCOMPATIBLE WITH

May be used concomitantly with aminoglycosides (e.g., amikacin [Amikin], gentamicin [Garamycin]), but these drugs must never be mixed in the same infusion (mutual inactivation). If given concurrently, administer at separate sites. Manufacturer recommends temporarily discontinuing other solutions infusing at the same site during intermittent infusion and states, "Do not add supplementary medications to premixed plastic IV containers" (e.g., Galaxy). Manufacturer lists gentamicin (Garamycin) and heparin as incompatible.

COMPATIBLE WITH **(Underline Indicates Conflicting Compatibility Information)**

Consult pharmacist; specific conditions may apply; see Compatibilities, p. xvi.

Y-site: Manufacturer lists amikacin (Amikin), aminophylline, ampicillin, atropine, cimetidine (Tagamet), digoxin (Lanoxin), dopamine (Intropin), doxycycline (Vibramycin), epinephrine (Adrenalin), erythromycin lactobionate (Erythrocin), furosemide (Lasix), kanamycin (Kantrex), mezlocillin (Mezlin), multivitamins (M.V.I.), oxytocin (Pitocin), penicillin G potassium, piperacillin (Pipracil), ticarcillin (Ticar), tobramycin (Nebcin). Other sources add allopurinol (Aloprim, Zyloprim), amifostine (Ethyol), aztreonam (Azactam), cisatracurium (Nimbex), diltiazem (Cardizem), docetaxel (Taxotere), etoposide phosphate (Etopophos), famotidine (Pepcid IV), filgrastim (Neupogen), fluconazole (Diflucan), fludarabine (Fludara), gatifloxacin (Tequin), gemcitabine (Gemzar), granisetron (Kytril), heparin, hetastarch in electrolytes (Hextend), insulin (regular), linezolid (Zyvox), melphalan (Alkeran), meperidine (Demerol), morphine, paclitaxel (Taxol), propofol (Diprivan), remifentanil (Ultiva), sargramostim (Leukine), tacrolimus (Prograf), teniposide (Vumon), theophylline, thiotepa (Thioplex), vancomycin (Vancocin).

RATE OF ADMINISTRATION

See Incompatible With. May be given through Y-tube or three-way stopcock of infusion set.

IV injection: A single dose equally distributed over 3 to 5 minutes.

Intermittent IV: A single dose over 30 minutes.

ACTIONS

A broad-spectrum, second-generation cephalosporin antibiotic. Bactericidal to selected gram-negative, gram-positive, and anaerobic organisms. Effective against many otherwise resistant organisms. Peak serum levels achieved at end of infusion. Widely distributed in most tissues, body fluids (CSF minimal), bone, gallbladder, myocardium, and skin and soft tissue. Primarily excreted in the urine. Crosses placental barrier. Secreted in breast milk.

INDICATIONS AND USES

Treatment of serious lower respiratory tract, urinary tract, skin and skin structure, gynecologic, intraabdominal, and bone and joint infections. Most effective against specific organisms (see literature). ■ Perioperative prophylaxis.

CONTRAINDICATIONS

Previous allergic reaction to cephalosporins or related antibiotics (penicillins). Absolute only if reaction was serious and in patients who have experienced a cephalosporin-associated hemolytic anemia.

PRECAUTIONS

Specific sensitivity studies are indicated to determine susceptibility of the causative organism to cefotetan. ■ Continue for at least 2 or 3 days after all symptoms of infection subside. ■ Avoid prolonged use of drug; superinfection caused by overgrowth of nonsusceptible organisms may result. ■ Use caution in patients with impaired renal function, a history of GI disease (especially colitis), bleeding disorders or allergies, and those receiving an extended course of cephalosporins. ■ Pseudomembranous colitis has been reported. May range from mild to life-threatening. Consider in patients that present with diarrhea during or after treatment with cefotetan. ■ Hemolytic anemia including fatalities has been reported. Discontinue cefotetan immediately if anemia develops during the course of therapy. May present within 2 to 3 weeks of therapy completion.

Monitor: Watch for early symptoms of allergic reaction. ■ Use extreme caution in the penicillin-sensitive patient; incidence of cross-sensitivity may range from 3% to 16%. ■ May cause hypoprothrombinemia (deficiency of prothrombin [Factor II]); 10 mg/week of prophylactic vitamin K may be indicated in elderly, debilitated, or other patients with vitamin K deficiency. Monitor PT. ■ May cause thrombophlebitis. Use small needles and large veins, and rotate infusion sites. ■ Observe for electrolyte imbalance and cardiac irregularities. Contains 3.5 mEq sodium per Gm. ■ Monitor CBC in patients receiving a prolonged course of therapy. ■ See Drug/Lab Interactions; additional monitoring may be indicated (e.g., renal function, drug serum levels, PT).

Patient Education: Avoid alcohol or alcohol-containing preparations; may cause abdominal cramps, flushing, headache, nausea and vomiting, shortness of breath, sweating, and tachycardia. ■ Report promptly any bleeding or bruising, diarrhea, symptoms of allergy (e.g., difficulty breathing, hives, itching, rash).

Maternal/Child: Category B: safety for use during pregnancy not established. Use only if clearly needed. ■ Use caution if breast-feeding. ■ Safety for use in children not established. Immature renal function of infants and small children will increase blood levels of all cephalosporins.

Elderly: Safety and effectiveness similar to younger adults; however, greater sensitivity of some older individuals cannot be ruled out. Consider age-related impaired organ function and nutritional status. ■ Monitoring of renal function suggested; reduced dose or extended intervals may be indicated.

DRUG/LAB INTERACTIONS

May produce symptoms of acute intolerance with alcohol (a disulfiram-like reaction with abdominal cramps, headache, flushing, nausea and vomiting, shortness of breath, sweating, tachycardia). Patient must abstain from alcohol during treatment and until at least 72 hours after discontinuation. ■ Risk of nephrotoxicity may be increased with aminoglycosides and other nephrotoxic agents (e.g., loop diuretics [furosemide (Lasix)]). ■ Sources differ on inhibition of excretion by probenecid. ■ May be antagonized by bacteriostatic antibiotics (e.g., chloramphenicol, erythomycin, tetracyclines); may interfere with bactericidal action. ■ Bleeding tendency increased with any medicine that affects blood clotting (e.g., heparin and oral anticoagulants [warfarin (Coumadin)], thrombolytic agents [e.g., alteplase (tPA)], salicylates, NSAIDs [e.g., ibuprofen (Advil, Motrin), naproxen (Aleve, Naprosyn)], sulfinpyrazone [Anturane]). ■ Large amounts of cephalosporins and/or salicylates may induce hypoprothrombinemia. ■ False increases in creatinine levels with Jaffe method. ■ False-positive for urine glucose except with enzyme-based tests (e.g., Chemstix). ■ Positive direct Coombs' test. ■ See Incompatible With and Side Effects.

SIDE EFFECTS

Full scope of allergic reactions, including anaphylaxis. Bleeding episodes; burning, discomfort, and pain at injection site; diarrhea; eosinophilia; elevated alkaline phosphatase, AST (SGOT), ALT (SGPT), and LDH; nausea; prolonged PT; pseudomembranous colitis; seizures (large doses); thrombocytosis. Hypoprothrombinemia (rare) and hemolytic anemia may occur. Serum sickness–like reactions have occurred (e.g., arthralgia, fever, polyarthritis, skin rashes), usually after a second course of therapy. Usually resolve after cephalosporins are discontinued.

ANTIDOTE

Notify physician of any side effects. Discontinue the drug if indicated. Treat allergic reaction as indicated and resuscitate as necessary. Mild cases of colitis may respond to discontinuation of cefotetan. Oral vancomycin (Vancocin) or metronidazole (Flagyl) is the treatment of choice for antibiotic-related pseudomembranous colitis. Bleeding episodes may respond to vitamin K or require discontinuation of drug. Fresh-frozen plasma, packed red cells, or platelet concentrates may be indicated in abnormal bleeding tendencies confirmed by lab evaluations. If bleeding is due to platelet dysfunction, discontinue and use an alternate antibiotic. Blood transfusions (e.g., packed red cells) may be indicated if hemolytic anemia develops. Hemodialysis is only slightly useful in overdose. Antihistamines and corticosteroids may be indicated to manage symptoms of serum sickness.

CEFOXITIN SODIUM

(se-fox'i-tin so'de-um)

Mefoxin

Antibacterial (cephalosporin)

pH 4.2 to 8

USUAL DOSE

1 to 2 Gm every 6 to 8 hours depending on severity of the infection, up to 12 Gm/24 hr. Maximum recommended dose is 2 Gm every 8 hours in the elderly (over 75 years of age) even if their SrCr is normal.

Uncomplicated infections: 1 Gm every 6 to 8 hours.

Moderately severe to severe infections: 1 Gm every 4 hours or 2 Gm every 6 to 8 hours.

Life-threatening infections: 2 Gm every 4 hours or 3 Gm every 6 hours.

Acute pelvic inflammatory disease (CDC recommendation [unlabeled]): 2 Gm every 6 hours. Given in combination with doxycycline (Vibramycin) 100 mg IV or PO every 12 hours.

Oral bacterial *Eikenella corrudens* (unlabeled): 1 to 2 Gm every 6 hours.

Perioperative prophylaxis: 2 Gm 30 minutes to 1 hour before incision. Follow with 2 Gm every 6 hours for 24 hours.

Prophylaxis during cesarean section: 2 Gm after clamping the umbilical cord. May repeat in 4 hours and again in 8 hours.

Prophylaxis during transurethral prostatectomy (unlabeled): 1 Gm before surgery. May be repeated every 8 hours for up to 5 days.

PEDIATRIC DOSE

Infants and children over 3 months of age: 13.3 to 26.7 mg/kg of body weight every 4 hours or 20 to 40 mg/kg every 6 hours. Do not exceed adult dose.

Perioperative prophylaxis in infants and children over 3 months of age: 30 to 40 mg/kg 30 minutes to 1 hour before incision and every 6 hours for 24 hours.

NEONATAL DOSE

Use sterile cefoxitin sodium USP only. Other formulations may contain benzyl alcohol.

Premature infants over 1,500 Gm and neonates to 1 week of age: 20 to 40 mg/kg every 12 hours.

Neonates 1 to 4 weeks of age: 20 to 40 mg/kg every 8 hours.

Infants 1 to 3 months of age: 20 to 40 mg/kg every 6 to 8 hours.

DOSE ADJUSTMENTS

In impaired renal function, the initial dose should be as above, but all remaining doses should be based on CrCl according to the following chart. See Drug/Lab Interactions.

Cefoxitin Maintenance Dose in Adults With Impaired Renal Function		
Creatinine Clearance (ml/min)	**Dose (grams)**	**Frequency**
30-50	1-2	q 8-12 hr
10-29	1-2	q 12-24 hr
5-9	0.5-1	q 12-24 hr
<5	0.5-1	q 24-48 hr

In pediatric patients, one source recommends reducing the dose and frequency consistent with the recommendations for adults. Another source recommends increasing the dosing interval based on CrCl according to the following chart.

Cefoxitin Maintenance Dose in Pediatric Patients With Impaired Renal Function	
Creatinine Clearance (ml/min)	**Frequency**
<50	q 8 hr
10-50	q 8-12 hr
<10	q 24-48 hr

DILUTION

Each 1 Gm or fraction thereof must be reconstituted with at least 10 ml of SW, D5W, or NS. A single dose may be further diluted in 50 to 100 ml of most common infusion solutions (see chart on inside back cover and literature). The use of butterfly needles and dilution in up to 1,000 ml of D5W, D5NS, or NS are preferred when administering larger doses as a continuous infusion. Available premixed, in piggyback vials, and in ADD-Vantage vials for use with ADD-Vantage infusion containers. May be given through a Y-tube, three-way stopcock, additive infusion set, or as a continuous infusion.

Storage: Reconstituted solutions are stable at CRT for 6 hours and 7 days if refrigerated. Solutions diluted in 50 to 1,000 ml diluent are stable for 24 hours at CRT and up to 9 days if refrigerated. Thaw frozen containers at CRT or under refrigeration. Do not force thaw. Stable for 21 days if refrigerated. Do not refreeze.

INCOMPATIBLE WITH

May be used concomitantly with aminoglycosides (e.g., amikacin [Amikin], gentamicin [Garamycin]), but these drugs must never be mixed in the same infusion (mutual inactivation). If given concurrently, administer at separate sites. Manufacturer recommends temporarily discontinuing other solutions infusing at the same site during intermittent infusion.

COMPATIBLE WITH (Underline Indicates Conflicting Compatibility Information)

Consult pharmacist; specific conditions may apply; see Compatibilities, p. xvi.

Additive: Aztreonam (Azactam), cimetidine (Tagamet), clindamycin (Cleocin), metronidazole (Flagyl IV), multivitamins (M.V.I.), sodium bicarbonate (Neut), verapamil (Isoptin).

Syringe: Heparin.

Y-site: Acyclovir (Zovirax), amifostine (Ethyol), amphotericin B cholesteryl (Amphotec), aztreonam (Azactam), cisatracurium (Nimbex), cyclophosphamide (Cytoxan), diltiazem (Cardizem), docetaxel (Taxotere), doxorubicin liposome (Doxil), etoposide phosphate (Etopophos), famotidine (Pepcid IV), fluconazole (Diflucan), foscarnet (Foscavir), gemcitabine (Gemzar), granisetron (Kytril), hetastarch in electrolytes (Hextend), hydromorphone (Dilaudid), linezolid (Zyvox), magnesium sulfate, meperidine (Demerol), morphine, ondansetron (Zofran), perphenazine (Trilafon), propofol (Diprivan), ranitidine (Zantac), remifentanil (Ultiva), teniposide (Vumon), thiotepa (Thioplex), vancomycin (Vancocin).

RATE OF ADMINISTRATION

See Incompatible With. Each 1 Gm or fraction thereof over 3 to 5 minutes or longer as indicated by amount of solution and condition of the patient. Rate of continuous infusion should be by physician order.

ACTIONS

A semisynthetic, second-generation cephalosporin antibiotic that is bactericidal to many gram-positive, gram-negative, and anaerobic organisms. Peak serum levels achieved by end of infusion. Widely distributed into most body tissues and fluids (CSF minimal), bone, gallbladder, myocardium, and skin and soft tissues. Crosses the placental barrier. Excreted rapidly in the urine. Secreted in breast milk.

INDICATIONS AND USES

Treatment of serious respiratory, GU, intraabdominal, gynecologic, bone and joint, skin and skin structure infections and septicemia. Effective only if the causative organism is susceptible. ▪ Perioperative prophylaxis.

Unlabeled uses: Treatment of acute pelvic inflammatory disease (CDC recommendation). ▪ Treatment of oral bacterial *Eikenella corrudens.* ▪ Prophylaxis during transurethral prostatectomy.

CONTRAINDICATIONS

Previous allergic reaction to cephalosporins or related antibiotics (penicillins). Absolute only if reaction was serious.

PRECAUTIONS

Sensitivity studies indicated to determine susceptibility of the causative organism to cefoxitin. ▪ Continue for at least 2 to 3 days after all symptoms of infection subside. ▪ Avoid prolonged use of drug; superinfection caused by overgrowth of nonsusceptible organisms may result. ▪ Use caution in patients with impaired renal function, allergies, or a history of GI disease (especially colitis). ▪ Pseudomembranous colitis has been reported. May range from mild to life-threatening. Consider in patients that present with diarrhea during or after treatment with cefoxitin. ▪ Continue treatment for group A beta-hemolytic streptococcal infections for 10 days or more to decrease the risk of rheumatic fever or glomerulonephritis.

Monitor: Watch for early symptoms of allergic reaction. ▪ Use extreme caution in the penicillin-sensitive patient; incidence of cross-sensitivity may range from 3% to 16%. ▪ Thrombophlebitis may result from prolonged or high dosage; use small needles, larger veins, and rotate infusion sites. ■ Observe for electrolyte imbalance or cardiac irregularities. Contains 2.3 mEq sodium/Gm. ■ See Drug/Lab Interactions; additional monitoring may be indicated (e.g., renal function, drug serum levels, PT).

Patient Education: Report promptly any bleeding or bruising, diarrhea, or symptoms of allergy (e.g., difficulty breathing, hives, itching, rash).

Maternal/Child: Category B: safety for use during pregnancy and breastfeeding not established. No problems documented. ■ Do not use formulations containing benzyl alcohol in infants and children under 3 months. ■ Immature renal function will increase blood levels. ■ Eosinophilia and elevated AST (SGOT) associated with higher doses in infants and children.

Elderly: No specific problems documented. Consider age-related impaired organ function and nutritional status; reduced dose or extended intervals may be indicated. ■ See Usual Dose.

DRUG/LAB INTERACTIONS

Risk of nephrotoxicity may be increased with aminoglycosides and other nephrotoxic agents (e.g., loop diuretics such as furosemide [Lasix]). ■ Probenecid inhibits excretion and may require reduction in dosage. ■ May be antagonized by bacteriostatic antibiotics (e.g., chloramphenicol, erythromycin, tetracyclines); may interfere with bactericidal action. ■ Large doses of cephalosporins and/or salicylates may induce hypoprothrombinemia (deficiency of prothrombin [Factor II]). The addition of agents that affect platelet aggregation and/or may have GI ulcerative potential (e.g., NSAIDs [ibuprofen (Advil, Motrin), naproxen (Aleve, Naprosyn)], or sulfinpyrazone [Anturane]) may increase risk of hemorrhage. ■ False-positive reaction for urine glucose except with enzyme-based tests (e.g., Chemstix). ■ Positive Coombs' test. ■ False increases in creatinine levels with Jaffe method. ■ See Incompatible With and Side Effects.

SIDE EFFECTS

Allergic reactions including anaphylaxis; anorexia; leukopenia; local site pain; nausea and vomiting; neutropenia; oral thrush; phlebitis; prolonged PT; proteinuria; pseudomembranous colitis; seizures (large doses); thrombophlebitis; and transient elevation of AST (SGOT), ALT (SGPT), BUN, and alkaline phosphatase. Hypoprothrombinemia (rare) and hemolytic anemia may occur. Serum sickness–like reactions have occurred (e.g., arthralgia, fever, polyarthritis, skin rashes), usually after a second course of therapy. Generally resolve after cephalosporins are discontinued.

ANTIDOTE

Notify physician of any side effects. Discontinue the drug if indicated. Oral vancomycin (Vancocin) or metronidazole (Flagyl) is the treatment of choice for antibiotic-related pseudomembranous colitis. Treat allergic reaction as indicated and resuscitate as necessary. Hemodialysis may be useful in overdose. Antihistamines and corticosteroids may be indicated to manage symptoms of serum sickness.

CEFTAZIDIME

(sef-taz'i-deem)

Antibacterial (cephalosporin)

Ceptaz, Fortaz, Tazicef, Tazidime

pH 5.5 to 8

USUAL DOSE

Range is from 250 mg to 2 Gm every 8 to 12 hours. Dosage based on severity of disease, condition of the patient, and susceptibility of the causative organism. Usual maximum dose for the elderly (over 75 years of age) is 1 Gm/24 hr, even if their SrCr is normal.

Uncomplicated GU infections: 250 mg every 12 hours.

Complicated GU infections: 500 mg every 8 to 12 hours.

Uncomplicated pneumonia and skin and skin structure infections: 500 mg to 1 Gm every 8 hours.

Bone and joint infections: 2 Gm every 12 hours.

Severe or life-threatening infections (especially in immunocompromised patients), meningitis, serious gynecologic and intraabdominal infections: 2 Gm every 8 hours.

Pseudomonal lung infections in cystic fibrosis patients (must have normal renal function): 30 to 50 mg/kg of body weight every 8 hours. Do not exceed 6 Gm/24 hr.

Melioidosis (unlabeled): 40 mg/kg every 8 hours.

PEDIATRIC DOSE

Use sodium carbonate formulation (Fortaz, Tazicef, Tazidime) only for infants and children under 12 years. Components of other formulations may be harmful. Reserve higher doses for immunocompromised pediatric patients or those with cystic fibrosis or meningitis. Do not exceed 6 Gm/24 hr.

Infants and children 1 month to 12 years: 30 to 50 mg/kg of body weight every 8 hours.

NEONATAL DOSE

Use sodium carbonate formulation only (Fortaz, Tazicef, Tazidime); components of other formulations may be harmful.

Neonates up to 4 weeks of age: 30 mg/kg every 12 hours.

The American Academy of Pediatrics suggests the following doses:

Less than 1 week of age weighing 2 kg or less: 50 mg/kg every 12 hours.

Less than 1 week of age weighing more than 2 kg: 50 mg/kg every 8 or 12 hours.

Neonates from 1 to 4 weeks of age: 50 mg/kg every 8 hours.

DOSE ADJUSTMENTS

In impaired renal function, the initial dose should be as above, but all remaining doses should be based on CrCl according to the following chart. If the normal dose would be lower than the doses in the chart, use the lower dose. Adjustment for pediatric patients is similar to adults; consider body surface or lean body mass and reduce dosing frequency.

Ceftazidime Maintenance Dose in Impaired Renal Function		
Creatinine Clearance (ml/min)	**Dose**	**Frequency**
31-50	1 Gm	q 12 hr
16-30	1 Gm	q 24 hr
6-15	500 mg	q 24 hr
<5	500 mg	q 48 hr
Hemodialysis patients	1 Gm	after each dialysis session
Peritoneal dialysis patients	500 mg	q 24 hr

In patients with impaired renal function who have severe infection (normally requiring a 6-Gm/24 hr dose), the dose in the chart above may be increased by 50% or the dosing frequency may be increased. In patients undergoing hemodialysis, give a loading dose of 1 Gm followed by 1 Gm after each dialysis. ■ Dose reduction not required in impaired hepatic function.

DILUTION

IV injection: Reconstitute 0.5 Gm with 5 ml of SW; 1 Gm or more with 10 ml of SW for injection. Shake well. Dilution generates CO_2. Invert vial and completely depress plunger of syringe. Insert needle through stopper and keep it within the solution. Expel bubbles from solution in syringe before injection.

Intermittent IV: A single dose may be further diluted in 50 to 100 ml of D5W, NS, or other compatible infusion solutions for injection (see literature or chart on inside back cover). Also available premixed, in infusion packs, in piggyback vials, and in ADD-Vantage vials for use with ADD-Vantage infusion containers.

Storage: Store unopened vials in carton at CRT. Protect from light. Administer within 18 hours of preparation, or refrigerate for up to 7 days. May be frozen for up to 3 months after initial dilution; thaw at room temperature (see instructions); do not refreeze. Will be light yellow to amber in color depending on concentration and diluent.

INCOMPATIBLE WITH

May be used concomitantly with aminoglycosides (e.g., amikacin [Amikin], gentamicin [Garamycin], and vancomycin), but these drugs must never be mixed in the same infusion (mutual inactivation). If given concurrently, administer at separate sites and flush IV line before and after administration. Manufacturer recommends temporarily discontinuing other solutions infusing at the same site during intermittent infusion and states, "Do not add supplementary medications to premixed plastic IV containers."

COMPATIBLE WITH **(Underline Indicates Conflicting Compatibility Information)**

Consult pharmacist; specific conditions may apply; see Compatibilities, p. xvi.

Additive: <u>Ciprofloxacin (Cipro IV)</u>, clindamycin (Cleocin), fluconazole (Diflucan), linezolid (Zyvox), metronidazole (Flagyl IV), ofloxacin (Floxin IV).

Syringe: Hydromorphone (Dilaudid).

Y-site: Acyclovir (Zovirax), allopurinol (Aloprim, Zyloprim), amifostine (Ethyol), aminophylline, aztreonam (Azactam), ciprofloxacin (Cipro IV), cisatracurium (Nimbex), diltiazem (Cardizem), docetaxel (Taxotere), enalaprilat (Vasotec IV), esmolol (Brevibloc), etoposide phosphate (Etopophos), famotidine (Pepcid IV), filgrastim (Neupogen), fludarabine (Fludara), foscarnet (Foscavir), gatifloxacin (Tequin), gemcitabine (Gemzar), granisetron (Kytril), heparin, hetastarch in electrolytes (Hextend), hydromorphone (Dilaudid), labetalol (Normodyne), linezolid (Zyvox), melphalan (Alkeran), meperidine (Demerol), morphine, ondansetron (Zofran), paclitaxel (Taxol), propofol (Diprivan), ranitidine (Zantac), remifentanil (Ultiva), sargramostim (Leukine), tacrolimus (Prograf), teniposide (Vumon), theophylline, thiotepa (Thioplex), vancomycin (Vancocin), vinorelbine (Navelbine), zidovudine (AZT, Retrovir).

RATE OF ADMINISTRATION

See Incompatible With. May be given through Y-tube or three-way stopcock of infusion set.

IV injection: A single dose equally distributed over 3 to 5 minutes.

Intermittent IV: A single dose over 30 minutes.

ACTIONS

A broad-spectrum, third-generation cephalosporin antibiotic. Bactericidal to selected gram-negative, gram-positive, and anaerobic organisms. Effective against many otherwise resistant organisms, including *Pseudomonas aeruginosa.* Peak serum levels achieved by end of infusion. Therapeutic levels distributed into many body fluids and tissues including CSF and aqueous humor. Excreted unchanged in the urine. Crosses placental barrier. Secreted in breast milk.

INDICATIONS AND USES

Treatment of serious lower respiratory tract, urinary tract, skin and skin structure, bone and joint, gynecologic, intraabdominal, CNS infections (including meningitis), and bacterial septicemia. Most effective against specific organisms (see literature).

Unlabeled uses: Treatment of melioidosis; empiric treatment of febrile neutropenia.

CONTRAINDICATIONS

Previous allergic reaction to cephalosporins or related antibiotics (penicillins). Absolute only if reaction was serious.

PRECAUTIONS

Specific sensitivity studies indicated to determine susceptibility of causative organism to ceftazidime. ■ Continue for at least 2 days after all symptoms of infection subside. ■ Use with caution in patients with renal impairment. Elevated levels of ceftazidime in these patients can lead to asterixis, coma, encephalopathy, myoclonia, neuromuscular excitability, and seizures; see Dose Adjustments. ■ May be associated with a fall in prothrombin activity. Patients at risk include those with renal or hepatic impairment, those with poor nutritional status, those receiving a protracted course of antimicrobial therapy, and/or those previously stabilized on anticoagulant therapy; see Monitor. ■ Avoid prolonged use of drug; superinfection caused by overgrowth of nonsusceptible organisms may result. ■ Use caution in patients with impaired renal function, allergies, or a history of GI disease (especially colitis). ■ Pseudomembranous colitis has been reported. May range from mild to life-threatening. Consider in patients that present with diarrhea during or after treatment with ceftazidime.

Monitor: Watch for early symptoms of allergic reaction. ■ Use extreme caution in the penicillin-sensitive patient; incidence of cross-sensitivity may range from 3% to 16%. ■ May cause thrombophlebitis. Use small needles and large veins, and rotate infusion sites. ■ Observe for electrolyte imbalance and cardiac irregularities. Contains 2.3 mEq of sodium/Gm. Ceptaz does not contain sodium. ■ Monitor PT and administer vitamin K as indicated; see Precautions. ■ See Drug/Lab Interactions; additional monitoring may be indicated (e.g., renal function, drug serum levels, PT).

Patient Education: Report promptly any bleeding or bruising, diarrhea, or symptoms of allergy (e.g., difficulty breathing, hives, itching, rash).

Maternal/Child: Category B: safety for use during pregnancy and breast-feeding not established. No problems documented. ■ Immature renal function of infants and small children will increase blood levels of all cephalosporins. ■ Only specific solutions can be used in children.

Elderly: No specific problems documented. Consider age-related impaired organ function and nutritional status; reduced dose or extended intervals may be indicated. ■ See Usual Dose.

DRUG/LAB INTERACTIONS

Risk of nephrotoxicity may be increased with aminoglycosides and other nephrotoxic agents (e.g., loop diuretics such as furosemide [Lasix]). ■ Probenecid does not increase blood levels as it does with other cephalosporins. ■ May be antagonized by bacteriostatic antibiotics (e.g., chloramphenicol, erythromycin, tetracyclines); may interfere with bactericidal action. ■ Large amounts of cephalosporins and/or salicylates may induce hypoprothrombinemia (deficiency of prothrombin [Factor II]). The addition of agents that affect platelet aggregation and/or may have GI ulcerative potential (e.g., NSAIDs [ibuprofen (Advil, Motrin), naproxen (Aleve, Naprosyn)], or sulfinpyrazone [Anturane]) may increase risk of hemorrhage. ■ False-positive Coombs' test. ■ May have a false-positive reaction for urine glucose except with enzyme-based tests (e.g., Chemstix). ■ See Incompatible With and Side Effects.

SIDE EFFECTS

Full scope of allergic reactions, including anaphylaxis and cardiopulmonary arrest. Aplastic anemia; burning, discomfort, and pain at injection site; diarrhea; elevated alkaline phosphatase, AST (SGOT), ALT (SGPT), GGT, and BUN; jaundice; nausea and vomiting; prolonged PT; pseudomembranous colitis; renal impairment; seizures (large doses); toxic nephropathy; urticaria. Hypoprothrombinemia (rare) and hemolytic anemia may occur. Serum sickness–like reactions have occurred (e.g., arthralgia, fever, polyarthritis, skin rashes), usually after a second course of therapy. Generally resolve after cephalosporins are discontinued.

Overdose: Asterixis, coma, encephalopathy, neuromuscular excitability, and seizures may occur in patients with renal impairment; see Precautions.

ANTIDOTE

Notify physician of any side effects. Discontinue the drug if indicated. Treat allergic reaction as indicated and resuscitate as necessary. Mild cases of colitis may respond to discontinuation of ceftazidime. Oral vancomycin (Vancocin) or metronidazole (Flagyl) is the treatment of choice for antibiotic-related pseudomembranous colitis. Hemodialysis may be useful in overdose. Antihistamines and corticosteroids may be indicated to manage symptoms of serum sickness.

CEFTIZOXIME SODIUM

(sef-ti-zox'eem so'de-um)

Cefizox

Antibacterial (cephalosporin)

pH 5.5 to 8

USUAL DOSE

Dependent on seriousness of infection. Range is 500 mg to 4 Gm every 8 to 12 hours. Usual maximum dose for the elderly (over 75 years of age) is 1.5 Gm even if their SrCr is normal.

Uncomplicated urinary tract infection: 500 mg every 12 hours.

Pelvic inflammatory disease: 2 Gm every 8 hours.

Other uncomplicated infections: 1 Gm every 8 to 12 hours.

Severe or refractory infections: 1 Gm every 8 hours or 2 Gm every 8 to 12 hours.

Life-threatening infections: 3 to 4 Gm every 8 hours. Another source suggests 2 Gm every 4 hours.

PEDIATRIC DOSE

Children over 6 months of age: 50 mg/kg of body weight every 6 to 8 hours. Up to 200 mg/kg/24 hr has been used, but do not exceed adult dose.

DOSE ADJUSTMENTS

Higher doses often reduced with positive clinical response. ■ In impaired renal function, give an initial dose of 500 mg to 1 Gm, reduce all subsequent doses according to the following chart. ■ See Drug/Lab Interactions.

Ceftizoxime Dose Guidelines in Impaired Renal Function		
Creatinine Clearance (ml/min)	**Less Severe Infections**	**Life-Threatening Infections**
50-79	500 mg q 8 hr	0.75-1.5 Gm q 8 hr
5-49	250-500 mg q 12 hr	0.5-1 Gm q 12 hr
0-4	500 mg q 48 hr or 250 mg q 24 hr	0.5-1 Gm q 48 hr or 0.5 Gm q 24 hr

No supplemental doses are required for patients undergoing dialysis. Time the prescribed dose to be given at the end of dialysis.

DILUTION

Each 1 Gm must be reconstituted with 10 ml SW. Shake well. May be further diluted in 50 to 100 ml of NS or other compatible solutions (see chart on inside back cover and literature) and given as an intermittent infusion. Available premixed, in piggyback vials, and in ADD-Vantage vials for use with ADD-Vantage infusion containers. Not given as a continuous infusion.

Storage: Store unopened vials at CRT. Protect from excess light. Administer within 24 hours of preparation, or within 48 to 96 hours if refrigerated.

INCOMPATIBLE WITH

May be used concomitantly with aminoglycosides (e.g., amikacin [Amikin], gentamicin [Garamycin]), but these drugs must never be mixed in the same infusion (mutual inactivation). If given concurrently, administer at separate sites.

COMPATIBLE WITH (Underline Indicates Conflicting Compatibility Information)

Consult pharmacist; specific conditions may apply; see Compatibilities, p. xvi.

Additive: Clindamycin (Cleocin), metronidazole (Flagyl IV).

Y-site: Acyclovir (Zovirax), allopurinol (Aloprim, Zyloprim), amifostine (Ethyol), amphotericin B cholesteryl (Amphotec), aztreonam (Azactam), <u>cisatracurium (Nimbex)</u>, docetaxel (Taxotere), doxorubicin liposome (Doxil), enalaprilat (Vasotec IV), esmolol (Brevibloc), etoposide phosphate (Etopophos), famotidine (Pepcid IV), fludarabine (Fludara), foscarnet (Foscavir), gatifloxacin (Tequin), gemcitabine (Gemzar), granisetron (Kytril), hetastarch in electrolytes (Hextend), hydromorphone (Dilaudid), labetalol (Normodyne), linezolid (Zyvox), melphalan (Alkeran), meperidine (Demerol), morphine, ondansetron (Zofran), propofol (Diprivan), ranitidine (Zantac), remifentanil (Ultiva), sargramostim (Leukine), teniposide (Vumon), thiotepa (Thioplex), <u>vancomycin (Vancocin)</u>, vinorelbine (Navelbine).

RATE OF ADMINISTRATION

May be given through Y-tube or three-way stopcock of infusion set.

IV injection: A single dose equally distributed over 3 to 5 minutes.

Intermittent IV: A single dose over 30 minutes.

ACTIONS

A broad-spectrum, third-generation cephalosporin antibiotic. Bactericidal to many gram-negative, gram-positive, and anaerobic organisms. Effective against many otherwise resistant organisms. Peak serum levels achieved by end of infusion. Widely distributed into most body tissues and fluids, including inflamed meninges and bone. Excreted in the urine. Crosses placental barrier. Secreted in breast milk.

INDICATIONS AND USES

Treatment of serious infections of the lower respiratory tract or urinary tract; intraabdominal, skin and skin structure, and bone and joint infections; gonorrhea; pelvic inflammatory disease; septicemia and meningitis. Most effective against specific organisms (see literature).

CONTRAINDICATIONS

Previous allergic reaction of cephalosporins or related antibiotics (penicillins). Absolute only if reaction was serious.

PRECAUTIONS

Specific sensitivity studies indicated to determine susceptibility of the causative organism to ceftizoxime. ■ Continue for at least 2 to 3 days after all symptoms of infection subside. ■ Avoid prolonged use of drug; superinfection caused by overgrowth of nonsusceptible organisms may result. ■ Use caution in patients with impaired renal function, allergies, or a history of GI disease (especially colitis). ■ Pseudomembranous colitis has been reported. May range from mild to life-threatening. Consider in patients that present with diarrhea during or after treatment with ceftizoxime.

Monitor: Watch for early symptoms of allergic reaction. ■ Use extreme caution in the penicillin-sensitive patient; incidence of cross-sensitivity may range from 3% to 16%. ■ May cause thrombophlebitis. Use small needles and large veins, and rotate infusion sites. ■ Observe for electrolyte imbalance or cardiac irregularities. Contains 2.6 mEq of sodium/Gm. ■ See Drug/Lab Interactions; additional monitoring may be indicated (e.g., renal function, drug serum levels, PT).

Patient Education: Report promptly any bleeding or bruising, diarrhea, or symptoms of allergy (e.g., difficulty breathing, hives, itching, rash).

Maternal/Child: Category B: safety for use during pregnancy and breast-feeding not established. No problems documented. ■ Not recommended for use in children under 6 months of age. ■ Transient elevation of eosinophils, ALT (SGPT), AST (SGOT), and CK have occurred in infants under 6 months of age; use not recommended; safety and efficacy not established.

Elderly: No specific problems documented. Consider age-related impaired organ function and nutritional status; reduced dose or extended intervals may be indicated. ■ See Usual Dose.

DRUG/LAB INTERACTIONS

Risk of nephrotoxicity may be increased with aminoglycosides and other nephrotoxic agents (e.g., loop diuretics such as furosemide [Lasix]). ■ Probenecid inhibits excretion and may require reduction in dosage. ■ May be antagonized by bacteriostatic antibiotics (e.g., chloramphenicol, erythromycin, tetracyclines); may interfere with bactericidal action. ■ Large amounts of cephalosporins and/or salicylates may induce hypoprothrombinemia (deficiency of prothrombin [Factor II]). The addition of agents that affect platelet aggregation and/or may have GI ulcerative potential (e.g., NSAIDs [ibuprofen (Advil, Motrin), naproxen (Aleve, Naprosyn)], or sulfinpyrazone [Anturane]) may increase risk of hemorrhage. ■ Positive Coombs' test. ■ See Incompatible With.

SIDE EFFECTS

Full scope of allergic reactions including anaphylaxis. Decreased hemoglobin or decreased hematocrit; decreased platelet functions; diarrhea; dyspnea; elevation of AST (SGOT), ALT (SGPT), total bilirubin, alkaline phosphatase, LDH, and BUN (transient); eosinophilia; fever; leukopenia; local site pain; nausea; oral thrush; prolonged PT; pseudomembranous colitis; seizures (large doses); thrombocytopenia; thrombophlebitis; vaginitis; vomiting. Hypoprothrombinemia (rare) and hemolytic anemia may occur. Serum sickness–like reactions have occurred (e.g., arthralgia, fever, polyarthritis, skin rashes), usually after a second course of therapy. Generally resolve after cephalosporins are discontinued.

ANTIDOTE

Notify the physician of any side effects. Discontinue the drug if indicated. Oral vancomycin (Vancocin) or metronidazole (Flagyl) is the treatment of choice for antibiotic-related pseudomembranous colitis. Treat allergic reaction as indicated and resuscitate as necessary. Hemodialysis may be somewhat useful in overdose. Antihistamines and corticosteroids may be indicated to manage symptoms of serum sickness.

CEFTRIAXONE SODIUM

(sef-try-ax'one so'de-um)

Rocephin

Antibacterial (cephalosporin)

pH 6.6 to 6.7

USUAL DOSE

Adults and children over 12 years: 1 to 2 Gm/24 hr. May be given as a single dose every 24 hours or equally divided into 2 doses and given every 12 hours. Do not exceed a total dose of 4 Gm/24 hr.

Meningitis: 2 Gm every 12 hours.

Empiric therapy in febrile neutropenic patients: 30 mg/kg/day in combination with amikacin 20 mg/kg/day.

Disseminated gonococcal infections (CDC recommendation): 1 Gm once daily for 7 days.

Gonococcal meningitis/endocarditis: 1 to 2 Gm every 12 hours for 10 to 14 days in meningitis, 4 weeks or more in endocarditis.

Lyme disease (unlabeled): 2 Gm daily for 10 to 30 days or 75 to 100 mg/kg/day for 14 to 30 days.

Endocarditis (unlabeled): 2 Gm once daily for 4 weeks (see literature for specific organisms).

Perioperative prophylaxis: 1 Gm IV 30 minutes to 2 hours before incision. Used primarily in patients undergoing coronary artery bypass surgery and in contaminated or potentially contaminated surgeries.

PEDIATRIC DOSE

Skin and soft tissue and other serious infections: 50 to 75 mg/kg of body weight/24 hr as a single dose or in equally divided doses every 12 hours (25 to 37.5 mg/kg every 12 hours). Do not exceed a total dose of 2 Gm/24 hr.

Lyme disease: 50 to 100 mg/kg daily for 10 to 21 days.

Acute PID in prepubertal children: 100 mg/kg/24 hr in combination with erythromycin or sulfisoxazole.

Bacterial meningitis: Begin with a loading dose of 100 mg/kg on day 1 (do not exceed a total dose of 4 Gm), follow with 100 mg/kg/day (not to exceed 4 Gm) as a single dose or in equally divided doses every 12 hours (50 mg/kg every 12 hours). An alternate regimen (American Academy of Pediatrics) begins with an 80- to 100-mg/kg loading dose (not over 4 Gm); follow with 80 mg/kg at 12-hour intervals for 2 doses, then 80 to 100 mg/kg every 24 hours. Continue for 7 to 14 days.

Empiric therapy in febrile neutropenic children over 1 year of age: 80 mg/kg/day in combination with amikacin 20 mg/kg/day.

NEONATAL DOSE

25 to 50 mg/kg/day as a single daily dose. Up to 75 mg/kg may be indicated ***in infants over 7 days old weighing over 2,000 Gm.*** Up to 100 mg/kg may be indicated in ***bacterial meningitis.*** Neonatal doses may also be given IM.

Infants born to mothers with gonococcal infections: 25 to 50 mg/kg one time only (do not exceed 125 mg).

DOSE ADJUSTMENTS

In adults with both hepatic and renal impairment, dose should not exceed 2 Gm daily unless serum concentrations of ceftriaxone are monitored. ■ See Drug/Lab Interactions.

DILUTION

Initially reconstitute each 250 mg with 2.4 ml (500 mg with 4.8 ml, etc.) of SW, NS, D5W, D10W, D5NS, or D5/½NS for injection (see chart on inside back cover or literature for additional diluents). Each ml will contain 100 mg. A single dose must be further diluted with 50 to 100 ml of the same solution and be given as an intermittent infusion. Shake well. Concentrations of 10 mg/ml to 40 mg/ml are recommended for intermittent infusion. Available premixed, in piggyback vials, and in ADD-Vantage vials for use with ADD-Vantage infusion containers.

Storage: Store vials at CRT and protect from light. Stable at room temperature for at least 24 hours in stated solutions or selected solutions up to 10 days if refrigerated. D5NS and D5/½NS should not be refrigerated. Stability and color (clear to yellow) depend on concentration and diluent. Thaw frozen solutions at room temperature before use. Discard unused portions; do not refreeze.

INCOMPATIBLE WITH

May be used concomitantly with aminoglycosides (e.g., amikacin [Amikin], gentamicin [Garamycin]), but these drugs must never be mixed in the same infusion (mutual inactivation). If given concurrently, administer at separate sites. Manufacturer lists vancomycin (Vancocin) and fluconazole (Diflucan) as incompatible and states, "May be given sequentially with thorough flushing of the IV line with compatible solution between the administrations."

COMPATIBLE WITH **(Underline Indicates Conflicting Compatibility Information)**

Consult pharmacist; specific conditions may apply; see Compatibilities, p. xvi.

Additive: Manufacturer lists metronidazole (Flagyl IV) not to exceed 5 to 7.5 mg/ml with ceftriaxone 10 mg/ml admixed in D5W or NS. Do not refrigerate; a precipitate will form.

Syringe: <u>Lidocaine</u>.

Y-site: Acyclovir (Zovirax), allopurinol (Aloprim, Zyloprim), amifostine (Ethyol), aztreonam (Azactam), cisatracurium (Nimbex), diltiazem (Cardizem), docetaxel (Taxotere), doxorubicin liposome (Doxil), etoposide phosphate (Etopophos), famotidine (Pepcid IV), fludarabine (Fludara), foscarnet (Foscavir), gatifloxacin (Tequin), gemcitabine (Gemzar), granisetron (Kytril), heparin, hetastarch in electrolytes (Hextend), linezolid (Zyvox), melphalan (Alkeran), meperidine (Demerol), methotrexate (Folex), morphine, paclitaxel (Taxol), propofol (Diprivan), remifentanil (Ultiva), sargramostim (Leukine), sodium bicarbonate, tacrolimus (Prograf), teniposide (Vumon), theophylline, thiotepa (Thioplex), <u>vancomycin (Vancocin)</u>, warfarin (Coumadin), zidovudine (AZT, Retrovir).

RATE OF ADMINISTRATION

Intermittent IV: A single dose over 30 minutes.

ACTIONS

A broad-spectrum, third-generation cephalosporin antibiotic. Bactericidal to selected gram-negative, gram-positive, and anaerobic organisms. Effective against many otherwise resistant organisms. Therapeutic concentrations achieved in many body fluids and tissues, including CSF. Has a long half-life (range is 5.8 to 8.7 hours); once-a-day dosing sufficient. Peak serum levels achieved by end of infusion. Excreted through bile and urine. Crosses placental barrier. Secreted in breast milk.

INDICATIONS AND USES

Treatment of serious lower respiratory tract, urinary tract, skin and skin structure, bone and joint, and intraabdominal infections. ■ Disseminated gonococcal infections. ■ Bacterial septicemia. ■ Meningitis. ■ Most effective against specific organisms (see literature). ■ Empiric therapy in febrile neutropenic patients. ■ Perioperative prophylaxis. ■ Given IM for additional indications (e.g., CDC recommendations for chancroid, gonorrhea, pelvic inflammatory disease [considered treatment of choice]).

Unlabeled uses: Treatment of Lyme disease, endocarditis, and numerous other infections.

CONTRAINDICATIONS

Previous allergic reaction to cephalosporins or related antibiotics (penicillins). Absolute only if reaction was serious.

PRECAUTIONS

Sensitivity studies are indicated to determine susceptibility of the causative organism to ceftriaxone. ■ Continue for at least 2 to 3 days after all symptoms of infection subside. Usual course of therapy 4 to 14 days; *S. pyogenes* requires treatment for 10 days. In serious invasive infection, continue for 5 to 7 days after cultures are negative. ■ Avoid prolonged use of drug; superinfection caused by overgrowth of nonsusceptible organisms may result. ■ Use caution in patients with both impaired renal and hepatic function, allergies, or a history of GI disease (especially colitis). ■ Pseudomembranous colitis has been reported. May range from mild to life-threatening. Consider in patients that present with diarrhea during or after treatment with ceftriaxone. ■ Prolonged use may lead to gallbladder disease.

Monitor: Watch for early symptoms of allergic reaction. ■ Use extreme caution in the penicillin-sensitive patient; incidence of cross-sensitivity may range from 3% to 16%. ■ Single daily dose reduces incidence of thrombophlebitis. Use of small needles, large veins, and rotation of infusion sites is preferred. ■ Observe for electrolyte imbalance and cardiac irregularities. Contains 3.6 mEq sodium per Gm. ■ See Dose Adjustments and Drug/Lab Interactions; additional monitoring may be indicated (e.g., renal function, drug serum levels, PT).

Patient Education: Report promptly any bleeding or bruising, diarrhea, or symptoms of allergy (e.g., difficulty breathing, hives, itching, rash).

Maternal/Child: Category B: safety for use during pregnancy and breast-feeding not established. No problems documented. ■ Immature renal function of infants and small children will increase blood levels of all cephalosporins. ■ Use with caution in hyperbilirubinemic neonates (especially premature infants); highly protein bound and may displace bilirubin from albumin.

Elderly: No specific problems documented.

DRUG/LAB INTERACTIONS

Risk of nephrotoxicity may be increased with aminoglycosides and other nephrotoxic agents (e.g., loop diuretics such as furosemide [Lasix]). ■ Probenecid does not increase blood levels as it does with other cephalosporins. ■ May be antagonized by bacteriostatic antibiotics (e.g., chloramphenicol, erythromycin, tetracyclines); may interfere with bactericidal action. ■ Large amounts of cephalosporins and/or salicylates may induce hypoprothrombinemia (deficiency of prothrombin [Factor II]). The addition of agents that affect platelet aggregation and/or may have GI ulcerative potential (e.g., NSAIDs [ibuprofen (Advil, Motrin), naproxen (Aleve, Naprosyn)], or sulfinpyrazone [Anturane]) may increase risk of hemorrhage. ■ False-positive Coombs' test. ■ May produce false-positive reaction for urine glucose except with enzyme-based tests (e.g., Chemstix). ■ See Incompatible With and Side Effects.

SIDE EFFECTS

Full scope of allergic reactions, including anaphylaxis, are possible. Agranulocytosis, "biliary sludge" or pseudolithiasis; bleeding episodes; burning, discomfort, and pain at injection site; casts in urine; diarrhea; dizziness; eosinophilia; elevated alkaline phosphatase, bilirubin, BUN, creatinine, AST (SGOT), and ALT (SGPT); headache; leukopenia; nephrolithiasis; prolonged PT; pseudomembranous colitis (may be life-threatening); renal precipitations; seizures (large doses); thrombophlebitis. Hypoprothrombinemia (rare) and hemolytic anemia may occur. Serum sickness–like reactions have occurred (e.g., arthralgia, fever, polyarthritis, skin rashes), usually after a second course of therapy. Generally resolve after cephalosporins are discontinued.

ANTIDOTE

Notify physician of any side effects. Discontinue the drug if indicated. Treat allergic reaction as indicated and resuscitate as necessary. Mild cases of colitis may respond to discontinuation of ceftriaxone. Oral vancomycin (Vancocin) or metronidazole (Flagyl) is the treatment of choice for antibiotic-related pseudomembranous colitis. Vitamin K may be useful in bleeding episodes, or drug may have to be discontinued. Not removed by hemodialysis. Antihistamines and corticosteroids may be indicated to manage symptoms of serum sickness.

CEFUROXIME SODIUM
(sef-yoor-ox′eem so′de-um)

Antibacterial (cephalosporin)

Kefurox, Zinacef

pH 5 to 8.5

USUAL DOSE

Dependent on seriousness of infection. Range is from 750 mg to 3 Gm every 8 hours for 5 to 10 days. Maximum dose is 3 Gm every 8 hours.
Uncomplicated infections (gonococcal, pneumonia, skin and soft tissue, urinary tract): 750 mg every 8 hours.
Severe or complicated infections and bone and joint infections: 1.5 Gm every 8 hours.
Life-threatening or infections due to less susceptible organisms: 1.5 Gm every 6 hours.
Bacterial meningitis: 3 Gm every 8 hours; see Precautions.
Perioperative prophylaxis: 1.5 Gm IV 30 minutes to 1 hour before incision; then 750 mg every 8 hours during prolonged procedures. 1.5 Gm at induction of anesthesia and every 12 hours to total dose of 6 Gm in open heart surgery.

PEDIATRIC DOSE

Do not exceed adult dose.
Infants and children 1 month of age or older: 12.5 to 33.3 mg/kg of body weight every 6 to 8 hours. Higher-end dosing used for more serious infections.
Bone and joint infections: 50 mg/kg every 8 hours. Up to 1.5 Gm/dose has been given.
Bacterial meningitis: 50 to 80 mg/kg every 6 to 8 hours; see Precautions.

NEONATAL DOSE

Infants under 1 month of age: 10 to 50 mg/kg every 8 to 12 hours. Other sources recommend 15 to 50 mg/kg every 12 hours or 10 to 25 mg/kg every 12 hours.
Bacterial meningitis: 33.3 to 50 mg/kg every 8 to 12 hours; see Precautions.

DOSE ADJUSTMENTS

Adults: Reduce total daily dose if renal function impaired according to the following chart. ■ See Drug/Lab Interactions.

Cefuroxime Dose Guidelines in Impaired Renal Function in Adults		
Creatinine Clearance (ml/min)	Dose	Frequency
>20	750 mg-1.5 Gm	q 8 hr
10-20	750 mg	q 12 hr
<10	750 mg	q 24 hr
Hemodialysis patients	750 mg	at end of each dialysis session

Children: In children with impaired renal function, reduce frequency as indicated in the chart for adults.

DILUTION

Each 750 mg must be reconstituted with 8 ml SW for injection, D5W, NS, or other compatible infusion solution (see chart on inside back cover and literature). Shake well. May be further diluted with compatible solutions to 50 or 100 ml and given as an intermittent infusion, or added to 500 to 1,000 ml and given as a continuous infusion. Available premixed, in piggyback vials, infusion packs, and in ADD-Vantage vials for use with ADD-Vantage infusion containers.

Storage: In dry state, store between 15° and 30° C (59° to 86° F); protect from light. Administer within 24 hours of preparation or within 48 hours if refrigerated.

INCOMPATIBLE WITH

May be used concomitantly with aminoglycosides (e.g., amikacin [Amikin], gentamicin [Garamycin]), but these drugs must never be mixed in the same infusion (mutual inactivation). If given concurrently, administer at separate sites. Manufacturer recommends temporarily discontinuing other solutions infusing at the same site during intermittent infusion and lists sodium bicarbonate incompatible as a diluent.

COMPATIBLE WITH (Underline Indicates Conflicting Compatibility Information)

Consult pharmacist; specific conditions may apply; see Compatibilities, p. xvi.

Additive: Manufacturer lists heparin (10 and 50 units/ml in NS) and potassium chloride (10 and 40 mEq/L in NS). Other sources list clindamycin (Cleocin), furosemide (Lasix), heparin, metronidazole (Flagyl IV), potassium chloride (KCl).

Y-site: Acyclovir (Zovirax), allopurinol (Aloprim, Zyloprim), amifostine (Ethyol), atracurium (Tracrium), aztreonam (Azactam), cisatracurium (Nimbex), cyclophosphamide (Cytoxan), diltiazem (Cardizem), docetaxel (Taxotere), etoposide phosphate (Etopophos), famotidine (Pepcid IV), fludarabine (Fludara), foscarnet (Foscavir), gemcitabine (Gemzar), granisetron (Kytril), hetastarch in electrolytes (Hextend), hydromorphone (Dilaudid), linezolid (Zyvox), melphalan (Alkeran), meperidine (Demerol), morphine, ondansetron (Zofran), pancuronium (Pavulon), perphenazine (Trilafon), propofol (Diprivan), remifentanil (Ultiva), sargramostim (Leukine), tacrolimus (Prograf), teniposide (Vumon), thiotepa (Thioplex), vancomycin (Vancocin), vecuronium (Norcuron).

RATE OF ADMINISTRATION

See Incompatible With. Injection or intermittent infusion may be given through Y-tube or three-way stopcock of infusion set.

IV injection: A single dose equally distributed over 3 to 5 minutes.

Intermittent IV: A single dose over 30 minutes.

Continuous infusion: 500 to 1,000 ml over 6 to 24 hours, depending on total dose and concentration.

ACTIONS

A broad-spectrum, second-generation cephalosporin antibiotic. Bactericidal to selected gram-negative, gram-positive, and anaerobic organisms. Effective against many otherwise resistant organisms. Widely distributed in most tissues, body fluids (including inflamed meninges), bone, skin, and soft tissue and aqueous humor. Peak serum levels achieved by end of infusion. Achieves therapeutic levels in CSF. Excreted in the urine. Crosses placental barrier. Secreted in breast milk.

INDICATIONS AND USES

Treatment of serious lower respiratory tract, urinary tract, bone and joint, skin and skin structure infections, septicemia, and meningitis. Most effective against specific organisms and when mixed organisms are present (see literature). ■ Perioperative prophylaxis. ■ Used IM to treat gonorrhea.

CONTRAINDICATIONS

Previous allergic reaction to cephalosporins or related antibiotics (penicillins). Absolute only if reaction was serious.

PRECAUTIONS

Sensitivity studies indicated to determine susceptibility of the causative organism to cefuroxime. ■ Continue for at least 2 to 3 days after all symptoms of infection subside. ■ Avoid prolonged use of drug; superinfection caused by overgrowth of nonsusceptible organisms may result. ■ Use caution in patients with impaired renal function, allergies, or a history of GI disease (especially colitis). ■ Pseudomembranous colitis has been reported. May range from mild to life-threatening. Consider in patients that present with diarrhea during or after treatment with cefuroxime. ■ May be associated with a fall in prothrombin activity. Patients at risk include those with renal or hepatic impairment, patients with poor nutritional status, patients receiving a protracted course of antimicrobial therapy, and patients previously stabilized on anticoagulant therapy; see Monitor. ■ No longer considered the drug of choice for treatment of bacterial meningitis due to poor coverage of penicillin-resistant *S. pneumoniae.*

Monitor: Watch for early symptoms of allergic reaction. ■ Use extreme caution in the penicillin-sensitive patient; incidence of cross-sensitivity may range from 3% to 16%. ■ May cause thrombophlebitis. Use small needles and large veins, and rotate infusion sites. ■ Observe for electrolyte imbalance and cardiac irregularities. Contains 2.4 mEq sodium/Gm. ■ Monitor PT and administer vitamin K as indicated. ■ See Drug/Lab Interactions; additional monitoring may be indicated (e.g., renal function, drug serum levels).

Patient Education: Report promptly any bleeding or bruising, diarrhea, or symptoms of allergy (e.g., difficulty breathing, hives, itching, rash).

Maternal/Child: Category B: safety for use during pregnancy and breast-feeding not established. No problems documented. ■ Is used in infants under 3 months of age, but safety not established; immature renal function will increase blood levels.

Elderly: No specific problems documented. Consider age-related impaired organ function and nutritional status; reduced dose or extended intervals may be indicated.

DRUG/LAB INTERACTIONS

Risk of nephrotoxicity may be increased with aminoglycosides and other nephrotoxic agents (e.g., loop diuretics such as furosemide [Lasix]). ■ Probenecid inhibits excretion and may require reduction in dosage. ■ May be antagonized by bacteriostatic antibiotics (e.g., chloramphenicol, erythromycin, tetracyclines); bactericidal action may be negated. ■ Large amounts of cephalosporins and/or salicylates may induce hypoprothrombinemia (deficiency of prothrombin [Factor II]). The addition of agents that affect platelet aggregation and/or may have GI ulcerative potential (e.g., NSAIDs [ibuprofen (Advil, Motrin), naproxen (Aleve, Naprosyn)], or sulfinpyrazone [Anturane]) may increase risk of hemorrhage. ■ May cause a false-negative reaction in specific blood glucose tests (ferricyanide). ■ False-positive reaction for urine glucose except with enzyme-based tests (e.g., Chemstix). ■ False-positive Coombs' test. ■ See Incompatible With and Side Effects.

SIDE EFFECTS

Full scope of allergic reactions including anaphylaxis. Decreased hemoglobin, hematocrit, or platelet functions; diarrhea; dyspnea; elevation of AST (SGOT), ALT (SGPT), total bilirubin, alkaline phosphatase, LDH, and BUN (transient); eosinophilia; fever; leukopenia; local site pain; nausea; oral thrush; prolonged PT; pseudomembranous colitis; seizures (large doses and decreased renal function); transient neutropenia; thrombocytopenia; thrombophlebitis; vaginitis; vomiting. Hypoprothrombinemia (rare) and hemolytic anemia may occur. Serum sickness–like reactions have occurred (e.g., arthralgia, fever, polyarthritis, skin rashes), usually after a second course of therapy. Generally resolve after cephalosporins are discontinued.

ANTIDOTE

Notify physician of any side effects. Discontinue the drug if indicated. Mild cases of colitis may respond to discontinuation of drug. Treat antibiotic-related pseudomembranous colitis with fluids, electrolytes, protein supplements, and oral vancomycin (Vancocin) or metronidazole (Flagyl). Treat allergic reaction and resuscitate as necessary. Hemodialysis may be somewhat useful in overdose. Antihistamines and corticosteroids may be indicated to manage symptoms of serum sickness.

CHLORAMPHENICOL SODIUM SUCCINATE

Antibacterial

(klor-am-fen′i-kole so′de-um suk′suh-nat)

Chloromycetin

pH 6.4 to 7

USUAL DOSE

For all age levels, determine baseline blood studies before administration. Avoid repeated courses of this drug if at all possible.

Adults and children with mature metabolic processes (e.g., normal kidney and liver function): 12.5 mg/kg every 6 hours. In exceptional cases, infections due to moderately resistant organisms may require up to 25 mg/kg every 6 hours. Severe infections (e.g., bacteremia or meningitis), especially when adequate cerebrospinal fluid concentrations are desired, may require up to 25 mg/kg every 6 hours. These increased doses must be reduced to 12.5 mg/kg every 6 hours as soon as possible. Maximum dose is 4 Gm/24 hr. Change to oral form as soon as practical.

NEONATAL DOSE

Infants 2 weeks of age or older with mature metabolic processes: 6.25 mg/kg every 6 hours. May increase to 12.5 mg/kg every 6 hours if indicated by severity of infection. See comments under Adult Dose.

Infants under 2 weeks of age or older infants with immature metabolic processes (e.g., premature infants): 6.25 mg/kg every 6 hours. Close monitoring of blood concentrations by microtechniques is recommended (information available from manufacturer).

Another source suggests a ***loading dose*** followed by ***maintenance doses*** based on age and weight. The first maintenance dose should be given 12 hours after the loading dose.

Loading dose: 20 mg/kg.

Maintenance dose: ***under 7 days of age or 7 days of age or older and under 2 kg:*** 25 mg/kg of body weight once daily.

Over 7 days of age and over 2 kg: 25 mg/kg every 12 hours.

DOSE ADJUSTMENTS

Reduce dose and/or initiate oral therapy as soon as feasible. ■ Reduce dose and/or extend intervals in infants and children with immature metabolic processes. See specific dose recommendations. Close monitoring of blood concentrations by microtechniques is recommended. ■ In patients with immature or impaired hepatic or renal function, dose reduction may be required.

DILUTION

Each 1 Gm should be reconstituted with 10 ml of SW for injection or D5W to prepare a 10% solution (100 mg/ml). May be further diluted in 50 to 100 ml of D5W for intermittent infusion. Give through Y-tube, three-way stopcock, or additive infusion set.

Storage: Administer within 24 hours of preparation.

COMPATIBLE WITH

Consult pharmacist; specific conditions may apply; see Compatibilities, p. xvi.

Solution: Most common infusion solutions.

Additive: Amikacin (Amikin), aminophylline, ascorbic acid, calcium chloride, calcium gluconate, colistimethate (Coly-Mycin M), dimenhydrinate (Dinate), dopamine (Intropin), ephedrine, heparin, hydrocortisone sodium succinate (Solu-Cortef), kanamycin (Kantrex), lidocaine, magnesium sulfate, methyldopate (Aldomet), methylprednisolone (Solu-Medrol), metronidazole (Flagyl IV), nafcillin (Nafcil), oxacillin (Bactocill), oxytocin (Pitocin), penicillin G potassium and sodium, pentobarbital (Nembutal), phenylephrine (Neo-Synephrine), phytonadione (Aquamephyton), plasma protein fraction (Plasmanate), potassium chloride (KCl), ranitidine (Zantac), sodium bicarbonate, thiopental (Pentothal), verapamil (Isoptin).

Syringe: Ampicillin, heparin, penicillin G sodium, selected agents used in radiology.

Y-site: Acyclovir (Zovirax), cyclophosphamide (Cytoxan), enalaprilat (Vasotec IV), esmolol (Brevibloc), foscarnet (Foscavir), hydromorphone (Dilaudid), labetalol (Normodyne), magnesium sulfate, meperidine (Demerol), morphine, perphenazine (Trilafon), tacrolimus (Prograf).

RATE OF ADMINISTRATION

IV injection: 1 Gm or fraction thereof over a minimum of 1 minute.

Intermittent infusion: A single dose over 10 to 30 minutes.

ACTIONS

Effective against many life-threatening organisms. Primarily bacteriostatic. May be bactericidal at high concentrations or against highly susceptible organisms. Acts by inhibiting protein synthesis. Well distributed in therapeutic doses throughout the body, especially in the liver and kidneys. Lowest concentrations are found in the brain and spinal fluid; however, chloramphenicol enters cerebrospinal fluid even in the absence of meningeal inflammation, appearing in concentrations about half of those found in the blood. Excreted in urine, bile, and feces. Crosses the placental barrier. Secreted in breast milk.

INDICATIONS AND USES

Only in serious infections in which potentially less dangerous drugs are ineffective or contraindicated; acute *Salmonella typhi* infections, meningeal infections (e.g., *Hemophilus influenzae*), bacteremia, rickettsia, lymphogranuloma psittacosis, and other serious gram-negative infections. ■ Cystic fibrosis regimens.

CONTRAINDICATIONS

Known chloramphenicol sensitivity. Must not be used in the treatment of trivial infections.

PRECAUTIONS

This is a lethal drug. Serious blood dyscrasias (e.g., aplastic anemia, hypoplastic anemia, thrombocytopenia, and granulocytopenia) resulting in irreversible bone marrow depression and death are known to occur. Aplastic anemia resulting in leukemia has been reported. Blood dyscrasias have occurred after both short-term and longer-term therapy. ■ Administration in a hospital with facilities for monitoring the patient and responding to any medical emergency is preferred. ■ Sensitivity studies mandatory to determine susceptibility of the causative organism not only to chloramphenicol but also to other less dangerous drugs. ■ Superinfection caused by overgrowth of nonsusceptible organisms, including fungi, is possible. Treatment should not be continued longer than required to produce a cure with little or no risk of relapse of the disease. ■ For IV use only. ■ A reversible type of bone marrow depression characterized by vacuolization of the erythroid cells, reduction of reticulocytes, and leukopenia is dose related and usually responds to withdrawal of chloramphenicol. ▪ Pseudomembranous colitis has been reported. May range from mild to life-threatening. Consider in patients that present with diarrhea during or after treatment with chloramphenicol.

Monitor: Obtain blood studies (CBC) before initiating therapy and approximately every 2 days during therapy; discontinue drug if blood studies show any indication of anemia, leukopenia, reticulocytopenia, thrombocytopenia, or any blood study findings attributable to chloramphenicol. ▪ Monitor chloramphenicol serum levels at least weekly, and more often if indicated (e.g., impaired liver or kidney function, immature metabolic processes, suspicion of beginning blood dyscrasias). ▪ Therapeutic levels range between 15 and 25 mcg/ml for meningitis; 10 and 20 mcg/ml for other infections. Trough levels should range between 5 and 15 mcg/ml for meningitis; 5 and 10 mcg/ml for other infections. ▪ Monitor hepatic and renal function as indicated. ▪ See Drug/Lab Interactions.

Patient Education: Promptly report fever, sore throat, tiredness, unusual bleeding, or bruising.

Maternal/Child: No studies documented. Use during pregnancy or breast-feeding with extreme caution; may have toxic effects on fetus/neonate/infant. ▪ Blood concentration in all premature and full-term neonates under 2 weeks of age differs from that of other neonates. Use caution, lower doses, and/or extended intervals in premature infants and newborns. May cause gray syndrome (e.g., abdominal distension with or without emesis, progressive pallid cyanosis, vasomotor collapse, irregular respiration, death within a few hours of onset of symptoms); monitor serum levels; see Precautions/Monitor.

DRUG/LAB INTERACTIONS

Decreases plasma clearance and prolongs duration of alfentanil (Alfenta). ▪ May cause irreversible bone marrow depression. Avoid concurrent therapy with drugs that cause blood dyscrasias (e.g., penicillins, hydantoins [phenytoin (Dilantin)]), other bone marrow depressants (e.g., cytotoxic drugs, radiation therapy). ▪ Increases serum levels of oral antidiabetics (e.g., chlorpropamide [Diabinase]) and increases hypoglycemic effects; dose reduction may be required. ▪ May antagonize effects of erythromycin, clindamycin, lincomycin, and penicillins. (Is used with ampicillin in pediatric patients.) ▪ Chloramphenicol can inhibit the P_{450} enzyme system; reduced metabolism and increased serum levels may occur in agents also metabolized by that route (e.g., cyclosporine, phenobarbitol, phenytoin, warfarin). ▪ May increase response to iron preparations in iron deficiency anemia. ▪ May delay response to antianemia drugs (e.g., iron preparations, vitamin B_{12}, folic acid). Avoid concurrent use in patients with anemia if possible. ▪ Phenobarbital may also increase metabolism and decrease effects of chloramphenicol. ▪ Rifampin increases chloramphenicol metabolism and decreases its effects. ▪ May decrease effectiveness of oral contraceptives; breakthrough bleeding and pregnancy may result.

SIDE EFFECTS

Blood dyscrasias (e.g., aplastic anemia, hypoplastic anemia, granulocytopenia, thrombocytopenia) may result in irreversible bone marrow depression and death. Allergic reactions (e.g., angioedema, anaphylaxis, fever, rashes, urticaria), confusion, depression, diarrhea, fever, gray syndrome of newborns and infants, headache, leukemia, nausea, optic and peripheral neuritis, paroxysmal nocturnal hemoglobinuria, pseudomembranous colitis, rashes, stomatitis, vomiting, and many others. ***May be fatal.***

ANTIDOTE

Notify the physician immediately of any adverse symptoms. Discontinue the drug upon appearance of anemia, leukopenia, reticulocytopenia, thrombocytopenia, or any other blood study findings attributable to chloramphenicol. Discontinue the drug for symptoms of optic and peripheral neuritis. Monitoring of plasma levels is imperative in all patients and especially in neonates. Treat allergic reaction as indicated, and resuscitate as necessary.

CHLORPROMAZINE HYDROCHLORIDE

(klor-proe′ma-zeen hye-droe-klor′id)

Phenothiazine
Antipsychotic
Antiemetic

Thorazine

pH 3 to 5

USUAL DOSE

Use of the IV route is reserved for the treatment of acute nausea and vomiting in surgery, intractable hiccups, and tetanus.

Acute nausea and vomiting in surgery: 2 mg. May repeat at 2-minute intervals as indicated. Do not exceed 25 mg. Usually given as an infusion.

Intractable hiccups: 25 to 50 mg diluted in 500 to 1,000 ml of NS. Given as a slow IV infusion with patient flat in bed. Monitor BP closely.

Tetanus: 25 to 50 mg as an infusion of at least 1 mg/ml. Individualize dose to patient response and tolerance. Repeat every 6 to 8 hours. Usually given in conjunction with barbiturates.

PEDIATRIC DOSE

See Maternal/Child. IV route rarely used for children. Not recommended for use in infants less than 6 months of age.

Acute nausea and vomiting in surgery, children 6 months of age or older: 1 mg. May repeat at 2-minute intervals as indicated. Monitor for hypotension. Another source suggests 2.5 to 4 mg/kg/24 hr in equally divided doses every 6 to 8 hours. Usual IV/IM dose does not exceed 2.5 to 4 mg/kg/24 hr or 40 mg/24 hr (whichever is less) in children 6 months to 5 years or up to 50 lbs, and 75 mg/24 hr in children 5 to 12 years.

Tetanus: 0.55 mg/kg of body weight (0.25 mg/lb) every 6 to 8 hours. Do not exceed 40 mg/24 hr for up to 23 kg (50 lbs) and 75 mg/24 hr for up to 50 kg (50 to 100 lbs), except in severe cases.

DOSE ADJUSTMENTS

Adjust dose to the individual and severity of condition. Reduce dose of any medication potentiated by phenothiazines by one fourth to one half. See Drug/Lab Interactions. ■ Reduce dose by one fourth to one half in the elderly, debilitated patients, or emaciated patients, and increase very gradually by response.

DILUTION

Each 25 mg (1 ml) must be diluted with 24 ml of NS for injection. 1 ml will equal 1 mg. May be further diluted in 500 to 1,000 ml of NS and given as an infusion. Handle carefully; may cause contact dermatitis. Sensitive to light. Slightly yellow color does not alter potency. Discard if markedly discolored.

Storage: Store at CRT. Protect from light and freezing.

COMPATIBLE WITH **(Underline Indicates Conflicting Compatibility Information)**

Consult pharmacist; specific conditions may apply; see Compatibilities, p. xvi.

Additive: Ascorbic acid (Cenolate), ethacrynate sodium (Edecrin), theophylline.

Syringe: Atropine, benztropine (Cogentin), butorphanol (Stadol), diphenhydramine (Benadryl), doxapram (Dopram), droperidol (Inapsine), fentanyl (Sublimaze), glycopyrrolate, hydromorphone (Dilaudid), meperidine (Demerol), metoclopramide (Reglan), midazolam (Versed), morphine, pentazocine (Talwin), perphenazine (Trilafon), prochlorperazine (Compazine), promethazine (Phenergan), ranitidine (Zantac), scopolamine.

Y-site: Cisatracurium (Nimbex), cisplatin (Platinol), cladribine (Leustatin), cyclophosphamide (Cytoxan), cytarabine (ARA-C), docetaxel (Taxotere), doxorubicin (Adriamycin), doxorubicin liposome (Doxil), famotidine (Pepcid IV), filgrastim (Neupogen), fluconazole (Diflucan), gatifloxacin (Tequin), gemcitabine (Gemzar), granisetron (Kytril), heparin, hetastarch in electrolytes (Hextend), hydrocortisone sodium succinate (Solu-Cortef), ondansetron (Zofran), potassium chloride (KCl), propofol (Diprivan), remifentanil (Ultiva), teniposide (Vumon), thiotepa (Thioplex), vinorelbine (Navelbine).

RATE OF ADMINISTRATION

Titrate to symptoms and vital signs. See Precautions.

IV injection: Each 1 mg or fraction thereof over 1 minute.

Infusion: Given very slowly. Do not exceed 1 mg/min.

Pediatric rate: Do not exceed 1 mg or fraction thereof over 2 minutes.

ACTIONS

A phenothiazine derivative with effects on the central, autonomic, and peripheral nervous systems. A psychotropic agent. Decreases anxiety and tension, relaxes muscles, produces sedation, and tranquilizes. Has an antiemetic effect and potentiates CNS depressants. Has strong antiadrenergic and anticholinergic activity. Also possesses slight antihistaminic and antiserotonin activity. Onset of action is prompt and of short duration in small IV doses. Extensively metabolized in liver and kidney and excreted primarily in urine. Crosses the placental barrier. Secreted in breast milk.

INDICATIONS AND USES

The IV route is used only for the treatment of acute nausea and vomiting in surgery, the treatment of intractable hiccups, and as an adjunct in the treatment of tetanus. ■ Used IM or PO for the treatment of schizophrenia and the management of psychotic disorders. ■ Also indicated IM, PO, or rectally to relieve restlessness and apprehension before surgery, to manage acute intermittent porphyria, to control manic episodes in manic-depressive illness, and to treat severe behavioral problems in children.

Unlabeled uses: Treatment of phencyclidine (PCP) psychosis. ■ Treatment of migraine headaches (IV or IM). ■ To reduce choreiform movements of Huntington's disease.

CONTRAINDICATIONS

Hypersensitivity to phenothiazines, comatose or severely depressed states, or the presence of large amounts of CNS depressants (e.g., alcohol, barbiturates, narcotics).

PRECAUTIONS

Use of the IV route is reserved for the treatment of acute nausea and vomiting in surgery, intractable hiccups, and tetanus. IM injection preferred. ■ Use caution in patients with bone marrow depression; glaucoma; cardiovascular, liver, renal, and chronic respiratory diseases; and acute respiratory diseases of children. ■ Reexposure of patients who have experienced jaundice, skin reactions, or blood dyscrasias with a phenothiazine is not recommended. Cross-sensitivity may occur. ■ May produce ECG changes (e.g., prolonged QT interval, changes in T waves). ■ Use with caution in patients with a history of seizure disorders; may lower seizure threshold. ■ Extrapyramidal symptoms caused by chlorpromazine may be confused with CNS signs of an undiagnosed disease (e.g., Reye's syndrome or encephalopathy). ■ May mask diagnosis of brain tumor, drug intoxication, and intestinal obstruction. ■ Tardive dyskinesia (potentially irreversible involuntary dyskinetic movements) may develop. Use smallest doses and shortest duration of therapy to minimize risk. ■ Neuroleptic malignant syndrome (NMS) characterized by hyperpyrexia, muscle rigidity, altered mental status, and autonomic instability has been reported; see Antidote. ■ May cause paradoxical excitation in children and the elderly. ■ Use phenothiazines with extreme caution in children with a history of sleep apnea, a family history of SIDS, or in the presence of Reye's syndrome. ■ May contain sulfites; use caution in patients with asthma. ■ Taper dose gradually following high dose or extended therapy to prevent possible occurrence of withdrawal symptoms (e.g., dizziness, gastritis, nausea, tremors, and vomiting).

Monitor: Keep patient in supine position throughout treatment and for at least ½ hour after treatment. Ambulate slowly and carefully; may cause postural hypotension. ■ Monitor BP and pulse before and during administration and between doses. ■ Cough reflex is often depressed; monitor closely if nauseated or vomiting to prevent aspiration. ■ Anticholinergic and cardiac effects may be troublesome during anesthesia. For patients receiving phenothiazines, taper and discontinue preoperatively if they will not be continued after surgery. ■ May discolor urine pink to reddish brown. ■ Photosensitivity of skin is possible. ■ See Drug/Lab Interactions.

Patient Education: Request assistance for ambulation; may cause dizziness or fainting. ■ Observe caution performing tasks that require alertness. ■ Avoid use of alcohol and other CNS depressants (e.g., diazepam [Valium], narcotics). ■ Possible eye and skin photosensitivity. Avoid unprotected exposure to sun. ■ Urine may discolor to pink or reddish brown.

Maternal/Child: See Precautions and Contraindications. ■ Category C: use during pregnancy only when clearly needed. Use near term may cause maternal hypotension and adverse neonatal effects (e.g., extrapyramidal syndrome, hyperreflexia, hyporeflexia, jaundice). ■ Fetuses and infants have a reduced capacity to metabolize and eliminate; may cause embryo toxicity, increase neonatal mortality, or cause permanent neurologic damage. May contain benzyl alcohol; use not recommended in neonates. ■ Not recommended during breast-feeding. Increases risk of dystonia and tardive dyskinesia. ■ Children metabolize antipsychotic agents more rapidly than adults and are at increased risk to develop extrapyramidal actions, especially during acute illness (e.g., chickenpox, CNS infections, dehydration, gastroenteritis, measles); monitor closely.

Elderly: See Dose Adjustments and Precautions. ■ Have a reduced capacity to metabolize and eliminate. May have increased sensitivity to postural hypotension, anticholinergic and sedative effects. ■ Increased risk of extrapyramidal side effects (e.g., tardive dyskinesia, parkinsonism).

DRUG/LAB INTERACTIONS

Use with epinephrine not recommended; may cause precipitous hypotension. ■ Use with agents that produce hypotension (e.g., antihypertensives, benzodiazepines, diuretics, lidocaine, paclitaxel) may produce severe hypotension. ■ Increased CNS, respiratory depression, and hypotensive effects with CNS depressants (e.g., narcotics, alcohol, anesthetics, and barbiturates); reduced doses of these agents usually indicated. ■ Chlorpromazine does not potentiate the anticonvulsant actions of barbiturates. Doses of anticonvulsant barbiturates should not be decreased if chlorpromazine is introduced. Instead begin chlorpromazine at a lower dose and titrate to effect. ■ Chlorpromazine may lower the seizure threshold. It may also interfere with phenytoin and valproic acid clearance, increasing potential for toxicity. Dose adjustment of anticonvulsants may be necessary. ■ Additive effects with MAO inhibitors (e.g., selegiline [Eldepryl]), anticholinergics, antihistamines, antihypertensives, hypnotics, muscle relaxants, rauwolfia alkaloids, and thiazide diuretics; dose adjustment may be necessary. ■ Barbiturates may also increase metabolism of chlorpromazine and reduce its effects. ■ Risk of cardiotoxicity increased with pimozide (Orap) and sparfloxacin (Zagam); concurrent use not recommended. ■ Risk of additive QT interval prolongation, cardiac depressant effects, and cardiac arrhythmias increased with cisapride (Propulsid), disopyramide (Norpace), erythromycin, probucol (Lorelco), procainamide (Pronestyl), and quinidine. ■ Concurrent use with antidepressants (e.g., fluoxetine [Prozac], paroxetine [Paxil]), tricyclic antidepressants (e.g., amitriptyline [Elavil]) or MAO inhibitors (e.g., selegiline [Eldepryl]) may increase effects of both drugs; risk of NMS may be increased. ■ Use with antithyroid drugs may increase risk of agranulocytosis. ■ May inhibit antiparkinson effects of levodopa. ■ May decrease pressor response to ephedrine. ■ May increase anticholinergic effect of orphenadrine (Norflex). ■ May decrease effects of oral anticoagulants. ■ Concurrent use with haloperidol, droperidol, or metoclopramide may cause increased extrapyramidal effects. ■ Use with metrizamide (Amipaque) may lower seizure threshold; discontinue chlorpromazine 48 hours before myelography and do not resume for 24 hours after test completed. ■ Metabolism and clearance of chlorpromazine is increased in cigarette smokers; decreased plasma levels and effectiveness may occur; dose adjustment of chlorpromazine may be indicated. ■ Decreased drowsiness may occur in cigarette smokers. May be offset by increased doses of chlorpromazine. ■ Use caution during anesthesia with barbiturates (e.g., methohexital, thiopental); may increase frequency and severity of hypotension and neuromuscular excitation. ■ Encephalopathic syndrome has been reported with concurrent use of lithium; monitor for S/S of neurologic toxicity. ■ Capable of innumerable other interactions. ■ May cause false-positive pregnancy test and false-positive amylase, PKU, and other urine tests.

SIDE EFFECTS

Usually transient if drug discontinued, but may require treatment if severe. Anaphylaxis, cardiac arrest, distorted Q and T waves, drowsiness, excitement, extrapyramidal symptoms (e.g., abnormal positioning, extreme restlessness, pseudoparkinsonism, weakness of extremities), fever, hematologic toxicities (e.g., agranulocytosis, aplastic anemia, leukopenia, thrombocytopenia), hypersensitivity reactions, hypertension, hypotension (occurs less frequently in smokers), melanosis, photosensitivity, tachycardia, tardive dyskinesia, and many others.

Overdose: Can cause convulsions, hallucinations, and death.

ANTIDOTE

Discontinue the drug at onset of any side effect and notify the physician. Discontinue chlorpromazine and all drugs not essential to concurrent therapy immediately if NMS occurs. Will require intensive symptomatic treatment, medical monitoring, and management of concomitant medical problems. Counteract hypotension with norepinephrine (Levophed) or phenylephrine (Neo-Synephrine) and IV fluids. Counteract extrapyramidal symptoms with benztropine (Cogentin) or diphenhydramine (Benadryl). Use diazepam (Valium) followed by phenytoin (Dilantin) for convulsions or hyperactivity. Maintain a clear airway and adequate hydration. Epinephrine is contraindicated for hypotension; further hypotension will occur. Phenytoin may be helpful in ventricular arrhythmias. Avoid analeptics such as caffeine and sodium benzoate in treating respiratory depression and unconsciousness; they may cause convulsions. Resuscitate as necessary. Not removed by dialysis.

CIDOFOVIR INJECTION

(si-doh-foh'veer in-jek'shun)

Vistide

Antiviral (nucleotide analog)

pH 7.4

USUAL DOSE

Preliminary lab work required before each dose; see Monitor.

A specific protocol is required; see chart, *Overview of the Treatment Regimen for Cidofovir*. A 4-Gm course of oral probenecid is required on the day of each infusion of cidofovir to reduce the risk of renal impairment. Hydration with 1 to 2 liters of NS is required to help reduce proteinuria and prevent increases in SrCr. Infrequent dosing schedule may eliminate need for an indwelling IV catheter, reducing discomfort and potential for infection.

Induction: 5 mg/kg in 100 ml NS once weekly for 2 weeks.

Maintenance: 5 mg/kg in 100 ml NS once every other week.

Overview of the Treatment Regimen for Cidofovir

Before Cidofovir Infusion	During Cidofovir Infusion	After Cidofovir Infusion
1. Patient takes 2 Gm of probenecid* (4 × 500 mg tablets) 3 hours before cidofovir infusion	1. Begin IV infusion of cidofovir (5 mg/kg body weight in 100 ml NS) at a constant rate over 1 hour†	1. Patient takes 1 Gm of probenecid (2 × 500 mg tablets) 2 hours after the *end* of cidofovir infusion
2. Infuse first liter of NS over 1 to 2 hours immediately before starting cidofovir infusion	2. For patients who can tolerate the extra fluid load, infuse a second liter of NS. If administered, initiate either at the start of the cidofovir infusion or immediately afterward, and infuse over a 1- to 3-hour period	2. Patient takes 1 Gm of probenecid (2 × 500 mg tablets) 8 hours after the *end* of cidofovir infusion

*Patients receiving concomitant probenecid and zidovudine should temporarily discontinue zidovudine or decrease the zidovudine dose by 50% on days of combined zidovudine and probenecid administration.

†The recommended dosage, frequency, or infusion rate must not be exceeded.

DOSE ADJUSTMENTS

Reduce dose to 3 mg/kg for the remainder of therapy, if SrCr increases by 0.3 to 0.4 mg/dl above baseline. ■ 5 mg/kg may be given to patients who develop a 2^+ proteinuria but have a stable SrCr. Encourage oral hydration; additional IV hydration may be appropriate. ■ Discontinue cidofovir if the SrCr increases by equal to or greater than 0.5 mg/dl above baseline or if proteinuria 3^+ or more develops. ■ Restarting cidofovir in patients whose renal function has returned to baseline after a SrCr elevation more than 0.5 mg/dl is not recommended. ■ Discontinue cidofovir in any patient who requires therapy with a nephrotoxic agent; see Contraindications. Cidofovir may be restarted after other nephrotoxic therapy is complete, an adequate washout period of at least 7 days has passed, and adequate renal function (SrCr less than 1.5 mg/dl) is confirmed.

DILUTION

Specific techniques required; see Precautions. A calculated dose must be diluted in 100 ml of NS.

Storage: Store unopened vials at CRT. May be refrigerated but must be used within 24 hours of dilution with NS. Allow to return to room temperature before administration. Discard partially used vials.

COMPATIBILITY

Manufacturer states, "Compatibility with Ringer's solution, LR, or bacteriostatic IV fluids not evaluated; no data available to support the addition of other drugs or supplements for concurrent administration."

RATE OF ADMINISTRATION

A single dose as an infusion at a constant rate over 1 hour. Use of an infusion pump is recommended.

ACTIONS

A nucleotide analog antiviral. Its active intracellular metabolite selectively inhibits CMV DNA synthesis. It is incorporated into the growing viral DNA chain, resulting in reductions in the rate of viral DNA synthesis. This action is independent of virus infection (acyclovir or ganciclovir require activation by a virally encoded enzyme). Elimination half-life is short (2.6 hours), but it has a long intracellular half-life, which permits infrequent dosing. Primarily excreted in urine (70% to 85% in 24 hours with concomitant doses of probenecid).

INDICATIONS AND USES

Treatment of newly diagnosed or relapsing CMV retinitis in patients with AIDS.

CONTRAINDICATIONS

Pre-existing renal dysfunction (e.g., baseline SrCr more than 1.5 mg/dl, calculated CrCl equal to or less than 55 ml/min, or a urine protein equal to or greater than 100 mg/dl [equivalent to a 2^+ or more proteinuria]). ■ Patients receiving agents with nephrotoxic potential (e.g., aminoglycosides, amphotericin B, foscarnet, NSAIDs [ibuprofen (Advil, Motrin), naproxen (Aleve, Naprosyn), IV pentamidine, vancomycin). No other nephrotoxic agent should be administered within 7 days of starting cidofovir or concomitantly during cidofovir therapy. ■ Hypersensitivity to cidofovir and/or a history of clinically severe hypersensitivity (e.g., hypotension, respiratory distress) to probenecid or other sulfa-containing medications (e.g., sulfamethoxazole-trimethoprim [Bactrim]).

PRECAUTIONS

Follow guidelines for handling cytotoxic agents. See Appendix A, p. 1142. ■ Administered by or under the direction of the physician specialist, preferably in an environment where emergency treatment is available. ■ This formulation is for IV use only; **DO NOT** use for intraocular injection. ■ Safety and effectiveness have not been established for treatment of other CMV infections (e.g., pneumonitis, gastroenteritis, congenital or neonatal CMV disease) or for CMV disease in non–HIV-infected individuals. ■ Calculated CrCl may not accurately estimate renal function in emaciated (e.g., patients with AIDS) or extremely muscular patients; a 24-hour urine collection may be required. ■ CMV resistant to ganciclovir may also be resistant to cidofovir, but may be sensitive to foscarnet (Foscavir). ▪ CMV resistant to foscarnet may be sensitive to cidofovir. ▪ Nephrotoxicity is dose limiting, the major toxicity of cidofovir. Do not exceed recommended doses, frequency, or rate of administration; may cause increased risk of renal toxicity. Acute renal failure requiring dialysis or contributing to death has occurred with as few as 1 or 2 doses of cidofovir. ▪ Renal function may not return to baseline after treatment with cidofovir. ▪ Proteinuria is an early indicator of nephrotoxicity; continued administration of cidofovir may lead to additional proximal tubular cell injury resulting in glycosuria, decreased serum phosphate, uric acid, and bicarbonate; increased SrCr; and/or acute renal failure, which may necessitate dialysis. ▪ May cause granulocytopenia (e.g., neutropenia). ▪ Although some reference sources have published doses for patients with impaired renal function, this drug is contraindicated in such patients and should be given only to those who meet specific dosing criteria; see Contraindications.

Monitor: 24 to 48 hours before each cidofovir infusion, obtain a SrCr, urine protein (via dipstick or quantitative urinalysis), and a CBC with differential (absolute neutrophil count [ANC]). Repeat between doses if indicated. ▪ Administration of probenecid as ordered and adequate hydration (oral and IV) are imperative. ▪ Antiretroviral therapy may be continued with the exception of zidovudine; see Drug/Lab Interactions. ▪ Probenecid frequently causes fever, flushing, headache, nausea with or without emesis, and rash. Use acetaminophen for prophylaxis or treatment of fever or headache. Encourage ingestion of food before each dose of probenecid to reduce nausea; prophylactic antiemetics (e.g., ondansetron [Zofran]) are appropriate. Consider use of antihistamines (e.g., diphenhydramine [Benadryl]) for prophylaxis or treatment in patients who develop mild hypersensitivity reactions (e.g., rash). Severe hypersensitivity reactions (e.g., laryngospasm, hypotension) have occasionally been reported with probenecid. Usually occur within several hours after patients have received probenecid even though they have received it before with no adverse reactions. Observe patient carefully for allergic reactions. Treatment for anaphylaxis (e.g., epinephrine, corticosteroids, and antihistamines) must be readily available. ▪ Monitor intraocular pressure, visual acuity, and ocular symptoms with a baseline ophthalmologic exam and periodically during therapy. Uveitis or iritis has been reported; may be treated with topical steroids. Risk of increased intraocular pressure and other visual problems may be increased in patients with pre-existing diabetes mellitus. ▪ If CrCl measurement is indicated, use of the Cockcroft-Gault formula is recommended to obtain a precise estimate.

Patient Education: Not a cure for CMV retinitis. Retinitis may recur during maintenance or after treatment; regular ophthalmologic exams imperative. ▪ Full compliance with regimen imperative (e.g., probenecid with food, increased IV and oral hydration, regular lab testing). ▪ Report diarrhea, eye pain or change in vision, fever, headache, loss of appetite, rash, nausea, and vomiting promptly. ▪ Report concomitant medication changes or additions. ▪ Notify all health care personnel of treatment with probenecid to avoid interactions. ▪ Consider birth control options; See Precautions/Maternal/Child.

Maternal/Child: Category C: should not be used during pregnancy; embryotoxic in animals. A potential carcinogen; knowledge of effects on women unknown. ▪ Women of childbearing age should use effective contraception during cidofovir therapy and for 1 month after completion. ▪ Men should use barrier contraception during cidofovir therapy and for 3 months after completion. ▪ Has caused reduced testical weight and hypospermia in animals. ▪ Do not administer to nursing mothers. HIV-infected mothers are advised not to breast-feed to avoid transmission to an uninfected child. ▪ Safety and effectiveness for use in children not established. Use in children with extreme caution and only if the benefits of treatment outweigh the risks of long-term carcinogenicity and reproductive toxicity. Consult physician specialist for adjustments in probenecid and hydration. **Elderly:** Effects have not been studied; monitor renal function carefully.

DRUG/LAB INTERACTIONS

Limited information available. Drug profile review by pharmacist imperative. ▪ Nephrotoxicity increased by other nephrotoxic agents (e.g., aminoglycosides [e.g., amikacin, gentamicin], amphotericin B [Fungizone, Abelcet], foscarnet [Foscavir], IV pentamidine, NSAIDs [e.g., ibuprofen (Motrin), vancomycin [Vancocin]); see Contraindications. ▪ Prior treatment with Foscavir may also increase the risk of nephrotoxicity; monitor renal function carefully. ▪ Probenecid decreases clearance of zidovudine; temporarily discontinue or reduce dose of zidovudine by 50% on days of combined zidovudine and probenecid administration. ▪ Probenecid may have interactions with numerous other drugs (e.g., acetaminophen, acyclovir [Zovirax], ACE inhibitors [e.g., enalaprilat (Vasotec)], aminosalicylic acid, barbiturates, benzodiazepines [e.g., diazepam, lorazepam (Ativan), midazolam], bumetamide, clofibrate, ddC, famotidine, furosemide, chlorpropamide [Diabinese], methotrexate, NSAIDs [e.g., ketoprofen (Orudis), ibuprofen (Advil, Motrin), naproxen (Aleve, Naprosyn)], theophyllines), usually decreasing their rate of excretion and increasing toxicity. Consider withholding any drug that may interact with probenecid on the day of cidofovir administration.

SIDE EFFECTS

Nephrotoxicity is dose limiting. Metabolic acidosis (Fanconi's syndrome), neutropenia, and ocular hypotony may be dose limiting and require prompt treatment. Anorexia, asthenia, decreased serum bicarbonate, chills, diarrhea, dyspnea, fever, headache, increased creatinine, infection, nausea and vomiting, ophthalmic effects (e.g., change in vision, eye pain, increased sensitivity to light, reddened eyes), pneumonia, proteinuria, and unusual tiredness or weakness may occur.

ANTIDOTE

There is no specific antidote. Keep physician informed. Adequate hydration, use of probenecid, and careful monitoring will help to reduce potential for renal impairment and may minimize other side effects. Filgrastim (Neupogen) may be used to treat neutropenia. See Monitor for management of probenecid side effects. Discontinue cidofovir based on criteria in Dose Adjustments. Treat overdose for 3 to 5 days with probenecid 1 Gm three times daily and vigorous IV hydration to tolerance. Treat anaphylaxis and resuscitate as indicated. Hemodialysis may be helpful in overdose. High-flux hemodialysis has reduced serum level of cidofovir by up to 75%.

CIMETIDINE
(sye-met'i-deen)

Antiulcer
(H_2 antagonist)
Gastric acid inhibitor
Adjunct urticaria therapy

Tagamet

pH 3.8 to 6

USUAL DOSE

Direct or intermittent IV: 300 mg every 6 hours. Increase frequency of dose, not amount, if necessary for pain relief. Do not exceed 2,400 mg/24 hr.

Continuous IV: 900 mg evenly distributed over 24 hours (37.5 mg/hr). May be preceded by a loading dose of 150 to 300 mg if indicated (total dose from 1,050 to 1,200 mg/24 hr). To maintain intragastric acid secretory rates at 10 mEq/hr or less, dose range may be higher in patients with pathologic hypersecretory states. Product insert mentions a study that used a range of 40 to 600 mg/hr averaging 160 mg/hr; well beyond usual doses. Any dose beyond the normal should be administered with extreme caution.

Additive for total parenteral nutrition (TPN): 70% to 100% of an average 24-hour dose has been used equally distributed over 24 hours as a continuous infusion. May be supplemented with intermittent doses as needed.

Prevention of upper GI bleeding: A continuous infusion of 37.5 to 50 mg/hr for up to 7 days. Maintain gastric pH at 3.5 to 4. May be preceded by a loading dose of up to 300 mg.

Prevention of aspiration pneumonitis: 300 mg 60 to 90 minutes before anesthesia.

Erosive gastroesophageal reflux disease (GERD): 1,600 mg/day (IV or PO) in divided doses every 6 hours (400 mg) or 12 hours (800 mg) for 12 weeks.

PEDIATRIC DOSE

5 to 10 mg/kg of body weight every 6 hours.

NEONATAL DOSE

2.5 to 5 mg/kg every 6 hours.

DOSE ADJUSTMENTS

Increase intervals between injections to achieve pain relief with least frequent dosage in impaired renal function. ■ Reduce dose by half in prevention of GI bleeding if CrCl is less than 30 ml/min.

DILUTION

IV injection: Each 300 mg must be diluted with 18 ml (total volume of 20 ml) of NS or other compatible solution for injection (see chart on inside back cover).

Intermittent infusion: Each 300 mg may be diluted in at least 50 ml of D5W or other compatible infusion solution and given piggyback. Available premixed. Do not use premixed plastic containers in series connections; may cause air embolism.

Continuous infusion: Total daily dose may be diluted in 100 to 1,000 ml of infusion solution. Compatible with most dextrose and saline solutions, lactated Ringer's solution, 5% sodium bicarbonate, and many others. Compatible in selected TPN solutions for 24 hours (consult pharmacist).

Storage: Stable at CRT for 48 hours after dilution.

INCOMPATIBLE WITH

Manufacturer states, "Do not add other drugs to premixed cimetidine in plastic containers."

COMPATIBLE WITH (Underline Indicates Conflicting Compatibility Information)

Consult pharmacist; specific conditions may apply; see Compatibilities, p. xvi.

Solution: Selected TNA and TPN solutions.

Additive: Acetazolamide (Diamox), amikacin (Amikin), aminophylline, atracurium (Tracrium), cefamandole (Mandol), cefazolin (Kefzol), cefoperazone (Cefobid), cefoxitin (Mefoxin), chlorothiazide (Diuril), clindamycin (Cleocin), colistimethate (Coly-Mycin M), dexamethasone (Decadron), digoxin (Lanoxin), epinephrine (Adrenalin), erythromycin lactobionate (Erythrocin), ethacrynate sodium (Edecrin), flumazenil (Romazicon), furosemide (Lasix), gentamicin (Garamycin), insulin (regular), isoproterenol (Isuprel), lidocaine, lincomycin (Lincocin), meropenem (Merrem IV), methylprednisolone (Solu-Medrol), metoclopramide (Reglan), nitroprusside sodium, norepinephrine (Levophed), penicillin G potassium, phytonadione (Aquamephyton), potassium chloride (KCl), protamine sulfate, quinidine gluconate, tacrolimus (Prograf), vancomycin (Vancocin), verapamil (Isoptin).

Syringe: Atropine, butorphanol (Stadol), diazepam (Valium), diphenhydramine (Benadryl), doxapram (Dopram), droperidol (Inapsine), fentanyl (Sublimaze), glycopyrrolate, heparin, hydromorphone (Dilaudid), lorazepam (Ativan), meperidine (Demerol), midazolam (Versed), morphine, nafcillin (Nafcil), nalbuphine (Nubain), penicillin G sodium, pentazocine (Talwin), perphenazine (Trilafon), prochlorperazine (Compazine), promethazine (Phenergan), scopolamine, sodium acetate, sodium chloride, sodium lactate, selected contrast agents used in radiology.

Y-site: Acyclovir (Zovirax), amifostine (Ethyol), aminophylline, atracurium (Tracrium), aztreonam (Azactam), cisatracurium (Nimbex), cisplatin (Platinol), cladribine (Leustatin), cyclophosphamide (Cytoxan), cytarabine (ARA-C), diltiazem (Cardizem), docetaxel (Taxotere), doxorubicin (Adriamycin), doxorubicin liposome (Doxil), enalaprilat (Vasotec IV), esmolol (Brevibloc), etoposide phosphate (Etopophos), filgrastim (Neupogen), fluconazole (Diflucan), fludarabine (Fludara), foscarnet (Foscavir), gatifloxacin (Tequin), gemcitabine (Gemzar), granisetron (Kytril), haloperidol (Haldol), heparin, hetastarch (Hespan and Hextend), idarubicin (Idamycin), inamrinone (Inocor), labetalol (Normodyne), levofloxacin (Levaquin), linezolid (Zyvox), melphalan (Alkeran), meropenem (Merrem IV), methotrexate (Folex), midazolam (Versed), milrinone (Primacor), ondansetron (Zofran), paclitaxel (Taxol), pancuronium (Pavulon), piperacillin/tazobactam (Zosyn), propofol (Diprivan), remifentanil (Ultiva), sargramostim (Leukine), tacrolimus (Prograf), teniposide (Vumon), theophylline, thiotepa (Thioplex), topotecan (Hycamtin), vecuronium (Norcuron), vinorelbine (Navelbine), zidovudine (AZT, Retrovir).

RATE OF ADMINISTRATION

IV injection: Each 300 mg or fraction thereof over a minimum of 5 minutes.

Intermittent infusion: Each 300-mg dose over 15 to 20 minutes.

Continuous infusion: Give loading dose at intermittent infusion rate and distribute balance of daily dose equally over 24 hours. Use of infusion pump preferred, especially with volumes of 250 ml or less, to avoid complications of overdose or too-rapid administration; see Side Effects.

ACTIONS

A histamine H_2 antagonist, it inhibits both daytime and nocturnal basal gastric acid secretion. It also inhibits gastric acid secretion stimulated by food, histamine, pentagastrin, caffeine, and insulin. Onset of action is prompt and effective for 4 to 5 hours. Excreted in the urine. Crosses placental barrier. Secreted in breast milk.

INDICATIONS AND USES

Short-term treatment of active duodenal ulcers and active benign gastric ulcers. ■ Pathologic hypersecretory conditions. ■ Erosive gastroesophageal reflux disease (GERD) diagnosed by endoscopy. ■ Prevention of GI bleeding in critically ill patients, especially those with potential for stress-related mucosal damage (e.g., erosive gastritis, stress ulcers). ■ Additive to TPN to simplify fluid and electrolyte management (decreases the volume and chloride content of gastric secretions).

Unlabeled uses: Preoperatively to prevent aspiration pneumonia. ■ Treatment of itching and flushing of anaphylaxis, pruritus, urticaria, and contact dermatitis. ■ Treatment of acetaminophen overdose (helps to reduce hepatotoxicity).

CONTRAINDICATIONS

Known hypersensitivity to cimetidine.

PRECAUTIONS

IV bolus administration has precipitated rare instances of cardiac arrhythmias, hypotension, and death. Gastric malignancy may be present even though patient is asymptomatic. ■ Gastric pain and ulceration may recur after medication stopped.

Monitor: Use antacids concomitantly to relieve pain. ■ Monitor PT. ■ See Drug/Lab Interactions. ■ Change to oral doses when appropriate; usually discontinued after 4 to 8 weeks.

Patient Education: Interacts with many medications. Check with pharmacist or physician before taking any other drugs. ■ Abstain from smoking; at least avoid smoking after the last dose of the day.

Maternal/Child: Category B: no adequate studies available; benefits must outweigh risks. ■ Discontinue breast-feeding. ■ Not recommended for children under 16, but 20 to 40 mg/kg/day has been used.

Elderly: Safety and effectiveness consistent with younger ages; renal clearance of cimetidine likely to be decreased.

DRUG/LAB INTERACTIONS

Interactions are numerous and potentially life threatening. Review of drug profile by pharmacist imperative. May potentiate warfarin-type anticoagulants; monitor PT. ■ Potentiates effects of alcohol, antimalarials (e.g., chloroquine), some benzodiazepines (e.g., diazepam [Valium]), beta blockers (e.g., propranolol [Inderal]), caffeine, calcium channel blockers (e.g., verapamil), carbamazepine, fluoroquinolones (e.g., ciprofloxacin [Cipro]), hydantoins (e.g., phenytoin [Dilantin]), lidocaine, metronidazole (e.g., Flagyl), pentoxifylline (Trental), procainamide (Pronestyl), quinidine, sulfonylureas, tricyclic antidepressants (e.g., imipramine [Tofranil]), theophyllines (e.g., aminophylline), and triamterene (Dyrenium). ■ May inhibit digoxin absorption. ■ Clinical effect (inhibition of nocturnal gastric secretion) reversed by cigarette smoking. ■ May precipitate apnea, confusion, and muscle twitching with morphine. ■ May cause increased myelosuppression with alkylating agents (e.g., carmustine). ■ Concurrent use with paroxetine (Paxil) may cause increased serum levels of paroxetine and an increase in BP. ■ May inhibit gastric absorption of ketoconazole (Nizoral). ■ Many unconfirmed reports of inhibiting pharmacologic action of other drugs.

SIDE EFFECTS

Bradycardia, confusion, diarrhea, delirium, dizziness, elevated AST (SGOT), fever, galactorrhea, gynecomastia, hallucinations, impotence, interstitial nephritis, muscular pain, rash.

Overdose: Cardiac arrhythmias, death, hypotension, respiratory failure, tachycardia.

ANTIDOTE

Notify physician of all side effects. May be treated symptomatically or may respond to decrease in frequency of dose. Physostigmine may be useful to reverse CNS toxicity. In overdose, assisted ventilation is indicated and beta blockers (e.g., metoprolol [Lopressor], propranolol [Inderal]) may control tachycardia.

CIPROFLOXACIN

(sip-ro-floks′a-sin)

Cipro I.V.

Antibacterial (fluoroquinolone)

pH 3.3 to 4.6

USUAL DOSE

Dose based on severity and nature of the infection, susceptibility of the causative organism, integrity of host-defense mechanisms, and renal and hepatic status. Range is from 200 to 400 mg according to the following chart. Continue for 7 to 14 days (at least 2 days after all symptoms of infection subside). Bone and joint infections may require treatment for 4 to 6 weeks or more. May be transferred to oral dosing when appropriate.

Ciprofloxacin Dose Guidelines

Infection	Type of Severity	Unit Dose	Frequency	Total 24-hr Dose	Duration
Urinary tract	Mild/moderate	200 mg	q 12 hr	400 mg	7-14 days
	Severe/ complicated	400 mg	q 12 hr	800 mg	
Lower respiratory tract	Mild/moderate	400 mg	q 12 hr	800 mg	7-14 days
	Severe/ complicated	400 mg	q 8 hr	1,200 mg	
Nosocomial pneumonia	Mild/moderate/ severe	400 mg	q 8 hr	1,200 mg	10-14 days
Skin and skin structure	Mild/moderate	400 mg	q 12 hr	800 mg	7-14 days
	Severe/ complicated	400 mg	q 8 hr	1,200 mg	
Bone and joint	Mild/moderate	400 mg	q 12 hr	800 mg	4-6 weeks
	Severe/ complicated	400 mg	q 8 hr	1,200 mg	
Septicemia (Canada)		400 mg	q 12 hr	800 mg	
Acute sinusitis	Mild/moderate	400 mg	q 12 hr	800 mg	10 days
Chronic bacterial prostatitis	Mild/moderate	400 mg	q 12 hr	800 mg	28 days
Inhalation[1] anthrax	Post-exposure	400 mg	q 12 hr	800 mg	60 days

[1]Begin drug administration as soon as possible after suspected or confirmed exposure.

Continued

Ciprofloxacin Dose Guidelines—cont'd					
Infection	**Type of Severity**	**Unit Dose**	**Frequency**	**Total 24-hr Dose**	**Duration**
Intraabdominal, complicated	Ciprofloxacin + metronidazole	400 mg 500 mg	q 12 hr q 6 hr	800 mg 2,000 mg	7-14 days
Empirical therapy in febrile neutropenic patients	Ciprofloxacin + piperacillin	400 mg 50 mg/kg	q 8 hr q 4 hr	1,200 mg Not to exceed 24 Gm/day or 300 mg/kg/24 hr	7-14 days

PEDIATRIC DOSE

Used only when alternate therapy cannot be used; see Precautions/Maternal/Child. 10 mg/kg of body weight every 12 hours. Do not exceed 400 mg/dose.

Inhalation anthrax (post-exposure): 10 mg/kg every 12 hours. Do not exceed 800 mg/24 hr. Administer for 60 days.

DOSE ADJUSTMENTS

Increase interval between doses (200 to 400 mg every 18 to 24 hours) if CrCl is less than 30 ml/min (see literature for additional information). ■ Dose reduction not required based on age; see Elderly. ■ See Drug/Lab Interactions.

DILUTION

Available prediluted in D5W in latex-free plastic infusion containers ready for use. A clear, colorless to slightly yellow solution. Do not hang plastic containers in a series; may cause air embolism. Also available in 20- and 40-ml vials containing 10 mg/ml (1% solution), which must be diluted with NS, D5W, SW, D10W, D5/¼NS, D5/½NS, or LR to a final concentration of 1 to 2 mg/ml.

Storage: Store at room temperature before dilution; protect from light, excessive heat, and freezing. Stable for up to 14 days refrigerated or at room temperature in the final diluted concentration.

INCOMPATIBLE WITH

Manufacturer recommends temporarily discontinuing other solutions infusing at the same site during intermittent infusion through a Y-site or volume control and that ciprofloxacin be administered separately and the IV line be flushed before and after administration of any other drug.

COMPATIBLE WITH **(Underline Indicates Conflicting Compatibility Information)**

Consult pharmacist; specific conditions may apply; see Compatibilities, p. xvi.

Additive: Amikacin (Amikin), aztreonam (Azactam), <u>ceftazidime (Fortaz)</u>, cyclosporine (Sandimmune), dopamine (Intropin), gentamicin (Garamycin), lidocaine, linezolid (Zyvox), <u>metronidazole (Flagyl IV)</u>, <u>piperacillin (Pipracil)</u>, potassium chloride (KCl), ranitidine (Zantac), tobramycin (Nebcin).

Y-site: Amifostine (Ethyol), amino acids with dextrose, aztreonam (Azactam), calcium gluconate, ceftazidime (Fortaz), cisatracurium (Nimbex), digoxin (Lanoxin), diltiazem (Cardizem), diphenhydramine (Benadryl), dobutamine (Dobutrex), docetaxel (Taxotere), dopamine (Intropin), doxorubicin liposome (Doxil), etoposide phosphate (Etopophos), gemcitabine (Gemzar), gentamicin (Garamycin), granisetron (Kytril), hetastarch in electrolytes (Hextend), LR, lidocaine, linezolid (Zyvox), lorazepam (Ativan), magnesium sulfate, metoclopramide (Reglan), midazolam (Versed), piperacillin (Pipracil), potassium acetate, potassium chloride (KCl), promethazine (Phenergan), ranitidine (Zantac), remifentanil (Ultiva), sodium bicarbonate, sodium chloride, tacrolimus (Prograf), teniposide (Vumon), thiotepa (Thioplex), tobramycin (Nebcin), verapamil (Isoptin).

RATE OF ADMINISTRATION

A single dose must be equally distributed over 60 minutes as an infusion. Too-rapid administration and/or the use of a small vein may increase incidence of anaphylaxis, local site inflammation, and other side effects. May be given through a Y-tube or three-way stopcock of infusion set. Temporarily discontinue other solutions infusing at the same site.

ACTIONS

A synthetic, broad-spectrum antimicrobial agent, a fluoroquinolone. Bactericidal to a wide range of aerobic gram-negative and gram-positive organisms through interference with the enzyme needed for synthesis of bacterial DNA. Onset of action is prompt, and serum levels are dose related. Half-life averages 5 to 6 hours. Readily distributed to body fluids (saliva, nasal and bronchial secretions, sputum, skin blister fluid, lymph, peritoneal fluid, bile and prostatic secretions). Found in lung, skin, fat, muscle, cartilage, and bone. Levels in cerebrospinal fluid and eye fluids are lower than plasma levels. Excreted primarily as unchanged drug in the urine, usually within 24 hours. Crosses placental barrier. Secreted in breast milk.

INDICATIONS AND USES

Treatment of mild, moderate, severe, and complicated infections of the urinary tract, lower respiratory tract, and skin and skin structure. ■ Treatment of mild, moderate, and severe nosocomial pneumonia. ■ Treatment of acute sinusitis, bone and joint infections, chronic bacterial prostatitis, and septicemia (Canada). ■ Treatment of complicated intraabdominal infections in combination with metronidazole (Flagyl). ■ Empirical therapy in febrile neutropenic patients in combination with piperacillin. ■ Reduce the incidence or progression of disease following exposure to aerosolized *Bacillus anthracis* (Anthrax). ■ Most effective against specific organisms (see literature). ■ Additional appropriate therapy required if anaerobic organisms are suspected of contributing to the infection. ■ Oral route of administration indicated for treatment of other infections (e.g., infectious diarrhea, typhoid fever, urethral and cervical gonococcal infections).

Unlabeled uses: Treatment of tuberculosis in combination with other antituberculosis agents (e.g., rifampin). ■ Treatment of *Mycobacterium avium* complex infection in AIDS patients.

CONTRAINDICATIONS

Known hypersensitivity to ciprofloxacin or any other quinolone antimicrobial agent (e.g., levofloxacin [Levaquin], norfloxacin [Noroxin]).

PRECAUTIONS

Specific culture and sensitivity studies indicated to determine susceptibility of the causative organism to ciprofloxacin. ■ *Pseudomonas aeruginosa* may develop resistance during treatment. Ongoing culture and sensitivity studies indicated. ■ Prolonged use may cause superinfection because of overgrowth of nonsusceptible organisms. Monitor carefully. ■ Mild to life-threatening pseudomembranous colitis has been reported. Consider this diagnosis in any patient with diarrhea during or after treatment. ■ Convulsions, increased intracranial pressure, and toxic psychosis have been reported in patients receiving quinolones, including ciprofloxacin. Ciprofloxacin may also cause CNS events, including confusion, depression, dizziness, hallucinations, and tremors. ■ Use caution in patients with impaired renal function and known CNS disorders (e.g., epilepsy, severe cerebral arteriosclerosis, or any other factors that predispose to seizures). ■ May cause ophthalmologic abnormalities (e.g., cataracts). Incidence increases with length of treatment. ■ Ruptures of shoulder, hand, and/or Achilles tendons that required surgical repair or resulted in prolonged disability have been reported in patients receiving quinolones. ■ Prolongation of the QT interval on ECG and infrequent cases of arrhythmia (including torsades de pointes) have been reported with the use of fluoroquinolones. The risk of arrhythmia may be reduced by avoiding their use in the presence of hypokalemia, significant bradycardia, cardiomyopathy, or concurrent treatment with class 1A antiarrhythmic agents (e.g., quinidine, procainamide [Pronestyl]) or with class III antiarrhythmic agents (e.g., amiodarone [Cordarone], sotalol [Betapace]).

Monitor: May cause anaphylaxis with the first or succeeding doses, even in patients without known hypersensitivity. Emergency equipment must always be available. ■ Maintain adequate hydration and acidity of urine throughout treatment. Will form crystals in alkaline urine. ■ Monitor hematopoietic, hepatic, and renal systems during prolonged treatment. ■ Use of large veins recommended to dilute toxicity, reduce incidence of allergic reactions, and reduce incidence of local irritation. Symptoms of local irritation do not preclude further administration of ciprofloxacin unless they recur or worsen. Generally resolve when infusion complete. ■ Concomitant use with theophylline may cause cardiac arrest, respiratory failure, seizures, and/or status epilepticus. If concomitant use cannot be avoided, monitor serum levels of theophylline and adjust dose as indicated. ■ Doses will increase slightly with transfer to oral ciprofloxacin (e.g., 200 mg to 250 mg, 400 mg to 500 mg). ■ See Drug/Lab Interactions.

Patient Education: Consider birth control options. ■ Avoid exposure to sunlight or artificial ultraviolet light; may cause severe sunburn. Wear dark glasses outdoors. ■ Request assistance for ambulation; may cause dizziness and lightheadedness. Use caution in tasks that require alertness. ■ Effects of caffeine- or theophylline-containing preparations may be increased. Limit or eliminate concurrent use. Monitor if concurrent use necessary. ■ Report tendon pain or inflammation promptly. ■ Report skin rash or any other hypersensitivity reaction promptly.

Maternal/Child: Category C: use during pregnancy only if benefits justify potential risk to fetus and mother. ■ Discontinue breast-feeding. ■ Safety for use in children under 18 years of age not established except for use post-exposure of inhalation anthrax. Appropriate based on risk/benefit assessment. ■ May erode cartilage of weight-bearing joints or cause other signs of arthropathy in infants and children.

Elderly: Safety and effectiveness similar to younger adults. Half-life may be slightly extended because of age-related renal impairment; see Dose Adjustments. Monitoring of renal function may be useful.

DRUG/LAB INTERACTIONS

May cause serious or fatal reactions with theophylline (e.g., cardiac arrhythmias or arrest, respiratory failure, or seizures). If must be used concomitantly, monitor serum levels of theophylline and decrease dose as appropriate. Observe closely with caffeine intake; has caused similar problems. ▪ Use with cyclosporine may cause an increase in SrCr and nephrotoxic effects. ▪ May potentiate oral anticoagulants (e.g., warfarin [Coumadin]); monitor PT/INR. ▪ Potentiated by probenicid; may require dose adjustment based on ciprofloxacin serum levels. ▪ Serum levels may be decreased with antineoplastic agents (e.g., cisplatin, doxorubicin [Adriamycin]). ▪ Serum levels may be increased with cimetidine (Tagamet). ▪ Severe hypoglycemia has been reported with concomitant use of glyburide (DiaBeta, Micronase), monitor serum glucose levels. ▪ May increase or decrease serum phenytoin levels; monitor phenytoin levels with concomitant use. ▪ Two case reports suggest concurrent administration with foscarnet (Foscavir) may cause seizures; monitor patient carefully. ▪ Risk of CNS stimulation and seizures may be increased with concurrent use of NSAIDs (e.g., ibuprofen [Advil, Motrin], naproxen [Aleve, Naprosyn]). ▪ May cause a false-positive when testing for opiates. ▪ See Side Effects.

SIDE EFFECTS

Allergic reactions (anaphylaxis, cardiovascular collapse, death, dyspnea, edema [facial or pharyngeal], eosinophilia, fever, hepatic necrosis, itching, jaundice, loss of consciousness, rash, urticaria); cardiac arrest; CNS stimulation (confusion, hallucinations, lightheadedness, restlessness, seizures, tingling, toxic psychosis, tremors); decreased hemoglobin, hematocrit, and platelet count; diarrhea; elevation of eosinophil and platelet counts, blood glucose, BUN, serum creatine, serum creatine phosphokinase, serum potassium, uric acid, and triglycerides; headache; hepatic enzyme abnormalities (elevation of alkaline phosphatase, AST [SGOT], ALT [SGPT], LDH, serum bilirubin); increased intracranial pressure; local site reactions; myalgias; nausea; photosensitivity and vision changes; postural hypotension; pseudomembranous colitis; respiratory failure; status epilepticus; tendinitis and tendon rupture. Capable of numerous other reactions in less than 1% of patients.

ANTIDOTE

Death may result from some of these side effects. Discontinue ciprofloxacin at the first appearance of a skin rash or any other sign of hypersensitivity, at the onset of any CNS symptom, or the onset of pseudomembranous colitis. Treat allergic reaction with epinephrine (Adrenalin), airway management, oxygen, IV fluids, antihistamines (diphenhydramine [Benadryl]), corticosteroids (Solu-Cortef), and pressor amines (dopamine [Intropin]) as indicated. Treat CNS symptoms as indicated. May require diazepam (Valium) for seizures. Mild cases of colitis may respond to discontinuation of ciprofloxacin. Oral vancomycin (Vancocin) or metronidazole (Flagyl) is the treatment of choice for antibiotic-related pseudomembranous colitis. Keep physician informed of all side effects. Many will require symptomatic treatment; monitor closely. Maintain hydration in overdose. No specific antidote; up to 10% may be excreted by hemodialysis or peritoneal dialysis. Maintain patient until drug excreted.

CISATRACURIUM BESYLATE

(sis-a-tra-kyoor′ee-um bes′uh-lat)

Neuromuscular blocking agent (nondepolarizing)
Anesthesia adjunct

Nimbex

pH 3.25 to 3.65

USUAL DOSE

Must be individualized based on previous drugs administered (e.g., fentanyl [Sublimaze], midazolam [Versed]), desired time to intubation, and anticipated length of surgery. Must be used with adequate anesthesia and/or sedation and after unconsciousness induced. Use of a peripheral nerve stimulator is indicated in all situations.

ADJUNCT TO PROPOFOL/N_2O/O_2 ANESTHESIA FOR ADULTS (IV BOLUS)

Initial dose: 0.15 to 0.2 mg/kg. 0.15 mg/kg should provide good to excellent conditions for intubation within 2 minutes and adequate muscle relaxation for 55 minutes (range 44 to 74 min). 0.2 mg/kg (7 ml [of a 2 mg/ml conc] for a 70-kg patient) should be effective within 1.5 minutes and last for 61 minutes (range 41 to 81 min). Up to 0.4 mg/kg has been used; has a dose-related length of effectiveness.

Maintenance dose: May be given by IV bolus or as a continuous infusion. Determine need for maintenance dose based on beginning symptoms of neuromuscular blockade reversal determined by a peripheral nerve stimulator. Usually required 40 to 60 minutes after a bolus dose. Do not administer before recovery begins. Repeated doses have no cumulative effect if recovery is allowed to begin before administration. See Dose Adjustments. ***IV bolus:*** 0.03 mg/kg (1 ml [of a 2 mg/ml conc] for a 70-kg patient) should provide an additional 20 minutes of muscle relaxation. Smaller or larger doses may be given based on expected duration of procedure. ***Continuous infusion:*** Begin infusion with 3 mcg/kg/min to rapidly counteract the spontaneous recovery, then decrease to 1 to 2 mcg/kg/min. Monitor maintenance infusion with a peripheral nerve stimulator.

SUPPORT OF INTUBATED, MECHANICALLY VENTILATED, OR RESPIRATORY CONTROLLED ADULT ICU PATIENTS

After intubation is accomplished (usually with succinylcholine), an initial bolus dose of 0.1 mg/kg provides adequate neuromuscular blockade. Maintain with 3 mcg/kg/min (range 0.5 to 10.2 mcg/kg/min). Published reports describe a wide interpatient variability in dosing requirements that may change from day to day. Adjust infusion rate according to clinical assessment of the patient's response. Use of a peripheral nerve stimulator is recommended. Do not increase dose until there is a definite response to nerve stimulation. If recovery from neuromuscular block has progressed, readministration of a bolus dose may be necessary. Long-term use (beyond 6 days) has not been studied.

PEDIATRIC DOSE

ADJUNCT TO HALOTHANE OR OPIOID ANESTHESIA FOR CHILDREN 2 TO 12 YEARS OF AGE

Initial dose: 0.1 mg/kg as an IV bolus. Should provide good to excellent conditions for intubation within 2.8 minutes and adequate muscle relaxation for 28 minutes (range 21 to 38 minutes). See all comments under Usual Dose and Maternal/Child.

Maintenance dose: Same as adult dosing; See all comments. *Continued*

DOSE ADJUSTMENTS

Reduce initial dose to 0.02 mg/kg in any condition that may result in a prolonged neuromuscular blockade (e.g., myasthenia gravis, myasthenic syndrome, carcinomatosis, debilitation, other drugs). Use a peripheral nerve stimulator to assess the level of neuromuscular block and to monitor dose requirements. See Drug/Lab Interactions. ▪ Increased initial and maintenance doses may be required in burn patients. Duration of action may be shortened. ▪ Half-life is extended but no dose adjustment is required in patients with renal or hepatic disease or in the elderly. Time of onset may be slightly faster in patients with liver disease and slower in the elderly and patients with renal disease. Slower onset may require a delay of an additional minute before intubation. ▪ Reduce maintenance dose by 30% to 40% in the presence of isoflurane or enflurane anesthesia. Larger reductions may be indicated in prolonged anesthesia. ▪ May need to reduce maintenance dose by 50% in patients undergoing coronary artery bypass surgery with induced hypothermia.

DILUTION

IV bolus: May be given undiluted.

Infusion: Further dilute in NS, D5W, or D5NS to a 0.1 mg/ml or 0.4 mg/ml solution. Using the 2 mg/ml solution, 10 mg diluted in 95 ml yields 0.1 mg/ml; 40 mg diluted in 80 ml yields 0.4 mg/ml.

ICU infusion: A 20-ml vial (10 mg/ml concentration) is available for use in ICU (200 mg/vial). 200 mg in 1,000 ml yields 0.2 mg/ml, in 500 ml yields 0.4 mg/ml.

Storage: Refrigerate in carton before use; protect from light; do not freeze. Use within 21 days if at room temperature even if it was rerefrigerated. Most diluted solutions are stable refrigerated or at room temperature for 24 hours.

INCOMPATIBLE WITH

Manufacturer lists propofol (Diprivan) and ketorolac (Toradol). Has an acid pH and may not be compatible with alkaline solutions having a pH greater than 8.5 (e.g., aminophylline, barbiturates, sodium bicarbonate).

COMPATIBLE WITH

(Underline Indicates Conflicting Compatibility Information)

Consult pharmacist; specific conditions may apply; see Compatibilities, p. xvi.

Manufacturer lists alfentanil (Alfenta), droperidol (Inapsine), fentanyl (Sublimaze), midazolam (Versed), and sufentanil (Sufenta) as compatible but does not specify additive or Y-site.

Y-site: Other sources list acyclovir (Zovirax), alfentanil (Alfenta), amikacin (Amikin), aminophylline, amphotericin B (Fungizone), ampicillin, ampicillin/sulbactam (Unasyn), aztreonam (Azactam), bretylium (Bretylate), bumetanide (Bumex), buprenorphine (Buprenex), butorphanol (Stadol), calcium gluconate, cefazolin (Kefzol), cefotaxime (Claforan), cefotetan (Cefotan), cefoxitin (Mefoxin), ceftazidime (Fortaz), ceftizoxime (Cefizox), ceftriaxone (Rocephin), cefuroxime (Zinacef), chlorpromazine (Thorazine), cimetidine (Tagamet), ciprofloxacin (Cipro IV), clindamycin (Cleocin), dexamethasone (Decadron), diazepam (Valium), digoxin (Lanoxin), diphenhydramine (Benadryl), dobutamine (Dobutrex), dopamine (Intropin), doxycycline (Vibramycin), droperidol (Inapsine), enalaprilat

(Vasotec IV), epinephrine (Adrenalin), esmolol (Brevibloc), famotidine (Pepcid IV), fentanyl (Sublimaze), fluconazole (Diflucan), furosemide (Lasix), ganciclovir (Cytovene), gatifloxacin (Tequin), gentamicin (Garamycin), haloperidol (Haldol), heparin, hetastarch in electrolytes (Hextend), hydrocortisone sodium succinate (Solu-Cortef), hydromorphone (Dilaudid), imipenem-cilastatin (Primaxin), inamrinone (Inocor), isoproterenol (Isuprel), lidocaine, linezolid (Zyvox), lorazepam (Ativan), magnesium sulfate, mannitol, meperidine (Demerol), methylprednisolone (Solu-Medrol), metoclopramide (Reglan), metronidazole (Flagyl IV), midazolam (Versed), minocycline (Minocin), morphine, nalbuphine (Nubain), nitroglycerin (Nitro-Bid IV), nitroprusside sodium, norepinephrine (Levophed), ofloxacin (Floxin IV), ondansetron (Zofran), phenylephrine (Neo-Synephrine), piperacillin (Pipracil), piperacillin/tazobactam (Zosyn), potassium chloride (KCl), procainamide (Pronestyl), prochlorperazine (Compazine), promethazine (Phenergan), ranitidine (Zantac), remifentanil (Ultiva), sodium bicarbonate, sufentanil (Sufenta), sulfamethoxazole-trimethoprim (Bactrim), theophylline, thiopental (Pentothal), ticarcillin (Ticar), ticarcillin/clavulanate (Timentin), tobramycin (Nebcin), vancomycin (Vancocin), zidovudine (AZT, Retrovir).

RATE OF ADMINISTRATION

IV bolus: A single dose over 5 to 10 seconds.

Infusion for anesthesia adjunct or ICU: Use of a microdrip (60 gtt/ml) or volume infusion pump required. Adjust rate to desired dose based on the following charts for 0.1 mg/ml and 0.4 mg/ml. For 0.2 mg/ml solution in ICU, multiply rates (ml/hr) of 0.1 mg/ml solution by 2 or divide rates (ml/hr) of 0.4 mg/ml solution in half.

Cisatracurium Infusion Rates for a Concentration of 0.1 mg/ml					
	Drug Delivery Rate (mcg/kg/min)				
Patient Weight (kg)	1	1.5	2	3	5
	Infusion Delivery Rate (ml/hr)				
10	6	9	12	18	30
45	27	41	54	81	135
70	42	63	84	126	210
100	60	90	120	180	300

Cisatracurium Infusion Rates for a Concentration of 0.4 mg/ml					
	Drug Delivery Rate (mcg/kg/min)				
Patient Weight (kg)	1	1.5	2	3	5
	Infusion Delivery Rate (ml/hr)				
10	1.5	2.3	3	4.5	7.5
45	6.8	10.1	13.5	20.3	33.8
70	10.5	15.8	21	31.5	52.5
100	15	22.5	30	45	75

ACTIONS

A nondepolarizing skeletal muscle relaxant with intermediate onset and duration of action. An isomer of atracurium (Tracrium) with three times its potency at a mg-for-mg dose. In contrast to most of the other neuromuscular blocking agents, cisatracurium has no clinically significant effect on HR or BP with usual doses even in patients with serious cardiovascular disease, and it also does not produce a dose-related histamine release. Causes paralysis by interfering with neural transmission at the myoneural junction. Produces maximum neuromuscular blockade within 1.5 to 3 minutes and lasts about 50 minutes in adults. Recovery to 75% usually occurs within 30 minutes. Metabolized by a process that mostly bypasses both the kidney and the liver. Forms specific metabolites (e.g., alcohol, laudanosine) that do not have neuromuscular blocking activity. Because of reduced dose requirements, laudanosine accumulation is lower than with atracurium, lowering the potential of seizures. Eliminated renally, primarily as metabolites.

INDICATIONS AND USES

Adjunctive to general anesthesia for inpatients and outpatients to facilitate endotracheal intubation and to relax skeletal muscles during surgery. ■ Relax skeletal muscles during mechanical ventilation in ICU.

CONTRAINDICATIONS

Known hypersensitivity to cisatracurium, other bis-benzylisoquinolinium compounds (e.g., atracurium), and benzyl alcohol (some preparations contain benzyl alcohol).

PRECAUTIONS

For IV use only. ■ Administered by or under the observation of the anesthesiologist. Adequate facilities, emergency resuscitation drugs and equipment, neuromuscular blocking antagonists (e.g., anticholinesterase agents [e.g., neostigmine, edrophonium]), and atropine must always be available. ■ Not recommended for rapid sequence intubation; succinylcholine is usually the drug of choice. ■ Myasthenia gravis and other neuromuscular diseases increase sensitivity to cisatracurium. Can cause critical reactions. ■ Sensitivity may be decreased in patients with burns or paralysis. See Dose Adjustments and Monitor. ■ In patients with renal or hepatic disease, half-life of metabolites is longer, and concentrations may be higher with long-term administration. ■ Did not trigger malignant hypertension (MH) in susceptible pigs at doses above those required for humans, but has not been studied in MH-susceptible humans. ■ Respiratory depression with propofol (Diprivan) or morphine may be preferred in some patients requiring mechanical ventilation. ■ Will not counteract the bradycardia produced by many anesthetic agents or vagal stimulation.

Monitor: This drug produces apnea. Controlled artificial ventilation with oxygen must be continuous and under direct observation at all times. Maintain a patent airway. ■ Use a peripheral nerve stimulator to monitor drug effect, determine the need for additional doses, confirm recovery from neuromuscular block, and avoid overdose. Place on a nonparalyzed limb in patients with paralysis. ■ Monitor vital signs and ECG continuously. ■ Has no analgesic properties or effect on consciousness. Use in conjunction with anesthesia, sedation, or analgesia as indicated. ■ Action potentiated by hypokalemia and some carcinomas. ■ Action may be potentiated or antagonized by dehydration, electrolyte imbalance, body temperature, or acid-base imbalance.

Maternal/Child: Category B: use in pregnancy only if clearly needed. Safety for use during labor and delivery not established. ■ Use caution during breast-feeding; probably best to defer breast-feeding until after full recovery. ■ Safety for use in infants under 2 years of age not established. ■ 10 ml (2 mg/ml) multiple dose vials contain benzyl alcohol; do not use in newborns. ■ In children 2 to 12 years of age, onset is faster, duration shorter, and recovery faster than in adults.

Elderly: Safely administered even in patients with significant cardiac disease. ■ Onset to complete neuromuscular block slightly slower; delay intubation until fully effective. Recovery may be slower.

DRUG/LAB INTERACTIONS

Potentiated by general anesthetics (e.g., enflurane, isoflurane), many antibiotics (e.g., aminoglycosides [kanamycin (Kantrex), gentamicin (Garamycin)], lincosamides [clindamycin (Cleocin)], polypeptides [bacitracin, colistimethate], tetracyclines), muscle relaxants, diuretics, lithium, local anesthetics, magnesium sulfate, procainamide (Pronestyl), quinidine, succinylcholine, and others. May need to reduce initial or maintenance dose of cisatracurium; use with caution. ■ Antagonized by acetylcholine and anticholinesterases. ■ Duration of neuromuscular block may be shorter and dose requirements may be higher during maintenance infusion in patients stabilized on carbamazepine (Tegretol) or phenytoin (Dilantin). ■ Time to onset of maximum block is faster when succinylcholine is given before cisatracurium. Succinylcholine must show signs of wearing off before cisatracurium is given. Use caution.

SIDE EFFECTS

Bradycardia, bronchospasm, flushing, hypotension, and rash occurred in fewer than 1% of patients. Both inadequate and/or prolonged neuromuscular blocks have been reported. Rare reports of seizures with similar agents in ICU could be caused by accumulated laudanosine, other conditions, or medications. Excessive dosing or prolonged action may result in respiratory insufficiency or apnea. Airway closure may be caused by relaxation of epiglottis, pharynx, and tongue muscles. Hypersensitivity reactions have been reported.

ANTIDOTE

Side effects can be medical emergencies. Treat symptomatically. Maintain a patent airway and continuous controlled artificial ventilation and oxygenation until full recovery is ensured. The more profound the neuromuscular block, the longer it will take until recovery begins. Recovery from neuromuscular block must be confirmed by a peripheral nerve stimulator before anticholinesterase agents (e.g., neostigmine [Prostigmin] or edrophonium [Enlon]) can be given with an anticholinergic agent (e.g., atropine) to reverse the muscle relaxation. Neostigmine 0.04 to 0.07 mg/kg at 10% recovery in conjunction with atropine should be effective in 9 to 10 minutes. Edrophonium 1 mg/kg at 25% recovery in conjunction with atropine (Enlon-Plus is edrophonium and atropine combined) should be effective in 3 to 5 minutes. Confirm recovery by 5-second head lift and grip strength. Recovery may be inhibited by cachexia, carcinomatosis, debilitation, or the concomitant use of certain drugs; see Drug/Lab Interactions. Resuscitate as necessary.

CISPLATIN

(sis′pla-tin)

CDDP, ✦Platinol, Platinol-AQ

Antineoplastic (alkylating agent)

pH 3.5 to 6

USUAL DOSE

Prehydration required; see Precautions and Monitor. See Dose Adjustments. May be given in combination with amifostine (Ethyol) to reduce nephrotoxicity and neurotoxicity of cisplatin. See amifostine monograph. Do not exceed 120 mg/M^2 as a total dose during each course of cisplatin (every 3 to 4 weeks).

Metastatic testicular tumors: 20 mg/M^2 daily for 5 days every 3 weeks for 3 courses. Bleomycin and vinblastine also indicated. Other combinations are in use.

Metastatic ovarian tumors: 75 to 100 mg/M^2 on day 1 every 4 weeks. Used in combination with cyclophosphamide (Cytoxan) 600 mg/M^2 IV on day 1 every 4 weeks. Another regimen uses paclitaxel 135 mg/M^2 (as a 24-hour infusion) followed by cisplatin 75 mg/M^2. Both agents are given once every 3 weeks for 6 courses. See paclitaxel monograph; premedication required. Used as a ***single agent,*** the dose of cisplatin is 100 mg/M^2 every 4 weeks.

First-line treatment of ovarian cancer: Given in combination with paclitaxel as follows: give paclitaxel (Taxol) 135 mg/M^2 as an infusion over 3 hours. Follow with cisplatin 75 mg/M^2 as an infusion over 24 hours. Repeat every 3 weeks. See paclitaxel monograph; premedication required. Other dose combinations and infusion times are being used.

Advanced bladder cancer: 50 to 70 mg/M^2 once every 3 to 4 weeks. 50 mg/M^2 is recommended once every 4 weeks for patients heavily pretreated with radiation or chemotherapy. Numerous other doses and combinations are used.

Non–small-cell lung cancer: Given in combination with gemcitabine as follows: gemcitabine (Gemzar) 1,000 mg/M^2 as an infusion on days 1, 8, and 15 of each 28-day cycle. Follow the gemcitabine infusion on day 1 with cisplatin 100 mg/M^2. See gemcitabine monograph; other dosing schedules are in use. Another regimen uses a combination of paclitaxel and cisplatin as follows: paclitaxel 135 mg/M^2 as an infusion over 24 hours followed by cisplatin 75 mg/M^2 over 6 to 8 hours. Repeat every 3 weeks. See paclitaxel monograph; premedication required. Recently approved for use with docetaxel 75 mg/M^2 infused over 1 hour followed immediately by an infusion of cisplatin 75 mg/M^2 over 30 to 60 minutes. Repeat every 3 weeks. See docetaxel monograph; premedication required.

Fallopian tube and peritoneal cancers of ovarian origin (unlabeled): Given in combination with paclitaxel as follows. Give paclitaxel 135 to 175 mg/M^2 as an infusion over 3 hours (extend to 24 hours as indicated by toxicity). Follow with cisplatin 50 to 75 mg/M^2. Repeat every 3 to 4 weeks. See paclitaxel monograph; premedication required.

Cancer with an unknown primary site (unlabeled): Cisplatin 60 to 80 mg/M^2 on day 1 or 20 mg/M^2/day for 5 consecutive days (days 1 through 5). Repeat every 3 weeks for 4 to 8 cycles. Usually given in combination with other agents (e.g., bleomycin [Blenoxane], docetaxel [Taxotere], etoposide [VePesid], fluorouracil [5-FU]).

DOSE ADJUSTMENTS

All doses adjusted based on prior radiation therapy or chemotherapy. ■ Initial or repeat doses may not be given unless SrCr is below 1.5 mg/100 ml and/or BUN is below 25 mg/100 ml; platelets should be 100,000/mm^3 and leukocytes 4,000/mm^3; verify auditory acuity as within normal limits. ■ Dosing should be cautious in the elderly. Lower-end initial doses may be indicated. Consider decrease in cardiac, hepatic, and renal function; concomitant disease; or other drug therapy; see Elderly.

DILUTION

Specific techniques required; see Precautions. Initially dilute each 10 (50) mg vial with 10 (50) ml of SW for injection (1 mg/ml). Platinol-AQ is prediluted to 1 mg/ml. Withdraw desired dose. Immediately before use, each one half of a single dose should be diluted in 1 liter of D5/¼NS, D5/½NS, or NS containing 12.5 to 25 Gm of mannitol (optional). Do not use D5W. Will decompose if adequate chloride ion not available. Is also diluted in smaller amounts of NS (100 to 500 ml). Do not use needles or IV tubing with aluminum parts to administer; a precipitate will form, and potency will decrease. See Monitor for additional optional additives.

Storage: Cisplatin remaining in multidose vial is stable at CRT for 28 days protected from light or 7 days under fluorescent light. Do not refrigerate. Diluted solution is stable at room temperature for at least 24 hours; protect from light if it will not be used within 6 hours. Use immediately if contains mannitol.

INCOMPATIBLE WITH

Manufacturer states, "Do not use needles, IV sets, or equipment containing aluminum." A black platinum precipitate will form if cisplatin comes in contact with aluminum. A precipitate will form if reconstituted solutions are refrigerated.

COMPATIBLE WITH **(Underline Indicates Conflicting Compatibility Information)**

Consult pharmacist; specific conditions may apply; see Compatibilities, p. xvi.

Additive: Carboplatin (Paraplatin), cyclophosphamide (Cytoxan), etoposide (VePesid), ifosfamide (Ifex), leucovorin calcium, magnesium sulfate, mannitol, ondansetron (Zofran), <u>paclitaxel (Taxol)</u>. Another source adds carmustine (BiCNU) and potassium chloride (KCl).

Syringe: Bleomycin (Blenoxane), cyclophosphamide (Cytoxan), doxapram (Dopram), doxorubicin (Adriamycin), droperidol (Inapsine), fluorouracil (5-FU), furosemide (Lasix), heparin, leucovorin calcium, methotrexate (Folex), metoclopramide (Reglan), mitomycin (Mutamycin), vinblastine (Velban), vincristine (Oncovin).

Y-site: Allopurinol (Aloprim, Zyloprim), aztreonam (Azactam), bleomycin (Blenoxane), carmustine (BiCNU), chlorpromazine (Thorazine), cimetidine (Tagamet), cladribine (Leustatin), cyclophosphamide (Cytoxan), dexamethasone (Decadron), diphenhydramine (Benadryl), doxorubicin (Adriamycin), doxorubicin liposome (Doxil), droperidol (Inapsine), etoposide (Etopophos, VePesid), famotidine (Pepcid IV), filgrastim (Neupogen), fludarabine (Fludara), fluorouracil (5-FU), furosemide (Lasix), ganciclovir (Cytovene), gatifloxacin (Tequin), gemcitabine (Gemzar), granisetron (Kytril), heparin, hydromorphone (Dilaudid), leucovorin calcium, linezolid (Zyvox), lorazepam (Ativan), melphalan (Alkeran), methotrexate

(Folex), methylprednisolone (Solu-Medrol), metoclopramide (Reglan), mitomycin (Mutamycin), morphine, ondansetron (Zofran), paclitaxel (Taxol), prochlorperazine (Compazine), promethazine (Phenergan), propofol (Diprivan), ranitidine (Zantac), sargramostim (Leukine), teniposide (Vumon), topotecan (Hycamtin), vinblastine (Velban), vincristine (Oncovin), vinorelbine (Navelbine).

RATE OF ADMINISTRATION

Each 1 liter of infusion solution over 3 to 4 hours. Give total dose (2 liters) over 6 to 8 hours. Rate must be sufficient to maintain hydration and diuresis. Solutions from 100 to 500 ml are sometimes given over 30 min. Infusion time has also been extended to 24 hours/dose. Too-rapid administration (5 min) increases nephrotoxicity and ototoxicity.

ACTIONS

A heavy metal complex (platinum and chloride atoms). Has properties similar to alkylating agents and is cell cycle nonspecific. Concentrates in liver, kidneys, large and small intestines. Little distributes into normal cerebrospinal fluid but can be detected in intracerebral tumors. Heavily protein bound. Only one fourth to one half of the drug is excreted in the urine by the end of 5 days. Secreted in breast milk.

INDICATIONS AND USES

Treatment of metastatic tumors of the testes, ovaries, and advanced bladder cancer. ■ First-line therapy for treatment of advanced cancer of the ovary in combination with paclitaxel. ■ First-line treatment of patients with inoperable, locally advanced, or metastatic non–small-cell lung cancer (NSCLC) in combination with gemcitabine, paclitaxel, or docetaxel. ■ Is used in specific combinations with other chemotherapeutic drugs.

Unlabeled uses: Treatment of cancers of the brain, adrenal cortex, breast, cervix, uterus, endometrium, head and neck, esophagus, lung, skin, prostate, and stomach; sarcomas; non-Hodgkins lymphoma; trophoblastic neoplasms; and numerous other malignancies. Treatment of fallopian tube and peritoneal cancers of ovarian origin and cancers with an unknown primary site.

CONTRAINDICATIONS

Hypersensitivity to cisplatin or other platinum-containing compounds, myelosuppressed patients, pre-existing impaired renal function, or hearing deficit.

PRECAUTIONS

Follow guidelines for handling cytotoxic agents. See Appendix A, p. 1142. ■ Administered by or under the direction of the physician specialist. ■ Adequate facilities and emergency resuscitation equipment and supplies must always be available. ■ Labeling changed to read "Doses greater than 100 mg/M^2/cycle once every 3 to 4 weeks are rarely used." This is an effort to eliminate serious errors resulting from confusion with carboplatin (Paraplatin). ■ Neuropathies may occur with higher doses, greater frequency of average doses, or prolonged therapy. ■ See Elderly.

Monitor: Hydrate patient with 1 to 2 liters of infusion fluid for 8 to 12 hours before injection. Urinary output should exceed 100 to 150 ml/hr. ■ Maintain adequate hydration and urinary output of at least 100 to 200 ml/hr for 24 hours after each dose. ■ The greater the dose, the more hydration is required (e.g., 20 mg/M^2, 1 liter; 40 mg/M^2, 2 liters). Potassium chloride (20 mEq) and magnesium sulfate (8 mEq) are frequently added to predosing fluids and/or cisplatin. ■ In addition to mannitol, furosemide

(Lasix) may be added to cisplatin if fluid overload is a concern. Avoid salt and water depletion. ■ Frequent kidney function tests, blood cell counts, and electrolytes are indicated. Repeat doses based on these studies; see Usual Dose. ■ Nausea and vomiting are frequently severe and prolonged (up to a week). Prophylactic administration of antiemetics recommended. Ondansetron (Zofran), metoclopramide (Reglan), or dexamethasone are effective in most patients. ■ Ototoxicity is cumulative; test hearing before administration and regularly during treatment. Ototoxicity increased in children. ■ Monitor uric acid levels before and during treatment and maintain hydration. Allopurinol may be indicated (preferred agent); see Drug/Lab Interactions. Alkalinization of urine may also be indicated. ■ Observe closely for signs of infection. Prophylactic antibiotics may be indicated pending results of C/S in a febrile neutropenic patient. ■ Monitor for thrombocytopenia (platelet count less than 50,000/mm^3). Initiate precautions to prevent excessive bleeding (e.g., inspect IV sites, skin, and mucous membranes; use extreme care during invasive procedures; test urine, emesis, stool, and secretions for occult blood).

Patient Education: Nonhormonal birth control recommended. ■ See Appendix D, p. 1148.

Maternal/Child: Avoid pregnancy; will produce teratogenic effects on the fetus. Has a mutagenic potential. ■ Discontinue breast-feeding. ■ Ototoxicity increased in children.

Elderly: Dose selection should be cautious; see Dose Adjustments. ■ Response (e.g., effectiveness) is similar to younger adults, but length of survival may be shorter. ■ Incidence of myelosuppression (e.g., severe leukopenia, neutropenia, thrombocytopenia), infectious complications, nephrotoxicity, and peripheral neuropathy may be increased.

DRUG/LAB INTERACTIONS

Ototoxicity and nephrotoxicity are potentiated with other ototoxic or nephrotoxic agents (e.g., aminoglycosides [e.g., gentamicin] and loop diuretics [e.g., furosemide (Lasix), ethacrynic acid (Edecrin)]). Concurrent use not recommended (Lasix is used to control fluid overload, use caution). ■ Serum levels of anticonvulsant agents (e.g., phenytoin [Dilantin]) may become subtherapeutic when used concurrently with cisplatin. Monitor anticonvulsant levels; increased doses may be indicated. ■ Bone marrow toxicity increased with other antineoplastic agents and/or radiation therapy. ■ Synergistic with etoposide (VePesid); may be beneficial. ■ Cisplatin may increase blood uric acid levels. Dose adjustment of antigout agents (e.g., allopurinol, colchicine, probenicid, sulfinpyrazone) may be indicated. Allopurinol may be preferred to uricosuric antigout agents to reduce risk of uric acid nephropathy. ■ May affect renal excretion and increase toxicity of many drugs (e.g., bleomycin, doxorubicin, fluorouracil, methotrexate). ■ Concurrent use with high-dose cytarabine may increase ototoxicity. ■ Myelotoxicity may be increased if administered before paclitaxel rather than after. Response duration may be shortened with concurrent use of pyridoxine (vitamin B_6) and altretamine (Hexalen). ■ Do not administer live-virus vaccines to patients receiving antineoplastic agents.

SIDE EFFECTS

Are frequent; can occur with the initial dose and will become more severe with succeeding doses. Alopecia, anaphylaxis (facial edema, hypotension, tachycardia, and wheezing within minutes of administration), asthenia, hyperuricemia, malaise, myelosuppression, nausea and vomiting, nephrotoxicity (often noted in the second week after a dose), ototoxicity including tinnitus and hearing loss in the high-frequency range, and peripheral neuropathy (may be irreversible).

ANTIDOTE

Notify physician of all side effects. Cisplatin may have to be discontinued permanently or until recovery. Symptomatic and supportive treatment is indicated. Administration of whole blood products (e.g., packed RBCs, platelets, leukocytes) and/or blood modifiers (e.g., darbepoetin alfa [Aranesp], epoetin alfa [Epogen, Procrit], filgrastim [Neupogen], pegfilgrastim [Neulasta], sargramostim [Leukine], oprelvekin [Neumega]) may be indicated to treat bone marrow toxicity. Pretreatment with amifostine may reduce nephrotoxic, neurotoxic, and hematologic effects. Treat anaphylaxis with epinephrine, corticosteroids, oxygen, and antihistamines. There is no specific antidote. Hemodialysis may be somewhat helpful in the first 1 to 1½ hours after administration.

CLADRIBINE

(kla'dri-been)

Antineoplastic (antimetabolite)

Leustatin

pH 5.7 to 6.9

USUAL DOSE

In all situations, may be administered on an outpatient basis with an appropriate pump and a central venous line in place. Administer any subsequent course with extreme caution. Hematologic recovery must be considered.

Hairy cell leukemia: 0.1 mg/kg/24 hr equally distributed as a continuous infusion over 24 hours. Repeat daily for 7 consecutive days. Usually only one course of treatment is given.

Chronic multiple sclerosis (orphan designation): Dose and process is the same as for hairy cell leukemia except the regimen is repeated once each month for 4 months.

Non-Hodgkin's lymphoma (unlabeled): Dose and process is the same as for hairy cell leukemia except regimen is repeated every 28 days.

DOSE ADJUSTMENTS

May be required in subsequent courses, with severe bone marrow impairment, with prior radiation or myelosuppressive agents. ■ May be required in severe renal insufficiency; effects of renal or hepatic impairment on excretion of cladribine not yet clarified for humans. ■ See Drug/Lab Interactions.

DILUTION

Specific techniques required; see Precautions. Available in single-use 10-ml vials containing 10 mg (1 mg/ml). Contains no preservatives; aseptic technique imperative. May develop a precipitate at low temperatures. Warm naturally to room temperature and shake vigorously. Do not heat or microwave.

Inpatient continuous infusion: A single daily calculated dose must be added to 500 ml of NS.

Outpatient continuous infusion: A total 7-day dose is added to a calculated amount of bacteriostatic NS to make a total volume of 100 ml. Specific equipment (i.e., a sterile medication reservoir and pump capable of delivering accurate minute amounts into a central venous line [presently using Pharmacia Deltec medication cassette with Pharmacia Deltec pump]) and a specific process including the use of a 0.22-micron syringe filter are required. Preparation of cassette usually done by pharmacist. Line of cassette remains clamped until attached to central venous line and pump is functional. See literature for details and follow all specific instructions for medication pump.

Storage: Protect from light. Refrigerate or freeze before reconstitution. Never refreeze. Discard any unused concentrate. ***500 ml dilution*** may be refrigerated for up to 8 hours after dilution. Immediate use preferred. ***100 ml dilution*** is stable in reservoir of medication cassette for 7 days if correctly diluted.

INCOMPATIBLE WITH

D5W will cause degradation of cladribine. Manufacturer states, "Adherence to the recommended diluents and infusion systems is advised."

COMPATIBLE WITH

Consult pharmacist; specific conditions may apply; see Compatibilities, p. xvi.

Y-site: Aminophylline, bumetanide (Bumex), buprenorphine (Buprenex), butorphanol (Stadol), calcium gluconate, carboplatin (Paraplatin), chlorpromazine (Thorazine), cimetidine (Tagamet), cisplatin (Platinol), cyclophosphamide (Cytoxan), cytarabine (ARA-C), dexamethasone (Decadron), diphenhydramine (Benadryl), dobutamine (Dobutrex), dopamine (Intropin), doxorubicin (Adriamycin), droperidol (Inapsine), enalaprilat (Vasotec IV), etoposide (VePesid), famotidine (Pepcid IV), furosemide (Lasix), granisetron (Kytril), haloperidol (Haldol), heparin, hydrocortisone (Hydrocortone, Solu-Cortef), hydromorphone (Dilaudid), idarubicin (Idamycin), leucovorin calcium, lorazepam (Ativan), mannitol, meperidine (Demerol), mesna (Mesnex), methylprednisolone (Solu-Medrol), metoclopramide (Reglan), mitoxantrone (Novantrone), morphine, nalbuphine (Nubain), ondansetron (Zofran), paclitaxel (Taxol), potassium chloride (KCl), prochlorperazine (Compazine), promethazine (Phenergan), ranitidine (Zantac), sodium bicarbonate, teniposide (Vumon), vincristine (Oncovin).

RATE OF ADMINISTRATION

Inpatient continuous infusion: A single dose properly diluted evenly distributed as an infusion over 24 hours.

Outpatient continuous infusion: Administered through a central venous line (very concentrated solution). Medication reservoir and pump required (presently using Pharmacia Deltec medication cassette and pump worn as a portable pack). Set rate for equal distribution of 100 ml over 7 days. Follow all specific instructions for pump.

ACTIONS

A synthetic antineoplastic agent. Mechanism of action is not known, but it is believed to be cytotoxic by inhibition of DNA synthesis and the accumulation of DNA strand breaks. Affects both dividing and resting cells. The 7-day course for hairy cell leukemia has resulted in complete remissions in a majority of patients with no evidence of persistent bone marrow disease. May potentially be a cure. Improvements in neurologic symptoms are occurring in patients with multiple sclerosis. In all situations time to response is about 4 months. Has immunosuppressant activity. Lymphocyte subsets (e.g., CD4, CD8 T cells) are affected; may take 6 to 12 months for full recovery. Crosses the blood-brain barrier. Average half-life is 5.4 hours. Metabolized in all cells. Specific methods of metabolism and routes of excretion are not known. Some drug does appear in urine.

INDICATIONS AND USES

Treatment of hairy cell leukemia (HCL). ■ Management of chronic multiple sclerosis *(orphan designation).*

Unlabeled uses: Treatment of non-Hodgkin's lymphoma.

CONTRAINDICATIONS

Hypersensitivity to cladribine or any of its components; neonates (7 day dilution contains benzyl alcohol).

PRECAUTIONS

Follow guidelines for handling cytotoxic agents. See Appendix A, p. 1142. ■ Administered by or under the direction of the physician specialist. ■ Anticipate severe suppression of bone marrow function, including neutropenia, anemia, and thrombocytopenia. ■ Because of the possibility of increased toxicity, use caution in known or suspected renal insufficiency, or any severe bone marrow impairment, or prior cytoxic or radiation therapy. ■ Appears to be no relationship between serum concentrations and ultimate clinical outcome. ■ Additional courses did not improve overall response. ■ Current studies suggest that overall response rate may be decreased in patients previously treated with splenectomy, deoxycoformycin (pentostatin), and in patients refractory to alpha-interferon. ■ May cause prolonged bone marrow hypocellularity; clinical significance not known.

Monitor: Obtain baseline CBC with differential (including CD4 and CD8 T cell counts) and platelets before therapy. May be repeated as indicated, but usually not required again until 7 or 8 days after treatment begins; then monitor as indicated for at least 4 to 8 weeks (anemia, neutropenia, thrombocytopenia, infection [bacterial, fungal, or viral], and bleeding are common and must be treated promptly). Monitoring schedule facilitates outpatient treatment; keep in close contact with patient. ■ Consider possibility of infection if fever occurs; appropriate lab tests, x-rays and broad-spectrum antibiotics may be indicated in suspected infection. ■ Monitor uric acid levels before and during treatment, maintain hydration; allopurinol may be indicated (preferred agent). Alkalinization of urine may also be indicated. ■ Monitor renal and hepatic function periodically. ■ Take precautions and limit invasive procedures in any patient with thrombocytopenia. Avoid constipation, and avoid alcohol and aspirin (risk of GI bleeding). ■ Platelet count usually returns to normal in 12 days (may be delayed if severe baseline thrombocytopenia was present), neutrophil count usually returns to normal in 5 weeks, and hemoglobin in 8 weeks. All should be normal by 9 weeks. ■ Complete response is indicated by an absence of hairy cells in bone marrow and peripheral blood and normalization of peripheral blood parameters. Confirm response with bone marrow aspiration and biopsy between 9 weeks and 4 months. ■ Prophylactic antiemetics may improve patient comfort. ■ Monitor for thrombocytopenia (platelet count less than 50,000/mm^3). Initiate precautions to prevent excessive bleeding (e.g., inspect IV sites, skin, and mucous membranes; use extreme care during invasive procedures; test urine, emesis, stool, and secretions for occult blood).

Patient Education: Avoid pregnancy; consider birth control options and future fertility. ■ Report fever, bleeding, cough, edema, injection site reactions, malaise, mouth sores, rashes, shortness of breath, stomach pain, and tachycardia promptly. Maintain hydration. ■ Manufacturer supplies a patient education booklet; review thoroughly and discuss with physician and nurse. ■ Review all literature provided with pump to deliver outpatient dosing. ■ See Appendix D, p. 1148.

Maternal/Child: Category D: avoid pregnancy; has potential to cause fetal harm. Has caused suppression of testicular cells in monkeys; effect on human fertility unknown. ■ Discontinue breast-feeding. ■ Safety for use in children not established. Investigationally used in higher doses to treat relapsed acute leukemia. Dose-limiting toxicity occurred.

Elderly: Geriatric-specific problems not encountered in studies to date. Consider age-related organ impairment.

DRUG/LAB INTERACTIONS

Increased toxicity with other myelosuppressive agents (e.g., methotrexate). ■ May raise concentration of blood uric acid, increased doses of antigout agents (e.g., allopurinol [Zyloprim]) may be indicated; avoid uricosurics (e.g., probenicid, sulfinpyrazone [Anturane]). ■ Do not administer live vaccines to patients receiving antineoplastic agents.

SIDE EFFECTS

Fever (69%) occurs first. Onset of thrombocytopenia (12%) begins in 7 to 10 days followed by anemia (severe [37%]) and neutropenia (severe [70%]). Fatigue (45%), headache (22%), injection site reactions (19%), infection (28%), nausea (28%), and rash (27%) are common. Many other side effects may or may not be related to cladribine; abdominal pain (6%), abnormal breath sounds (11%), abnormal chest sounds (9%), anorexia (17%), arthralgia (5%), chills (9%), constipation (9%), cough (10%), diaphoresis (9%), diarrhea (10%), dizziness (9%), edema (6%), epistaxis (5%), erythema (6%), insomnia (7%), malaise (7%), myalgia (7%), pain (6%), petechiae (8%), pruritus (6%), purpura (10%), shortness of breath (7%), tachycardia (6%), trunk pain (6%), weakness (9%), vomiting (13%).

Overdose: Acute nephrotoxicity, irreversible neurologic toxicity (paraparesis/quadriparesis), severe bone marrow depression (anemia, neutropenia, and thrombocytopenia).

ANTIDOTE

Keep physician informed of all side effects; many will be treated symptomatically as indicated. Platelet or RBC transfusions are frequently required to treat anemia or thrombocytopenia, especially during the first month. Filgrastim (Neupogen) or pegfilgrastim [Neulasta] may be used to increase neutrophil count, although recovery is usually spontaneous. Use specific antibiotics to combat infection. Discontinue cladribine if renal toxicity, neurotoxicity, or overdose occurs. No specific antidote for overdose. Supportive therapy as indicated will help sustain the patient in toxicity. Resuscitate if indicated.

CLINDAMYCIN PHOSPHATE
(klin-da-mye'sin fos'fat)

Antibacterial
Antiprotozoal
(lincosamide)

Cleocin Phosphate

pH 5.5 to 7

USUAL DOSE

Doses based on susceptibility of specific organisms; see literature.

Serious infections: 600 to 1,200 mg/24 hr in 2, 3, or 4 equally divided doses (300 to 600 mg every 12 hours, 200 to 400 mg every 8 hours, or 150 to 300 mg every 6 hours).

More severe infections: 1,200 to 2,700 mg/24 hr in 2, 3, or 4 equally divided doses (600 to 1,350 mg every 12 hours, 400 to 900 mg every 8 hours, or 300 to 675 mg every 6 hours).

Life-threatening infections: Up to 4.8 Gm/24 hr has been given.

Acute pelvic inflammatory disease (unlabeled): 900 mg every 8 hours for at least 4 days. Concurrent administration of 2 mg/kg of gentamicin as an initial dose and 1.5 mg/kg every 8 hours thereafter is recommended. Continue both drugs for at least 48 hours after patient improves. Complete 10- to 14-day treatment program with oral doxycycline or clindamycin.

CNS toxoplasmosis in AIDS (unlabeled): 1,200 to 2,400 mg/24 hr in divided doses (e.g., 300 to 600 mg every 6 hours). Up to 4.8 Gm has been required. Used in combination with pyrimethamine (Daraprim).

***Pneumocystis carinii* pneumonia (unlabeled):** 600 mg every 6 hours or 900 mg every 8 hours. Used in combination with primaquine.

Babesiosis (unlabeled): 1,200 to 2,400 mg/24 hr in 4 equally divided doses (300 to 600 mg every 6 hours). Continue for 7 to 10 days. Used in combination with quinine.

Prophylaxis of bacterial endocarditis: 300 mg IV or PO 30 minutes before procedure and 150 mg IV or PO in 6 hours.

PEDIATRIC DOSE

Minimum recommended dose regardless of weight is 300 mg/24 hr for severe infections.

Children over 1 month of age: 15 to 40 mg/kg of body weight/24 hr in 3 or 4 equally divided doses for serious infections. Alternately 350 mg/M^2/24 hr may be used. 450 mg/M^2/24 hr may be used for more serious infections if necessary.

Bone infections: 7.5 mg/kg every 6 hours.

Babesiosis (unlabeled): A suggested dose is 20 mg/kg/24 hr. Continue for 7 to 10 days. Used in combination with 25 mg/kg/24 hr of oral quinine.

Prophylaxis of bacterial endocarditis: 10 mg/kg IV or PO 30 minutes before procedure. Give 5 mg/kg IV or PO in 6 hours.

NEONATAL DOSE

Under 1 month of age, full term: 3.75 to 5 mg/kg every 6 hours or 5 to 6.7 mg/kg every 8 hours. Another source suggests:

Infants under 7 days of age weighing less than 2 kg: 5 mg/kg every 12 hours.

Infants under 7 days of age weighing over 2 kg: 5 mg/kg every 8 hours.

Infants over 7 days of age weighing less than 1.2 kg: 5 mg/kg every 12 hours.

Infants over 7 days of age weighing 1.2 to 2 kg: 5 mg/kg every 8 hours.

Infants over 7 days of age weighing over 2 kg: 5 mg/kg every 6 hours.

DOSE ADJUSTMENTS

May be required in severely impaired liver or renal function.

DILUTION

Available prediluted in 300-, 600-, and 900-mg ready-to-use Galaxy bags or ADD-Vantage vials for use with ADD-Vantage infusion containers, or each 18 mg must be reconstituted with a minimum of 1 ml of D5W, NS, or other compatible infusion solution (300 mg with 17 ml diluent, 600 mg with 34 ml, and 900 mg with 50 ml). See chart on inside back cover or product insert for additional diluents. Additional diluent (50 to 100 ml) may be used to decrease concentration, but never exceed a concentration greater than 18 mg/ml. May be further diluted in larger amounts of compatible infusion solutions and given as a continuous infusion after the initial dose.

Storage: Stable at CRT for 24 hours in compatible diluents and infusion solutions.

INCOMPATIBLE WITH

Manufacturer lists aminophylline, ampicillin, barbiturates, calcium gluconate, magnesium sulfate, phenytoin (Dilantin).

COMPATIBLE WITH **(Underline Indicates Conflicting Compatibility Information)**

Consult pharmacist; specific conditions may apply; see Compatibilities, p. xvi.

Solution: Isolyte H, D5/Isolyte M, D5/Isolyte P, Normosol R; see chart on inside back cover.

Additive: Manufacturer states no incompatibility has been demonstrated with gentamicin (Garamycin), kanamycin (Kantrex), or penicillin. Other sources list amikacin (Amikin), <u>ampicillin</u>, aztreonam (Azactam), cefamandole (Mandol), cefazolin (Kefzol), cefepime (Maxipime), cefoperazone (Cefobid), cefotaxime (Claforan), cefoxitin (Mefoxin), ceftazidime (Fortaz), ceftizoxime (Cefizox), cefuroxime (Zinacef), cimetidine (Tagamet), fluconazole (Diflucan), <u>gentamicin (Garamycin)</u>, heparin, hydrocortisone sodium succinate (Solu-Cortef), kanamycin (Kantrex), methylprednisolone (Solu-Medrol), metoclopramide (Reglan), metronidazole (Flagyl IV), ofloxacin (Floxin IV), penicillin G, piperacillin (Pipracil), potassium chloride (KCl), <u>ranitidine (Zantac)</u>, sodium bicarbonate, tobramycin (Nebcin), verapamil (Isoptin).

Syringe: Amikacin (Amikin), aztreonam (Azactam), gentamicin (Garamycin), heparin.

Y-site: Amifostine (Ethyol), amiodarone (Cordarone), amphotericin B cholesteryl (Amphotec), aztreonam (Azactam), cisatracurium (Nimbex), cyclophosphamide (Cytoxan), diltiazem (Cardizem), docetaxel (Taxotere), doxorubicin liposome (Doxil), enalaprilat (Vasotec IV), esmolol (Brevibloc), etoposide phosphate (Etopophos), fludarabine (Fludara), foscarnet (Foscavir), gatifloxacin (Tequin), gemcitabine (Gemzar), granisetron (Kytril), heparin, hetastarch in electrolytes (Hextend), hydromorphone (Dilaudid), labetalol (Normodyne), levofloxacin (Levaquin), linezolid (Zyvox), magnesium sulfate, melphalan (Alkeran), meperidine (Demerol), midazolam (Versed), morphine, multivitamins (M.V.I.), ondansetron (Zofran), perphenazine (Trilafon), piperacillin/tazobactam (Zosyn), propofol (Diprivan), remifentanil (Ultiva), sargramostim (Leukine), tacrolimus (Prograf), teniposide (Vumon), theophylline, thiotepa (Thioplex), vinorelbine (Navelbine), zidovudine (AZT, Retrovir).

RATE OF ADMINISTRATION

Severe hypotension and cardiac arrest can occur with too-rapid injection.

Intermittent infusion: 30 mg or fraction thereof over at least 1 minute (each 300 mg over a minimum of 10 minutes/1,200 mg over a minimum of 40 to 60 minutes). Do not give more than 1,200 mg in single 1-hour infusion.
Continuous infusion: Administer initial dose at 10 (15 or 20) mg/min over 30 minutes. Will result in serum levels above 4 (5 or 6) mg/ml. To maintain these serum levels, continue infusion at 0.75 (1 or 1.25) mg/min.

ACTIONS

A semisynthetic antibiotic that quickly converts to active clindamycin. It inhibits protein synthesis in the bacterial cell, producing irreversible changes in the protein-synthesizing ribosomes. Widely distributed in most body fluids, tissues, and bones. There is no clinically effective distribution to cerebrospinal fluid. Excreted in urine and feces in small amounts. Most excreted in inactive form in the urine. Crosses placental barrier. Secreted in breast milk.

INDICATIONS AND USES

Treatment of serious infections caused by susceptible anaerobic bacteria; or susceptible aerobic bacterial infections in penicillin-allergic patients; or infections that do not respond or are resistant to other less toxic antibiotics, such as penicillins or cephalosporins. ■ Treatment of acute pelvic inflammatory disease. ■ Prophylaxis of bacterial endocarditis.
Unlabeled uses: Alternative to sulfonamides with pyrimethamine to treat CNS toxoplasmosis in AIDS patients. ■ Treat *Pneumocystis carinii* pneumonia in combination with primaquine. ■ Treatment of babesiosis.

CONTRAINDICATIONS

Known hypersensitivity to clindamycin or lincomycin. Treatment of minor bacterial or viral infections.

PRECAUTIONS

A highly toxic drug, to be used only when absolutely necessary and when an alternate drug (e.g., erythromycin) is not acceptable. ■ Sensitivity studies indicated to determine susceptibility of the causative organism to clindamycin. ■ Avoid prolonged use; superinfection caused by overgrowth of nonsusceptible organisms may result. ■ Use caution with a history of GI, severe renal, or liver disease, and in patients with a history of asthma or significant allergies. ■ Pseudomembranous colitis has been reported. May range from mild to life-threatening. Consider in patients that present with diarrhea during or after treatment with clindamycin. ■ Not appropriate to treat meningitis.
Monitor: Capable of causing severe, even fatal, colitis; observe for symptoms of diarrhea. ■ Periodic blood cell counts and liver and kidney studies are indicated in prolonged therapy. ■ Each ml contains 9.45 mg benzyl alcohol. Monitor organ system functions if used in infants.
Patient Education: Do not treat diarrhea without notifying physician.
Maternal/Child: Safety for use in pregnancy not established. ■ Best to discontinue breast-feeding, even though considered acceptable by pediatricians. ■ See Monitor before using in infants.
Elderly: Monitor carefully for changes in bowel frequency; may not tolerate diarrhea well.

DRUG/LAB INTERACTIONS

May potentiate other neuromuscular blocking agents (e.g., kanamycin, streptomycin, tubocurarine, mivacurium) and cause profound respiratory depression. ■ Antagonized by erythromycin. ■ May decrease cyclosporine (Sandimmune) levels. Monitor and adjust dose if necessary.

SIDE EFFECTS

Abdominal pain, agranulocytosis, allergic reactions, anaphylaxis, anorexia, azotemia, cardiac arrest, diarrhea, elevated ALT (SGPT), eosinophilia (transient), erythema multiforme, esophagitis, hypotension, jaundice, leukopenia, metallic taste, nausea, neutropenia (transient), oliguria, polyarthritis (rare), pseudomembranous colitis, skin rashes, tenesmus (straining at stool), thrombocytopenic purpura, thrombophlebitis, urticaria, vomiting.

ANTIDOTE

Notify the physician of any side effects. Discontinue the drug if indicated (colitis, diarrhea, allergic reactions, etc.), treat allergic reaction as indicated, and resuscitate as necessary. Do not treat diarrhea with opiates or diphenoxylate with atropine (Lomotil); condition will worsen. Mild cases may respond to discontinuation of drug. Treat antibiotic-related pseudomembranous colitis with fluids, electrolytes, protein supplements, and oral vancomycin or metronidazole (Flagyl IV) as indicated. Stagger administration times to prevent inappropriate binding of vancomycin. Hemodialysis or CAPD will not decrease blood levels in toxicity.

COAGULATION FACTOR VIIa (RECOMBINANT)

Antihemorrhagic

(ko-ag-yew-la′shun fak′ter sev′en a [re-kom′be-nant])

NovoSeven **pH 5.5**

USUAL DOSE

90 mcg/kg every 2 hours until hemostasis is achieved, or until the treatment has been judged to be inadequate. In clinical studies, a decision on outcome was reached for a majority of patients with joint or muscle bleeds within eight doses, although more doses were required for severe bleeds. Doses between 35 and 120 mcg/kg have been used successfully. Minimum effective dose has not been established. For severe bleeds, dosing should continue at 3- to 6-hour intervals after hemostasis is achieved to maintain the hemostatic plug. The appropriate duration of post-hemostatic dosing has not been studied and should be minimized; see Precautions. If a new bleeding episode or rebleeding occurs, return to 2-hour dosing intervals.

PEDIATRIC DOSE

See Usual Dose. Clinical studies were conducted with dosing determined according to body weight and not according to age.

DOSE ADJUSTMENTS

Dose and administration interval may be adjusted based on the severity of the bleeding and the degree of hemostasis achieved. If patient develops intravascular coagulation or thrombosis, dosage should be reduced or treatment stopped; see Monitor.

DILUTION

Aseptic technique is imperative. Available in 1.2- and 4.8-mg vials. Bring vial and SW to CRT. Inject 2.2 ml SW into 1.2-mg vial or 8.5 ml SW into 4.8-mg vial, aiming the needle against the side so that the stream of water runs down the vial wall. Do not inject SW directly onto the powder. Gently swirl vial until powder is completely dissolved. Final concentration following reconstitution is approximately 0.6 mg/ml (600 mcg/ml). Withdraw calculated dose into a syringe for administration by IV injection. **Storage:** Refrigerate before reconstitution. Avoid exposure to direct sunlight. After reconstitution, store at CRT or refrigerate. Should be used within 3 hours. Do not freeze reconstituted product or store in syringe. Discard unused product.

COMPATIBILITY

Manufacturer states, "Intended for IV injection only and should not be mixed with infusion solutions. Do not store reconstituted solution in syringes."

RATE OF ADMINISTRATION

A single dose as a slow IV injection over 2 to 5 minutes, depending on dose administered.

ACTIONS

A vitamin K–dependent glycoprotein structurally similar to human plasma–derived Factor VIIa. Produced by recombinant DNA technology. Promotes hemostasis by activating the extrinsic pathway of the coagulation cascade. When complexed with tissue factor, can activate coagulation Factor X to Factor Xa, and coagulation Factor IX to Factor IXa. Factor Xa, in complex with other factors, then converts prothrombin to thrombin. This leads to the formation of a hemostatic plug by converting fibrinogen to fibrin. Half-life is 2.3 hours. Duration of action is 3 hours.

INDICATIONS AND USES

Treatment of bleeding episodes in hemophilia A or B patients with inhibitors to Factor VIII or Factor IX.

CONTRAINDICATIONS

Hypersensitivity to coagulation factor VIIa (recombinant), any of its components, and in patients with known hypersensitivity to mouse, hamster, or bovine proteins.

PRECAUTIONS

Should be administered to patients only under the direct supervision of a physician experienced in the treatment of hemophilia. ■ The extent of the risk of thrombotic adverse events after treatment is not known, but is considered to be low. Patients with disseminated intravascular coagulation (DIC), advanced atherosclerotic disease, crush injury, or septicemia may have an increased risk of developing thrombotic events due to circulating tissue factor or predisposing coagulopathy. ■ Biologic and clinical effects of prolonged elevated levels of Factor VIIa have not been studied; therefore, the duration of post-hemostatic dosing should be minimized, and patients should be appropriately monitored by a physician experienced in the treatment of hemophilia during this time period.

Monitor: Evaluation of hemostasis should be used to determine the effectiveness of therapy and to provide a basis for modification of the treatment schedule; coagulation parameters do not necessarily correlate with or predict the effectiveness of therapy. Coagulation parameters (e.g., PT, aPTT, plasma FVII clotting activity [FVII:C]) may be used as an adjunct to the clinical evaluation of hemostasis in monitoring the effectiveness and treatment schedule, although these parameters have shown no direct correlation to achieving hemostasis. ■ Monitor patients if they develop signs or symptoms of activation of the coagulation system or thrombosis. When there is laboratory confirmation of intravascular coagulation or presence of clinical thrombosis, dosage should be reduced or the treatment stopped, depending on the patient's symptoms; see Dose Adjustments.

Patient Education: Discuss benefits versus risk of therapy and signs of hypersensitivity reactions including hives, urticaria, chest tightness, wheezing, hypotension, and anaphylaxis.

Maternal/Child: Category C: safety for use during pregnancy and breast-feeding not established. Use only if clearly indicated and benefit justifies potential risk to the fetus. ■ A decision should be made whether to discontinue nursing or to discontinue the drug. ■ The safety and effectiveness was not determined to be different in various age-groups from infants to adolescents (0 to 16 years of age); see Pediatric Dose.

Elderly: Geriatric patients were not enrolled in clinical trials.

DRUG/LAB INTERACTIONS

The risk of potential interaction between Factor VIIa and coagulation factor concentrates has not been adequately evaluated. Simultaneous use of activated prothrombin complex concentrates (e.g., anti-inhibitor coagulant complex [Autoplex-T, Feiba VH]) or prothrombin complex concentrates (e.g., Factor IX [AlphaNine, Benefix]) should be avoided. ■ Although specific drug interactions were not studied in clinical trials, coagulation factor VIIa (recombinant), has been used concomitantly with antifibrinolytic therapies (e.g., tranexamic acid [Cyclokapron], aminocaproic acid [Amicar]).

SIDE EFFECTS

Generally well tolerated. The majority of patients reporting side effects received more than 12 doses. Allergic reaction, arthrosis, bradycardia, coagulation disorder, DIC, edema, fever, decreased fibrinogen plasma, decreased prothrombin, decreased therapeutic response, headache, hemarthrosis, hemorrhage, hypertension, hypotension, increased fibrinolysis, injection site reaction, pain, pneumonia, pruritus, purpura, rash, renal function abnormalities, thrombosis, vomiting.

ANTIDOTE

Discontinue drug and notify physician of any major side effects. Treat allergic reactions as indicated. For thrombosis or DIC, anticoagulation with heparin may be indicated.

CONJUGATED ESTROGENS

(kon′jyou-gay-ted es′troh-jens)

Hormone (estrogen) Antihemorrhagic

Premarin Intravenous — **pH 7.2 to 7.4**

USUAL DOSE

25 mg in 1 injection. May be repeated in 6 to 12 hours if indicated.

DILUTION

Withdraw all air from the vial of powder. Carefully withdraw contents from ampule of sterile diluent provided. Direct flow of diluent gently against the side of the vial of powder. Mix solution by rotating the vial between the palms of the hands. Do not shake. Do not use if discolored or precipitate present.

Storage: Must be refrigerated before and after reconstitution. Most frequently used promptly, but it is stable for up to 60 days if protected from light.

INCOMPATIBLE WITH

Manufacturer lists ascorbic acid (Cenolate), protein hydrolysate, or any solution with an acid pH.

COMPATIBLE WITH

According to the manufacturer, infusion with other agents is not generally recommended. May be given at Y-tube if compatible solutions are infusing.

RATE OF ADMINISTRATION

5 mg or fraction thereof over 1 minute. Must be given direct IV or through IV tubing close to needle site. Infusion solution must be compatible (normal saline, dextrose, and invert sugar solutions). Perineal or vaginal burning may be caused by too-rapid injection.

ACTIONS

Produces a prompt increase in circulating prothrombin and accelerator globulin and decrease in antithrombin activities of the blood. The coagulability of the blood, especially in capillary beds, is enhanced. Promptly corrects bleeding due to estrogen deficiency. Metabolized primarily in the liver and excreted in the urine. Secreted in breast milk.

INDICATIONS AND USES

Dysfunctional uterine bleeding caused by hormonal imbalance in the absence of organic pathology.

Unlabeled uses: Postcoital contraception.

CONTRAINDICATIONS

Breast cancer (except selected metastatic disease), estrogen-dependent neoplasia, pregnancy, thrombophlebitis or thromboembolic disorders, undiagnosed abnormal genital bleeding. Other specific contraindications for estrogens must be considered.

PRECAUTIONS

Dilution in an IV infusion is not recommended. ■ Even though bleeding is controlled, the etiology of the bleeding must be determined and definitive therapy instituted. ■ Follow immediately with oral estrogens as recommended for dysfunctional uterine bleeding. ■ Use with caution in epilepsy, hypercalcemia, migraine, asthma, or cardiac, hepatic, or renal disease; induces salt and water retention. ■ Estrogens may be carcinogenic; use only for specific indications.

Monitor: Monitor VS; may cause a temporary BP elevation.

Maternal/Child: Category X: avoid pregnancy. Safety for use in children not established. Has adverse effects on epiphyseal closure of bone.

DRUG/LAB INTERACTIONS

May decrease effects of oral antidiabetics. ■ Barbiturates (e.g., phenobarbital), phenytoin (Dilantin), and rifampin (Rifadin) increase metabolism and decrease serum levels and effects. ■ May decrease metabolism and increase serum levels of cyclosporine. May increase risk of cyclosporine toxicity. ■ Increased risk of hepatotoxicity with other hepatotoxic agents (e.g., dantrolene [Dantrium]). ■ May increase blood glucose levels and serum lipids.

SIDE EFFECTS

Rare when used as directed; flushing, nausea, vomiting.

ANTIDOTE

No toxicity has been reported throughout years of clinical use. Discontinue if jaundice occurs.

COSYNTROPIN

(koe-sin-troe′pin)

Cortrosyn

Diagnostic agent (adrenocorticotropic)

pH 5.5 to 7.5

USUAL DOSE

250 mcg (0.25 mg). Up to 750 mcg (0.75 mg) has been used.

PEDIATRIC DOSE

Children over 2 years of age: May use adult dose, but 125 mcg (0.125 mg) is usually adequate.

Children under 2 years of age: 125 mcg (0.125 mg). Usually given IM.

DILUTION

Dilute vial with a minimum of 1.1 ml NS. May dilute with 2 to 5 ml of NS. May be given directly IV after this initial dilution or further diluted in D5W or NS and given as an infusion (250 mcg in 250 ml equals 1 mcg/ml).

Storage: Discard unused reconstituted cosyntropin.

COMPATIBILITY

Manufacturer states, "Should not be added to blood or plasma; may be inactivated by enzymes." Consider specific use.

RATE OF ADMINISTRATION

IV injection: A single dose over 2 minutes.

Infusion: A single dose evenly distributed over 4 to 8 hours.

ACTIONS

A synthetic form of adrenocorticotropic hormone (ACTH). Stimulates the adrenal cortex to secrete adrenocortical hormone. Does not increase cortisol secretion in patients with primary adrenocortical insufficiency. Peak plasma cortisol levels occur in 1 hour after cosyntropin dose in patients with normal renal function.

INDICATIONS AND USES

Diagnostic aid for adrenocortical insufficiency.

CONTRAINDICATIONS

Hypersensitivity to cosyntropin.

PRECAUTIONS

Preferable to ACTH because it is less likely to cause allergic reactions. ■ May be used in patients who have had an allergic reaction to ACTH. ■ Infusion method used if greater stimulus needed to effect results. ■ May be used IM as a rapid screening test for adrenal function; see package insert.

Monitor: Continuous observation for at least the first 30 minutes is mandatory. Observe frequently thereafter. ■ Check BP frequently; may cause elevated BP and salt water retention. ■ Diabetes may require increased insulin or oral hypoglycemics. ■ Monitor correct collection of specimens. ■ See Drug/Lab Interactions.

Patient Education: May mask signs of infection. ■ May decrease resistance. ■ Avoid immunization with live vaccines.

Maternal/Child: Use caution in pregnancy and breast-feeding.

DRUG/LAB INTERACTIONS

Plasma cortisol may be falsely elevated for patients taking spironolactone when fluorometric procedure used; patients receiving corticosteroids; and individuals with increased plasma bilirubin levels or free hemoglobin in the plasma. ■ Many drug reactions are possible with corticosteroids, but usually not a concern with specific diagnostic use.

SIDE EFFECTS

Bradycardia, dizziness, dyspnea, fainting, fever, flushing, irritability, rash, seizures, urticaria.

ANTIDOTE

Notify the physician of any side effect. Keep epinephrine and diphenhydramine available to treat anaphylaxis. Resuscitate as necessary.

CYCLOPHOSPHAMIDE

(sye-kloe-foss′fa-mide)

Antineoplastic (alkylating agent/ nitrogen mustard)

Cytoxan Lyophilized, Neosar, ✱Procytox

pH 3 to 7.5

USUAL DOSE

Although effective alone in susceptible malignancies, cyclophosphamide is more frequently used concurrently or sequentially with other antineoplastic agents. See Monitor section.

Malignant diseases: ***As a single agent:*** The initial dose may be 40 to 50 mg/kg of body weight, usually given in divided doses (10 to 20 mg/kg/24 hr) over 2 to 5 days. Induction doses may range as high as 100 mg/kg. Alternate dosing schedules are: 3 to 5 mg/kg twice weekly, or 10 to 15 mg/kg every 7 to 10 days, or 1.5 to 3 mg/kg/24 hr. Higher doses have been used, based on the condition being treated. ***Combination protocols:*** Numerous combination therapies are in use. Has been used with bleomycin, busulfan, carboplatin, carmustine, cisplatin, cytarabine, dacarbazine, dexamethasone, doxorubicin, etoposide, fluorouracil, methotrexate, mitoxantrone, prednisone, and vincristine.

Polymyositis (unlabeled): 500 mg every 1 to 3 weeks as an IV infusion over 1 hour.

Polyarteritis nodosa (unlabeled): Begin with 4 mg/kg/24 hr. Adjust dose based on patient response.

PEDIATRIC DOSE

Induction: 2 to 8 mg/kg/day or 60 to 250 mg/M^2/day in divided doses. Repeat for 6 or more days. Alternately, a total 7-day dose may be given once a week.

Maintenance: 10 to 15 mg/kg every 7 to 10 days or 30 mg/kg at 3- to 4-week intervals or when bone marrow recovery occurs.

DOSE ADJUSTMENTS

Dose based on average weight in presence of edema or ascites. ▪ Dose is reduced by one third to one half if hematologic disease is present or there has been extensive radiation therapy. ▪ Reduced dose may be required in the adrenalectomized patient and in impaired hepatic function. ▪ Often used with other antineoplastic drugs in reduced doses to achieve tumor remission.

DILUTION

Specific techniques required; see Precautions. Each 100 mg must be diluted with 5 ml of SW or bacteriostatic water for injection (paraben preserved only); yields 20 mg/ml. Shake solution gently and allow to stand until clear. Further dilution with up to 250 ml D5W, NS, D5NS, ½NS, LR, or D5R is recommended to reduce side effects. Do not use heat to facilitate dilution.

Storage: Diluted solution without preservative must be used within 6 hours; with preservative use within 24 hours. Stable up to 6 days if refrigerated. Do not store cyclophosphamide in temperatures over 37° C (90° F).

COMPATIBLE WITH

Consult pharmacist; specific conditions may apply; see Compatibilities, p. xvi.

Additive: Bleomycin (Blenoxane), cisplatin (Platinol), dacarbazine (DTIC), doxorubicin (Adriamycin), fluorouracil (5-FU), mesna (Mesnex), methotrexate (Folex), mitoxantrone (Novantrone), ondansetron (Zofran).

Syringe: Bleomycin (Blenoxane), cisplatin (Platinol), doxapram (Dopram), doxorubicin (Adriamycin), droperidol (Inapsine), fluorouracil (5-FU), furosemide (Lasix), heparin, leucovorin calcium, methotrexate (Folex), metoclopramide (Reglan), mitomycin (Mutamycin), vinblastine (Velban), vincristine (Oncovin).

Y-site: Allopurinol (Aloprim, Zyloprim), amifostine (Ethyol), amikacin (Amikin), ampicillin, aztreonam (Azactam), bleomycin (Blenoxane), cefamandole (Mandol), cefazolin (Kefzol), cefepime (Maxipime), cefoperazone (Cefobid), cefotaxime (Claforan), cefoxitin (Mefoxin), cefuroxime (Zinacef), chloramphenicol (Chloromycetin), chlorpromazine (Thorazine), cimetidine (Tagamet), cisplatin (Platinol), cladribine (Leustatin), clindamycin (Cleocin), dexamethasone (Decadron), diphenhydramine (Benadryl), doxorubicin (Adriamycin), doxorubicin liposome (Doxil), doxycycline (Vibramycin), droperidol (Inapsine), erythromycin lactobionate

(Erythrocin), etoposide phosphate (Etopophos), famotidine (Pepcid IV), filgrastim (Neupogen), fludarabine (Fludara), fluorouracil (5-FU), furosemide (Lasix), ganciclovir (Cytovene), gatifloxacin (Tequin), gemcitabine (Gemzar), gentamicin (Garamycin), granisetron (Kytril), heparin, hydromorphone (Dilaudid), idarubicin (Idamycin), kanamycin (Kantrex), leucovorin calcium, linezolid (Zyvox), lorazepam (Ativan), melphalan (Alkeran), methotrexate (Folex), methylprednisolone (Solu-Medrol), metoclopramide (Reglan), metronidazole (Flagyl IV), minocycline (Minocin), mitomycin (Mutamycin), morphine, nafcillin (Nafcil), ondansetron (Zofran), oxacillin (Bactocill), paclitaxel (Taxol), penicillin G potassium, piperacillin (Pipracil), piperacillin/tazobactam (Zosyn), prochlorperazine (Compazine), promethazine (Phenergan), propofol (Diprivan), ranitidine (Zantac), sargramostim (Leukine), sodium bicarbonate, sulfamethoxazole-trimethoprim (Bactrim), teniposide (Vumon), thiotepa (Thioplex), ticarcillin (Ticar), ticarcillin/clavulanate (Timentin), tobramycin (Nebcin), topotecan (Hycamtin), vancomycin (Vancocin), vinblastine (Velban), vincristine (Oncovin), vinorelbine (Navelbine).

RATE OF ADMINISTRATION

Each 100 mg or fraction thereof over 15 minutes or longer. May be given by IV push, as an intermittent infusion, or through the Y-tube or three-way stopcock if the IV solution is dextrose or saline.

ACTIONS

An alkylating agent of the nitrogen mustard group with antitumor activity; cell cycle phase nonspecific, but most effective in S phase. It is an inert compound but is activated by hepatic microsomal enzymes to produce regression in the size of malignant tumors. Elimination half-life is 3 to 10 hours. Metabolized in the liver, it or its metabolites are excreted in the urine. Secreted in breast milk.

INDICATIONS AND USES

To suppress or retard neoplastic growth. Has been used in lymphomas such as Hodgkin's disease, non-Hodgkin's, leukemias, and multiple myeloma; in mycosis fungoides and in numerous other malignancies (e.g., bladder, breast, neuroblastoma, ovarian, retinoblastoma, sarcomas [bony and soft tissue], small-cell lung cancer). Used in pediatric patients for acute and chronic leukemias, Hodgkin's or non-Hodgkin's lymphomas, neuroblastoma, and retinoblastoma. Used orally to treat many other indications including biopsy-proven nephrotic syndrome in children when disease fails to respond to primary therapy or primary therapy causes intolerable side effects.

Unlabeled uses: Severe rheumatologic conditions. ■ Polyarteritis nodosa. ■ Alone or in combination with corticosteroids to treat polymyositis.

CONTRAINDICATIONS

Previous hypersensitivity, severely depressed bone marrow function.

PRECAUTIONS

Follow guidelines for handling cytotoxic agents. See Appendix A, p. 1142. ■ Administered by or under the direction of the physician specialist. ■ Use caution in cases of leukopenia, thrombocytopenia, bone marrow infiltrated with malignant cells, previous radiation therapy, previous cytotoxic therapy, and severe hepatic or renal disease. ■ Wait 5 to 7 days after a major surgical procedure before beginning treatment. May interfere with normal wound healing. ■ Do not administer any live vaccine to patients receiving antineoplastic drugs. ■ May cause syndrome of inappropriate antidiuretic hormone (SIADH) with normal doses because of fluid loading. ■ May result in reversible hemorrhagic ureteritis or renal tubular necrosis. ■ One incident of cross-sensitivity with other alkylating agents has been reported. ■ Anaphylaxis resulting in death has been reported. ■ Pseudomembranous colitis has been reported. May range from mild to life-threatening. Consider in patients that present with diarrhea during or after treatment with cyclophosphamide. ■ Stevens-Johnson syndrome and toxic epidermal necrolysis have occurred rarely.

Monitor: Prehydration with 500 to 1,000 ml NS recommended, especially with higher doses. ■ Marked leukopenia will occur after the initial dose. Recovery should begin in 7 to 10 days. ■ Monitor neutrophils and platelets and examine urine for RBCs on a regular basis. ■ Maintenance doses are regulated by an acceptable leukocyte count (2,500 to 4,000 cells/mm^3) and the absence of serious side effects. The maximum effective maintenance dose should be used. ■ Observe continuously for infection. Prophylactic antibiotics may be indicated pending results of C/S in a febrile neutropenic patient. ■ Use antiemetics for patient comfort. ■ Acute hemorrhagic cystitis occurs in 7% to 12% of patients; administer before 4 PM to decrease amount of drug remaining in bladder overnight. Encourage fluid intake and frequent voiding to prevent cystitis. ■ Monitor for thrombocytopenia (platelet count less than 50,000/mm^3). Initiate precautions to prevent excessive bleeding (e.g., inspect IV sites, skin, and mucous membranes; use extreme care during invasive procedures; test urine, emesis, stool, and secretions for occult blood).

Patient Education: Nonhormonal birth control recommended. ■ Increase fluid intake and void frequently. ■ See Appendix D, p. 1148.

Maternal/Child: Category D: may produce teratogenic effects on the fetus. Has a mutagenic potential. ■ Discontinue breast-feeding. ■ When given in remission, has been effective in prolonging the duration of the remission in children with acute lymphoblastic (stem-cell) leukemia. ■ Safety profile in children similar to that of adults.

Elderly: Consider age-related organ impairment; toxicity may be increased.

DRUG/LAB INTERACTIONS

Half-life increased and metabolic concentrations decreased with chloramphenicol. ■ Thiazide diuretics (e.g., chlorothiazide [Diuril]) may prolong leukopenia. ■ Increased risk of bleeding with anticoagulants (e.g., warfarin [Coumadin]); dose reduction of anticoagulant may be indicated. ■ May reduce serum digoxin levels. ■ Can potentiate doxorubicin-induced cardiotoxicity. ■ May prolong neuromuscular blockade and prolonged respiratory depression caused by succinylcholine. These effects are dose dependent and may occur up to several days after cyclophosphamide is discontinued. ■ May decrease effectiveness of quinolone antibiotics (e.g., ciprofloxacin [Cipro]). ■ Risk of bleeding or infection may be increased with allopurinol (Zyloprim). ■ Chronic administration of high doses of phenobarbital may increase metabolism of cyclophosphamide and decrease its effectiveness. ■ Capable of many other interactions.

SIDE EFFECTS

Alopecia (regrowth may be slightly darker), amenorrhea, asthenia, gonadal suppression, leukopenia (see Precautions), malaise, mucosal ulcerations, nausea and vomiting, darkening of skin and fingernails, susceptibility to infection.

Major: Anaphylaxis (death), bone marrow depression, hemorrhagic ureteritis (reversible), interstitial pneumonitis, pulmonary fibrosis, pseudomembranous colitis, renal tubular necrosis (reversible), secondary neoplasia, SIADH, sterile hemorrhagic cystitis (which can be fatal).

ANTIDOTE

Minor side effects will be treated symptomatically if necessary. Discontinue the drug and notify the physician of hematuria immediately. Formalin bladder instillation may control cystitis. Mesna has decreased incidence of cystitis. Administration of whole blood products (e.g., packed RBCs, platelets, leukocytes) and/or blood modifiers (e.g., darbepoetin alfa [Aranesp], epoetin alfa [Epogen, Procrit], filgrastim [Neupogen], pegfilgrastim [Neulasta], sargramostim [Leukine], oprelvekin [Neumega]) may be indicated to treat bone marrow toxicity. There is no specific antidote. Supportive therapy as indicated will help sustain the patient in toxicity. Approximately 36% can be removed by hemodialysis.

CYCLOSPORINE

Immunosuppressant

(sye-kloe-spor′in)

Sandimmune

USUAL DOSE

5 to 6 mg/kg of body weight as a single dose 4 to 12 hours before transplantation. Repeat once each day until oral solution can be tolerated. Individualized adjustment is imperative and may be required on a daily basis. Administered at ⅓ of the oral dose in patients temporarily unable to take oral cyclosporine.

PEDIATRIC DOSE

Same as adult dose; however, higher doses may be required. See Maternal/Child.

DOSE ADJUSTMENTS

Reduced dose may be required in impaired renal function. ■ Higher doses may be required in children. ■ See Monitor and Drug/Lab Interactions.

DILUTION

Each 50 mg should be diluted immediately before use with 20 to 100 ml of NS or D5W and given as an infusion. May leach phthalate from polyvinylchloride containers; use diluents in glass infusion bottles. Dilute immediately before use and discard unused portion.

Storage: Discard diluted solution after 24 hours.

COMPATIBLE WITH

Consult pharmacist; specific conditions may apply; see Compatibilities, p. xvi. Leaches out plasticizers, including DEHP from PVC infusion bags and IV tubing; use of non-PVC containers and IV tubing recommended.

Additive: Ciprofloxacin (Cipro IV).

Y-site: Alatrofloxacin (Trovan IV), gatifloxacin (Tequin), linezolid (Zyvox), propofol (Diprivan), sargramostim (Leukine).

RATE OF ADMINISTRATION

A single dose properly diluted over 2 to 6 hours.

ACTIONS

A potent immunosuppressive agent. Interferes with IL-2 production and blocks T-cell proliferative signals during early T-cell activation. Prolongs survival of kidney, liver, and heart allogeneic transplants in the human. Measured by specific or nonspecific assays. Extensively metabolized by the cytochrome P_{450} hepatic enzyme system metabolites and excreted in bile and urine. Crosses the placental barrier. Secreted in breast milk.

INDICATIONS AND USES

Prophylaxis of organ rejection in kidney, liver, and heart allogeneic transplants in conjunction with adrenocortical steroids. ■ Treatment of chronic rejection in patients previously treated with other immunosuppressive agents if oral administration not feasible.

Unlabeled uses: Prophylaxis of organ rejection in pancreas, bone marrow, and heart/lung transplantation. ■ Severe ulcerative colitis.

CONTRAINDICATIONS

Hypersensitivity cyclosporine or polyoxyethylated castor oil.

PRECAUTIONS

Oral dosage preferred; begin as soon as feasible. ■ Usually administered in the hospital by or under the direction of a physician experienced in immunosuppressive therapy and management of organ transplant patients. ■ Adequate laboratory and supportive medical resources must be available. ■ All formulations may be given concomitantly with adrenocortical steroids. Manufacturer has a black box warning. ***Do not administer IV cyclosporine with any other immunosuppressive agent except adrenocortical steroids.*** Only the oral emulsified form (Neoral) may be given with other immunosuppressive agents. ■ In impaired renal function, if rejection is severe, try other immunosuppressive therapy or allow rejection and removal of the kidney rather than increase dose of cyclosporine. ■ May cause lymphomas. ■ Encephalopathy has been reported. May be manifest as impaired consciousness, convulsions, visual disturbances, loss of motor function, movement disorders, and psychiatric disturbances. Predisposing factors may include hypertension, hypomagnesemia, hypocholesterolemia, high-dose corticosteroids, high cyclosporine blood levels, and graft-versus-host disease. Patients receiving liver transplants may be more susceptible to encephalopathy than patients receiving kidney transplants. Reversal of encephalopathy has occurred after discontinuation or dose reduction of cyclosporine. ■ See Drug/Lab Interactions.

Monitor: Monitor BUN, SrCr, serum bilirubin, and liver enzymes frequently. Timing and amount of rise in BUN and creatinine and degree of nephrotoxicity or hepatotoxicity distinguish between need for dose reduction or symptoms of organ rejection. ■ Monitor cyclosporine blood levels. Measured by specific or nonspecific assay. 24-hour specific trough values of 100 to 200 ng/ml of whole blood or 24-hour nonspecific trough values of 250 to 800 ng/ml of whole blood minimize side effects and rejection events. Nonspecific assays trough values are higher because they include metabolites. Confirm assay method to evaluate appropriately. ■ Observe constantly for signs of infection (fever, sore throat, tiredness) or unusual bleeding or bruising. ■ Prophylactic antibiotics may be indicated pending results of C/S in a febrile neutropenic patient. ■ Monitor BP. ■ See Drug/Lab Interactions.

Patient Education: Use nonhormonal birth control. Do not use oral contraceptives. See Appendix D, p. 1148. ■ Do not make any changes in formulation (e.g., IV, capsules, oral solution) without physician direction. May require dose adjustment.

Maternal/Child: Category C: safety for use in pregnancy and in men and women capable of conception not established. Embryotoxic and fetotoxic in rats. ■ Discontinue breast-feeding. ■ Safety for use in children not established but has been used in patients as young as 6 months. Hypertension occurs more frequently in children.

DRUG/LAB INTERACTIONS

Interactions are numerous and potentially life threatening. Review of drug profile by pharmacist imperative. ■ Nephrotoxicity may be increased because of additive nephrotoxic effects with amphotericin B, aminoglycosides (e.g., gentamicin), colchicine, diclofenac (Cataflam), foscarnet (Foscavir), H_2 antagonists (e.g., cimetidine, ranitidine), ketoconazole (Nizoral), melphalan (Alkeran), NSAIDs (e.g., ibuprofen [Advil, Motrin], naproxen [Aleve, Naprosyn], sulindac [Clinoril]), quinolones (e.g., ciprofloxacin [Cipro]), sulfamethoxazole-trimethoprim (Bactrim); use extreme caution and monitor renal function closely. ■ Concurrent use with melphalan may cause acute renal failure. May occur after the first dose of each drug. ■ Concurrent administration with colchicine may cause cyclosporine toxicity (e.g., GI, hepatic, renal, and neuromuscular toxicity). ■ Cyclosporine plasma levels may be increased with concurrent use of chloramphenicol or protease inhibitors (e.g., indinavir [Crixivan], ritonavir [Norvir]); use caution. ■ Metabolism decreased and serum levels increased by amiodarone (Cordarone), bromocriptine (Parlodel), calcium channel blockers (e.g., diltiazem [Cardizem], verapamil [Isoptin]), carvedilol (Coreg), colchicine, danozole (Danocrine), erythromycin, fluconazole (Diflucan), itraconazole (Sporanox), ketoconazole (Nizoral), metoclopramide (Reglan), methylprednisolone (Solu-Cortef), quinupristin/dalfopristin (Synercid). Monitor blood levels with concurrent use to avoid cyclosporine toxicity. ■ Cyclosporine blood levels and effectiveness may be decreased by barbiturates (e.g., phenobarbital), carbamazepine (Tegretol), clindamycin, famotidine (Pepcid), hydantoins (e.g., phenytoin [Dilantin]), oxcarbazepine (Trileptal), rifampin (Rifadin), sulfamethoxazole-trimethoprim (Bactrim), St. John's wort; transplant rejection may occur. ■ Rifabutin (Mycobutin) may increase metabolism of cyclosporine; use care with concomitant use. ■ Concurrent use with nafcillin may decrease or increase cyclosporine levels. Monitor blood levels. ■ Cyclosporine reduces clearance and may increase blood levels of digoxin, etoposide (oral), lovastatin, methotrexate, and prednisolone; in addition it may increase the volume distribution of digoxin and cause toxicity rather quickly. Monitor digoxin levels. ■ May decrease mycophenolate mofetil (CellCept) levels. Monitor levels closely when cyclosporine is added or removed from a drug regimen containing mycophenolate. ■ Imipenem-cilastatin (Primaxin) may increase cyclosporine blood levels resulting in CNS toxicity. ■ Potentiates nondepolarizing muscle relaxants (e.g., tubocurarine, doxacurium [Nuromax]); will prolong neuromuscular blockade. ■ Do not use potassium-sparing diuretics (e.g., spironolactone [Aldactone]); may increase risk of hyperkalemia. ■ May cause convulsions with methylprednisolone. Has additive effects with other immunosuppressive agents (except steroids); may increase risk of lymphoma. ■ Serum levels may increase with chloroquine (Aralen). ■ Avoid vaccinations and do not use live vaccines in patients receiving cyclosporine. ■ Grapefruit juice may affect certain enzymes of the P_{450} enzyme system and should be avoided.

SIDE EFFECTS

Acne, convulsions, cramps, diarrhea, encephalopathy, gum hyperplasia, headache, hepatotoxicity, hirsutism, hyperkalemia, hypertension (more severe in children), hyperuricemia, infection, leukopenia, lymphoma, nausea and vomiting, paresthesia, renal dysfunction, skin rash, and tremor. Mild allergic reactions have occurred. Stevens-Johnson syndrome and toxic epidermal necrolysis have occurred rarely.

ANTIDOTE

Notify physician of all side effects. Most can be treated symptomatically. Drug may be decreased or discontinued or other immunosuppressive agents utilized. Nephrotoxicity, hepatotoxicity, or hematopoietic depression may require temporary reduction of dosage or permanent withholding of treatment. Dialysis is not effective in overdose.

CYTARABINE

(sye-tare′a-been)

Antineoplastic (antimetabolite)

ARA-C, ✱Cytosar, Cytosar-U

pH 5

USUAL DOSE

Acute non-lymphocytic leukemia in adults and children: ***Single agent:*** 200 mg/M²/24 hr as a continuous infusion for 5 days. Repeat every 2 weeks. ***Combination chemotherapy:*** Dose is variable depending on specific regimen or protocol. Examples are 100 mg/M²/24 hr as a continuous infusion or 100 mg/M² as an IV injection every 12 hours. Repeat daily on days 1 through 7. Another regimen uses 100 to 200 mg/M² or 2 to 6 mg/kg/24 hr as a continuous infusion or equally divided into 2 or 3 doses and given by IV injection or intermittent infusion. Given for 5 to 10 days. Maintain treatment until therapeutic effect or toxicity occurs. Modify on a day-to-day basis for maximum individualized effectiveness.

Acute myelocytic leukemia or erythroleukemia in adults and children: As a single agent, 100 to 200 mg/M²/24 hr or 3 mg/kg/24 hr for 5 to 10 days as a continuous infusion or in divided doses by IV injection. Total dose is 1,000 mg/M². Repeat every 2 weeks.

Refractory or secondary leukemia in adults and children: As a single agent, 3 Gm/M² as an IV infusion over 2 to 3 hours every 12 hours for 4 to 12 doses. Repeat at 2- to 3-week intervals.

DOSE ADJUSTMENTS

Dose (mg/kg) based on average weight in presence of edema or ascites. ■ Dose reduction may be indicated in impaired hepatic or renal function. ■ See Precautions/Monitor. ■ Usually used with other antineoplastic drugs in specific doses to achieve tumor remission. ■ Withhold or modify dose based on degree of bone marrow depression; see Monitor.

DILUTION

Specific techniques required; see Precautions. Some preparations are liquid and do not require reconstitution or each 100 mg must be reconstituted with 5 ml (500 mg with 10 ml) of SW for injection with benzyl alcohol 0.9%. Solution pH about 5. May be given by IV injection as is or further diluted in 50 to 100 ml or more of NS or D5W and given as an infusion. IV injection should be through a free-flowing IV tubing. Use only clear solutions.

Storage: Stable at room temperature for 48 hours.

COMPATIBLE WITH **(Underline Indicates Conflicting Compatibility Information)**

Consult pharmacist; specific conditions may apply; see Compatibilities, p. xvi.

Additive: Daunorubicin (Cerubidine), etoposide (VePesid), gentamicin (Garamycin), hydrocortisone sodium succinate (Solu-Cortef), lincomycin (Lincocin), magnesium sulfate, methotrexate (Folex), methylprednisolone (Solu-Medrol), mitoxantrone (Novantrone), ondansetron (Zofran), potassium chloride (KCl), sodium bicarbonate, vincristine (Oncovin).

Syringe: Metoclopramide (Reglan).

Y-site: Amifostine (Ethyol), aztreonam (Azactam), cefepime (Maxipime), chlorpromazine (Thorazine), cimetidine (Tagamet), cladribine (Leustatin), dexamethasone (Decadron), diphenhydramine (Benadryl), doxorubicin liposome (Doxil), droperidol (Inapsine), etoposide phosphate (Etopophos), famotidine (Pepcid IV), filgrastim (Neupogen), fludarabine (Fludara), furosemide (Lasix), gatifloxacin (Tequin), gemcitabine (Gemzar), gentamicin (Garamycin), granisetron (Kytril), heparin, hydrocortisone sodium succinate (Solu-Cortef), hydromorphone (Dilaudid), idarubicin (Idamycin), linezolid (Zyvox), lorazepam (Ativan), melphalan (Alkeran), methotrexate (Folex), methylprednisolone (Solu-Medrol), metoclopramide (Reglan), morphine, ondansetron (Zofran), paclitaxel (Taxol), piperacillin/tazobactam (Zosyn), prochlorperazine (Compazine), promethazine (Phenergan), propofol (Diprivan), ranitidine (Zantac), sargramostim (Leukine), sodium bicarbonate, teniposide (Vumon), thiotepa (Thioplex), vinorelbine (Navelbine).

RATE OF ADMINISTRATION

IV injection: Each 100 mg or fraction thereof over 1 to 3 minutes.

IV infusion: Single daily dose properly diluted over 30 minutes to 24 hours, depending on amount of infusion solution and dosage regimen.

ACTIONS

An antimetabolite and pyrimidine antagonist that interferes with the synthesis of DNA. Cell cycle specific for S phase. Through various chemical processes this deprivation acts more quickly on rapidly growing cells and causes their death. Cytotoxic and cytostatic. A potent bone marrow depressant. Crosses the blood-brain barrier. Serum half-life averages 1 to 3 hours. Metabolized in the liver and excreted in the urine.

INDICATIONS AND USES

Induction and maintenance of remission in acute non-lymphocytic leukemia in adults and children. Also used for treatment of acute lymphocytic leukemia (ALL), the blast phase of chronic myelocytic leukemia, and acute myelocytic leukemia (AML). ■ Is used intrathecally in the treatment of meningeal leukemia. A liposomal formulation (DepoCyt) is available for intrathecal use only, lipofoam molecules contained in this product are much too large for IV use.

CONTRAINDICATIONS

Hypersensitivity to cytarabine, pre-existing drug-induced bone marrow depression.

PRECAUTIONS

Follow guidelines for handling cytotoxic agents. See Appendix A, p. 1142. ■ Administered by or under the direction of the physician specialist. ■

Remissions induced by cytarabine are brief unless followed by maintenance therapy. ■ Use caution with impaired liver or renal function. ■ Severe GI, pulmonary, or CNS toxicity has occurred with experimental cytarabine regimens. Toxicities are different (e.g., reversible corneal toxicity, hemorrhagic conjunctivitis, cerebral and cerebellar dysfunction, severe GI ulceration) from those seen with conventional therapy. Deaths have been reported. ■ Benzyl alcohol may cause a fatal "gasping syndrome" in premature infants.

Monitor: Leukocyte and platelet counts should be monitored daily. ■ During induction therapy, WBC depression is biphasic with the first nadir occurring at days 7 to 9 and a deeper fall at days 15 to 24. Platelet depression begins around day 5 and reaches a nadir at days 12 to 15. ■ Hold or modify therapy for platelet count less than 50,000 or polymorphonuclear granulocytes less than 1,000 cells/mm^3. Restart therapy when bone marrow recovery is confirmed. ■ Monitor bone marrow, liver, and renal function at regular intervals during therapy. ■ Higher doses tolerated by IV injection compared with IV infusion, but the incidence and intensity of nausea and vomiting are increased. ■ Prophylactic administration of antiemetics recommended. ■ Be alert for signs of bone marrow depression, bleeding, infection, or neurotoxicity. These side effects are dose- and schedule-dependent. ■ Monitor for thrombocytopenia (platelet count less than 50,000/mm^3). Initiate precautions to prevent excessive bleeding (e.g., inspect IV sites, skin, and mucous membranes; use extreme care during invasive procedures; test urine, emesis, stool, and secretions for occult blood). ■ Prophylactic antibiotics may be indicated pending results of C/S in a febrile neutropenic patient. ■ Monitor uric acid levels; maintain hydration; allopurinol may be indicated.

Patient Education: Nonhormonal birth control recommended. ■ See Appendix D, p. 1148. ■ Promptly report early signs of neurotoxicity (e.g., ataxia, confusion, lethargy).

Maternal/Child: Category D: avoid pregnancy. May produce teratogenic effects on the fetus, especially during the first trimester. ■ Discontinue breast-feeding. ■ See Drug/Lab Interactions.

Elderly: Consider age-related organ impairment; toxicity may be increased.

DRUG/LAB INTERACTIONS

May inhibit digoxin absorption. ■ Do not administer any live vaccines to patients receiving antineoplastic drugs. ■ May cause acute pancreatitis in patients who previously received L-asparaginase. ■ May antagonize action of gentamicin against *Klebsiella*. ■ May antagonize antifungal actions of flucytosine (Ancobon). ■ Clearance decreased and toxicity increased with nephrotoxic agents (e.g., aminoglycosides [gentamicin]), may cause neurotoxic symptoms (e.g., ataxia, confusion, lethargy). ■ Concurrent use of high doses of cytarabine with cisplatin may increase ototoxicity.

SIDE EFFECTS

Abdominal pain, bone marrow depression (e.g., anemia, leukopenia, thrombocytopenia), bone pain, cardiomyopathy, chest pain, conjunctivitis, diarrhea, esophagitis, fever, hepatic dysfunction, hypersensitivity reactions, hyperuricemia, malaise, megaloblastosis, mucosal bleeding, myalgia, nausea, oral ulceration, pancreatitis, peripheral motor and sensory neuropathies, rash, stomatitis, thrombophlebitis, vomiting. Higher than usual dose regimens may cause severe coma, GI ulcerations and peritonitis, personality changes, pulmonary toxicity, somnolence, or death.

ANTIDOTE

Notify the physician of all side effects. Most will be treated symptomatically. Some toxicity is necessary to produce remission. Discontinue the drug for serious bone marrow depression. Administration of whole blood products (e.g., packed RBCs, platelets, leukocytes), and/or blood modifiers (e.g., darbepoetin alfa [Aranesp], epoetin alfa [Epogen, Procrit], filgrastim [Neupogen], pegfilgrastim [Neulasta], sargramostim [Leukine], oprelvekin [Neumega]) may be indicated to treat bone marrow toxicity. Drug must be restarted as soon as signs of bone marrow recovery occur, or its effectiveness will be lost. Use corticosteroids for cytarabine syndrome (fever, myalgia, bone pain, occasional chest pain, maculopapular rash, conjunctivitis, malaise). Usually occurs in 6 to 12 hours after administration. Continue cytarabine if patient responds to corticosteriods. There is no specific antidote; supportive therapy as indicated will help to sustain the patient in toxicity.

CYTOMEGALOVIRUS IMMUNE GLOBULIN INTRAVENOUS (HUMAN)

(si-to-meg-uh-lo-vi-rus uh-mun′ glob′u-lin)

Passive immunizing agent
Antibacterial
Antiviral

CMV-IGIV, CytoGam

USUAL DOSE

150 mg/kg is the maximum recommended dose per infusion.

Kidney transplant: 150 mg/kg of body weight as an IV infusion. This initial dose must be given within 72 hours of transplant. Additional infusions of 100 mg/kg are given at 2, 4, 6, and 8 weeks post-transplant, then reduced to 50 mg/kg at 12 and 16 weeks post-transplant.

Heart, liver, lung, and pancreas transplants: 150 mg/kg of body weight as an IV infusion. This initial dose must be given within 72 hours of transplant. Consider use in combination with ganciclovir (Cytovene) 10 mg/kg/day for 14 days. Additional infusions of cytomegalovirus IGIV containing 150 mg/kg are given at 2, 4, 6, and 8 weeks post-transplant, then reduced to 100 mg/kg at 12 and 16 weeks post-transplant.

DILUTION

Absolute sterile technique required; contains no preservatives. Available in 20- and 50-ml vials (50 mg/ml); multiple vials may be required. Use only if clear and colorless. Enter vial only once and initiate infusion within 6 hours. Must be completely infused within 12 hours of dilution. See Rate of Administration.

Storage: Store dry powder in refrigerator between 2° and 8° C (35° to 46° F).

COMPATIBILITY

Administration through a separate infusion line recommended. If absolutely necessary, may be piggybacked in a pre-existing line containing NS, ½NS, dextrose 2.5%, 5%, 10%, or 20% in water or saline. Do not dilute CMV-IGIV more than one part to two parts of any of these solutions.

RATE OF ADMINISTRATION

Use of an in-line filter (pore size 15 microns [0.2 microns acceptable]) and a constant infusion pump (e.g., IVAC) is required. Begin with a rate of 15 mg/kg/hr. May be increased to 30 mg/kg/hr in 30 minutes if no discomfort or adverse effects. May be increased in another 30 minutes to 60 mg/kg/hr if no discomfort or adverse effects. Do not exceed the 60 mg/kg/hr rate or allow the volume infused to exceed 75 ml/hr regardless of mg/kg/hr dose. Slow rate of infusion at onset of patient discomfort or any adverse reactions. Infusion must be complete within 12 hours of dilution. Subsequent doses may be increased at 15-minute intervals using the same mg/kg/hr rates and adhering to the volume maximum of 75 ml/hr.

ACTIONS

A sterile solution of immunoglobulin Gm (IgG). Derived from pooled adult human plasma selected for high titers of antibody for cytomegalovirus (CMV). Purified by a specific process. Can raise the relevant antibody levels sufficiently to attenuate or reduce the incidence of serious CMV disease. Antibody levels will last 2 to 3 weeks. Recent studies of combined prophylaxis with CMV-IGIV and ganciclovir have shown reductions in the incidence of serious CMV-associated disease in CMV-seronegative recipients of CMV-seropositive organs below that expected from one drug alone.

INDICATIONS AND USES

Prophylaxis of CMV disease associated with transplantation of kidney, heart, liver, lung, and pancreas. In transplants of these organs other than kidney from CMV-seropositive donors to seronegative recipients, prophylactic CMV-IGIV should be considered in combination with ganciclovir.

CONTRAINDICATIONS

History of a prior severe reaction associated with any human immunoglobulin preparations. Individuals with selective immunoglobulin A deficiency may develop antibodies to IgA and are at risk for anaphylaxis.

PRECAUTIONS

75% of untreated recipients would be expected to develop CMV disease. Use of CMV-IGIV has effected a 50% reduction in this disease rate. Effective results have been obtained with a variety of immunosuppressive regimens (e.g., combinations of azathioprine, cyclosporine, prednisone). ■ A fatal CMV infection occurred even with ganciclovir treatment in one patient, who inadvertently missed a single injection.

Monitor: Continuous monitoring of vital signs is preferred. Must be monitored before infusion, at every rate change, the midpoint, at the conclusion, and several times after completion. ■ All supplies for emergency treatment of acute anaphylatic reaction must be available; see Antidote.

Patient Education: Adherence to the prescribed regimen is imperative.

Maternal/Child: Category C: safety for use during pregnancy or breast-feeding not established. Use only if clearly needed.

DRUG/LAB INTERACTIONS

Defer vaccination with any live-virus vaccine (e.g., measles, mumps, rubella) until 3 months after CMV-IGIV administration.

SIDE EFFECTS

Incidence related to rate of administration; back pain, chills, fever, flushing, hypotension, muscle cramps, nausea, vomiting, wheezing. Allergic reactions, including anaphylaxis, are possible.

ANTIDOTE

With onset of any minor side effect, reduce rate of infusion immediately or discontinue temporarily. Discontinue CMV-IGIV if symptoms persist and notify the physician. May be treated symptomatically and infusion resumed at a slower rate if symptoms subside. Discontinue CMV-IGIV if hypotension or anaphylaxis occur and treat immediately. Epinephrine (Adrenalin), diphenhydramine (Benadryl), oxygen, vasopressors (e.g., dopamine [Intropin]), corticosteroids, and ventilation equipment must always be available. Resuscitate as necessary.

DACARBAZINE

(da-kar′ba-zeen)

Antineoplastic (miscellaneous)

DTIC, DTIC-Dome

pH 3 to 4

USUAL DOSE

Malignant melanoma: 2 to 4.5 mg/kg of body weight/24 hr for 10 days. May be repeated at 4-week intervals. May administer 250 mg/M^2 daily for 5 days. Repeat in 3 weeks. Has proved as effective in lesser doses as in larger doses. Individualized response determines dosage of subsequent treatments.

Hodgkin's disease: 150 mg/M^2/24 hr for 5 days. Repeat every 4 weeks. Used in combination with other drugs in a specific regimen. An alternate regimen is 375 mg/M^2 on day one in combination with a specific protocol. Repeat every 15 days.

DOSE ADJUSTMENTS

Dose (mg/kg) based on average weight in presence of edema or ascites. ■ Used with other antineoplastic drugs and radiation therapy in reduced doses to achieve tumor remission. ■ Dose reduction may be required in impaired liver and renal function.

DILUTION

Specific techniques required; see Precautions. Each 100-mg vial is diluted with 9.9 ml (200 mg with 19.7 ml) of SW for injection (10 mg/ml). Further dilution in 50 to 250 ml of D5W or NS for infusion is preferred. May be given through Y-tube or three-way stopcock of infusion set through a free-flowing IV.

Storage: Discard in 6 to 8 hours if kept at room temperature. Reconstituted solution stable for 72 hours, diluted solution for 24 hours if refrigerated at 4° C (39° F).

COMPATIBLE WITH

(Underline Indicates Conflicting Compatibility Information)

Consult pharmacist; specific conditions may apply; see Compatibilities, p. xvi.

Additive: Bleomycin (Blenoxane), carmustine (BiCNU), cyclophosphamide (Cytoxan), cytarabine (ARA-C), dactinomycin (Cosmegen), doxorubicin (Adriamycin), fluorouracil (5-FU), methotrexate (Folex), ondansetron (Zofran), vinblastine (Velban).

Y-site: Amifostine (Ethyol), aztreonam (Azactam), doxorubicin liposome (Doxil), etoposide phosphate (Etopophos), filgrastim (Neupogen), fludarabine (Fludara), granisetron (Kytril), heparin, melphalan (Alkeran), ondansetron (Zofran), paclitaxel (Taxol), sargramostim (Leukine), teniposide (Vumon), thiotepa (Thioplex), vinblastine (Velban), vinorelbine (Navelbine).

RATE OF ADMINISTRATION

Total dose over 30 to 60 minutes. More rapid rate may cause severe venous irritation.

ACTIONS

An antineoplastic agent. Exact mechanism of action is not known; may inhibit DNA and RNA synthesis. It is an alkylating agent, cell cycle phase nonspecific. Probably localizes in the liver and is excreted in the urine.

INDICATIONS AND USES

Metastatic malignant melanoma. ▪ Hodgkin's disease. ▪ Soft-tissue sarcomas.

Unlabeled uses: Treatment of malignant pheochromocytoma with cyclophosphamide and vincristine. ▪ Treatment of metastatic malignant melanoma with tamoxifen.

CONTRAINDICATIONS

Known hypersensitivity to dacarbazine.

PRECAUTIONS

Follow guidelines for handling cytotoxic agents. See Appendix A, p. 1142. ▪ Administered by or under the direction of the physician specialist. ▪ Use caution in impaired liver and renal function.

Monitor: Determine absolute patency of vein; a stinging or burning sensation indicates extravasation; severe cellulitis and tissue necrosis will result. Discontinue injection; use another vein. ▪ Monitor bone marrow function, white and RBC count, and platelet count frequently. ▪ Nausea and vomiting may be reduced by restricting oral intake of fluid and foods for 4 to 6 hours before administration. Use prophylactic antiemetics. ▪ Be alert for signs of bone marrow depression, bleeding, or infection. ▪ Monitor for thrombocytopenia (platelet count less than 50,000/mm^3). Initiate precautions to prevent excessive bleeding (e.g., inspect IV sites, skin, and mucous membranes; use extreme care during invasive procedures; test urine, emesis, stool, and secretions for occult blood). ▪ Prophylactic antibiotics may be indicated pending results of C/S in a febrile neutropenic patient.

Patient Education: Protect skin surfaces; may cause photosensitive skin reactions. ▪ Nonhormonal birth control recommended. ▪ Report burning or stinging at IV site promptly. ▪ See Appendix D, p. 1148.

Maternal/Child: Category C: safety for use in pregnancy or breast-feeding and in men and women capable of conception not established. ▪ Discontinue breast-feeding.

Elderly: Consider age-related organ impairment; toxicity may be increased.

DRUG/LAB INTERACTIONS

Do not administer any live vaccines to patients receiving antineoplastic drugs. ▪ Inhibited by phenobarbital and phenytoin (Dilantin). ▪ Potentiates allopurinol.

SIDE EFFECTS

Leukopenia and thrombocytopenia may be serious enough to cause death. Alopecia, anaphylaxis, anorexia, facial flushing, facial paresthesias, fever, hepatotoxicity, malaise, myalgia, nausea, skin necrosis, vomiting.

ANTIDOTE

Notify physician of all side effects. Most will be treated symptomatically. Bone marrow depression may require temporary or permanent withholding of treatment. Administration of whole blood products (e.g., packed RBCs, platelets, leukocytes) and/or blood modifiers (e.g., darbepoetin alfa [Aranesp], epoetin alfa [Epogen, Procrit], filgrastim [Neupogen], pegfilgrastim [Neulasta], sargramostim [Leukine], oprelvekin [Neumega]) may be indicated to treat bone marrow toxicity. There is no specific antidote. Supportive therapy as indicated will help sustain the patient in toxicity. For extravasation, elevate extremity; consider injection of long-acting dexamethasone (Decadron LA) throughout extravasated tissue. Use a 27- or 25-gauge needle. Apply moist, warm compresses.

DACLIZUMAB

(dah-kliz'uh-mab)

Recombinant monoclonal antibody
Immunosuppressant

Zenapax

pH 6.9

USUAL DOSE

Used concurrently with cyclosporine (Sandimmune) and corticosteroids. **Organ rejection prophylaxis in renal transplant:** 1 mg/kg as an infusion for a total of 5 doses. Administer the first dose no more than 24 hours before transplantation. Give the 4 remaining doses at intervals of 14 days.

PEDIATRIC DOSE

Safety for use in children not established; studies not complete but preliminary data suggest the use of the same 1 mg/kg dose and regimen as used in adults. See Maternal/Child.

DOSE ADJUSTMENTS

No dose adjustments indicated in severe renal impairment or based on age, gender, race, or degree of proteinuria. ■ No data available in patients with severe impaired liver function.

DILUTION

Each single dose must be diluted with 50 ml of NS. Do not shake; gently invert to avoid foaming. Sterile technique is imperative. Discard any unused portion.

Storage: Store unopened vials in the refrigerator (2° to 8° C [36° to 45° F]). Do not shake or freeze. Protect from light. Should be used within 4 hours of dilution. If necessary, may be refrigerated for up to 24 hours. Discard prepared solution after 24 hours.

COMPATIBILITY

Manufacturer states, "Other drug substances should not be added or infused simultaneously through the same IV line." No incompatibilities have been observed with PVC or polyethylene bags or infusion sets.

RATE OF ADMINISTRATION

A single dose, properly diluted, must be given as an infusion over 15 minutes. May be given through a peripheral or central vein.

ACTIONS

An immunosuppressive agent. A humanized IgG_1 monoclonal antibody produced by recombinant DNA technology. Acts as an IL-2 receptor antagonist that binds to the Tac subunit of the high-affinity IL-2 receptor complex and inhibits IL-2 mediated activation of lymphocytes, a critical pathway in the cellular immune response involved in allograft rejection. Blocks only those immune cells (T-cells) that are activated by a foreign substance, impairing the response of the immune system to antigenic challenges. During studies, trough levels of 5 to 10 mcg/ml were considered necessary for saturation of the Tac subunit to block the responses of activated T-lymphocytes. Does not suppress the entire immune system, which would increase the risk of infection. Has reduced the incidence of kidney rejection episodes without increasing most side effects and may improve survival rates. Estimated terminal half-life is 20 days (range 11 to 38 days). May cross the placental barrier. May be secreted in breast milk.

INDICATIONS AND USES

Prophylaxis of acute organ rejection in patients receiving renal transplants. Used as part of an immunosuppressive regimen that includes cyclosporine and corticosteroids.

CONTRAINDICATIONS

Known hypersensitivity to daclizumab or any of its components (composite of human [90%] and murine [10%] antibodies).

PRECAUTIONS

Usually administered by or under the direction of a physician experienced in immunosuppressive therapy and management of organ transplant patients. Adequate laboratory and supportive medical resources must be available. ■ Use caution; allergic reactions have not been observed, but this is a protein substance—emergency equipment and drugs for treatment of severe hypersensitivity reactions must be immediately available. ■ Readministration after an initial course of therapy has not been studied in humans, but other monoclonal antibodies have precipitated anaphylactoid reactions. ■ Potential for causing lymphoproliferative disorders and opportunistic infections is unknown. ■ Use with caution in patients with diabetes mellitus, infections, or malignancies. ■ It is not known whether daclizumab use will have a long-term effect on the ability of the immune system to respond to antigens first encountered during induced immunosuppression. ■ Low titers of anti-idiotype antibodies to daclizumab have been detected in some patients during treatment; no adverse effects have been noted.

Monitor: Obtain baseline CBC with differential and platelets and baseline renal and liver tests if not already completed for other immunosuppressant agents. ■ Monitor vital signs. ■ Observe closely for signs of infection (e.g., fever, sore throat, tiredness) or unusual bleeding or bruising. ■ Prophylactic antibiotics may be indicated pending results of C/S in a febrile neutropenic patient. ■ Symptoms of cytokine release syndrome (e.g., chills, fever, dyspnea, and malaise) have not been reported but may occur; observe carefully. ■ See Precautions and Drug/Lab Interactions.

Patient Education: Report difficulty in breathing, swallowing, rapid heart beat, rash, itching, swelling of lower extremities, or weakness immediately. ■ Avoid pregnancy; nonhormonal birth control preferred. Women with childbearing potential should use effective contraception before beginning daclizumab therapy, during therapy, and for 4 months after completion. ■ See Appendix D, p. 1148.

Maternal/Child: Category C: use during pregnancy only if benefits justify the potential risk to the fetus. Avoid pregnancy; effective contraception required. See Patient Education. ■ Discontinue breast-feeding. ■ Has been used in children from 11 months to 17 years of age (average age 12 years), but safety not established; studies still in progress. Somewhat higher rates of hypertension and dehydration occurred in pediatric patients.

Elderly: Specific information not available. Use caution and observe closely.

DRUG/LAB INTERACTIONS

Has been administered concurrently with acyclovir (Zovirax), azathioprine (Imuran), corticosteroids, cyclosporine, ganciclovir (Cytovene), and mycophenolate mofetil (CellCept); no additional adverse reactions noted. ■ Limited experience with concurrent use of antithymocyte globulin, antilymphocyte globulin, muromonab-CD3 (Orthoclone), and tacrolimus (Prograf). ■ May increase fasting blood glucose.

SIDE EFFECTS

Daclizumab did not appear to alter the pattern, frequency, or severity of known side effects associated with the use of immunosuppressive drugs. Whereas 95% of a placebo-treated group reported side effects from concurrent immunosuppressants, 96% of the daclizumab group (also being treated with concurrent immunosuppressants) reported similar side effects. Side effects seen in patients receiving immunosuppressive therapy may include abdominal distention, abdominal pain, back pain, bleeding, cellulitis, chest pain, constipation, coughing, dehydration, diarrhea, dizziness, dyspepsia, dyspnea, dysuria, edema, epigastric pain (not food related), fatigue, fever, headache, heartburn, hypertension, hypotension, impaired wound healing without infection, insomnia, lymphocele, musculoskeletal pain, nausea, oliguria, postoperative pain, pulmonary edema, renal tubular necrosis, tachycardia, thrombosis, tremor, vomiting, and wound infections. Daclizumab did not increase the number of posttransplant lymphomas.

ANTIDOTE

Notify physician of all side effects. Most will be treated symptomatically. Daclizumab may be discontinued or alternate immunosuppressive agents substituted. Discontinue immediately if anaphylaxis occurs and treat with oxygen, epinephrine, corticosteroids, and/or antihistamines (e.g., diphenhydramine [Benadryl]). Resuscitate as necessary.

DACTINOMYCIN

(dak-ti-noe-mye'sin)

Cosmegen

Antineoplastic (antibiotic)

pH 5.5 to 7

USUAL DOSE

Dose will depend on tolerance of the patient, the size and location of the tumor, and the use of other forms of therapy. Calculation of the dose for obese or edematous patients should be based on body surface area. The dose intensity per 2 week cycle for adults and pediatric patients should not exceed 15 mcg/kg/day (0.015 mg/kg/day) or 400 to 600 mcg/M^2/day (0.4 to 0.5 mg/M^2/day) for 5 days.

Wilm's tumor, childhood rhabdomyosarcoma, and Ewing's sarcoma: 15 mcg/kg/day for 5 days. May be administered in various combinations and schedules with other chemotherapeutic agents.

Metastatic nonseminomatous testicular cancer: 1,000 mcg/M^2 (1 mg/M^2) on day 1 as part of a combination regimen with bleomycin, cisplatin, cyclophosphamide, and vinblastine.

Gestational trophoblastic neoplasia: 12 mcg/kg/day for 5 days as a single agent or 500 mcg on days 1 and 2 as part of a combination regimen with cisplatin, cyclophosphamide, etoposide, leucovorin calcium, methotrexate, and vincristine.

PEDIATRIC DOSE

Same as Usual Dose for adults.

DOSE ADJUSTMENTS

Calculate dose based on body surface area in presence of edema or ascites. ■ Used with other antineoplastic drugs in reduced doses to achieve tumor remission. ■ Reduce dose of dactinomycin and radiation therapy when used concurrently, if either has been used previously, or if previous chemotherapy has been employed. ■ Dose selection should be cautious in the elderly. Consider potential for decreased cardiac, hepatic, and renal function, and concomitant disease or drug therapy; see Elderly.

DILUTION

Specific techniques required; see Precautions. Dilute each 0.5 mg vial with 1.1 ml of preservative-free SW for injection (0.5 mg/ml). SW with preservative (benzyl alcohol or paraben) will cause precipitation. Use 2.2 ml to yield 0.25 mg/ml (vent vial to relieve pressure). Very corrosive to soft tissue. Use sterile two-needle technique if given by IV injection; one needle to dilute and withdraw and one needle to inject into the vein (rinse with blood or IV solution before removing). May be given by IV injection, through the Y-tube or three-way stopcock of a free-flowing infusion of D5W or NS, or further diluted in 50 ml of the above solutions for infusion. Do not use a filter smaller than 5 microns; loss of potency will occur. Discard any unused portion.

Storage: Store at 25° C (77° F), excursion permitted to 15° to 30° C (59° to 86° F). Protect from light and humidity.

INCOMPATIBLE WITH

Will form a precipitate with SW that contains preservatives. Cellulose ester membrane filters may result in a reduced dose by partial removal of dactinomycin.

COMPATIBLE WITH

Consult pharmacist; specific conditions may apply; see Compatibilities, p. xvi.

Additive: Dacarbazine (DTIC).

Y-site: Allopurinol (Aloprim, Zyloprim), amifostine (Ethyol), aztreonam (Azactam), cefepime (Maxipime), etoposide phosphate (Etopophos), fludarabine (Fludara), gemcitabine (Gemzar), granisetron (Kytril), melphalan (Alkeran), ondansetron (Zofran), sargramostim (Leukine), teniposide (Vumon), thiotepa (Thioplex), vinorelbine (Navelbine).

RATE OF ADMINISTRATION

IV injection: A single dose over 2 to 3 minutes.

IV infusion: A single dose over 20 to 30 minutes.

ACTIONS

A highly toxic antibiotic antineoplastic agent, cell cycle phase nonspecific. Cytotoxic, it interferes with cell division by binding DNA to slow production of RNA. Found in high concentrations in the kidney, liver, and spleen. Minimally metabolized. Elimination half-life is 30 to 40 hours. Excreted as unchanged drug in bile and urine.

INDICATIONS AND USES

As part of a combination chemotherapy and/or multi-modality for treatment of Wilms' tumor, childhood rhabdomyosarcoma, Ewing's sarcoma, and metastatic nonseminomatous testicular cancer. ■ Alone or in combination with other chemotherapeutic agents for the treatment of gestational trophoblastic neoplasia.

Unlabeled uses: Kaposi's sarcoma, osteosarcoma.

CONTRAINDICATIONS

Exposure to chickenpox, herpes zoster, known sensitivity to dactinomycin, infants under 6 to 12 months of age.

PRECAUTIONS

Follow guidelines for handling cytotoxic agents. See Appendix A, p. 1142. ■ Highly toxic and both the powder and solution must be handled and administered with care. Inhalation of dust or vapors and contact with skin or mucous membranes, especially those of the eyes, must be avoided. If eye contact occurs, rinse for at least 15 minutes with water, saline or a balanced salt ophthalmic solution and then seek immediate ophthalmologic consultation. If skin contact occurs, remove contaminated clothing and rinse area for 15 minutes. Medical attention should be sought immediately and clothes should be destroyed. ■ Administered by or under the direction of the physician specialist. ■ In general, dactinomycin should not be administered concomitantly with radiation therapy in the treatment of Wilms' tumor unless the benefit outweighs the risk. Hepatomegaly and elevated AST (SGOT) levels have been reported. ■ May have increased incidence of second primary tumors following treatment with dactinomycin and radiation. Long-term followup of cancer survivors is indicated.

Monitor: Determine absolute patency of vein. A stinging or burning sensation indicates extravasation; severe cellulitis and tissue necrosis will result. Discontinue injection; use another vein. ■ Monitor renal, hepatic, and bone marrow function frequently. ■ Except for immediate nausea and vomiting, side effects may not appear for 2 to 4 days and may not peak for one to two weeks. Always observe closely. Use prophylactic antiemetics. ■ If stomatitis, diarrhea, or severe hematopoietic depression appears, discontinue therapy until the patient has recovered. ■ An increased incidence of GI toxicity, bone marrow depression, and skin and mucosal reactions has been reported when dactinomycin is administered in combination with radiation therapy. ■ Monitor for thrombocytopenia (platelet count less than 50,000/mm^3). Initiate precautions to prevent excessive bleeding (e.g., inspect IV sites, skin, and mucous membranes; use extreme care during invasive procedures; test urine, emesis, stool, and secretions for occult blood). ■ Allopurinol, increased fluid intake, and alkalinization of the urine may be required to reduce uric acid levels. ■ Observe closely for signs of infection. Prophylactic antibiotics may be indicated pending results of C/S in a febrile neutropenic patient.

Patient Education: Nonhormonal birth control recommended. ■ Report burning or stinging at IV site promptly. ■ See Appendix D, p. 1148.

Maternal/Child: Category D: avoid pregnancy. May produce teratogenic effects on the fetus; use caution in men and women capable of conception. ■ Discontinue breast-feeding. ■ See Contraindications.

Elderly: Response similar to that in younger adults; however, recent studies suggest elderly may be at increased risk for myelosuppression; see Dose Adjustments.

DRUG/LAB INTERACTIONS

Radiation therapy potentiates dactinomycin. ■ Dactinomycin alone may reactivate erythema from previous radiation therapy. ■ Do not administer live vaccines to patients receiving antineoplastic drugs. ■ Inhibits action of penicillin. ■ See Dose Adjustments. ■ May interfere with bioassay procedures used in determining antibacterial drug levels.

SIDE EFFECTS

Abdominal pain, acne, alopecia, anaphylaxis, anemia, anorexia, ascites, cheilitis, diarrhea, dysphagia, erythema flare-up, esophagitis, fatigue, fever, GI ulceration, hepatitis, hepatomegaly, hypocalcemia, lethargy, leukopenia, liver function test abnormalities, malaise, myalgia, nausea, pharyngitis, pneumonitis, proctitis, skin eruptions, thrombocytopenia, ulcerative stomatitis, vomiting.

ANTIDOTE

Any side effect can result in death. Notify the physician of all side effects. Most will be treated symptomatically. Bone marrow depression may require withholding dactinomycin until recovery occurs. There is no specific antidote. Supportive therapy as indicated will help sustain the patient in toxicity. Administration of whole blood products (e.g., packed RBCs, platelets, leukocytes) and/or blood modifiers (e.g., darbepoetin alfa [Aranesp], epoetin alfa [Epogen, Procrit], filgrastim [Neupogen], pegfilgrastim [Neulasta], sargramostim [Leukine], oprelvekin [Neumega]) may be indicated to treat bone marrow toxicity. For extravasation, discontinue immediately and elevate extremity. Apply ice to the site q.i.d. for 3 days. Close observation and reconstructive surgery consultation recommended.

DANTROLENE SODIUM

(dan′troe-leen so′de-um)

Dantrium Intravenous

Skeletal muscle relaxant (direct acting)

pH 9.5

USUAL DOSE

In patients known to be susceptible to malignant hyperthermia, oral dantrolene is indicated prophylactically preoperatively and postoperatively for 1 to 3 days following therapeutic IV treatment. Postoperative dosing is indicated after emergency treatment.

Prophylactic dose: 2.5 mg/kg as an infusion administered over 1 hour before anesthesia. Oral dantrolene may be used.

Therapeutic or emergency dose: 1 mg/kg of body weight as an initial dose. Repeat as necessary until symptoms subside or a cumulative dose of 10 mg/kg is reached. Entire regimen may be repeated if symptoms reappear. Dose required depends on degree of susceptibility to malignant hyperthermia, length of time of exposure to triggering agent, and time lapse between onset of crisis and beginning of treatment.

Post-crisis follow-up: An oral dose of 4 to 8 mg/kg/day for 1 to 3 days to prevent recurrences. If oral dosing not feasible, begin IV dose at 1 mg/kg and individualize by increasing based on patient response.

PEDIATRIC DOSE

Prophylactic, therapeutic, and post-crisis follow-up doses are the same as for adults.

DOSE ADJUSTMENTS

Dose selection should be cautious in the elderly. Reduced doses may be indicated based on the potential for decreased organ function and concomitant disease or drug therapy.

DILUTION

Each 20 mg must be diluted with 60 ml SW for injection without a bacteriostatic agent. Shake until solution is clear. May be administered through a Y-tube or three-way stopcock of infusion tubing. If large volumes will be used, transfer to plastic infusion bags; do not use glass bottles; see Compatibility. Protect diluted solution from direct light and discard after 6 hours.

Storage: Store undiluted vials between 15° and 30° C (59° and 86° F).

COMPATIBILITY

Manufacturer states, "D5W, NS, and acidic solutions are not compatible and should not be used." May form a precipitate with glass bottles; use of plastic IV bags recommended.

RATE OF ADMINISTRATION

Prophylactic dose: A single dose as an infusion distributed over 1 hour.

Therapeutic or emergency dose: Each single dose should be given by rapid continuous IV push. Follow immediately with subsequent doses as indicated.

Follow-up dose: Each single dose over 2 to 3 minutes.

ACTIONS

A direct-acting skeletal muscle relaxant. Inhibits excitation-contraction coupling by interfering with the release of the calcium ion from the sarcoplasmic reticulum to reverse the physiologic cause of malignant hyperthermia. Has no appreciable effect on cardiovascular or respiratory function. Onset of action is prompt and lasts about 5 hours. Metabolized in the liver and excreted in urine.

INDICATIONS AND USES

Perioperatively to prevent, treat, or minimize the severity of clinical and laboratory signs of malignant hyperthermia in individuals who may be or are known to be susceptible.

CONTRAINDICATIONS

None when used as indicated.

PRECAUTIONS

Use caution in patients with impaired pulmonary or cardiac function or history of liver disease. ■ Discontinue all anesthetic agents immediately when onset of malignant hyperthermia is recognized. S/S of the fulminant hypermetabolism of skeletal muscle characteristic of malignant hyperthermia crisis are tachycardia, tachypnea, central venous desaturation, hypercapnia, metabolic acidosis, skeletal muscle rigidity, cyanosis, mottling of skin, fever, increased use of anesthesia circuit CO_2 absorber.

Monitor: Monitor ECG, vital signs, electrolytes, and urine output continuously. ■ Oxygen needs are increased. ■ Manage metabolic acidosis. ■ Institute cooling measures. ■ Confirm absolute patency of vein; avoid extravasation.

Patient Education: May experience decreased grip strength, weakness in leg muscles, and lightheadedness postoperatively. May persist for 48 hours. ■ Request assistance for ambulation. ■ Use caution when eating; choking and difficulty swallowing has been reported on day of administration. ■ Avoid alcohol and other CNS depressants (e.g., diazepam [Valium]). ■ Avoid tasks that require alertness. ■ Photosensitivity may occur; sunscreens or protective clothing may be required. ■ May cause diarrhea, fatigue, nausea, and weakness. Notify physician if they persist. ■ Promptly report bloody or tarry stools, itching, jaundice (yellow color) of eyes and skin, or skin rash.

Maternal/Child: Category C: embryocidal with larger doses in rats. Benefits must outweigh risks. ■ Discontinue breast-feeding. ■ Use caution in children under 5 years; safety not established.

Elderly: Dose selection should be cautious; see Dose Adjustments.

DRUG/LAB INTERACTIONS

Ability to bind to plasma proteins inhibited by warfarin and clofibrate; increased by tolbutamide. ■ Avoid concurrent use of calcium channel blockers (e.g., diltiazem [Cardizem]) and dantrolene. Myocardial depression, arrhythmias, and hyperkalemia have been reported. ■ May cause hepatotoxicity with estrogens, especially in women over 35 years of age.

SIDE EFFECTS

Erythema, pulmonary edema, urticaria, thrombophlebitis.

ANTIDOTE

No specific antidote is available or needed when used correctly. Notify physician and initiate supportive measures (adequate airway and ventilation, monitor ECG) in overdosage. Large amounts of IV fluids may be needed to prevent crystalluria. Treat anaphylaxis and resuscitate as necessary.

DARBEPOETIN ALFA

(dar-beh-poe′ee-tin al′fa)

Antianemic agent

Aranesp

pH 5.7 to 6.4

USUAL DOSE

Rate of hemoglobin increase is dose dependent and varies among patients. Availability of iron stores, baseline hemoglobin, and concurrent medical problems affect the rate and extent of response. If a patient fails to respond or maintain a response, other etiologies should be considered and evaluated. See Monitor and Precaution.

Starting dose: May be given by IV or SC injection. 0.45 mcg/kg of body weight once per week. Adjust dose to achieve and maintain a target hemoglobin not to exceed 12 Gm/dl. See Dose Adjustment.

Conversion from epoetin alfa to darbepoetin alfa: Estimate starting dose of darbepoetin based on the weekly dose of epoetin alfa at the time of substitution as shown in the following chart. Administer darbepoetin once per week in patients who were receiving epoetin alfa 2 to 3 times a week and once every 2 weeks in patients who were receiving epoetin alfa once per week. Titrate to maintain the target hemoglobin. The route of administration (IV or SC) should remain the same.

Darbepoetin Alfa Starting Dose Based on Previous Epoetin Alfa Dose	
Previous Weekly Epoetin Alfa Dose (units/week)	**Weekly Darbepoetin Alfa Dose (mcg/week)**
<2,500	6.25
2,500 to 4,999	12.5
5,000 to 10,999	25
11,000 to 17,999	40
18,000 to 33,999	60
34,000 to 89,999	100
>90,000	200

PEDIATRIC DOSE

Safety and effectiveness for use in pediatric patients not established.

DOSE ADJUSTMENTS

Based on hemoglobin. Dose should be started slowly and adjusted for each patient to achieve and maintain a target hemoglobin level not to exceed 12 Gm/dl. Allow sufficient time before adjusting a dose; increased hemoglobin levels may not be observed for 2 to 6 weeks. Dose adjustments should not be made more frequently than once a month.

Reduce dose by 25%

If the hemoglobin is increasing and approaching 12 Gm/dl.

If the hemoglobin continues to increase after dose reduction by 25%, ***withhold doses*** until hemoglobin begins to decrease, then resume dosing at 25% below the previous dose.

If the hemoglobin increases by more than 1 Gm/dl in any 2-week period.

Increase dose by 25%

If the hemoglobin increases by less than 1 Gm/dl in a 4-week period. Further increases may be made at 4-week intervals until the specified hemoglobin is obtained.

Many patients may be maintained on a dose that is lower than the starting dose. Predialysis patients, in particular, may require lower doses. Some patients may be adequately maintained with an SC dose administered once every 2 weeks.

DILUTION

Available in numerous concentrations and in two formulations (polysorbate or albumin solutions); check vial carefully. Must be given undiluted as an IV injection. Do not administer in conjunction with other drug solutions. Do not shake; will render solution biologically inactive. Single-dose vial contains no preservatives. Use only 1 dose per vial, then discard.

Storage: Store at 2° to 8° C. Do not freeze. Protect from light.

COMPATIBILITY

Manufacturer states, "Do not administer in conjunction with other drug solutions."

RATE OF ADMINISTRATION

A single dose over at least 1 minute.

ACTIONS

An erythropoiesis-stimulating protein produced by recombinant DNA technology. Closely related to human erythropoietin. Production of endogenous erythropoietin is impaired in patients with chronic renal failure, and erythropoietin deficiency is the primary cause of their anemia. Darbepoetin has the same biologic effects as erythropoietin produced naturally by the kidneys. Stimulates bone marrow to produce RBCs, increasing the reticulocyte count within 10 days and the red cell count, hemoglobin, and hematocrit within 2 to 6 weeks. Normal iron stores are necessary because it steps up RBC production to a rate above what the body usually makes. New cells need iron, which is quickly depleted. Distribution is confined to the vascular space. Half-life is approximately 21 hours. Continued therapy will maintain improved RBC levels and decrease the need for transfusions.

INDICATIONS AND USES

Treatment of anemia associated with chronic renal failure, including patients receiving dialysis and patients not receiving dialysis.

CONTRAINDICATIONS

Known hypersensitivity to albumin, polysorbate, or darbepoetin. Uncontrolled hypertension.

PRECAUTIONS

May be given IV or SC to patients not receiving dialysis. ■ May increase risk of cardiovascular events. Higher risk may be associated with a higher hemoglobin and/or a higher rate of rise of hemoglobin. Do not exceed target hemoglobin of 12 Gm/dl or a rate of rise of more than 1 Gm/dl in a 2-week period. ■ Increases in hemoglobin of greater than 1 Gm/dl during any 2-week period have been associated with an increased incidence of cardiac arrest, neurologic events (e.g., seizures, stroke), exacerbations of hypertension, congestive heart failure (CHF), vascular thrombosis/ischemia/infarction, acute MI, and fluid overload/edema. See Dose Adjustment. ■ BP may increase during therapy with darbepoetin. Hypertensive encephalopathy and seizures have been observed. ■ Patients with uncontrolled hypertension should not be treated with darbepoetin until BP has been adequately controlled. ■ In addition to low baseline hemoglobin and inadequate iron stores, delayed or diminished response may result from concurrent medical problems (e.g., infections, inflammatory or malignant processes, occult blood loss, underlying hematologic disease, folic acid or vitamin B_{12} deficiency, hemolysis, aluminum intoxication, osteofibrosis cystica, bone marrow fibrosis). ■ Safety and efficacy have not been established in patients with underlying hematologic diseases (e.g., hemolytic anemia, sickle cell anemia, thalassemia, porphyria). ■ Therapy results in an increase in RBCs and a decrease in plasma volume, which could reduce dialysis efficiency; adjustment of dialysis prescription may be necessary. ■ Not intended for use in anemias caused by iron or folate deficiencies, hemolysis, or GI bleeding. ■ Not a substitute for emergency transfusion in patients requiring immediate correction of severe anemia. ■ As with all proteins, there is a potential for immunogenicity. The incidence of antibody development in patients receiving darbepoetin has not been determined. Use caution; allergic reactions and/or anaphylaxis can occur. ■ The formulation containing albumin carries a risk for transmission of viral diseases or Creutzfeldt-Jakob disease. However, donor screening and manufacturing processes make this risk extremely remote.

Monitor: Monitor hemoglobin weekly following initiation or adjustment of therapy. Once stabilized, continue to monitor at least monthly. ■ Monitor BP routinely. Initiation or intensification of antihypertensive therapy and dietary restrictions may be necessary. If BP is difficult to control by pharmacologic or dietary measures, the dose of darbepoetin should be reduced or withheld. ■ Monitor for the presence of premonitory neurologic symptoms during initiation of therapy or when dose is adjusted. Seizures have been reported; see Precautions. ■ Predialysis patients may be more responsive to the effects of therapy. Monitor BP, hemoglobin, renal function, and fluid and electrolyte balance. ■ Normal iron stores required to support epoetin-stimulated erythropoiesis. Transferrin saturation should be at least 20% and ferritin at least 100 ng/ml (100 mcg/L). Monitor before and during therapy. Supplemental iron (ferrous sulfate 325 mg PO 3 times a day) is usually required to increase and maintain transferrin saturation. Administration of parenteral iron may be necessary in some patients.

Patient Education: Risk of seizures, especially for first several months of therapy. Do not drive or operate heavy equipment. ■ Stress the importance of compliance with diet, iron and vitamin (e.g., folic acid, B_{12}) supplementation, and dialysis regimen. ■ Close monitoring of BP and hemoglobin is imperative. ■ Menses may resume; possibility of pregnancy. Contraception may be indicated. ■ Additional instruction (e.g., equipment, techniques) will be required in patients who will self-administer (manufacturer supplies brochure).

Maternal/Child: Category C: may present risk to fetus; benefits must justify risk. ■ Use caution in nursing mothers.

Elderly: Response similar to that found in younger patients; however, the elderly may have a greater sensitivity to its effects. ■ Monitor blood chemistry and BP carefully due to increased risk of renal and/or cardiovascular complications.

DRUG/LAB INTERACTIONS

Specific information not available.

SIDE EFFECTS

Commonly reported ***serious*** adverse reactions include cardiac arrhythmia, CHF, sepsis, vascular access thrombosis. Other commonly reported side effects were chest pain, diarrhea, fever, headache, hypertension, hypotension, infection (e.g., abscess, bacteremia, peritonitis, pneumonia, sepsis), myalgia, nausea. Less commonly reported side effects include abdominal pain, allergic reactions (e.g., rash, urticaria), angina, arthralgia, asthenia, back pain, constipation, dizziness, fatigue, flu-like symptoms, fluid overload, injection site reactions (infection, hemorrhage), limb pain, peripheral edema, vomiting. Cardiac arrest and death have been reported.

ANTIDOTE

Notify physician of all side effects; most will be treated symptomatically. Excessive hypertension may require discontinuation of darbepoetin until BP is controlled or may respond to a reduction in dose of darbepoetin or to an increase in antihypertensive therapy. Reduce dose of darbepoetin in patients with an increase in hemoglobin of more than 1 Gm/dl in 2 weeks or in patients with hemoglobin over 12 Gm/dl. May need to withhold darbepoetin until hemoglobin falls to 12 Gm/dl. Consider phlebotomy in the event of overdose or polycythemia. Adjustments in dialysis prescription may be required during dialysis to prevent clotting. Treat minor allergic reactions symptomatically. Discontinue drug and treat anaphylaxis as indicated; resuscitate as necessary.

DAUNORUBICIN HYDROCHLORIDE ■ DAUNORUBICIN CITRATE LIPOSOME INJECTION

(daw-noe-roo′bi-sin hye-droe-klor′id)

Antineoplastic (antibiotic)

Cerubidine ■ DaunoXome

pH 4.5 to 6.5 ■ 4.9 to 6

USUAL DOSE

CONVENTIONAL DAUNORUBICIN

Adult acute nonlymphocytic leukemia: 45 mg/M^2/day on days 1, 2, and 3 in adults under age 60 (adults over age 60 may require reduction to 30 mg/M^2/day). Used in specific protocol combination therapy (e.g., cytarabine 100 mg/M^2/day for 7 days). Repeat daunorubicin, 30 to 45 mg/M^2/day depending on age for only 2 days in subsequent courses and cytarabine for only 5 days every 3 to 4 weeks. To obtain a normal-appearing bone marrow may require up to 3 courses.

Adult acute lymphocytic leukemia: 45 mg/M^2/day on days 1, 2, and 3. Used in combination therapy (e.g., vincristine, prednisone, and L-asparaginase).

In all situations, when remission is complete, an individual maintenance program should be established.

DAUNOXOME (LIPOSOME INJECTION)

Advanced, HIV-associated Kaposi's sarcoma: 40 mg/M^2 as an IV infusion. Repeat every 2 weeks. Continue treatment until there is evidence of disease progression (specifics outlined in package insert).

PEDIATRIC DOSE

CONVENTIONAL DAUNORUBICIN

Acute lymphocytic leukemia in children 2 years of age and older: 25 mg/M^2/day on day 1 each week, vincristine 1.5 mg/M^2 on day 1 each week, and prednisone 40 mg/M^2 PO daily. Remission should be obtained in 4 weeks. If a partial remission is obtained after 4 weeks, 1 or 2 more weeks of treatment may produce a complete remission.

Acute lymphocytic leukemia in infants and children less than 2 years of age or less than 0.5 M^2 body surface: Calculate dose based on weight instead of body surface area. 1 mg/kg.

See Maternal/Child.

DAUNOXOME: Safety for use in children not established.

DOSE ADJUSTMENTS

ALL DAUNORUBICINS: See Precautions/Monitor.

CONVENTIONAL DAUNORUBICIN: Profound suppression of bone marrow is usually required to eradicate the leukemic cells and induce a complete remission. Evaluate bone marrow and peripheral blood to determine need for additional courses. ■ See Usual Dose for adults over 60 years of age. ■ Reduce dose in impaired liver or renal function according to the following chart.

Daunorubicin Dosing in Impaired Hepatic or Renal Function		
Serum Bilirubin	Serum Creatinine	Dose Reduction
1.2 to 3.0 mg	—	25%
>3 mg	—	50%
—	>3 mg	50%

DAUNOXOME: Reduce dose to 75% of normal (30 mg/M^2) if serum bilirubin is 1.2 to 3 mg/dl. Reduce dose to 50% of normal (20 mg/M^2) if serum bilirubin or creatinine is greater than 3 mg/dl. ▪ Withhold dose if absolute granulocyte count is less than 750 cells/mm^3.

DILUTION

Specific techniques required; see Precautions.

CONVENTIONAL DAUNORUBICIN: Each 20 mg must be diluted with 4 ml of SW for injection (5 mg/ml). Agitate gently to dissolve completely. Further dilute each dose with 10 to 15 ml of NS. Usually given through Y-tube or three-way stopcock of a free-flowing infusion of D5W or NS. May be added to 100 ml NS and given as an infusion. Use extreme caution.

DAUNOXOME: A single dose must be diluted with an equal amount of D5W. Available as a 2 mg/ml preservative-free solution. Withdraw the calculated volume (dose of DaunoXome) from the vial and transfer to a sterile infusion bag that contains an equal volume of D5W. Desired concentration is 1 mg/ml. Do not use any other diluent. A translucent red liposomal dispersion; do not use if opaque. Do not use in-line filters for infusion. See Incompatible With.

Storage: ***Conventional daunorubicin:*** Protect from sunlight. Diluted solution stable 24 hours at room temperature, 48 hours if refrigerated; then discard. ***Daunoxome:*** Refrigerate unopened vials; avoid freezing. Protect from light. Discard unused drug. Reconstituted solutions may be refrigerated for a maximum of 6 hours.

INCOMPATIBLE WITH

CONVENTIONAL DAUNORUBICIN

Manufacturer states, "Should not be administered mixed with other drugs or heparin."

DAUNOXOME

Manufacturer states, "The only fluid that may be mixed with daunoxome is D5W. Must not be mixed with saline, bateriostatic agents such as benzyl alcohol, or any other solution."

COMPATIBLE WITH

Consult pharmacist; specific conditions may apply; see Compatibilities, p. xvi.

CONVENTIONAL DAUNORUBICIN

Additive: ***Not recommended by manufacturer.*** Cytarabine (ARA-C), etoposide (VePesid), hydrocortisone sodium succinate (Solu-Cortef).

Y-site: Amifostine (Ethyol), etoposide phosphate (Etopophos), filgrastim (Neupogen), gemcitabine (Gemzar), granisetron (Kytril), melphalan (Alkeran), methotrexate (Folex), ondansetron (Zofran), sodium bicarbonate, teniposide (Vumon), thiotepa (Thioplex), vinorelbine (Navelbine).

RATE OF ADMINISTRATION

CONVENTIONAL DAUNORUBICIN

IV injection: A single dose of properly diluted medication over 3 to 5 minutes.

IV infusion: A single dose evenly distributed over 30 to 45 minutes.

DAUNOXOME

A single dose as an infusion evenly distributed over 60 minutes. Do not use an in-line filter. Back pain, flushing, and chest tightness may occur. Usually subsides if infusion is stopped, and usually does not recur if infusion is restarted at a slower rate after symptoms subside.

ACTIONS

CONVENTIONAL DAUNORUBICIN: A highly toxic antibiotic antineoplastic agent. Rapidly cleared from plasma, it inhibits synthesis of DNA. Cell cycle specific for S phase; exact method of action is unknown; antimitotic, cytotoxic, and immunosuppressive. Widely distributed in tissues, with the highest concentrations occurring in the spleen, kidneys, liver, lungs, and heart. Does not cross blood-brain barrier. Metabolized in the liver and other tissues. Elimination half-life is 18 to 30 hours. Slowly excreted in bile and urine.

DAUNOXOME: A liposomal preparation of daunorubicin formulated to maximize selectivity for solid tumors. In the circulation, the liposomal preparation protects the entrapped daunorubicin from chemical and enzymatic degradation, minimizes protein binding, and generally decreases uptake by normal (non–reticuloendothelial system) tissues. The mechanism of delivery is not known, but may be through the often altered and/or compromised vasculature of tumors. In animals, it has been shown to accumulate in tumors to a greater extent than conventional daunorubicin. Released over time within the cells of the solid tumor. Persists at high levels within tumor tissue for several days. It differs from conventional daunorubicin because it mostly confines itself to vascular fluid volume. Plasma clearance is slower and the AUC (area under the curve) is larger.

INDICATIONS AND USES

CONVENTIONAL DAUNORUBICIN: Treatment of acute nonlymphocytic leukemia in adults (myelogenous, monocytic, erythroid). ▪ Combination therapy for induction of remission in acute lymphocytic leukemia in adults and children.

DAUNOXOME: Currently approved only for first-line cytotoxic therapy for advanced HIV-associated Kaposi's sarcoma.

CONTRAINDICATIONS

CONVENTIONAL DAUNORUBICIN: Hypersensitivity to daunorubicin or any of its components. ***Not absolute;*** pre-existing bone marrow suppression, impaired cardiac function, pre-existing infection; see Precautions.

DAUNOXOME: History of hypersensitivity reaction to previous treatment with DaunoXome or any of its components (includes conventional daunorubicin). Not recommended in patients with less than advanced HIV-related Kaposi's sarcoma.

PRECAUTIONS

ALL DAUNORUBICINS: Follow guidelines for handling cytotoxic agents. See Appendix A, p. 1142. ▪ Administered by or under the direction of the physician specialist with facilities for monitoring the patient and responding to any medical emergency. ▪ Bone marrow suppression will occur in all patients given a therapeutic dose. ▪ Urine may be reddish color (from dye, not hematuria). ▪ Use extreme caution in pre-existing drug-induced bone marrow suppression, existing heart disease, previous treatment with other anthracyclines (e.g., doxorubicin [Adriamycin]), or radiation therapy encompassing the heart.

Monitor: ALL DAUNORUBICINS: Monitor CBC including differential and platelet count before each dose. ▪ Monitoring of liver function, kidney function, ECG, chest x-ray, echocardiography, and systolic ejection fraction indicated before and during therapy; recommended before each course. ▪ Evaluation of cardiac function by medical history and physical exam is recommended before each dose. ▪ Monitor closely for S/S of hemorrhage or infection, may be life-threatening. ▪ Prophylactic antibiotics may be indicated pending results of C/S in a febrile neutropenic patient. ▪ Determine absolute patency of vein. A stinging or burning sensation indicates extravasation; discontinue injection and use another vein. Severe cellulitis and tissue necrosis will result from extravasation with conventional daunorubicins; has not been observed with DaunoXome. ▪ Prophylactic antiemetics may reduce nausea and vomiting and increase patient comfort. ▪ Monitor uric acid levels; maintain hydration; allopurinol may be indicated. ▪ Monitor for thrombocytopenia (platelet count less than 50,000/mm^3). Initiate precautions to prevent excessive bleeding (e.g., inspect IV sites, skin, and mucous membranes; use extreme care during invasive procedures; test urine, emesis, stool, and secretions for occult blood).

CONVENTIONAL DAUNORUBICIN: May cause acute congestive heart failure with total cumulative doses over 550 mg/M^2 in adults (400 mg/M^2 if previous treatment with doxorubicin or radiation therapy in area of heart), 300 mg/M^2 in children over 2 years, and 10 mg/kg in children under 2 years.

DAUNOXOME: May also cause cardiomyopathy. Monitoring of LVEF recommended at total cumulative doses of 320 mg/M^2, 480 mg/M^2, and every 240 mg/M^2 thereafter.

Patient Education: Nonhormonal birth control recommended. ▪ Report IV site burning or stinging promptly. ▪ Secondary leukemias have been reported. ▪ See Appendix D, p. 1148.

Maternal/Child: ALL DAUNORUBICINS: Category D: can cause fetal harm. Avoid pregnancy. ▪ Safety for use in breast-feeding not established; discontinue breast-feeding. ▪ Cardiotoxicity may be more frequent and occur at lower cumulative doses in children. ▪ See Monitor.

DAUNOXOME: Safety for use in children not established.

Elderly: Cardiotoxicity and myelotoxicity may be more severe. Consider age-related renal impairment. Safety of DaunoXome for use in the elderly has not been established.

DRUG/LAB INTERACTIONS

Concurrent use with cyclophosphamide (Cytoxan) may increase cardiotoxicity. ▪ Dose reduction may be required with concurrent use of other myelosuppressive agents. ▪ Concurrent use with hepatotoxic agents (e.g., high-dose methotrexate) may increase risk of toxicity. ▪ Risk of cardiotoxicity increased in patients previously treated with maximum cumulative doses of other anthracyclines (e.g., doxorubicin [Adriamycin], idarubicin [Idamycin]) and/or radiation encompassing the heart. ▪ Do not administer vaccines or chloroquine to patients receiving antineoplastic drugs. ▪ See Precautions.

SIDE EFFECTS

All Daunorubicins: Bone marrow suppression and cardiotoxicity are dose related and dose limiting.

Conventional Daunorubicin: Acute congestive heart failure, alopecia (reversible), bone marrow suppression (marked with average doses), chills, decrease in systolic ejection fraction, depressed QRS voltage, diarrhea, fever, gonadal suppression, mucositis, myocarditis, nausea, pericarditis, skin rash, vomiting.

DaunoXome: Granulocytopenia is most common. Symptoms common to conventional daunorubicin may also occur. Infusion related back pain, chest tightness, and flushing may be related to liposomal formulation.

Overdose: Will cause increased severity of myelosuppression, fatigue, nausea, and vomiting.

ANTIDOTE

Most side effects will be tolerated or treated symptomatically. Keep physician informed. Close monitoring of cumulative dosage, bone marrow, ECG, chest x-ray, echocardiography, and systolic ejection fraction may prevent most serious and potentially fatal side effects. There is no specific antidote. Supportive therapy as indicated will help sustain the patient in toxicity. Administration of whole blood products (e.g., packed RBCs, platelets, leukocytes) and/or blood modifiers (e.g., darbepoetin alfa [Aranesp], epoetin alfa [Epogen, Procrit], filgrastim [Neupogen], pegfilgrastim [Neulasta], sargramostim [Leukine], oprelvekin [Neumega]) may be indicated to treat bone marrow toxicity. For extravasation, aspirate as much infiltrated drug as possible, flood site with normal saline, and inject hydrocortisone sodium succinate (Solu-Cortef) or hyaluronidase (Wydase) throughout extravasated tissue. Use a 27- or 25-gauge needle. Cold, moist compresses may be helpful; elevate extremity. Site should be observed promptly by a reconstructive surgeon.

DEFEROXAMINE MESYLATE

(de-fer-ox′a-meen mes′uh-lat)

Antidote
Chelating agent

Desferal

pH 4 to 6

USUAL DOSE

Available on an allocation basis from the manufacturer. Hospitals and selected health facilities are allowed to keep four boxes on hand. See Precautions for ordering process.

Acute iron intoxication: 15 mg/kg/hr may be given up to a total dose of 90 mg/kg every 8 hours. ***Do not exceed 6 Gm in 24 hours by way of any or all routes—IV, IM, clysis, or oral.***

Chronic iron overload: In addition to IM dose given with each unit of blood, give 2 Gm IV at a rate not to exceed 15 mg/kg/hr. Use a separate vein.

Aluminum toxicity: Dose must be individualized. 100 mg can bind 4.1 mg of aluminum.

Diagnosis of aluminum toxicity: 1 Gm infused at a rate not to exceed 15 mg/kg/hr. Usually given post-dialysis, but may be given during the last 2 hours of dialysis.

PEDIATRIC DOSE

Acute iron intoxication in children over 3 years of age: A continuous infusion of 50 mg/kg of body weight up to 2 Gm every 6 hours or 90 mg/kg every 8 hours. ***Do not exceed a rate of 15 mg/kg/hr or a total dose of 6 Gm in 24 hours.***

Acute iron intoxication in children under 3 years of age: 15 mg/kg/hr as a continuous infusion.

Chronic iron overload: 50 mg/kg/dose every 6 hours at a rate not to exceed 15 mg/kg/hr. Maximum 2 Gm/dose or 6 Gm in 24 hours.

Diagnosis of aluminum toxicity: 15 to 20 mg/kg at a rate not to exceed 15 mg/kg/hr. See comment under Usual Dose.

DILUTION

Each 500 mg must be diluted in 2 ml of SW for injection. When completely dissolved, deferoxamine must be further diluted in an IV solution; NS, D5W, D10W, and LR are compatible.

Storage: Under sterile conditions, deferoxamine diluted with sterile water may be stored at room temperature for 1 week. Protect from light.

COMPATIBILITY

Manufacturer states, "Reconstituting in solvents or under conditions other than indicated may result in precipitation. Turbid solutions should not be used."

RATE OF ADMINISTRATION

In all situations the fully diluted solution must not exceed a rate of 15 mg/kg of body weight/hr; see Side Effects; Overdose.

ACTIONS

An iron-chelating agent, deferoxamine complexes with iron to form ferrioxamine, a stable chelate that prevents the iron from entering into further chemical reactions. Readily soluble in water, it passes easily through the kidney, giving the urine a characteristic reddish color. It will remove iron from free serum iron, ferritin, and transferrin, but not from hemoglobin or cytochromes. Metabolized by plasma enzymes.

INDICATIONS AND USES

To facilitate the removal of iron in the treatment of acute iron intoxication or chronic iron overload from multiple transfusions.

Unlabeled uses: Diagnosis and management of aluminum accumulation in bone of renal failure patients and in aluminum-induced dialysis encephalopathy.

CONTRAINDICATIONS

Severe renal disease or anuria.

PRECAUTIONS

IM administration is preferred. May be given SC by hypodermoclysis. IV administration should be used only in a state of cardiovascular shock or chronic iron overload. ■ For long-term therapy, check for cataract development. ■ See Maternal/Child. ■ To order from manufacturer (Novartis), fax request to 1-973-781-5508 (24-hour line). Include a copy of the prescription or doctor's order, a written request for a 2-week supply, and the name and address of a wholesaler for billing purposes. Questions? Telephone 1-888-669-6682.

Monitor: Deferoxamine is adjunctive therapy. Standard measures for treating acute iron intoxication are also indicated: induction of emesis and/or gastric lavage; suction and maintenance of a clear airway; control of shock with IV fluids, blood, oxygen, and vasopressors; correction of acidosis. Monitor serum ferritin or iron concentration. ■ In acute iron intoxication, larger-than-normal amounts of IV fluids are required to maintain intravascular volume and prevent kidney damage. Monitor blood gases, central venous pressure (CVP), and cardiac output frequently to assess effects of absorbed iron. Monitor renal function.

Patient Education: Report any hearing or vision changes. ■ Do not take vitamin C unless prescribed by physician.

Maternal/Child: Category C: use only if clearly needed during early pregnancy or during child-bearing years. ■ Use in children under 3 years only if there is iron mobilization greater than 1 mg/24 hr.

Elderly: See Drug/Lab Interactions. ■ Risk of cardiac decompensation increased.

DRUG/LAB INTERACTIONS

Risk of cardiac decompensation from increased tissue iron toxicity increased when given concurrently with ascorbic acid (Cenolate).

SIDE EFFECTS

Occur more frequently with too-rapid administration; abdominal discomfort, allergic type of reactions including anaphylaxis, blurring of vision, diarrhea, flushing of the skin, fever, hypotension, leg cramps, shock, tachycardia, urticaria. Blood dyscrasias (e.g., leukopenia, thrombocytopenia) have been reported.

Overdose: Acute transient loss of vision, acute renal failure, agitation, aphasia, bradycardia, CNS depression including coma, headache, hypotension, GI disturbances, nausea, and tachycardia may occur with too rapid administration, inadvertent IV bolus, or overdose.

ANTIDOTE

At first sign of side effects, decrease rate of administration. If side effects persist, discontinue drug and notify physician. Further dilution and decrease in rate of administration may be necessary. Readily dialyzable. Resuscitate as indicated.

DENILEUKIN DIFTITOX

(den-ih-loo′kin dif′tih-tox)

Antineoplastic
Biological response modifier

Ontak

pH 6.9 to 7.2

USUAL DOSE

Pretesting indicated and premedication suggested; see Monitor.

9 or 18 mcg/kg/day administered as an IV infusion for 5 consecutive days. Repeat course every 21 days. The optimal duration of therapy has not been determined. However, in studies, only 2% of patients who did not demonstrate at least a 25% decrease in tumor burden by the initiation of the fourth course of treatment subsequently responded.

DOSE ADJUSTMENTS

In patients with hypoalbuminemia, administration of denileukin diftitox should be delayed until serum albumin levels are at least 3 Gm/dl; see Monitor.

DILUTION

Each 2-ml vial contains 300 mcg (150 mcg/ml) of frozen recombinant denileukin diftitox. Bring to CRT before preparing dose. Thaw in refrigerator (2° to 8° C) for not more than 24 hours or at CRT for 1 to 2 hours. Do not heat. Gently swirl contents of vial. Do not shake. Solution may be hazy initially. Haze should clear as solution reaches CRT. The concentration of denileukin diftitox must be at least 15 mcg/ml during all steps in the preparation of the infusion solution. This is best accomplished by aseptically withdrawing the calculated dose of denileukin diftitox and injecting it into an empty infusion bag. For each 1 ml of denileukin diftitox from the vial(s), no more than 9 ml of sterile NS without preservative should then be added to the bag. For example: A 70-kg patient receiving a 9-mcg/kg dose would require 630 mcg of denileukin diftitox (or 4.2 ml). Withdraw 4.2 ml of denileukin diftitox from vials and inject into an empty infusion bag. Add no more than 37.8 ml (9 × 4.2 ml) of preservative-free NS to infusion bag. The final solution will be 630 mcg in 42 ml of solution, which equals the desired concentration of 15 mcg/ml. Diluted denileukin diftitox must be prepared and stored in a plastic syringe or soft plastic IV infusion bag. Do not use a glass container; see Compatibility.

Storage: Store unopened vials in freezer at −10° C. Prepared solutions should be administered within 6 hours. Discard unused solution. Do not refreeze.

COMPATIBILITY

Manufacturer states, "Do not physically mix denileukin diftitox with other drugs." Do not mix in glass. Adsorption to glass may occur in the dilute state.

RATE OF ADMINISTRATION

A single dose evenly distributed over at least 15 minutes. Administer via peripheral or central vein by a pump device or IV infusion bag. Do not administer through an in-line filter. Some evidence suggests that infusion over 25 to 30 minutes may be better tolerated. If adverse reactions occur during the infusion, the infusion should be discontinued or the rate should be reduced depending on the severity of the reaction. There is no clinical experience with infusion times lasting more than 80 minutes.

ACTIONS

A recombinant DNA–derived cytotoxic protein. A fusion protein that utilizes both the cytotoxic action of diphtheria toxin and the cell-targeting ability of interleukin-2 (IL-2) to kill certain leukemia and lymphoma cells. Targets specific receptors (IL-2 receptors) on malignant cells while minimizing damage to normal cells that do not express the receptor. Human IL-2 receptors exist in three forms, low (CD25), intermediate (CD122/CD132), and high (CD25/CD122/CD132) affinity. The high-affinity form of this receptor is usually found only on activated T lymphocytes, activated B lymphocytes, and activated macrophages. Malignant cells expressing one or more of the subunits of the IL-2 receptor are found in certain leukemias and lymphomas, including cutaneous T-cell lymphoma (CTCL [a low-grade non-Hodgkin's lymphoma]). Ex vivo studies suggest that denileukin diftitox interacts with the high-affinity IL-2 receptor on the cell surface and inhibits cellular protein synthesis, resulting in cell death within hours. No differences in pharmacologic action noted based on age, gender, and/or race. Studies in rats show the liver and kidneys to be the primary sites of distribution and accumulation of denileukin diftitox outside of the vasculature. In these studies, denileukin diftitox was metabolized by proteolytic degradation. Excreted material was less than 25% of the total injected dose and consisted of low-molecular-weight breakdown products. Half-life in lymphoma patients is 70 to 80 minutes. Development of antibodies to denileukin diftitox has been shown to increase clearance; see Precautions.

INDICATIONS AND USES

Treatment of patients with persistent or recurrent cutaneous T-cell lymphoma whose malignant cells express the CD25 component of the IL-2 receptor. The safety and efficacy of denileukin diftitox in patients with CTCL whose malignant cells do not express the CD25 component of the IL-2 receptor have not been examined.

CONTRAINDICATIONS

Hypersensitivity to denileukin diftitox, any of its components, diphtheria toxin, or interleukin-2.

PRECAUTIONS

Administered under the supervision of a physician experienced in the use of antineoplastic therapy and the management of patients with cancer. Administer in a facility equipped and staffed for cardiopulmonary resuscitation and where the patient can be properly monitored. ■ Acute hypersensitivity reactions were reported in 69% of study patients during or within 24 hours of infusion; approximately one half of the reactions occurred on the first day of dosing regardless of the treatment cycle. Pretreatment with acetaminophen or a NSAID (e.g., ibuprofen [Motrin]) and antihistamines (e.g., diphenhydramine) may reduce acute infusion-related events. ■ Vascular leak syndrome, characterized by at least two of the following three symptoms (edema, hypoalbuminemia [2.8 or less], hypotension), was reported in 27% of study patients. Onset usually occurs within 2 weeks of the infusion. Patients with edema or pre-existing low serum albumin levels may be predisposed to this syndrome. Use special caution in patients with pre-existing cardiovascular disease. ■ Before therapy, 39% of patients had low titers of antibody that cross-reacted with the diphtheria toxin domains of the denileukin diftitox, presumably due to prior diphtheria immunization. Development of anti–denileukin diftitox antibodies was observed in 41 of 49 patients after a single course and in 33 of 34 patients after three courses of therapy. Following anti–denileukin diftitox antibody formation, there was a significant increase in clearance of the drug. The antibody response in all such patients was directed against the diphtheria toxin domain. A low titer of antibodies to the IL-2 portion of the denileukin diftitox molecule also developed in approximately 50% of patients. The presence of antibodies did not affect the ability of the patient to respond to therapy. The presence or absence of antibodies did not correlate with the risk of immediate hypersensitivity-type infusional adverse events.

Monitor: Before administration of denileukin diftitox, the patient's malignant cells should be tested for CD25 expression. A testing service for the assay of CD25 on skin biopsy samples is available. For information on this service, call 800-964-5836. ■ Pretreatment with acetaminophen or NSAIDs and antihistamines (e.g., diphenhydramine [Benadryl]) 30 to 60 minutes before each infusion may reduce infusion-related events; see Precautions. ■ Monitor CBC and a blood chemistry panel, including liver and renal function, before therapy and weekly during therapy. ■ Monitor serum albumin levels before each course of therapy. Hypoalbuminemia was reported in 83% of study patients with lymphoma. Nadir occurs 1 to 2 weeks after administration. Delay administration if necessary until serum albumin levels are at least 3 Gm/dl. Note Dose Adjustments. ■ Monitor weight, edema, BP, and serum albumin levels on an outpatient basis. Onset of vascular leak syndrome may be delayed, usually occurring within the first two weeks of infusion. Symptoms may persist or worsen after discontinuation of therapy. ■ Monitor for signs and symptoms of infection. Patients with CTCL have a predisposition to cutaneous infections, and binding of denileukin diftitox to activated lymphocytes and macrophages may lead to cell death and may impair patient's immune system. ■ Monitor for thrombocytopenia (platelet count less than 50,000/mm^3). Initiate precautions to prevent excessive bleeding (e.g., inspect IV sites, skin, and mucous membranes; use extreme care during invasive procedures; test urine, emesis, stool, and secretions for occult blood). ■ Monitor injection site. To minimize occurrence or phlebitis, change the injection site frequently. ■ See Precautions, Side Effects, and Antidote.

Patient Education: Report weight gain, edema, or signs of a hypersensitivity reaction promptly. Keep physician informed of all side effects.

Maternal/Child: Category C: safety for use in pregnancy not established. Use only if clearly needed. ■ Discontinue breast-feeding. ■ Safety and effectiveness in children not established.

Elderly: Response rates similar to those seen in younger patients. Adverse events that tended to be more frequent and/or severe in lymphoma patients who were 65 years of age or older include anemia, anorexia, confusion, hypotension, nausea and/or vomiting, rash.

DRUG/LAB INTERACTIONS

Drug interaction studies have not been conducted.

SIDE EFFECTS

All patients experienced at least one adverse event. The occurrence of side effects tended to diminish in frequency and severity after the first two courses of therapy. ■ Most frequent reasons for discontinuation of therapy were systemic flu-like symptoms (e.g., anorexia, asthenia, chills, fever, malaise, nausea, and vomiting), hypoalbuminemia, infection, rash, respiratory events (e.g., dyspnea, apnea, pulmonary edema, or pneumonia), and vascular leak syndrome. ■ Most frequent reasons for therapy-related hospitalization were evaluation of fever, management of vascular leak syndrome, or dehydration secondary to gastrointestinal toxicity. ■ There were two distinct infusion-related reactions: The first is an acute hypersensitivity-type symptom complex that occurred in 69% of study patients and included one or more of the following symptoms: allergic reaction, anaphylaxis, back pain, chest pain or tightness, dysphagia or laryngismus, dyspnea, hypotension, rash, syncope, tachycardia, and vasodilation; see Precautions. The second is a flu-like syndrome that occurred in 91% of study patients. Symptoms developed within hours to days following infusion and included one or more of the following: asthenia, arthralgias, digestive symptoms, fever and/or chills, and myalgias. ■ Other reported side effects included acute renal insufficiency; albuminuria; anemia; anorexia; confusion; creatinine increase; decreased serum levels of albumin, calcium, and potassium; dehydration; deep venous thrombosis; diarrhea (may be delayed and prolonged); dizziness; headache; hematuria; hypertension; hyperthyroidism; hypocalcemia; hypokalemia; hypothyroidism; hypotension; increased SrCr; injection site reaction; insomnia; leukopenia; nervousness; pancreatitis; paresthesia; pharyngitis; pruritus; pulmonary embolism; pyuria; rash; rhinitis; sweating; thrombocytopenia; thrombotic events; transient hepatic transaminase elevations (ALT, [SGPT], AST [SGOT]); and vomiting.

ANTIDOTE

Notify physician of any side effects. If adverse reactions occur during administration, the infusion should be discontinued or the rate should be reduced depending on the severity of the reaction. IV antihistamines, corticosteroids, and/or epinephrine may be required. Most symptoms of the flu-like syndrome will respond to treatment with antipyretics and/or antiemetics (e.g., promethazine [Phenergan] or prochlorperazine [Compazine]). Premedication with acetaminophen and an antihistamine 30 to 60 minutes before each infusion may help reduce the frequency and/or severity of symptoms. While on therapy, patients may continue to receive acetaminophen every 4 to 6 hours while awake. Fever, chills, and/or pain not controlled with acetaminophen alone may be treated with a NSAID. Rigors may be treated with meperidine. Skin rashes may require treatment with topical and/or oral corticosteroids. Treatment of vascular leak syndrome depends on whether edema or hypotension is the primary clinical problem. Patients who present with dehydration should be considered for IV fluid replacement therapy. If BP is still not adequate after replacement therapy, pressor agents (e.g., dopamine [Intropin]) should be considered. Use of diuretics should be avoided in patients whose intravascular depletion has not been corrected. However, patients who present primarily with edema may benefit from diuretic therapy. Continuous monitoring of fluid status, weight, and BP is essential. If overdose occurs, hepatic and renal function and overall fluid status should be closely monitored. Resuscitate as necessary.

DESMOPRESSIN ACETATE
(des-moe-press′in as′ah-tat)

Hormone
Antidiuretic
Antihemorrhagic

DDAVP, 1-Deamino-8-D-Arginine Vasopressin **pH 3.5 to 4**

USUAL DOSE

Diabetes insipidus: 2 to 4 mcg daily in 2 divided doses. Adjust each dose individually for an adequate diurnal rhythm of water turnover. IV dose has 10 times the antidiuretic effect of intranasal desmopressin. Available as a tablet to manage cranial central diabetes insipidus.

Hemophilia A and von Willebrand's disease (type 1): 0.3 mcg/kg of body weight. Administer 30 minutes preoperatively.

DOSE ADJUSTMENTS

Many specific requirements depending on diagnosis; see Precautions, Monitor. ■ Reduce dose accordingly when transferring from intranasal to IV administration.

DILUTION

Diabetes insipidus: May be given undiluted.

Hemophilia A and von Willebrand's disease (type 1): Dilute a single dose in 10 ml of NS for children under 10 kg; 50 ml for adults and children over 10 kg. Must be given as an infusion.

Storage: Refrigerate at 2° to 8° C (36° to 46° F). Use diluted product promptly.

COMPATIBILITY

Specific information not available. Consider specific use; consult pharmacist.

RATE OF ADMINISTRATION

Diabetes insipidus: A single dose by IV injection over 1 minute.

Hemophilia A and von Willebrand's disease (type 1): A single dose as an infusion over 15 to 30 minutes.

ACTIONS

A synthetic analog of the natural hormone arginine vasopressin (human antidiuretic hormone—ADH). It is more potent than arginine vasopressin in increasing plasma levels of factor VIII activity in patients with hemophilia A and von Willebrand's disease (Type I). Produces dose-related increase in factor VIII levels within 30 minutes and peaks in 90 to 120 minutes. Onset of action as an antidiuretic is prompt and lasts from 8 to 20 hours. Increases water resorption in the kidney, increases urine osmolality, and decreases urine output. Clinically effective antidiuretic doses are usually below the levels needed to affect vascular or visceral smooth muscle.

INDICATIONS AND USES

Antidiuretic replacement therapy in the management of central (cranial) diabetes insipidus. ■ Management of the temporary polyuria and polydipsia following head trauma or surgery in the pituitary region. ■ Maintenance of hemostasis in patients with hemophilia A or von Willebrand's disease during surgical procedures and postoperatively. ■ To stop bleeding in patients with hemophilia A or von Willebrand's disease with episodes of spontaneous or trauma-induced injuries.

CONTRAINDICATIONS

Infants under 3 months in hemophilia A or von Willebrand's disease, known hypersensitivity to desmopressin.

PRECAUTIONS

Use caution in patients with coronary artery insufficiency or hypertension. ■ Excessive fluid intake may result in an extreme decrease in plasma osmolality. May lead to seizures and coma. ■ Use with caution in patients predisposed to thrombus formation. ■ Use with caution in patients with conditions associated with fluid and electrolyte imbalance (e.g., cystic fibrosis).

Monitor: ***Diabetes insipidus:*** ■ Not effective for the treatment of nephrogenic diabetes insipidus. ■ Confirm diagnosis of diabetes insipidus by the water deprivation test, the hypertonic saline infusion test, and the response to ADH. Monitor continued response by measuring urine volume and osmolality. Plasma osmolality may be needed. Monitor serum electrolytes in therapy lasting longer than 7 days. Accuracy and effectiveness of dose measured by duration of sleep and adequate, not excessive, water turnover.

Hemophilia A: May be considered for use in patients with factor VIII activity levels from 2% to 5% with careful monitoring. Generally used only when the factor VIII activity level is above 5%. ■ Not indicated in patients with hemophilia B or those with factor VIII antibodies. ■ Monitor factor VIII coagulant, factor VIII antigen, factor VIII ristocetin cofactor, and aPTT.

Von Willebrand's disease (type I): Most effective when factor VIII activity level above 5%. ■ Monitor bleeding time, factor VIII activity levels, ristocetin cofactor activity, and von Willebrand factor antigen during therapy to ensure adequate levels. ■ Not indicated for treatment of severe classic von Willebrand's disease (Type I), Type IIB von Willebrand's disease (will induce platelet aggregation), or if there is evidence of an abnormal molecular form of factor VIII antigen.

Hemophilia and von Willebrand's disease: Sometimes used with aminocaproic acid. ■ Monitor BP and pulse during infusion.

Patient Education: When antidiuretic effect is not needed, caution patients (especially the young and the elderly) to limit fluid intake to satisfy thirst needs only; this decreases potential occurrence of water intoxication and hyponatremia.

Maternal/Child: Use only when clearly indicated in pregnancy and breast-feeding. ■ Risk of hyponatremia and water intoxication increased in children. Restrict fluid intake. ■ Safety for use in children under 12 years with diabetes insipidus not established. ■ See Contraindications.

Elderly: Risk of hyponatremia and water intoxication increased. Use caution and careful fluid intake restriction.

DRUG/LAB INTERACTIONS

May produce hypertension with other vasopressors (e.g., dopamine [Intropin]). ■ May be potentiated by chlorpropamide, clofibrate, or carbamazepine.

SIDE EFFECTS

Are infrequent. High doses may produce facial flushing, headache, hypertension (slight), mild abdominal cramps, nausea, and vulval pain. May cause burning, local erythema, and swelling at site of injection; hyponatremia; and water intoxication. Anaphylaxis has been reported.

ANTIDOTE

Notify physician of all side effects. Most will respond to reduction of dose or rate of administration, or symptomatic treatment. May need to discontinue drug. Resuscitate as necessary.

DEXAMETHASONE SODIUM PHOSPHATE

(dex-a-meth′a-sone so′de-um fos′fat)

Hormone (adrenocorticoid/glucocorticoid)
Antiinflammatory, Antiemetic
Immunosuppressant, Diagnostic agent

Decadron, Decadron Phosphate

pH 7 to 8.5

USUAL DOSE

Average dose range is 0.5 to 24 mg daily. May be divided into 2 to 4 doses. IV dexamethasone is usually given in an emergency situation or when oral dosing is not feasible. Larger doses may be justified by patient condition. Repeat until adequate response, then decrease dose as indicated. Total dose usually does not exceed 80 mg/24 hr. Dosage must be individualized. High-dose treatment is utilized until patient condition stabilizes, usually no longer than 48 to 72 hours. Doses similar by IV or oral route.

Antiinflammatory: See average dose range above.

Shock: Several regimens have been suggested:

1 to 6 mg/kg as a single injection; *or*

40 mg. Repeat every 2 to 6 hours as needed; *or*

20 mg as a ***loading dose,*** followed by a continuous infusion of 3 mg/kg equally distributed over 24 hours.

Cerebral edema: ***Loading dose:*** 10 mg. ***Maintenance dose:*** 4 mg every 6 hours (usually given IM). Reduce dose after 2 to 4 days. Discontinue gradually over 5 to 7 days. A brain tumor requiring treatment before dexamethasone can be discontinued is the exception.

Cerebral edema (ICP) in recurrent or inoperable brain tumors: 2 mg every 8 to 12 hours (usually given IM). Adjust based on patient response.

Antiemetic in management of emesis-inducing chemotherapy: Several regimens have been used:

10 to 20 mg before chemotherapy. Lower doses may be given over the next 24 to 72 hours if necessary; *or*

Give a loading dose of 4 to 8 mg/M^2. May repeat 2 to 4 mg/M^2 every 6 hours; *or*

20 mg combined with 8 mg of ondansetron (Zofran) in 50 ml D5W before chemotherapy; *or*

20 mg 40 minutes before administration of chemotherapeutic agent. Given concurrently with metoclopramide and lorazepam or diphenhydramine; *or*

10 mg 30 minutes before administration of chemotherapeutic agent. Given concurrently with oral dexamethasone 8 mg beginning prior evening, 4 mg every 4 to 6 hours continuing through treatment day, with droperidol or haloperidol.

Airway edema: ***Adults and children:*** 0.25 to 0.5 mg/kg every 6 hours for croup or beginning 24 hours before elective extubation. Repeat for 4 to 6 doses. Up to 1 mg/kg/24 hr may be given in divided doses before and after extubation.

Allergic conditions: (Usually given IM or PO) 4 to 8 mg on the first day, then PO in decreasing doses (1.5 mg every 12 hours on day 2 and 3; 0.75 mg every 12 hours on day 4; and 0.75 mg on day 5 and 6).

Meningitis: ***Adults and children:*** 0.15 mg/kg/dose every 6 hours for 4 days.
Primary or secondary adrenocortical insufficiency (physiologic replacement): 0.03 to 0.15 mg/kg/24 hr or 0.6 to 0.75 mg/M^2/24 hr given in divided doses every 6 to 12 hours (0.015 to 0.075 mg/kg every 12 hours, or 0.0075 to 0.0375 mg/kg every 6 hours, or 0.3 to 0.375 mg/M^2 every 12 hours, or 0.15 to 0.1875 mg/M^2 every 6 hours). Usually given IM. Dexamethasone has minimal mineralocorticoid properties; may require a concomitant mineralocorticoid (e.g., hydrocortisone IV or fludrocortisone [Florinef] PO). Hydrocortisone is the drug of choice for this indication.

PEDIATRIC DOSE

See Maternal/Child.
Cerebral edema: ***Loading dose:*** 0.5 to 1.5 mg/kg of body weight.
Maintenance dose: 0.2 to 0.5 mg/kg/24 hr in equally divided doses every 6 hours (0.05 to 0.125 mg/kg every 6 hours) for 5 days, then gradually decrease.
Airway edema: See Usual Dose.
Antiemetic: ***Loading dose:*** 4 to 8 mg/M^2. May repeat 2 to 4 mg/M^2 every 6 hours.
Antiinflammatory: 0.03 to 0.15 mg/kg/24 hr in equally divided doses every 6 to 12 hours (0.015 to 0.075 mg/kg every 12 hours or 0.0075 to 0.0375 mg/kg every 6 hours).
Meningitis: See Usual Dose.

DOSE ADJUSTMENTS

Reduced dose may be required in the elderly and with cyclophosphamide. ■ See Drug/Lab Interactions.

DILUTION

May be given undiluted or added to IV glucose or saline solutions and given as an infusion. 24 mg/ml product for IV use only; 4 mg/ml may be used IM/IV.
Storage: Use diluted solutions within 24 hours. Sensitive to heat. Protect from freezing.

COMPATIBLE WITH **(Underline Indicates Conflicting Compatibility Information)**

Consult pharmacist; specific conditions may apply; see Compatibilities, p. xvi.
Additive: Amikacin (Amikin), aminophylline, bleomycin (Blenoxane), cimetidine (Tagamet), furosemide (Lasix), granisetron (Kytril), lidocaine, meropenem (Merrem IV), mitomycin (Mutamycin), nafcillin (Nafcil), ondansetron (Zofran), prochlorperazine (Compazine), ranitidine (Zantac), verapamil (Isoptin).
Syringe: Diphenhydramine (Benadryl), granisetron (Kytril), hydromorphone (Dilaudid), metoclopramide (Reglan), ondansetron (Zofran), ranitidine (Zantac), sufentanil (Sufenta).
Y-site: Acyclovir (Zovirax), allopurinol (Aloprim, Zyloprim), amifostine (Ethyol), amikacin (Amikin), amphotericin B cholesteryl (Amphotec), aztreonam (Azactam), cefepime (Maxipime), cisatracurium (Nimbex), cisplatin (Platinol), cladribine (Leustatin), cyclophosphamide (Cytoxan), cytarabine (ARA-C), docetaxel (Taxotere), doxorubicin (Adriamycin), doxorubicin liposome (Doxil), etoposide phosphate (Etopophos), famotidine (Pepcid IV), fentanyl (Sublimaze), filgrastim (Neupogen), fluconazole (Diflucan), fludarabine (Fludara), foscarnet (Foscavir), gatifloxacin (Tequin), gemcitabine (Gemzar), granisetron (Kytril), heparin, hetastarch in electrolytes (Hextend), hydromorphone (Dilaudid), levofloxacin (Levaquin), linezolid (Zyvox), lorazepam (Ativan), melphalan (Alkeran), me-

peridine (Demerol), meropenem (Merrem IV), methotrexate (Folex), morphine, ondansetron (Zofran), paclitaxel (Taxol), piperacillin/tazobactam (Zosyn), potassium chloride (KCl), propofol (Diprivan), remifentanil (Ultiva), sargramostim (Leukine), sodium bicarbonate, sufentanil (Sufenta), tacrolimus (Prograf), teniposide (Vumon), theophylline, thiotepa (Thioplex), vinorelbine (Navelbine), zidovudine (AZT, Retrovir).

RATE OF ADMINISTRATION

A single dose over 1 minute or less if necessary. As an IV infusion, give at prescribed rate.

ACTIONS

An antiinflammatory glucocorticoid. A synthetic adrenocortical steroid with little sodium retention. Very soluble in water. Seven times as potent as prednisolone and 20 to 30 times as potent as hydrocortisone. Has minimal mineralocorticoid activity. Primarily used for antiinflammatory and immunosuppressive effects. May be used in conjunction with other forms of therapy, such as epinephrine for acute allergic reactions or antibiotics for acute infections. Metabolized primarily in the liver and excreted as inactive metabolites in urine. Crosses the placental barrier. Excreted in urine and breast milk.

INDICATIONS AND USES

Supplementary therapy for severe allergic reactions. ■ Reduction of acute edematous states (cerebral edema, airway edema). ■ Shock unresponsive to conventional therapy. ■ Acute exacerbations of disease for patients receiving steroid therapy. ■ Adrenocortical insufficiency; total, relative, and operative. ■ Antiemetic for chemotherapy-induced vomiting (e.g., cisplatin). Has numerous other uses by other routes of administration (e.g., IM, intraarticular, intralesional, intrasynovial, soft-tissue injection, oral inhalant).

Unlabeled uses: Adjunct to treatment of meningitis with antibiotics (to reduce incidence of ototoxicity). ■ Dexamethasone or betamethasone are given IM to the mother to accelerate the production of lung surfactant in utero in the prevention of respiratory distress syndrome of premature infants.

CONTRAINDICATIONS

Hypersensitivity to any product component including sulfites, systemic fungal infections.

Relative contraindications: Active or latent peptic ulcer, acute or healed tuberculosis, acute or chronic infections (especially chickenpox), acute psychoses, diabetes mellitus, diverticulitis, fresh intestinal anastomoses, myasthenia gravis, ocular herpes simplex, osteoporosis, pregnancy, psychotic tendencies, renal insufficiency, thromboembolic tendencies.

PRECAUTIONS

Withdrawal from therapy should be gradual to avoid precipitation of symptoms of adrenal insufficiency. The patient is observed, especially under stress, for up to 2 years. ■ Prophylactic antacids may prevent peptic ulcer complications. ■ Use with caution in hypothyroidism and cirrhosis. **Monitor:** May increase insulin needs in diabetes. ■ Monitor electrolytes periodically. May cause sodium retention and potassium and calcium excretion. May cause hypertension secondary to fluid and electrolyte disturbances. ■ May mask signs of infection. ■ Administer a single dose before 9 AM to reduce suppression of individual's adrenocortical activity. ■

Periodic ophthalmic exams may be necessary with prolonged treatment. ■ See Drug/Lab Interactions.

Patient Education: Report edema, tarry stools, or weight gain promptly. Anorexia, diarrhea, dizziness, fatigue, low blood sugar, nausea, weakness, weight loss, and vomiting promptly. May indicate adrenal insufficiency after dose reduction or discontinuing therapy; report any of these symptoms. ■ May mask signs of infection and/or decrease resistance. ■ Diabetics may have an increased requirement for insulin or oral hypoglycemics. ■ Avoid immunization with live vaccines. ■ Carry ID stating steroid dependent if receiving prolonged therapy.

Maternal/Child: Category C: has caused birth defects; benefits must outweigh risks. ■ Observe newborn for hypoadrenalism if mother has received large doses. ■ Monitor growth and development of children receiving prolonged treatment. ■ Use of a preservative-free solution recommended for neonates.

Elderly: Reduced muscle mass and plasma volume may necessitate a reduced dose. Monitor BP, blood glucose, and electrolytes carefully. ■ Increased risk of hypertension. ■ Higher risk of glucocorticoid-induced osteoporosis. ■ Avoid aluminum-based antacids (risk of Alzheimer's disease).

DRUG/LAB INTERACTIONS

Aminoglutethimide (Cytadren) and mitotane (Lysodren) suppress adrenal function and increase metabolism of dexamethasone two-fold. Not recommended for concurrent use, or dexamethasone dose may require doubling to be effective. Use of hydrocortisone suggested. ■ Metabolism increased and effects reduced by hepatic enzyme inducing agents (e.g., alcohol, barbiturates [e.g., phenobarbital], hydantoins [e.g., phenytoin (Dilantin)], rifampin [Rifadin]); dose adjustments may be required when adding or deleting from drug profile. ■ Risk of hypokalemia increased with amphotericin B or potassium-depleting diuretics (e.g., thiazides, furosemide, ethacrynic acid). Monitor potassium levels and cardiac function. ■ Increased risk of digitalis (e.g., digoxin) toxicity secondary to hypokalemia. ■ May also decrease effectiveness of potassium supplements; monitor serum potassium. ■ Diuretics decrease sodium and fluid retention effects of corticosteroids; corticosteroids decrease sodium excretion and diuretic effects of diuretics. ■ Clearance increased and effects decreased with ephedrine. ■ May antagonize effects of anticholinesterases (e.g., neostigmine), isoniazid, salicylates, and somatrem; dose adjustments may be required. ■ Clearance decreased and effects increased with estrogens, oral contraceptives, and ketoconazole (Nizoral). ■ May interact with anticoagulants, nondepolarizing muscle relaxants (e.g., doxacurium [Nuromax]) or theophyllines; may inhibit or potentiate action; monitor carefully. ■ Monitor patients receiving insulin or thyroid hormones carefully; dose adjustments of either or both agents may be required. ■ Use with ritodrine (Yutopar) has caused pulmonary edema in the mother; discontinue both agents with onset of S/S of pulmonary edema. ■ Do not vaccinate with attenuated-virus vaccines (smallpox, etc.) during therapy. ■ Altered protein binding capacity will impact effectiveness of this drug. ■ Smoking may antagonize therapeutic effects. ■ See Precautions. ■ Decreases uptake of radioactive material in cerebral edema; will alter brain scan.

SIDE EFFECTS

Do occur but are usually reversible: burning, Cushing's syndrome, electrolyte imbalance, embolism, euphoria, glycosuria, headache, hyperglycemia, hypersensitivity reactions including anaphylaxis, hypertension, menstrual irregularities, peptic ulcer, perforation and hemorrhage, protein catabolism, sweating, thromboembolism, tingling, weakness, and many others.

ANTIDOTE

Notify the physician of any side effect. Will probably treat the side effect. Resuscitate as necessary for anaphylaxis and notify physician. Keep epinephrine immediately available.

DEXMEDETOMIDINE HYDROCHLORIDE

(dex-med′ih-tom′ih-deen hye-droe-klor′id)

Alpha$_2$-adrenoceptor agonist
Sedative-hypnotic

Precedex

pH 4.5-7.0

USUAL DOSE

Loading dose: 1 mcg/kg as an infusion over 10 minutes.

Maintenance infusion: 0.2 to 0.7 mcg/kg/hr. Adjust rate to achieve the desired level of sedation; see Monitor. Dexmedetomidine is ***not*** indicated for infusions lasting longer than 24 hours. Has been infused in mechanically ventilated patients before, during, and after extubation provided the infusion does not exceed 24 hours.

DOSE ADJUSTMENTS

Reduced doses may be required in patients with renal or hepatic impairment and in the elderly. ■ Dose reduction may be required when co-administered with anesthetics, sedatives, hypnotics, or opioids; see Drug Interactions.

DILUTION

Supplied in single-use vials containing 200 mcg/2 ml. Must be diluted before administration. Preparation of the solution is the same, whether for loading dose or maintenance infusion. Withdraw 2 ml of dexmedetomidine and add to 48 ml of NS for a final concentration of 4 mcg/ml. Shake gently.

Storage: Store unopened vials at CRT.

INCOMPATIBLE WITH

According to the manufacturer, the compatibility of dexmedetomidine with blood, serum, or plasma has not been established; avoid co-administration. Adsorption of dexmedetomidine to some types of natural rubbers may occur. Although dexmedetomidine is dosed to effect, it is advisable to use administration components that are made with synthetic or coated natural rubber gaskets.

COMPATIBLE WITH

Consult pharmacist; specific conditions may apply; see Compatibilities, p. xvi.

Y-site: Manufacturer lists atracurium (Tracrium), atropine, D5W, etomidate (Amidate), fentanyl (Sublimaze), glycopyrrolate, LR, mannitol 20%, midazolam (Versed), mivacurium (Mivacron), morphine, NS, pancuronium

(Pavulon), phenylephrine (Neo-Synephrine), plasma substitute (manufacturer does not identify a specific product), succinylcholine, thiopental (Pentothal), vercuronium (Norcuron).

RATE OF ADMINISTRATION

Administer using a controlled infusion device. Rapid IV or bolus administration may result in bradycardia and sinus arrest.

Loading dose: Infuse over 10 minutes.

Maintenance infusion: See Usual Dose. Titrate to desired clinical effect.

ACTIONS

A relatively selective alpha$_2$-adrenoceptor agonist with sedative properties. In animal studies, the desired alpha$_2$ selectivity is seen following slow IV infusions of low and medium doses (10 to 300 mcg/kg), but both alpha$_1$ and alpha$_2$ activity are seen following slow IV infusion of high doses (equal to or greater than 1,000 mcg/kg) or with rapid IV administration. Appears to have both sedative and moderate analgesic activity and may decrease the requirement for concomitant sedation and analgesia when used as a short term infusion in the ICU setting. Other actions include reduced BP, HR, and reduced salivation. Highly protein bound. Almost completely metabolized in the liver via direct glucuronidation and cytochrome P_{450}-mediated metabolism. Metabolites excreted primarily in urine and to a small extent in feces. Half-life is approximately 2 hours. Pharmacokinetics not altered by age or gender.

INDICATIONS AND USES

Sedation of initially intubated and mechanically ventilated patients during treatment in an intensive care setting. Should be administered by continuous infusion not to exceed 24 hours.

Unlabeled uses: Premedication before thiopental induction in minor GYN surgery. ■ Analgesic following laparoscopic tubal ligation. ■ Adjunct in coronary artery bypass graft (CABG) surgery. ■ Adjunct in ophthalmic surgery. ■ Treatment of shivering. ■ To decrease severity of cardiostimulatory and postanesthetic delirium of ketamine (Ketalar).

CONTRAINDICATIONS

None noted.

PRECAUTIONS

Administered by persons skilled in the management of patients in the intensive care setting. ■ Clinically significant episodes of bradycardia and sinus arrest have been reported in young, healthy volunteers with high vagal tone or with different routes of administration, including rapid intravenous or bolus administration; see Rate of Administration. ■ Hypotension and bradycardia have been reported. Decreases sympathetic nervous system activity. Use caution in patients with advanced heart block, severe ventricular dysfunction, diabetes mellitus, chronic hypertension, hypovolemia, and the elderly; hypotension and/or bradycardia may be more pronounced. Clinical intervention may be required; see Antidote. ■ Patients may be arousable and alert when stimulated. This alone should not be considered as evidence of lack of effectiveness in the absence of other clinical signs and symptoms. ■ Dexmedetomidine should not be administered for longer than 24 hours. Although not specifically studied, if dexmedetomidine is chronically administered and then discontinued abruptly, withdrawal symptoms similar to those seen with another alpha$_2$ agonist, clonidine (Catapres), could result. Symptoms include nervousness, agitation, headache, rapid rise in blood pressure, and elevated catecholamine concentrations in the plasma. ■ Use with caution in patients with hepatic impairment. Clearance of dexmedetomidine is decreased; see Dose Adjustments. Use caution in patients with impaired renal function. Accumulation of metabolites may occur; see Dose Adjustments.

Monitor: Continuous monitoring of VS, oxygenation, and cardiac and fluid status imperative. ■ Hypovolemia may increase risk of hypotension. ■ Use of a sedation scale (e.g., Ramsay) recommended for monitoring of sedative effect. ■ Transient hypertension has been observed primarily during the loading dose in association with initial peripheral vasoconstrictive effects. Treatment is generally not required; see Antidote. ■ See Precautions.

Maternal/Child: Category C: Safety for use in pregnancy and breast-feeding not established. Use only when clearly indicated. ■ Not recommended for use in obstetric procedures, including cesarean section; no assurance of safety for fetus. ■ Safety and effectiveness in children less than 18 years of age not established.

Elderly: In patients older than 65 years, a higher incidence of bradycardia and hypotension was observed following administration of dexmedetomidine. ■ Consider age-related organ impairment and history of previous or concomitant disease or drug therapy. ■ See Dose Adjustments.

DRUG/LAB INTERACTIONS

In vitro studies showed no evidence of cytochrome P_{450}-mediated drug interactions that are likely to be of clinical significance. ■ Potentiated by anesthetics (e.g., enflurane, isoflurane, sevoflurane), sedatives or hypnotics (e.g., barbiturates, benzodiazepines [e.g., diazepam (Valium), midazolam (Versed)], propofol [Diprivan]), and opioids (e.g., alfentanil, meperidine, morphine). Reduced doses of both drugs may be indicated. See Dose Adjustments. ■ Concurrent use with other vasodilators (e.g., amiodarone [Cordarone], nitroprusside sodium) or negative chronotropic agents (e.g., beta blockers [e.g., metoprolol (Lopressor)], calcium channel blockers [e.g., diltiazem (Cardizem)]) may have an additive effect; use with caution.

SIDE EFFECTS

Most frequently reported side effects requiring treatment were anemia, bradycardia, fever, hypertension, hypotension, hypoxia, nausea, tachycardia, and vomiting. Less frequently reported side effects include abnormal vision, acidosis, agitation, apnea, arrhythmia (e.g., atrial fibrillation), bronchospasm, confusion, delirium, dizziness, dyspnea, hallucination, headache, heart block, hypercapnia, hyperkalemia, hypoventilation, increased alkaline phosphatase, increased GGT (gamma glutamyltransferase), increased ALT (SGOT), increased AST (SGPT), increased sweating, infection, light anesthesia, neuralgia, neuritis, pain, pleural effusion, pulmonary edema, rigors, somnolence, and speech disorder.

Overdose: Bradycardia, cardiac arrest, first-degree AV block, hypotension, second-degree heart block.

ANTIDOTE

Keep physician informed of all side effects. Hypotension and bradycardia may be treated by slowing or stopping the dexmedetomidine infusion, increasing the rate of IV fluid administration, elevation of the lower extremities, or use of pressor amines (e.g., dopamine [Intropin]). Administration of anticholinergic agents (e.g., atropine or glycopyrrolate) may be considered to modify vagal tone. Transient hypertension during loading dose may be treated by decreasing the rate of the infusion. Resuscitate as necessary.

DEXRAZOXANE

(dex-rah-zox'ayn)

Antidote
Antineoplastic adjunct
Chelating agent

Zinecard

pH 3.5 to 5.5

USUAL DOSE

Administered in conjunction with doxorubicin. Dose ratio of dexrazoxane to doxorubicin (Adriamycin) is 10:1 (500 mg/M^2 dexrazoxane to 50 mg/M^2 doxorubicin). Doxorubicin dose must be given within 30 minutes of starting the dexrazoxane injection, but only after the full dose of dexrazoxane is administered.

PEDIATRIC DOSE

Safety for use in children not established. One source indicates that 3,500 mg/M^2/24 hr for 3 days is the maximum tolerated dose based on coagulation parameters.

DOSE ADJUSTMENTS

No specific adjustments recommended. Dose of dexrazoxane is dependent on dose of doxorubicin. When dose of doxorubicin is reduced (e.g., patients with hyperbilirubinemia), adjust dexrazoxane dose accordingly. Maintain 10:1 ratio. ■ See Antidote. ■ Has not been evaluated in renal or hepatic insufficiency.

DILUTION

Specific techniques required; see Precautions. Initially reconstitute each 250 mg (500 mg) with 25 ml (50 ml) of ⅙ M sodium lactate diluent provided by manufacturer (10 mg/ml). May be further diluted with D5W or NS. Concentration should range from 1.3 to 5 mg/ml. An additional 25 ml (50 ml) of diluent would yield 5 mg/ml; 75 ml (150 ml) would yield 2.5 mg/ml.

Storage: Store unopened vials at CRT. Reconstituted or diluted solution stable for 6 hours at CRT or refrigerated. Discard unused solutions.

COMPATIBILITY

Manufacturer states, "Should not be mixed with other drugs"; degrades rapidly at a pH above 7.

RATE OF ADMINISTRATION

A single dose may be given by slow IV push or rapid infusion (given over 10 to 15 minutes in one study). Complete dexrazoxane dose but begin doxorubicin within 30 minutes of beginning dexrazoxane.

ACTIONS

A cardioprotective agent. A potent intracellular chelating agent that readily penetrates cell membranes and interferes with iron-mediated free radical generation thought to be, in part, responsible for anthracycline-induced cardiomyopathy. Reduces the incidence of doxorubicin cardiomyopathy. Rapidly distributed, at least partly metabolized. Elimination half-life is 2.5 hours. Primarily excreted in urine. See Drug/Lab Interactions.

INDICATIONS AND USES

Reduce the incidence and severity of cardiomyopathy associated with cumulative doses of doxorubicin exceeding 300 mg/M^2. May allow higher doses of doxorubicin and improved response rates and duration. Currently approved only for use in women with metastatic breast cancer who would benefit from continuing doxorubicin therapy above this cumulative dose.

CONTRAINDICATIONS

Do not use with chemotherapy regimens that do not contain an anthracycline or in the initiation of doxorubicin therapy.

PRECAUTIONS

Follow guidelines for handling cytotoxic agents. See Appendix A, p. 1142. Usually administered by or under the direction of the physician specialist. ■ May cause coagulation abnormalities (e.g., increased PT, PTT, and decreased levels of fibrinogen and clotting factors).

Monitor: Obtain baseline ECG, serum levels of iron and zinc, and liver and renal function tests. Monitor at intervals. Baseline left ventricular ejection fraction (LVEF) helpful. ■ Obtain baseline CBC, PT, and PTT and monitor frequently for increased bone marrow depression and coagulation abnormalities. ■ Reduces but does not eliminate the risk of doxorubicin-induced cardiotoxicity. Monitor for signs of congestive heart failure (e.g., basilar rales, S_3 gallop, paroxysmal nocturnal dyspnea, significant dyspnea on exertion, cardiomegaly by x-ray, or progressive decline from baseline of LVEF). A decline in QRS voltage on a 6-lead ECG of more than 30% may indicate cardiomyopathy. ■ Use of prophylactic antiemetics may be indicated.

Patient Education: Nonhormonal birth control recommended. ■ Report pain at injection site promptly.

Maternal/Child: Category C: safety for use in pregnancy, breast-feeding, and children not established. ■ Embryotoxic and teratogenic in rats at doses lower than required for humans. May cause testicular atrophy. ■ Discontinue breast-feeding.

Elderly: No specific recommendations. Response similar to that seen in younger patients. Consider age-related impaired organ function and concomitant disease or drug therapy.

DRUG/LAB INTERACTIONS

Not indicated for use in initiation of doxorubicin therapy; may interfere with antitumor effects of combination regimens. ■ May have additive bone marrow depressant effects with other bone marrow depressants (e.g., fluorouracil [5-FU], cyclophosphamide [Cytoxan]). ■ Does not affect pharmacokinetics of doxorubicin.

SIDE EFFECTS

Increased myelosuppression (e.g., granulocytopenia, leukopenia, and thrombocytopenia); may be dose limiting. Coagulation abnormalities, decreased serum zinc, increased serum iron, increased AST and ALT, increased serum triglycerides, pain at injection site do occur. Alopecia, anorexia, diarrhea, and nausea and vomiting, as well as other side effects, do occur but are most likely caused by chemotherapeutic regimen.

ANTIDOTE

Keep physician informed of side effects; most will be treated symptomatically. Recovery from myelosuppression similar with or without dexrazoxane. A reduced dose may be indicated if coagulation abnormalities develop. Hemodialysis or peritoneal dialysis may be useful in overdose.

DEXTRAN HIGH MOLECULAR WEIGHT

Plasma volume expander

(deks′tran hi mo-lek′u-ler)

Dextran 70, Dextran 75, Gentran 75, Macrodex **pH 3 to 7**

USUAL DOSE

Variable, depending on amount of fluid loss and resultant hemoconcentration. Initially 30 Gm (500 ml). Total dose should not exceed 1.2 Gm/kg (20 ml/kg) of body weight in the first 24 hours for adults and children. May give 0.6 Gm/kg (10 ml/kg) every 24 hours thereafter if indicated. ***Use of Dextran 1 is indicated for prophylaxis of serious anaphylactic reactions.***

DILUTION

Available as a 6% solution in 500-ml bottles properly diluted in NS or D5W and ready for use. Dextran 70 (Cutter) is available in a 250-ml bottle. Use only clear solution. Crystallization of dextran can occur at low temperatures. Submerge in warm water and dissolve all crystals before administration.

Storage: Store at constant temperature not above 25° C (76° F). Discard partially used solution; no preservative added.

COMPATIBILITY

One source suggests that drugs should not be added to a dextran solution.

RATE OF ADMINISTRATION

Variable, depending on indication, present blood volume, and patient response. Initial 500 ml may be given at 20 to 40 ml/min if hypovolemic. If additional high molecular weight dextran is required, reduce flow to lowest rate possible to maintain hemodynamic status desired. In normovolemic patients, rate should not exceed 4 ml/min.

ACTIONS

A glucose polymer that approximates colloidal properties of human albumin. Provides hemodynamically significant plasma volume expansion in excess of the amount infused for about 24 hours. Dilutes total serum proteins and hematocrit values. Smaller dextran molecules are eliminated in urine; larger molecules are degraded to glucose.

INDICATIONS AND USES

Adjunct in treatment of shock or impending shock caused by burns, hemorrhage, surgery, or trauma.

Unlabeled uses: Treatment of nephrosis, toxemia of late pregnancy, and prevention of postoperative deep vein thrombosis.

CONTRAINDICATIONS

Severe bleeding disorders; marked hemostatic defects (e.g., thrombocytopenia, hypofibrinogenemia), even if drug-induced (e.g., heparin, warfarin); known hypersensitivity to dextran; breast-feeding and pregnancy unless a lifesaving measure; severe congestive cardiac failure; renal failure.

PRECAUTIONS

For IV use only. ■ Used when whole blood or blood products are not available. Not a substitute for whole blood or plasma proteins. ■ Use extreme caution in heart disease, impaired hepatic or renal function, congestive heart failure, pulmonary edema, in patients with edema and sodium retention of pathologic abdominal conditions, and in patients receiving anticoagulants or corticosteroids.

Monitor: Monitor pulse, BP, central venous pressure, and urine output every 5 to 15 minutes for the first hour and hourly thereafter while indicated. ■ Maintain hydration of patient with additional IV fluids; dextran promotes tissue dehydration. Avoid overhydration with dilution of electrolyte balance. ■ Change IV tubing or flush well with normal saline before infusing blood. Dextran will promote coagulation of blood in the tubing (glucose content). ■ May reduce coagulability of the circulating blood. Observe patient for increased bleeding; maintain hematocrit above 30%. ■ Hemoglobin, hematocrit, electrolyte, and serum protein evaluations are necessary during therapy. ■ 500 ml contains 77 mEq of sodium and chloride. ■ See Drug/Lab Interactions.

Maternal/Child: Category C: safety for use in pregnancy and breast-feeding not established.

DRUG/LAB INTERACTIONS

Draw blood for laboratory tests and type and cross-match before giving dextran, or notify laboratory of its use. May alter type and cross-match, blood sugar, total protein, and total bilirubin evaluation. ■ May produce elevated urine specific gravity (also symptom of dehydration) and increase AST (SGOT) and ALT (SGPT). ■ See Monitor for interaction with blood.

SIDE EFFECTS

Bleeding, dehydration, fever, hypotension, joint pain, nausea, overhydration, tightness of the chest, urticaria, vomiting, wheezing. Severe anaphylaxis and death have occurred. Excessive doses have caused wound hematoma, seroma, and bleeding; distant bleeding (hematuria, melena); and pulmonary edema.

ANTIDOTE

Notify physician of any side effect. Discontinue the drug immediately at the first sign of an allergic reaction, provided other means of sustaining the circulation are available. Use epinephrine (Adrenalin) and/or antihistamines (diphenhydramine [Benadryl]) as indicated. Factor VIII infusion may reverse excessive bleeding. Resuscitate as necessary.

DEXTRAN LOW MOLECULAR WEIGHT

(deks′tran lo mo-lek′u-ler)

Plasma volume expander

Dextran 40, Gentran 40, L.M.D. 10%, Rheomacrodex

pH 3 to 7

USUAL DOSE

Adjunct in shock: Variable, depending on amount of fluid loss and resultant hemoconcentration. Do not exceed 2 Gm/kg (20 ml) of body weight total over first 24 hours and 1 Gm/kg (10 ml) total over each succeeding 24 hours. Discontinue infusion after 5 days of therapy. ***Dextran 1 is indicated for prophylaxis of serious anaphylactic reactions.***

Prophylaxis of venous thrombosis and/or pulmonary embolism: 10 mg/kg of body weight on day of surgery. 500 ml daily for 2 to 3 days, then 500 ml every 2 to 3 days up to 2 weeks. Length of treatment based on risk of thromboembolic complication. ***Note previous comment on use of dextran 1.***

As priming fluid: 10 to 20 ml/kg of body weight. Do not exceed this dose. May be used in conjunction with other priming fluids.

DILUTION

Available as a 10% solution in 500-ml bottles properly diluted in NS or D5W and ready for use. Use only clear solution. Crystallization of dextran can occur at low temperatures. Submerge in warm water and dissolve all crystals before administration.

Storage: Store at constant temperature not above 25° C (76° F). Discard partially used solution; no preservative added.

COMPATIBILITY

Consult pharmacist; specific conditions may apply; see Compatibilities, p. xvi. One source suggests that drugs should not be added to a dextran solution.

Y-site: Another source suggests compatibility with enalaprilat (Vasotec IV) and famotidine (Pepcid IV).

RATE OF ADMINISTRATION

Initial 500 ml may be given rapidly. Remainder of any desired daily dose should be evenly distributed over 8 to 24 hours depending on use. Slow rate or discontinue dextran for rapid increase of central venous pressure.

ACTIONS

A low–molecular-weight, rapid, but short-acting plasma volume expander. A colloid hypertonic solution, it increases plasma volume by once or twice its own volume. Helps to restore normal circulatory dynamics, increasing arterial and pulse pressure, central venous pressure, and cardiac output. Improves microcirculatory flow and prevents sludging in venous channels. Mobilizes water from body tissues and increases urine output.

INDICATIONS AND USES

Adjunctive therapy in the treatment of shock caused by hemorrhage, burns, trauma, or surgery. ■ Prophylaxis during surgical procedures with a high incidence of venous thrombosis and pulmonary embolism. ■ Pump priming during extracorporeal circulation.

CONTRAINDICATIONS

Severe bleeding disorders, marked hemostatic defects (e.g., thrombocytopenia, hypofibrinogenemia) even if drug-induced (e.g., heparin, warfarin), known hypersensitivity to dextran, breast-feeding and pregnancy unless a lifesaving measure, severe congestive cardiac failure, renal failure.

PRECAUTIONS

For IV use only. ■ Use caution in heart disease, renal shutdown, congestive heart failure, pulmonary edema, patients with edema and sodium retention, and patients taking corticosteroids.

Monitor: Monitor pulse, BP, central venous pressure (if possible), and urine output every 5 to 15 minutes for the first hour and hourly thereafter while indicated. ■ Slow rate or discontinue dextran for rapid increase of central venous pressure (normal 7 to 14 mm H_2O pressure). ■ If anuric or oliguric after 500 ml of dextran, discontinue the dextran. Mannitol may help increase urine flow. ■ Maintain hydration of patient with additional IV fluids; dextran promotes tissue dehydration. Avoid overhydration and dilution of serum electrolytes. ■ Change IV tubing or flush well with normal saline before superimposing blood. Dextran will promote coagulation of blood in the tubing (glucose content). ■ May reduce coagulability of the circulating blood slightly. Observe for bleeding complications, particularly following surgery or if patient is being anticoagulated. Maintain hematocrit above 30%. ■ 500 ml contains 77 mEq of sodium and chloride. ■ See Drug/Lab Interactions.

Maternal/Child: Category C: safety for use in pregnancy and breast-feeding not established.

DRUG/LAB INTERACTIONS

Draw blood for laboratory tests and type and cross-match before giving dextran, or notify laboratory of its use. May alter type and cross-match, blood sugar, total protein, and total bilirubin evaluation. ■ May produce elevated urine specific gravity (also a symptom of dehydration) and increase AST (SGOT) and ALT (SGPT). ■ See Monitor for interaction with blood.

SIDE EFFECTS

Bleeding, dehydration, fever, hypotension, joint pain, nausea, overhydration, tightness of chest, urticaria, vomiting, wheezing. Severe anaphylaxis and death can occur. Excessive doses have caused wound hematoma, wound seroma, wound bleeding, distant bleeding (hematuria, melena), and pulmonary edema.

ANTIDOTE

Notify the physician of any side effect. Discontinue the drug immediately at the first sign of an allergic reaction, provided other means of sustaining the circulation are available. Use epinephrine (Adrenalin) and/or antihistamines (diphenhydramine [Benadryl]) as indicated. Factor VIII infusion may reverse excessive bleeding. Resuscitate as necessary.

DEXTRAN 1

(deks′tran)

Promit

Dextran adjunct
Antidote

USUAL DOSE

20 ml (150 mg/ml) 1 to 2 minutes before every IV clinical dextran infusion. If 15 minutes or more elapses before the clinical dextran infusion is started, a full dose of dextran 1 must be repeated before the infusion.

PEDIATRIC DOSE

0.3 ml/kg of body weight. To be given in same manner as adult dose.

DILUTION

May be given undiluted. May be given through Y-tube or three-way stopcock of an infusion set if there is minimum dilution with the primary IV. May not be diluted with or administered through an IV tubing containing clinical dextran infusion.

COMPATIBILITY

According to the manufacturer, dextran 1 should not be diluted or admixed with clinical dextran (high molecular weight or low molecular weight) and should not be given through an IV set used to infuse clinical dextran. Use of a heparin lock is suggested.

RATE OF ADMINISTRATION

IV injection: A single dose over 1 minute.

ACTIONS

A monovalent hapten, it binds one of two available sites on dextran-reacting antibodies. An adequate dose (molar excess) given just before the IV administration of clinical dextran solution prevents the formation of immune complexes with the polyvalent clinical dextrans and helps prevent severe anaphylaxis. Incidence of anaphylaxis is 15 to 20 times less. Rapidly excreted in urine.

INDICATIONS AND USES

Prophylaxis of serious anaphylactic reactions associated with IV infusion of clinical dextran solutions.

CONTRAINDICATIONS

Do not give if clinical dextran is contraindicated (severe bleeding disorders; marked hemostatic defects [e.g., thrombocytopenia, hypofibrinogenemia], even if drug-induced [e.g., heparin, warfarin]; breast-feeding and pregnancy unless a life-saving measure; severe congestive cardiac failure; renal failure).

PRECAUTIONS

For IV use only. ■ Will not prevent mild allergic reactions induced by clinical dextran solutions. ■ If any reaction occurs to dextran 1, ***do not administer clinical dextran infusion.***

Monitor: May cause severe hypotension and bradycardia.

Maternal/Child: Category B: see Contraindications.

DRUG/LAB INTERACTIONS

See Precautions and Dilution.

SIDE EFFECTS

Bradycardia, cutaneous reactions, hypotension (moderate to severe), nausea, pallor, shivering.

ANTIDOTE

Discontinue drug immediately and notify physician at the first sign of allergic reaction or side effect. Do not administer clinical dextran solution. Use epinephrine (Adrenalin) and/or antihistamines (diphenhydramine [Benadryl]) as indicated. Resuscitate as necessary.

DEXTROSE

(dek′stros)

Glucose

Nutritional (carbohydrate)

pH 3.5 to 6.5

USUAL DOSE

Depends on use and age, weight, and clinical condition of the patient.

2½% (25 Gm/L) or 5% (50 Gm/L) dextrose: 50 to 1,000 ml. May be repeated as indicated. Consider total amount of fluid.

10% dextrose (100 Gm/L): 5 ml. May repeat as necessary or 500 to 1,000 ml once or twice every 24 hours as indicated.

20% dextrose (200 Gm/L): 500 ml once or twice every 24 hours as indicated.

50% dextrose (500 Gm/L): 20 ml (10 Gm) to 50 ml (25 Gm). May repeat if indicated in ***insulin-induced hypoglycemia.***

10% (100 Gm/L), 20% (200 Gm/L), 30% (300 Gm/L), 38.5% (385 Gm/L), 40% (400 Gm/L), 50% (500 Gm/L), 60% (600 Gm/L), 70% (700 Gm/L): 500 to 1,500 ml/24 hr as an infusion after admixture with other solutions such as amino acids or fat emulsion. Used for nutritional support.

NEONATAL DOSE

Acute symptomatic hypoglycemia: 250 to 500 mg/kg of body weight of 10% to 25% dextrose. See Rate of Administration and Precautions.

DOSE ADJUSTMENTS

Dosing should be cautious in the elderly. Lower-end initial doses may be indicated. Consider decrease in cardiac, hepatic, and renal function; concomitant disease; or other drug therapy. ▪ See Rate of Administration, Precautions, and Monitor.

DILUTION

May be given undiluted in prepared solutions or further diluted to achieve desired final concentration. Check label for aluminum content; see Precautions. Dextrose solutions are excellent media for bacterial growth. Do not use unless the solution is entirely clear and the vial is sterile. Do not store after adding additives.

COMPATIBILITY

Will cause pseudoagglutination of red blood cells if administered simultaneously with whole blood. Consult pharmacist or refer to individual drug monograph before admixing with other drugs or solutions.

RATE OF ADMINISTRATION

2½% and 5% solution, rate dependent on amount.

10% solution, 5 ml over 10 to 15 seconds.

10% solution, 1,000 ml over at least 3 hours.

20% solution, 500 ml over 30 to 60 minutes.

50% solution, 3 ml over 1 minute.

500 ml of 30% to 70% solution over 4 to 12 hours, depending on body weight. A rate of 0.5 Gm/kg/hr will not cause glycosuria. At 0.8 Gm/kg/hr 95% is retained and will cause glycosuria. May cause hyperosmolar syndrome.

Excessive or rapid administration in very-low-birth-weight infants may cause hyperglycemia, hypoglycemia, or increased serum osmolality and possible intracerebral hemorrhage.

ACTIONS

A monosaccharide, it provides glucose calories for metabolic needs. Metabolized to CO_2 and water. Its oxidation provides water to sustain volume and may help lower excess ketone production and prevent protein loss. Hypertonic solutions (20% to 50%) act as diuretics and reduce CNS edema. Readily excreted by the kidneys, producing diuresis.

INDICATIONS AND USES

Provide calories and fluid by peripheral infusion when calories and fluid are required (2½%, 5%, 10%). ■ Provide calories by central IV infusion in conditions requiring a minimum volume of fluid (20%). ■ Provide calories by central IV infusion in combination with other amino acid solutions as total parenteral nutrition (10% to 70%). ■ Treatment of insulin-induced hypoglycemia (50%). ■ Treatment of acute symptomatic episodes of hypoglycemia in the neonate and infant (25%). ■ Shock (sustain blood volume). ■ Diuresis (20% to 50% solution). ■ Hyperkalemia (20% solution). ■ As a diluent for IV administration of medications (2½% to 10% solutions usually). A sclerosing solution (25% to 50% solution, 3 to 20 ml).

CONTRAINDICATIONS

Delirium tremens with dehydration; diabetic coma while blood sugar is excessive; hepatic coma intracranial or intraspinal hemorrhage; glucose-galactose malabsorption syndrome. Solutions containing dextrose may be contraindicated in patients with known allergies to corn or corn products.

PRECAUTIONS

Use caution in severe kidney damage. ■ 50% dextrose can be used as a sclerosing agent and will cause thrombosis. ■ Use caution in infants of diabetic mothers, in patients with carbohydrate intolerance or subclinical or overt diabetes, and in patients receiving corticosteroids. ■ Use dextrose with extreme caution in low-birth-weight or septic infants. May cause severe hyperglycemia, may increase serum osmolality, and may cause intracerebral hemorrhage. ■ Some solutions may contain aluminum. In impaired kidney function, aluminum may reach toxic levels. Premature neonates are particularly at risk because of their immature kidneys and requirement for calcium and phosphate, which also contain aluminum. Research indicates that patients with impaired renal function who receive greater than 4 to 5 mcg/kg/day of parenteral aluminum are at risk for developing CNS or bone toxicity associated with aluminum accumulation.

Monitor: Do not use as a diluent for blood or administer simultaneously through the same infusion set; dextrose in any dilution causes clumping of RBCs unless sodium chloride is added. ■ For concentrations over 12.5% (hypertonic) very large (central) veins and slow administration are absolutely necessary. ■ Confirm patency of vein; avoid extravasation. ■ Insulin requirements may be increased. Monitor blood glucose. ■ Potassium and vitamins are readily depleted. Watch for any signs of beginning deficiency and replace as needed. Add other electrolytes and minerals as required by fluid and electrolyte status. ■ Can cause fluid or solute overload. May result in dilution of serum electrolyte concentrations, overhydration, congested states, or pulmonary edema. ■ Rapid administration of hypertonic solutions will cause hyperglycemia (over 0.5 Gm/kg/hr) and may cause hyperosmolar syndrome. ■ Concentrated dextrose solutions must not be withdrawn abruptly. Will cause reactive hypoglycemia. Reduce rate of administration gradually and then follow with administration of 5% or 10% dextrose solution. ■ See Precautions.

Maternal/Child: Category C: safety for use in pregnancy and breast-feeding not established. Benefits must outweigh risks. ■ See Precautions.

Elderly: Lower-end initial doses may be indicated; see Dose Adjustments. Specific age-related differences in response have not been identified.

DRUG/LAB INTERACTIONS

See Monitor.

SIDE EFFECTS

Rare in small doses administered slowly: acidosis, alkalosis, fluid overload (congested states, pulmonary edema, overhydration, dilution of serum electrolyte concentrations), hyperglycemia (during infusion), hyperosmolar syndrome (mental confusion, loss of consciousness), hypokalemia, hypovitaminosis, reactive hypoglycemia (after infusion), thrombosis.

ANTIDOTE

Discontinue the drug and notify the physician of the side effect. Symptomatic treatment is probable.

DIAZEPAM

(dye-az′e-pam)

Benzodiazepine
Sedative-hypnotic
Antianxiety agent
Anticonvulsant
Amnestic
Skeletal muscle relaxant (adjunct)

Valium ■ ✤Diazemuls

pH 6.2 to 6.9 ■ pH 8

USUAL DOSE

Maximum dose except in status epilepticus is 30 mg in 8 hours. Note some changes in times of administration between conventional diazepam (Valium) and emulsified forms (e.g., Diazemuls). The emulsified form is no longer available in the United States.

Preoperative Medication

Conventional diazepam (Valium): 5 to 10 mg before surgery.

Emulsified diazepam (Diazemuls): 10 mg 1 to 2 hours before surgery.

Moderate Anxiety Disorders and Symptoms of Anxiety

All formulations: 2 to 5 mg. Repeat in 3 to 4 hours if necessary.

Severe Anxiety Disorders and Symptoms of Anxiety

All formulations: 5 to 10 mg. Repeat in 3 to 4 hours if necessary.

Acute Alcohol Withdrawal

All formulations: 10 mg initially, then 5 to 10 mg in 3 to 4 hours if necessary.

Status Epilepticus

All formulations: 5 to 10 mg. May be repeated at intervals of 10 to 15 minutes up to a total dose of 30 mg. May repeat in 2 to 4 hours. Another source suggests 0.2 to 0.5 mg/kg every 15 to 30 minutes for 2 or 3 doses. Some specialists start with 20 mg and titrate the total dose over 10 minutes or until seizures stop. Maximum dose in 24 hours is 100 mg.

Cardioversion

Conventional diazepam (Valium): 5 to 15 mg 5 to 10 minutes before procedure begins.

Emulsified diazepam (Diazemuls): 5 to 15 mg 10 to 20 minutes before procedure begins.

Endoscopy

Conventional diazepam (Valium): 10 mg or less is usually effective given immediately before procedure begins; titrate to desired sedation (e.g., slurred speech). Up to 20 mg may be indicated if a narcotic is not used. **Emulsified diazepam (Diazemuls):** 5 to 10 mg 30 minutes before the procedure begins; titrate to desired sedation (e.g., slurred speech). Up to 20 mg may be indicated if a narcotic is not used.

Muscle Spasm

All formulations: 5 to 10 mg. Repeat in 3 to 4 hours if necessary. Larger doses may be required in tetanus.

PEDIATRIC DOSE

Safety for use in neonates not established but is used. Neonates have reduced or immature organ function; may be susceptible to prolonged CNS depression. Avoid small veins (e.g., dorsum of hand or wrist); see Monitor. Use in infants and children is most frequent in tetany, status epilepticus, or allergic reactions. Use of longer-acting anticonvulsants (e.g., phenobarbital, phenytoin) following diazepam may be indicated. Not recommended but is used for other general indications.

Sedative/Muscle Relaxant

All formulations: 0.04 to 0.2 mg/kg every 2 to 4 hours. Maximum dose 0.6 mg/kg in 8 hours.

Tetanus in Infants 30 Days to 5 Years of Age or Younger

Respiratory assistance must be available.

All formulations: 1 to 2 mg every 3 to 4 hours.

Conventional diazepam (Valium): One source suggests a maximum single dose not to exceed 0.25 mg/kg; repeat in 15 to 30 minutes if necessary. A third dose may be given, but if it does not relieve symptoms, consider alternative therapy.

Tetanus in Children 5 Years of Age or Older

Respiratory assistance must be available.

All formulations: 5 to 10 mg every 3 to 4 hours.

Conventional diazepam (Valium): One source suggests a maximum single dose not to exceed 0.25 mg/kg; repeat in 15 to 30 minutes if necessary. A third dose may be given, but if it does not relieve symptoms, consider alternative therapy.

Status Epilepticus in Neonates (unlabeled)

All formulations: 0.3 to 0.75 mg/kg every 15 to 30 minutes for 2 to 3 doses. Maximum total dose is 5 mg.

Status Epilepticus in Infants Over 30 Days

All formulations: 0.2 to 0.5 mg every 2 to 5 minutes to a maximum 5-mg dose. May repeat in 2 to 4 hours. Another source suggests 0.2 to 0.5 mg/kg every 15 to 30 minutes to a maximum 5-mg dose.

Status Epilepticus in Children 5 Years or Older

All formulations: 1 mg every 2 to 5 minutes to a maximum 10-mg dose. May repeat in 2 to 4 hours. Another source suggests 0.2 to 0.5 mg/kg every 15 to 30 minutes to a maximum 10-mg dose.

DOSE ADJUSTMENTS

Reduce dose by one half for the elderly or debilitated, in impaired liver or renal function, in patients with limited pulmonary reserve, and in the presence of other CNS depressants. Begin with a small dose and increase in gradual increments. ■ See Drug/Lab Interactions.

DILUTION

All formulations: Do not dilute or mix with any other drug. Should be given directly into the vein. Inject into IV tubing close to vein site only when direct IV injection is not feasible. Consider heparin lock for frequent injection. Change site every 2 to 3 days. Some precipitation or adsorption into plastic tubing may occur.

Conventional diazepam: ***Not soluble in any solution.*** If dilution is imperative, add dilution solution to diazepam, not diazepam to solution; consult pharmacist. Direct IV administration is preferred but can be administered at a Y-tube injection site.

Emulsified diazepam: May be diluted with their emulsion base [Intralipid or Nutralipid]). Mixture should be used within 6 hours. In any other solution, ***emulsion may be destabilized and may not be visually apparent.*** Incompatible with polyvinylchloride infusion sets. If a filter is used for emulsified forms, it must have a pore size of 5 microns or more so as not to break down the emulsion. Emulsified forms eliminate the use of nonphysiologic, potentially irritating solvents.

Storage: ***Conventional diazepam (Valium):*** Store at CRT in cartons to protect from light. Do not freeze.

Emulsified diazepam (Diazemuls): Store below 25° C (77° F) unless manufacturer suggests refrigeration. Do not freeze. Protect from light. Note expiration date.

INCOMPATIBLE WITH

Manufacturers for all preparations recommend not mixing with any other drug or solution in syringe or solution. Precipitation can occur. Emulsified forms are incompatible with polyvinylchloride infusion sets. ***Emulsion may be destabilized and may not be visually apparent.*** See Dilution.

COMPATIBLE WITH

(Underline Indicates Conflicting Compatibility Information)

Not recommended by manufacturers. Consult pharmacist; specific conditions may apply; see Compatibilities, p. xvi.

CONVENTIONAL DIAZEPAM

Additive: Verapamil (Isoptin).

Syringe: Cimetidine (Tagamet), <u>ranitidine (Zantac)</u>.

Y-site: <u>Cisatracurium (Nimbex)</u>, dobutamine (Dobutrex), fentanyl (Sublimaze), <u>hydromorphone (Dilaudid)</u>, morphine, nafcillin (Nafcil), quinidine gluconate, <u>remifentanil (Ultiva)</u>, sufentanil (Sufenta).

EMULSIFIED DIAZEPAM

Additive: Intralipid, Nutralipid; see Dilution.

RATE OF ADMINISTRATION

If a filter is used for emulsified forms, it must have a pore size of 5 microns or more so as not to break down the emulsion.

Adults: 5 mg (1 ml) or fraction thereof over 1 minute.

Infants and children: Give total dose over a minimum of 3 minutes, but do not exceed a rate of 0.25 mg/kg over 3 minutes.

ACTIONS

A benzodiazepine that depresses the central, autonomic, and peripheral nervous systems in an undetermined manner. Exerts antianxiety, sedative/hypnotic, amnesic, anticonvulsant, skeletal muscle relaxant, and antitremor effects. Diminishes patient recall. Metabolized in the liver; stays in the body in appreciable amounts for several days and is excreted very slowly in the urine. Crosses the placental barrier. Secreted in breast milk.

INDICATIONS AND USES

Management of moderate to severe anxiety disorders or short-term relief of symptoms of anxiety. ■ Acute alcohol withdrawal. ■ Acute stress reactions. ■ Muscle spasm. ■ Status epilepticus and severe recurrent convulsive seizures, including tetany. ■ Preoperative medication, including endoscopic procedures. ■ Cardioversion.

Unlabeled uses: Conscious sedation in dental procedures, treatment of panic disorders.

CONTRAINDICATIONS

Known hypersensitivity, open-angle glaucoma unless receiving appropriate therapy, shock, coma, acute alcoholic intoxication with depression of vital signs. Emulsion in Dizac contains soybean oil; do not use in patients with known hypersensitivity to soy protein.

PRECAUTIONS

Check label carefully. Some preparations are for IV use only (e.g., Diazemuls); others can be given IM/IV (e.g., Valium). ■ Drug of choice for initial treatment of status epilepticus or seizures resulting from drug overdose or poisoning. Some specialists administer phenytoin simultaneously to facilitate long-term control (onset of action is not as immediate as diazepam). Oral phenytoin or phenobarbital may be used for maintenance. ■ May not be effective if seizures are due to acute brain lesions. ■ Not recommended for treatment of petit mal or petit mal variant seizures; may cause tonic state epilepticus. ■ Use caution in the elderly, those who are very ill, and those with limited pulmonary reserve (e.g., chronic lung disease) or unstable cardiac status.■ Withdrawal symptoms will occur for several weeks after extended or large doses. ■ Hypoalbuminemia may increase the incidence of side effects. ■ Intended for short-term use only. ■ Available PO and as a rectal gel.

Monitor: See Dilution. ■ To reduce the incidence of thrombophlebitis, avoid smaller veins. Extravasation or arterial administration hazardous. ■ Oxygen, respiratory assistance, and flumazenil (Romazicon) must always be available. ■ Bed rest required for a minimum of 3 hours after IV injection.

Patient Education: May produce drowsiness or dizziness. Request assistance with ambulation and use caution performing tasks that require alertness. Do not drive or operate hazardous machinery until all effects have subsided. ■ Avoid use of alcohol or other CNS depressants (e.g., antihistamines, barbiturates). ■ May be habit-forming with long-term use or high-dose therapy. ■ Has amnestic potential; may impair memory. ■ Consider birth control options.

Maternal/Child: Category D: has caused birth deformities, especially in the first trimester. ■ Not recommended during pregnancy, childbirth, or while breast-feeding.

Elderly: See Dose Adjustments. Start with a small dose and increase gradually based on response. ■ More sensitive to therapeutic and adverse effects (e.g., ataxia, dizziness, oversedation). ■ IV injection may be more likely to cause apnea, bradycardia, hypotension, and cardiac arrest. ■ See Precautions and Drug/Lab Interactions.

DRUG/LAB INTERACTIONS

Concurrent use with other CNS depressants (e.g., alcohol, antihistamines, barbiturates, MAO inhibitors [e.g., selegiline (Eldepryl)], narcotics [e.g., morphine, meperidine (Demerol), fentanyl], phenothiazines [e.g., prochlorperazine (Compazine)], tricyclic antidepressants [e.g., imipramine (Tofranil-PM)]) may result in additive effects for up to 48 hours. Reduced doses of both drugs may be indicated. ■ May increase serum concentrations of digoxin and phenytoin (Dilantin); monitor digoxin and phenytoin serum levels. ■ Ritonavir (Norvir) may increase risk of prolonged sedation and respiratory depression. Concurrent use not recommended. Benzodiazepines metabolized by alternate routes may be safer (e.g., lorazepam [Ativan], oxazepam [Serax], temazepam [Restoril]). ■ Concurrent use with beta-blockers (e.g., metoprolol [Lopressor], propranolol [Inderal]), cimetidine (Tagamet), disulfiram (Antabuse), estrogen-containing oral contraceptives, fluoxetine (Prozac), isoniazid (Nydrazid), itraconazole (Sporanox), ketoconazole (Nizoral), omeprazole (Prilosec), probenecid, and valproic acid (Depakene) may inhibit hepatic metabolism, resulting in increased plasma concentrations of benzodiazepines. ■ Diazepam decreases clearance and increases toxicity of zidovudine (AZT). ■ May increase clearance and decrease effectiveness of levodopa. ■ Hypotensive effects of benzodiazepines may be increased by any agent that induces hypotension (e.g., antihypertensives, bretylium, CNS depressants, diuretics, lidocaine, paclitaxel). ■ Use with rifampin (Rifadin) increases clearance and reduces effects of diazepam. ■ Theophyllines (Aminophylline) antagonize sedative effects of benzodiazepines. ■ Smoking increases metabolism and clearance of diazepam, decreasing plasma levels and sedative effects. ■ Clozapine (Leponex) has caused respiratory distress or cardiac arrest in a few patients; use concurrently with extreme caution. ■ Decreased drowsiness may occur in cigarette smokers, especially if elderly. ■ Grapefruit juice may affect certain enzymes of the P_{450} enzyme system and should be avoided.

SIDE EFFECTS

Apnea, ataxia, blurred vision, bradycardia, cardiac arrest, cardiovascular collapse, coma, confusion, coughing, depressed respiration, depression, diminished reflexes, drowsiness, dyspnea, headache, hiccups, hyperexcited states, hyperventilation, laryngospasm, neutropenia, nystagmus, somnolence, syncope, venous thrombosis and phlebitis at injection site, vertigo.

ANTIDOTE

Notify the physician of all side effects. Reduction of dosage may be required. Discontinue the drug for major side effects or paradoxical reactions, including hyperexcitability, hallucinations, and acute rage. Flumazenil (Romazicon) will reverse all sedative effects of benzodiazepines. A patent airway, artificial ventilation, oxygen therapy, and other symptomatic treatment must be instituted promptly. May cause emesis; observe closely. Treat allergic reaction, or resuscitate as necessary.

DIAZOXIDE
(dye-az-ox′ide)

Antihypertensive (vasodilator)

Hyperstat IV

pH 11.6

USUAL DOSE

1 to 3 mg/kg of body weight up to a maximum dose of 150 mg (10 ml). Another source suggests a dose of 50 to 100 mg. May be repeated every 5 to 15 minutes until an adequate response is obtained. Desired BP reduction should be achieved slowly over several hours to 1 to 2 days. Repeat as indicated at intervals of 4 to 24 hours to maintain desired BP. For short-term use until a regimen of oral antihypertensive medication is effective. Use for more than 4 or 5 days is rarely indicated. Do not use for more than 10 days.

Hypertensive emergency: Applies to rare situations in which some BP decrease (not all the way to a normal range) is required to prevent or limit target organ damage. Examples are acute left ventricular failure with pulmonary edema, acute MI, dissecting aortic aneurysm, eclampsia, hypertensive encephalopathy, intracranial hemorrhage, unstable angina. Initial reduction in BP should be no greater than 25% within minutes to 2 hours. Within the next 2 to 6 hours, gradually reduce toward 160/100 mm Hg. Avoid excessive declines; may precipitate cerebral, coronary, or renal ischemia. Has been administered by continuous IV infusion at 7.5 to 30 mg/min (unlabeled).

Hypertensive emergencies of pregnancy (e.g., preeclampsia, eclampsia): 30 mg. Repeat every few minutes until an adequate response is obtained. See comments above and Maternal/Child.

PEDIATRIC DOSE

1 to 3 mg/kg of body weight up to 150 mg/dose. See instructions in Usual Dose.

DOSE ADJUSTMENTS

See Drug/Lab Interactions.

DILUTION

Should be given undiluted.

Storage: Protect from light and freezing. Store at CRT.

COMPATIBILITY

Specific information not available; consider specific use and patient assessment requirements. Is incompatible at Y-site with hydralazine and propranolol (Inderal); see Drug/Lab Interactions.

RATE OF ADMINISTRATION

Rapidly as a single dose over 10 to 30 seconds. Not as effective when administered at a slower rate.

ACTIONS

A potent, rapid-acting, antihypertensive agent. Produces vasodilation by relaxing the smooth muscle of peripheral arterioles. Increases cardiac output while maintaining coronary and cerebral blood flow. Effects on renal blood flow not significant. Effective in patients not responsive to other antihypertensive agents. Acts within 1 to 5 minutes with a duration of 2 to 12 hours (range is 30 minutes to 72 hours). Usually no further decrease in BP after 30 minutes, but a gradual increase over the above duration to pretreatment levels. Crosses placental barrier; probably secreted in breast milk.

INDICATIONS AND USES

Severe hypertension (e.g., malignant and nonmalignant hypertensive emergencies).

CONTRAINDICATIONS

Compensatory hypertension (e.g., arteriovenous shunt or coarctation of the aorta), known sensitivity to thiazides or other sulfonamide-derived drugs (e.g., furosemide [Lasix], sulfamethoxazole-trimethoprim [Bactrim]), labor and delivery. Not effective in pheochromocytoma.

PRECAUTIONS

Avoid rapid decrease in BP. May precipitate cerebral, coronary, or renal ischemia. Has caused angina and myocardial and cerebral infarction. ■ Use caution in patients with impaired cerebral or cardiac circulation. ■ Use with other antihypertensive agents may cause profound hypotension; see Drug/Lab Interactions.

Monitor: Give only into a peripheral vein; avoid extravasation. ■ Maintain patient in recumbent position during injection and for at least 1 hour after injection. Should remain supine for 8 to 10 hours when used in conjunction with furosemide (Lasix). ■ Check BP every 5 minutes until stabilized and hourly thereafter. ■ Take BP with patient in standing position before ambulation. ■ Use caution in diabetes; monitor blood glucose levels. May cause hyperglycemia; difficult to assess. ■ Diuresis may be required to reverse sodium and water retention before diazoxide can be effective. Causes sodium and water retention and may precipitate edema and CHF. ■ May cause hyperuricemia; difficult to assess. ■ See Drug/Lab Interactions.

Maternal/Child: Category C: safety for use in pregnancy, breast-feeding, and children not established. ■ Has been used in preeclampsia and eclampsia. Use restricted to situations in which delivery is imminent or more commonly used agents (e.g., hydralazine) have not been effective. ■ See Contraindications. May stop uterine contractions if given during labor. Oxytoxics may be required. ■ May produce fetal or neonatal hyperbilirubinemia, thrombocytopenia, altered carbohydrate metabolism, and other adverse reactions if given before delivery. ■ Discontinue breast-feeding.

DRUG/LAB INTERACTIONS

Potentiates coumarin and its derivatives; a reduced dose of anticoagulant may be required. ■ May increase hypotensive, hyperglycemic, and hyperuricemic effects of thiazides and other diuretics (e.g., furosemide [Lasix]); see Monitor. ■ May decrease phenytoin (Dilantin) levels, reducing anticonvulsant effect. ■ Do not administer within 6 hours of beta-adrenergic blocking agents (e.g., atenolol [Tenormin], propranolol [Inderal]), hydralazine, methyldopate (Aldomet), minoxidil (Loniten), nitrites, prazosin (Minipress), reserpine, or papaverine-like compounds. Profound hypotension will result. ■ Use with sulfonyureas (e.g., tolbutamide [Orinase]) may cause hyperglycemia. ■ Interferes with assessment of hyperglycemia and hyperuricemia. ■ Will cause a false-negative insulin response to glucagon.

SIDE EFFECTS

Abdominal discomfort, cerebral ischemia, confusion, congestive heart failure, convulsions, edema, flushing, headache, hyperglycemia, hypotension (severe), ileus, lightheadedness, myocardial ischemia, nausea, orthostatic hypotension, palpitations, paralysis, sensations of warmth, sensitivity reactions, sodium and water retention, supraventricular tachycardia, sweating, vomiting, weakness.

ANTIDOTE

Notify the physician of all side effects. Some will subside spontaneously; others will require symptomatic treatment. Treat sensitivity reaction as indicated and resuscitate as necessary. If hypotension occurs, place patient in a Trendelenburg position. Treat undesirable hypotension with dopamine (Intropin) or norepinephrine (Levophed); if no response, diazoxide is probably not the cause of the hypotension. Excessive hyperglycemia may be treated with insulin. Hemodialysis or peritoneal dialysis may be required in overdose.

DIGOXIN IMMUNE FAB (OVINE)

(di-jox′in uh-mun′ fab)

Antidote (digitalis intoxication)

Digibind, DigiFab

pH 6 to 8

USUAL DOSE

Testing for sensitivity to sheep serum and/or premedication may be indicated; see Contraindications and Monitor.

Acute toxicity in adults and children: Determine dose by symptoms and clinical findings. Serum concentration may not reflect actual toxicity for 6 to 12 hours. Symptoms of life-threatening toxicity due to digoxin overdose include severe arrhythmias (e.g., VT, VF), progressive bradycardia, second- or third-degree heart block not responsive to atropine, and/or serum potassium levels exceeding 5 to 5.5 mEq/L in adults and 6 mEq/L in children.

Dose in numbers of vials based on ingested dose is calculated by dividing the body load of digoxin or digitoxin in milligrams by 0.5. Each vial of ***Digibind*** contains 38 mg/vial and will bind 0.5 mg digoxin or digitoxin. Each vial of ***DigiFab*** contains 40 mg/vial and will bind 0.5 mg of digoxin (data with reference to digitoxin is not available). Dose may also be based on serum digoxin levels (see package insert; has charts for adults and children).

An initial dose of up to 20 vials has been used. 20 vials will bind approximately 50 (0.25 mg) tablets of Lanoxin and should provide adequate treatment of most life-threatening ingestions in adults and children. If ingested substance is unknown, if serum digoxin level is not available, or if there is concern about sensitivity to the serum, consider giving 10 vials. Observe clinical response and repeat if indicated. In clinical trials of Digibind the average dose was 10 vials. A single dose may be repeated in several hours if toxicity has not reversed or appears to recur. Febrile reactions are dose related.

Toxicity in chronic therapy: ***Adults:*** 6 vials should be adequate to reverse most cases of toxicity in adults in acute distress or if a serum digoxin concentration is not available.

Children: less than 20 kg: 1 vial should be adequate if signs of toxicity are present.

DILUTION

Each vial must be diluted with 4 ml of SW for injection (results in 9.5 mg/ml for Digibind and 10 mg/ml for DigiFab). Mix gently. May be given in this initial dilution or may be further diluted with any desired amount of NS (with ***Digibind,*** 34 ml NS/vial yields 1 mg/ml; with ***DigiFab,*** 36 ml NS/vial yields 1 mg/ml). Consider volume overload in children when further diluting in NS. Administer to infants after initial dilution using a tuberculin syringe to deliver an accurate dose with less volume; for extremely small doses, dilute to 1 mg/ml before administration.

Storage: Refrigerate unreconstituted vials. Use reconstituted solution promptly or store in refrigerator for up to 4 hours.

COMPATIBILITY

Specific information not available. Consider specific use; consult pharmacist.

RATE OF ADMINISTRATION

Decrease the rate of infusion or discontinue temporarily if an infusion reaction occurs. Do not give as an IV bolus injection unless cardiac arrest is imminent. Be prepared to treat anaphylaxis.

Digibind: Must be given through a 0.22-micron membrane filter. A single dose as an IV infusion equally distributed over 15 to 30 minutes.

DigiFab: A single dose as an infusion over 30 minutes.

ACTIONS

Antigen-binding fragments (Fab) prepared from specific antidigoxin antibodies produced in sheep are isolated and purified. Fab fragments bind molecules of digoxin and make them unavailable for binding at their site of action. Freely distributed in extracellular space. Reduces the level of free digoxin in the serum. Onset of action is prompt, with improvement in symptoms of toxicity within 30 minutes. Fab-digoxin complexes are cleared by the kidney. DigiFab is also cleared in the reticuloendothelial system.

INDICATIONS AND USES

Digibind: Treatment of patients with life-threatening digitalis intoxication or overdose (digoxin or digitoxin).

DigiFab: Treatment of patients with life-threatening or potentially life-threatening digoxin toxicity or overdose. Not indicated for milder cases of digitalis toxicity.

All formulations: Indicated for known suicidal or accidental consumption of fatal doses of digoxin, including ingestion of 10 mg or more of digoxin in previously healthy adults, 4 mg (or more than 0.1 mg/kg) in previously healthy children, or ingestion causing steady-state serum concentrations greater than 10 ng/ml. ▪ Indicated for chronic ingestions causing steady-state serum digoxin concentrations exceeding 6 ng/ml in adults or 4 ng/ml in children. ▪ Indicated for manifestations of life-threatening toxicity due to digoxin overdose, including severe ventricular arrhythmias (such as VT or VF), progressive bradycardia, or third-degree heart block not responsive to atropine. ▪ Also indicated when potassium concentrations are above 5 to 5.5 mEq/L in adults or 6 mEq/L in children with rapidly progressive S/S of digoxin toxicity. ▪ See Precautions and Maternal/Child.

CONTRAINDICATIONS

None known when used for specific indications. If hypersensitivity exists and treatment is necessary, premedicate with corticosteroids and diphenhydramine and prepare to treat anaphylaxis.

PRECAUTIONS

Administered under the direction of the physician specialist with facilities for monitoring the patient and responding to any medical emergency. Cardiac arrest can result from ingestion of more than 10 mg digoxin by healthy adults, 4 mg digoxin by healthy children, or serum digoxin levels above 10 ng/ml. ■ Larger doses of digoxin immune Fab act more quickly but increase the possibility of febrile or allergic reaction. ■ Use caution in impaired cardiac function. Inability to use cardiac glycosides may endanger patient. Support with dopamine (Intropin) or vasodilators. ■ The clinical problem may not be caused by digitalis toxicity if the patient fails to respond to digoxin immune Fab. ■ Consider that multiple drugs may have been used and are producing toxicity in suicide attempts. ■ See Monitor.

Monitor: Although allergy testing is not required before treating life-threatening digitalis toxicity, patients allergic to ovine proteins or those who have previously received antibodies or Fab fragments produced from sheep are at risk. Determine patient response to any previous injections of serum of any type and history of any allergic-type reactions. In addition, ***DigiFab*** considers that patients with allergies to papain, chymopapain, other papaya extracts, or the pineapple enzyme bromelain may be at risk. ***Digibind*** provides the information below on sensitivity testing; that information is not included in the package insert for ***DigiFab.*** ■ Test for sensitivity if indicated. Make a 1:100 solution by diluting 0.1 ml of reconstituted solution (10 mg/ml) with 9.9 ml sterile NS (100 mcg/ml).

Scratch test: Make a ¼-inch skin scratch through a drop of 1:100 dilution in NS. Inspect the site in 20 minutes. An urticarial wheal surrounded by a zone of erythema is a positive reaction.

Skin test: Inject 0.1 ml (10 mcg) of 1:100 dilution intradermally. Inspect the site in 20 minutes. A urticarial wheal surrounded by a zone of erythema is a positive reaction. Concomitant use of antihistamines may interfere with sensitivity tests. If skin testing causes a systemic reaction, place a tourniquet above the testing site and treat anaphylaxis.

■ Standard treatment of digitalis intoxication includes withdrawal of the intoxicating agent, correction of electrolyte disturbances (especially hyperkalemia), acid-base imbalances, hypoxia, and treatment of cardiac arrhythmias. ■ Monitor VS, ECG, and potassium concentration frequently during and after drug administration. ■ Monitor for S/S of an acute allergic reaction (e.g., angioedema, bronchospasm with wheezing or cough, erythema, hypotension, laryngeal edema, pruritus, stridor, tachycardia, urticaria). ■ Obtain serum digoxin concentrations if possible. High margin of error will occur if drawn soon after ingestion. 6 to 8 hours are required after the last digitalis dose to obtain an accurate serum concentration. ■ Potassium may be shifted from inside to outside the cell, causing increased renal excretion. May appear to have hyperkalemia while there is a total body deficit of potassium. When the digitalis effect is reversed, hypokalemia may develop rapidly. ■ Do not redigitalize until all Fab fragments have been eliminated from the body. May take several days. May take longer in severe renal impairment, and reintoxication may occur by release of newly unbound digoxin into the blood. ■ See Precautions and Drug/Lab Interactions.

Maternal/Child: Category C: use only when clearly indicated and benefits outweigh risks in pregnancy, breast-feeding, and infants. ■ ***Digibind*** indicates that it should be used in infants and children if more than 0.3 mg of digoxin is ingested, if serum digoxin levels equal to or greater than 6.4 nmol/L, or if there is underlying heart disease.

Patient Education: Contact the physician immediately if S/S of a delayed allergic reaction or serum sickness occur (e.g., rash, pruritus, urticaria).

Elderly: Consider age-related impaired renal function; monitor closely for recurrent toxicity; see Monitor.

DRUG/LAB INTERACTIONS

Will cause a precipitous rise in total serum digoxin, but most will be bound to the Fab fragment. Will interfere with digitalis immunoassay measurements until Fab fragment is completely eliminated. ■ Catecholamines (e.g., epinephrine) may aggravate digitalis arrhythmias. ■ See skin test in Monitor.

SIDE EFFECTS

Acute anaphylaxis with urticaria, respiratory distress, and vascular collapse are possible. Exacerbation of congestive heart failure and low cardiac output states and increased ventricular response in atrial fibrillation may occur due to withdrawal of digitalis effects. Hypokalemia may be life threatening.

ANTIDOTE

Notify the physician of all side effects. Discontinue the drug and treat anaphylaxis immediately. Corticosteroids, epinephrine (Adrenalin [see Drug/Lab Interactions]), diphenhydramine (Benadryl), oxygen, IV fluids, vasopressors (dopamine), and ventilation equipment must always be available. Resuscitate as necessary. Treat hypokalemia cautiously when necessary. Support exacerbated cardiac conditions as necessary.

DIGOXIN INJECTION

(di-jox′in in-jek′shun)

Cardiac glycoside
Antiarrhythmic
Inotropic agent

Lanoxin, Lanoxin Pediatric

pH 6.8 to 7.2

USUAL DOSE

Calculate dose based on lean body weight (LBW), CrCl, age, as well as concomitant disease states, concurrent medications, and other factors that may alter the effects of digoxin.

0.25 to 0.5 mg (1 to 2 ml) as the **initial dose,** followed by 0.25 to 0.5 mg (1 to 2 ml) at 4- to 6-hour intervals until digitalized (approximately 4 to 6 hours). Assess clinical response (e.g., serum digoxin levels) before each additional dose. 0.5 to 1 mg (2 to 4 ml) is usually required for digitalization. AHA guidelines recommend a loading dose of 10 to 15 mcg/kg LBW. Maintenance dose is usually 0.125 to 0.5 mg daily.

PEDIATRIC DOSE

Use 0.1 mg/ml pediatric injection (100 mcg/ml).

Digitalizing dose: Give one half of total daily dose initially, then two doses of one fourth total daily dose at 8-hour intervals. Assess clinical response before each additional dose. If using a tuberculin syringe to measure a pediatric dose, do not flush syringe with parenteral solution after contents are injected, may result in an overdose.

Usual Digitalizing and Maintenance Dosages of Digoxin		
Age	**Digitalizing Dose (mcg/kg)***	**Daily IV Maintenance Dose (mcg/kg)†**
Premature	15-25	20%-30% of IV loading dose‡ divided and given every 12 hours
Full-term	20-30	
1-24 months	30-50	
2-5 years	25-35	25%-35% of IV loading dose‡
5-10 years	15-30	
Over 10 years	8-12	

*IV digitalizing doses are 80% of oral digitalizing doses; see Pediatric Dose for correct division of digitalizing dose.
†Divided daily dosing is recommended for children under 10 years of age.
‡Projected or actual digitalizing dose providing clinical response.

DOSE ADJUSTMENTS

Reduce dose in partially digitalized patients and patients with impaired renal function. ■ Dose reduction may be required before cardioversion. ■ See Drug/Lab Interactions; adjustments may be required with numerous drugs. ■ Reduced doses may be indicated in advanced heart failure, myocardial infarction, severe carditis, or severe pulmonary disease. ■ Adjustments may be required in thyroid disease. ■ 0.125 mg maintenance dose suggested for patients over 70 years of age or with impaired renal function and 0.0625 mg is suggested for marked renal impairment. ■ See Precautions.

DILUTION

May be given undiluted or each 1 ml may be diluted in 4 ml SW, NS, D5W, or LR for injection. Less diluent will cause precipitation. Use diluted solution immediately. Give through Y-tube or three-way stopcock of IV infusion set. See Pediatric Dose.

Storage: Store unopened vials at CRT protected from light.

INCOMPATIBLE WITH

Manufacturer recommends not mixing with other drugs in the same container and not administering simultaneously via the same IV line.

COMPATIBLE WITH

(Underline Indicates Conflicting Compatibility Information)

See Incompatible With. Consult pharmacist; specific conditions may apply; see Compatibilities, p. xvi.

Additive: Bretylium (Bretylate), cimetidine (Tagamet), furosemide (Lasix), lidocaine, ranitidine (Zantac), verapamil (Isoptin).

Syringe: Heparin, milrinone (Primacor).

Y-site: Ciprofloxacin (Cipro IV), cisatracurium (Nimbex), diltiazem (Cardizem), famotidine (Pepcid IV), gatifloxacin (Tequin), hetastarch in electrolytes (Hextend), inamrinone (Inocor), insulin (regular), linezolid (Zyvox), meperidine (Demerol), meropenem (Merrem IV), midazolam (Versed), milrinone (Primacor), morphine, potassium chloride (KCl), remifentanil (Ultiva), tacrolimus (Prograf).

RATE OF ADMINISTRATION

Each single dose over a minimum of 5 minutes.

ACTIONS

A crystalline cardiac glycoside obtained from *Digitalis lanata;* this is a fast-acting hydrolytic product of lanatoside C. Onset of action is within 5 to 30 minutes and lasts 2 to 3 days. It has positive inotropic action, increasing the strength of myocardial contraction. It also alters the electric behavior of heart muscle through actions on myocardial automaticity, conduction velocity, and refraction. Results are a slower, stronger beat with increased cardiac output. Venous pressure falls, coronary circulation is increased, and heart size may become more normal. Widely distributed throughout the body and rapidly excreted in the urine. Secreted in breast milk.

INDICATIONS AND USES

Congestive heart failure. ■ Atrial fibrillation; see Precautions. ■ Atrial flutter. ■ Selected paroxysmal tachycardia or AV junctional rhythm. ■ Selected supraventricular tachycardias. ■ Cardiogenic shock. ■ Selected situations in myocardial infarction. ■ Preoperative, intraoperative, and postoperative need for digitalis because of stress on the heart.

CONTRAINDICATIONS

Beriberi heart disease, digitalis intoxication or previous toxic response, hypersensitivity to digoxin, selected cases of hypersensitive carotid sinus syndrome, ventricular fibrillation, ventricular tachycardia unless heart failure occurs after a protracted episode and the etiology is not digitalis intoxication.

PRECAUTIONS

IV administration is the preferred parenteral route. Used only when oral therapy is not feasible or rapid therapeutic effect is necessary. ■ Diltiazem (Cardizem) or verapamil (Isotopin) generally preferred to treat atrial fibrillation; adenosine (Adenocard) preferred to treat PSVT. ■ Some clinicians suggest stopping digoxin 12 hours before surgery to reduce risk of perioperative arrhythmias in digitalized patients. The exception is patients with supraventricular tachyarrhythmias; they should receive a dose the morning of surgery. ■ Use with caution in patients with hypercalcemia or liver or kidney disease. ■ Hypocalcemia may nullify effect of digoxin. If calcium levels need to be restored to normal, give calcium slowly and in small amounts. Death has occurred in digitalized patients receiving calcium. ■ Plasma levels in thyroid disease are inversely proportional to thyroid status. Dose may be increased in thyrotoxic patients and decreased in patients with myxedema. ■ Use caution in patients with first- or second-degree heart block; may precipitate complete heart block. ■ Use caution in patients with advanced heart failure, myocardial infarction, severe carditis, or severe pulmonary disease. May be sensitive to digoxin-induced arrhythmia. Initiate therapy with lower doses. ■ If countershock is necessary (last-resort treatment of life-threatening arrhythmias), begin with low voltage levels and increase gradually to avoid ventricular arrhythmias. ■ See Drug/Lab Interactions.

Monitor: Hypomagnesemia, hypokalemia, and hypercalcemia may predispose patient to digitalis toxicity. Monitor electrolytes frequently during therapy. Avoid rapid changes. Supplements indicated to maintain normal serum electrolyte levels. ■ Monitor HR and BP. ■ Baseline and periodic ECG monitoring suggested. ■ ECG monitoring recommended in children to avoid intoxication. ■ Monitor digoxin levels. Draw at least 6 to 8 hours after last dose, preferably just before next dose. Therapeutic effects usually achieved with serum levels in a range from 0.8 to 1.5 ng/ml. Toxic threshold is equal to or greater than 2 ng/ml. ■ Monitor renal function. ■ See Precautions and Drug/Lab Interactions.

Maternal/Child: Category C: use only if clearly needed. ■ Has been used to treat fetal tachycardia. ■ Safety for use in nursing mothers not established.

Elderly: Monitor carefully. Reduced dose may be indicated. Consider reduced body mass and reduced kidney function.

DRUG/LAB INTERACTIONS

Monitor serum levels carefully and adjust doses as indicated. ■ Digoxin serum levels increased by amiodarone, atorvastatin (Lipitor), benzodiazepines (e.g., diazepam [Valium]), calcium channel blockers (e.g., verapamil [Isoptin], diltiazem [Cardizem] to a lesser extent), cyclosporine (Sandimmune), esmolol (Brevibloc), flecanide (Tambocor), ibuprofen (Motrin), indomethacin (Indocin), itraconazole (Sporanox), macrolides (e.g., erythromycin), nifedipine (Procardia), quinidine, spironolactone (Aldactone), telmisartan (Micardis), tetracyclines (e.g., doxycycline), tolbutamide, and many others; may increase therapeutic effects or cause toxicity. ■ Synergistic with beta blockers (e.g., atenolol [Tenormin], metoprolol [Lopressor]); both drugs slow AV conduction and can cause complete heart block. ■ Digitalis toxicity may be precipitated by potassium-depleting corticosteroids and diuretics (e.g., furosemide [Lasix], chlorodiazide [Diuril]), calcium, sympathomimetic amines (e.g., epinephrine), reserpine, succinylcholine, amphotericin B. ■ Increased risk of arrhythmias with nondepolarizing muscle relaxants (e.g., pancuronium [Pavulon]), reserpine, sympathomimetic amines (e.g., epinephrine), succinylcholine. ■ Initiation of thyroid treatment may require an increase in digoxin dose; treatment with thioamines (propylthiouracil [PTU]) may require a decreased dose. ■ Potassium-sparing diuretics (e.g., spironolactone [Aldactone]), cimetidine (Tagamet) may increase or decrease toxic effects. ■ Serum levels and therapeutic effects may be reduced by antineoplastic agents (e.g., bleomycin, carmustine, cyclophosphamide, cytarabine, doxorubicin, methotrexate, procarbazine, vincristine), rifampin (Rifadin), topiramate (Topamax), and many others. When these drugs are discontinued, digitalis toxicity may occur. ■ See Precautions and Monitor.

SIDE EFFECTS

Seldom last more than 3 days after drug is discontinued. Any form of digitalis may cause partial or AV block and almost any arrhythmia, including paroxysmal tachycardia, atrial tachycardia, fibrillation, or standstill. ***First ECG signs of toxicity*** are ST segment sagging, PR prolongation, and possible bigeminal rhythm. ***Clinical signs of toxicity*** are mostly abdominal discomfort or pain, anorexia, blurred vision, confusion, diarrhea, disturbed color (yellow) vision, headache, nausea, photopsia (points of light in peripheral vision), vomiting, and weakness.

ANTIDOTE

Discontinue the drug at the first sign of toxicity and notify the physician. Dosage may be decreased or discontinued. For severe toxicity, digoxin immune Fab is a specific antidote. Depending on symptoms, one or more of the following may be required: atropine, phenytoin (Dilantin), potassium salts (potassium chloride), procainamide (Pronestyl), or disodium edetate (EDTA disodium). See Precautions. Peritoneal dialysis or hemodialysis not effective in overdose.

DIHYDROERGOTAMINE MESYLATE

(dye-hye-droe-er-got'a-meen mes'uh-lat)

D.H.E. 45

Ergot alkaloid
Migraine agent

pH 3.2 to 4

USUAL DOSE

Abort or prevent headaches: 1 mg (1 ml). May be repeated in 1 hour. No more than 2 doses (2 mg total) may be given IV in 24 hours. Do not exceed 6 mg in 1 week; see Precautions. Administration of an antiemetic (e.g., metoclopramide [Reglan] 10 mg) PO 1 hour before dihydroergotamine is recommended.

Chronic intractable headache: 0.5 mg (0.5 ml). Administer an antiemetic IV (e.g., metoclopramide) about 10 minutes before injection.

Prevention of orthostatic hypotension associated with spinal or epidural anesthesia (unlabeled): 0.5 mg (0.5 ml). Give a few minutes before anesthetic.

PEDIATRIC DOSE

See Maternal/Child. Administration of an antiemetic (e.g., metoclopramide, prochlorperazine), usually PO, 1 hour before dihydroergotamine is recommended.

Children 6 to 9 years of age: 100 to 150 mcg (0.1 to 0.15 mg).

Children 9 to 12 years of age: 200 mcg (0.2 mg).

Children 12 to 16 years of age: 250 to 500 mcg (0.25 to 0.5 mg).

For all age ranges, repeat up to 2 doses at 20-minute intervals if necessary. Another source suggests 250 mcg (0.25 mg) at the start of the attack. Repeat in 1 hour if necessary.

DILUTION

May be given undiluted.

Storage: Protect ampules from light and heat.

COMPATIBILITY

Specific information not available. Consider specific use; consult pharmacist.

RATE OF ADMINISTRATION

1 mg or fraction thereof over 1 minute.

ACTIONS

An alpha-adrenergic blocking agent that causes constriction of both peripheral and cerebral blood vessels and produces depression of central vasomotor centers. Metabolized by the liver. Metabolites eliminated primarily in feces. Secreted in breast milk.

INDICATIONS AND USES

To abort or prevent vascular headaches (migraine, histamine cephalalgia). Used when rapid control is desired or other routes not feasible. ■ Treatment of chronic intractable headache.

Unlabeled uses: To prevent orthostatic hypotension associated with spinal or epidural anesthesia. Use SC to enhance heparin effects in preventing postoperative deep vein thrombosis after abdominal, thoracic, or pelvic surgeries or total hip replacement and IM or SC to treat orthostatic hypotension.

CONTRAINDICATIONS

Breast-feeding, coronary artery disease, hepatic or renal disease, hypersensitivity, uncontrolled hypertension, peripheral vascular disease, pregnancy or women who may become pregnant, sepsis. ■ Co-administration with potent CYP3A4 inhibitors, including protease inhibitors and macrolide antibiotics, is contraindicated; see Drug/Lab Interactions.

PRECAUTIONS

IM or SC use is preferred but may be given IV to obtain a more rapid effect. ■ Co-administration with potent CYP3A4 inhibitors, including protease inhibitors and macrolide antibiotics, increases the risk of vasospasm leading to cerebral ischemia and/or ischemia of the extremities (peripheral). May be serious and/or life threatening; see Contraindications and Drug/Lab Interactions. ■ Use only when a clear diagnosis of migraine has been established. Do not exceed dosing guidelines or use for chronic daily administration; see Usual Dose.

Monitor: Monitor vital signs; observe closely. ■ See Drug/Lab Interactions.

Patient Education: Consider birth control options. ■ Take only as directed. ■ Report ineffectiveness or an increase in frequency or severity of headaches. ■ Report chest pain, increased HR, itching, muscle pain or weakness of arms or legs, numbness or tingling of extremities, or swelling.

Maternal/Child: Category X: avoid pregnancy. See Contraindications. ■ Safety for use in children not established. Severe side effects (e.g., extrapyramidal reactions may occur). Pretreatment with an antiemetic may be helpful. Limit pediatric use to patients who have not responded to less toxic treatment.

Elderly: Increased risk of hypothermia and ischemic complications (e.g., cardiac, peripheral). ■ Consider age-related renal impairment.

DRUG/LAB INTERACTIONS

Contraindicated with potent CYP3A4 inhibitors, including antifungals (itraconazole [Sporanox], ketoconazole [Nizoral]), protease inhibitors (ritonavir [Norvir], nelfinavir [Viracept], and indinavir [Crixivan]), and macrolide antibiotics (clarithromycin [Biaxin], erythromycin, and troleandomycin [TAO]); see Contraindications and Precautions. ■ Administer less potent CYP3A4 inhibitors with caution as vasospasm may occur. Less potent inhibitors include, but are not limited to, saquinavir (Invirase), nefazodone (Serzone), fluconazole (Diflucan), grapefruit juice, fluoxetine (Prozac), fluvoxamine (Luvox), zileuton (Zyflo), and clotrimazole (Gyne-Lotrimin, Mycelex). ■ Opposes vasodilating effects of nitrates (e.g., nitroglycerin), decreasing their effectiveness. ■ May cause hypertensive crisis in combination with other vasopressors (e.g., epinephrine). ■ May cause peripheral vasoconstriction with ischemia and/or cyanosis with beta-adrenergic blockers (e.g., propranolol [Inderal]) and nicotine.

SIDE EFFECTS

Rare in therapeutic doses, but may include angina pectoris, blindness, gangrene, muscle pains, muscle weakness, nausea, numbness and tingling of the fingers and toes, pleural and retroperitoneal fibrosis, thirst, uterine bleeding, and vomiting.

ANTIDOTE

Discontinue the drug and notify the physician of any side effects. Another drug will probably be chosen if further treatment is indicated. Vasodilators (nitroprusside sodium) and CNS stimulants (e.g., caffeine and sodium benzoate) are indicated as an antidote. Heparin and low molecular weight dextran may be used to reduce thrombosis due to excessive vasoconstriction. Hemodialysis may be indicated. Resuscitate as necessary.

DILTIAZEM HYDROCHLORIDE

(dil-tye′a-zem hye-droe-klor′id)

Calcium channel blocker
Antiarrhythmic

Cardizem

pH 3.7 to 4.1

USUAL DOSE

0.25 mg/kg of body weight initially (20 mg for the average patient). A second dose of 0.35 mg/kg may be given in 15 minutes if needed to achieve HR reduction (25 mg for the average patient). Any additional bolus doses used to achieve an appropriate response must be individualized to each patient. Patients with PSVT will probably respond to bolus doses and may not require an infusion, but to maintain reduction in HR in patients with atrial fibrillation or atrial flutter, immediately follow with an intravenous infusion at an initial rate of 10 mg/hr. May only be used for up to 24 hours. Some patients may maintain response with an initial rate of 5 mg/hr. Infusion may be increased by 5 mg/hr increments to a maximum dose of 15 mg/hr. Discontinue infusion within 24 hours. Oral antiarrhythmic agents (e.g., digoxin, quinidine, procainamide, calcium channel blockers [e.g., diltiazem, verapamil], beta blockers [e.g., atenolol, metoprolol, propranolol]) to maintain reduced HR are usually started within 3 hours of initial bolus of diltiazem.

DOSE ADJUSTMENTS

Specific mg/kg dose must be used for patients with low body weights. ■ Reduced dose may be indicated in impaired hepatic or renal function. ■ See Drug/Lab Interactions.

DILUTION

Available as a solution in 25- or 50-mg vials (5 mg/ml), as a powder with supplied diluent (Lyo-ject syringe 25 mg [5 mg/ml]), and in a piggyback monovial containing 100 mg (with transfer needle set to facilitate preparation of an infusion).

Cardizem Injectable or Cardizem Lyo-Ject Syringe				
Diluent Volume	Quantity of Cardizem (Diltiazem) Injection	Final Concentration	Administration: Dose	Administration: Infusion Rate
100 ml	125 mg (25 ml)	1 mg/ml	5 mg/hr 10 mg/hr 15 mg/hr	5 ml/hr 10 ml/hr 15 ml/hr
250 ml	250 mg (50 ml)	0.83 mg/ml	5 mg/hr 10 mg/hr 15 mg/hr	6 ml/hr 12 ml/hr 18 ml/hr
500 ml	250 mg (50 ml)	0.45 mg/ml	5 mg/hr 10 mg/hr 15 mg/hr	11 ml/hr 22 ml/hr 33 ml/hr

Cardizem Monovial				
Diluent Volume	Quantity of Cardizem Monovial to Add	Final Concentration	Administration	
			Dose	Infusion Rate
100 ml	100 mg (1 monovial)	1 mg/ml	5 mg/hr 10 mg/hr 15 mg/hr	5 ml/hr 10 ml/hr 15 ml/hr
250 ml	200 mg (2 monovials)	0.8 mg/ml	5 mg/hr 10 mg/hr 15 mg/hr	6.25 ml/hr 12.5 ml/hr 18.8 ml/hr
500 ml	200 mg (2 monovials)	0.4 mg/ml	5 mg/hr 10 mg/hr 15 mg/hr	12.5 ml/hr 25 ml/hr 37.5 ml/hr

IV injection: May be given undiluted through Y-tube or three-way stopcock of tubing containing NS, D5W, or D5/½NS.
Infusion: May be further diluted for infusion in any of the above solutions.
Storage: Vials may be stored at room temperature for up to 1 month, then discarded. Refrigeration before and after dilution preferred. Use within 24 hours of dilution. Discard unused medication and/or solution. Do not freeze.

INCOMPATIBLE WITH

Manufacturer recommends that **all formulations** not be mixed with any other drugs in the same container and, if possible, that they not be co-infused in the same IV line.
Cardizem Lyo-Ject Syringe is listed by the manufacturer as incompatible at the ***Y-site*** with acetazolamide (Diamox), acyclovir (Zovirax), aminophylline, ampicillin (Polycillin-N), ampicillin/sulbactam (Unasyn), cefamandole (Mandol), cefoperazone (Cefobid), diazepam (Valium), furosemide (Lasix), hydrocortisone sodium succinate (Solu-Cortef), methylprednisolone (Solu-Medrol), mezlocillin (Mezlin), nafcillin (Nafcil), phenytoin (Dilantin), rifampin (Rifadin), sodium bicarbonate. **Cardizem** is listed as incompatible with all of the above and insulin (regular).
Cardizem Monovial is listed by the manufacturer as incompatible at the ***Y-site*** with acetazolamide (Diamox), acyclovir (Zovirax), cefoperazone (Cefobid), diazepam (Valium), furosemide (Lasix), phenytoin (Dilantin), rifampin (Rifadin).

COMPATIBLE WITH **(Underline Indicates Conflicting Compatibility Information)**

Consult pharmacist; specific conditions may apply; see Compatibilities, p. xvi.
Manufacturer lists **Cardizem Lyo-Ject Syringe** as compatible at the ***Y-site*** with insulin (regular) and lists the **Cardizem Monovial** (1 mg/ml) in NS as compatible at the ***Y-site*** with aminophylline, ampicillin, ampicillin/sulbactam (Unasyn), cefamandole (Mandol), hydrocortisone sodium succinate (Solu-Cortef), insulin (regular), methylprednisolone (Solu-Medrol), mezlocillin (Mezlin), nafcillin (Nafcil), sodium bicarbonate.
Other sources list the following but do not differentiate formulations.
Y-site: Albumin, amikacin (Amikin), amphotericin B (Fungizone), aztreonam (Azactam), bretylium (Bretylate), bumetanide (Bumex), cefazolin (Kefzol), cefotaxime (Claforan), cefotetan (Cefotan), cefoxitin (Mefoxin), ceftazidime (Fortaz), ceftriaxone (Rocephin), cefuroxime (Zinacef), cimet-

idine (Tagamet), ciprofloxacin (Cipro IV), clindamycin (Cleocin), digoxin (Lanoxin), dobutamine (Dobutrex), dopamine (Intropin), doxycycline (Vibramycin), epinephrine (Adrenalin), erythromycin lactobionate (Erythrocin), esmolol (Brevibloc), fentanyl (Sublimaze), fluconazole (Diflucan), gentamicin (Garamycin), heparin, hetastarch in electrolytes (Hextend), hetastarch in NS (Hespan), hydromorphone (Dilaudid), imipenem-cilastatin (Primaxin), labetalol (Normodyne), lidocaine, lorazepam (Ativan), meperidine (Demerol), metoclopramide (Reglan), metronidazole (Flagyl IV), midazolam (Versed), milrinone (Primacor), morphine, multivitamins (M.V.I.), nicardipine (Cardene IV), nitroglycerin (Nitro-Bid IV), nitroprusside sodium, norepinephrine (Levophed), oxacillin (Bactocill), penicillin G potassium, pentamidine, piperacillin (Pipracil), potassium chloride (KCl), potassium phosphates, procainamide (Pronestyl), ranitidine (Zantac), sulfamethoxazole-trimethoprim (Bactrim), theophylline, ticarcillin (Ticar), ticarcillin/clavulanate (Timentin), tobramycin (Nebcin), vancomycin (Vancocin), vecuronium (Norcuron).

RATE OF ADMINISTRATION

IV injection: Each single dose equally distributed over 2 minutes.

Infusion: 5 mg to 15 mg/hr based on patient response. See charts under Dilution for diluent, dose, and infusion rate information. Use of a metriset (60 gtt/min) required; volumetric infusion pump preferred.

ACTIONS

Directly inhibits the influx of calcium ions through slow channels during membrane depolarization of cardiac and vascular smooth muscle. Effective in supraventricular tachycardias because it slows conduction through the AV node, prolongs the effective refractory period, reduces ventricular rates, and helps to prevent embolic complications. Prevents reentry phenomena through the AV node. Reduces HR (10% with a single dose, 20% at peak effectiveness), systolic and diastolic BP, systemic vascular resistance, pulmonary artery systolic and diastolic BPs, and coronary vascular resistance with no significant effect on contractility, left ventricular end diastolic pressure, right atrial pressure, or pulmonary capillary wedge pressure. Increases cardiac output and stroke volume. Has little or no effect on normal AV nodal conduction at normal HRs. Produces less myocardial depression than verapamil. Effective within 3 minutes; maximum effect should occur within 7 to 11 minutes and last for 1 to 3 hours. 70% to 80% bound to plasma proteins. Metabolized in the liver. Excreted in urine and bile. Secreted in breast milk.

INDICATIONS AND USES

Temporary control of rapid ventricular rate in atrial fibrillation or atrial flutter unless associated with an accessory bypass tract (e.g., Wolff-Parkinson-White syndrome or short PR syndrome). ■ Rapid conversion of paroxysmal supraventricular tachycardia (PSVT) to normal sinus rhythm including AV nodal reentrant tachycardias and reciprocating tachycardias associated with an extranodal accessory pathway (e.g., Wolff-Parkinson-White syndrome or short PR syndrome). ■ Narrow complex PSVT not responsive to adenosine (Adenocard).

Unlabeled uses: Decrease refractory angina and pulse rates in unstable angina.

CONTRAINDICATIONS

Atrial fibrillation or flutter when associated with an accessory bypass tract (e.g., Wolff-Parkinson-White or short PR syndrome), cardiogenic shock, congestive heart failure (severe) unless secondary to supraventricular tachyarrhythmia treatable with diltiazem, known sensitivity to diltiazem, second- or third-degree AV block or sick sinus syndrome (unless functioning ventricular pacemaker in place), severe hypotension, patients receiving IV beta-adrenergic blocking agents (e.g., atenolol [Tenormin], propranolol [Inderal]) within 2 to 4 hours, ventricular tachycardia. Not recommended for wide QRS tachycardias of uncertain origin or for tachycardias induced by drugs or poisons.

PRECAUTIONS

For short-term use only. ■ While diltiazem will effectively decrease HR, cardioversion will probably be required to convert atrial fibrillation or atrial flutter to a normal sinus rhythm. ■ Valsalva maneuver recommended before use of diltiazem in all paroxysmal supraventricular tachycardias if clinically appropriate. ■ Use IV diltiazem with caution in patients with pre-existing impaired ventricular function (e.g., congestive heart failure, acute myocardial infarction or pulmonary congestion documented by x-ray); may exacerbate disease. Use of oral diltiazem in these patients is contraindicated. ■ May cause second- or third-degree AV block in sinus rhythm; discontinue diltiazem if AV block occurs. ■ Can cause life-threatening tachycardia with severe hypotension in atrial fibrillation or flutter in patients with an accessory bypass tract and periods of asystole in patients with sick sinus syndrome. ■ Use with caution in impaired renal or hepatic function. ■ Ventricular premature beats (VPBs) may occur on conversion of PSVT to sinus rhythm; considered to have no clinical significance. ■ Continue regular dosing on day of OR and thereafter unless otherwise specified by physician. If discontinued, may cause severe angina or MI.

Monitor: Accurate pretreatment diagnosis differentiating wide-complex QRS tachycardia of supraventricular origin from ventricular origin is imperative. ■ ECG monitoring during administration preferred; must be available. ■ Monitor BP closely. ■ Emergency resuscitation drugs and equipment must always be available. ■ See Drug/Lab Interactions.

Maternal/Child: Category C: large doses (5 to 10 times mg/kg dose) have resulted in embryo and fetal death and skeletal abnormalities in animals. ■ Discontinue breast-feeding. ■ Safety for use in children not established.

Elderly: Half-life may be prolonged. ■ May cause tinnitus.

DRUG/LAB INTERACTIONS

Do not give concomitantly (within a few hours) with IV beta-adrenergic blocking agents (e.g., atenolol [Tenormin], propranolol [Inderal]); see Contraindications. May result in bradycardia, AV block, and/or depression of contractility. Use extreme caution if these drugs are administered orally or if patient has received before admission; usually tolerated. ■ May result in additive effects with any agent known to affect cardiac contractility and/or SA or AV node conduction (e.g., digoxin [Lanoxin], disopyramide (Norpace), procainamide [Pronestyl], beta-blockers [e.g., propranolol], quinidine). ■ Is used with digitalis, but monitor for excessive slowing of HR and/or AV block. ■ May potentiate anesthetics; titrate both drugs carefully. ■ May decrease metabolism and increase serum concentrations and toxicity of drugs metabolized by the cytochrome P_{450} enzyme system (e.g., amlodipine [Norvasc], carbamazepine [Tegretol], cyclosporine [Sandimmune], quinidine, theophylline, valproate [Depacon]). ■ Metabolism may be decreased and serum concentrations increased by cimetidine

(Tagamet) and ranitidine (Zantac). ■ May cause severe hypotension with fentanyl (Sublimaze). ■ Concurrent administration with cisapride (Propulsid) may cause syncope and prolongation of the QT interval. ■ Any drug metabolized in the liver may cause competitive inhibition of metabolism (e.g., insulin).

SIDE EFFECTS

Arrhythmia (junctional rhythm or isorhythmic dissociation), flushing, hypotension (asymptomatic and symptomatic), and injection site reactions (burning, itching) occurred most frequently and were most often mild and transient but could have serious potential. Amblyopia, asthenia, atrial flutter, AV block (first- or second-degree), bradycardia, chest pain, congestive heart failure, constipation, dizziness, dry mouth, dyspnea, edema, elevated alkaline phosphatase and AST (SGOT), headache, hyperuricemia, nausea, paresthesia, pruritus, sinus node dysfunction, sinus pause, sweating, syncope, ventricular arrhythmias, ventricular fibrillation, ventricular tachycardia, and vomiting have occurred.

ANTIDOTE

Discontinue diltiazem if a high-degree AV block occurs in sinus rhythm. Notify physician promptly of all side effects. Treatment will depend on clinical situation; maintain IV fluids as indicated. Rapid ventricular response in atrial flutter/fibrillation should respond to cardioversion, procainamide, and/or lidocaine. Treat bradycardia, AV block, and asystole with standard AHA protocol (atropine, isoproterenol, pacing). Treat cardiac failure with inotropic agents (isoproterenol, dopamaine, or dobutamine) and diuretics. Calcium chloride will reverse effects of verapamil; may be useful with diltiazem. Dopamine or norepinephrine (levarterenol) and Trendelenburg position should reverse hypotension. Treat allergic reactions or resuscitate as necessary.

DIPHENHYDRAMINE HYDROCHLORIDE

(dye-fen-hye′dra-meen hye-droe-klor′id)

Antihistamine
Antidyskinetic/antiparkinsonism
Antiemetic
Antivertigo agent
Sedative-hypnotic

Benadryl

pH 5 to 6

USUAL DOSE

10 to 50 mg. Up to 100 mg may be given. Individualize dose based on patient symptoms and response. Total dosage should not exceed 400 mg/24 hr.

PEDIATRIC DOSE

See Contraindications and Maternal/Child.

Children after neonatal period: 1.25 mg/kg/dose every 6 hours as needed or 150 mg/M^2/24 hr in equally divided doses given every 6 hours. Never exceed a total dosage of 300 mg/24 hr.

Anaphylaxis or phenothiazine overdose: 1 to 2 mg/kg IV slowly.

DOSE ADJUSTMENTS

Reduce dose for the elderly or debilitated. ■ See Drug/Lab Interactions.

DILUTION

May be given undiluted.

COMPATIBLE WITH (Underline Indicates Conflicting Compatibility Information)

Consult pharmacist; specific conditions may apply; see Compatibilities, p. xvi.

Additive: Amikacin (Amikin), aminophylline, ascorbic acid (Cenolate), bleomycin (Blenoxane), buprenorphine (Buprenex), colistimethate (Coly-Mycin M), erythromycin lactobionate (Erythrocin), hydrocortisone sodium succinate (Solu-Cortef), lidocaine, methyldopate (Aldomet), nafcillin (Nafcil), penicillin G potassium and sodium.

Syringe: Atropine, butorphanol (Stadol), chlorpromazine (Thorazine), cimetidine (Tagamet), dexamethasone (Decadron), dimenhydrinate (Dinate), droperidol (Inapsine), fentanyl (Sublimaze), glycopyrrolate, hydromorphone (Dilaudid), meperidine (Demerol), metoclopramide (Reglan), midazolam (Versed), morphine, nalbuphine (Nubain), pentazocine (Talwin), perphenazine (Trilafon), prochlorperazine (Compazine), promethazine (Phenergan), ranitidine (Zantac), scopolamine, sufentanil (Sufenta), and selected contrast agents used in radiology.

Y-site: Acyclovir (Zovirax), aldesleukin (Proleukin), amifostine (Ethyol), aztreonam (Azactam), ciprofloxacin (Cipro IV), cisatracurium (Nimbex), cisplatin (Platinol), cladribine (Leustatin), cyclophosphamide (Cytoxan), cytarabine (ARA-C), docetaxel (Taxotere), doxorubicin (Adriamycin), doxorubicin liposome (Doxil), etoposide phosphate (Etopophos), famotidine (Pepcid IV), fentanyl (Sublimaze), filgrastim (Neupogen), fluconazole (Diflucan), fludarabine (Fludara), gatifloxacin (Tequin), gemcitabine (Gemzar), granisetron (Kytril), heparin, hetastarch in electrolytes (Hextend), hydrocortisone sodium succinate (Solu-Cortef), hydromorphone (Dilaudid), idarubicin (Idamycin), linezolid (Zyvox), melphalan (Alkeran), meperidine (Demerol), meropenem (Merrem IV), methotrexate (Folex), morphine, ondansetron (Zofran), paclitaxel (Taxol), piperacillin/tazobactam (Zosyn), potassium chloride (KCl), propofol (Diprivan), remifentanil (Ultiva), sargramostim (Leukine), sufentanil (Sufenta), tacrolimus (Prograf), teniposide (Vumon), thiotepa (Thioplex), vinorelbine (Navelbine).

RATE OF ADMINISTRATION

25 mg or fraction thereof over 1 minute. Extend injection time in non-emergency situations and children. See Maternal/Child.

ACTIONS

A potent antihistamine, it is capable of blocking the effects of histamines at various receptor sites, either eliminating allergic reaction or greatly modifying it. It also has anticholinergic (antispasmodic), antiemetic, and sedative effects. It has rapid onset of action and is widely distributed throughout the body. A portion of this drug is metabolized in the liver; the rest is excreted unchanged in the urine. Some secretion may occur in breast milk.

INDICATIONS AND USES

Allergic reactions to blood or plasma. ■ Supplemental therapy to epinephrine in anaphylaxis and other uncomplicated allergic reactions requiring prompt treatment. ■ Preoperative or generalized sedation. ■ Management of parkinsonism, including drug-induced (e.g., phenothiazines [e.g., prochlorperazine (Compazine)]). ■ Severe nausea and vomiting. ■ Motion sickness. ■ To replace oral therapy when it is impractical or contraindicated.

CONTRAINDICATIONS

Breast-feeding, hypersensitivity to antihistamines, newborn or premature infants.

PRECAUTIONS

IV route used only in emergency situations. ■ Avoid SC or perivascular injection. ■ Use with extreme caution in infants, children, elderly or debilitated individuals, asthmatic attack, bladder neck obstruction, narrow-angle glaucoma, lower respiratory tract infections, prostatic hypertrophy, pyloroduodenal obstruction, and stenosing peptic ulcer.

Monitor: Will induce drowsiness. ■ Monitor vital signs; observe closely. ■ See Drug/Lab Interactions.

Patient Education: Do not drive or operate hazardous equipment until effects wear off. ■ May cause drowsiness and dizziness; request help to ambulate. ■ Avoid alcohol and other CNS depressants (e.g., diazepam [Valium], narcotics).

Maternal/Child: See Contraindications, Precautions, Monitor, and Side Effects. ■ Category B: use only when clearly needed. May increase risk of abnormalities during the first trimester. ■ Use extreme caution in infants and children; may cause hallucinations, convulsions, or death. May also reduce mental alertness and cause excitation.

Elderly: See Dose Adjustments, Precautions, Monitor, and Side Effects. ■ May cause confusion, dizziness, hyperexcitability, hypotension and/or sedation. ■ Sensitivity to cholinergic effects increased (e.g., dry mouth, urinary retention).

DRUG/LAB INTERACTIONS

Increases effectiveness of epinephrine and is often used in conjunction with it. ■ Potentiates anticholinergics (e.g., atropine); alcohol, beta blockers (e.g., metoprolol [Lopressor], propranolol [Inderal]), hypnotics, itraconazole (Sporanox), sedatives, tranquilizers, and other CNS depressants (e.g., reserpine, antipyretics); thioridazine (Mellaril); procarbazine (Matulane); and others. Reduced dose of potentiated drug may be indicated. ■ Anticholinergic and CNS sedative effects prolonged by MAO inhibitors (e.g., selegiline [Eldepryl]). Concurrent use not recommended. ■ Effectiveness of many drugs is reduced in combination with diphenhydramine because of increased metabolism. ■ May inhibit the wheal and flare reaction to antigen skin tests.

SIDE EFFECTS

Rare when used as indicated: anaphylaxis; blurring of vision; confusion; constipation; diarrhea; difficulty in urination; diplopia; drowsiness; drug rash; dryness of mouth, nose, and throat; epigastric distress; headache; hemolytic anemia; hypotension; insomnia; nasal stuffiness; nausea; nervousness; palpitations; photosensitivity; rapid pulse; restlessness; thickening of bronchial secretions; tightness of the chest and wheezing; tingling, heaviness, weakness of hands; urticaria; vertigo; vomiting. Overdose may cause convulsions, hallucinations, and death in children.

ANTIDOTE

For exaggerated drowsiness or other disturbing side effects, discontinue the drug and notify the physician. Side effects will usually subside within a few hours or may be treated symptomatically. Treat hypotension promptly; may lead to cardiovascular collapse. Use dopamine (Intropin), norepinephrine, or phenylephrine. Epinephrine is contraindicated for hypotension; further hypotension will occur. Propranolol (Inderal) is the drug of choice for ventricular arrhythmias. Treat convulsions with diazepam (Valium) 0.1 mg/kg IV slowly. Some central anticholinergic effects may require physostigmine. Avoid analeptics (e.g., caffeine); will cause convulsions. Epinephrine must be available to treat anaphylaxis. Resuscitate as necessary.

DIPHTHERIA ANTITOXIN

(dif-ther′e-ah an′ti-tok′sin)

Immunizing agent (active)

USUAL DOSE

Testing for sensitivity to horse serum required before use; see Precautions/Monitor. Suggested ranges for adults and children to be given as a single dose.

Pharyngeal or laryngeal disease of 48 hours duration: 20,000 to 40,000 units.

Nasopharyngeal lesions: 40,000 to 60,000 units.

Extensive disease (3 or more days duration or anyone with brawny swelling of the neck): 80,000 to 120,000 units.

DILUTION

Each 1 ml should be diluted with 19 ml D5W or NS and given as an infusion. Warm to 32° to 35° C (90° to 95° F).

Storage: Refrigerate before dilution.

COMPATIBILITY

Specific information not available. Consider specific use; consult pharmacist.

RATE OF ADMINISTRATION

To be given as a slow IV infusion, 1 ml/min. Titrate carefully to patient reaction.

ACTIONS

A sterile solution of purified antitoxic substances prepared from the blood serum of horses immunized against diphtheria toxin. Neutralizes the toxins produced by *Corynebacterium diphtheriae.*

INDICATIONS AND USES

Passive transient protection against or treatment of patients with clinical symptoms of diphtheria.

CONTRAINDICATIONS

Hypersensitivity to horse serum unless only treatment available for a life-threatening situation. Several techniques including preload of antihistamines and/or desensitization may be considered (see literature).

PRECAUTIONS

In the United States, diphtheria antitoxin may be obtained from the CDC diphtheria duty officer. The physician is asked to call (404)639-2888 during EST business hours or (404)639-2889 during nonbusiness hours. The CDC phone number is (404)639-3311. Read drug literature supplied with antitoxin completely before use. Essential to evaluate symptoms and individual status of each patient. ■ Determine patient response to any previous injections of serum of any type and history of any allergic-type reactions. ■ Hospitalize patient if possible. ■ If diphtheria is suspected, bacteriologic confirmation of the disease is not necessary to initiate treatment. Begin treatment as soon as possible. Each hour delay increases dosage requirements and decreases effectiveness.

Monitor: Test every patient without exception for sensitivity to horse serum (1-ml vial of 1:10 dilution horse serum supplied). Conjunctival test and skin test recommended for maximum safety.

Conjunctival test: Instill 1 drop 1:10 horse serum in conjunctival sac for adults (1 drop 1:100 dilution for children). Itching, redness, burning, and/or lacrimation within 30 minutes is a positive reaction. A drop of normal saline in the opposite eye is used as a control and should be asymptomatic. Reverse adverse effects of positive reaction with 1 drop epinephrine ophthalmic solution.

Skin test: Inject 0.1 ml of 1:100 horse serum intradermally. In patients with a history of allergies use 0.05 ml of a 1:1,000 solution. A like injection of normal saline can be used as a control. An urticarial wheal surrounded by a zone of erythema is a positive reaction. Compare in 20 minutes.

■ Other testing methods may be used. Use at least two. ■ Continue treatment until all symptoms controlled or bacteriologic confirmation of another disease entity confirmed. ■ Use of full therapeutic doses of antimicrobial agents recommended in conjunction with diphtheria antitoxin. ■ All contacts must be evaluated. Prophylactic antibiotics and immunization may be indicated. ■ See Drug/Lab Interactions.

DRUG/LAB INTERACTIONS

Concomitant use of antihistamines may interfere with sensitivity tests.

SIDE EFFECTS

Acute anaphylaxis with urticaria, respiratory distress, and vascular collapse. Serum sickness may occur. Usually appears in 7 to 12 days. Local pain, local erythema, and urticaria without systemic reaction can occur.

ANTIDOTE

Discontinue the drug and notify the physician of all side effects. Treat anaphylaxis immediately. Epinephrine (Adrenalin) and diphenhydramine (Benadryl), oxygen, vasopressors (dopamine), corticosteroids, and ventilation equipment must always be available. Salicylates, antihistamines, and/or corticosteroids may be useful in serum sickness. Resuscitate as necessary.

DIPYRIDAMOLE
(dye-peer-id'a-mole)

Coronary vasodilator
Diagnostic agent
Platelet aggregation inhibitor

Persantine IV

pH 2.2 to 3.2

USUAL DOSE

Myocardial perfusion imaging: 0.57 mg/kg of body weight equally distributed over 4 minutes (0.142 mg/kg/min). A 70-kg adult would receive a total dose of 39.9 mg (10 mg/min). Never exceed 0.57 mg/kg dose. Thallium should be injected within 5 minutes following the 4-minute infusion of dipyridamole.

Platelet aggregation inhibitor (unlabeled): 250 mg/24 hr as an infusion.

DILUTION

Each 1 ml (5 mg) must be diluted with a minimum of 2 ml D5W, D5/½NS, or D5NS. Total volume should range from a minimum of 20 ml to 50 ml (39.9 mg [8 ml] would be diluted in a minimum of 16 ml for a total infusion of 24 ml; additional diluent can be used to facilitate titration). May not be given undiluted; will cause local irritation.

Platelet aggregation inhibitor: Each 250-mg dose should be diluted with 250 ml D5W (1 mg/ml). Concentration may be increased if larger doses required.

Storage: Undiluted drug should be stored at CRT and protected from direct light; avoid freezing.

COMPATIBILITY

Specific information not available. Consider specific use; consult pharmacist.

RATE OF ADMINISTRATION

A single dose must be equally distributed over 4 minutes (0.142 mg/kg/min).

Platelet aggregation inhibitor: 10 mg/hr as a continuous infusion. Use of a microdrip (60 gtt/ml) or infusion pump recommended.

ACTIONS

A coronary vasodilator that will cause an increase in coronary blood flow velocity of from 3.8 to 7 times greater than resting velocity. Action may result from the inhibition of adenosine uptake. Peak velocity is reached in 2.5 to 8.7 minutes. Will cause a 20% increase in HR and a mild but significant decrease in systolic and diastolic BP in the supine position. Vital signs may take up to 30 minutes to return to baseline measurements. Used in combination with thallium, visualization shows dilation with sustained enhanced flow of intact vessels, leaving reduced pressure and flow across areas of hemodynamically important coronary vascular constriction. Results achieved are comparable to exercise-induced thallium imaging. Metabolized in the liver. Excreted in bile. Secreted in breast milk.

INDICATIONS AND USES

An alternative to exercise in thallium myocardial perfusion imaging for the evaluation of coronary artery disease in patients who cannot exercise adequately.

Unlabeled uses: Prophylactic inhibition of platelet aggregation in thromboembolism and myocardial infarction.

CONTRAINDICATIONS

Hypersensitivity to dipyridamole.

PRECAUTIONS

Administered by or under the direction of the cardiologist. ■ Full facilities for treatment of any airway, allergic, or cardiac emergency, including laboratory analysis, must be available. ■ Theophylline (aminophylline) and other emergency drugs must be immediately available. ■ Patients with a history of unstable angina or a history of asthma may be at greater risk; use extreme caution. ■ This drug has caused two fatal myocardial infarctions as well as other serious side effects in a small percentage of patients; clinical information to be gained must be weighed against risk to the patient.

Monitor: An IV line with a Y-tube or three-way stopcock must be in place. ■ Monitor vital signs continuously during infusion and for at least 15 minutes after or until return to baseline. ■ ECG monitoring using at least 1 chest lead should be continuous. ■ Patient is usually in a supine position, but tests have been conducted in a sitting position. Lower to supine with head tilted down (Trendelenburg) if hypotension occurs.

Maternal/Child: Category B: safety for use during pregnancy not established. Use only if clearly needed. ■ Temporarily discontinue breast-feeding. ■ Safety for use in children not established.

DRUG/LAB INTERACTIONS

Theophylline bronchodilators (e.g., aminophylline, oxtriphylline [Choledyl], theophylline) reverse the effect of dipyridamole on myocardial blood flow. Interferes with dipyridamole-assisted myocardial perfusion studies. Withhold bronchodilators for 36 hours before testing.

SIDE EFFECTS

BP lability, chest pain/angina pectoris, dizziness, dyspnea, ECG abnormalities (e.g., extrasystoles, ST-T changes, tachycardia), fatigue, flushing, headache, hypertension, hypotension, nausea, pain (unspecified), paresthesia. Numerous other side effects occur in less than 1% of patients.

Major: Bronchospasm, cerebral ischemia (transient), fatal and nonfatal myocardial infarction, ventricular fibrillation, ventricular tachycardia (symptomatic) occurred in 0.3% of patients.

ANTIDOTE

Physician will be present throughout test administration. Theophylline (aminophylline) is an adenosine receptor antagonist and will reverse the adenosine-mediated effects of dipyridamole (e.g., angina pectoris, bronchospasm, severe hypotension, ventricular arrhythmias). If bronchospasm or chest pain occur, administer 50 to 250 mg of theophylline at a rate not to exceed 50 mg over 30 seconds. If symptoms are not relieved by 250 mg of theophylline, sublingual nitroglycerin may be helpful. Persistent chest pain may indicate impending potentially fatal myocardial infarction. If patient condition permits, thallium may be injected and allowed to circulate for 1 minute before injection of theophylline (aminophylline); this will permit initial thallium perfusion imaging before reversal of vasodilatory effects of dipyridamole on coronary circulation. Use head-down supine position for hypotension before administering theophylline (aminophylline). After reversal of vasodilatory action, treat arrhythmias as indicated. Resuscitate as necessary.

DOBUTAMINE HYDROCHLORIDE

(doe-byoo′ta-meen hye-droe-klor′id)

Inotropic agent
Cardiac stimulant

Dobutrex

pH 2.5 to 5.5

USUAL DOSE

0.5 to 1 mcg/kg/min initially in patients likely to respond to minimum treatment. The usual effective initial dose ranges from 2.5 to 15 mcg/kg of body weight/min. AHA guidelines suggest 2 to 20 mcg/kg/min. Gradually adjust rate at 2- to 10-minute intervals to effect desired response. AHA guidelines recommend titrating so HR does not increase by more than 10% of baseline. Up to 40 mcg/kg/min has been used in some instances; increases potential for toxicity (e.g., myocardial ischemia). U.S. experience in controlled trials does not extend beyond 48 hours of therapy.

PEDIATRIC DOSE

2 to 20 mcg/kg/min. Initial dose usually 5 to 10 mcg/kg/min. Adjust rate to effect desired response.

DOSE ADJUSTMENTS

Lower-end initial doses may be appropriate in the elderly based on potential for decreased organ function, concomitant disease, or other drug therapy. See Drug/Lab Interactions.

DILUTION

Available prediluted in D5W, or each 250-mg (20-ml) vial must be further diluted to at least 50 ml. Any amount of infusion solution desired above 50 ml may be used (250 mg in 1 L equals 250 mcg/ml; 250 mg in 500 ml equals 500 mcg/ml; 250 mg in 250 ml equals 1,000 mcg/ml). Adjust to fluid requirements of the patient. Compatible with D5W, D10W, D5/½NS, D5NS, D5/Isolyte M, LR, D5LR, Normosol-M in D5W, 20% Osmitrol in water, NS, or sodium lactate.

Pediatric dilution: 6 mg/kg in 100 ml diluent. 1 ml/hr equals 1 mcg/kg/min.

Storage: When mixed in infusion solution, use within 24 hours. Pink coloring of solution does not affect potency; will crystallize if frozen.

INCOMPATIBLE WITH

Manufacturer states, "Do not add to sodium bicarbonate or any other strongly alkaline solution" (e.g., aminophylline, barbiturates [e.g., thiopental (Pentothal)]). Manufacturer recommends not using other drugs as additives, not using in conjunction with other agents, and not using with diluents containing both sodium bisulfate and ethanol.

COMPATIBLE WITH

(Underline Indicates Conflicting Compatibility Information)

See Incompatible With. Consult pharmacist; specific conditions may apply; see Compatibilities, p. xvi.

Additive: ***Not recommended by manufacturer.*** Amiodarone (Cordarone), atracurium (Tracrium), atropine, <u>bretylium (Bretylate)</u>, <u>calcium chloride</u>, dopamine (Intropin), enalaprilat (Vasotec IV), epinephrine (Adrenalin), flumazenil (Romazicon), <u>heparin</u>, hydralazine, isoproterenol (Isuprel), lidocaine, meperidine (Demerol), meropenem (Merrem IV), morphine, nitroglycerin (Nitro-Bid IV), norepinephrine (Levophed), phentolamine (Regitine), phenylephrine (Neo-Synephrine), <u>potassium chloride (KCl)</u>, procainamide (Pronestyl), propranolol (Inderal), ranitidine (Zantac), <u>verapamil (Isoptin)</u>.

Syringe: ***Not recommended by manufacturer.*** Heparin, ranitidine (Zantac). **Y-site:** Amifostine (Ethyol), amiodarone (Cordarone), atracurium (Tracrium), aztreonam (Azactam), bretylium (Bretylate), calcium chloride, calcium gluconate, ciprofloxacin (Cipro IV), cisatracurium (Nimbex), cladribine (Leustatin), diazepam (Valium), diltiazem (Cardizem), docetaxel (Taxotere), dopamine (Intropin), doxorubicin liposome (Doxil), enalaprilat (Vasotec IV), epinephrine (Adrenalin), etoposide phosphate (Etopophos), famotidine (Pepcid IV), fentanyl (Sublimaze), fluconazole (Diflucan), furosemide (Lasix), gatifloxacin (Tequin), gemcitabine (Gemzar), granisetron (Kytril), haloperidol (Haldol), heparin, hetastarch in electrolytes (Hextend), hydromorphone (Dilaudid), inamrinone (Inocor), insulin (regular), labetalol (Normodyne), levofloxacin (Levaquin), lidocaine, linezolid (Zyvox), lorazepam (Ativan), magnesium sulfate, meperidine (Demerol), midazolam (Versed), milrinone (Primacor), morphine, nicardipine (Cardene IV), nitroglycerin (Nitro-Bid IV), nitroprusside sodium, norepinephrine (Levophed), pancuronium (Pavulon), potassium chloride (KCl), propofol (Diprivan), ranitidine (Zantac), remifentanil (Ultiva), streptokinase, tacrolimus (Prograf), thiotepa (Thioplex), vecuronium (Norcuron), verapamil (Isoptin), zidovudine (AZT, Retrovir).

RATE OF ADMINISTRATION

Begin with recommended dose for body weight and seriousness of condition. Gradually increase to effect desired response. May take up to 10 minutes to achieve peak effect of a specific dose. Maintain at correct therapeutic level with microdrip (60 gtt/ml) or infusion pump. Half-life of dobutamine is only about 2 minutes. See Maternal/Child.

Infusion Rate (ml/hr) for Dobutamine 500 mcg/ml												
	Patient's Weight (kg)											
Drug Delivery Rate (mcg/kg/min)	5	10	20	30	40	50	60	70	80	90	100	110
0.5	0.3	0.6	1.2	1.8	2.4	3	3.6	4.2	4.8	5.4	6	6.6
1	0.6	1.2	2.4	3.6	4.8	6	7.2	8.4	9.6	10.8	12	13.2
2.5	1.5	3	6	9	12	15	18	21	24	27	30	33
5	3	6	12	18	24	30	36	42	48	54	60	66
7.5	4.5	9	18	27	36	45	54	63	72	81	90	99
10	6	12	24	36	48	60	72	84	96	108	120	132
12.5	7.5	15	30	45	60	75	90	105	120	135	150	165
15	9	18	36	54	72	90	108	126	144	162	180	198
17.5	10.5	21	42	63	84	105	126	147	168	189	210	231
20	12	24	48	72	96	120	144	168	192	216	240	264

Infusion Rate (ml/hr) for Dobutamine 1000 mcg/ml												
	Patient's Weight (kg)											
Drug Delivery Rate (mcg/kg/min)	5	10	20	30	40	50	60	70	80	90	100	110
0.5	0.15	0.3	0.6	0.9	1.2	1.5	1.8	2.1	2.4	2.7	3	3.3
1	0.3	0.6	1.2	1.8	2.4	3	3.6	4.2	4.8	5.4	6	6.6
2.5	0.75	1.5	3	4.5	6	7.5	9	10.5	12	13.5	15	16.5
5	1.5	3	6	9	12	15	18	21	24	27	30	33
7.5	2.25	4.5	9	13.5	18	22.5	27	31.5	36	40.5	45	49.5
10	3	6	12	18	24	30	36	42	48	54	60	66
12.5	3.75	7.5	15	22.5	30	37.5	45	52.5	60	67.5	75	82.5
15	4.5	9	18	27	36	45	54	63	72	81	90	99
17.5	5.25	10.5	21	31.5	42	52.5	63	73.5	84	94.5	105	115.5
20	6	12	24	36	48	60	72	84	96	108	120	132

Infusion Rate (ml/hr) for Dobutamine 2000 mcg/ml												
	Patient's Weight (kg)											
Drug Delivery Rate (mcg/kg/min)	5	10	20	30	40	50	60	70	80	90	100	110
0.5	0.08	0.15	0.3	0.45	0.6	0.75	0.9	1.05	1.2	1.35	1.5	1.65
1	0.15	0.3	0.6	0.9	1.2	1.5	1.8	2.1	2.4	2.7	3	3.3
2.5	0.38	0.75	1.5	2	3	4	4.5	5	6	7	7.5	8
5	0.75	1.5	3	4.5	6	7.5	9	10.5	12	13.5	15	16.5
7.5	1.13	2.25	4.5	7	9	11	13.5	16	18	20	22.5	25
10	1.5	3	6	9	12	15	18	21	24	27	30	33
12.5	1.88	3.75	7.5	11	15	19	22.5	26	30	34	37.5	41
15	2.25	4.5	9	13.5	18	22.5	27	31.5	36	40.5	45	49.5
17.5	2.63	5.25	10.5	15.75	21	26.25	31.5	36.75	42	47.25	52.50	57.75
20	3	6	12	18	24	30	36	42	48	54	60	66

ACTIONS

A synthetic catecholamine chemically related to dopamine, it is a direct-acting inotropic agent possessing beta-stimulator activity. Induces short-term increases in cardiac output by improving stroke volume with minimum increases in rate and BP, minimum rhythm disturbances, and decreased peripheral vascular resistance. Usually most effective for only a few hours. May improve atrioventricular conduction. Peak effect obtained in 2 to 10 minutes. Has a very short duration of action. Half-life is 2 minutes; may be up to 5 minutes in preterm infants. Metabolized in the liver and other tissues. Metabolites are primarily excreted in the urine.

INDICATIONS AND USES

Short-term inotropic support in cardiac decompensation resulting from depressed contractility (organic heart disease or cardiac surgical procedures).

Unlabeled uses: Increase cardiac output in children with congenital heart disease undergoing cardiac catheterization.

CONTRAINDICATIONS

Hypersensitivity to any components (contains sulfites), idiopathic hypertrophic subaortic stenosis, shock without adequate fluid replacement.

PRECAUTIONS

Use extreme caution in myocardial infarction; increases in HR of more than 10% may increase myocardial ischemia and size of infarction. ■ Contains sulfites; use caution in patients with allergies. ■ Precipitous hypotension occurs rarely; usually reverses with a decrease in rate of administration; see Antidote. ■ Ineffective if marked mechanical obstruction (e.g., severe valvular aortic stenosis) is present. ■ Use beyond 48 hours has been associated with increased risks of hospitalization and death.

Monitor: Correct hypovolemia and acidosis as indicated before initiating treatment. ■ Observe patient's response continuously; monitor HR, ectopic activity, BP, and urine flow. Measure pulmonary wedge pressure, central venous pressure, and cardiac output if possible. ■ May cause significant increase in BP or HR, especially systolic pressure. Patients with preexisting hypertension may be at increased risk of developing an increased pressor response. ■ Monitor for changes in fluid balance, electrolytes, and acid-base balance. ■ Use digitalis preparation before starting dobutamine in patients with atrial fibrillation with rapid ventricular response. ■ See Drug/Lab Interactions.

Maternal/Child: Category B: use only if benefits outweigh risks. Safety for use in pregnancy, breast-feeding, and children not established. ■ Increases cardiac output and systemic BP in pediatric patients of every age group, usually at infusion rates that are lower than those that cause significant tachycardia. Less effective than dopamine (Intropin) in premature neonates.

Elderly: Lower-end initial doses may be indicated; see Dose Adjustments. ■ Differences in response between the elderly and younger patients have not been identified, but greater sensitivity of some elderly cannot be ruled out.

DRUG/LAB INTERACTIONS

May be ineffective if beta-blocking drugs (e.g., propranolol [Inderal]) have been given. ■ Produces higher cardiac output and lower pulmonary wedge pressure when given concomitantly with nitroprusside sodium. ■ May cause serious arrhythmias in presence of cyclopropane or halogen anesthetics, severe hypertension with oxytocic drugs, or guanethidine (Ismelin). ■ Pressor response increased with tricyclic antidepressants (e.g., amitriptyline [Elavil]) and rauwolfia alkaloids (e.g., reserpine [Serpasil]); may cause hypertension. ■ May cause arrhythmias with bretylium. ■ Has been given concurrently without evidence of drug interaction with acetaminophen (Tylenol), atropine, digitalis preparations, folic acid, furosemide, glyceryl trinitrate (nitroglycerin), heparin, isosorbide dinitrate (Iso-Bid), lidocaine, morphine, potassium chloride, protamine, and spironolactone (Aldactone).

SIDE EFFECTS

Anginal pain, chest pain, headache, hypertension, hypokalemia, increased ventricular ectopic activity, myocardial ischemia, nausea, palpitations, shortness of breath, tachycardia. Allergic reactions (e.g., bronchospasm, eosinophilia, fever, skin rash) have been reported. Local inflammatory changes may occur with infiltration.

Overdose: In addition to all of the above, overdose may cause anorexia, anxiety, excessive hypertension or hypotension, myocardial ischemia, tremor, ventricular tachycardia, and/or fibrillation.

ANTIDOTE

Notify physician of all side effects. Decrease infusion rate and notify physician immediately if number of PVCs increases or there is a marked increase in pulse rate (30 or more beats) or BP (50 or more mm Hg systolic). For accidental overdose, reduce rate or temporarily discontinue until condition stabilizes. Maintain a patent airway with adequate oxygenation and ventilation. Treat ventricular tachyarrhythmias with propranolol (Inderal) or lidocaine. Hypertension usually responds to a reduced rate or temporarily discontinuing dobutamine. Reduce rate or discontinue dobutamine if hypotension occurs. May require treatment with vasopressors (e.g., dopamine, norepinephrine). See Precautions.

DOCETAXEL

(doh-seh-tax'ell)

Antineoplastic agent (miscellaneous)

Taxotere

USUAL DOSE

Premedication: Must be pretreated with oral corticosteroids for 3 days to reduce the incidence and severity of fluid retention and hypersensitivity reactions. Usual regimen is dexamethasone (Decadron) 8 mg PO twice a day for 3 days. Begin 1 day before each docetaxel infusion. One source suggests that pretreatment with diphenhydramine (Benadryl) and/or an H_2 antagonist (e.g., famotidine [Pepcid], ranitidine [Zantac]) given IV 30 minutes before docetaxel infusion may help reduce hypersensitivity reactions and cutaneous toxicity.

Breast cancer: 60 to 100 mg/M^2 as an infusion. Repeat every 3 weeks.

First-line treatment of non–small-cell lung cancer (NSCLC): 75 mg/M^2 as an infusion over 1 hour. Follow immediately with cisplatin 75 mg/M^2 as an infusion over 30 to 60 minutes. Repeat every 3 weeks.

NSCLC after failure of prior chemotherapy: 75 mg/M^2 as an infusion. Repeat every 3 weeks. Larger doses increased toxicity, infection, and treatment-related mortality.

Treatment of small-cell lung cancer and ovarian cancer (unlabeled): 100 mg/M^2 as an infusion. Repeat every 3 weeks.

Head and neck cancer (unlabeled): 60 to 100 mg/M^2 as an infusion. Repeat every 3 to 4 weeks for an average of 2 to 6 cycles.

Esophageal or gastric cancer (unlabeled): In ***combination*** with other agents (e.g., gemcitabine [Gemzar], cisplatin, fluorouracil, leucovorin calcium), docetaxel 60 to 85 mg/M^2 every 21 to 28 days. As a ***single agent,*** 100 mg/M^2 every 21 days.

Prostate cancer (unlabeled): 40 to 80 mg/M^2 as an infusion. Repeat every 3 weeks.

Bladder cancer (unlabeled): 75 to 100 mg/M^2 as an infusion. Repeat every 3 weeks for up to 6 treatment cycles.

PEDIATRIC DOSE

Safety for use in children not established.

DOSE ADJUSTMENTS

All diagnoses: Withhold therapy if neutrophils below 1,500/mm^3 or platelets below 100,000 cells/mm^3. ■ Discontinue therapy in patients who develop grade 3 or higher peripheral neuropathy. ■ See Precautions.

Breast cancer: Reduce dose to 75 mg/M^2 or discontinue docetaxel for patients initially dosed at 100 mg/M^2 who experience febrile neutropenia, severe neutropenia (neutrophils below 500/mm^3 for more than 1 week), severe or cumulative cutaneous reaction, severe (grade 4) infection, or severe peripheral neuropathy. Further reduce to 55 mg/M^2 or discontinue docetaxel if any of the above reactions persist. ■ Patients receiving the lower dose of docetaxel (60 mg/M^2) may have the dose increased gradually if lower dose was well tolerated.

Non–small-cell lung cancer: In NSCLC patients who experience either febrile neutropneia, neutrophils less than 500 cells/mm^3 for more than 1 week, severe or cumulative cutaneous reactions, or other grade 3 or 4 non-hematologic toxicities, withhold docetaxel until resolution of toxicity, then resume at 55 mg/M^2.

Head and neck cancer: Reduced dose may be indicated with dose-limiting toxicities (e.g., febrile neutropenia, neutrophils less than 500 cell/mm^3 for more than 1 week, severe or cumulative cutaneous reactions, or other grade 3 or 4 nonhematologic toxicities) or when used in combination with other chemotherapeutic agents (e.g., cisplatin, fluorouracil). Regimens used include docetaxel 20 to 80 mg/M^2 once every 7 to 17 days for 6 cycles or 25 to 90 mg/M^2 in combination with cisplatin, fluorouracil, and leucovorin calcium (if indicated) once every 4 weeks for a maximum of 3 cycles.

Prostate cancer: Reduced dose may be indicated with dose-limiting toxicities (e.g., febrile neutropenia, neutrophils less than 500 cells/mm^3 for more than 1 week, severe or cumulative cutaneous reactions, or other grade 3 or 4 nonhematologic toxicities) or when used in combination with other chemotherapeutic agents (e.g., estramustine [Emcyt]). Regimens used include docetaxel 20 to 40 mg/M^2 once a week for 2 weeks with a 1-week rest or for 6 weeks with a 2-week rest.

DILUTION

Specific techniques required; see Precautions. More than one vial of docetaxel and diluent may be required. Repeat procedure for reconstitution of each vial required. Allow vials to stand at room temperature for 5 minutes. Withdraw entire contents of diluent vial (provided by manufacturer) in a syringe and transfer to vial of docetaxel concentrate (10 mg/ml). Mix the diluted solution by repeated inversions for at least 45 seconds to ensure full mixture. Do not shake. Allow to stand for several minutes to allow most of the foam to dissipate. Total dose must be further diluted in a minimum of 250 ml of NS or D5W, manually rotated to mix thoroughly, and given as an infusion; see Incompatible With. Should be administered through polyethylene-lined administration sets. Desired concentration should be between 0.3 and 0.74 mg/ml (100 mg in 250 ml = 0.4 mg/ml). If a dose greater than 240 mg is required, use a larger volume of NS or D5W so that a final concentration of 0.74 mg/ml is not exceeded. Solution should be clear.

Storage: Unopened vials of docetaxel and diluent in cartons may be refrigerated or stored at CRT (2° C [36° F] to 25° C [77° F]). Protect from light. Reconstituted or premixed solutions are stable for up to 8 hours, and fully diluted solutions are stable for up to 4 hours (includes 1 hour for administration) either refrigerated or at room temperature. Use immediately after preparation is preferred.

INCOMPATIBLE WITH

Leaches out plasticizers, including DEHP, from PVC infusion bags and administration sets. Use glass or polypropylene bottles or plastic (polypropylene or polyolefin) bags and polyethylene-lined administration sets to minimize patient exposure to leached DEHP. Do not allow concentrate to come into contact with plasticized PVC equipment or devices used to prepare solutions.

COMPATIBLE WITH

Consult pharmacist; specific conditions may apply; see Compatibilities, p. xvi.

Y-site: Acyclovir (Zovirax), amifostine (Ethyol), amikacin (Amikin), aminophylline, ampicillin, ampicillin/sulbactam (Unasyn), aztreonam (Azactam), bumetanide (Bumex), buprenorphine (Buprenex), butorphanol

(Stadol), calcium gluconate, cefazolin (Kefzol), cefepime (Maxipime), cefoperazone (Cefobid), cefotaxime (Claforan), cefotetan (Cefotan), cefoxitin (Mefoxin), ceftazidime (Fortaz), ceftizoxime (Cefizox), ceftriaxone (Rocephin), cefuroxime (Zinacef), chlorpromazine (Thorazine), cimetidine (Tagamet), ciprofloxacin (Cipro IV), clindamycin (Cleocin), dexamethasone (Decadron), diphenhydramine (Benadryl), dobutamine (Dobutrex), dopamine (Intropin), doxycycline (Vibramycin), droperidol (Inapsine), enalaprilat (Vasotec IV), famotidine (Pepcid IV), fluconazole (Diflucan), furosemide (Lasix), ganciclovir (Cytovene), gemcitabine (Gemzar), gentamicin (Garamycin), granisetron (Kytril), haloperidol (Haldol), heparin, hydrocortisone (Hydrocortone, Solu-Cortef), hydromorphone (Dilaudid), imipenem-cilastatin (Primaxin), leucovorin calcium, lorazepam (Ativan), magnesium sulfate, mannitol, meperidine (Demerol), meropenem (Merrem IV), mesna (Mesnex), metoclopramide (Reglan), metronidazole (Flagyl IV), minocycline (Minocin), morphine, ofloxacin (Floxin IV), ondansetron (Zofran), piperacillin (Pipracil), piperacillin/tazobactam (Zosyn), potassium chloride (KCl), prochlorperazine (Compazine), promethazine (Phenergan), ranitidine (Zantac), sodium bicarbonate, sulfamethoxazole-trimethoprim (Bactrim), ticarcillin (Ticar), ticarcillin/clavulanate (Timentin), tobramycin (Nebcin), vancomycin (Vancocin), zidovudine (AZT, Retrovir).

RATE OF ADMINISTRATION

A single dose, properly diluted, equally distributed over 1 hour. Room temperature should be cool and lighting should be low. Extended infusion rates (e.g., 6 to 24 hours) or frequently repeated infusions (e.g., several days in a row) seem to increase the risk of dose-limiting mucositis.

ACTIONS

An antineoplastic. A novel, semisynthetic, antimicrotubule agent derived from the needles of the yew plant. It inhibits cancer cell division by acting on the cells' internal skeleton, which is made of elements called microtubules. Microtubules assemble and disassemble during the cell cycle. Docetaxel promotes the assembly and blocks the disassembly of microtubules, preventing the cancer cells from dividing. The end result is cancer cell death. May be up to twice as potent as paclitaxel; cross-resistance between docetaxel and paclitaxel does not occur consistently. Highly protein bound. Probably metabolized in the liver by isoenzymes of the P_{450} family. Half-life is 11.1 hours. Eliminated primarily through feces and bile.

INDICATIONS AND USES

Treatment of locally advanced or metastatic breast cancer after failure of prior chemotherapy. ■ As a single agent in the treatment of locally advanced or metastatic NSCLC after failure of platinum-based chemotherapy (e.g., cisplatin). ■ In combination with cisplatin for first-line treatment of unresectable, locally advanced NSCLC.

Unlabeled uses: First-line treatment as a single agent or in combination with other chemotherapy agents to treat breast cancer. Treatment of small-cell lung cancer and ovarian cancer after first-line or platinum-based chemotherapy has failed. ■ Treatment of bladder cancer; esophageal, gastric, or gastroesophageal cancers; head and neck cancer; melanoma; non-Hodgkin's lymphoma; ovarian cancer; prostate cancer; small-cell lung cancer; and soft-tissue sarcoma.

CONTRAINDICATIONS

Baseline neutropenia less than 1,500 cells/mm^3, history of hypersensitivity reactions to docetaxel or other drugs formulated with polysorbate 80, severe impaired liver function. In the United States docetaxel is not recommended for patients with a bilirubin above the upper limits of normal, or in patients with ALT and/or AST greater than 1.5 times upper limit of normal range and increases in alkaline phosphatase greater than 2.5 times the upper limits of normal range; see Precautions.

PRECAUTIONS

Follow guidelines for handling cytotoxic agents. See Appendix A, p. 1142. ■ Usually administered by or under the direction of the physician specialist. ■ Adequate diagnostic and treatment facilities must be readily available. ■ Patients hypersensitive to paclitaxel may also be hypersensitive to docetaxel. ■ Myelosuppression may be more frequent and more severe in patients who have received prior cytotoxic drug therapy or radiation therapy. ■ Incidence of mortality increased in patients with abnormal liver function and in those receiving higher doses. Not recommended for patients with hepatic impairment; see Contraindications. If docetaxel is considered essential for a patient with mild hepatic impairment, initial doses of 60 to 75 mg/M^2 should be used. Risk of toxicity and death significant. ■ Use with caution in patients with pleural effusion; may be exacerbated by docetaxel-induced fluid retention. ■ See Drug/Lab Interactions.

Monitor: Obtain baseline CBC with differential and platelets; monitor frequently during therapy and before each dose. See Dose Adjustments. ■ Obtain baseline bilirubin, AST, ALT, and alkaline phosphatase; monitor as indicated during therapy (recommended before each dose). ■ Determine absolute patency of vein. A stinging or burning sensation indicates extravasation; severe cellulitis and tissue necrosis may result. Discontinue injection; use another vein. ■ Obtain baseline vital signs, monitor during and for at least 1 hour following infusion. ■ Monitor for hypersensitivity reactions; may occur within minutes. Discontinue docetaxel if severe (e.g., bronchospasm, hypotension, generalized rash/erythema). Continue monitoring for a minimum of 1 hour following the infusion, especially during the first two treatment cycles. ■ Monitor for localized erythema of the palms of the hands and soles of the feet with or without desquamation. A reduced dose may be indicated if severe. ■ Monitor for fluid retention. Severe salt restriction and treatment with oral diuretics may be indicated. ■ Observe for signs of peripheral neurotoxicity; docetaxel may need to be discontinued; see Dose Adjustments. ■ Observe for signs of infection. Use of prophylactic antibiotics may be indicated pending C/S in a febrile, neutropenic patient. ■ Not highly emetogenic; routine prophylaxis with antiemetics may not be required. ■ Monitor for thrombocytopenia (platelet count less than 50,000/mm^3). Initiate precautions to prevent excessive bleeding (e.g., inspect IV sites, skin, and mucous membranes; use extreme care during invasive procedures; test urine, emesis, stool, and secretions for occult blood).

Patient Education: Avoid pregnancy; nonhormonal birth control recommended. ■ Review of monitoring requirements and adverse events before therapy imperative. ■ Report pain or burning at injection site and any unusual or unexpected symptoms or side effects as soon as possible. ■ May produce significant hypotension. Effects may be additive with current medications. Review all medications (prescription and nonprescription) with nurse and/or physician. ■ See Appendix D, p. 1148. ■ Obtain name and telephone number of a contact person for emergencies, questions, or problems. ■ Seek resources for counseling or supportive therapy.

Maternal/Child: Category D: avoid pregnancy, may cause fetal harm. ■ Discontinue breast-feeding. ■ Safety for use in children not established, but clinical studies have shown that the maximum tolerated dose is lower in children than in adults, especially if they have been treated with prior courses of chemotherapy. A colony-stimulating factor (e.g., filgrastim, sargramostim) has been used to reduce neutropenia and increase tolerance of the maximum dose.

Elderly: No specific recommendations at this time. Monitor hepatic function carefully.

DRUG/LAB INTERACTIONS

Metabolism inhibited and serum levels increased with ketoconazole (Nizoral). ■ Monitor drug profile carefully to avoid problems with other agents that may affect or be affected by cytochrome P_{450} processes (e.g., cyclosporine [Sandimmune], erythromycin, itraconazole [Sporanox], ketoconazole [Nizoral], midazolam [Versed], testosterone, troleandomycin [TAO]). ■ Additive bone marrow depression may occur with radiation therapy and/or other bone marrow–depressing agents (e.g., azathioprine [Imuran], chloramphenicol, melphalan [Alkeran]). Dose reduction may be required. ■ Leukopenic and/or thrombocytopenic effects may be increased with drugs that cause blood dyscrasias (e.g., anticonvulsants [e.g., carbamazepine (Tegretol), phenytoin (Dilantin)], NSAIDs [e.g., ibuprofen (Advil, Motrin), naproxen (Aleve, Naprosyn)]). Adjust dose based on differential and platelet count. ■ Risk of infection is increased with concurrent use of other immunosuppressants (e.g., azathioprine, chlorambucil [Leukeran], cyclophosphamide [Cytoxan], cyclosporine [Sandimmune], glucocorticoid corticosteroids [e.g., dexamethasone], muromonab CD-3 [Orthoclone], tacrolimus [Prograf]). ■ Docetaxel metabolism is inhibited by paclitaxel and, to a lesser extent, paclitaxel may be inhibited by docetaxel. Docetaxel may also be inhibited by other agents metabolized by the CYP 3A isoenzyme. ■ Do not administer live vaccines to patients receiving antineoplastic agents.

SIDE EFFECTS

Generally reversible but can be fatal. Bone marrow suppression is dose dependent and can be dose limiting (anemia, leukopenia, neutropenia, thrombocytopenia). Abdominal pain; alopecia; anorexia; bleeding episodes; cardiac arrhythmias; colitis; conjunctivitis; cutaneous reactions (e.g., localized rash on hands, feet, arms, face, thorax); diarrhea; erythema multiforme of Stevens-Johnson syndrome; hepatitis; increased ALT, AST, and bilirubin; infections; febrile neutropenia; fever without infection; fluid retention (e.g., ascites, edema, pericardial effusion, pleural effusion); hypersensitivity reactions (e.g., back pain, chest tightness, chills, drug fever, dyspnea, flushing, hypotension, pruritus, rash); infusion site reactions; lacrimation; nausea; paresthesias (e.g., pain, burning sensation); seizures or transient loss of consciousness; stomatitis; vomiting.

Overdose: Bone marrow suppression, mucositis, peripheral neurotoxicity.

ANTIDOTE

Keep physician informed of all side effects. Most will be treated symptomatically as indicated. Most hypersensitivity reactions will subside with temporary discontinuation of docetaxel, and incidence seems to decrease with subsequent doses. Severe reactions may require epinephrine (Adrenalin), antihistamines (e.g., diphenhydramine [Benadryl]), corticosteroids (e.g., dexamethasone [Decadron]), or bronchodilators (e.g., albuterol [Ventolin], theophylline [aminophylline]). Rechallenge may be considered if there is objective tumor response and no other options. Aggressive premedication (adding cromolyn 400 mg PO 4 times daily has helped some patients) and reduction in rate of administration may allow continued treatment. Neutropenia can be profound and the nadir usually occurs about day 8. Recovery is generally rapid and spontaneous but may be treated with filgrastim (G-CSF, Neupogen) or pegfilgrastim (Neulasta). Severe thrombocytopenia may require platelet transfusions or treatment with oprelvekin (Neumega) may be indicated. Severe anemia (less than 8 Gm/dl) may require packed cell transfusions; moderate anemia (less than 11 Gm/dl) may be treated with darbepoetin alfa [Aranesp] or epoetin alfa (Epogen). Hypotension and bradycardia do not usually occur at the same time except in hypersensitivity. Treat only if symptomatic. Treat any serious or symptomatic arrhythmia (e.g., conduction abnormalities, ventricular tachycardia) promptly and monitor continuously during subsequent doses. Serious cutaneous reactions with desquamation (rare), serious fluid retention (more frequent with cumulative doses of 1,300 mg/M^2), persistent febrile neutropenia, severe peripheral neuropathy, or severe liver impairment may require discontinuation of docetaxel. Cutaneous reactions (palmar-plantar erythrodysesthesia) that occur despite prophylaxis may respond to pyridoxine 50 mg three times daily. There is no specific antidote for overdose. Supportive therapy will help sustain the patient in toxicity. Resuscitate if indicated.

DOLASETRON MESYLATE

(doe-lass′eh-tron mes′uh-lat)

Antiemetic
(5 HT_3 receptor antagonist)

Anzemet

pH 3.2 to 3.8

USUAL DOSE

Prevention of chemotherapy-induced nausea and vomiting: 1.8 mg/kg as a single dose 30 minutes before chemotherapy. Alternatively, a fixed dose of 100 mg may be used for most patients.

Prevention of postoperative nausea and/or vomiting: 12.5 mg as a single dose 15 minutes before cessation of anesthesia.

Treatment of postoperative nausea and/or vomiting: 12.5 mg as a single dose as soon as nausea or vomiting presents.

Radiotherapy-induced nausea and vomiting (unlabeled use): 40 mg or 0.3 mg/kg at time of treatment or when nausea or vomiting presents.

PEDIATRIC DOSE

Doses are those recommended for ***pediatric patients 2 to 16 years of age.*** Safety and effectiveness in children under 2 years of age have not been established. Dolasetron solution for injection may be mixed with apple or apple-grape juice for oral administration to pediatric patients.

Prevention of chemotherapy-induced nausea and vomiting: 1.8 mg/kg up to a maximum of 100 mg as a single dose 30 minutes before chemotherapy.

Prevention of postoperative nausea and/or vomiting: 0.35 mg/kg up to a maximum dose of 12.5 mg as a single dose 15 minutes before cessation of anesthesia.

Treatment of postoperative nausea and/or vomiting: 0.35 mg/kg up to a maximum dose of 12.5 mg as a single dose as soon as nausea or vomiting presents.

DOSE ADJUSTMENTS

No dose adjustments required for the elderly, renal failure, or impaired hepatic function.

DILUTION

IV injection: A single dose may be given undiluted.

IV infusion: A single dose may be further diluted up to 50 ml in NS, D5W, D5/½NS, D5LR, LR, or 10% mannitol.

Storage: Store vials at CRT; protect from light. Stable after dilution at CRT for 24 hours or 48 hours if refrigerated.

COMPATIBILITY

Manufacturer states, "Should not be mixed with other drugs. Flush the infusion line with a compatible IV solution before and after administration." One source lists as compatible at the Y-site with hetastarch in electrolytes (Hextend).

RATE OF ADMINISTRATION

Flush infusion line before and after administration. May cause bradycardia, severe hypotension, and syncope during or shortly after administration.

IV injection: A single dose over 30 seconds.

IV infusion: A single dose over up to 15 minutes.

ACTIONS

An antinauseant and antiemetic agent. A selective antagonist of specific serotonin ($5HT_3$) receptors, similar to granisetron and ondansetron. Chemotherapeutic agents such as cisplatin increase the release of serotonin from specific cells in the GI tract, causing emesis. By antagonizing these receptors, chemotherapy-induced nausea and vomiting are prevented. Rapidly and completely metabolized to its active metabolite, hydrodolasetron. Hydrodolasetron is widely distributed throughout the body. Maximum concentration occurs 0.6 hours after injection or infusion. Average half-life is 7.3 hours. Plasma clearance increased and half-life reduced in children, more so in younger children. Excreted in urine and feces. Not known if dolasetron is secreted in breast milk.

INDICATIONS AND USES

Prevention of nausea and vomiting associated with initial and repeat courses of emetogenic cancer chemotherapy, including high-dose cisplatin. ▪ Prevention of postoperative nausea and vomiting when indicated. ▪ Treatment of postoperative nausea and/or vomiting. Also available in tablet form.

Unlabeled uses: Prophylaxis and treatment of radiotherapy-induced nausea and vomiting.

CONTRAINDICATIONS

Known hypersensitivity to dolasetron.

PRECAUTIONS

Use with caution in patients who have or may develop prolongation of cardiac conduction intervals, particularly QT intervals (e.g., patients with hypokalemia, hypomagnesemia, congenital QT syndrome, cumulative high-dose anthracycline therapy [e.g., doxorubicin (Adriamycin)], patients taking diuretics with potential for inducing electrolyte abnormalities [e.g., furosemide, hydrochlorothiazide] or antiarrhythmic drugs or other drugs that lead to QT prolongation [amiodarone, procainamide, quinidine]). ▪ Cross-sensitivity has been reported between dolasetron and other $5HT_3$-receptor agonists (e.g., granisetron [Kytril], ondansetron [Zofran]). ▪ Available in tablet form. See Drug/Lab Interactions and Side Effects.

Monitor: Observe closely. Monitor VS. Any patient found to have a second-degree or higher AV conduction block should be monitored continuously. ▪ Ambulate slowly to avoid orthostatic hypotension. ▪ Does not influence anesthesia recovery time.

Patient Education: Request assistance for ambulation. ▪ Report promptly if nausea persists. ▪ Maintain adequate hydration. ▪ Review prescription medications with health care provider.

Maternal/Child: Category B: no evidence of impaired fertility or harm to fetus. Use during pregnancy only if clearly needed. ▪ Use caution if required during breast-feeding. ▪ Safety and effectiveness for use in children under 2 years of age have not been established. ▪ Plasma clearance increased and half-life reduced in children, more so in younger children.

Elderly: Response similar to other age groups. No dose adjustment required.

DRUG/LAB INTERACTIONS

Does not induce or inhibit the cytochrome P_{450} drug metabolizing system, but plasma levels increased when given concurrently with cimetidine (Tagamet [inhibitor of cytochrome P_{450}]), and decreased when given concurrently with rifampin (Rifadin [inducer of cytochrome P_{450}]); clinical significance not known. ■ Clearance decreased when given concurrently with atenolol (Tenormin). ■ See Precautions and use extreme caution with diuretics with potential for inducing electrolyte abnormalities (e.g., furosemide [Lasix], hydrochlorothiazide [Hydrodiuril]) or antiarrhythmic drugs or other drugs that lead to prolonged QT intervals (e.g., amiodarone [Cordarone], procainamide [Pronestyl], quinidine). ■ Clearance not affected by ACE inhibitors (e.g., enalaprilat), calcium channel blockers (e.g., diltiazem [Cardizem], nifedipine [Procardia], verapamil [Isoptin]), glyburide (DiaBeta), propranolol (Inderal), and various chemotherapy agents. ■ Has been safely coadministered with drugs used in chemotherapy and surgery (recovery time not affected). ■ Has not inhibited the antitumor activity of cisplatin, fluorouracil, doxorubicin, or cyclophosphamide in murine models.

SIDE EFFECTS

May cause bradycardia, severe hypotension, and syncope during or shortly after administration. Can cause ECG interval changes (PR, QT, JT prolongation, and QRS widening). While these changes have rarely been reported, they may lead to cardiovascular consequences (e.g., cardiac arrhythmias, heart block). Usually self-limiting with declining blood levels, but may last as long as 24 hours.

Average dose: Abdominal pain, abnormal liver function tests (transient increased AST, ALT), chills, diarrhea, dizziness, fatigue, fever, headache, hypertension, local pain or burning at injection site, shivering. Numerous other side effects may occur in less than 2% of patients.

Overdose: Severe hypotension and dizziness.

ANTIDOTE

Most side effects will be treated symptomatically. Keep physician informed. Overdose in one patient was treated with plasma expanders (e.g., albumin, dextran), dopamine (Intropin), atropine, and continuous BP and ECG monitoring. Epinephrine, atropine, and/or cardiac pacing may be required to treat ECG interval changes. Prolonged QT interval may lead to VT or other ventricular arrhythmias. There is no specific antidote. Treat anaphylaxis and resuscitate as necessary.

DOPAMINE HYDROCHLORIDE

(doe′pa-meen hye-droe-klor′id)

Inotropic agent
Cardiac stimulant
Vasopressor

Intropin, ✦Revimine

pH 2.5 to 5

USUAL DOSE

Adults: 2 to 5 mcg/kg of body weight/min initially in patients likely to respond to minimum treatment. 5 to 10 mcg/kg/min may be required initially to correct hypotension in the seriously ill patient. Gradually increase by 5 to 10 mcg/kg/min at 10- to 30-minute intervals until optimum response occurs. Average dose is 20 mcg/kg/min; over 50 mcg/kg/min has been required in some instances but is not recommended. If more than 20 mcg/kg/min is required to maintain BP, consider use of norepinephrine (Levophed) in addition. Doses over 20 mcg/kg/min decrease renal perfusion.

PEDIATRIC DOSE

See Maternal/Child. Note comments in Usual Dose and those under another source below. Usual starting dose is 1 to 5 mcg/kg/min. Dose increments range from 2.5 to 5 mcg/kg/min. Usual maximum dose is 15 to 20 mcg/kg/min. Doses up to 50 mcg/kg/min have been administered. Titrate dose gradually to desired effect.

Another source suggests:

Low dose: 2 to 5 mcg/kg/min; increases renal blood flow with minimal effect on HR and cardiac output.

Intermediate dose: 5 to 15 mcg/kg/min; increases HR, cardiac contractility, cardiac output and, to a lesser extent, renal blood flow.

High dose: Doses equal to or greater than 20 mcg/kg/min; alpha adrenergic effects are prominent; decreases renal perfusion. Maximum dose recommended is 50 mg/kg/min.

DOSE ADJUSTMENTS

Reduce dose to one tenth of the calculated amount for individuals being treated with MAO inhibitors (e.g., selegiline [Eldepryl]) and drugs with MAO-inhibiting effects (e.g., furazolidone [Furoxone]). ■ Lower-end initial doses may be appropriate in the elderly based on potential for decreased organ function and concomitant disease or drug therapy. ■ See Drug/Lab Interactions.

DILUTION

Each 5- or 10-ml (200-mg, 400-mg, or 800-mg) ampule must be diluted in 250 to 500 ml of the following IV solutions and given as an infusion: NS, D5W, D5NS, D5/½NS, D5LR, ⅙ M sodium lactate, or LR injection.

mcg/ml of Dopamine Concentrations of 40 mg/ml and 80 mg/ml in Various Volumes of Diluent

Concentration of Dopamine	40 mg/ml		80 mg/ml
Volume of Dopamine	**5 ml (200 mg)**	**10 ml (400 mg)**	**10 ml (800 mg)**
250 ml diluent	800 mcg/ml	1,600 mcg/ml	3,200 mcg/ml
500 ml diluent	400 mcg/ml	800 mcg/ml	1,600 mcg/ml
1,000 ml diluent	200 mcg/ml	400 mcg/ml	800 mcg/ml

Available prediluted in 250 ml or 500 ml of D5W. Dopamine content varies: choose 0.8 mg/ml, 1.6 mg/ml, 3.2 mg/ml, or 6.4 mg/ml. More concentrated solutions may be used if absolutely necessary to reduce fluid volume. Also available as 160 mg/ml to be added to 100 ml of diluent (1,600 mcg/ml); may be used in patients with fluid retention or those requiring a very slow rate of infusion.

Pediatric dilution: 6 mg/kg in 100 ml D5W. 1 ml/hr equals 1 mcg/kg/min.

Storage: Discard diluted solution after 24 hours.

INCOMPATIBLE WITH

Manufacturer states, "Do not add to sodium bicarbonate or any other strongly alkaline solution" (e.g., aminophylline, barbiturates [e.g., thiopental (Pentothal)]), oxidizing agents, or iron salts. Dopamine is inactivated in alkaline solution."

COMPATIBLE WITH **(Underline Indicates Conflicting Compatibility Information)**

See Incompatible With. Consult pharmacist; specific conditions may apply; see Compatibilities, p. xvi.

Additive: Aminophylline, atracurium (Tracrium), bretylium (Bretylate), calcium chloride, chloramphenicol (Chloromycetin), ciprofloxacin (Cipro IV), dobutamine (Dobutrex), enalaprilat (Vasotec IV), flumazenil (Romazicon), gentamicin (Garamycin), heparin, hydrocortisone sodium succinate (Solu-Cortef), kanamycin (Kantrex), lidocaine, meropenem (Merrem IV), methylprednisolone (Solu-Medrol), nitroglycerin (Nitro-Bid IV), oxacillin (Bactocill), potassium chloride (KCl), ranitidine (Zantac), verapamil (Isoptin).

Syringe: Doxapram (Dopram), heparin, ranitidine (Zantac).

Y-site: Alatrofloxacin (Trovan IV), aldesleukin (Proleukin), amifostine (Ethyol), amiodarone (Cordarone), atracurium (Tracrium), aztreonam (Azactam), ciprofloxacin (Cipro IV), cisatracurium (Nimbex), cladribine (Leustatin), diltiazem (Cardizem), dobutamine (Dobutrex), docetaxel (Taxotere), doxorubicin liposome (Doxil), enalaprilat (Vasotec IV), epinephrine (Adrenalin), esmolol (Brevibloc), etoposide phosphate (Etopophos), famotidine (Pepcid IV), fentanyl (Sublimaze), fluconazole (Diflucan), foscarnet (Foscavir), furosemide (Lasix), gatifloxacin (Tequin), gemcitabine (Gemzar), granisetron (Kytril), haloperidol (Haldol), heparin, hetastarch in electrolytes (Hextend), hydrocortisone sodium succinate (Solu-Cortef), hydromorphone (Dilaudid), inamrinone (Inocor), labetalol (Normodyne), levofloxacin (Levaquin), lidocaine, linezolid (Zyvox), lorazepam (Ativan), meperidine (Demerol), methylprednisolone (Solu-Medrol), metronidazole (Flagyl IV), midazolam (Versed), milrinone (Primacor), morphine, nicardipine (Cardene IV), nitroglycerin (Nitro-Bid IV), nitroprusside sodium, norepinephrine (Levophed), ondansetron (Zofran), pancuronium (Pavulon), piperacillin/tazobactam (Zosyn), potassium chloride (KCl), propofol (Diprivan), ranitidine (Zantac), remifentanil (Ultiva), sargramostim (Leukine), streptokinase, tacrolimus (Prograf), theophylline, thiotepa (Thioplex), tirofiban (Aggrastat), vecuronium (Norcuron), verapamil (Isoptin), warfarin (Coumadin), zidovudine (AZT, Retrovir).

RATE OF ADMINISTRATION

Begin with recommended dose for body weight and seriousness of condition. Gradually increase by 5 to 10 mcg/kg of body weight/min to effect desired response. Use slowest possible rate to maintain adequate or preset systolic BP. Use a microdrip (60 gtt/ml) or an infusion pump for accuracy. Optimum urine flow determines correct evaluation of dosage. Decrease dose gradually; may cause marked hypotension if discontinued suddenly. Expansion of blood volume with IV fluids may be indicated.

ACTIONS

Dopamine is a chemical precursor of norepinephrine, possessing alpha, beta, and dopaminergic receptor–stimulating actions. Increases cardiac output with minimum increase in myocardial oxygen consumption. Dilates renal and mesenteric blood vessels at doses lower than those required to elevate systolic BP. Therapeutic doses effect little change on diastolic BP. Doses over 10 mcg/kg/min may cause peripheral vasoconstriction and marked increases in pulmonary occlusive pressure. Has short duration of action. Metabolized by monoamine oxidase (MAO) catechol *O*-methyltransferase (COMT) to inactive metabolites and is promptly excreted in the urine.

INDICATIONS AND USES

To correct hemodynamic imbalances, including hypotension resulting from shock syndrome of myocardial infarction, trauma, endotoxic septicemia, open heart surgery, renal failure, and chronic cardiac decompensation. ▪ Drug of choice for hypotension and shock. ▪ AHA guidelines recommend dopamine as the second drug of choice after atropine to treat symptomatic bradycardia.

Unlabeled uses: Chronic obstructive pulmonary disease (4 mcg/kg/min), congestive heart failure (2 to 5 mcg/kg/min), infant respiratory distress syndrome (begin at 5 mcg/kg/min). Low-dose dopamine has been used postoperatively to protect the kidneys of surgical patients from inflammatory insults, ischemia, and nephrotoxicity.

CONTRAINDICATIONS

Hypersensitivity to any components (contains sulfites), pheochromocytoma, uncorrected tachyarrhythmias, ventricular fibrillation.

PRECAUTIONS

Some preparations contain sulfites; use caution in patients with allergies. ▪ Use caution in patients with a history of occlusive vascular disease.

Monitor: Recognition of signs and symptoms and prompt treatment with dopamine will improve prognosis. ▪ Check BP every 2 minutes until stabilized at the desired level. Check every 5 minutes thereafter during therapy. Avoid hypertension. If possible, check central venous pressure or pulmonary wedge pressure before administration and as ordered thereafter. ▪ Use larger veins (antecubital fossa) and avoid extravasation; may cause necrosis and sloughing of tissue. Central vein preferred for continuous infusions. ▪ If possible, correct hypovolemia with IV fluids, whole blood or plasma as indicated; correct acidosis if present. ▪ Monitor for decreased urine output, increased tachycardia, or new arrhythmias. ▪ With high-dose administration, palpate pulses and monitor extremities for signs of peripheral vasoconstriction (e.g., coldness, paresthesias). ▪ Therapy may be continued until the patient can maintain hemodynamic and renal functions. ▪ See Maternal/Child and Drug/Lab Interactions.

Maternal/Child: Category C: safety for use in pregnancy and breast-feeding not established. If used benefits must outweigh risks. ▪ Safety for use in children not established. Has been used, but experience is limited. ▪ Clearance is affected by age, renal and hepatic function. In younger children, particularly neonates, clearance is highly variable. Newborn infants may be more sensitive to the vasoconstrictive effects of dopamine. Close hemodynamic monitoring required. ▪ Do not administer into an umbilical arterial catheter. Vasospastic events have been reported when dopamine is infused through an umbilical vessel.

Elderly: Lower-end initial doses may be appropriate; see Dose Adjustments. ▪ Response of elderly versus younger patients not documented.

DRUG/LAB INTERACTIONS

Alkaline solutions, including sodium bicarbonate, inactivate dopamine. ▪ May cause serious arrhythmias in presence of cyclopropane or halogen anesthetics, severe hypertension with oxytocic drugs (e.g., methylergonovine [Methergine] or oxytocin). ▪ May cause hypertensive crisis with MAO inhibitors (e.g., selegiline [Eldepryl]). ▪ Antagonizes effects of guanethidine (Ismelin). ▪ Some effects may be antagonized by alpha- or beta-blocking agents (e.g., labetalol [Trandate], propranolol [Inderal]). ■ Pressor response may be decreased by tricyclic antidepressants; increased doses of dopamine may be required. ■ Will cause severe bradycardia and hypotension with phenytoin (Dilantin). ■ See Dose Adjustments.

SIDE EFFECTS

Aberrant conduction, anginal pain, azotemia, bradycardia, dyspnea, ectopic beats, headache, hypertension, hypotension, nausea, palpitation, piloerection, tachycardia, vasoconstriction, vomiting, widened QRS complex.

ANTIDOTE

Notify the physician of all side effects. Decrease infusion rate and notify the physician immediately for decrease in established urine flow rate, disproportionate rise in diastolic BP, increasing tachycardia, or new arrhythmias. For accidental overdosage with hypertension, reduce rate or temporarily discontinue until condition stabilizes. Phentolamine may be required. To prevent sloughing and necrosis in areas where extravasation has occurred, with a fine hypodermic needle inject 5 to 10 mg of phentolamine (Regitine) diluted in 10 to 15 ml normal saline liberally throughout the tissue in the extravasated area. Begin as soon as extravasation recognized.

DOXAPRAM HYDROCHLORIDE

(dox′a-pram hye-droe-klor′id)

Respiratory stimulant
Analeptic

Dopram

pH 3.5 to 5

USUAL DOSE

Specific testing may be indicated before administration; see Precautions.

Postanesthesia respiratory depression: 0.5 to 1 mg/kg of body weight. Up to 1.5 mg/kg may be given as a single injection, or up to 2 mg/kg may be divided and given as several injections at 5-minute intervals. Repeat every 1 to 2 hours as necessary to maintain respiration or follow with an infusion. 4 mg/kg or a total dose of 300 mg for the average adult is the recommended total dose by infusion. ***Do not exceed 3 Gm/24 hr. Minimum effective dosage is recommended. Repetitive doses are to be used only if the initial dose elicits a positive response.***

Chronic obstructive pulmonary disease: 1 to 2 mg/min. Maximum dose is 3 mg/min (360 mg) over no more than 2 hours. Repeat doses not recommended.

DILUTION

May be given undiluted or diluted with equal parts of SW for injection; or dilute 250 mg (12.5 ml) in 250 ml D5W, D10W, D5NS, D10NS, or NS and give as an infusion.

Chronic obstructive pulmonary disease: Dilute 400 mg in 180 ml infusion fluid (2 mg/ml). May be given by slow IV injection or infusion.

INCOMPATIBLE WITH

Manufacturer states, "Admixture with alkaline solutions such as aminophylline, sodium bicarbonate, or thiopental (Pentothal) will result in precipitation or gas formation."

COMPATIBLE WITH

See Incompatible With. Consult pharmacist; specific conditions may apply; see Compatibilities, p. xvi.

Syringe: Amikacin (Amikin), bumetanide (Bumex), chlorpromazine (Thorazine), cimetidine (Tagamet), cisplatin (Platinol), cyclophosphamide (Cytoxan), dopamine (Intropin), doxycycline (Vibramycin), epinephrine (Adrenalin), lincomycin (Lincocin), methotrexate (Folex), phytonadione (Aquamephyton), pyridoxine (vitamin B_6), tobramycin (Nebcin), vincristine (Oncovin).

RATE OF ADMINISTRATION

Postanesthesia respiratory depression: Total desired dose of undiluted medication over 5 minutes. Infusion rate may start at 5 mg/min; decrease to 1 to 3 mg/min with observance of respiratory response. If an infusion is used after the initial priming dose, rate may start at 1 to 3 mg/min depending on patient response. Discontinue use after 2 hours, wait 1 to 2 hours, and repeat entire process. Use an infusion pump or microdrip (60 gtt/ml) for accuracy. See Monitor.

Chronic obstructive pulmonary disease: Specific dose over a 2-hour period. Begin at 1 to 2 mg/min. May be titrated to response by injection or infusion. ***Never*** exceed 3 mg/min.

ACTIONS

An analeptic CNS stimulant. Affects medullary respiratory center to increase the depth of respiration and to slightly increase the rate. Achieves maximum effect in 2 minutes and lasts about 10 to 12 minutes with a single dose. Elevates BP and HR. Rapidly metabolized. See Precautions.

INDICATIONS AND USES

To pharmacologically stimulate deep breathing in the postoperative patient. ■ As a temporary measure in hospitalized patients with acute respiratory insufficiency superimposed on chronic obstructive pulmonary disease (COPD). Its use should be for a short period of time as an aid in the prevention of elevation of arterial CO_2 tension during administration of O_2. Do not use in conjunction with mechanical ventilation.

Unlabeled uses: Has been used for the treatment of neonatal apnea when methylxanthines (e.g., caffeine, theophyllines) have failed. Begin at 0.1 to 0.2 mg/kg/hr and increase up to 1.5 mg/kg/hr as needed.

CONTRAINDICATIONS

Cerebrovascular accidents, convulsive states of any etiology, coronary artery disease, head injury, severe hypertension, inadequate ventilation capacity, known hypersensitivity to doxapram, neonates, severe pulmonary dysfunction.

PRECAUTIONS

Rule out airway obstruction, hypoxia, and/or apnea due to muscle relaxants before use. ■ Not an antagonist to muscle relaxant drugs or a specific narcotic antagonist. Specific tests (e.g., peripheral nerve stimulation, pulse oximetry, end tidal carbon dioxide) to assess adequacy of ventilation are recommended before administration. ■ Anticonvulsants such as IV short-acting barbiturates (e.g., pentobarbital [Nembutal]), oxygen, and resuscitative equipment must be available. ■ Adjunctive therapy only. Does not inhibit depressant drug metabolism. ■ Stimulates systemic epinephrine increase. ■ Use care in agitation, asthma, cardiac arrhythmias or disease, cerebral edema, gastric surgery, hyperthyroidism, increased intracranial pressure, pheochromocytoma, tachycardia, and ulcers.

Monitor: Maintain an adequate airway at all times. Oxygen and facilities for controlled ventilation must be available. ■ Observe patient continuously and monitor BP, pulse, and deep tendon reflexes during therapy until 1 hour after doxapram is discontinued. Adjust rate if indicated. ■ Arterial blood gas measurements are desirable to determine effective ventilation. ■ Failure to respond to treatment may indicate CNS source for sustained coma; requires neurologic evaluation; repeat doses are not indicated. ■ Confirm patency of vein; vascular extravasation and thrombophlebitis can result from extended use. ■ In chronic obstructive pulmonary disease, arterial blood gases before administration and every 30 minutes thereafter are mandatory; do not use in conjunction with mechanical ventilation. Adjust rate of infusion and oxygen delivery as indicated by arterial blood gases and patient response. Consider increased work of breathing. Observe for CO_2 retention and acidosis. Repeat infusions not recommended. ■ See Drug/Lab Interactions.

Maternal/Child: Category B: safety for use in pregnancy, breast-feeding, and children under 12 years not established. ■ Contains benzyl alcohol, which has been associated with a fatal "gasping syndrome" in neonates. ■ See Contraindications.

DRUG/LAB INTERACTIONS

Sympathomimetics (e.g., epinephrine), MAO inhibitors (e.g., selegiline [Eldepryl]), and vasopressors (e.g., dobutamine, isoproterenol) may increase pressor effects when used concurrently with doxapram and produce excessive hypertension. ■ In patients who have received a volatile anesthetic agent (e.g., cyclopropane, halothane) known to sensitize the myocardium to catecholamines, delay administration of doxapram until the volatile agent has been excreted to reduce the potential for cardiac arrhythmias. ■ May temporarily mask the residual effects of muscle relaxants (e.g., cisatracurium [Nimbex], diazepam [Valium]).

SIDE EFFECTS

Albuminuria; chest pain or tightness; confusion; cough; decreased hemoglobin, hematocrit, and RBCs; diaphoresis; dizziness; dyspnea; elevated BUN; fever; hiccups; hyperactivity; nausea; phlebitis; salivation; urinary retention or urgency; vomiting; warmth.

Major: Aggravated deep tendon reflexes, arrhythmias (e.g., VT, VF), bilateral Babinski sign, bronchospasm, convulsions, hypertension, hypotension, laryngospasm, PVCs, respiratory alkalosis, skeletal muscle spasm, tachycardia.

Chronic obstructive pulmonary disease: Acidosis and CO_2 retention.

ANTIDOTE

Notify physician of any side effect. Depending on severity, physician may elect to continue the drug at a reduced rate of administration or discontinue it. Discontinue doxapram with onset of sudden hypotension or dyspnea. IV diazepam (Valium) or pentobarbital sodium (Nembutal) may be useful in overdose. Discontinue doxapram if blood gases deteriorate. Resuscitate as necessary.

DOXERCALCIFEROL

Vitamin D analog

(dox′err-kal-sif-er-ol)

Hectorol Injection

USUAL DOSE

Optimal dose of doxercalciferal must be individualized. The dose is adjusted in an attempt to achieve intact parathyroid hormone (iPTH) levels within a targeted range of 150 to 300 pg/ml. See Precautions and Monitor. Recommended initial dose is 4 mcg administered as a bolus dose three times weekly at the end of dialysis (approximately every other day). Total weekly dose is 12 mcg/week. Maximum dose was limited to 18 mcg/week in clinical studies.

DOSE ADJUSTMENTS

Adjust dosing based on patient response in order to lower blood iPTH into the range of 150 to 300 pg/ml. The chart below is a suggested approach to dose titration. Doses higher than 18 mcg weekly have not been studied. During titration monitor iPTH, serum calcium, phophorus, and calcium × phosphorus product (Ca × P) weekly. Maximize iPTH suppression while maintaining serum calcium and phosphorous levels in prescribed ranges; see Monitor. ■ Immediately suspend dosing if hypercalcemia, hyperphosphatemia, or a Ca × P product of greater than 70 is noted. Reinitiate therapy at a dose that is 1 mcg lower when parameters have normalized. ■ Patients with impaired hepatic function may not metabolize doxercalciferol appropriately, see Precautions.

Suggested Dose Adjustment Guidelines for Doxercalciferol	
Decreased by <50% and above 300 pg/ml	Increase by 1.0 to 2.0 mcg at eight-week intervals as necessary
150-300 pg/ml	Maintain
<100 pg/ml	Suspend for one week, then resume at a dose that is at least 1.0 mcg lower

DILUTION

May be given undiluted. Available as 2 mcg/ml solution in 1- and 2-ml vials.

Storage: Store unopened vials at 25° C (77° F); range: 15° to 30° C (59° to 86° F). Protect from light. Discard unused portion.

COMPATIBILITY

Specific information not available. Consider specific use; consult pharmacist.

RATE OF ADMINISTRATION

Administer as a bolus dose at the end of dialysis.

ACTIONS

A synthetic vitamin D analog. Metabolizes to a naturally occurring, biologically active form of vitamin D_2 that regulates blood calcium at levels required for essential body functions (i.e., intestinal absorption of dietary calcium, tubular reabsorption of calcium by the kidney, and, in conjunction with the parathyroid hormone [PTH]), the mobilization of calcium from the skeleton). Acts directly on bone cells (osteoblasts) to stimulate skeletal growth, and on the parathyroid glands to suppress PTH synthesis and secretion. In uremic patients, deficient production of biologically active vitamin D metabolites leads to secondary hyperparathyroidism, which contributes to the development of metabolic bone disease. Doxercalciferol is activated in the liver. Peak blood levels are reached in 2.1 to 13.9 hours. Mean half-life range is 32 to 96 hours.

INDICATIONS AND USES

Reduction of elevated iPTH levels in the management of secondary hyperparathyroidism in patients undergoing chronic renal dialysis.

CONTRAINDICATIONS

Evidence of vitamin D toxicity, hypercalcemia, hyperphosphatemia, or known hypersensitivity to any ingredient in this product; see Precautions.

PRECAUTIONS

Overdose of any form of vitamin D, including doxercalciferol, is dangerous. Progressive hypercalcemia due to overdose of vitamin D and its metabolites may require emergency attention. Acute hypercalcemia may exacerbate tendencies for cardiac arrhythmias and seizures and may potentiate the action of digitalis drugs. Chronic administration may place patient at risk of hypercalcemia, elevated Ca × P product, and generalized vascular and other soft-tissue calcification. If clinically significant hypercalcemia develops, dose should be reduced or held. Do not allow the Ca × P product to exceed 70. See Side Effects and Antidote. ■ To avoid possible additive effects and hypercalcemia, phosphate or vitamin D-related compounds should not be taken concomitantly with doxercalciferol. ■ Oversuppression of iPTH levels may lead to adynamic bone syndrome. ■ Hyperphosphatemia can exacerbate hyperparathyroidism. ■ Use caution in patients with impaired hepatic function. More frequent monitoring of iPTH, calcium, and phosphorus levels is recommended. ■ Patients with higher pre-treatment serum levels of calcium (more than 10.5 mg/dl) or phosphorus (more than 6.9 mg/dl) may be more likely to experience hypercalcemia or hyperphosphatemia; see Contraindications.

Monitor: During initiation of therapy, obtain baseline serum iPTH, calcium and phosphorus levels and determine levels weekly during the early phase of treatment (i.e., first 12 weeks). For dialysis patients, serum or plasma iPTH and serum calcium, phosphorus, and alkaline phosphatase should be determined periodically. See Dose Adjustments. ■ Calculate Ca × P (should be less than 70). ■ Monitor serum calcium levels weekly after all dose changes and during subsequent dose titration. ■ Monitor for signs and symptoms of hypercalcemia. See Side Effects. Radiographic evaluation of suspect anatomical regions may be useful in the early detection of generalized vascular or other soft-tissue calcification. ■ Oral calcium-based or other non–aluminum-containing phosphate binders and a low phosphate diet are indicated to control serum phosphorus levels in dialysis patients. Hyperphosphatemia can lessen the effectiveness of doxercalciferol in reducing blood PTH levels. After initiating doxercalciferol therapy, the dose of phosphate binders should be decreased to correct persistent mild hypercalcemia (10.6 to 11.2 mg/dl for 3 consecutive determinations), or increased to correct persistent mild hyperphosphatemia (7 to 8 mg/dl for 3 consecutive determinations). ■ Persistent or markedly elevated serum calcium levels may be corrected by dialysis against a reduced calcium or calcium-free dialysate. ■ See Precautions and Drug/Lab Interactions.

Patient Education: Report symptoms of hypercalcemia promptly. Dose adjustment or treatment may be required. Strict adherence to dietary supplementation of calcium and restriction of phosphorus is required to ensure optimal effectiveness of therapy. Phosphate-binding compounds (e.g., calcium acetate [Phos-lo]) may be needed to control serum phosphorus levels in patients with CRF, but excessive use of aluminum-containing products (e.g., aluminum hydroxide gel [Alternagel]) should be avoided. ■ Review all non-prescription drugs with physician.

Maternal/Child: Category B: safety for use in pregnancy not established, use only if clearly needed. ■ Discontinue breast-feeding. ■ Safety and effectiveness have not been established for use in pediatric patients.

Elderly: No overall differences in effectiveness or safety observed.

DRUG/LAB INTERACTIONS

Specific interaction studies have not been performed. ■ Digitalis toxicity is potentiated by hypercalcemia. Use caution when doxercalciferol is prescribed concomitantly with digitalis compounds. ■ Phosphate or vitamin D–related compounds should not be taken concomitantly with doxercalciferol. ■ May reduce serum total alkaline phosphatase levels. ■ Magnesium-containing antacids may cause hypermagnesemia, concomitant use is not recommended. ■ Concomitant use with enzyme inducers (e.g., glutethimide, phenobarbital [Luminal], phenytoin [Dilantin], rifampin [Rifadin]) may affect hydroxylation of doxercalciferol and require dose adjustments.

SIDE EFFECTS

Dose-limiting side effects are hypercalcemia, hyperphosphatemia, and oversuppression of iPTH (less than 150 pg/ml). Overdose or chronic administration may lead to hypercalcemia. Signs and symptoms of vitamin D intoxication associated with hypercalcemia include: ***Early:*** bone pain, constipation, dry mouth, headache, metallic taste, muscle pain, nausea, somnolence, vomiting, and weakness. ***Late:*** Albuminuria, anorexia, cardiac arrhythmias, conjunctivitis (calcific), death, decreased libido, ectopic calcification, elevated AST and ALT, elevated BUN, hypercholesterolemia, hypertension, hyperthermia, overt psychosis (rare), pancreatitis, photophobia, pruritus, rhinorrhea, somnolence, and weight loss.

Overdose: Hypercalcemia, hypercalciuria, hyperphosphatemia, and oversuppression of PTH secretion leading in certain cases to adynamic bone disease. High intake of calcium and phosphate concomitant with doxercalciferol may lead to similar abnormalities. High levels of calcium in the dialysate bath may contribute to hypercalcemia.

ANTIDOTE

Notify physician of any side effects. Treatment of patients with clinically significant hypercalcemia (more than 1 mg/dl above the upper limit of normal range) consists of immediate dose reduction or interruption of the therapy and includes a low-calcium diet, withdrawal of calcium supplements, patient mobilization, attention to fluid and electrolyte imbalances, assessment of electrocardiographic abnormalities (critical in patients receiving digitalis), and hemodialysis or peritoneal dialysis against a calcium-free dialysate, as warranted. Monitor serum calcium levels frequently until calcium levels return to within normal limits. Not removed from blood during hemodialysis. When serum calcium levels return to within normal limits (usually 2 to 7 days), therapy may be restarted at a dose that is at least 1 mcg lower than prior therapy.

DOXORUBICIN HYDROCHLORIDE ▪ DOXORUBICIN HYDROCHLORIDE LIPOSOME INJECTION

(dox-oh-roo′bi-sin hye-droe-klor′id)

Antineoplastic (anthracycline antibiotic)

ADR, Adriamycin PFS, Adriamycin RDF, Rubex ▪ Doxil

pH 3.8 to 6.5 ▪ pH 6.5

USUAL DOSE

Assessment required before dosing; see Precautions and Monitor.

CONVENTIONAL DOXORUBICIN

60 to 75 mg/M^2 once every 21 days as a ***single agent.*** An alternate dose schedule is 30 mg/M^2 once each day for 3 days. Repeat every 4 weeks. When used in ***combination*** with other agents, the most common dose of doxorubicin is 40 to 60 mg/M^2 every 21 to 28 days. Recent studies suggest that cardiotoxicity may be reduced and doses may be increased by administration of 20 mg/M^2 on a weekly basis or by giving larger doses (60 to 75 mg/M^2) as a prolonged infusion (48 to 96 hours). A central venous catheter or infuse-a-port would be necessary. Dexrazoxane (Zinecard) is now available to reduce the incidence and severity of cardiomyopathy for women with metastatic breast cancer who have received 300 mg/M^2 of doxorubicin (see product insert).

DOXIL (LIPOSOME DOXORUBICIN)

AIDS-related Kaposi's sarcoma: 20 mg/M^2 once every 3 weeks. Continue as long as response is satisfactory and treatment is tolerated. 20 mg/M^2 every 2 weeks has also been used.

Ovarian cancer: 40 to 50 mg/M^2 as an infusion every 4 weeks for as long as the patient does not progress, shows no evidence of cardiotoxicity, and continues to tolerate treatment. A minimum of four courses is recommended.

Breast cancer (unlabeled): 30 to 50 mg/M^2 once every 2 to 4 weeks.

PEDIATRIC DOSE

CONVENTIONAL DOXORUBICIN: 30 mg/M^2 once each day for 3 days. Repeat every 4 weeks. See Maternal/Child.

DOXIL: Safety for use in children not established.

DOSE ADJUSTMENTS

ALL DOXORUBICINS: ***Elevated serum bilirubin:*** Give 50% of above doses for serum bilirubin from 1.2 to 3 mg/ml and 25% for serum bilirubin above 3 mg/ml. ▪ See Precautions.

CONVENTIONAL DOXORUBICIN: Reduce dose in impaired liver and kidney function. ▪ Lower-end doses are appropriate for the elderly (inadequate marrow reserves) and those with prior therapy or neoplastic marrow infiltration.

DOXIL: Dose adjustments are required in hematologic toxicity (see the following chart) and in patients with stomatitis or palmar-plantar erythrodysesthesia (see product literature for guidelines).

Doxil Dosing Based on Hematologic Toxicity			
Grade	ANC (cells/mm^3)	Platelets (cells/mm^3)	Modification
1	1,500-1,900	75,000-150,000	Resume treatment with no dose reduction
2	1,000-<1,500	50,000-<75,000	Wait until ANC ≥1,500 and platelets ≥75,000; redose with no dose reduction
3	500-999	25,000-<50,000	Wait until ANC ≥1,500 and/or platelets ≥75,000; redose with no dose reduction
4	<500	<25,000	Wait until ANC ≥1,500 and/or platelets ≥75,000; redose at 25% dose reduction or continue full dose with cytokine support

DILUTION

Specific techniques required; see Precautions.

Conventional Doxorubicin: Each 10 mg must be diluted with 5 ml of NS. Do not use bacteriostatic diluent. An additional 5 ml of diluent for each 10 mg is recommended (2 mg/ml). Shake to dissolve completely. Also available in preservative-free solutions. May be further diluted in 50 ml or more D5W or NS and given as a continuous infusion through a central venous line.

Doxil: Each dose must be diluted in 250 ml D5W. Not a clear solution, but a translucent red liposomal dispersion. Do not use in-line filters. Maximum dose for dilution in 250 ml is 90 mg. See Incompatible With.

Storage: ***Conventional doxorubicin:*** Refrigerate unopened vials; protect from light. Reconstituted solution stable for 7 days at CRT and 15 days refrigerated. Diluted solution stable 24 hours at room temperature, 48 hours if refrigerated; then discard. Protect from sunlight.

Doxil: Refrigerate unopened vials; avoid freezing for longer than 1 month. Refrigerate diluted solution and use within 24 hours.

INCOMPATIBLE WITH

Conventional Doxorubicin

Manufacturer lists fluorouracil and heparin and states mixing with other drugs is not recommended unless specific compatibility data available.

Doxil

Specific information not available. Manufacturer states, "Do not mix with other drugs unless specific compatibility data available. Do not use any other diluent (use D5W only). Do not use any bacteriostatic agents (e.g., benzyl alcohol)."

COMPATIBLE WITH (Underline Indicates Conflicting Compatibility Information)

See Incompatible With. Consult pharmacist; specific conditions may apply; see Compatibilities, p. xvi. Other sources suggest the following compatibilities.

CONVENTIONAL DOXORUBICIN

Additive: Bleomycin (Blenoxane), cyclophosphamide (Cytoxan), dacarbazine (DTIC), ondansetron (Zofran), paclitaxel (Taxol), vinblastine (Velban), vincristine (Oncovin).

Syringe: Bleomycin (Blenoxane), cisplatin (Platinol), cyclophosphamide (Cytoxan), droperidol (Inapsine), leucovorin calcium, methotrexate (Folex), metoclopramide (Reglan), mitomycin (Mutamycin), vinblastine (Velban), vincristine (Oncovin).

Y-site: Amifostine (Ethyol), aztreonam (Azactam), bleomycin (Blenoxane), chlorpromazine (Thorazine), cimetidine (Tagamet), cisplatin (Platinol), cladribine (Leustatin), cyclophosphamide (Cytoxan), dexamethasone (Decadron), diphenhydramine (Benadryl), droperidol (Inapsine), etoposide phosphate (Etopophos), famotidine (Pepcid IV), filgrastim (Neupogen), fludarabine (Fludara), furosemide (Lasix), gatifloxacin (Tequin), gemcitabine (Gemzar), granisetron (Kytril), hydromorphone (Dilaudid), leucovorin calcium, linezolid (Zyvox), lorazepam (Ativan), melphalan (Alkeran), methotrexate (Folex), methylprednisolone (Solu-Medrol), metoclopramide (Reglan), mitomycin (Mutamycin), morphine, ondansetron (Zofran), paclitaxel (Taxol), prochlorperazine (Compazine), promethazine (Phenergan), ranitidine (Zantac), sargramostim (Leukine), sodium bicarbonate, teniposide (Vumon), thiotepa (Thioplex), topotecan (Hycamtin), vinblastine (Velban), vincristine (Oncovin), vinorelbine (Navelbine).

DOXIL

Y-site: Acyclovir (Zovirax), allopurinol (Aloprim, Zyloprim), aminophylline, ampicillin, aztreonam (Azactam), bleomycin (Blenoxane), butorphanol (Stadol), calcium gluconate, carboplatin (Paraplatin), cefazolin (Kefzol), cefepime (Maxipime), cefoxitin (Mefoxin), ceftizoxime (Cefizox), ceftriaxone (Rocephin), chlorpromazine (Thorazine), cimetidine (Tagamet), ciprofloxacin (Cipro IV), cisplatin (Platinol), clindamycin (Cleocin), cyclophosphamide (Cytoxan), cytarabine (ARA-C), dacarbazine (DTIC), dexamethasone (Decadron), diphenhydramine (Benadryl), dobutamine (Dobutrex), dopamine (Intropin), droperidol (Inapsine), enalaprilat (Vasotec IV), etoposide (VePesid), famotidine (Pepcid IV), fluconazole (Diflucan), fluorouracil (5-FU), furosemide (Lasix), ganciclovir (Cytovene), gentamicin (Garamycin), granisetron (Kytril), haloperidol (Haldol), heparin, hydrocortisone sodium succinate (Solu-Cortef), hydromorphone (Dilaudid), ifosfamide (Ifex), leucovorin calcium, lorazepam (Ativan), magnesium sulfate, mesna (Mesnex), methotrexate (Folex), methylprednisolone (Solu-Medrol), metronidazole (Flagyl IV), ondansetron (Zofran), piperacillin (Pipracil), potassium chloride (KCl), prochlorperazine (Compazine), ranitidine (Zantac), sulfamethoxazole-trimethoprim (Bactrim), ticarcillin (Ticar), ticarcillin/clavulanate (Timentin), tobramycin (Nebcin), vancomycin (Vancocin), vinblastine (Velban), vincristine (Oncovin), vinorelbine (Navelbine), zidovudine (AZT, Retrovir).

RATE OF ADMINISTRATION

CONVENTIONAL DOXORUBICIN

IV injection: A single dose of properly diluted medication over a minimum of 3 to 5 minutes. Should be given through Y-tube or three-way stopcock of a free-flowing infusion of NS or D5W. Slow injection rate further for erythematous streaking along the vein or facial flushing.

Continuous infusion: Central venous line required. Equally distributed over 24 hours.

Doxil

Rapid infusion may increase risk of acute infusion-related reactions (e.g., apnea, asthma, back pain, bronchospasm, chills, cyanosis, facial swelling, fever, flushing, headache, hypotension, pruritus, rash, shortness of breath, syncope, tachycardia, tightness in the chest or throat). Primarily occurs during the first infusion; may resolve with a reduced rate or may take up to a day after infusion completed to resolve.

AIDS-related Kaposi's sarcoma: A single dose as an infusion evenly distributed over 30 minutes.

Ovarian or breast cancer: Begin with an initial rate of 1 mg/minute to minimize the risk of infusion reactions. If no adverse infusion-related effects, the rate may be increased to evenly distribute and complete infusion in 1 to 2 hours.

ACTIONS

Conventional Doxorubicin: A highly toxic antibiotic antineoplastic agent that is cell cycle specific for the S phase. Widely distributed and rapidly cleared from plasma, it interferes with cell division by binding with DNA to slow production of nucleic acid synthesis. Tissue levels remain constant for 7 to 10 days. Metabolized in the liver. Elimination half-life is 18 to 30 hours. Does not cross blood-brain barrier. Slowly excreted in bile and urine. Secreted in breast milk.

Doxil: Doxorubicin encapsulated in long-circulating STEALTH liposomes (phospholipids). The small size of these liposomes and their persistence in the circulation enable them to evade immune system detection and penetrate the often altered and/or compromised vasculature of tumors. Once distributed to tumor tissue, the doxorubicin is released by an unknown mechanism. It differs from conventional doxorubicin because it mostly confines itself to vascular fluid volume. Metabolized and eliminated renally. Plasma clearance is slower. Half-life is extended to 55 hours. Concentration in Kaposi's sarcoma lesions is much higher than in normal skin (range is 3 to 53 times higher).

INDICATIONS AND USES

Conventional Doxorubicin: To suppress or retard neoplastic growth. Regression has been produced in soft tissue, osteogenic, and other sarcomas; Hodgkin's disease; non-Hodgkin's lymphomas; acute leukemias; breast, GU, thyroid, lung, and stomach carcinoma; neuroblastoma; and many other carcinomas.

Doxil: Treatment of AIDS-related Kaposi's sarcoma in patients whose disease has progressed on prior combination chemotherapy or who are intolerant to combination chemotherapy. ▪ Treatment of metastatic carcinoma of the ovary in patients with disease that is refractory to both paclitaxel and platinum-based chemotherapy regimens (e.g., cisplatin [Platinol], carboplatin [Paraplatin]).

Unlabeled uses: Doxil: In various combinations for late-stage malignancies. ▪ Treatment of locally advanced and metastatic breast cancer.

CONTRAINDICATIONS

Conventional Doxorubicin: Myelosuppression resulting from treatment with other antineoplastic agents, radiotherapy, impaired cardiac function, or previous treatment with complete cumulative doses of doxorubicin, daunorubicin, idarubicin, and/or other anthracyclines and anthracenes.

ALL DOXORUBICINS: History of hypersensitivity to conventional or liposomal formulations of doxorubicin or to their components.

PRECAUTIONS

ALL DOXORUBICINS: Follow guidelines for handling cytotoxic agents and patient excreta. Precautions recommended for up to 5 days after a dose. See Appendix A, p. 1142. ▪ Usually administered by or under the direction of the physician specialist, with facilities for monitoring the patient and responding to any medical emergency. ▪ For IV use only. Do not give IM or SC. ▪ ***Do Not Substitute*** Doxil for conventional doxorubicin on a mg/mg basis. Severe side effects have resulted. Differences in liposomal products as well as conventional products can substantially affect the functional properties of these agents; do not substitute one agent for another. ▪ Use extreme caution in pre-existing drug-induced bone marrow suppression, existing heart disease, previous treatment with other anthracyclines (e.g., daunorubicin), other cardiotoxic agents (e.g., bleomycin), concurrent cyclophosphamide therapy, or radiation therapy encompassing the heart; risk of cardiotoxicity increased and may occur at lower doses. ▪ All forms of doxorubicin may cause cardiotoxicity. Life-threatening or fatal congestive heart failure may occur during therapy or months after therapy is completed. The current recommended total cumulative dose is 550 mg/M^2. This dose recommendation is reduced to 400 mg/M^2 in patients who have received radiotherapy to the mediastinal area or concomitant therapy with other cardiotoxic agents (e.g., bleomycin, cyclophosphamide, daunorubicin, mitoxantrone, mitomycin C). These recommendations may change in specific situations now that dexrazoxane is available to reduce the incidence and severity of cardiomyopathy; however, cardiac toxicity may occur at lower cumulative doses even if cardiac risk factors are not present. ▪ May have cross-sensitivity with lincomycin. ▪ Not considered effective in the treatment of brain tumors, cancers of the kidney or large bowel, CNS metastasis, or malignant melanoma. ▪ Pseudomembranous colitis has been reported. May range from mild to life-threatening. Consider in patients that present with diarrhea during or after treatment with doxorubicin. ▪ See Maternal/Child and Side Effects.

CONVENTIONAL DOXORUBICIN: Used cautiously with other antineoplastic drugs to achieve tumor remission. ▪ Secondary acute myelogenous leukemia (AML) has been reported; the occurrence of refractory secondary AML is more common when doxorubicin is given in combination with DNA-damaging antineoplastic agents, in patients heavily pretreated with cytotoxic drugs, or when doses of doxorubicin have been escalated.

DOXIL: Benefits must outweigh risks if Doxil is used in patients with a history of cardiovascular disease. ▪ Has caused palmar-plantar erythrodysesthesia. Incidence may be increased with higher doses or increased frequency. May be severe and require discontinuation of Doxil. ▪ Severe, additive myelosuppression may occur in Kaposi's sarcoma patients and may be dose limiting.

Monitor: ALL DOXORUBICINS: Monitoring of CBC including differential and platelet count, uric acid levels, liver function (AST, ALT, alkaline phosphatase, and bilirubin), kidney function, ECG, chest x-ray, and echocardiogram is necessary before and during therapy. At a minimum, recommended before each dose. ▪ Observe for S/S of cardiotoxicity (e.g., fast or irregular HR, shortness of breath, swelling of the feet or lower legs). Endomyocardial biopsy or gated radionuclide scans have been used to monitor potential cardiac toxicity. ▪ Maintain adequate hydration. ▪ Allopurinol may prevent formation of uric acid crystals. ▪ Be alert for signs of bone marrow depression, bleeding, or infection. ▪ Monitor for thrombocytopenia (platelet count less than 50,000/mm^3). Initiate precautions to prevent excessive bleeding (e.g., inspect IV sites, skin, and mucous membranes; use extreme care during invasive procedures; test urine, emesis, stool, and secretions for occult blood). ▪ Use of prophylactic antibiotics may be indicated pending C/S in a febrile, neutropenic patient. Sepsis in a neutropenic patient has resulted in discontinuation of treatment and in rare cases, death. ▪ Prophylactic antiemetics are indicated. ▪ See Drug/Lab Interactions.

CONVENTIONAL DOXORUBICIN: Use only large veins. Avoid veins over joints or in extremities with compromised venous or lymphatic drainage. Determine absolute patency of vein. A stinging or burning sensation indicates extravasation; severe cellulitis and tissue necrosis will result. ***Extravasation may occur with or without stinging or burning and even if blood returns well on aspiration of infusion needle.*** Observe and touch site frequently to feel air and/or liquid under the skin. If extravasation occurs discontinue injection; use another vein.

DOXIL: Extravasation may cause irritation at infusion site. Discontinue, use another vein.

Patient Education: ALL DOXORUBICINS: Urine will be reddish for several days (from dye, not hematuria). ▪ Nonhormonal birth control recommended. ▪ Effects may be additive with current medications. Review all medications (prescription and nonprescription) with nurse and/or physician. ▪ Report promptly shortness of breath and/or swelling of the feet or lower legs. ▪ Report S/S of infection (e.g., chills, fever, painful urination) and any unusual bleeding (e.g., bruising, tarry stools). ▪ Report IV site burning, stinging, puffiness, or the feeling of liquid under the skin and any other side effects promptly. ▪ Report tingling, burning, redness, flaking, swelling, blisters or small sores on the palms of hands or soles of feet. ▪ See Precautions. ▪ See Appendix D, p. 1148.

Maternal/Child: ALL DOXORUBICINS: Category D: avoid pregnancy; can cause fetal harm. ▪ Has been used only when benefits outweigh risks. ▪ Discontinue breast-feeding. ▪ Treatment during childhood may result in abnormal cardiac function, especially in females. ▪ Infants and children are at increased risk for developing delayed cardiotoxicity; follow-up cardiac evaluation is recommended; see Precautions. ▪ Infants and children may be at greater risk for developing acute myelogenous leukemia (AML) and other neoplasms. ▪ Infants and children may develop S/S of acute "recall" pneumonitis with concomitant use of doxorubicin and dactinomycin (Actinomycin-D) after local radiation therapy. ▪ In infants under 2 years of age, doxorubicin clearance is similar to adults, but clearance may be increased in children over 2 years of age. ▪ May contribute to prepubertal growth failure and/or gonadal impairment (which is usually temporary). ▪ See Precautions, extended recommendations for handling patient excreta.

Elderly: ALL DOXORUBICINS: Cardiotoxicity and myelotoxicity may be more severe in patients over 70 years of age. ▪ Consider age-related organ impairment and concomitant disease and/or drug therapy; see Dose Adjustments.

DRUG/LAB INTERACTIONS

Studies not yet completed for Doxil; interactions may be similar to conventional doxorubicins. ▪ May exacerbate cyclophosphamide-induced hemorrhagic cystitis or increase hepatotoxicity of 6-mercaptopurine. ▪ May increase bone marrow toxicity of other chemotherapeutic agents and radiation. ▪ Barbiturates increase clearance and decrease effects. ▪ May decrease serum levels of digoxin. ▪ May decrease serum levels of anticonvulsants (e.g., phenytoin [Dilantin], carbamazepine [Tegretol], valproate [Depacon]) when given concurrently with cisplatin. ▪ Risk of cardiotoxicity increased in patients previously treated with maximum cumulative doses of other anthracyclines (e.g., doxorubicin [Adriamycin], idarubicin [Idamycin]) and/or radiation encompassing the heart. ▪ Concurrent use with hepatotoxic agents (e.g., methotrexate) may increase risk of toxicity. ▪ Cyclosporine (Sandimmune) and streptozocin (Zanosar) may decrease clearance and increase toxicity of doxorubicin. ▪ Paclitaxel (Taxol) appears to decrease the clearance of doxorubicin. Administration of doxorubicin before paclitaxel is recommended to prevent increased toxicity. ▪ Co-administration with high-dose progesterone may increase doxorubicin toxicity. ▪ Many drug interactions possible; observe patient closely. ▪ Do not administer live vaccines to patients receiving antineoplastic drugs. ▪ Increased toxicity to mucosa, myocardium, skin (including redness and exfoliative changes), and liver possible when given concurrently with or after radiation. ▪ Dexrazoxane is given with doxorubicin to reduce cardiotoxic effects. May also decrease antitumor effectiveness if given before a cumulative dose of doxorubicin 300 mg/M^2 is reached or other chemotherapeutic agents are included in the protocol (e.g., fluorouracil). ▪ See Precautions.

SIDE EFFECTS

All Doxorubicins: Abdominal pain, acute cardiac failure, allergic reactions (including life-threatening or fatal anaphylaxis), alopecia (complete), anorexia, asthenia, bone marrow depression (e.g., anemia, hypochromic anemia, leukopenia, neutropenia [ANC less than 1,000/mm^3], thrombocytopenia) may be dose-limiting; constipation, decreased serum calcium, depressed QRS voltage, diarrhea, dry skin, esophagitis, fever, gonadal suppression, headache, hyperpigmentation of nail beds and dermal creases, hyperuricemia, increase in alkaline phosphatase, ALT (SGPT), AST (SGOT), bilirubin, BUN, glucose, SrCr; mucositis, nausea, oral moniliasis, paresthesia, prolonged PT, pseudomembranous colitis, stomatitis, weakness, vomiting.

Doxil: In addition to all of the above, acute infusion reactions, palmar-plantar erythrodysesthesia. ***Kaposi's sarcoma*** patients may be taking numerous other drugs that may confuse the overall side effect picture (e.g., didanosine [ddI], stavudine [D4T], sulfamethoxazole-trimethoprim [Bactrim], zalcitabine [ddC], zidovudine [AZT]).

Overdose: All Doxorubicins: Increase in bone marrow suppression and mucositis.

ANTIDOTE

All Doxorubicins: Most side effects will either be tolerated or treated symptomatically. Keep the physician informed. Bone marrow toxicity may require cessation of therapy. Administration of whole blood products (e.g., packed RBCs, platelets, leukocytes) and/or blood modifiers (e.g., darbepoetin alfa [Aranesp], epoetin alfa [Epogen, Procrit], filgrastim [Neupogen], pegfilgrastim [Neulasta], sargramostim [Leukine], oprelvekin [Neumega]) may be indicated to treat bone marrow toxicity. Acute cardiac failure occurs suddenly (most common when total cumulative dosage approaches 550 mg/M^2) and frequently does not respond to currently available treatment (digoxin, diuretics [e.g., furosemide (Lasix)], ACE inhibitors [e.g., enalaprilat]). Close monitoring of accumulated dosage, bone marrow, ECG, chest x-ray, echocardiography, and systolic ejection fraction may prevent most serious and potentially fatal cardiac side effects. There is no specific antidote. Supportive therapy as indicated will help sustain the patient in toxicity. Treat allergic reactions as required; discontinue therapy if severe.

Conventional Doxorubicin: For extravasation flood the area with normal saline. Use a 27- or 25-gauge needle. Elevate the extremity, apply cold compresses, and ice for 30 minutes four times a day for 3 days. Site should be observed promptly by a reconstructive surgeon.

Doxil: In addition to all of the above, treatment may have to be interrupted or discontinued for severe palmar-plantar erythrodysesthesia or acute infusion reactions. May be able to control palmar-plantar erythrodysesthesia by allowing it to resolve and increasing intervals between subsequent cycles.

DOXYCYCLINE HYCLATE

(dox-i-sye′kleen hi′klat)

Antibacterial (tetracycline)
Antiprotozoal
Antimalarial

Doxy 100, Doxy 200, Vibramycin IV

pH 1.8 to 3.3

USUAL DOSE

Adults and Children Over 45 kg

200 mg the first day in one or two infusions followed by 100 to 200 mg/24 hr on subsequent days in one or two infusions. Depends on severity of the infection.

Primary and secondary syphilis: 150 mg every 12 hours for at least 10 days.

Acute pelvic inflammatory disease: 100 mg every 12 hours. Used in combination with cefoxitin 2 Gm every 6 hours.

Prevention and/or treatment of anthrax post-exposure: 100 mg every 12 hours.

PEDIATRIC DOSE

Children 45 kg or Less (But Over 8 Years)

4.4 mg/kg of body weight/24 hr in one or two equally divided doses (2.2 mg/kg every 12 hours). Follow on subsequent days with 2.2 to 4.4 mg/kg/24 hr given once daily or in two equally divided doses (1.1 to 2.2 mg/kg every 12 hours). Do not exceed adult dose.

Prevention and/or treatment of anthrax post-exposure: 2.2 mg/kg every 12 hours.

DOSE ADJUSTMENTS

Reduction may be indicated in impaired liver function. ▪ See Drug/Lab Interactions.

DILUTION

Check expiration date. Outdated ampules may cause nephrotoxicity. Each 100 mg or fraction thereof is diluted with 10 ml of SW or NS. Further dilute each 10 ml with 100 to 1,000 ml of a compatible infusion solution such as NS, D5W, R, LR, D5LR, 10% invert sugar in water, Normosol-M or Normosol-R in 5% dextrose in water, or other compatible solutions (see literature). Recommended concentrations 0.1 to 1 mg/ml. 1,000 ml diluent equals 0.1 mg/ml, 100 ml equals 1 mg/ml. Protect from direct sunlight during infusion.

Storage: Store at CRT; protect from light. After reconstitution, must be refrigerated and used within 72 hours.

COMPATIBLE WITH **(Underline Indicates Conflicting Compatibility Information)**

Consult pharmacist; specific conditions may apply; see Compatibilities, p. xvi.

Additive: Meropenem (Merrem IV), ranitidine (Zantac).

Syringe: Doxapram (Dopram).

Y-site: Acyclovir (Zovirax), amifostine (Ethyol), amiodarone (Cordarone), aztreonam (Azactam), cisatracurium (Nimbex), cyclophosphamide (Cytoxan), diltiazem (Cardizem), docetaxel (Taxotere), etoposide phosphate (Etopophos), filgrastim (Neupogen), fludarabine (Fludara), gemcitabine (Gemzar), granisetron (Kytril), hetastarch in electrolytes (Hextend), hetastarch in NS (Hespan), hydromorphone (Dilaudid), linezolid (Zyvox), magnesium sulfate, melphalan (Alkeran), meperidine (Demerol), meropenem (Merrem IV), morphine, ondansetron (Zofran), perphenazine (Trilafon), propofol (Diprivan), remifentanil (Ultiva), sargramostim (Leukine), tacrolimus (Prograf), teniposide (Vumon), theophylline, thiotepa (Thioplex), vinorelbine (Navelbine).

RATE OF ADMINISTRATION

Each 100 mg or fraction thereof, properly diluted, over a minimum of 1 to 4 hours. 100 mg diluted in 100 ml equals 1 mg/ml and must be given over a minimum of 2 hours. 100 mg diluted in 200 ml equals 0.5 mg/ml and can be given in 1 hour if absolutely necessary. Infusion must be completed in 6 hours when diluted in LR injection with or without dextrose 5% and in 12 hours when diluted in other compatible solutions.

ACTIONS

A broad-spectrum tetracycline antibiotic, bacteriostatic against many gram-positive and gram-negative organisms and protozoa. Thought to interfere with the protein synthesis of microorganisms. Doxycycline is well distributed in most body tissues and is highly bound to plasma protein. Doxycycline may penetrate normal meninges, the eye, and the prostate more easily than most tetracyclines. Half-life is 12 to 22 hours. Partially metabolized in the liver and excreted in bile, urine, and feces. Crosses the placental barrier. Excreted in breast milk.

INDICATIONS AND USES

Infections caused by susceptible strains or organisms, such as rickettsiae, spirochetal agents, viruses, and many other gram-negative and gram-positive bacteria. Types of infections treated may include GU infections, including those caused by *Chlamydia trachomatis* and *Neisseria gonorrhoeae;* respiratory tract infections, including mycoplasmal pneumonia, skin and soft tissue infections, and others. ■ To substitute for contraindicated penicillin or sulfonamide therapy. ■ Drug of choice when a tetracycline is indicated for treatment of an extrarenal infection in patients with renal impairment. ■ Adjunct to amebicides in acute intestinal amebiasis. ■

Prevention and/or treatment of anthrax in all its forms, including cutaneous and inhalation anthrax post-exposure.

CONTRAINDICATIONS

Known hypersensitivity to tetracyclines; pregnancy, breast-feeding. Not recommended in children under 8 years.

PRECAUTIONS

Sensitivity studies indicated to determine susceptibility of the causative organism to doxycycline. ■ Continue for at least 2 to 3 days after all symptoms of infection subside. ■ Avoid prolonged use of drug; superinfection caused by overgrowth of nonsusceptible organisms may result. ■ Use caution in impaired liver function. Doxycycline serum concentrations and liver function tests are indicated. ■ Pseudomembranous colitis has been reported. May range from mild to life-threatening. Consider in patients that present with diarrhea during or after treatment with doxycycline. ■ Initiate oral therapy as soon as possible. ■ Organisms resistant to one tetracycline are usually resistant to others. ■ If syphilis is suspected, perform a darkfield examination before initiating tetracyclines.

Monitor: Determine absolute patency of vein and avoid extravasation; thrombophlebitis may occur. ■ Monitor blood glucose; may reduce insulin requirements. ■ See Drug/Lab Interactions.

Patient Education: May cause dizziness or lightheadedness; request assistance for ambulation. ■ Alert patient to photosensitive skin reaction. ■ Consider birth control options.

Maternal/Child: Category D: avoid pregnancy; see Contraindications. ■ May cause skeletal retardation in the fetus and infants and permanent tooth discoloration in children under 8 years, including in utero or through mother's milk. ■ Discontinue breast-feeding.

DRUG/LAB INTERACTIONS

Inhibits oral contraceptives; may result in pregnancy or breakthrough bleeding. ■ May alter lithium levels. ■ Interferes with bactericidal action of all penicillins (e.g., ampicillin, oxacillin, methicillin). May be toxic with sulfonamides. ■ Serum levels decreased by barbiturates, carbamazepine (Tegretol), hydantoins (e.g., phenytoin), and others. ■ May depress plasma prothrombin activity; a reduction in anticoagulant dose may be indicated.

SIDE EFFECTS

Relatively nontoxic in average doses. More toxic in large doses or if given too rapidly. Anogenital lesions, anorexia, blood dyscrasias, CNS toxicity (e.g., dizziness, lightheadedness), diarrhea, dysphagia, enterocolitis, nausea, skin rashes, vomiting.

Major: Hypersensitivity reactions including anaphylaxis; blurred vision and headache (benign intracranial hypertension); bulging fontanels in infants; hepatotoxicity; pancreatitis; photosensitivity, pseudomembranous colitis, systemic candidiasis; thrombophlebitis.

ANTIDOTE

Notify the physician of all side effects. If minor side effects are progressive or any major side effect occurs, discontinue the drug, treat allergic reaction, or resuscitate as necessary. Mild cases of colitis may respond to discontinuation of doxycycline. Treat antibiotic-related pseudomembranous colitis with fluid, electrolytes, protein supplements, and oral vancomycin or metronidazole (Flagyl). Not removed by hemodialysis.

DROPERIDOL
(droe-per′i-dole)

Inapsine

Antiemetic
Anesthesia adjunct

pH 3 to 3.8

USUAL DOSE

May cause serious proarrhythmic effects and death; reserve use to patients for whom other treatments are ineffective or inappropriate. Dose should be individualized and initiated at a low dose. Adjust upward, with caution, to achieve the desired effect. Consider age, body weight, physical status, underlying pathological conditions, use of other drugs, type of anesthesia to be used, and surgical procedure involved; see Precautions. Maximum recommended initial dose is 2.5 mg. Additional 1.25-mg doses may be given to achieve the desired effect but should be used only if the potential benefit outweighs the potential risk.

Prevention of perioperative nausea and vomiting: 2.5 mg by slow IV injection. Additional 1.25-mg doses may be given with caution to achieve desired effect only if benefits outweigh potential risk. 0.625 to 1.25 mg has been shown to have an effect similar to ondansetron (Zofran) 4 mg.

PEDIATRIC DOSE

Prevention of perioperative nausea and vomiting, children 2 to 12 years: The maximum recommended dose is 0.1 mg/kg (100 mcg/kg). Another source suggests 0.03 to 0.07 mg/kg/dose (30 to 70 mcg/kg/dose) over 2 minutes or up to 0.1 mg/kg/dose with caution to achieve desired effect only if benefits outweigh potential risk and total dose does not exceed 2.5 mg. May be given IM or IV.

DOSE ADJUSTMENTS

Initiate at a low dose and adjust upward with caution to achieve the desired effect. ▪ Reduce dose of narcotics and all CNS depressants to one fourth or one third of usual dose before, during, and for 24 hours after injection of droperidol. ▪ If other CNS depressants (e.g., narcotics) have been given previously, reduce dose of droperidol. ▪ Reduce dose for elderly, debilitated, and poor-risk patients and those with impaired kidney or liver function.

DILUTION

May be given undiluted. Give through Y-tube or three-way stopcock of the infusion set. May be added to a convenient volume of selected infusion solutions (D5W, NS, or LR).

Storage: Store vials at CRT; protect from light. Diluted solutions stable at CRT for at least 48 hours (up to 7 days in selected solutions; see literature).

INCOMPATIBLE WITH

Manufacturer states, "Will precipitate if mixed with barbiturates" (e.g., phenobarbital [Luminal], thiopental [Pentothal]).

COMPATIBLE WITH **(Underline Indicates Conflicting Compatibility Information)**

Consult pharmacist; specific conditions may apply; see Compatibilities, p. xvi.

Syringe: Manufacturer lists atropine, butorphanol (Stadol), chlorpromazine (Thorazine), diphenhydramine (Benadryl), fentanyl (Sublimaze), glycopyrrolate, meperidine (Demerol), morphine, perphenazine (Trilafon), promethazine (Phenergan), scopolamine. Other sources add bleomycin (Blenoxane), cimetidine (Tagamet), cisplatin (Platinol), cyclophosphamide

(Cytoxan), dimenhydrinate (Dinate), doxorubicin (Adriamycin), metoclopramide (Reglan), midazolam (Versed), mitomycin (Mutamycin), nalbuphine (Nubain), pentazocine (Talwin), prochlorperazine (Compazine), vinblastine (Velban), vincristine (Oncovin).

Y-site: Alatrofloxacin (Trovan IV), amifostine (Ethyol), aztreonam (Azactam), bleomycin (Blenoxane), buprenorphine (Buprenex), cisatracurium (Nimbex), cladribine (Leustatin), cisplatin (Platinol), cyclophosphamide (Cytoxan), cytarabine (ARA-C), docetaxel (Taxotere), doxorubicin (Adriamycin), doxorubicin liposome (Doxil), etoposide phosphate (Etopophos), famotidine (Pepcid IV), filgrastim (Neupogen), fluconazole (Diflucan), fludarabine (Fludara), gatifloxacin (Tequin), gemcitabine (Gemzar), granisetron (Kytril), heparin, hetastarch in electrolytes (Hextend), hydrocortisone sodium succinate (Solu-Cortef), idarubicin (Idamycin), linezolid (Zyvox), melphalan (Alkeran), meperidine (Demerol), methotrexate (Folex), metoclopramide (Reglan), mitomycin (Mutamycin), ondansetron (Zofran), paclitaxel (Taxol), potassium chloride (KCl), propofol (Diprivan), remifentanil (Ultiva), sargramostim (Leukine), teniposide (Vumon), thiotepa (Thioplex), vinblastine (Velban), vincristine (Oncovin), vinorelbine (Navelbine).

RATE OF ADMINISTRATION

IV injection: ***Adults:*** 2.5 mg or fraction thereof over 1 to 2 minutes. ***Children:*** A single dose or fraction thereof over a minimum of 2 minutes.

Infusion: Titrate by dose and desired patient response. Do not exceed rate for IV injection.

ACTIONS

An antianxiety agent that produces marked tranquilization and sedation. Has an antiemetic action also. It produces mild alpha-adrenergic blockade and produces peripheral vascular dilation. May decrease an abnormally high pulmonary arterial pressure. A dose-dependent and significant QT prolongation at all dose levels (0.1, 0.175, and 0.25 mg/kg) has been observed within 10 minutes of administration in patients without known cardiac disease. Effective in 3 to 10 minutes with maximum results in 30 minutes. Lasts 2 to 4 hours. Some effects persist for 12 hours. Metabolized in the liver. Excreted in urine and feces. Crosses placental barrier very slowly. Secreted in breast milk.

INDICATIONS AND USES

To reduce the incidence of nausea and vomiting associated with surgical and diagnostic procedures.

Unlabeled uses: Antiemetic in cancer chemotherapy including potent emetic agents (e.g., cisplatin). ■ Antiemetic in Meniere's disease. ■ Treatment of acute psychotic episodes manifested by severe agitation and combativeness.

CONTRAINDICATIONS

Known hypersensitivity to droperidol and patients with known or suspected QT prolongation, including those with congenital long QT syndrome.

PRECAUTIONS

Use of agents other than droperidol is recommended. ■ QT prolongation and torsades de pointes have been reported with doses at or below those recommended. Some cases have occurred in patients with no known risk factors for QT prolongation, and some cases have been fatal. ■ Primarily used by or under direct observation of the anesthesiologist. ■ Use with extreme caution in patients who may be at risk for development of prolonged QT syndrome (e.g., clinically significant bradycardia [less than 50 bpm]; any clinically significant cardiac disease; treatment with class 1A antiarrhythmics and/or class III antiarrhythmics; treatment with MAO inhibitors [e.g., selegiline (Eldepryl)]; concomitant treatment with other drug products known to prolong the QT interval; electrolyte imbalance, in particular hypokalemia or hypomagnesemia; or concomitant treatment with drugs that may cause electrolyte imbalance or hypovolemia). See Drug Interactions. ■ Other risk factors may include patients over 65 years of age, alcohol abuse, Parkinson's disease, pheochromocytoma, and the use of agents such as benzodiazepines, volatile anesthetics, and IV opiates. ■ Correct hypokalemia and/or hypomagnesemia before administration. ■ When used without a general anesthetic, topical anesthesia is still required when appropriate (e.g., bronchoscopy).

Monitor: A potent drug. Obtain a baseline ECG on all patients. Do not administer droperidol if a prolonged QT interval exists (QTc greater than 440 msec for males or 450 msec for females). ■ Monitor VS and ECG closely. Monitor for palpitations, syncope, and/or other symptoms of irregular cardiac rhythm and evaluate promptly. ■ Resuscitation equipment, a narcotic antagonist (if a narcotic has been used concurrently), IV infusion line, IV fluids, and equipment and drugs to manage emergency situations must be readily available. ■ In patients for whom the benefit is believed to outweigh the risks of potentially serious arrhythmias, monitor for arrhythmias during the treatment and for 2 to 3 hours after treatment. ■ Orthostatic hypotension is common; move and position patients with care. ■ EEG pattern may be slow in returning to normal postoperatively. See Precautions.

Patient Education: Avoid activities that require alertness for 24 hours after receiving droperidol. ■ Do not drink alcoholic beverages or take other CNS depressants (e.g., antihistamines, pain meds, sleeping pills) for 24 hours after receiving droperidol.

Maternal/Child: Category C: safety for use during pregnancy not established; is rarely used. Exceptions are selected use during cesarean section. ■ Is secreted in breast milk; avoid breast-feeding. ■ Children may be more susceptible to extrapyramidal side effects. ■ Safety for use in children under 2 years not established.

Elderly: See Dose Adjustments. ■ More likely to experience hypotension and excessive sedation.

DRUG/LAB INTERACTIONS

Concurrent use with fentanyl (Sublimaze) may cause hypotension and decrease pulmonary arterial pressure. ■ May cause precipitous hypotension with epinephrine. ■ Use caution with other CNS depressant drugs (e.g., barbiturates, tranquilizers, opioids, and general anesthetics); may have additive or potentiating effects with droperidol; see Dose Adjustments. ■ Increased risk of QT prolongation and torsades de pointes with other drugs known to increase the QT interval (e.g., class 1A antiarrhythmics [e.g., disopyramide (Norpace), procainamide (Pronestyl), quinidine] and/or class III antiarrhythmics [e.g., amiodarone (Cordarone), bretylium, dofetilide (Tikosyn), ibutilide (Corvert), sotalol (Betapace)], anticonvulsants [e.g., fosphenytoin (Cerebyx)], antidepressants [e.g., amitriptyline (Elavil)], antihistamines [e.g., diphenhydramine (Benadryl)], antimalarials [e.g., chloroquine], antineoplastics [e.g., doxorubicin (Adriamycin)], azole antifungal agents [e.g., itraconazole (Sporanox)], calcium channel blockers [e.g., nicardipine (Cardene)], fluoroquinolones [e.g., gatifloxacin (Tequin)], other neuroleptics [e.g., haloperidol, lithium], and many others); see Precautions. ■ Concomitant treatment with diuretics (e.g., furosemide [Lasix)]), laxatives, steroids with mineralocorticoid potential (e.g., hydrocortisone) may cause electrolyte imbalance, hypovolemia, and/or induce hypokalemia or hypomagnesemia. ■ See Dose Adjustments and Precautions.

SIDE EFFECTS

Common: Abnormal EEG, chills, dizziness, hallucinations, hypotension, restlessness, shivering, tachycardia.

Major/overdose: Apnea; cardiac arrest; extrapyramidal symptoms; hypotension (severe); neuroleptic malignant syndrome (altered consciousness, muscle rigidity, and autonomic instability); palpitations, syncope, or other symptoms of irregular cardiac rhythm; QT prolongation and torsades de pointes; respiratory depression; ventricular tachycardia; death.

ANTIDOTE

Notify the physician of any side effect. Minor side effects will probably be transient; for major side effects discontinue the drug, treat symptomatically, and notify the physician. Treat hypotension with fluid therapy (rule out hypovolemia) and vasopressors such as dopamine (Intropin) or levarterenol (Levophed). Epinephrine is contraindicated for hypotension. Further hypotension will occur. Treat extrapyramidal symptoms with benztropine mesylate (Cogentin) or diphenhydramine (Benadryl). Treat cardiac arrhythmias as indicated (e.g., magnesium sulfate for torsades de pointes, lidocaine for ventricular tachycardia). An increase in temperature, HR, or CO_2 production may be symptoms of neuroleptic malignant syndrome or malignant hyperpyrexia. Consider prompt treatment with dantrolene (Dantrium). Resuscitate as necessary.

DROTRECOGIN ALFA (ACTIVATED)

Thrombolytic

(droh′treh-koh-jin al′fah)

Xigris

USUAL DOSE

24 mcg/kg/hr as an infusion for a total duration of 96 hours. Dose adjustment based on clinical or laboratory parameters is not recommended. If the infusion is interrupted, it should be restarted at the 24 mcg/kg/hr infusion rate. Dose escalation or bolus doses are not recommended.

PEDIATRIC DOSE

Safety and effectiveness for use in pediatric patients not established; see Maternal/Child.

DOSE ADJUSTMENTS

Dose adjustments are not indicated based on age, gender, hepatic dysfunction, or renal dysfunction. ■ Patients with end-stage renal disease (ESRD) were excluded from the study, but clearance rates did not meaningfully differ from those in normal healthy subjects.

DILUTION

Available in 5-mg and 20-mg vials. Calculate the number of vials needed. Infusion must be complete within 12 hours of preparation. A 70-kg patient would require 20.16 mg over 12 hours. Reconstitute each 5-mg vial with 2.5 ml of SW (10 ml SW for the 20-mg vial). Add diluent slowly and avoid inverting or shaking the vial. Swirl gently until completely dissolved. Yields a 2 mg/ml concentration. Must be further diluted in NS. Slowly withdraw the desired reconstituted dose of drotrecogin alfa. When further diluting in NS, minimize agitation of the solution by directing the stream to the side of the IV bag or bottle. Gently invert this diluted solution several times to ensure mixing without agitation. Manufacturer states "Do not transport the diluted solution between locations using mechanical delivery systems." Dilution of 20 mg in 200 ml yields 100 mcg/ml, in 100 ml yields 200 mcg/ml, and in 20 ml yields 1,000 mcg/ml (1 mg/ml). Dilution for use in an ***IV infusion pump*** is usually between 100 and 200 mcg/ml. Dilution for use in a ***syringe pump*** is usually between 100 and 1,000 mcg/ml; see Rate of Administration.

Storage: Vials should be refrigerated in the carton until use. Protect from light. Do not freeze or use beyond the expiration date on the vial. Contains no preservatives; use immediately after reconstitution and dilution preferred. Reconstituted solutions are considered stable for 3 hours at CRT but must be used within the 3 hours, and the infusion must be completed within 12 hours of preparation.

COMPATIBILITY

Manufacturer states, "Administer via a dedicated IV line or a dedicated lumen of a multilumen central venous catheter. The only solutions that can be administered through the same line are NS, LR, dextrose, or dextrose and saline mixtures." No incompatibilities have been observed with glass infusion bottles or infusion bags and syringes made of polyvinylchloride, polyethylene, polypropylene, or polyolefin.

RATE OF ADMINISTRATION

Avoid exposure of diluted solution to heat and/or direct sunlight.

Infusion: 24 mcg/kg/hr for a total duration of 96 hours. *When using low concentrations (less than approximately 200 mcg/ml) at low flow rates (less than approximately 5 ml/hr), the infusion set must be primed for approximately 15 minutes at a flow rate of approximately 5 ml/hr to reduce the amount of adsorption of drotrecogin alfa by the IV tubing.*

ACTIONS

A recombinant form of human Activated Protein C. Has the same amino acid sequence as human plasma–derived Activated Protein C. Activated Protein C exerts an antithrombotic effect by inhibiting factors Va and VIIIa. It inhibits plasminogen activator inhibitor-1 (PAI-1) and limits the generation of activated thrombin–activatable fibrinolysis inhibitor. May exert an antiinflammatory effect by inhibiting human tumor necrosis factor production, blocking selected leukocyte adhesion, and limiting selected thrombin-induced inflammatory responses. Mechanisms of effect on survival in patients with severe sepsis are not completely understood. Produces dose-dependent declines in D-dimer and IL-6. Also produces declines in thrombin-antithrombin levels, prothrombin F1.2, and IL-6, more rapid increases in protein C and antithrombin levels, and normalization of plasminogen. Rapidly produces steady-state concentrations proportional to infusion rates, with maximum effects on D-dimer levels occurring at the end of the 96-hour infusion. Plasma clearance is 50% higher in patients with severe sepsis than in healthy subjects. During clinical studies, mortality rates were significantly lower for patients receiving drotrecogin than for patients receiving a placebo. Mortality reduction was greater in patients with severe physiologic disturbances, those with serious underlying disease predating sepsis, and in older patients.

INDICATIONS AND USES

Reduction of mortality in adult patients with severe sepsis (sepsis associated with acute organ dysfunction) who have a high risk of death (as determined by APACHE II criteria). Effectiveness in adult patients with severe sepsis and lower risk of death has not been established.

CONTRAINDICATIONS

Conditions in which bleeding could be associated with a high risk of death or significant morbidity, such as active internal bleeding, intracranial neoplasm or mass lesion or evidence of cerebral herniation, presence of an epidural catheter, recent (within 3 months) hemorrhagic stroke, recent (within 2 months) intracranial or intraspinal surgery or severe head trauma, trauma with an increased risk of life-threatening bleeding, and known hypersensitivity to drotrecogin alfa or any of its components.

PRECAUTIONS

Safety and effectiveness for use longer than 96 hours not established. ▪ Administered by or under the direction of a physician experienced in its use and in a facility equipped to monitor the patient and respond to any medical emergency. ▪ Bleeding is the most common serious adverse effect; evaluate each patient carefully and weigh the anticipated benefits against the potential risks. Risk of bleeding may be increased in patients with severe sepsis who have one or more of the following conditions:

Concurrent therapeutic heparin (equal to or greater than 15 units/kg/hr); platelet count less than 30,000/mm^3, even if the platelet count is increased after transfusions

Prothrombin time-INR more than 3

Recent (within 6 weeks) gastrointestinal bleeding

Recent (within 3 days) thrombolytic therapy

Recent (within 7 days) oral anticoagulants (e.g., warfarin [Coumadin]) or glycoprotein GPIIb/IIIa inhibitors (e.g., abciximab [ReoPro], eptifibatide [Integrilin], tirofiban [Aggrastat])

Recent (within 7 days) aspirin more than 650 mg/day or other platelet inhibitors (e.g., dipyridamole [Persantine], plicamycin [Mithracin], sulfinpyrazone [Anturane], ticlopidine [Ticlid], valproic acid [e.g., Depakene, Depacon])

Recent (within 3 months) ischemic stroke, intracranial arteriovenous malformation, or aneurysm

Known bleeding diathesis

Chronic severe hepatic disease

Any condition in which bleeding constitutes a significant hazard or would be particularly difficult to manage because of its location.

▪ As with all proteins, there is a potential for immunogenicity. Antibody development has been reported rarely. Drotrecogin has not been readministered to patients with severe sepsis. ▪ Use caution; allergic reactions and/or anaphylaxis can occur. ▪ Risk of intracranial bleeding may be increased in patients with severe coagulopathy and/or severe thrombocytopenia. ▪ May prolong the aPTT so it is not a reliable test to assess the status of coagulopathy. Has minimal effect on PT, and PT can be used to monitor status of coagulopathy. ■ See Drug/Lab Interactions.

Monitor: Patients with severe sepsis and organ failure require intensive and diagnosis-specific monitoring. ■ Obtain appropriate baseline clotting studies (e.g., PT, TT, PTT, aPTT, CBC, fibrinogen levels, platelets). ■ Baseline assessment (patient condition, pain, hematomas, petechiae, or recent wounds) should be completed. ■ Type and cross-match may also be ordered. ■ Monitor PT as indicated. ■ Maintain strict bed rest; monitor the patient carefully and frequently for pain and signs of bleeding; observe catheter sites and apply pressure dressings to any recently invaded site; watch for hematuria, hematemesis, bloody stool, petechiae, hematoma, flank pain, muscle weakness; and do neuro checks as indicated. ■ Discontinue drotrecogin alfa 2 hours before the patient undergoes an invasive surgical procedure or procedures with an inherent risk of bleeding. When hemostasis has been achieved, use may be reconsidered 12 hours after major invasive procedures or surgery or restarted immediately after uncomplicated, less invasive procedures. ■ See Precautions and Drug/Lab Interactions.

Maternal/Child: Category C: use during pregnancy only if clearly needed. ■ Discontinue breast-feeding. ■ Literature states that although the pharmacokinetics appear to be similar in adult and pediatric patients with severe sepsis, effectiveness cannot be extrapolated to pediatric patients.

Elderly: Response similar to that found in younger patients.

DRUG/LAB INTERACTIONS

Specific drug interactions have not been studied. ■ Concomitant use of prophylactic low-dose heparin did not appear to affect safety; effect on efficacy not evaluated. ■ Use caution; risk of bleeding may be increased by any medicine that affects blood clotting, including anticoagulants (e.g., heparin, lepirudin [Refludan], warfarin [Coumadin]); GPIIb/IIIa receptor antagonists (e.g., abciximab [ReoPro], eptifibatide [Integrilin], tirofiban [Aggrastat]); any medication that may cause hypoprothrombinemia, thrombocytopenia, or GI ulceration or bleeding (e.g., selected antibiotics [e.g., cefamandole (Mandol), cefoperazone (Cefobid), cefotetan (Cefotan), ticarcillin (Ticar)], aspirin, NSAIDs [e.g., ibuprofen (Advil, Motrin), naproxen (Aleve, Naprosyn), phenylbutazone (Butazolidin)]); and/or any other medication that inhibits platelet aggregation (e.g., dipyridamole [Persantine], plicamycin [Mithracin], sulfinpyrazone [Anturane], ticlopidine [Ticlid], valproic acid [e.g., Depakene, Depacon]); see Precautions. ■ May interfere with coagulation assays based on aPTT (e.g., factor VIII, IX, and XI assays); factor concentration will be lower than true concentration. Does not interfere with assays based on PT (e.g., factor II, V, VII, X assays).

SIDE EFFECTS

Bleeding is most common. The majority of bleeding events were ecchymoses or GI tract bleeding, but intra-abdominal, intra-thoracic, retroperitoneal, intracranial, GU, and skin and soft tissue bleeding have been reported. Allergic reactions and anaphylaxis may occur.

ANTIDOTE

Notify physician of all side effects. Note even the most minute bleeding tendency. Oozing at IV sites may occur. Control minor bleeding by local pressure. If clinically important bleeding occurs, discontinue the infusion of drotrecogin alfa. Carefully assess other agents that may contribute to the bleeding. Continued use of drotrecogin alfa may be reconsidered when adequate hemostasis is achieved. For severe bleeding in a critical location or suspected intracranial bleeding, discontinue drotrecogin alfa and any heparin therapy immediately. Obtain PT, platelet count, and fibrinogen level. Draw blood for type and cross-match. Platelets, cryoprecipitate, whole blood, packed RBCs, fresh-frozen plasma, desmopressin, tranexamic acid (Cyklokapron), and aminocaproic acid (Amicar) may be indicated. Topical preparations of aminocaproic acid may stop minor bleeding. Consider protamine if heparin has been used. No known antidote; if overdose occurs, stop the infusion and monitor for signs of hemorrhagic complications. Treat minor allergic reactions symptomatically. Discontinue drug and treat anaphylaxis as indicated; resuscitate as necessary.

EDETATE CALCIUM DISODIUM

(ed′e-tate kal′se-um di′so-de-um)

Antidote
Chelating agent
Lead mobilization

Calcium Disodium Edetate, Calcium Disodium Versenate, Calcium EDTA

pH 6.5 to 8

USUAL DOSE

Specific fluid requirements indicated; see Monitor.

Asymptomatic adults and children with blood lead levels over 20 mcg/dl but under 70 mcg/dl: 1,000 mg/M^2/24 hr for 3 to 5 days. After a rest period of 2 to 4 days (preferably up to 2 weeks) to allow for redistribution of lead, repeat the process, if indicated, based on severity of lead toxicity and patient tolerance. Do not exceed 50 mg/kg/24 hr.

Symptomatic adults and children with blood levels over 70 mcg/dl: Dimercaprol (BAL) will be given IM in divided doses every 4 hours for 5 days. 4 hours after the first dose of BAL begin edetate calcium disodium 1,000 mg/M^2/24 hr (50 mg/kg/24 hr) for 5 days. BAL may be stopped after the first 3 days if the blood lead concentration has decreased to less than 50 mcg/dl. After a rest period of 7 to 14 days edetate calcium disodium should be repeated for blood lead concentrations above 45 mcg/dl.

DOSE ADJUSTMENTS

Reduce dose in pre-existing renal disease and/or adults with lead nephropathy. In adults with lead nephropathy dose is based on serum creatinine levels and repeated monthly until lead excretion is reduced towards normal.

Dose Adjustments in Impaired Renal Function and/or Adults With Lead Nephropathy	
Serum Creatinine Level	**Dose**
<2 mg/dl	1,000 mg/M^2/24 hr for 5 days
2-3 mg/dl	500 mg/M^2/24 hr for 5 days
3-4 mg/dl	500 mg/M^2/48 hr for 3 doses
>4 mg/dl	500 mg/M^2/week

DILUTION

Add total daily dose to 250 to 500 ml of D5W or NS for infusion.

Storage: Before use, store at CRT.

COMPATIBILITY

Manufacturer lists amphotericin B (Fungizone), hydralazine, D10W, 10% invert sugar in NS, LR, Ringer's solution, ⅙ M lactate as incompatible. Must be diluted in specific IV solutions; see Dilution.

RATE OF ADMINISTRATION

References vary greatly. Manufacturer recommends the total daily dose be evenly distributed over 8 to 12 hours. Others recommend infusing over 2 hours for symptomatic patients and over 1 hour for asymptomatic patients. Physician should order a specific rate. May cause hypocalcemic tetany and/or an increase in intracranial pressure with too-rapid injection.

ACTIONS

Helps to remove metals, especially lead, from the body. Will form a stable chelate with metals that have the ability to displace calcium (e.g., lead, zinc, cadmium). These stable compounds are then excreted in urine; up to 50% in 1 hour and 95% in 24 hours. Mostly chelates from bone.

INDICATIONS AND USES

Acute and chronic lead poisoning and lead encephalopathy.

CONTRAINDICATIONS

Anuria, active renal disease, or hepatitis.

PRECAUTIONS

Patients with lead encephalopathy and cerebral edema may have a lethal increase in intracranial pressure with IV infusion; IM injection preferred. ■ Usually given IM in children, unless given concurrently with BAL (insufficient IM injection sites). ■ May produce toxic and fatal effects. Produces the same renal damage as lead poisoning (e.g., proteinuria and microscopic hematuria). ■ Use with caution in mild renal disease; see Dose Adjustments. ■ The patient must be removed from the source of contamination promptly. ■ Animal studies verify lead excretion from urine and decreased blood levels, but lead in the brain may increase due to internal redistribution. After a 5-day course of treatment, lead levels in animal brains did not decrease. ■ Use for diagnosis of lead poisoning as a lead mobilization test is controversial; see literature. ■ Do not confuse with edetate disodium (Endrate), which does not chelate lead but actually removes calcium from the body and can be very dangerous. ■ Not effective in mercury, gold, or arsenic poisoning.

Monitor: Urine flow must be established before drug is administered. IV fluids may be used. Avoid excessive fluid in patients with cerebral edema or lead encephalopathy. Once urine flow is established, further IV fluid is restricted in all patients to basal water and electrolyte requirements. ■ Monitor urinalysis, urine sediment, renal and hepatic function, and electrolyte levels before treatment; repeat daily in serious cases and on the second and fifth day in less serious cases. Daily urine specimens are recommended to determine status of renal function. ■ Monitor ECG and vital signs. ■ Excretion of calcium is not increased, but excretion of zinc and other essential metals is; monitor and replace as indicated. ■ Obtain specific fluid orders from the physician.

Patient Education: If no urine output for 12 hours, report immediately.

Maternal/Child: Category B: safety for use during pregnancy not established; benefits must outweigh risks. ■ Use caution in nursing mothers.

Elderly: Consider age-related organ damage.

DRUG/LAB INTERACTIONS

Steroids will increase renal toxicity. ■ Inhibits the action of zinc insulin preparations by chelating the zinc.

SIDE EFFECTS

Acute renal tubular necrosis, anemia, anorexia, cardiac rhythm irregularities, chills, excessive thirst, fever, headache, hematuria, hypercalcemia, hypersensitivity (e.g., sneezing, nasal congestion), hypotension, increases in liver function tests (mild), leg and other muscle cramps, malaise, nausea, numbness, proteinuria, tetany, tingling, transient bone marrow depression, tremors, vomiting, weakness, zinc deficiency.

ANTIDOTE

Notify the physician of any side effects. Most will improve with a decrease in rate of the infusion or will be treated symptomatically. Discontinue if urine flow stops to avoid high tissue levels of the drug. Discontinue at the first sign of renal toxicity (e.g., presence of large renal epithelial cells or increasing numbers of RBCs). Treat cerebral edema with repeated doses of mannitol.

EDETATE DISODIUM
(ed'e-tate di'so-de-um)

Antihypercalcemic agent
Calcium chelating agent

EDTA Disodium, Endrate

pH 6.5 to 7.5

USUAL DOSE
50 mg/kg of body weight/24 hr or in equally divided doses every 12 hours (25 mg/kg every 12 hours). Total dose should not exceed 3 Gm/24 hr. Usually given for 5 days, held for 2 days. Regimen may be repeated to a total of 15 doses.

PEDIATRIC DOSE
40 mg/kg of body weight/24 hr in equally divided doses every 6 to 12 hours (20 mg/kg every 12 hours, 10 mg/kg every 6 hours). Do not exceed 70 mg/kg/24 hr or adult dose, whichever is less. See instructions in Usual Dose.

DOSE ADJUSTMENTS
Dose selection should be cautious in the elderly. Reduced doses may be indicated based on potential for decreased organ function and concomitant disease or drug therapy.

DILUTION
Recommended dose must be diluted in 500 ml D5W or NS and given as an infusion. A 0.5% solution will reduce the risk of thrombophlebitis. Do not exceed cardiac reserve in any patient. Use less diluent if necessary in children. Must be diluted to at least a 3% solution.

Storage: Store at room temperature.

COMPATIBILITY
Specific information not available. Consider specific use; consult pharmacist.

RATE OF ADMINISTRATION
Must not exceed more than 15 mg of actual medication over 1 minute. Total dose usually given over 3 to 4 hours. Rapid IV infusion may cause a sudden drop in serum calcium, resulting in tetany, convulsions, arrhythmias, and death. Reduce rate and further dilute solution for pain at injection site.

ACTIONS
A calcium-chelating agent. Also forms chelates with other polyvalent metals (e.g., magnesium, zinc). Attracts calcium ions immediately on injection and becomes calcium disodium edetate. Capable of severely depleting the body of calcium stores. Exerts a negative inotropic effect on the heart. It is well distributed in extracellular fluids and rapidly excreted in the urine.

INDICATIONS AND USES
Treatment of cardiac arrhythmias (atrial and ventricular, especially when caused by digitalis toxicity). ■ Hypercalcemia.

CONTRAINDICATIONS
Anuria, known sensitivity to edetate disodium, renal disease.

PRECAUTIONS
Used only when the severity of disease indicates necessity. ■ May produce hypocalcemia quickly, especially if used for purposes other than chelating

calcium. ■ Use repeatedly with caution because of potential for nephrotoxicity and mobilization of extracirculatory calcium stores. ■ Use caution in cardiac disease (may adversely affect myocardial contractility), diabetes (lower blood sugar may require less insulin), severe renal disease, liver disease, congestive heart failure (1 Gm of sodium in each 5 Gm), limited cardiac reserve and patients with a history of seizures or intracranial lesions.

Monitor: Monitor vital signs and ECG before and during therapy. ■ Confirm patency of vein, avoid extravasation; can cause tissue necrosis. ■ Routine electrolyte panel (potassium deficiency) and urine specimens for casts and cells necessary during therapy. Magnesium, zinc, and other trace element deficiencies can occur. ■ Keep patient in supine position during and after administration (15 to 30 minutes) to avoid postural hypotension. ■ Obtain blood for serum calcium levels just before beginning a new infusion; specific lab methods required. ■ Inhibits coagulation of blood (transient). Liver function tests may be indicated. ■ See Drug/Lab Interactions.

Maternal/Child: Category C: safety for use in pregnancy or breast-feeding not established. Use with extreme caution and only if clearly needed.

Elderly: Reduced doses may be indicated; see Dose Adjustments. Monitoring of renal function is suggested.

DRUG/LAB INTERACTIONS

Inhibits mannitol. ■ Potentiates neuromuscular blocking antibiotics (e.g., gentamicin [Garamycin]). ■ Inhibits coagulation of blood (transient). ■ A sudden drop in calcium levels may decrease effects of digoxin. ■ Obtain blood for serum calcium levels just before beginning a new infusion. Specific laboratory methods must be used for accurate evaluation.

SIDE EFFECTS

Anorexia, arthralgia, circumoral paresthesias, diarrhea, fatigue, fever, glycosuria, headache, hyperuricemia, hypotension, malaise, nasal congestion, nausea, numbness, sneezing, tearing, thirst, thrombophlebitis, urinary urgency, vomiting.

Major: Anaphylaxis, anemia, cardiac arrhythmias, dermatitis, hemorrhage, hypocalcemic tetany, prolonged QT interval, renal tubular destruction (reversible), seizures, death.

ANTIDOTE

Notify the physician of any side effect. For progression of minor side effects or any major side effect, discontinue drug immediately and notify the physician. Calcium gluconate is the antidote of choice and should be available for infusion at all times (use extreme caution if patient is digitalized). Treat mild hypotension by maintaining in supine position until recovery. Additional hydration indicated with S/S of nephrotoxicity. Treat anaphylaxis and resuscitate as necessary.

EDROPHONIUM CHLORIDE

(ed-roe-foe′nee-um klor′id)

Cholinergic
Cholinesterase inhibitor
Antidote
Diagnostic agent

Enlon, Reversol, Tensilon

pH 5.4

USUAL DOSE

1 to 10 mg (0.1 to 1 ml) at specified intervals depending on usage. Maximum dose should never exceed 40 mg (4 doses of 10 mg each).

Myasthenia gravis diagnosis: 10 mg (1 ml) in tuberculin syringe. Give 2 mg (0.2 ml). If no reaction occurs in 45 seconds, give remaining 8 mg (0.8 ml). Test may be repeated after 30 minutes.

Myasthenia treatment evaluation: 1 to 2 mg (0.1 to 0.2 ml) 1 hour after oral intake of drug being used for treatment. Package insert has a chart differentiating myasthenic and nonmyasthenic responses.

Myasthenia crisis evaluation: 2 mg (0.2 ml) in tuberculin syringe. Give 1 mg (0.1 ml). If the patient's condition does not deteriorate, give 1 mg (0.1 ml) after 60 seconds. Improvement in cardiac status and respiration should occur.

Antagonist to curare and other nondepolarizing muscle relaxants: 10 mg (1 ml). May be repeated as necessary up to 4 doses. (Available in combination with atropine [Enlon-Plus] for use in reversal of nondepolarizing muscle relaxants.)

Terminate paroxysmal atrial tachycardia (unlabeled): 5 to 10 mg as a bolus injection. See Dose Adjustments. Repeat once in 10 minutes if necessary.

Slow supraventricular tachycardias (unlabeled): 2 mg as a test dose. Repeat 2 mg every 1 minute until arrhythmia controlled or total dose of 10 mg is given. If HR decreases, may begin an infusion of 0.25 mg/min. May be increased to 2 mg/min if necessary.

PEDIATRIC DOSE

May be given IM if the IV route is not available; however, doses are different; check literature.

Myasthenia gravis diagnosis: ***Neonates:*** 0.1 mg (0.01 ml). ***Infants:*** 0.5 mg (0.05 ml).

Children less than 34 kg: 1 mg (0.1 ml); if no response in 30 to 45 seconds, give 1 mg every 30 to 45 seconds up to 5 mg (0.5 ml). ***34 kg or more,*** give 2 mg (0.2 ml); if no response in 30 to 45 seconds, give 1 mg (0.1 ml) every 30 to 45 seconds up to 10 mg. Another source has the same dose for neonates but recommends 0.2 mg/kg/dose (0.02 ml/kg/dose) for ***infants and children*** with 20% of a dose given as a test dose slowly. If no response in 1 minute, give in 1-mg increments to a maximum calculated dose or 10 mg, whichever is less.

DOSE ADJUSTMENTS

Reduce antiarrhythmic dose to 5 to 7 mg in the elderly.

DILUTION

May be given undiluted. In the treatment of myasthenia crisis, this drug may be diluted in D5W or NS and given as a continuous IV. Use an infusion pump or microdrip (60 gtt/ml).

COMPATIBLE WITH

Consult pharmacist; specific conditions may apply; see Compatibilities, p. xvi.

Y-site: Heparin, hydrocortisone sodium succinate (Solu-Cortef), potassium chloride (KCl).

RATE OF ADMINISTRATION

2 mg (0.2 ml) or fraction thereof over 15 to 30 seconds.

Curare antagonist: A single dose over 30 to 45 seconds.

Antiarrhythmic: See Usual Dose.

ACTIONS

An anticholinesterase and antagonist of nondepolarizing neuromuscular-blocking agents. Inhibits the enzyme acetylcholinesterase, allowing acetylcholine to accumulate at the myoneural junction. Restores normal transmission of nerve impulses. Acts within 30 to 60 seconds and has an extremely short duration of action, seldom exceeding 10 minutes. Produces vagal stimulation, shortens refractory period of atrial muscle, and slows conduction through the AV node.

INDICATIONS AND USES

Diagnosis of myasthenia gravis. ■ Evaluation of adequate treatment of myasthenia gravis. ■ Evaluation of emergency treatment of myasthenia crisis. ■ An antagonist to nondepolarizing muscle relaxants (e.g., tubocurarine [Curare], gallamine triethiodide [Flaxedil], doxacurium [Nuromax]). ■ Adjunct in treatment of respiratory depression caused by Curare overdosage.

Unlabeled uses: Termination of supraventricular tachycardia unresponsive to cardiac glycosides. Adenosine is the drug of choice. ■ Diagnosis of supraventricular tachycardia. ■ Evaluate function of a demand pacemaker.

CONTRAINDICATIONS

Apnea, known hypersensitivity to anticholinesterase agents, mechanical intestinal and urinary obstructions of mechanical type.

PRECAUTIONS

A physician should be present when this drug is used. ■ The term ***crisis*** is used when severe respiratory distress with ventilatory inadequacy occurs. The crisis may be secondary to a sudden increase in severity of myasthenia gravis (myasthenic crisis) or to overtreatment with anticholinesterase drugs (cholinergic crisis). If apnea is present, controlled ventilation must be secured before any testing with edrophonium. ■ Use caution when administering to patients being treated with anticholinesterase drugs (e.g., neostigmine [Prostigmin]). S/S of cholinergic crisis may mimic those of myasthenic weakness, and the patient's condition may worsen with administration of edrophonium. ■ Use caution in patients with bronchial asthma, cardiac arrhythmias, or myasthenia gravis treated with anticholinesterase drugs. ■ Isolated cases of respiratory or cardiac arrests have been reported. ■ Contains sulfites; use caution in patients with allergies.

Monitor: Atropine 1 mg must be available and ready for injection at all times. ■ Continuously observe patient reactions. ■ Anticholinesterase insensitivity may develop; withhold drugs and support respiration as necessary. ■ See Drug/Lab Interactions.

Maternal/Child: Safety for use during pregnancy and breast-feeding not established. Use during pregnancy only if benefit justifies potential risk to mother and fetus. ■ Discontinue breast-feeding. ■ Safety and effectiveness in reversing neuromuscular blockade in pediatric patients not established.

However, doses of 0.1 to 1.43 mg/kg have been used; effects (antagonism) were more rapid than in adults.

DRUG/LAB INTERACTIONS

Muscarinic effects antagonized by atropine; see Antidote. ■ May be inhibited by corticosteroids and magnesium. ■ May cause bradycardia with digitalis glycosides. ■ Briefly antagonizes the effects of nondepolarizing neuromuscular blocking agents (e.g., atracurium, pancuronium, vecuronium). ■ Prolongs muscle relaxant effect of succinylcholine.

SIDE EFFECTS

Abdominal cramps, anorexia, anxiety, bradycardia, bronchiolar spasm, cardiac arrhythmias and arrest, cold moist skin, contraction of the pupils, convulsions, diarrhea, dysphagia, fainting, increased lacrimation, increased pulmonary secretion, increased salivation, insomnia, irritability, laryngospasm, muscle weakness, nausea, perspiration, ptosis, respiratory arrest (either muscular or central), urinary frequency and incontinence, vomiting.

ANTIDOTE

If side effects occur, discontinue the drug and notify the physician. Atropine sulfate in doses of 0.4 to 0.5 mg IV will counteract most side effects and may be repeated every 3 to 10 minutes. Endotracheal intubation or tracheostomy is considered prophylactic in anesthesia or crises. Artificial ventilation, oxygen therapy, cardiac monitoring, adequate suctioning, and treatment of shock or convulsions must be instituted and maintained as necessary. Treat allergic reactions with epinephrine.

EDROPHONIUM CHLORIDE AND ATROPINE SULFATE

(ed-roe-foe′nee-um, a′troe-peen)

Cholinergic
Cholinesterase inhibitor
Antidote

Enlon-Plus

pH 4.4 to 4.6

USUAL DOSE

0.05 to 0.1 ml/kg (0.5 to 1 mg/kg of edrophonium with 0.007 to 0.014 mg/kg of atropine). Each 1 ml of prepared solution contains 10 mg edrophonium and 0.14 mg atropine. Must be administered at a point of at least 5% recovery of twitch response to neuromuscular stimulation. Use of peripheral nerve stimulator recommended. A total dose of 1 mg/kg of edrophonium is rarely exceeded. Length of action is usually sufficient to cover effects of commonly used short- and medium-acting nondepolarizing muscle relaxants (e.g., atracurium [Tracrium], mivacurium [Mivacron], vecuronium [Norcuron]).

DOSE ADJUSTMENTS

None required, even though elderly patients and those with impaired renal or hepatic function may have a prolonged half-life and reduced clearance.

DILUTION

May be given undiluted through Y-tube or three-way stopcock of infusion set.

Storage: Available in vials containing 5 ml or 15 ml. Store at room temperature 15° to 26° C (59° to 78° F).

COMPATIBILITY

Specific information not available. Consider specific use; consult pharmacist.

RATE OF ADMINISTRATION

A single dose over 45 to 60 seconds.

ACTIONS

A combination of anticholinesterase agent and a parasympatholytic (anticholinergic) drug. Edrophonium antagonizes the effect of nondepolarizing neuromuscular blocking agents by inhibiting or inactivating acetylcholinesterase. Acetylcholine is not hydrolyzed as rapidly by acetylcholinesterase and accumulates, improving transmission of impulses across the myoneural junction. Unavoidable accumulation of acetylcholine at muscarinic cholinergic sites may cause bradycardia, bronchoconstriction, increased secretions, and other parasympathomimetic effects. Magnitude of effects varies depending on vagal nerve activity present. Atropine counteracts these side effects. Edrophonium is effective immediately with maximum antagonism within 1 to 2 minutes and lasts for 70 minutes. Atropine affects HR immediately, peaks in 2 to 16 minutes, and lasts for over 2 hours. With this combination agent, full reversal is usually accomplished before patient leaves recovery, muscarinic effects are minimized, and patient evaluation can be accomplished in OR. Some hepatic metabolism. Primarily excreted in urine, with some excretion in bile.

INDICATIONS AND USES

Reversal agent or antagonist of nondepolarizing neuromuscular blocking agents. Not effective against depolarizing neuromuscular blocking agents (e.g., succinylcholine). ■ Adjunctive treatment of respiratory depression of curare overdose.

CONTRAINDICATIONS

Acute glaucoma, adhesions between the iris and lens of the eye, known hypersensitivity to either component or sulfites, mechanical intestinal and urinary obstructions, and pyloric stenosis.

PRECAUTIONS

Administer only by or under the direct observation of the anesthesiologist. ■ May contain sulfites; use caution in patients with allergies. ■ Use caution in patients with bronchial asthma, cardiac arrhythmias, myasthenia gravis (or symptoms of myasthenic weakness) treated with anticholinesterase drugs, prostatic hypertrophy, and debilitated patients with chronic lung disease. ■ Recurarization has not been reported after satisfactory reversal obtained. ■ See Drug/Lab Interactions.

Monitor: An additional supply of atropine 1 mg must be available and ready for injection at all times. ■ Continuously observe patient reactions and monitor responses. Monitor ECG, vital signs, and reversal with a peripheral nerve stimulator. Ventilation (assisted or controlled) must be secured. ■ Anticholinesterase insensitivity may develop; reduce or withhold drugs and support respiration as necessary until sensitivity returns. ■ Confirm patency of vein; will cause tissue irritation. ■ See Drug/Lab Interactions.

Maternal/Child: Category C: use during pregnancy only if benefits outweigh risks. ■ Safety for use during breast-feeding or in children not established. ■ Pediatric patients may have increased vagal tone with greater variance in effects. ■ Atropine rate of clearance decreased in children less than 2 years of age but dose adjustment not indicated.

Elderly: Prolonged plasma half-life and reduced clearance but dose adjustment not indicated; elimination of nondepolarizing muscle relaxants is similarly decreased.

DRUG/LAB INTERACTIONS

Never administer before any nondepolarizing muscle relaxant (e.g., mivacurium [Mivacron]). ■ May cause symptoms of anticholinesterase overdose (cholinergic crisis) with anticholinesterase drugs (e.g., pyridostigmine [Mestinon], neostigmine [Prostigmin], glaucoma agents). ■ Frequency and duration of bradycardia increased with narcotic analgesics unless given with a potent inhalant anesthetic. ■ Excessive bradycardia may develop with beta-adrenergic blocking agents (e.g., atenolol [Tenormin], esmolol [Brevibloc], timolol [Timpotic]); atropine alone should be given before Enlon-Plus in these patients. ■ Bradycardia and first-degree heart block may be increased when muscle relaxants with no vagolytic effects (e.g., vecuronium [Norcuron]) are reversed. ■ Cardiac arrest has occurred in digitalized patients and jaundiced patients receiving anticholinesterase drugs (e.g., pyridostigmine [Mestinon], neostigmine [Prostigmin], glaucoma agents); all side effects could be additive. ■ Prolongs muscle relaxant effect of succinylcholine. ■ Actions of atropine may interfere with absorption of other medications. ■ Concomitant use of atropine with other cholinergic drugs (e.g., antihistamines, antiparkinson agents, antipsychotics, tricyclic antidepressants) will increase mouth dryness and other side effects (e.g., decreased GI motility).

SIDE EFFECTS

Allergic reactions including anaphylaxis; arrhythmias in up to 10% of patients (e.g., bradycardia, first-, second-, and third-degree AV block, junctional rhythms, PACs, prolonged R-R interval, PVCs, P wave changes, tachycardia). All side effects of atropine and edrophonium can occur; refer to individual monographs.

Overdose: Cholinergic crisis due to overdose or concomitant use of other anticholinesterase drugs (bradycardia, diarrhea, increased bronchial and salivary secretions, nausea, sweating, vomiting), convulsions, delirium, fever, shock, tachycardia. In atropine poisoning (delirium, fever, tachycardia), death is usually due to medullary center paralysis.

ANTIDOTE

If side effects occur, discontinue drug and notify physician. Atropine sulfate in doses of 0.4 to 0.5 mg IV will counteract most side effects of edrophonium and may be repeated every 3 to 10 minutes. Endotracheal intubation or tracheostomy is considered prophylactic in anesthesia or crisis. In all situations treatment is symptomatic and includes artificial ventilation, oxygen therapy, cardiac monitoring, adequate suctioning, and treatment of fever, shock, or convulsions. Institute and maintain as necessary. Treat allergic reactions with diphenhydramine (Benadryl) and epinephrine (Adrenalin).

ENALAPRILAT

(en-al′ah-prill-at)

ACE inhibitor
Antihypertensive
Vasodilator

Vasotec IV

pH 6.5 to 7.5

USUAL DOSE

1.25 mg every 6 hours. Doses up to 5 mg every 6 hours have been tolerated for up to 36 hours, but clinical studies have not shown a need for dosage over 1.25 mg. Additional doses of 1.25 mg may be given every 6 hours except in dialysis patients. Dosage is the same when converting from oral to IV therapy. Resume oral therapy as soon as tolerated. See Precautions.

PEDIATRIC DOSE

0.625 to 1.25 mg every 6 hours. See Maternal/Child.

DOSE ADJUSTMENTS

Reduce initial dose to 0.625 mg in patients taking diuretics, patients with CHF, hyponatremia, severe volume or salt depletion, a CrCl less than 30 ml/min (SrCr greater than 3 mg/dl), and dialysis patients; see Rate of Administration. If the 0.625 dose is not clinically effective after 1 hour, it may be repeated. Reduce additional dose of 1.25 mg by one half for dialysis patients. ■ Blood levels markedly increased in the elderly; dose selection should be cautious. Consider decreased cardiac, hepatic, and renal function; concomitant disease; or other drug therapy. ■ See Drug/Lab Interactions and Precautions.

DILUTION

May be given undiluted through the port of a free-flowing infusion of NS, D5W, D5NS, D5LR, or Isolyte E. May also be diluted in up to 50 ml of any of the same solutions and given as an infusion.

Storage: Store at CRT. Stable for up to 24 hours after dilution.

COMPATIBLE WITH

(Underline Indicates Conflicting Compatibility Information)

Consult pharmacist; specific conditions may apply; see Compatibilities, p. xvi.

Additive: Dobutamine (Dobutrex), dopamine (Intropin), heparin, meropenem (Merrem IV), nitroglycerin (Nitro-Bid IV), nitroprusside sodium, potassium chloride (KCl).

Y-site: Allopurinol (Aloprim, Zyloprim), amifostine (Ethyol), amikacin (Amikin), aminophylline, ampicillin, ampicillin/sulbactam (Unasyn), aztreonam (Azactam), butorphanol (Stadol), calcium gluconate, cefazolin (Kefzol), cefoperazone (Cefobid), ceftazidime (Fortaz), ceftizoxime (Cefizox), chloramphenicol (Chloromycetin), cimetidine (Tagamet), cisatracurium (Nimbex), cladribine (Leustatin), clindamycin (Cleocin), dextran 40, dobutamine (Dobutrex), docetaxel (Taxotere), dopamine (Intropin), doxorubicin liposome (Doxil), erythromycin lactobionate (Erythrocin), esmolol (Brevibloc), etoposide phosphate (Etopophos), famotidine (Pepcid IV), fentanyl (Sublimaze), filgrastim (Neupogen), ganciclovir (Cytovene), gatifloxacin (Tequin), gemcitabine (Gemzar), gentamicin (Garamycin), granisetron (Kytril), heparin, hetastarch in electrolytes (Hextend), hetastarch in NS (Hespan), hydrocortisone sodium succinate (Solu-Cortef), labetalol (Normodyne), lidocaine, linezolid (Zyvox), magnesium sulfate, melphalan (Alkeran), meropenem (Merrem IV), methylprednisolone (Solu-Medrol), metronidazole (Flagyl IV), morphine, nafcillin (Nafcil), nicardipine

(Cardene IV), nitroprusside sodium, penicillin G potassium, phenobarbital (Luminal), piperacillin (Pipracil), piperacillin/tazobactam (Zosyn), potassium chloride (KCl), potassium phosphates, propofol (Diprivan), ranitidine (Zantac), remifentanil (Ultiva), sodium acetate, sulfamethoxazole-trimethoprim (Bactrim), teniposide (Vumon), thiotepa (Thioplex), tobramycin (Nebcin), vancomycin (Vancocin), vinorelbine (Navelbine).

RATE OF ADMINISTRATION

A single dose must be evenly distributed over 5 minutes. Extend rate of infusion up to 1 hour in patients at risk for severe hypotension (e.g., heart failure, hyponatremia, high-dose diuretic therapy, recent intensive diuresis or increase in diuretic dose, renal dialysis, or severe volume and/or salt depletion of any etiology).

ACTIONS

An antihypertensive agent. An angiotensin-converting enzyme inhibitor that prevents conversion of angiotensin I to angiotensin II. Peripheral arterial resistance is reduced in hypertensive patients. In patients with heart failure, significant reduction in pulmonary capillary wedge pressure (preload), peripheral vascular resistance (afterload), BP, and heart size occurs, as well as an increase in cardiac output (stroke index) and exercise tolerance time. Initial response may take 15 minutes to 1 hour. Peak BP reduction occurs in 1 to 4 hours, and effects last up to 6 hours. Peak effects of subsequent doses may be greater than the initial dose. Excreted in urine. Crosses placental barrier. Secreted in breast milk.

INDICATIONS AND USES

Treatment of hypertension when oral therapy is not practical. ■ Heart failure not adequately responsive to diuretics and digitalis. Enalaprilat is used in addition to digitalis and diuretics. ■ Hypertensive emergencies (effects are variable).

Unlabeled uses: Treatment of hypertension or renal crisis in scleroderma.

CONTRAINDICATIONS

Hypersensitivity to enalaprilat or its components, a history of angioedema related to previous treatment with an ACE inhibitor, or hereditary or idiopathic angioedema.

PRECAUTIONS

Has been used IV for up to 7 days. ■ Use caution in patients with a history of angioedema, aortic stenosis or hypertrophic cardiomyopathy. ■ Use caution in patients with collagen vascular disease and renal disease; neutropenia and/or agranulocytosis have been reported. Monitoring of WBC may be indicated. ■ Use caution in surgery, with anesthesia, or with agents that produce hypotension. ■ May rarely cause a syndrome that starts with cholestatic jaundice, progresses to hepatic necrosis, and may progress to death. Discontinue in patients who develop elevated liver enzymes or jaundice. ■ ACE inhibitors often cause a persistent, nonproductive cough, which should resolve when drug is discontinued. ■ Average dose for conversion to oral therapy is 5 mg/day as a single dose. When a reduced dose of enalaprilat IV has been indicated (e.g., diuretics, impaired renal function, dialysis), reduce initial oral dose to 2.5 mg/day as a single dose. Adjust either by patient response. ■ Patients sensitive to one ACE inhibitor may be sensitive to another. ■ See Monitor and Drug/Lab Interactions.

Monitor: Monitor vital signs very frequently. May cause precipitous drop in BP following the first dose. ■ Use extreme caution in fluid-depleted patients. Patients with congestive heart failure may become hypotensive at any time. Arrhythmias or conduction defects may occur. ■ Monitor BUN and SrCr. An increase in either may require a decrease in dose of enalaprilat or discontinuation of a diuretic. ■ Diuretics given concomitantly may cause a precipitous drop in BP within the first hour of the initial dose; observe the patient closely. Severe dietary salt restriction or dialysis will aggravate this effect. ■ May cause oliguria or progressive azotemia in patients with severe congestive heart failure whose renal function is dependent on the activity of the renin-angiotensin-aldosterone system. Acute renal failure and death are possible. ■ May cause hyperkalemia. May cause a significant increase in serum potassium with potassium-sparing diuretics or potassium supplements. Use with caution and only in documented hypokalemia. Use salt substitutes with caution. Monitor serum potassium levels. ■ Monitoring of WBC may be indicated in patients with collagen vascular disease or renal disease. ■ See Drug/Lab Interactions.

Patient Education: Consider birth control options. ■ May cause dizziness; avoid sudden changes in posture and request assistance for ambulation if necessary.

Maternal/Child: Avoid pregnancy; Category C (first trimester) and Category D (second and third trimester). Can cause fetal and neonatal morbidity and death. If pregnancy occurs, discontinue immediately; many alternate antihypertensive agents. ■ Observe any infant with in utero exposure for hypotension, oliguria, and hyperkalemia. ■ Has caused reversible acute renal failure in a premature infant whose mother received enalaprilat. ■ Safety for use in breast-feeding not established. ■ Safety for use in children not established but has been used. ■ May contain benzyl alcohol, which has been associated with a fatal "gasping syndrome" in neonates.

Elderly: Dose selection should be cautious; see Dose Adjustments and Precautions/Monitor. ■ May be less sensitive to effects due to a decrease in plasma renin activity or more sensitive to hypotensive effects due to increased blood levels (decreased renal excretion).

DRUG/LAB INTERACTIONS

Use caution in surgery, with anesthesia, or with any agents that produce hypotension. ■ May be used concomitantly with other antihypertensive agents (e.g., thiazide diuretics [chlorothiazide (Diuril)]). Effects are additive. ■ Diuretics given concomitantly may cause a precipitous drop in BP. ■ May cause hyperkalemia with potassium-sparing diuretics (e.g., spironolactone [Aldactone], triamterene [Dyrenium], amiloride [Midamor]), potassium supplements, potassium-containing salt substitutes, or low-salt milk. ■ Use caution and consider lower doses when administering nitroglycerin, nitroprusside sodium, other nitrates, or other vasodilators (e.g., hydralazine). ■ In patients with compromised renal function, concurrent use with NSAIDs (e.g., ibuprofen [Advil, Motrin], naproxen [Aleve, Naprosyn]) may result in further deterioration of renal function. ■ Concurrent use with NSAIDs may also decrease the hypotensive effects of enalaprilat by inhibiting the renal prostaglandin synthesis and/or by causing sodium and fluid retention. ■ May increase lithium concentration, resulting in lithium toxicity. ■ Interaction with some imaging agents (e.g., iodohippurate, technetium) may render diagnostic renal function tests inconclusive. ■ May decrease hemoglobin and hematocrit slightly. ■ See Precautions and Monitor.

SIDE EFFECTS

Abdominal pain, angioedema, anosmia (absence of sense of smell), atrial fibrillation, bradycardia, chest pain, conjunctivitis, cough (persistent dry), diarrhea, dizziness, dry eyes, dyspnea, eosinophilic pneumonitis, fatigue, flank pain, gynecomastia, headache, hepatotoxicity, herpes zoster, hoarseness, hyperkalemia, hypotension (severe), impotence, insomnia, muscle cramps, nausea, palpitations, paresthesias, photosensitivity, pneumonia, pruritus, pulmonary edema, pulmonary embolism and infarction, pulmonary infiltrates, rash, Raynaud's phenomenon, renal failure (reversible), rhinorrhea, somnolence, sore throat, taste disturbances, tearing, toxic epidermal necrolysis, vomiting. Anaphylaxis has been reported.

ANTIDOTE

For minor side effects, notify the physician. Most will be tolerated or treated symptomatically. If symptoms progress or any major side effect occurs (angioedema, precipitous hypotension, hyperkalemia), discontinue drug and notify the physician immediately. Hypotension should respond to IV fluids if the patient's condition allows their use. Other drugs in the regimen may need to be discontinued or the dosage reduced. Epinephrine, diphenhydramine (Benadryl), and hydrocortisone may be used to treat angioedema. Maintain the patient as indicated. If cardiac arrhythmias occur, treat appropriately. Hemodialysis may be useful in toxicity.

EPHEDRINE SULFATE

(e-fed′rin sul′fat)

Bronchodilator
Vasopressor

pH 4.5 to 7

USUAL DOSE

5 to 25 mg; may be repeated as needed based on patient response. 150 mg/24 hr is the maximum total dose.

PEDIATRIC DOSE

3 mg/kg of body weight/24 hr or 25 to 100 mg/M^2/24 hr divided into four to six doses. Rarely used IV in children.

DOSE ADJUSTMENTS

See Drug/Lab Interactions.

DILUTION

May be given undiluted. Not usually added to IV solutions. May be injected through Y-tube or three-way stopcock of infusion set. Compatible at Y-site with most commonly used infusion solutions.

COMPATIBLE WITH (Underline Indicates Conflicting Compatibility Information)

Consult pharmacist; specific conditions may apply; see Compatibilities, p. xvi.

Additive: Chloramphenicol (Chloromycetin), lidocaine, nafcillin (Nafcil), penicillin G potassium, <u>thiopental (Pentothal)</u>.

Syringe: Pentobarbital (Nembutal).

Y-site: Etomidate (Amidate), hetastarch in electrolytes (Hextend), propofol (Diprivan).

RATE OF ADMINISTRATION

Each 10 mg or fraction thereof over 1 minute.

ACTIONS

A sympathomimetic drug that stimulates both alpha- and beta-adrenergic receptors. It is less potent but longer acting than epinephrine. It has positive inotropic action, increasing the strength of myocardial contraction. It increases the HR and elevates the BP. Some arteriolar vasoconstriction occurs. It stimulates the CNS, relaxes the smooth muscle of the bronchi and GI tract, and dilates the pupils. Metabolic rate and respiratory rate are increased. Widely distributed in body fluids, ephedrine crosses the blood-brain barrier. It is excreted in urine. Secreted in breast milk.

INDICATIONS AND USES

Bronchospasm. ▪ Hypotension. ▪ Bradycardia caused by atrioventricular block. ▪ Pressor agent during spinal anesthesia. ▪ Stokes-Adams syndrome. ▪ Allergic disorders (epinephrine preferred). ▪ Narcotic, barbiturate, and alcohol poisoning. Generally replaced by more effective agents for all uses.

CONTRAINDICATIONS

Hypersensitivity to ephedrine; labor and delivery if maternal BP exceeds 130/80 mm Hg (may cause prolonged uterine atony with hemorrhage); narrow-angle glaucoma; psychoneurosis. Do not use to treat overdosage of phenothiazines (e.g., chlorpromazine [Thorazine]). A further drop in BP and irreversible shock may result. One manufacturer states that it is contraindicated during anesthesia with halogenated anesthetics (e.g., halothane).

PRECAUTIONS

See label; only specific solutions can be given IV. ▪ Use caution in heart disease, angina, diabetes, hyperthyroidism, and prostatic hypertrophy. ▪ Has a cumulative effect.

Monitor: Check BP every 5 minutes. ▪ See Drug/Lab Interactions.

Maternal/Child: Category C: may cause anoxia in fetus. ▪ Safety for use in breast-feeding not established. ▪ See Contraindications.

DRUG/LAB INTERACTIONS

Do not use concomitantly with other sympathomimetic agents (e.g., dopamine [Intropin], dobutamine [Dobutrex], epinephrine). Additive effects may cause toxicity. ▪ MAO inhibitors (e.g., selegiline [Eldepryl]) and furazolidone (Furoxone) increase pressor response and may cause hypertensive crisis and intracranial hemorrhage. ▪ May cause severe hypertension with oxytocics (e.g., oxytocin [Pitocin]). ▪ Cyclopropane or halogenated anesthetics (e.g., halothane, isoflurane) and digoxin may sensitize myocardium and increase risk of arrhythmias. ▪ Reserpine (Hydropres), methyldopa (Aldomet), and tricyclic antidepressants (e.g., amytriptyline [Elavil]) may decrease pressor response and decrease effectiveness. ▪ Atropine blocks reflex bradycardia enhancing pressor effect; observe for hypertension. ▪ Antihypertensive effect of guanethidine (Ismelin) may be decreased; monitor carefully. ▪ Urinary alkalinizers (e.g., acetazolamide, sodium bicarbonate) decrease ephedrine elimination and increase risk of toxicity with prolonged use. ▪ Alpha- and beta-blocking drugs (e.g., phentolamine [Regitine], propranolol [Inderal]) antagonize effects of ephedrine. ▪ Use with theophylline may increase CNS and GI side effects. ▪ Interacts with many other drugs. ▪ See Contraindications.

SIDE EFFECTS

Rare in therapeutic doses; anorexia, cardiac arrhythmias, headache, insomnia, nausea, nervousness, painful urination, palpitations, precordial pain, sweating, tachycardia, urinary retention, vertigo, vomiting. Confusion, delirium, euphoria, and hallucinations may occur with higher doses. Convulsions, pulmonary edema, and respiratory failure may occur with overdose.

ANTIDOTE

If side effects occur, discontinue drug and notify physician. Side effects may be treated symptomatically. Treat hypotension with IV fluids; vasopressors (e.g., dopamine [Intropin]) are contraindicated. Treat hypertension with phentolamine (Regitine) and convulsions with diazepam (Valium). Treat cardiac arrhythmias with beta blockers (e.g., propranolol [Inderal]). Resuscitate as necessary.

EPINEPHRINE HYDROCHLORIDE

(ep-i-nef′rin hi-dro-klor′id)

Cardiac stimulant
Bronchodilator
Antiallergic
Vasopressor

Adrenalin Chloride

pH 2.5 to 5

USUAL DOSE

Hypersensitivity reactions or bronchospasm: 0.1 to 0.25 mg (1 to 2.5 ml of a 1:10,000 concentration). Start with a small dose, giving only as much as required to alleviate undesirable symptoms, and repeat as necessary (usually every 20 to 30 minutes), gradually increasing dose depending on need. Another source suggests 0.2 to 0.5 mg of 1:10,000 concentration. May be repeated as necessary.

Cardiac arrest: AHA guidelines recommend 1 mg (10 ml of a 1:10,000 concentration) IV; may repeat every 3 to 5 minutes. Follow each dose with a 20-ml IV flush to ensure delivery to systemic circulation. See Incompatible With. If the 1-mg dose is not effective, up to 0.2 mg/kg may be used to treat ventricular fibrillation, pulseless ventricular tachycardia, asystole, or pulseless electrical activity. Alternately, may be given as a continuous infusion by adding 30 mg (30 ml of a 1:1,000 concentration) to 250 ml NS or D5W. Infuse at 100 ml/hr and titrate to response.

Endotracheal: A diluted solution may be given through the endotracheal tube before an IV is established. AHA guidelines recommend 2 to 2.5 mg diluted in 10 ml NS.

Vasopressor or maintenance dose: 1 to 10 mcg/min titrated to desired response, AHA guidelines recommend that epinephrine be used to treat symptomatic bradycardia after atropine, dopamine, and transcutaneous pacing. For profound bradycardia or hypotension 2 to 10 mcg/min may be given as an infusion (1 mg of 1:1,000 concentration in 500 ml NS) at a rate of 1 to 5 ml/min.

PEDIATRIC DOSE

See Maternal/Child.

Hypersensitivity reactions or bronchospasm in infants and children: 0.01 mg/kg (0.1 ml/kg of a 1:10,000 concentration). May repeat at 20-minute to 4-hour intervals. One source suggests a maximum dose of 0.3 mg, another 0.5 mg. Usually given SC as a 1:1,000 concentration.

Severe anaphylactic shock in infants and children: One source suggests 0.1 mg IV of a 1:100,000 concentration (0.1 ml of 1:1,000 concentration diluted in 10 ml NS) given over 5 to 10 minutes. Another source suggests 0.01 ml/kg of a 1:1,000 concentration SC. Maximum 0.3 ml/dose. Repeat every 15 minutes as needed.

Bradycardia in infants and children: AHA guidelines recommend 0.01 mg/kg (0.1 ml/kg of 1:10,000 concentration) to treat symptomatic bradycardia. May be given as an infusion. Begin with 0.1 to 1 mcg/kg/minute then titrate to response. AHA guidelines recommend 0.1 mg/kg (0.1 ml/kg) of a 1:1,000 concentration via ET.

Asystolic or pulseless arrest in infants and children: AHA guidelines recommend 0.01 mg/kg (0.1 ml/kg of a 1:10,000 concentration). Repeat every 3 to 5 minutes during arrest. Up to 0.1 to 0.2 mg/kg may be used if initial doses are ineffective. May be given via ET (0.1 mg/kg [0.1 ml/kg of a 1:1,000 concentration]) every 3 to 5 minutes until IV established, then begin with first IV dose. Another source suggests 0.01 to 0.03 mg/kg of 1:10,000 concentration initially. May repeat every 3 to 5 minutes in neonates. In infants and children subsequent doses of 0.1 mg/kg every 3 to 5 minutes may be given if needed. Prepare an infusion and titrate from 0.1 to 1 mcg/kg/min to desired effect. Use upper dosing range if asystole present. With higher dose, be aware of preservative content to avoid toxicity.

DOSE ADJUSTMENTS

See Drug/Lab Interactions. ■ Doses larger than 1 mg may not be indicated in patients over 65 years of age and patients in ventricular fibrillation.

DILUTION

Check label. Not all epinephrine solutions can be given IV.

IV Injection: Available prediluted (0.1 mg/ml [1:10,000 solution]) in 3-ml and 10-ml syringes. Each 1 mg (1 ml) of 1:1,000 solution must be diluted in at least 10 ml of NS to prepare a 1:10,000 solution. Available in a 30-ml vial (30 mg [1:1,000 solution]) to facilitate larger doses or continuous infusion.

Infusion: For occasional use as a vasopressor or for maintenance, epinephrine may be further diluted in 250 to 500 ml D5W. Give through Y-tube or three-way stopcock of infusion set. See chart on inside back cover for additional compatible solutions.

Epinephrine HCl Infusion Rates*

Desired Dose	1 mg in 500 ml D5W (2 mcg/ml)			1 mg in 250 ml D5W 2 mg in 500 ml D5W (4 mcg/ml)		
mcg/min	mcg/hr	ml/min	ml/hr	mcg/hr	ml/min	ml/hr
1	60	0.5	30	60	0.25	15
2	120	1	60	120	0.5	30
3	180	1.5	90	180	0.75	45
4	240	2	120	240	1	60
5	300	2.5	150	300	1.25	75

Continued

Epinephrine HCl Infusion Rates*—cont'd						
Desired Dose	1 mg in 500 ml D5W (2 mcg/ml)			1 mg in 250 ml D5W 2 mg in 500 ml D5W (4 mcg/ml)		
mcg/min	mcg/hr	ml/min	ml/hr	mcg/hr	ml/min	ml/hr
6	360	3	180	360	1.5	90
7	420	3.5	210	420	1.75	105
8	480	4	240	480	2	120
*Pediatric infusion: 0.6 mg/kg in 100 ml D5W – 1 ml/hr = 0.1 mcg/kg/min						

In ***cardiac arrest,*** 30 mg is sometimes added to 250 ml of NS or D5W (120 mcg/ml).

Storage: Do not use if brown or if a sediment is present. Deteriorates rapidly. Protect from light.

INCOMPATIBLE WITH

Manufacturer states, "Readily destroyed and precipitate forms with alkalis, alkaline solutions (e.g., sodium bicarbonate and oxidizing agents)." ***If co-administration with sodium bicarbonate is indicated, give at separate sites.*** Unstable in any solution with a pH over 5.5 (e.g., aminophylline, ampicillin, lidocaine, thiopental [Pentothal], warfarin [Coumadin]).

COMPATIBLE WITH **(Underline Indicates Conflicting Compatibility Information)**

See Incompatible With. Consult pharmacist; specific conditions may apply; see Compatibilities, p. xvi.

Additive: Amikacin (Amikin), cimetidine (Tagamet), dobutamine (Dobutrex), furosemide (Lasix), ranitidine (Zantac), verapamil (Isoptin).

Syringe: Doxapram (Dopram), heparin, milrinone (Primacor), and selected contrast agents used in radiology.

Y-site: Atracurium (Tracrium), calcium chloride, calcium gluconate, cisatracurium (Nimbex), diltiazem (Cardizem), dobutamine (Dobutrex), dopamine (Intropin), famotidine (Pepcid IV), fentanyl (Sublimaze), furosemide (Lasix), heparin, hetastarch in electrolytes (Hextend), hydrocortisone sodium succinate (Solu-Cortef), hydromorphone (Dilaudid), inamrinone (Inocor), labetalol (Normodyne), levofloxacin (Levaquin), lorazepam (Ativan), midazolam (Versed), milrinone (Primacor), morphine, nicardipine (Cardene IV), nitroglycerin (Nitro-Bid IV), norepinephrine (Levophed), pancuronium (Pavulon), phytonadione (Aquamephyton), potassium chloride (KCl), propofol (Diprivan), ranitidine (Zantac), remifentanil (Ultiva), vecuronium (Norcuron), warfarin (Coumadin).

RATE OF ADMINISTRATION

IV injection: Each 1 mg or fraction thereof over 1 minute or longer. May be given more rapidly in cardiac resuscitation; follow with 20-ml IV flush.

Infusion: Vasopressor or maintenance: 1 to 10 mcg/min titrated to desired patient response.

Cardiac arrest: Titrated to deliver a single dose over 3 to 5 minutes based on patient response. Must be delivered by central venous access. Use an infusion pump to control rate.

ACTIONS

A naturally occurring hormone secreted by the adrenal glands. A sympathomimetic drug, it imitates almost all actions of the sympathetic nervous system. It is a vasoconstrictor and delays the absorption of many drugs; a potent cardiac stimulant, it strengthens the myocardial contraction (positive inotropic effect) and increases cardiac rate (positive chronotropic effect). Increases myocardial and cerebral blood flow during CPR. A potent dilator or relaxant of smooth muscle, especially bronchial muscle. Decreases blood supply to the abdomen and increases blood supply to skeletal muscles. Elevates systolic BP, lowers diastolic BP, and increases pulse pressure. Seldom used as a vasopressor because of its short duration of action. It is rapidly inactivated in the body by various enzymes and excreted in changed form in the urine. Crosses placental barrier. Secreted in breast milk.

INDICATIONS AND USES

Cardiac resuscitation. First-line drug of choice when initial CPR, intubation, ventilation, and initial defibrillation have failed to achieve response in ventricular fibrillation, pulseless ventricular tachycardia, asystole, or pulseless electrical activity. ■ Drug of choice for anaphylactic shock. ■ Antidote of choice for histamine overdose and allergic reactions including bronchial asthma, urticaria, and angioneurotic edema. ■ Stokes-Adams syndrome. ■ Occasionally used as a vasopressor (e.g., symptomatic bradycardia).

CONTRAINDICATIONS

Anesthesia with halogenated hydrocarbons or cyclopropane; cerebral arteriosclerosis, hypertension, labor and delivery if maternal BP exceeds 130/80 mm Hg (may cause prolonged uterine atony with hemorrhage), hyperthyroidism, narrow-angle glaucoma, nervous instability, organic brain damage, patients receiving high doses of digitalis, shock. Do not use to treat overdosage of adrenergic blocking agents (e.g., phenoxybenzamine [Dibenzyline]), phenothiazines (e.g., chlorpromazine [Thorazine]), methotrimeprazine (Levoprome); a further drop in BP will occur and irreversible shock may result. Do not use concurrently with esmolol (Brevibloc).

PRECAUTIONS

Usual route is SC except in cardiac resuscitation or as a vasopressor infusion. ■ Give intracardiac only if no other route is available. ■ Use caution in the elderly, diabetics, in hypotension (except in anaphylactic shock), patients receiving thyroid preparations, and those with long-term emphysema or bronchial asthma with degenerative heart disease. ■ Often used with corticosteroids in treatment of anaphylactic shock. ■ Increasing BP and HR may cause myocardial ischemia, angina, and increased myocardial oxygen demand. ■ Larger doses in cardiac arrest are based on optimal response range of epinephrine (0.045 to 0.2 mg/kg). May not improve survival or neurologic outcome and may cause postresuscitation myocardial dysfunction. ■ Higher doses may be required to treat poison-induced shock.

Monitor: Check BP every 5 minutes. ■ Vasoconstriction-induced tissue sloughing can occur. Avoid administering in areas of limited blood supply (e.g., fingers, toes) or if peripheral vascular disease is present. ■ Infusion during cardiac arrest must be administered by central venous access to ensure delivery to systemic circulation and to avoid extravasation. ■ Intracardiac injection or IV injection in cardiac arrest must be accompanied by cardiac massage to perfuse drug into the myocardium and permit effective defibrillation. ■ Correct acidosis, hypoxemia. ■ See Drug/Lab Interactions.

Maternal/Child: Category C: may cause anoxia in fetus. ■ Discontinue breast-feeding. May produce tachyarrhythmias in pediatric patients. ■ High dose infusions may produce profound vasoconstriction compromising perfusion. Even lower doses may compromise renal and splanchnic blood flow. ■ Contraindicated in treatment of VT secondary to cocaine. ■ See Contraindications.

Elderly: See Dose Adjustments and Precautions.

DRUG/LAB INTERACTIONS

May be used alternately with isoproterenol (Isuprel), but they may not be used together. Both are direct cardiac stimulants and death may result. Adequate interval between doses must be maintained. ■ Simultaneous use with oxytocics (e.g., ergonovine), MAO inhibitors (e.g., isocarboxazid [Marplan]), furazolidone (Furoxone), or guanethidine (Ismelin) may cause hypertensive crisis. ■ Pressor response increased by anesthetics (e.g., halothane, cyclopropane), tricyclic antidepressants (e.g., amitriptyline [Elavil]), antihistamines (e.g., diphenhydramine [Benadryl]), rauwolfia alkaloids (e.g., reserpine [Serpasil]), sodium levothyroxine, and urinary alkalizers; may cause hypertension. ■ May cause hypertension with beta-adrenergic blockers (e.g., propranolol [Inderal]) and alpha-adrenergic blockers (e.g., phentolamine [Regitine]). ■ Inhibited by ergot alkaloids and phenothiazines (e.g., prochlorperazine [Compazine]). ■ Inhibits insulin and oral hypoglycemic agents; increased dose may be required. ■ May cause arrhythmias with bretylium. ■ Interacts with many other drugs. ■ See Contraindications for additional drug interactions.

SIDE EFFECTS

Often transitory; sometimes occur with average doses.

Anxiety, dizziness, dyspnea, glycosuria, pallor, palpitations.

Overdose (frequently caused by too-rapid injection): Cerebrovascular hemorrhage, collapse (rapid), fibrillation, headache (severe), hypertension, hypotension (irreversible), pulmonary edema, pupillary dilation, restlessness, tachycardia, weakness, death.

ANTIDOTE

If side effects from the average dose become progressively worse, discontinue the drug and notify the physician. IM or SC route may be preferable. For a severe reaction caused by toxicity, treat the patient for shock and administer an antihypertensive agent such as phentolamine (Regitine) or nitroprusside sodium. Treat cardiac arrhythmias with a beta-adrenergic blocker (propranolol [Inderal]). Resuscitate as necessary.

EPIRUBICIN HYDROCHLORIDE

(ep′e-roo′buh-sin hye-droe-klor′id)

Antineoplastic (anthracycline antibiotic)

Ellence ▪ ✤Pharmorubicin PFS

pH 3 ▪ pH 4 to 5.5

USUAL DOSE

In combination therapies, epirubicin is used instead of doxorubicin in the combination regimen. Usually given on the same days and at the same intervals as the doxorubicin it replaces.

Ellence

Recommended starting dose is 100 to 120 mg/M^2. Patients receiving the 120-mg/M^2 dose should also receive prophylactic antibiotic therapy with sulfamethoxazole-trimethoprim (e.g., Bactrim, Septra) or a fluoroquinolone (e.g., ciprofloxacin [Cipro]). Ellence is usually given in repeated 3- to 4-week cycles. Total dose may be given on day 1 of each cycle or equally divided and given on days 1 and 8 of each cycle.

Another regimen used is 60 mg/M^2 as an infusion on days 1 and 8 given in a regimen with oral cyclophosphamide 75 mg/M^2 on days 1 to 14 and fluorouracil 500 mg/M^2 on days 1 and 8. Repeat every 28 days for six cycles.

✤Pharmorubicin PFS

Metastatic breast cancer: ***Single agent:*** 75 to 90 mg/M^2 once every 21 days. This dose may be divided and given on day 1 and day 2. An alternative weekly dose schedule of 12.5 to 25 mg/M^2 has been used and has been reported to produce less clinical toxicity than higher doses given every 3 weeks. ***Combination therapy:*** 50 mg/M^2. Used in combination with cyclophosphamide and fluorouracil.

Early-stage breast cancer (Stage II-IIIA): 50 to 60 mg/M^2 given on days 1 and 8 every 4 weeks. Used in combination with cyclophosphamide and fluorouracil.

Small-cell lung cancer: ***Single agent:*** 90 to 120 mg/M^2 once every 3 weeks. ***Combination therapy:*** 50 to 90 mg/M^2. Several combinations have been used (e.g., with either cisplatin or ifosfamide; with cyclophosphamide and vincristine; with cyclophosphamide and etoposide, or with cisplatin and etoposide).

Non–small-cell lung cancer: ***Single agent:*** 120 to 150 mg/M^2 on day 1 every 3 to 4 weeks. ***Combination therapy:*** 90 to 120 mg/M^2 on day 1 every 3 to 4 weeks. Used in combination with cisplatin, etoposide, mitomycin, vinblastine, and vindesine.

Non-Hodgkin's lymphoma: ***Single agent:*** 75 to 90 mg/M^2 once every 3 weeks. ***Combination therapy:*** 60 to 75 mg/M^2. Used in combination with cyclophosphamide, prednisone, and vincristine with or without bleomycin for the treatment of newly diagnosed non-Hodgkin's lymphoma.

Hodgkin's disease: ***Combination therapy:*** 35 mg/M^2 once every 2 weeks or 70 mg/M^2 once every 3 to 4 weeks. Used in combination with bleomycin, dacarbazine, and vinblastine.

Ovarian cancer: ***Single agent:*** 50 to 90 mg/M^2 once every 3 or 4 weeks in patients who have had prior therapy. ***Combination therapy:*** 50 to 90 mg/M^2 once every 3 or 4 weeks can be added to their regimen in patients who have had prior therapy; or the same dose in combination with cisplatin and cyclophosphamide is used for initial therapy of ovarian cancer.

Locally unresectable or metastatic gastric cancer: ***Single agent:*** 75 to 100 mg/M^2 once every 3 weeks. ***Combination therapy:*** 80 mg/M^2 once every 3 to 4 weeks. Used in combination with fluorouracil.

ALL FORMULATIONS

Soft tissue sarcoma (unlabeled): 45 to 60 mg/M^2/day for 2 to 3 days of a 21- or 28-day treatment cycle. Up to 150 to 180 mg/M^2 has been given on day 1 of a 21-day treatment cycle for 8 cycles. This higher dose has not proven to be more effective but is more toxic; G-CSF support required.

Esophageal and esophagogastric junction cancers (unlabeled): 50 mg/M^2 on day 1 of a 21-day treatment cycle. Use in conjunction with cisplatin on day 1 and a continuous infusion of fluorouracil for up to 8 cycles. An alternate regimen uses epirubicin 50 to 60 mg/M^2 on day 1 or 20 mg/M^2 on days 1 to 3 of a 28-day treatment cycle in conjunction with cisplatin and fluorouracil for up to 6 cycles.

PEDIATRIC DOSE

Specific information on safety for use in children not available. See Maternal/Child.

DOSE ADJUSTMENTS

ALL FORMULATIONS: Reduced dose required with elevated serum bilirubin. Give 50% of a dose for serum bilirubin from 1.2 to 3 mg/dl or AST 2 to 4 times upper limit of normal. Give 25% of a dose for serum bilirubin greater than 3 mg/ml or AST greater than 4 times upper limit of normal. **ELLENCE:** Reduce dose to 75 to 90 mg/M^2 in heavily pretreated patients, those with pre-existing bone marrow depression, or in the presence of neoplastic bone marrow infiltration. ▪ Consider reduced dose in patients with severe renal impairment (SrCr greater than 5 mg/dl). ▪ Base dose adjustments after the first treatment cycle on hematologic response during treatment cycle nadir and nonhematologic toxicities. In patients who received the full dose on day 1, reduce dose to 75% of initial first dose in subsequent cycles for platelet count less than 50,000/mm^3, absolute neutrophil count (ANC) less than 250/mm^3, neutropenic fever, or grades 3 or 4 nonhematologic toxicity. Delay dose in subsequent treatment cycles until platelet count recovers to at least 100,000/mm^3, ANC recovers to at least 1,500/mm^3, and nonhematologic toxicities have recovered to equal to or less than grade 1. For patients receiving a divided dose, reduce the day-8 dose to 75% of the day-1 dose if platelet counts are 75,000 to 100,000/mm^3 and ANC is 1,000 to 1,499/mm^3. Omit the day-8 dose if platelet counts are less than 75,000/mm^3, ANC less than 1,000/mm^3, or grade 3 or 4 nonhematologic toxicity has occurred.

✤PHARMORUBICIN PFS: Use lower dose in range for patients with inadequate marrow reserves due to old age, prior therapy, or neoplastic marrow infiltration. ▪ Reduced dose, delay, or suspension of epirubicin may be required based on hematologic toxicity; manufacturer provides no specific recommendations. ▪ No dose adjustment required in impaired renal function.

DILUTION

Specific techniques required; see Precautions.

Ellence: Available as 2 mg/ml in 25-ml and 100-ml vials. A ready-to-use, preservative-free solution; further dilution not required. Must be given through Y-tube or three-way stopcock of a free-flowing infusion of NS or D5W.

Pharmorubicin PFS: Available as 2 mg/ml in 5-ml, 25-ml, and 100-ml vials. Use of the 100-ml vial should be restricted to a pharmacy admixture program using a sterile transfer or dispensing device. Enter any vial only once and withdraw desired dose into a syringe. No further dilution is required.

Storage: ***Ellence:*** Refrigerate vials at 2° to 8° C (34° to 46° F); protect from light. Do not freeze. Must be used within 24 hours of first penetration of vial. Discard unused solution.

Pharmorubicin: Store unopened PFS vials in refrigerator; keep in original cartons to protect from light. Use any filled syringe within 24 hours if stored at room temperature and within 48 hours if refrigerated. Syringes prepared from the pharmacy bulk vial must be used within 24 or 48 hours of the initial puncture of that vial based on method of storage. Once the transfer set has been inserted in the bulk vial, any remaining undispensed drug must be discarded in 8 hours.

INCOMPATIBLE WITH

Manufacturers recommend not mixing with other drugs in the same syringe. Avoid prolonged contact with alkaline solutions; will result in hydrolysis of all forms of epirubicin. Do not mix with heparin or fluorouracil (5-FU); may precipitate. Incompatible with ifosfamide (Ifex) when combined in syringe or solution with mesna (Mesnex).

COMPATIBLE WITH

See Incompatible With. Consult pharmacist; specific conditions may apply; see Compatibilities, p. xvi.

Syringe: Ifosfamide (Ifex).

RATE OF ADMINISTRATION

IV injection: ***All formulations:*** A single dose over a minimum of 3 to 5 minutes. Must be given through Y-tube or three-way stopcock of a free-flowing infusion of NS or D5W. Slow injection rate further for erythematous streaking along the vein or facial flushing.

ACTIONS

A semisynthetic, anthracycline, antineoplastic antibiotic agent. Exact method of action is unknown. Rapidly penetrates cell and interferes with cell division by binding with DNA to slow production of nucleic acid synthesis. Free radicals cause further cytotoxic activity. Metabolized in the liver, the process of glucuronidation distinguishes epirubicin from doxorubicin and may account for its faster elimination and reduced toxicity. It is less toxic and in particular less cardiotoxic than doxorubicin. Has the same antitumor effect at equal doses. WBC nadir is reached in 10 to 14 days and should return to normal by day 21. Elimination half-life is 30 to 40 hours. Does not cross blood-brain barrier. Primarily excreted in bile; some excretion in urine.

INDICATIONS AND USES

Ellence: Used in combination with other agents in the treatment of patients with evidence of axillary-node tumor involvement following resection in primary breast cancer. **Pharmorubicin:** Treatment of metastatic as well as early stage breast cancer, small-cell lung cancer (both limited and extensive disease), advanced non–small-cell lung cancer, non-Hodgkin's lymphoma, Hodgkin's disease, Stage III and IV ovarian cancer, and metastatic and locally unresectable gastric cancers. May be used as a single agent or in combination with other chemotherapeutic agents.

Unlabeled uses: ***All formulations:*** Treatment of soft-tissue sarcomas in combination with other agents. Treatment of esophageal and esophagogastric junction cancers in combination with other agents. Ellence has been used in place of Pharmorubicin for various indications.

CONTRAINDICATIONS

History of severe cardiac disease, recent MI, or severe hepatic disease. Baseline neutrophil count less than 1,500 cells/mm^3 or myelosuppression resulting from treatment with other antineoplastic agents or radiation therapy. Contraindicated in patients who have received previous treatment with maximum recommended cumulative doses of daunorubicin (Cerubidine), doxorubicin (Adriamycin), idarubicin (Idamycin), mitoxantrone (Novantrone), or mitomycin C. Hypersensitivity to epirubicin, other anthracyclines, or anthracenediones.

PRECAUTIONS

Follow guidelines for handling cytotoxic agents. See Appendix A, p. 1142. In addition to standard precautions, treat spills or leakage with 1% sodium hypochlorite. For accidental contact with eyes or skin, flush with copious amounts of water, soap and water, or sodium bicarbonate. ■ Administered by or under the direction of the physician specialist, with facilities for monitoring the patient and responding to any medical emergency. ■ For IV use only. Do not give IM or SC. ■ May cause serious, irreversible myocardial toxicity with congestive heart failure and/or cardiomyopathy as the cumulative dose approaches 900 mg/M^2. Cardiotoxicity may be acute or delayed, occurring months to years after treatment. ■ Use extreme caution in pre-existing drug-induced bone marrow suppression, existing heart disease, previous treatment with other anthracyclines (e.g., daunorubicin, doxorubicin, idarubicin), other cardiotoxic agents (e.g., bleomycin), or radiation therapy encompassing the heart; cardiac toxicity may occur at lower cumulative doses and may be additive. ■ Administration of epirubicin after previous radiation therapy may induce an inflammatory recall reaction at the irradiation site. ■ Incidence of secondary leukemia may be increased.

Monitor: Use only large veins. Avoid veins over joints or in extremities with compromised venous or lymphatic drainage. Determine absolute patency of vein. Extravasation may occur with or without stinging or burning along the injection site even if blood returns well on aspiration of the infusion needle. Observe site frequently. Extravasation can result in severe cellulitis and tissue necrosis; if it occurs, discontinue injection; use another vein. ■ Obtain baseline CBC including differential and platelet count, serum calcium and potassium, SrCr, uric acid level, liver function tests (AST, ALT, alkaline phosphatase, and serum bilirubin), ECG, chest x-ray, and echocardiogram. Monitor lab values during therapy, especially before each dose. Monitor ECG, chest x-ray, echocardiogram, and/or radionuclide angiography in patients who have had mediastinal radiation, other anthracycline or anthracene therapy, those with pre-existing cardiac disease, or S/S of impending heart disease, or those who have received prior epirubicin cumulative doses exceeding 550 mg/M^2. ■ Monitor for signs of cardiac toxicity (e.g., rapid or irregular HR, shortness of breath, swelling of abdomen, feet, and lower legs); early signs usually include sinus tachycardia and non-specific ST-T wave changes in the ECG. ■ Prevention and treatment of hyperuricemia due to tumor lysis syndrome may be accomplished with adequate hydration, and if necessary, allopurinol and alkalinization of urine. ■ Be alert for signs of bone marrow depression, bleeding, or infection. ■ Use of prophylactic antibiotics may be indicated pending C/S in a febrile, neutropenic patient. ■ Monitor for thrombocytopenia (platelet count less than 50,000/mm^3). Initiate precautions to prevent excessive bleeding (e.g., inspect IV sites, skin, and mucous membranes; use extreme care during invasive procedures; test urine, emesis, stool, and secretions for occult blood). ■ Prophylactic antiemetics are indicated. ■ See Drug/Lab Interactions.

Patient Education: Urine will be reddish for several days (from drug, not hematuria). ■ Nonhormonal birth control recommended. May induce chromosomal damage in sperm. Effective contraception suggested for men receiving epirubicin. ■ Report IV site burning, stinging, or puffiness promptly. ■ Report rapid or irregular HR, shortness of breath, and swelling of the abdomen, feet, or lower legs. ■ Review side effects; may be severe (e.g., nausea and vomiting, cardiotoxicity). ■ See Appendix D, p. 1148.

Maternal/Child: Category D: can cause fetal harm. Avoid pregnancy. May cause testicular atrophy. ■ Discontinue breast-feeding. ■ Information on safety for use in children not available. Some studies suggest that children may be at greater risk for anthracycline-induced acute cardiotoxicity and/or chronic CHF.

Elderly: Cardiotoxicity and myelotoxicity may be more severe; monitor closely for dose-related toxicities. ■ See Dose Adjustments. ■ There is a major decrease in plasma clearance of epirubicin in women over 70 years of age; monitor closely for signs of toxicity. ■ See Dose Adjustments.

DRUG/LAB INTERACTIONS

May increase bone marrow toxicity of other chemotherapeutic agents. ■ Increased toxicity including skin redness and exfoliative changes possible when given concurrently with or after radiation. ■ Monitoring of cardiac function may be indicated in patients taking medications that may cause heart failure (e.g., calcium channel blockers such as verapamil [Isoptin]), beta-blockers (e.g., propranolol [Inderal]). ■ Plasma clearance decreased and serum levels increased by cimetidine (Tagamet), discontinue cimetidine. ■ Hepatic toxicity may be increased with concurrent use of other hepatotoxic agents (e.g., methotrexate, isoniazid [INH]). ■ Risk of cardiotoxicity increased in patients previously treated with maximum cumulative doses of other anthracyclines (e.g., doxorubicin [Adriamycin], idarubicin [Idamycin]) and/or radiation encompassing the heart. ■ Leukopenic and/or thrombocytopenic effects may be increased with drugs that cause blood dyscrasias (e.g., anticonvulsants [e.g., carbamazepine (Tegretol), phenytoin (Dilantin)], NSAIDs [e.g., ibuprofen (Advil, Motrin), naproxen (Aleve, Naprosyn)]). Adjust dose based on differential and platelet count. ■ Do not administer live vaccines to patients receiving antineoplastic agents. ■ See Precautions.

SIDE EFFECTS

Dose-limiting toxicities are infection, myelosuppression (anemia, leukopenia, neutropenia, thrombocytopenia), and cardiotoxicity (usually delayed manifested by reduced LVEF and/or S/S of CHF [e.g., ascites, dependent edema, dyspnea, gallop rhythm, hepatomegaly, pleural effusion, pulmonary edema, tachycardia]). Severe cellulitis, vesication, local pain, and tissue necrosis can occur with extravasation. Venous sclerosis may result from injection into small veins or repeated injection into the same vein. Other side effects are alopecia, amenorrhea, anorexia, arrhythmias (transient), conjunctivitis, diarrhea, febrile neutropenia, fever, hot flashes, itching, keratosis, malaise, mucositis (esophagitis, stomatitis), nausea and vomiting, phlebitis, rash, recall of skin reaction associated with prior radiation. Hypersensitivity reactions have been reported.

Overdose: May cause an acute myocardial dysfunction within 24 hours. Pronounced mucositis, leukopenia, and thrombocytopenia may occur within 7 to 14 days.

ANTIDOTE

Most side effects will either be tolerated or treated symptomatically. Keep the physician informed. Hematopoietic toxicity (leukopenia, thrombocytopenia) may require dose reduction or cessation of therapy, antibiotics, platelet and granulocyte transfusions, oprelvekin (Neumega), darbepoetin alfa [Aranesp], epoetin alfa (Epogen, Procrit), filgrastim (Neupogen), pegfilgrastim (Neulasta), or sargramostim (Leukine). Acute cardiac failure occurs suddenly (most common when total cumulative doses approach 900 mg/M^2) and frequently does not respond to currently available treatment. Close monitoring of accumulated dose, bone marrow, ECG, chest x-ray, echocardiography, and systolic ejection fraction may prevent most serious and potentially fatal cardiac side effects. There is no specific antidote. Supportive therapy as indicated will help sustain the patient in toxicity. Dexrazoxane is currently available to prevent cardiotoxicity of doxorubicin in specific situations; in the future it may be considered with epirubicin. If extravasation occurs, attempt aspiration of the infiltrated epirubicin. Elevate the extremity and apply local intermittent ice compresses for up to 3 days. Observe the site frequently. Should be seen by a reconstructive surgeon if local pain persists or skin changes progress after 3 to 4 days. Ulceration may require early wide excision of the involved area. Treat hypersensitivity reactions as indicated.

EPOETIN ALFA

(e-poi'ah-tin al'fah)

Recombinant human erythropoietin
Antianemic agent

EPO, Epogen, ♣Eprex, Erythropoietin, Procrit **pH 6.6 to 7.2**

USUAL DOSE

In all situations rate of hematocrit increase is dose dependent and varies among patients. Availability of iron stores, baseline hematocrit, and concurrent medical problems affect the rate and extent of response. See Monitor.

Anemia of chronic renal failure in adults: May be given by IV or SC injection. 50 to 100 units/kg of body weight 3 times a week initially. Range is from 15 to 500 units/kg/dose. Median dose is 75 to 100 units/kg. A 55-kg (120-lb) individual would receive 2,750 units at 50 units/kg, 4,125 units at 75 units/kg, and 5,500 units at 100 units/kg. Entire contents of a vial (2,000, 3,000, or 4,000 units) has been used instead of an exact calculated dose. Predialysis patients usually require doses in the average range, peritoneal dialysis patients respond rapidly to lower doses, and higher-end doses may be required, especially in dialysis patients (see literature). Reduce dose by 25 units/kg when the hemoglobin concentration reaches 10 Gm/dl or the hematocrit reaches the target range (30% to 36%) or rises more than 4 points in any 2-week period. Increase dose by 25 units/kg if the hematocrit does not increase by 5 to 6 points after 8 weeks of therapy and is below target range. Continue to increase by 25 units/kg/dose at 4- to 6-week intervals until target range is reached.

Maintenance dose: Individually titrated. After reaching target range, reduce by 25 units/kg. Median maintenance dose is 75 units/kg 3 times/week; range is 12.5 to 525 units/kg 3 times weekly. Adjust dose by 10 to 25 units/kg increments at 2- to 6-week intervals to keep hematocrit in target range. Evaluate iron stores if hematocrit falls; see Monitor.

Anemia in HIV-infected patients, including zidovudine-induced: May be given IV or SC. 100 units/kg 3 times a week for 8 weeks. Obtain endogenous serum erythropoietin level (before transfusion) before initiating therapy; see Monitor. After 8 weeks of therapy, the dose may be increased by 50 to 100 units/kg 3 times a week (total dose of 150 to 200 units/kg). Evaluate response every 4 to 8 weeks and adjust dose accordingly by 50 to 100 units/kg (total dose of 200 to 300 units/kg). Not likely to be effective if doses of 300 units/kg 3 times a week have not corrected the anemia.

Maintenance dose: When desired response is attained (i.e., reduced transfusion requirements or increased hematocrit), titrate dose to maintain the response. Consider variations in zidovudine (AZT) dose and presence of infectious or inflammatory episodes. If the hematocrit exceeds 40%, discontinue until the hematocrit drops to 36%. Reduce dose by 25% when treatment is resumed and titrate carefully to maintain desired hematocrit.

Anemia associated with cancer patients on chemotherapy: SC injection recommended. 100 to 150 units/kg 3 times a week. May be given with or without concomitant antineoplastic drug therapy. Obtain endogenous serum erythropoietin level (before transfusion) before initiating therapy; see Monitor. If adequate response has not occurred after 8 weeks, increase the dose up to 300 units/kg 3 times a week. Not likely to be effective if doses of 300 units/kg 3 times a week have not corrected the anemia. If the hematocrit exceeds 40%, discontinue until the hematocrit drops to 36%. Reduce dose by 25% when treatment is resumed, and titrate carefully to maintain desired hematocrit.

Reduction of allogenic blood transfusions in surgery patients: SC injection recommended. Obtain hemoglobin before initiating therapy. Should be greater than 10 Gm/dl but less than 13 Gm/dl. 300 units/kg/day for 10 days before surgery, on the day of surgery, and for 4 days after surgery. Has been given concurrently with anticoagulant prophylaxis. An alternate dose schedule is 600 units/kg once each week on days 21, 14, and 7 before surgery and again on the day of surgery. Begin iron supplementation no later than the beginning of treatment with epoetin alfa and continue throughout the course of therapy.

PEDIATRIC DOSE

May be given by IV or SC injection.

Anemia of chronic renal failure requiring dialysis: ***Initial:*** 50 units/kg of body weight 3 times a week. Increase dose if after 8 weeks, the hematocrit has not increased by 5 to 6 points and is still below the desired range (30% to 36%). Decrease dose if the hematocrit approaches 36% or increases by more than 4 points in any 2-week period. See all comments in the similar section under Usual Dose.

Maintenance: Gradually decrease to the lowest dose that will maintain the hematocrit at the desired level (30% to 36%). See all comments in the similar section under Usual Dose.

Anemia of chronic renal failure not requiring dialysis, children ages 3 months to 20 years: Doses of 50 to 250 units/kg 1 to 3 times a week have been reported. See comments under anemia of chronic renal failure requiring dialysis including maintenance dose and comments in the similar section under Usual Dose.

Anemia in zidovudine treated HIV-infected children, children 8 months to 17 years: Doses of 50 to 400 units/kg 2 to 3 times a week have been reported. See all comments under the similar section in Usual Dose.

Anemia in cancer patients on chemotherapy, children 6 months to 18 years: Doses of 25 to 300 units/kg 3 to 7 times a week have been reported. See all comments under the similar section in Usual Dose.

NEONATAL DOSE

Anemia of prematurity (unlabeled): 25 to 100 units/kg/dose SC 3 times a week or 200 units/kg/dose IV/SC every day or every other day for 2 to 6 weeks.

DOSE ADJUSTMENTS

Based on hematocrit. See Usual Dose for each indication. ■ Dose based on average weight if edema is present. ■ An increase in dose may be necessary in patients with aluminum toxicity. ■ See Precautions and Monitor.

DILUTION

Available in numerous concentrations; check dose on vial carefully. May be given undiluted as an IV injection. Do not shake during preparation; will render it biologically inactive. Single-dose vial contains no preservatives. Use only 1 dose per vial, then discard. Never reenter vial. Now available in multidose vial with preservative; sterile technique imperative.

Storage: Refrigerate single and multidose vials before use, multidose vial after initial use. Discard in 21 days.

COMPATIBILITY

Manufacturers state, "Do not dilute or administer in conjunction with other drug solutions." One source indicates there may be protein loss from adsorption to PVC containers and tubing. Manufacturer suggests it may be mixed 1-to-1 with bacteriostatic NS in a syringe when prepared from a single-dose vial for SC injection; see literature.

RATE OF ADMINISTRATION

A single dose over at least 1 minute.

ACTIONS

An amino acid glycoprotein manufactured by recombinant DNA technology. Has the same biologic effects as erythropoietin produced naturally by the kidneys. Stimulates bone marrow to produce RBCs, increasing the reticulocyte count within 10 days and the red cell count, hemoglobin, and hematocrit within 2 to 6 weeks. Normal iron stores are necessary because it steps up RBC production to a rate above what the body usually makes. New cells need iron, which is quickly depleted. Half-life is 4 to 13 hours. Continued therapy will maintain improved RBC levels and decrease need for transfusions. Within 2 months most patients are transfusion independent. Considered replacement therapy as insulin is to diabetics.

INDICATIONS AND USES

To treat anemia associated with chronic renal failure in adults and children and decrease the need for transfusions in patients receiving dialysis (end-stage renal disease) and those not receiving dialysis. ▪ Treatment of anemias related to zidovudine (AZT, Retrovir) therapy in HIV-infected patients. ▪ Treatment of anemia in cancer patients on chemotherapy. ▪ Treatment of anemic patients scheduled to undergo noncardiac, nonvascular surgery to reduce the need for allogenic blood transfusions, especially in patients at high risk for perioperative transfusions with significant anticipated blood loss. ▪ Not indicated for anemic patients who are willing to donate autologous blood.

Unlabeled uses: Other drug-induced anemias; rheumatoid arthritis and other chronic inflammatory diseases; sickle cell anemia; and anemia of prematurity.

CONTRAINDICATIONS

Known hypersensitivity to albumin (human) or to mammalian cell-derived products, uncontrolled hypertension.

PRECAUTIONS

All patients: May be given IV or SC in patients not receiving dialysis. May be given to dialysis patients into the venous line at the end of the dialysis procedure to eliminate additional venous access. ▪ In addition to low baseline hematocrit and inadequate iron stores, delayed or diminished response may result from concurrent medical problems (infections, inflammatory or malignant processes, occult blood loss, underlying hematologic disease, folic acid or vitamin B_{12} deficiency, hemolysis, aluminum intoxication, osteitis fibrosa cystica). ▪ Not intended for use in anemias caused by iron or folate deficiencies, hemolysis, or GI bleeding. ▪ Use caution in patients with porphyria; may exacerbate disease. ▪ Not a substitute for emergency transfusion in patients requiring immediate correction of severe anemia. ***Chronic renal failure:*** 98% of previously transfusion-dependent patients are able to maintain a stable hematocrit greater than 30% with epoetin alfa therapy. ▪ Epoetin alfa, with or without phlebotomy, has reduced iron and ferritin stores in hemodialysis patients with iron overload and associated hemosiderosis secondary to multiple RBC transfusions. ▪ Some authorities believe epoetin should be discontinued 2 weeks before planned renal engraftment to prevent risk of excessive erythrocytosis and resultant adverse effects (renal artery thrombosis with loss of graft occurred in one patient). ▪ Epoetin alfa reduces need for blood transfusions and decreases exposure to foreign histocompatibility; potential for finding a compatible graft may be increased. ***HIV infection:*** Epoetin has no effect on HIV disease process; primarily improves quality of life. ▪ Used concomitantly with filgrastim (G-CSF, Neupogen) to control granulocytopenia; filgrastim increases the neutrophil count while epoetin alfa increases the hemoglobin concentration. Helps maintain somewhat more normal counts in zidovudine therapy, but additional blood transfusions will probably be required. ***Cancer patients on chemotherapy:*** Treatment of patients with grossly elevated serum erythropoietin levels (e.g., greater than 200 mU/ml) is not recommended. ***Surgery patients:*** Safety established only for patients receiving anticoagulation prophylaxis.

Monitor: ***All patients:*** Hypertension must be controlled before initiation of therapy. Monitor BP frequently and control aggressively; generally rises when hematocrit is increasing rapidly. 25% of renal patients require an increase in antihypertensive therapy and dietary restrictions. Exacerbation of hypertension has not been observed in patients being treated with epoetin alfa for other indicated anemias; however, any indication may require a decrease in dose of epoetin if BP difficult to control or withhold epoetin until BP is controlled. ▪ CBC with differential and platelet counts; BUN; uric acid; creatinine; phosphorus; sodium; and potassium are required before treatment is initiated and at regular intervals during therapy. Modest increases are expected. Changes in dialysis treatment may be required. ▪ Normal iron stores required to support epoetin-stimulated erythropoiesis. Transferrin saturation should be at least 20% and ferritin at least 100 ng/ml. Monitor before and during therapy. Supplemental iron (ferrous sulfate 325 mg PO 3 times daily) is usually required to increase and maintain transferrin saturation. Administration of IV iron dextran may be necessary in some patients. ▪ Seizures rare, but more occur in the first 90 days. Observe BP and neurologic symptoms. Caution against driving or operating heavy machinery. ▪ Monitor patients with pre-existing vascular disease carefully (especially those with chronic renal failure); increase in hematocrit may precipitate a cerebrovascular accident, transient ischemic attack, or myocardial infarction. ▪ As anemia is corrected, elevated bleeding time decreases toward normal with epoetin treatment as it does with transfusion. ***Chronic renal failure:*** Can cause polycythemia. Baseline hematocrit required. Repeat twice weekly until stabilization in the target range (30% to 36%). Continue monitoring at regular intervals. After any dose adjustment, twice-weekly hematocrit is required for 2 to 6 weeks to evaluate outcome and make further dose adjustments. If hematocrit exceeds 36%, withhold doses and check hematocrit twice weekly until it reaches 33%. Reduce dose as indicated in Usual Dose. ▪ Dialysis patients may require additional anticoagulation with heparin to prevent clotting of artificial kidney or clotting of the vascular access (AV shunt) and to maintain efficiency of the dialysis procedure. ▪ Compliance with dialysis and/or dietary restrictions is mandatory. ▪ Monitor fluid and electrolyte balance carefully in patients not receiving dialysis. Improved sense of well-being may mask need for dialysis. ***HIV infection:*** Effectiveness in

HIV-infected patients seems to be dependent on an endogenous serum erythropoietin level less than 500 mU/ml (normal levels are 4 to 26 mU/ml) and a dose of zidovudine (AZT, Retrovir) of less than 4,200 mg/wk. ***Cancer patients on chemotherapy:*** Monitor hematocrit weekly until stable. ***Surgery patients:*** Monitor iron supplementation and anticoagulant therapy.

Patient Education: Risk of seizures, especially during first 90 days of therapy. Do not drive or operate heavy equipment. ■ Menses may resume; possibility of pregnancy. Contraception may be indicated. ■ Additional instruction (e.g., equipment, techniques) will be required in patients on home dialysis who will self-administer (manufacturer supplies brochure). ■ Stress importance of compliance with diet, iron, and vitamin (e.g., folic acid, B_{12}) supplementation.

Maternal/Child: Category C: may present risk to fetus; benefits must justify risk. ■ Use caution in nursing mothers. ■ Safety for use in children not established for diagnoses other than anemia of renal disease. ■ Limited data available for use in neonates. May contain benzyl alcohol, do not use in neonates.

Elderly: Monitor blood chemistry and BP carefully due to increased risk of renal and/or cardiovascular complications.

DRUG/LAB INTERACTIONS

Specific information not available.

SIDE EFFECTS

Generally well tolerated. Occur most frequently in patients with chronic renal failure. Increased hypertension is common, and hypertensive encephalopathy and seizures can occur. Clotted vascular access (AV shunt) and clotting of the artificial kidney may occur during dialysis. Too-rapid increase in hematocrit (over 4 points in 2 weeks) or a hematocrit over 36% (polycythemia) often occurs. Allergic reactions have been reported. Other reported side effects are those common to the underlying disease and not necessarily attributable to epoetin and include: arthralgias, asthenia, bone marrow fibrosis, cerebrovascular accident or transient ischemic attack, chest pain, cough, CVA/TIA, diarrhea, dizziness, edema, fatigue, fever, headache, hyperkalemia, myocardial infarction, nausea, rash, respiratory congestion, shortness of breath, tachycardia, and vomiting.

ANTIDOTE

Notify physician of all side effects; most will be treated symptomatically. Excessive hypertension may require discontinuation of epoetin until BP is controlled or may respond to reduction in dose of epoetin or to an increase in antihypertensive therapy. Reduce dose of epoetin in patients with an increase in hematocrit over 4 points in 2 weeks or any patient with a hematocrit over 36% (renal patients) to 40% (others). May need to withhold epoetin until hematocrit falls to 33%. Consider phlebotomy in toxicity. Additional heparin may be required during dialysis to prevent clotting. Treat minor allergic reactions symptomatically. Discontinue drug and treat anaphylaxis as indicated; resuscitate as necessary.

EPOPROSTENOL SODIUM

(e-poe-pros′ten-ol so′de-um)

Flolan

Vasodilating agent
Antihypertensive (pulmonary)

pH 10.2 to 10.8

USUAL DOSE

Acute dose ranging: May or may not take place during cardiac catheterization. May be administered through a peripheral line. Begin infusion at 2 ng/kg/min. Increase in increments of 2 ng/kg/min every 15 minutes or longer until dose-limiting pharmacologic effects occur. Flushing, headache, hypotension, nausea, vomiting are most common. See Side Effects for others. Average mean dose range in trials before side effects occurred was 8.3 to 8.9 ng/kg/min. Usually given concomitantly with anticoagulant therapy; see Monitor.

Chronic continuous infusion: May be given through a peripheral line on a temporary basis until a central venous line is established. A central venous catheter should be in place as soon as possible and must be used for continuous long-term 24-hour administration with an ambulatory infusion pump. Begin at 4 ng/kg/min less than the maximum-tolerated infusion rate determined during acute dose ranging. If the maximum-tolerated rate is less than 5 ng/kg/min, begin at one half of that rate. Average mean dose range during trials was 5 ng/kg/min.

PEDIATRIC DOSE

Safety for use in children not established. In one study, the mean maximum dose used during acute dose titration was 25 ng/kg/min. Children seemed to tolerate slightly higher long-term doses than adults.

DOSE ADJUSTMENTS

Changes in the chronic infusion rate are to be expected. If symptoms of primary pulmonary hypertension (PPH) persist, recur, or worsen, increase infusion rate promptly by 1 to 2 ng/kg/min. Wait at least 15 minutes to assess clinical response. Observe patient for several hours to confirm patient tolerance and take BP and HR in supine and standing positions. In trials most patients progressed to a dose a little less than their acute dose-ranging intolerable dose within 12 weeks. ■ Occurrence of dose-related side effects that do not resolve may require a decrease in the chronic infusion rate. Begin with 2 ng/kg/min and wait at least 15 minutes to assess clinical response. Use extreme caution if decreasing the dose; abrupt withdrawal or sudden large reductions may cause a rapid return of PPH symptoms and may precipitate death. ■ In patients receiving lung transplants, doses were tapered after the initiation of cardiopulmonary bypass. ■ Dose selection for the elderly should be cautious. ■ Asymptomatic increases in pulmonary artery pressure with increases in cardiac output may occur during acute dose-ranging; consider dose adjustment. ■ See Precautions.

DILUTION

Infusion pump required. It must be small and lightweight; able to adjust infusion rates in 2-ng/kg/min increments; have occlusion, end of infusion, and low battery alarms; be accurate to ±6% of the programmed rate; be positive-pressure driven (continuous or pulsatile) with intervals between pulses not exceeding 3 minutes at rates required to deliver drug; and have a disposable reservoir cassette made of polyvinyl chloride, polypropylene, or glass with a capacity of at least 100 ml. Pumps used during trials were manufactured by Pharmacia Deltec, Medfusion, Inc., and Baxter Health Care. Sterile diluent for epoprostenol is provided by the manufacturer. Do not use any other diluent. Concentration will be determined by desired dose/kg/min and parameters of ambulatory infusion pump to be used. See Rate of Administration. Two vials of provided sterile diluent will be required to prepare each 24-hour dose in each of the concentrations in the chart below:

Guidelines for Dilution of Epoprostenol to Various Concentrations	
To Make 100 ml of Solution with Final Concentration (ng/ml) of:	**Directions**
3,000 ng/ml	Dissolve contents of one 0.5-mg vial with 5 ml of STERILE DILUENT for epoprostenol. Withdraw 3 ml and add to sufficient STERILE DILUENT for epoprostenol to make a total of 100 ml.
5,000 ng/ml	Dissolve contents of one 0.5-mg vial with 5 ml of STERILE DILUENT for epoprostenol. Withdraw entire vial contents and add sufficient STERILE DILUENT for epoprostenol to make a total of 100 ml.
10,000 ng/ml	Dissolve contents of two 0.5-mg vials each with 5 ml of STERILE DILUENT for epoprostenol. Withdraw entire vial contents and add sufficient STERILE DILUENT for epoprostenol to make a total of 100 ml.
15,000 ng/ml	Dissolve contents of one 1.5-mg vial with 5 ml of STERILE DILUENT for epoprostenol. Withdraw entire vial contents and add sufficient STERILE DILUENT for epoprostenol to make a total of 100 ml.

Acute dose-ranging may require more than one solution strength. 3,000 ng/ml and 10,000 ng/ml concentrations should be satisfactory to deliver between 2 and 16 ng/kg/min in adults. A maximum 2-day supply can be diluted at one time (200 ml). For use at room temperature, withdraw 33.3 ml and deposit in pump reservoir cassette or sterile infusion bag for each 8-hour period. If used with cold pouches and frozen gel packs, 100 ml can be placed in the pump reservoir cassette or a 100-ml sterile infusion bag for each 24-hour period. Frozen gel packs must be changed every 12 hours. Reservoir cassettes are disposable. Most patients prepare a 24-hour dose in a new reservoir cassette before a new dose is required and use cold pouches to maintain temperature.

Storage: Unopened vials of epoprostenol may be stored at CRT in the carton to protect from light. Diluent may be stored at CRT. Protection from light not required. See expiration dates on both. Before use, reconstituted solutions must be refrigerated and protected from light. Do not freeze. Reconstituted solution must be discarded after 48 hours or if accidentally frozen. While in use, must not be exposed to direct sunlight or temperatures above 25° C (77° F) or below 0° C (32° F). Stable in pump reservoir for only 8 hours at CRT. Use of cold pouches with frozen gel packs can extend reservoir life to 24 hours. Time stored in refrigerator and in reservoir of pump must be included in maximum 48-hour time frame.

COMPATIBILITY

Manufacturer states, "Stable only when reconstituted with the provided diluent. Must not be reconstituted or mixed with any other parenteral medications or solutions prior to or during administration."

RATE OF ADMINISTRATION

Administered by a continuous IV infusion based on rate determined for acute dose-ranging, continuous chronic infusion, or dose adjustments. Flow must not be interrupted for longer than 2 to 3 minutes. Time to completion of administration must never exceed more than 8 hours at room temperature, more than 24 hours with use of cold pouches and changing frozen gel packs every 12 hours, or more than 48 hours from time of initial reconstitution. The infusion rate may be calculated using the following formula:

$$\text{Infusion rate (ml/hr)} = \frac{\text{Dose (ng/kg/min)} \times \text{Weight in kg} \times 60 \text{ min/hr}}{\text{Final concentration (ng/ml)}}$$

The following chart may be used for infusion rates at a final concentration of 3,000 ng/ml. See package insert for tables at additional concentrations:

Infusion Rates for Epoprostenol at a Concentration of 3,000 ng/ml

Patient Weight (kg)	Dose or Drug Delivery Rate (ng/kg/min)							
	2	4	6	8	10	12	14	16
	Infusion Delivery Rate (ml/hr)							
10	—	—	1.2	1.6	2	2.4	2.8	3.2
20	—	1.6	2.4	3.2	4	4.8	5.6	6.4
30	1.2	2.4	3.6	4.8	6	7.2	8.4	9.6
40	1.6	3.2	4.8	6.4	8	9.6	11.2	12.8
50	2	4	6	8	10	12	14	16
60	2.4	4.8	7.2	9.6	12	14.4	16.8	19.2
70	2.8	5.6	8.4	11.2	14	16.8	19.6	22.4
80	3.2	6.4	9.6	12.8	16	19.2	22.4	25.6
90	3.6	7.2	10.8	14.4	18	21.6	25.2	28.8
100	4	8	12	16	20	24	28	32

ACTIONS

A naturally occurring prostaglandin. It directly vasodilates pulmonary and systemic arterial vascular beds and inhibits platelet aggregation. Right and left ventricle afterload is reduced, and cardiac output and stroke volume are increased. Effect on HR is dose related. Produces dose-related increases in cardiac index and stroke volume and dose-related decreases in pulmonary vascular resistance, total pulmonary resistance, and mean systemic arterial pressure. Has been shown to increase exercise capacity, improve hemodynamic status, and extend survival. Onset of action is immediate. Half-life is approximately 6 minutes at body pH of 7.4. Metabolized to two primary metabolites by rapid hydrolyzation and enzymatic degradation.

INDICATIONS AND USES

Long-term IV treatment of primary pulmonary hypertension (PPH) and pulmonary hypertension associated with the scleroderma spectrum of diseases in New York Heart Association Class III and IV patients who do not respond adequately to conventional treatment.

Unlabeled uses: Treatment of pulmonary hypertension secondary to congenital diaphragmatic hernia and congenital heart disease. ■ Also being used for the treatment of pulmonary hypertension after cardiac surgery; improving ulcer healing and other symptoms (e.g., pain) occurring in patients with peripheral vascular disease; decreasing severity, frequency, and duration of symptoms in Raynaud's phenomenon; treatment of pulmonary hypertension in children; improvement of arterial oxygenation in patients with acute respiratory distress syndrome.

CONTRAINDICATIONS

Congestive heart failure due to severe left ventricular systolic dysfunction, known hypersensitivity to epoprostenol or related compounds (e.g., alprostadil [Prostin VR Pediatric], prostaglandin E_1 [Alprostadil]).

PRECAUTIONS

Administered by or under the direction of the physician specialist. ■ During dose-ranging, facilities for monitoring the patient and responding to any medical emergency must be available. ■ Causes of secondary pulmonary hypertension should be eliminated and diagnosis of PPH carefully established. ■ Abrupt withdrawal, interruptions in drug delivery, or sudden large reductions in dose may result in rebound pulmonary hypertension, including dyspnea, dizziness, and weakness. Death of one patient was attributed to these causes. Backup medication and equipment must always be available. ■ Use of a multilumen catheter should be considered if other IV therapy is used. ■ Not recommended for patients who develop pulmonary edema during acute dose-ranging; may develop pulmonary veno-occlusive disease. ■ Asymptomatic increases in pulmonary artery pressure with increases in cardiac output may occur during acute dose-ranging; consider dose adjustment. ■ Cardiac catheterization used during trials for acute dose-ranging, but is not necessary; consider benefit versus risk. In patients undergoing lung transplants, it is recommended that the dose of epoprostenol be tapered after initiation of cardiopulmonary bypass. ■ See Monitor, Patient Education, Drug/Lab Interactions.

Monitor: ECG monitoring and frequent monitoring of vital signs recommended during acute dose-ranging. ■ Observe for dose-limiting side effects. ■ Thrombocytopenia has been reported; periodic platelet counts may be indicated. ■ To reduce the risk of pulmonary thromboembolism or systemic embolism, anticoagulant therapy is recommended concomitantly unless contraindicated. ■ Therapy may be required for months or years; consideration must be given to the ability of the patient and family to manage this care. ■ Monitor standing and supine HR and BP for several hours after any adjustment. ■ Thorough patient teaching and continued support services are imperative to facilitate a good clinical outcome. ■ See Precautions, Patient Education, Drug/Lab Interactions.

Patient Education: After initial dose titration and training, this is a self-administered drug. Must assume responsibility for drug reconstitution, drug administration, and care of the permanent central venous catheter. ■ Aseptic technique during reconstitution and with routine care of permanent indwelling central venous catheter is imperative to prevent infection. ■ Report fever or any sign of infection at catheter site (e.g., redness, warmth). ■ Delivery of medication cannot be interrupted. Interruption will cause a rapid return of PPH symptoms. ■ Should have access to a backup infusion pump and intravenous infusion sets to avoid potential interruption in drug delivery. ■ Dose adjustments should be made only under the direction of the physician except in an emergency situation (e.g., unconsciousness, collapse).

Maternal/Child: Category B: use only if clearly needed. No evidence of fetal harm in animal studies to date. ■ Safety for use during labor and delivery not established. ■ Use caution in nursing mothers; safety not established. ■ Safety for use in children not established. ■ Some studies suggest children may tolerate higher doses than adults.

Elderly: See Dose Adjustments. Decreased organ function (cardiac, hepatic, renal), concomitant disease, and other drug therapy may cause concern. Response of younger patients versus the elderly not documented.

DRUG/LAB INTERACTIONS

Hypotension may be increased with diuretics, antihypertensive agents, or other vasodilators. ■ Risk of bleeding may be increased with antiplatelet agents, anticoagulants, or NSAIDs (e.g., ibuprofen [Advil, Motrin], naproxen [Aleve, Naprosyn]). ■ Epoprostenol may increase the bioavailability of oral digoxin. May decrease clearance of furosemide (Lasix), and digoxin, monitor digoxin levels.

SIDE EFFECTS

Acute dose-ranging: Flushing, headache, hypotension, nausea, and vomiting are most common and are dose-limiting. Abdominal pain, anxiety/nervousness, back pain, bradycardia, chest pain, constipation, dizziness, dyspnea, dyspepsia, musculoskeletal pain, paresthesia, sweating, tachycardia, and many other side effects may occur.

Chronic continuous infusion: Any of the above and anemia, chills, diarrhea, fever, flu-like symptoms, hypersplenism, hyperthyroidism, infection (may be local at site of catheter insertion), jaw pain, pancytopenia, splenomegaly, thrombocytopenia.

Overdose: Hypotension, hypoxemia, respiratory arrest, and death.

ANTIDOTE

Continuous maintenance of drug flow imperative. Keep physician informed of all side effects. Most will be treated with dose reduction; some may require symptomatic treatment. Marketed through Glaxo Wellcome Inc. Flolan Lifeline Services program. Call 1-800-9-FLOLAN for drug or pump problems.

EPTIFIBATIDE

(ep-tih-fib'ah-tide)

Platelet aggregation inhibitor

Integrilin

pH 5.25

USUAL DOSE

Used in combination with heparin and aspirin. Serum creatinine less than 2 mg/dl required in patients receiving the following doses.

ACUTE CORONARY SYNDROME

Eptifibatide: 180 mcg/kg as an IV bolus as soon as possible following diagnosis. Follow with a continuous infusion of 2 mcg/kg/min until hospital discharge or initiation of coronary artery bypass graft (CABG) surgery for up to 72 hours. Alternately, if a patient is to undergo a percutaneous coronary intervention (PCI) while receiving eptifibatide, the infusion should be continued up to hospital discharge, or for 18 to 24 hours after the procedure, whichever comes first. Patient may receive up to 96 hours of therapy. See Dosing Charts by Weight and Dose Adjustments. Dose in patients with a SrCr less than 2 mg/dl weighing more than 121 kg should not exceed a bolus of 22.6 mg or an infusion rate of 15 mg/hr.

Aspirin: 160 to 325 mg PO initially and daily thereafter.

Heparin: ***Medical management:*** Suggested heparin dose to achieve the target aPTT of 50 to 70 seconds during medical management is ***Weight 70 kg or more,*** 5,000 units as an IV bolus followed by an infusion of 1,000 units/hr. ***Weight less than 70 kg,*** 60 units/kg as an IV bolus followed by an infusion of 12 units/kg/hr.

Patients undergoing PCI: Target ACT is 200 to 300 seconds during PCI. If heparin is initiated before PCI, give additional boluses during PCI as needed to keep ACT in range. Heparin infusion after PCI is discouraged.

PERCUTANEOUS CORONARY INTERVENTION (PCI)

Eptifibatide: 180 mcg/kg as an IV bolus immediately before initiation of PCI followed by a continuous infusion of 2 mcg/kg/min. Repeat bolus of 180 mcg/kg 10 minutes after the first bolus. Continue infusion until hospital discharge or for up to 18 to 24 hours, whichever comes first. A minimum of 12 hours of infusion is recommended. See Dosing Charts by Weight and Dose Adjustments. Dose in patients with a SrCr less than 2 mg/dl weighing more than 121 kg should not exceed a bolus of 22.6 mg or an infusion rate of 15 mg/hr.

Aspirin: 160 to 325 mg PO 1 to 24 hours before PCI and daily thereafter.

Heparin: Target ACT is 200 to 300 seconds during PCI. In patients not treated with heparin within 6 hours of PCI, give 60 units/kg as a bolus. Give additional boluses as needed during PCI to keep ACT in range. Heparin infusion is discouraged after PCI. Discontinue eptifibatide infusions in patients requiring thrombolytic therapy.

Eptifibatide Dosing Charts by Weight					
	180 mcg/kg Bolus Volume	2 mcg/kg/min Infusion Rate		1 mcg/kg/min Infusion Rate	
Patient Weight (kg)	From 2 mg/ml Vial	From 2 mg/ml 100-ml Vial	From 0.75 mg/ml 100-ml Vial	From 2 mg/ml 100-ml Vial	From 0.75 mg/ml 100-ml Vial
37-41	3.4 ml	2 ml/hr	6 ml/hr	1 ml/hr	3 ml/hr
42-46	4 ml	2.5 ml/hr	7 ml/hr	1.3 ml/hr	3.5 ml/hr
47-53	4.5 ml	3 ml/hr	8 ml/hr	1.5 ml/hr	4 ml/hr
54-59	5 ml	3.5 ml/hr	9 ml/hr	1.8 ml/hr	4.5 ml/hr
60-65	5.6 ml	3.8 ml/hr	10 ml/hr	1.9 ml/hr	5 ml/hr
66-71	6.2 ml	4 ml/hr	11 ml/hr	2 ml/hr	5.5 ml/hr
72-78	6.8 ml	4.5 ml/hr	12 ml/hr	2.3 ml/hr	6 ml/hr
79-84	7.3 ml	5 ml/hr	13 ml/hr	2.5 ml/hr	6.5 ml/hr
85-90	7.9 ml	5.3 ml/hr	14 ml/hr	2.7 ml/hr	7 ml/hr
91-96	8.5 ml	5.6 ml/hr	15 ml/hr	2.8 ml/hr	7.5 ml/hr
97-103	9 ml	6 ml/hr	16 ml/hr	3 ml/hr	8 ml/hr
104-109	9.5 ml	6.4 ml/hr	17 ml/hr	3.2 ml/hr	8.5 ml/hr
110-115	10.2 ml	6.8 ml/hr	18 ml/hr	3.4 ml/hr	9 ml/hr
116-121	10.7 ml	7 ml/hr	19 ml/hr	3.5 ml/hr	9.5 ml/hr
>121	11.3 ml	7.5 ml/hr	20 ml/hr	3.7 ml/hr	10 ml/hr

DOSE ADJUSTMENTS

Acute coronary syndrome: Discontinue eptifibatide infusion before CABG surgery. ■ In patients with SrCr between 2 and 4 mg/dl, give a bolus of 180 mcg/kg. Decrease rate of the continuous infusion to 1 mcg/kg/min. In patients with SrCr between 2 and 4 mg/dl and weighing more than 121 kg, a maximum bolus of 22.6 mg followed by a maximum infusion rate of 7.5 mg/hr should be administered.

PCI: In patients with SrCr between 2 and 4 mg/dl, give a bolus of 180 mcg/kg. Decrease rate of the continuous infusion to 1 mcg/kg/min. Repeat bolus of 180 mcg/kg 10 minutes after the first bolus. In patients with SrCr between 2 and 4 mg/dl and weighing more than 121 kg, a maximum bolus of 22.6 mg followed by a maximum infusion rate of 7.5 mg/hr should be administered.

All diagnoses: Dose adjustments are not required in patients with SrCr between 1 and 2 mg/dl. ■ Dose reduction may be indicated in patients over 75 years of age weighing less than 50 kg. ■ See Dosing Charts by Weight in Usual Dose. ■ See Contraindications.

DILUTION

The 10-ml vial contains 20 mg of eptifibatide; the 100-ml vials contain 75 mg or 200 mg of eptifibatide.

IV bolus: Given undiluted. Withdraw total bolus dose (usually from the 10-ml vial) into a syringe.

Infusion: Usually given undiluted directly from the 75 mg/100 ml (0.75 mg/ml) or the 200 mg/100 ml (2 mg/ml) vials using an IV infusion pump. The 100-ml vial should be spiked with a vented infusion set. Center the spike within the circle on the stopper top. May be diluted with NS or D5NS. Use of a metriset or infusion pump appropriate.

Storage: Refrigerate vials at 2° to 8° C (36° to 46° F) or they may be kept at CRT for up to 2 months. Protect from light until administration. Do not use beyond the expiration or discard date. Discard any unused portion left in the vial.

INCOMPATIBLE WITH

Manufacturer lists furosemide (Lasix). Any solution or drug not mentioned under Compatible With.

COMPATIBLE WITH

Manufacturer lists as compatible at **Y-site** with NS or D5NS with or without up to 60 mEq/L of potassium chloride as well as with alteplase (t-PA), atropine sulfate, dobutamine (Dobutrex), heparin, lidocaine, meperidine (Demerol), metoprolol (Lopressor), midazolam (Versed), morphine, nitroglycerin (Nitro-Bid IV), verapamil (Isoptin).

RATE OF ADMINISTRATION

IV bolus: A single dose IV push over 1 to 2 minutes.

Infusion: See Dosing Charts by Weight under Usual Dose.

ACTIONS

A cyclic heptapeptide (amino acid) that binds to the platelet receptor glycoprotein GP IIb/IIIa of human platelets and inhibits platelet aggregation by preventing the binding of fibrinogen, von Willebrand factor, and other adhesive ligands to GP IIb/IIIa. Inhibits platelet aggregation in a dose- and concentration-dependent manner. Recovery of platelet function after termination of the eptifibatide infusion is rapid. Administered alone, eptifibatide has no measurable effect on PT or aPTT. Does not exert a pharmacologic effect on other integrins. Recommended regimens of a bolus followed by an infusion produce immediate inhibition of platelet aggregation and an early peak level, followed by a small decline, with steady state achieved within 4 to 6 hours. Plasma elimination half-life is approximately 2.5 hours. 50% cleared from plasma by the kidneys. Balance of clearance is by non-renal mechanisms. Has been shown to reduce clinical events (e.g., acute MI, need for urgent intervention) in patients undergoing PCI during drug administration and in those receiving medical management alone.

INDICATIONS AND USES

Used in combination with heparin, aspirin and, in selected situations, a thienopyridine (ticlopidine [Ticlid] or clopidogrel [Plavix]). ■ Treatment of patients with acute coronary syndrome (unstable angina or non–Q-wave MI), including those who are to be managed medically and those undergoing PCI. In this setting has been shown to decrease the rate of a combined endpoint of death or new MI. ■ Treatment of patients undergoing PCI, including those undergoing intracoronary stenting. In this setting has been shown to decrease the rate of a combined endpoint of death, new MI, or need for urgent intervention.

CONTRAINDICATIONS

Known hypersensitivity to any component of the product. ■ Current or planned administration of another parenteral GP IIb/IIIa inhibitor (e.g., abciximab [ReoPro], tirofiban [Aggrastat]). ■ Dependency on renal dialysis. ■ History of bleeding diathesis or evidence of active abnormal bleeding within the previous 30 days. ■ History of stroke within 30 days or any history of hemorrhagic stroke. ■ Major surgery within the preceding 6 weeks. ■ Severe hypertension (systolic BP greater than 200 mm Hg or diastolic BP greater than 110 mm Hg) not adequately controlled on antihypertensive therapy.

PRECAUTIONS

Use with caution in patients with platelet count less than 100,000/mm^3 and in patients with hemorrhagic retinopathy. ■ Use caution when given with drugs that affect hemostasis (e.g., warfarin [Coumadin]). Safety when used in combination with thrombolytic agents (e.g., alteplase [t-PA, Activase]), reteplase [Retavase], urokinase [Abbokinase], streptokinase [Streptase]) has not been established. See Drug/Lab Interactions. ■ Use with caution in patients with renal insufficiency; see Dose Adjustments. There is no experience in patients with SrCr greater than 4 mg/dl. ■ Bleeding is the most common complication encountered during therapy. ■ Major bleeding was unusual in patients not undergoing a cardiac revascularization procedure (PCI or CABG). ■ Risk of major bleeding increased inversely with patient weight, especially for patients weighing less than 70 kg. ■ Most major bleeding occurs at the arterial access site for cardiac catheterization or from the GI or GU tracts. Care should be taken when attempting vascular access that only the anterior wall of the femoral artery is punctured. ■ In all studies, eptifibatide was less beneficial in women than in men. The reason is unclear. Differences in race have not been studied. ■ Because eptifibatide is readily reversible, procedures such as emergency CABG may be performed safely shortly after discontinuation of an infusion without the need for platelet transfusions.

Monitor: Before therapy obtain platelet count, hemoglobin or hematocrit, SrCr, and PT/aPTT. Obtain ACT in patients undergoing PCI. ■ Maintain target aPTT between 50 and 70 seconds unless PCI is to be performed. During PCI, the ACT should be maintained between 200 and 300 seconds. ■ The aPTT or ACT should be checked before sheath removal. The sheath should not be removed unless the aPTT is less than 45 seconds or the ACT is less than 150 seconds. In patients treated with heparin, bleeding can be minimized by close monitoring of the aPTT. ■ If the platelet count drops to less than 100,000/mm^3, heparin and eptifibatide should be discontinued. Monitor closely and initiate appropriate therapy as indicated. ■ Monitor the patient for signs of bleeding; take vital signs (avoiding automatic BP cuffs); observe any invaded sites at least every 15 minutes (e.g., sheaths, IV sites, cutdowns, punctures, Foleys, NGs); watch for hematuria, hematemesis, bloody stool, petechiae, hematoma, flank pain, muscle weakness. Perform neuro checks frequently. If during therapy, bleeding cannot be controlled with pressure, heparin and eptifibatide should be discontinued. ■ Use care in handling patient; minimize use of urinary catheters, nasotracheal intubation, and nasogastric tubes. Avoid arterial puncture, venipuncture, and IM injection. Use extreme precautionary methods and only compressible sites if these procedures are absolutely necessary (i.e., avoid subclavian or jugular veins). Apply pressure for 30 minutes to any invaded site and then apply pressure dressings. Saline or heparin locks suggested to facilitate blood draws.

Additional monitoring for patients receiving PCI: Patients receiving PCI who have a sheath in place should be maintained on complete bed rest with the head of the bed elevated 30 degrees and the affected limb restrained in a straight position. Monitor sheath insertion site(s) and distal pulses of affected leg(s) frequently while sheath is in place and for 6 hours after removal. Measure any hematoma and monitor for enlargement. ■ After PCI, eptifibatide should be continued until hospital discharge or for up to 18 to 24 hours, whichever comes first. See suggested time frames under each dose. Heparin use is discouraged after the PCI procedure. The femoral artery sheath may be removed during eptifibatide infusion, but only after heparin has been discontinued and its effects largely reversed. Heparin should be discontinued 3 to 4 hours before pulling the sheath, and an aPTT less than 45 seconds or an ACT of less than 150 seconds should be documented. ■ Care should be taken to obtain proper hemostasis after removal of the sheath using standard compressive techniques followed by close observation. Sheath hemostasis should be achieved at least 4 hours before hospital discharge.

Patient Education: Compliance with all measures to minimize bleeding (e.g., strict bed rest, positioning) is imperative. ■ Avoid use of razors, toothbrushes, and other sharp items. ■ Use caution while moving to avoid excessive bumping. ■ Report all episodes of bleeding and apply local pressure if indicated. ■ Expect oozing from IV sites.

Maternal/Child: Category B: safety for use in pregnancy not established; use only if clearly needed. ■ It is not known whether eptifibatide is excreted in breast milk; use caution if administered to a nursing mother. ■ Safety and effectiveness have not been established for children.

Elderly: Dose adjusted by weight; see Dosing Charts by Weight in Usual Dose. ■ Clearance decreased and plasma levels increased in older patients; incidence of bleeding complications was higher and eptifibatide-associated bleeding was greater in the elderly during studies. ■ No apparent difference in effectiveness between older and younger patients.

DRUG/LAB INTERACTIONS

All studies with eptifibatide included the use of aspirin and heparin. In the ESPRIT study, clopidogrel (Plavix) or ticlopidine (Ticlid) were administered routinely, starting the day of PCI. Concomitant use, although indicated, increases the risk of bleeding. ■ Use caution when given with drugs that affect hemostasis such as thrombolytics (e.g., alteplase [t-PA, Activase], reteplase [Retavase], urokinase [Abbokinase], streptokinase [Streptase]), oral anticoagulants (e.g., warfarin [Coumadin]), NSAIDs (e.g., ibuprofen [Advil, Motrin], naproxen [Aleve, Naprosyn], dipyridamole [Persantine], ticlopidine [Ticlid], clopidogrel [Plavix]), selected antibiotics (e.g., cefamandole [Mandol], cefoperazone [Cefobid]). ■ Avoid concomitant treatment with other inhibitors of platelet receptor GP IIb/IIIa (e.g., abciximab [ReoPro], tirofiban [Aggrastat]) may have potentially serious additive effects. See Contraindications.

SIDE EFFECTS

Bleeding is the most frequent adverse event; may occur more frequently in patients undergoing CABG or PCI, or in the elderly or those weighing less than 70 kg. Bleeding is usually reported as mild oozing, but major bleeding (e.g., intracranial hemorrhage and stroke) may occur. Fatal bleeding events have been reported. Laboratory findings related to bleeding include decrease in hemoglobin, hematocrit, and platelet count and occult blood in urine and feces. Other side effects that have been reported include allergic reactions, hypotension, and thrombocytopenia. Incidence in studies similar to that seen with placebo.

Acute toxicity: Specific information not available for humans, but decreased muscle tone, dyspnea, loss of righting reflex, petechial hemorrhages in the femoral and abdominal areas, and ptosis occurred in animals.

ANTIDOTE

Keep physician informed of laboratory values and side effects. Discontinue the infusion of eptifibatide and heparin if any serious bleeding not controllable with pressure occurs, if CABG surgery is initiated, and/or if patient requires thrombolytic therapy. If platelet count drops to below 100,000/mm^3, discontinue heparin and eptifibatide. Monitor closely; platelet transfusion may be required. If a hypersensitivity reaction should occur, discontinue the infusion and treat as indicated by severity (e.g., epinephrine, dopamine [Intropin], theophylline, antihistamines such as diphenhydramine [Benadryl]) and/or corticosteroids as necessary. No specific antidote is available. Platelet inhibition reverses rapidly when infusion is discontinued. Hemodialysis may be useful in an overdose situation.

ERGONOVINE MALEATE

(er-gone-o′veen ma′le-at)

Uterine stimulant (oxytocic)
Diagnostic agent

Ergotrate Maleate

pH 2.7 to 3.5

USUAL DOSE

Uterine stimulant: 1 ml (0.2 mg). Repeat in 2 to 4 hours if necessary. A maximum of 5 doses is usually not exceeded.

Diagnosis of Prinzmetal's angina (unlabeled): 0.05 mg IV during coronary angiography (see Precautions). Repeat every 5 minutes until onset of chest pain or a total dose of 0.4 mg.

DILUTION

May be given undiluted. Some clinicians recommend dilution with 5 ml of NS. Do not add to IV solutions. Give through Y-tube or three-way stopcock of infusion set.

Storage: Should be refrigerated; may not be stored at room temperature more than 60 days. Check expiration date on vial; deteriorates with age.

COMPATIBLE WITH

Consult pharmacist; specific conditions may apply; see Compatibilities, p. xvi.

Additive: Amikacin (Amikin), sodium bicarbonate.

RATE OF ADMINISTRATION

0.2 mg or fraction thereof over 1 minute. Too-rapid injection may cause severe nausea and vomiting.

ACTIONS

An oxytocic, it exerts a direct stimulation on the smooth muscle of the uterus, causing contraction of the uterus. Produces vasoconstriction, increases central venous pressure, elevates BP, and may rarely produce peripheral ischemia. In therapeutic doses the prolonged initial contraction is followed by periods of relaxation and contraction. Effective within 1 minute for up to 3 hours. The least toxic of the ergot derivatives, it is probably metabolized in the liver and excreted in feces. Secreted in breast milk.

INDICATIONS AND USES

Prevents or controls postpartum or postabortal hemorrhage.

Unlabeled uses: Diagnosis of Prinzmetal's angina.

CONTRAINDICATIONS

Known hypersensitivity to ergot alkaloids; pregnancy before the third stage of labor (delivery of placenta).

PRECAUTIONS

Not recommended for use before the delivery of the placenta. ■ IV administration is for emergency use only. IM or PO route is preferred and should be used after the initial IV dose. ■ Use caution in patients with cardiac, renal, or liver disease and in febrile or septic states. ■ Simulates spontaneous coronary arterial spasms responsible for Prinzmetal's angina when injected during coronary arteriography. These spasms are reversible with nitroglycerin. This use has precipitated arrhythmias including ventricular tachycardia and myocardial infarction.

Monitor: Monitor BP, pulse, and uterine response. Observe for vaginal bleeding and frequent periods of uterine relaxation. ■ Uterine response may be poor in calcium-deficient patients and will require calcium replacement for effective response. Avoid or use extreme caution if calcium replacement is needed in patients taking digoxin. ■ See Drug/Lab Interactions.

Maternal/Child: See Contraindications. Do not administer before delivery of the placenta; it may cause hypoxia and intracranial hemorrhage in the infant, captivation of the placenta, or missed diagnosis of a second infant. ■ May decrease prolactin levels and inhibit breast-feeding.

DRUG/LAB INTERACTIONS

Severe hypertension and cerebrovascular accidents can result with ephedrine, epinephrine, methoxamine (Vasoxyl), and other vasopressors. Chlorpromazine (Thorazine) IV will reduce this hypertension.

SIDE EFFECTS

Rare in therapeutic doses, but may include the following:

Allergic phenomena, blindness, chest pain, confusion, diarrhea, dilated pupils, dizziness, headache, hypertension, hypotension, nausea, numb and/or cold extremities, ringing in the ears, shortness of breath, vomiting, weakness.

Overdose: Abortion, convulsions, excitement, gangrene, hypercoagulability, severe nausea and vomiting, shock, tachycardia, thirst, tremor, uterine bleeding.

ANTIDOTE

Discontinue the drug immediately at the onset of any side effect and notify the physician. Most side effects are transient unless there is severe toxicity and will be treated symptomatically. Use antiemetics (e.g., prochlorperazine [Compazine], ondansetron [Zofran]) for nausea and vomiting. Treat cardiac ischemia with nitroglycerin, seizures with diazepam (Valium) or phenytoin (Dilantin). Treat peripheral ischemia with nitroprusside sodium, tolazoline (Priscoline), or phentolamine (Regitine). Treat hypertension with nitroprusside sodium, chlorpromazine (Thorazine), or hydralazine. Severe poisoning is treated with vasodilator drugs, sedatives, calcium gluconate to relieve muscular pain, and other supportive treatment. Heparin is used to control hypercoagulability.

ERTAPENEM

(er-tah-pen′em)

Antibacterial (carbapenem)

Invanz

pH 7.5

USUAL DOSE

1 Gm once per day. Duration of therapy is based on diagnosis as listed in the chart below.

Ertapenem Dosing Guidelines

Infection*	Daily Dose	Duration
Complicated intra-abdominal infections	1 Gm	5-14 days
Complicated skin and skin structure infections	1 Gm	7-14 days
Community-acquired pneumonia	1 Gm	7-14 days†
Complicated urinary tract infections, including pyelonephritis	1 Gm	10-14 days†
Acute pelvic infections, including postpartum endomyometritis, septic abortion, and post-surgical gynecologic infections.	1 Gm	3-10 days

*Due to designated pathogens.
†Duration includes a possible switch to an appropriate oral therapy, after at least 3 days of parenteral therapy, once clinical improvement has been demonstrated.

PEDIATRIC DOSE

Safety and effectiveness for use in pediatric patients and adolescents under 18 years of age not established.

DOSE ADJUSTMENTS

Reduce dose to 0.5 Gm (500 mg) daily in patients with a CrCl at or less than 30 ml/min/1.73 M^2. No dose adjustment is indicated in patients with a CrCl at or more than 31 ml/min/1.73.M^2. Give a supplementary dose of 150 mg to a patient who received the daily dose within 6 hours of a dialysis session. ■ No dose adjustment is indicated based on age, gender, or impaired hepatic function; however, dosing should be cautious in the elderly, and reduced doses may be indicated based on potential for decreased organ function.

DILUTION

Reconstitute each 1 Gm of ertapenem with 10 ml SW, NS, BWFI. Shake well to dissolve. Must be further diluted in 50 ml of NS.

Storage: Store unopened vials at or below 25° C (77° F). Use reconstituted and diluted solution within 6 hours when stored at CRT. May refrigerate for up to 24 hours and use within 4 hours after removal.

COMPATIBILITY

Manufacturer states, "Do not mix or co-infuse ertapenem with other medications. Do not use diluents containing dextrose."

RATE OF ADMINISTRATION

A single dose as an infusion equally distributed over 30 minutes.

ACTIONS

A unique, synthetic 1-beta-methyl-carbapenem structurally related to beta-lactam antibiotics. Effective against gram-positive and gram-negative aerobic and anaerobic bacteria. May effectively replace some combination therapies. Does not cover *Pseudomonas* and *Acinetobacter* species. Bactericidal activity results from inhibition of bacterial cell wall synthesis. Stable against hydrolysis by a variety of beta-lactamases, including penicillinases, cephalosporinases, and extended spectrum beta-lactamases. Hydrolyzed by metallo-beta-lactamases. Widely distributed throughout the body into many body tissues and fluids. Highly protein bound. Average half-life is 4 hours. Primarily excreted in urine (some as unchanged drug). Some excretion in feces. May cross the placental barrier. Secreted in breast milk.

INDICATIONS AND USES

Treatment of adults with moderate to severe infections caused by susceptible strains of microorganisms in conditions that include complicated intra-abdominal infections; complicated skin and skin structure infections; community-acquired pneumonia; complicated urinary tract infections, including pyelonephritis; and acute pelvic infections, including postpartum endomyometritis, septic abortion, and post-surgical gynecologic infections.

CONTRAINDICATIONS

Known hypersensitivity to any component of ertapenem or other drugs in the same class (e.g., imipenem-cilastatin), or in patients who have had anaphylactic reactions to beta-lactams (e.g., piperacillin/tazobactam [Zosyn]). ■ The IM preparation is reconstituted with 1% lidocaine and is contraindicated for IV use and in patients with a known hypersensitivity to amide-type local anesthetics.

PRECAUTIONS

Confirm proper dilution for IV use; see Contraindications. ■ Culture and sensitivity studies indicated to determine susceptibility of the causative organism to ertapenem. ■ Prolonged use may cause superinfection because of overgrowth of nonsusceptible organisms. ■ CNS stimulation and seizures have been reported. Use with caution in patients with CNS disorders (e.g., brain lesions or history of seizures) and/or compromised renal function. ■ Pseudomembranous colitis has been reported and may range in severity from mild to life-threatening. Consider this diagnosis in patients who present with diarrhea during or after treatment with ertapenem. ■ See Monitor.

Monitor: Serious and occasionally fatal hypersensitivity reactions have been reported in patients receiving therapy with beta-lactams. More likely in patients with a history of sensitivity to multiple allergens; obtain a careful history and watch for early symptoms of allergic reaction. Emergency equipment must be readily available. ■ Obtain baseline CBC with differential and platelets, and baseline kidney and liver studies (e.g., CrCl, serum creatinine, ALT, AST, serum bilirubin). Monitor periodically during prolonged therapy. ■ Monitor patients who are at risk for CNS stimulation or are receiving anticonvulsant therapy for focal tremors, myoclonus, or seizures. If these symptoms occur, neurologic evaluation is indicated and dose reduction or discontinuation of ertapenem may be indicated. ■ Monitor IV site carefully and rotate as indicated. ■ See Precautions.

Patient Education: Report promptly: fever, rash, sore throat, unusual bleeding or bruising, severe stomach cramps and/or diarrhea, seizures, and pain or discomfort at the injection site.

Maternal/Child: Category B: use during pregnancy only if clearly needed. ■ Safety for use during breast-feeding not established; is found in breast milk. Benefits must outweigh risks to infant (e.g., diarrhea, candidiasis, or allergic response). Undetectable in breast milk 5 days after ertapenem is discontinued.

Elderly: Dosing should be cautious in the elderly; see Dose Adjustments. ■ Response similar to that seen in younger patients, but may be more sensitive to side effects. ■ Monitoring of renal function may be indicated.

DRUG/LAB INTERACTIONS

Probenicid reduces the renal clearance of ertapenem, but this is not clinically significant. ■ Probably does not inhibit the action of digoxin or vinblastine (Velban). ■ Probably does not inhibit metabolism mediated by most of the cytochrome P_{450} isoenzyme system. ■ No other drug interaction studies have been conducted.

SIDE EFFECTS

Diarrhea, headache, pain at the injection site, nausea, phlebitis/thrombophlebitis, vaginitis in females and vomiting were most common and described as mild to moderate. Numerous other side effects occurred in less than 1% of patients.

Major: Allergic reactions (e.g., anaphylaxis, cardiovascular collapse, death, dyspnea, edema [facial, laryngeal, or pharyngeal], hypotension, itching, shock, urticaria), CNS stimulation (e.g., anxiety, confusion, depression, hallucinations, insomnia, nightmares, paranoia, restlessness, seizures, tremor), and pseudomembranous colitis.

ANTIDOTE

Keep physician informed of all side effects. Most minor side effects will be treated symptomatically. Discontinue ertapenem at the first sign of hypersensitivity (e.g., skin rash). Treat allergic reactions as indicated with epinephrine, airway management, oxygen, IV fluids, antihistamines (e.g., diphenhydramine [Benadryl]), corticosteroids (e.g., hydrocortisone sodium succinate [Solu-Cortef]), and pressor amines (e.g., dopamine [Intropin]). Treat CNS symptoms as indicated; may require dose reduction and/or anticonvulsants (e.g., phenytoin [Dilantin], diazepam [Valium]) for seizures. Mild cases of colitis may respond to discontinuation of the drug. Treat antibiotic-related pseudomembranous colitis with fluid, electrolytes, protein supplements, and oral vancomycin (Vancocin) or metronidazole (Flagyl). Ertapenem is partially removed by hemodialysis.

ERYTHROMYCIN LACTOBIONATE

(eh-rih'throw-my'sin lak-to-by-o-nate)

Erythrocin IV

Antibacterial (macrolide)

pH 6.5 to 7.7

USUAL DOSE

Antibacterial: 15 to 20 mg/kg of body weight/24 hr in equally divided doses every 6 hours (350 to 500 mg every 6 hours). Continuous infusion over 24 hours is preferred. Up to 4 Gm/24 hr has been given. See Elderly.

Legionnaires' disease: 1 Gm every 6 hours as a continuous infusion.

Pelvic inflammatory disease: 500 mg every 6 hours as a continuous infusion for 3 days. Follow with oral erythromycin 250 mg every 6 hours for 7 days.

Diabetic gastroparesis (unlabeled): 200 mg immediately before each meal. When practical, continue treatment with oral erythromycin 3 times daily, 30 minutes before meals, for 4 weeks.

PEDIATRIC DOSE

15 to 20 mg/kg of body weight/24 hr in equally divided doses every 6 hours is recommended (3.75 to 5 mg/kg every 6 hours). Another source recommends 20 to 50 mg/kg/24 hr in equally divided doses every 6 hours (5 to 12.5 mg/kg every 6 hours).

DOSE ADJUSTMENTS

Reduced dose may be required in impaired liver function.

DILUTION

Each 500 mg or fraction thereof must be reconstituted with 10 ml of SW without preservatives to avoid precipitation. Forms a 5% solution. Shake well to ensure dilution.

Continuous infusion (preferred): Further dilute to a 1 to 5 mg/ml solution (e.g., each 1 Gm in 200 to 1,000 ml of NS or LR. If a dextrose solution is used, add sodium bicarbonate (Neut) 1 ml for each 100 ml of solution.

Intermittent infusion: Dilute to a maximum concentration of 5 mg/ml (1 Gm in 200 ml). Available in ADD-Vantage vials for use with ADD-Vantage infusion containers.

Storage: Reconstituted solution stable for 14 days if refrigerated or for 24 hours at room temperature. Diluted and/or buffered solution stable for 8 hours at CRT or 24 hours if refrigerated.

COMPATIBLE WITH

(Underline Indicates Conflicting Compatibility Information)

Consult pharmacist; specific conditions may apply; see Compatibilities, p. xvi, and Dilution.

Additive: Aminophylline, ampicillin, ascorbic acid (Cenolate), chloramphenicol (Chloromycetin), cimetidine (Tagamet), diphenhydramine (Benadryl), hydrocortisone sodium succinate (Solu-Cortef), lidocaine, penicillin G potassium and sodium, pentobarbital (Nembutal), potassium chloride (KCl), prochlorperazine (Compazine), ranitidine (Zantac), sodium bicarbonate, verapamil (Isoptin).

Y-site: Acyclovir (Zovirax), amiodarone (Cordarone), cyclophosphamide (Cytoxan), diltiazem (Cardizem), enalaprilat (Vasotec IV), esmolol (Brevibloc), famotidine (Pepcid IV), foscarnet (Foscavir), heparin, hetastarch in electrolytes (Hextend), hydromorphone (Dilaudid), idarubicin (Idamycin), labetalol (Normodyne), lorazepam (Ativan), magnesium sulfate, meperidine (Demerol), midazolam (Versed), morphine, multivitamins (M.V.I.), perphenazine (Trilafon), tacrolimus (Prograf), theophylline, zidovudine (AZT, Retrovir).

RATE OF ADMINISTRATION

Administer with a volume control set. Slow infusion rate for pain along injection site.

Continuous infusion (preferred): A 0.1% to 0.2% solution equally distributed over 6 to 24 hours.

Intermittent infusion: 1 Gm or fraction thereof in at least 100 ml over 20 to 60 minutes.

Diabetic gastroparesis (unlabeled): 1 to 3 mg/kg/hr, usually approximately over 15 minutes.

ACTIONS

Macrolide antibiotic, bactericidal and bacteriostatic, used as a substitute for penicillin or tetracyclines. Effective against a number of gram-positive and some gram-negative organisms as well as chlamydia trachomatis, mycoplasmas, and spirochetes. Metabolized by the liver and excreted in urine and bile. Crosses placental barrier. Secreted in breast milk.

INDICATIONS AND USES

Treatment of mild to moderate infections of the upper and lower respiratory tract, skin and skin structures, and gynecologic infections caused by susceptible organisms. ■ Alternative treatment in several sexually transmitted diseases in females with a history of penicillin sensitivity. ■ Legionnaires' disease.

Unlabeled uses: Diabetic gastroparesis.

CONTRAINDICATIONS

Known erythromycin sensitivity. See Drug/Lab Interactions. ■ Coadministration with ritonavir (Norvir) is contraindicated.

PRECAUTIONS

Sensitivity studies indicated to determine susceptibility of the causative organism to erythromycin. ■ Begin oral therapy as soon as practical. ■ Superinfection caused by overgrowth of nonsusceptible organisms is rare unless this drug is given in combination with other antibacterial agents. ■ Use caution in impaired liver function or a history of cardiac disease (may induce torsades de pointes). ■ Pseudomembranous colitis has been reported. May range from mild to life-threatening. Consider in patients that present with diarrhea during or after treatment with erythromycin.

Monitor: Monitor vital signs. ■ Monitor IV site for redness and inflammation. ■ See Drug/Lab Interactions.

Maternal/Child: Category B: use only if clearly needed. ■ Considered safe for use in breast-feeding; use caution. ■ Some products contain benzyl alcohol; not recommended for use in neonates.

Elderly: Risk of developing erythromycin-induced hearing loss is increased in elderly patients, particularly those with impaired renal or hepatic function, when doses of 4 Gm/day or higher are used. ■ May be more susceptible to development of torsades de pointes. ■ May experience increased effects of oral anticoagulation; see Drug/Lab Interactions.

DRUG/LAB INTERACTIONS

Contraindicated with ritonavir. ■ Bacterial activity is antagonized by coadministration of clindamycin. ■ May inhibit penicillins. ■ Will increase serum levels and potentiate effects of alfentanil, anticoagulants (e.g., warfarin [Coumadin]), bromocriptine (Parlodel), carbamazepine (Tegretol), cisapride (Propulsid), cyclosporine (Sandimmune), digoxin, disopyramide (Norpace), ergot alkaloids (e.g., Hydergine), itraconazole (Sporanox), lovastatin (Mevacor), methylprednisolone, midazolam (Versed), phenytoin (Dilantin), theophyllines, and triazolam (Halcion); serious toxicity may result. ■ Concomitant administration with cisapride is contraindicated. May cause serious cardiotoxicity. ■ Severe vinblastine toxicity has been reported in conjunction with erythromycin. ■ May increase serum levels of sildenafil (Viagra). ■ Concurrent use with aminophylline may decrease plasma levels of erythromycin. ■ Serotonin syndrome has been reported with co-administration of erythromycin and serotonin-uptake inhibitors (e.g., sertraline [Zoloft], fluoxetine [Prozac]).

SIDE EFFECTS

Relatively free from side effects when given as directed. Nausea and vomiting, urticaria, and mild local venous discomfort. Increased incidence of usually reversible ototoxicity with larger doses. Pseudomembranous colitis has been reported. Torsades de pointes has been reported; see Elderly. Anaphylaxis may occur.

ANTIDOTE

Notify the physician of early or mild symptoms. For severe symptoms, discontinue the drug, treat allergic reactions, or resuscitate as necessary and notify physician.

ESMOLOL HYDROCHLORIDE

(ess′moe-lol hye-droe-klor′id)

Beta-adrenergic blocking agent
Antiarrhythmic

Brevibloc

pH 4.5 to 5.5

USUAL DOSE

Supraventricular tachycardia: 100 mcg/kg (0.1 mg/kg) of body weight/min is an average dose. Range is 50 to 200 mcg/kg/min (0.05 to 0.2 mg/kg/min). Dosage must be individualized by titration. Each step in the process consists of a loading dose followed by a maintenance dose. Begin with a ***loading dose*** of 500 mcg/kg/min (0.5 mg/kg/min) for 1 minute only. Follow with a ***maintenance infusion*** of 50 mcg/kg/min (0.05 mg/kg/min) for 4 minutes. If desired therapeutic effect has not occurred, repeat the loading dose and increase the maintenance infusion to 100 mcg/kg/min (0.1 mg/kg/min). Continue this two-step process by repeating the same loading dose while increasing the maintenance infusion by 50 mcg/kg/min (0.05 mg/kg/min). As the desired HR is approached or a safety end-point (decreasing BP) occurs, omit the loading dose and titrate the maintenance dose up or down in 25- to 50-mcg/kg/min (0.025 to 0.05 mg/kg/min) increments to desired HR. Interval between titration steps may be increased from 5 to 10 minutes if desired. Hypotension is common and is dose related. Doses greater than 200 mcg/kg/min (0.2 mg/kg/min) are not recommended. AHA guidelines recommend a loading dose of 0.5 mg/kg over 1 minute followed by a maintenance infusion at 0.05 mg/kg/min to a maximum rate of 0.3 mg/kg/min. Titrate to effect.

Intraoperative and postoperative tachycardia and/or hypertension: For immediate control 80 mg (approximately 1 mg/kg) over 30 seconds. Follow with an infusion of 150 mcg/kg/minute (0.15 mg/kg/min) if necessary. Adjust as required up to 300 mcg/kg/min (0.3 mg/kg/min) to maintain desired HR and/or BP. For gradual control, use procedure listed for SVT. Higher doses (250 to 300 mcg/kg/min [0.25 to 0.3 mg/kg/min]) may be required to control BP. Another source recommends 250 to 500 mcg (0.25 to 0.5 mg) over 1 minute as a loading dose, followed with a maintenance dose of 50 mcg/kg/min (0.05 mg/kg/min) for 4 minutes. Repeat loading dose and increase maintenance dose by 50 mcg/kg/min (0.05 mg/kg/min).

PEDIATRIC DOSE

Safety for use in children not established. 50 mcg/kg/min (0.05 mg/kg/min), titrate every 10 minutes in 25 to 50 mcg/kg/min (0.025 to 0.05 mg/kg/min) increments up to 300 mcg/kg/min (0.3 mg/kg/min). Another source recommends a loading dose of 100 to 500 mcg/kg (0.1 to 0.5 mg/kg) administered over 1 minute. Follow with a maintenance infusion of 25 to 100 mcg/kg/min (0.025 to 0.1 mg/kg/min). If inadequate response, repeat loading dose and/or increase maintenance dose in 25- to 50-mcg/kg/min (0.025 to 0.05 mg/kg/min) increments every 5 to 10 minutes. Titrate to individual desired response. Usual range may be from 50 to 500 mcg/kg/min (0.05 to 0.5 mg/kg/min).

DOSE ADJUSTMENTS

Reduced dose may be required in impaired renal function. ■ Reduction required with transfer to alternate agent; see Monitor. ■ See Drug/Lab Interactions.

DILUTION

Available premixed as 10 mg/ml in 250 ml NS or 20 mg/ml in 100 ml NS (double strength) and as a 10 mg/ml single-dose vial. 10 mg/ml single-dose vial may be given by IV injection without further dilution or may be further diluted in D5W, D5R, D5LR, D5NS, D5/½NS, NS, LR, or ½NS. Premixed solutions have a medication port (for withdrawing the initial bolus) and a delivery port.

Storage: Store vials and premix at CRT; diluted solution stable at room temperature for 24 hours.

INCOMPATIBLE WITH

Manufacturer lists sodium bicarbonate and states, "Should not be admixed with other drugs prior to dilution in suitable IV fluid, and do not introduce additives to Brevibloc premixed injection."

COMPATIBLE WITH **(Underline Indicates Conflicting Compatibility Information)**

Consult pharmacist; specific conditions may apply; see Compatibilities, p. xvi.

Solution: D5W with 40 mEq KCl; see Dilution.

Additive: Aminophylline, atracurium (Tracrium), bretylium (Bretylate), <u>digoxin (Lanoxin)</u>, <u>dopamine (Intropin)</u>, heparin, <u>lidocaine</u>.

Y-site: Amikacin (Amikin), aminophylline, amiodarone (Cordarone), ampicillin, atracurium (Tracrium), butorphanol (Stadol), calcium chloride, cefazolin (Kefzol), cefoperazone (Cefobid), ceftazidime (Fortaz), ceftizoxime (Cefizox), chloramphenicol (Chloromycetin), cimetidine (Tagamet), cisatracurium (Nimbex), clindamycin (Cleocin), diltiazem (Cardizem), dopamine (Intropin), enalaprilat (Vasotec IV), erythromycin lactobionate (Erythrocin), famotidine (Pepcid IV), fentanyl (Sublimaze), gatifloxacin (Tequin), gentamicin (Garamycin), heparin, hetastarch in electrolytes (Hextend), hydrocortisone sodium succinate (Solu-Cortef), insulin (regular), labetalol (Normodyne), linezolid (Zyvox), magnesium sulfate, methyldopate (Aldomet), metronidazole (Flagyl IV), midazolam (Versed), morphine, nafcillin (Nafcil), nitroglycerin (Nitro-Bid IV), nitroprusside sodium, norepinephrine (Levophed), pancuronium (Pavulon), penicillin G potassium, phenytoin (Dilantin), piperacillin (Pipracil), potassium chloride (KCl), potassium phosphates, propofol (Diprivan), ranitidine (Zantac), remifentanil (Ultiva), sodium acetate, streptomycin, sulfamethoxazole-trimethoprim (Bactrim), tacrolimus (Prograf), tobramycin (Nebcin), vancomycin (Vancocin), vecuronium (Norcuron).

RATE OF ADMINISTRATION

IV injection: See Usual Dose.

Infusion: Titrate infusion according to procedure outlined in Usual Dose.

ACTIONS

A short-acting, B_1-selective adrenergic blocking agent with antiarrhythmic effects. Decreases HR and BP in a dose-related titratable manner. Hemodynamically similar to propranolol, but vascular resistance is not increased. Onset of action occurs within 1 to 2 minutes and lasts about 20 to 30 minutes. Metabolized via esterases in RBCs and excreted in urine.

INDICATIONS AND USES

Management of supraventricular tachycardia (atrial fibrillation or atrial flutter) in situations requiring short-term control of ventricular rate with a short-acting agent (perioperative, postoperative, or other emergent circumstances). ■ Management of noncompensatory tachycardia when HR requires specific intervention. ■ Management of intraoperative and postoperative tachycardia and/or hypertension.

CONTRAINDICATIONS

Not intended for use in chronic settings when transfer to another agent is anticipated. ■ Do not use concurrently with epinephrine. ■ Bradycardia, cardiogenic shock, congestive heart failure not secondary to a tachycardia responsive to beta-adrenergic blockers, overt cardiac failure, second- or third-degree heart block.

PRECAUTIONS

For IV use only. ■ Use with extreme caution in asthmatics, diabetics, impaired renal function, or patients with a history of hypoglycemia. ■ If patient is scheduled for surgery, administer esmolol before, during, and after without interruption. May cause arrhythmia, angina, MI, or death if stopped abruptly. ■ Although it has not been a problem with esmolol, it is recommended that the dose of beta-adrenergic blockers be reduced gradually to avoid rebound angina, MI, or ventricular arrhythmias. Use caution, especially in patients with coronary artery disease.

Monitor: Continuous observation of the patient and ECG and BP monitoring are mandatory during administration. Hypotension should reverse within 30 minutes after decreasing the infusion rate or discontinuing the drug. ■ Well tolerated if administered through a central vein. Incidence of infusion site inflammation. Incidence of inflammation or thrombophlebitis increases with dilutions greater than 10 mg/ml. ■ Intended for short-term use only. Transfer to an alternative antiarrhythmic agent (e.g., propranolol [Inderal], digoxin [Lanoxin], verapamil [Isoptin]) is required after stable clinical status and HR control are obtained. Thirty minutes after first dose of alternative agent, reduce dose of esmolol by 50%. Monitor patient carefully. One hour after the second dose of alternative agent, discontinue esmolol infusion if condition remains satisfactory. ■ May cause hypoglycemia and mask the symptoms. ■ See Drug/Lab Interactions and Contraindications.

Maternal/Child: Category C: safety for use in pregnancy, breast-feeding, and children not established. Use only when clearly indicated. Has caused fetal problems during delivery.

Elderly: Potential risk of increased cardiac depression; monitor and reduce dose if indicated.

DRUG/LAB INTERACTIONS

Epinephrine concurrently is contraindicated. ■ Use with calcium channel blockers (e.g., diltiazem [Cardizem], verapamil [Isoptin]) may potentiate both drugs and result in severe depression of myocardium and AV conduction and severe hypotension. ■ Increases digoxin blood levels, synergistic with digoxin; both drugs slow AV conduction. ■ IV morphine increases esmolol steady-state levels by 50%. ■ Esmolol should not be used in patients receiving vasoconstrictive or inotropic drugs (e.g., dopamine [Intropin], epinephrine, norepinephrine [Levophed], digoxin) because of the potential for blocked cardiac contractility when the supraventricular rate is high. ■ Concomitant use with catecholamine-depleting drugs (e.g., reserpine [Serpasil]) may produce additive effects. Monitor for hypotension and bradycardia. ■ May prolong neuromuscular blockade produced by succinylcholine. ■ Warfarin (Coumadin) may increase esmolol concentrations. ■ Warfarin is not affected. ■ May mask S/S of developing hypoglycemia in patients on insulin or oral antidiabetic agents. ■ Concurrent use with xanthines (e.g., aminophylline, theophyllines) may result in mutual inhibition of therapeutic effect. ■ See Contraindications.

SIDE EFFECTS

Hypotension and inflammation or induration of the infusion site are the major side effects. Asthenia, bronchospasm, congestive heart failure, confusion, fever, flushing, lightheadedness, midscapular pain, nausea and vomiting, pallor, paresthesia, rhonchi, somnolence, speech disorders, taste disorders, and urinary retention have occurred. One grand mal seizure has been reported.

ANTIDOTE

Notify the physician of all side effects. Decrease rate or discontinue drug if hypotension occurs, and notify physician immediately. Hypotension should reverse within 30 minutes. Trendelenburg position may be appropriate. May require treatment with IV fluids or vasopressors (e.g., dopamine [Intropin], norepinephrine [levarterenol]), but protracted severe hypotension may result. Unresponsive hypotension and bradycardia may be reversed by glucagon 5 to 10 mg over 30 seconds followed by a continuous infusion of 5 mg/hr. Reduce rate as condition improves. Use atropine for bradycardia; digitalis and diuretics for cardiac failure. Treat other side effects symptomatically and resuscitate as necessary.

ETIDRONATE DISODIUM

(ee-tid′roe-nate di′so-de-um)

Didronel IV

Antihypercalcemic (bisphosphonate)

pH 4 to 5.5

USUAL DOSE

7.5 mg/kg of body weight/24 hr daily for 3 days. In selected situations, patients have been treated for 7 days during the first course of therapy. If hypercalcemia recurs, a second course of therapy limited to 3 days may be given. Begin at least 7 days after completion of first course. The day after the last infusion, begin follow-up treatment with oral etidronate 20 mg/kg/day. Usually continues for 30 days but may be extended up to 90 days if serum calcium levels remain normal or within clinically acceptable parameters. See Monitor.

DOSE ADJUSTMENTS

Reduce dose in patients with a SrCr between 2.5 to 4.9 mg/dl; see Contraindications.

DILUTION

Must be diluted in 250 ml or more of NS and given as an infusion according to the manufacturer. Another source states, "May be diluted in D5W."

Storage: Stable at room temperature for 48 hours.

COMPATIBILITY

Specific information not available. Consider specific use; consult pharmacist.

RATE OF ADMINISTRATION

250 ml of diluted solution over a minimum of 2 hours. Extend infusion time if larger amounts of fluid are used.

ACTIONS

A bisphosphonate; reduces normal and abnormal bone resorption and bone formation. Does not appear to alter renal tubular reabsorption of calcium. Not effective in hyperparathyroidism where increased renal tubular reabsorption may contribute to the cause of hypercalcemia. In hypercalcemia of malignancy the renal tubules become less able to concentrate urine, and this reduces the ability of the kidneys to eliminate excess calcium. By reducing excess bone resorption, etidronate interrupts this process. Not metabolized. Within 24 hours about half of this drug is chemically absorbed to bone and the remainder is excreted in the urine. Half-life in bone is 3 to 6 months.

INDICATIONS AND USES

Hypercalcemia of malignancy inadequately managed by dietary modification or oral hydration or persisting after adequate hydration has been restored. ■ Oral form has other uses. ■ Newer antihypercalcemic agents available (e.g., gallium nitrate [Ganite], pamidronate disodium [Aredia]).

Unlabeled uses: Prevent or decrease bone loss in women undergoing chemotherapy.

CONTRAINDICATIONS

Hypersensitivity to bisphosphonates (e.g., pamidronate [Aredia]), SrCr greater than 5 mg/dl.

PRECAUTIONS

Use caution in patients with enterocolitis. ■ Delay treatment in patients with fractures until callus is evident (especially fractures of long bones). ■ Hypercalcemia of hyperparathyroidism may coexist in patients with malignancy. Etidronate will probably not be effective. ■ Hyperphosphatemia may occur with higher doses. Serum phosphate usually returns to normal levels 2 to 4 weeks posttherapy.

Monitor: Increased risk of hypocalcemia in patients treated over 3 days IV. ■ Monitor serum calcium, serum phosphates, and albumin. ■ Monitor renal function with SrCr. ■ Must be adequately hydrated and have adequate urine output. Pretreatment and simultaneous treatment with IV saline and loop diuretics (e.g., furosemide [Lasix]) is recommended and will increase calcium excretion. Rate of renal calcium excretion is directly related to renal sodium excretion. ■ Avoid overhydration in the elderly and in cardiac failure. ■ Maintain adequate nutrition including calcium and vitamin D.

Patient Education: Regular visits and assessment of lab tests imperative. ■ Restriction of dietary calcium and vitamin D may be required. ■ Take only prescribed medications. ■ Report abdominal cramps, chills, confusion, muscle spasms, sore throat, and/or any new medical problems promptly.

Maternal/Child: Category C: safety for use in pregnancy or breast-feeding not established. Use only when clearly indicated. ■ Safety for use in children not established.

Elderly: See Precautions and Monitor.

DRUG/LAB INTERACTIONS

Renal toxicity may be potentiated by nephrotoxic drugs (e.g., aminoglycosides [gentamicin]).

SIDE EFFECTS

Diarrhea, elevated SrCr and BUN, hyperphosphatemia, hypersensitivity reactions (angioedema, pruritus, rash, urticaria), hypocalcemia, loss of taste or metallic taste (temporary), nausea, renal insufficiency. Bleeding and ECG changes have occurred in animals with too-rapid injection or excessive doses (27 mg/kg).

ANTIDOTE

Notify the physician of any side effect. May respond to symptomatic treatment or to decrease in rate of infusion. Hypocalcemia is rare but can be treated with IV calcium gluconate. Treatment is symptomatic and supportive. Resuscitate as necessary.

ETOPOSIDE

(eh-toh′-poh-syd)

Antineoplastic (mitotic inhibitor)

Etopophos, Etoposide Phosphate, Toposar, VePesid, VP-16-213

pH 2.9 to 4

USUAL DOSE

Testicular cancer: 50 to 100 mg/M^2 daily for 5 days or 100 mg/M^2/day on days 1, 3, and 5. Repeat at 3- to 4-week intervals.

Small-cell lung cancer: 35 mg/M^2/day for 4 days to 50 mg/M^2/day for 5 days. Repeat at 3- to 4-week intervals. Used in combination with other chemotherapy agents.

Kaposi's sarcoma (unlabeled): 150 mg/M^2/day for 3 consecutive days every 4 weeks. Repeat cycles based on patient response.

Unlabeled uses: High-dose regimens of 400 to 800 mg/M^2/day for 3 days have been given for one or two courses in conjunction with autogenous bone marrow transplantation for the treatment of advanced malignancies.

DOSE ADJUSTMENTS

Modify dose if indicated based on myelosuppressive effects of other drugs administered in combination and any previous radiation therapy or chemotherapy (compromised bone marrow reserve). Frequently given in combination with cisplatin, bleomycin, and doxorubicin. ■ Withhold dose if platelets less than 50,000/mm^3 or absolute neutrophil count less than 500/mm^3. Do not restart until adequate recovery. ■ Dose selection should be cautious in the elderly. Reduced doses may be indicated based on potential for decreased organ function and concomitant disease or drug therapy; see Elderly. ■ Reduce dose by 25% if CrCl is 15 to 50 ml/minute. ■ Dose reduction may be required in impaired hepatic function.

DILUTION

Specific techniques required; see Precautions. **Nonphosphate products (e.g., VePesid):** Each 100 mg (5 ml) must be diluted in at least 250 ml of D5W or NS and given as an infusion (0.4 mg/ml). 500 ml of solution will yield 0.2 mg/ml. Maximum concentration to prevent precipitation is 0.4 mg/ml. Monitor closely for precipitation from dilution to completion of infusion. One source suggests dilution with LR or 10% mannitol, but cautions that crystals may form. Discard crystallized solution. Undiluted etoposide has caused acrylic or ABS plastic devices to crack and leak; handle carefully during dilution process.

Phosphate product (e.g., Etopophos): Reconstitute each 100-mg vial with 5 or 10 ml of SW, D5W, or NS (with or without benzyl alcohol). 5 ml of diluent will yield 20 mg/ml, 10 ml will yield 10 mg/ml. May be given without further dilution (to reduce possibility of fluid overload) or may be further diluted to concentrations as low as 0.1 mg/ml with D5W or NS. A 1-mg/ml solution has a pH of 2.9. The water solubility of Etopophos decreases the potential for precipitation following dilution and during administration.

Storage: ***Nonphosphate Products (e.g., VePesid):*** May be stored at CRT before dilution. Stable after dilution at CRT for 96 hours (0.2 mg/ml solution) or 24 hours (0.4 mg/ml) in D5W or NS. Stability reduced to 8 hours in LR or 10% mannitol. ***Phosphate Products (e.g., Etopophos):*** Refrigerate in carton until use. Store reconstituted or diluted solutions in glass or plastic containers at CRT or refrigerate for up to 24 hours. When returned to room temperature from refrigeration, use Etopophos solutions immediately.

INCOMPATIBLE WITH

NONPHOSPHATE PRODUCTS (E.G., VEPESID)

Hydrolysis may occur in alkaline solutions.

COMPATIBLE WITH

Consult pharmacist; specific conditions may apply; see Compatibilities, p. xvi.

NONPHOSPHATE PRODUCTS (E.G., VEPESID)

Additive: Carboplatin (Paraplatin), cisplatin (Platinol), cytarabine (ARA-C), daunorubicin (Cerubidine), fluorouracil (5-FU), ifosfamide (Ifex), ondansetron (Zofran); another source adds mesna (Mesnex).

Y-site: Allopurinol (Aloprim, Zyloprim), amifostine (Ethyol), aztreonam (Azactam), cladribine (Leustatin), doxorubicin liposome (Doxil), fludarabine (Fludara), gemcitabine (Gemzar), granisetron (Kytril), melphalan (Alkeran), methotrexate (Folex), mitoxantrone (Novantrone), ondansetron (Zofran), paclitaxel (Taxol), piperacillin/tazobactam (Zosyn), sargramostim (Leukine), sodium bicarbonate, teniposide (Vumon), thiotepa (Thioplex), topotecan (Hycamtin), vinorelbine (Navelbine).

PHOSPHATE PRODUCTS (E.G., ETOPOPHOS)

Additive: Specific information not available; consult pharmacist.

Y-site: Acyclovir (Zovirax), amikacin (Amikin), aminophylline, ampicillin, ampicillin/sulbactam (Unasyn), aztreonam (Azactam), bleomycin (Blenoxane), bumetanide (Bumex), buprenorphine (Buprenex), butorphanol (Stadol), calcium gluconate, carboplatin (Paraplatin), carmustine (BiCNU), cefazolin (Kefzol), cefoperazone (Cefobid), cefotaxime (Claforan), cefotetan (Cefotan), cefoxitin (Mefoxin), ceftazidime (Fortaz), ceftizoxime (Cefizox), ceftriaxone (Rocephin), cefuroxime (Zinacef), cimetidine (Tagamet), ciprofloxacin (Cipro IV), cisplatin (Platinol), clindamycin (Cleocin), cyclophosphamide (Cytoxan), cytarabine (ARA-C), dacarbazine (DTIC), dactinomycin (Cosmegen), daunorubicin (Cerubidine), dexamethasone (Decadron), diphenhydramine (Benadryl), dobutamine (Dobutrex), dopamine (Intropin), doxorubicin (Adriamycin), doxycycline (Vibramycin), droperidol (Inapsine), enalaprilat (Vasotec IV), famotidine (Pepcid IV), fluconazole (Diflucan), fludarabine (Fludara), fluorouracil (5-FU), furosemide (Lasix), ganciclovir (Cytovene), gatifloxacin (Tequin), gemcitabine (Gemzar), gentamicin (Garamycin), granisetron (Kytril), haloperidol (Haldol), heparin, hydrocortisone (Hydrocortone, Solu-Cortef), hydromorphone (Dilaudid), idarubicin (Idamycin), ifosfamide (Ifex), leucovorin calcium, linezolid (Zyvox), lorazepam (Ativan), magnesium sulfate, mannitol, meperidine (Demerol), mesna (Mesnex), methotrexate (Folex), metoclopramide (Reglan), metronidazole (Flagyl IV), minocycline (Minocin), mitoxantrone (Novantrone), morphine, nalbuphine (Nubain), ofloxacin (Floxin IV), ondansetron (Zofran), paclitaxel (Taxol), piperacillin (Pipracil), piperacillin/tazobactam (Zosyn), plicamycin (Mithracin), potassium chloride (KCl), promethazine (Phenergan), ranitidine (Zantac), sodium bicarbonate, streptozocin (Zanosar), sulfamethoxazole-trimethoprim (Bactrim), teniposide (Vumon), thiotepa (Thioplex), ticarcillin (Ticar), ticarcillin/clavulanate (Timentin), tobramycin (Nebcin), vancomycin (Vancocin), vinblastine (Velban), vincristine (Oncovin), zidovudine (AZT, Retrovir).

RATE OF ADMINISTRATION

Nonphosphate products (e.g., VePesid): Total desired dose, properly diluted (0.2 to 0.4 mg/ml) and evenly distributed over at least 30 to 60 minutes. Rapid infusion may cause marked hypotension. May be extended if fluid volume is a concern.

Phosphate products (e.g., Etopophos): Total desired dose, properly reconstituted or diluted, may be given evenly distributed over as little as 5 minutes or up to 210 minutes.

ACTIONS

A semisynthetic derivative of podophyllotoxin. Cell cycle–specific for the G_2 phase, it inhibits DNA synthesis. Etopophos (phosphate) is a water-soluble ester of etoposide that promptly converts to etoposide in plasma. Half-life is from 3 to 12 hours (average is 7 hours). Highly protein-bound to human plasma proteins. Metabolized in the liver. Primarily excreted through urine and bile (feces). Secreted in breast milk.

INDICATIONS AND USES

To suppress or retard neoplastic growth in refractory testicular tumors (used in combination with other agents after previous surgery, chemotherapy, and radiotherapy). ■ Suppress or retard small-cell lung cancer (used in combination with other chemotherapeutic agents as first-line treatment).

Unlabeled uses: High-dose regimens before bone marrow transplantation. Treatment of acute nonlymphocytic leukemias, Hodgkin's disease, non-Hodgkin's lymphomas, carcinoma of the breast, Kaposi's sarcoma, and neuroblastoma. Additional tumors have shown up to 20% response. Used alone or in combination with other agents.

CONTRAINDICATIONS

Hypersensitivity to etoposide, etoposide phosphate, or any other component of the formulations.

PRECAUTIONS

Follow guidelines for handling cytotoxic agents. See Appendix A, p. 1142. ■ Usually administered by or under the direction of the physician specialist. ■ A low serum albumin may result in an increase of free (active) etoposide, resulting in an increased risk of toxicity. Occurs more frequently in children. ■ Oral dose of nonphosphate product (e.g., etoposide) is usually twice the IV dose.

Monitor: Determine absolute patency and quality of vein and adequate circulation of extremity. Avoid extravasation; necrosis and venous induration have occurred. ■ Use caution to prevent bone marrow depression. Platelet count, hemoglobin, WBC count, and differential must be completed before start of therapy and before each dose. See Dose Adjustments. Monitor between courses also. ■ Examine patient's mouth for ulceration before each dose. ■ Monitor hepatic and renal function before and during therapy. ■ Bone marrow recovery from a course is usually complete within 20 days. No cumulative toxicity has been reported as yet. ■ Be alert for signs of bone marrow depression or infection. ■ Monitor for thrombocytopenia (platelet count less than 50,000/mm^3). Initiate precautions to prevent excessive bleeding (e.g., inspect IV sites, skin, and mucous membranes; use extreme care during invasive procedures; test urine, emesis, stool, and secretions for occult blood). ■ Prophylactic antibiotics may be indicated pending results of C/S in a febrile neutropenic patient. ■ Maintain adequate hydration. ■ Prophylactic antiemetics may increase patient comfort.

Patient Education: Nonhormonal birth control recommended. ■ Report IV site burning or stinging promptly. ■ Report chills, difficult breathing, fever, and rapid heartbeat promptly. See Appendix D, p. 1148.

Maternal/Child: Category D: avoid pregnancy. Can cause fetal harm. ■ Discontinue breast-feeding. ■ Has been used in children, but safety and effectiveness not established. Anaphylactic reactions have been reported. See Precautions. ■ Depending on the preparation, VePesid may contain benzyl alcohol or polysorbate 80; do not use in neonates or premature infants.

Elderly: Monitor renal, hepatic, and hematologic function closely. ■ See Dose Adjustments. ■ Incidence of anorexia, asthenia, dehydration, elevated BUN levels, granulocytopenia, leukopenia (Grade III or IV), mucositis, and somnolence occur more frequently in the elderly. ■ May also be more sensitive to expected side effects (e.g., alopecia, gastrointestinal effects, infectious complications, and myelosuppression). Potential for greater sensitivity increased if renal function impaired.

DRUG/LAB INTERACTIONS

All products: Concurrent or consecutive use with other bone marrow depressants (e.g., bleomycin, cisplatin, doxorubicin) and/or radiation therapy may produce additive bone marrow depression. See Dose Adjustments. ■ Do not administer live vaccines to patients receiving antineoplastic drugs. ■ Clearance decreased and toxicity increased by cyclosporine. **Nonphosphate products (e.g., VePesid):** May potentiate warfarin; monitor PT. **Phosphate product (e.g., Etopophos):** Use caution with drugs that are known to inhibit phosphatase activities (e.g., levamisole [Ergamisol]).

SIDE EFFECTS

Bone marrow toxicity (e.g., leukopenia, neutropenia, thrombocytopenia) can be severe, is dose related, and may be dose limiting. Side effects are usually reversible: abdominal pain, alopecia, anaphylactic reactions (bronchospasm, chills, dyspnea, fever, hypotension), anemia, anorexia, constipation, diarrhea, dizziness, elevated liver function tests (e.g., AST, ALT), hypotension, mucositis, nausea, neuritic pain, paralytic ileus, peripheral neurotoxicity, stomatitis, thrombophlebitis, vomiting. Hepatic toxicity and metabolic acidosis have occurred with higher-than-recommended doses.

ANTIDOTE

Notify the physician of all side effects; symptomatic treatment is often indicated, dose reduction may be necessary. For extravasation, discontinue the drug immediately and administer into another vein. Consider injection of long-acting dexamethasone (Decadron LA) throughout extravasated tissue. Use a 27- or 25-gauge needle. Elevate extremity; moist heat may be helpful. Hypotension is usually due to a rapid infusion rate. Discontinue infusion. Trendelenburg position and IV fluids should reverse the hypotension; vasopressors (e.g., dopamine [Intropin]) may be required. After recovery, restart at slower rate. Administration of whole blood products (e.g., packed RBCs, platelets, leukocytes) and/or blood modifiers (e.g., darbepoetin alfa [Aranesp], epoetin alfa [Epogen, Procrit], filgrastim [Neupogen], pegfilgrastim [Neulasta], sargramostim [Leukine], oprelvekin [Neumega]) may be indicated to treat bone marrow toxicity. Discontinue infusion at first sign of allergic reaction; resuscitate as necessary.

FACTOR IX (HUMAN) ■ FACTOR IX COMPLEX (HUMAN)

Antihemorrhagic

AlphaNine SD, Mononine ■ Bebulin VH, Konyne 80, Profinine SD, Proplex T

pH 7 to 7.4 ■ pH 7 to 7.4

USUAL DOSE

Completely individualized based on patient's circumstances, condition, degree of deficiency, and desired blood level percentage. Specific products may be indicated or preferred in some situations; see Indications and Uses. Range is 10 to 75 IU/kg of body weight. May be repeated every 12 hours in some situations, required only every 2 or 3 days in others. Actual number of international units contained shown on each bottle or vial. Units required to raise blood level percentages can be calculated as follows:

Body weight (kg) × Desired increase (% of normal) × 1 Unit/kg

(70 kg × 40% increase × 1 IU/kg equals 2,800 IU). To maintain levels above 25%, calculate each dose to raise level to 40% to 60% of normal.

Minor hemorrhage: A single injection calculated to increase plasma level to 20% to 30%. May be repeated in 24 hours if indicated.

Major trauma or surgery: Increase plasma level to 25% to 50% and maintain at that level for a minimum of 1 week or as indicated. May require daily injections (every 18 to 30 hours).

Dental extraction: Increase plasma level to 50% before procedure; repeat if indicated.

Reversal of coumarin effect: **FACTOR IX COMPLEX:** 15 IU/kg.

Prophylaxis: 10 to 20 IU/kg once or twice a week or increase plasma level to 20% to 30%.

DILUTION

Diluent usually provided. Some preparations also supply double-ended needles for dilution and filter needle for aspiration into a syringe. Sterile technique imperative. Confirm expiration date. Use plastic syringes to prevent binding to glass surfaces. Factor IX and diluent should be at room temperature. Direct diluent from above to side of vial to gently moisten all contents. Swirl gently to dissolve; avoid foaming. Do not shake. May take 1 to 5 minutes. Should be clear and colorless. Must be used within 3 hours to avoid bacterial contamination. The addition of 2 to 3 units of heparin/ml factor IX complex may reduce the incidence of thrombosis. May be given through an IV administration set (often provided) if multiple vials are required. Discard any unused contents. Discard all administration equipment after single use; do not attempt to resterilize.

AlphaNine: Follow general directions above. After diluent is drawn through double-ended needle, remove diluent bottle first; then remove double-ended needle. ***Do not invert concentrate vial until ready to withdraw contents!*** Air from syringe into vial required to withdraw contents. Withdraw through filter.

Mononine: Follow general directions above. After diluent is drawn through double-ended needle, remove diluent bottle first; then remove double-ended needle. ***Use only the provided self-venting filter spike to transfer***

Mononine to a syringe! Do not inject any air into Mononine vial; could cause product loss. Discard filter and use only provided wing needle and micropore tubing to administer.

Storage: Store lyophilized powder at 2° to 8° C (36° to 46° F); do not freeze. Do not refrigerate after dilution. ***Mononine*** may be stored at room temperature before dilution for up to 30 days.

COMPATIBILITY

Specific information not available. Consider specific use; consult pharmacist.

RATE OF ADMINISTRATION

Average rate is 2 to 3 ml or 100 units/min. Completely individualized according to patient's condition. Decrease rate of administration for side effects such as burning or pain at injection site, chills, fever, flushing, headache, tingling, or changes in BP or pulse. Never exceed 10 ml/min.

ACTIONS

A lyophilized concentrate of human coagulation factors: IX (plasma thromboplastin and antihemophilic factor B), II (prothrombin), VII (proconvertin), and X (Stuart-Prower factor). In contrast to other products, AlphaNine and Mononine are highly purified factor IX and contain only minimal amounts of the other factors. All products are obtained from fresh human plasma and prepared, irradiated, and dried by specific processes. Konyne 80 is dry heat–treated at 80° C for 72 hours. Additional processes are used to prepare AlphaNine and Mononine that markedly reduce the possibility of viral contamination. Concentration of 25 units/ml is 25 times greater than normal plasma. Preparations contain varying amounts of total protein in each vial. Half-life extends beyond 24 hours.

INDICATIONS AND USES

All factor IX products: Prevention and control of bleeding in patients with Factor IX deficiency due to hemophilia B. May be required to correct or prevent a dangerous bleeding episode or to perform surgery. ▪ Prophylaxis to prevent spontaneous bleeding in patients with proven specific congenital deficiency (hemophilia B). **Factor IX (human):** Preferred for surgical coverage; treatment of crush injuries, treatment; of large IM hemorrhages requiring several days of replacement therapy; and treatment in neonates, individuals with severe hepatocellular dysfunction, or those with a history of thrombotic complications associated with factor IX complex. **Factor IX complex:** Prevention and control of bleeding in patients with hemophilia A who have inhibitors to Factor VIII. ▪ Reversal of coumarin effect (fresh-frozen plasma preferred unless risk of hepatitis transfer would be life threatening). ▪ Hemorrhage caused by hepatitis-induced lack of production of liver-dependent coagulation factors. ▪ Proplex T is used for prevention or control of bleeding episodes in patients with Factor VII deficiency.

CONTRAINDICATIONS

Factor IX complex: Known liver disease with suspicion of intravascular coagulation or fibrinolysis. ▪ Factor VII deficiency except for Proplex T. **Mononine:** Known hypersensitivity to mouse protein. ▪ No other known contraindications for **AlphaNine, Bebulin VH,** or **Konyne 80. AlphaNine, Alpha-Nine SD, Bebulin VH,** and **Mononine** are not indicated for replacement of any other coagulation factors.

PRECAUTIONS

Used when plasma infusions would result in hypervolemia and/or proteinemia or when blood volume or RBC replacement is not indicated. ▪ Use extreme caution in newborns, infants, postoperative patients, and patients with liver disease. Factor IX (human) (e.g., AlphaNine, Mononine) would be preferred because studies show no incidence of thrombin generation. ▪ Fresh-frozen plasma may be required in addition to factor IX complex when prompt reversal is required. ▪ Danger of thromboembolic episodes (DIC, myocardial infarction, pulmonary embolism, venous thrombosis) increases with plasma levels over 50%. ▪ Large or frequently repeated doses of factor IX complex may cause intravascular hemolysis in patients with type A, B, or AB blood.

Monitor: Monitor the patient's levels of coagulation factors before, after, and between administrations. ***Do not overdose;*** see Side Effects. ▪ AIDS or hepatitis is possible for the recipient. Health professionals should exercise caution in handling. Possibility markedly reduced with additional preparation process of AlphaNine, AlphaNine SD, Konyne 80, and Mononine. ▪ Observe for signs and symptoms of postoperative thrombosis or disseminated intravascular coagulation (DIC). Risk multiplies with repeated administrations except for AlphaNine, AlphaNine SD, and Mononine.

Patient Education: Alert to possible risk of HIV virus and hepatitis. ▪ Report early signs of hypersensitivity promptly (burning or pain along injection site, hives, rash, tightness of chest, wheezing). ▪ Notify physician if medication seems less effective. May be developing antibodies to factor IX. ▪ Carry identification card. ▪ Proper preparation and administration imperative if given in home.

Maternal/Child: Category C: safety for use during pregnancy not established; use only if clearly indicated; see Precautions. ▪ Use extreme caution in neonates with hepatitis; high rate of morbidity.

DRUG/LAB INTERACTIONS

Concurrent use of aminocaproic acid (Amicar) may increase risk of thrombosis.

SIDE EFFECTS

Burning or pain along injection site, changes in BP, chills, fever, flushing, headache, nausea, tingling, urticaria, vomiting.

Major: Anaphylaxis, DIC, hepatitis, myocardial infarction, postoperative thrombosis (rare with pure factor IX [Human] products), pulmonary embolism. Consider risk potential of contracting AIDS and hepatitis; markedly reduced with pure factor IX (Human) products (AlphaNine, AlphaNine SD, Mononine), and Konyne 80.

ANTIDOTE

Temporarily discontinue or decrease rate of administration for minor side effects. If any major symptoms appear, discontinue drug and notify physician. Treat allergic reactions as indicated; a different lot may not cause the reaction. For thrombosis or DIC, anticoagulation with heparin may be indicated.

FACTOR IX (RECOMBINANT)

Antihemorrhagic

BeneFIX

USUAL DOSE

Adults and children: Completely individualized based on the degree of deficiency, location and extent of bleeding, and the patient's clinical condition, age, and recovery of factor IX. All doses should be titrated to the patient's clinical response. Actual number of international units contained shown on each bottle or vial. Units required to raise blood level percentages are somewhat increased with this recombinant product compared to other factor IX products and can be calculated as follows:

Number of Factor IX IU Required =
Body Weight (in kg) × Desired Factor IX Increase (%) × 1.2 IU/kg

In the presence of an inhibitor, higher doses may be required.
The following chart may be used to guide dosing in bleeding episodes and surgery:

Factor IX (Recombinant) Dosing Guidelines

Type of Hemorrhage	Circulating Factor IX Activity Required (%)	Frequency of Doses (hours)	Duration of Therapy (days)
Minor Uncomplicated hemarthroses, superficial muscle, or soft tissue	20-30	12-24	1-2
Moderate Intramuscle or soft tissue with dissection, mucous membranes, dental extractions, or hematuria	25-50	12-24	Treat until bleeding stops and healing begins, about 2 to 7 days
Major Pharynx, retropharynx, retroperitoneum, CNS, surgery	50-100	12-24	7-10

Source: Roberts and Eberst

DILUTION

Sterile diluent, double-ended needle, filter spike, and infusion set provided. Sterile technique imperative. Confirm expiration date. Use plastic syringes to prevent binding to glass surfaces. Factor IX and diluent should be at room temperature. After removing the vial caps on Factor IX and diluent, wipe with antiseptic and allow to dry. Insert short end of the double-ended needle in the diluent vial. Insert long end in the Factor IX vial with the tip directed to the side of the wall to prevent excessive foaming. Fully invert the diluent vial to a vertical position and allow the diluent to run completely into the Factor IX vial. If the diluent does not transfer completely,

do not use (a very small amount remaining is permissible). Remove transfer needle. Gently rotate the vial to dissolve. Should be clear and colorless. Attach filter spike to the plastic syringe and insert in the reconstituted solution; invert and withdraw contents. ***Do not*** inject air into the vial; may cause partial loss of product. Multiple vials may be drawn in the same syringe, but a new sterile filter spike must be used for each vial. Must be used within 3 hours of reconstitution.

Storage: Refrigerate packaged product (2° to 8° C [36° to 46° F]). Packaged product may be stored at room temperature not exceeding 25° C (77° F) for up to 6 months (mark date removed from refrigerator on carton). Avoid freezing. Do not use after the expiration date.

COMPATIBILITY

Specific information not available. Consider specific use; consult pharmacist.

RATE OF ADMINISTRATION

A single dose over several minutes. Average rate during studies was 50 units/kg infused over 10 minutes. Individualized according to patient's condition and comfort level. Decrease rate for side effects such as burning or pain at injection site, chills, fever, flushing, headache, tingling, or changes in BP or pulse.

ACTIONS

An antihemorrhagic. A purified protein produced by recombinant DNA technology for use in the treatment of factor IX deficiency. Its primary amino acid sequence is identical to a form of plasma-derived factor IX, and it has structural and functional characteristics similar to those of endogenous factor IX. Inherently free from the risk of transmission of human bloodborne pathogens such as HIV, hepatitis viruses, and parvovirus. Factor IX is the specific clotting factor deficient in patients with hemophilia B and in patients with acquired factor IX deficiencies. Factor IX (Recombinant) increases plasma levels of factor IX and can temporarily correct the coagulation defect in these patients. Half-life ranges from 11 to 26 hours.

INDICATIONS AND USES

Control and prevention of hemorrhagic episodes in patients with hemophilia B (congenital factor IX deficiency or Christmas disease), including control and prevention of bleeding in surgical settings.

CONTRAINDICATIONS

Known history of hypersensitivity to hamster protein. ■ Not indicated for the treatment of other factor deficiencies (e.g., factors II, VII, and X). ■ Not indicated for the treatment of hemophilia A patients with inhibitors to factor VIII. ■ Not indicated for the reversal of coumarin-induced anticoagulation. ■ Not indicated for the treatment of bleeding due to low levels of liver-dependent coagulation factors.

PRECAUTIONS

Usually administered under the supervision of a physician experienced in the treatment of hemophilia B. ■ Allergic-type hypersensitivity reactions are possible. ■ BeneFIX contains only coagulation factor IX, but thromboembolic episodes (e.g., disseminated intravascular coagulation [DIC], myocardial infarction, pulmonary embolism, venous thrombosis) have been reported with other factor IX concentrates. These episodes increase with plasma levels over 50%. May be hazardous in patients with signs of fibrinolysis or DIC. ■ Because of potential thromboembolic problems, use caution in patients with liver disease, patients in the postoperative period, neonates, or in patients at risk of thromboembolic phenomena or DIC. Benefit must be weighed against risk.

Monitor: To ensure desired factor IX activity levels, precise monitoring using the factor IX activity assay is recommended, especially during surgical intervention. ***Do not overdose;*** see Side Effects. ■ Monitor for development of factor IX inhibitors. Patients dosed with high-purity factor IX products who develop inhibitors are at increased risk of anaphylaxis with repeat doses.

Patient Education: Allergic reactions can occur. Report difficulty breathing, hives, itching, tightness of the chest, and/or wheezing promptly. If self-administering, discontinue use and contact physician immediately.

Maternal/Child: Category C: use during pregnancy or during breast-feeding only if clearly indicated. ■ To this date, no adverse reactions related to treatment have been reported in children.

Elderly: Response similar to other age-groups.

DRUG/LAB INTERACTIONS

Specific information not available.

SIDE EFFECTS

Allergic rhinitis, altered taste, burning or pain along injection site, burning sensation in jaw and skull, changes in BP, chills, dizziness, drowsiness, dry cough, fever, flushing, headache, lethargy, lightheadedness, nausea, phlebitis at injection site, rash, tightness in the chest, tingling, urticaria, vomiting.

Major: Anaphylaxis, DIC, myocardial infarction, postoperative thrombosis (rare with pure factor IX products), pulmonary embolism.

ANTIDOTE

Temporarily discontinue or decrease rate of administration for minor side effects. If any major symptoms appear, discontinue drug and notify physician. Treat allergic reactions as indicated. For thrombosis or DIC, anticoagulation with heparin may be indicated.

FAMOTIDINE

(fam-o'tah-deen)

Antiulcer agent
(H_2 antagonist)
Gastric acid inhibitor

Pepcid IV

pH 5 to 5.6

USUAL DOSE

20 mg (2 ml) every 12 hours. Increase frequency of dose, not amount, if necessary for pain relief.

PEDIATRIC DOSE

Age 1 to 16 years: Starting dose is 0.25 mg/kg every 12 hours. Treatment duration and dose must be individualized based on clinical response, pH determination, and/or endoscopy. Doses up to 0.5 mg/kg every 12 hours may be required for gastric acid suppression. Another source suggests 0.6 to 0.8 mg/kg/24 hr (0.3 to 0.4 mg/kg every 12 hours or 0.2 to 0.27 mg/kg every 8 hours). May need to reduce interval to every 8 hours because of increased elimination. Maximum dose is 40 mg/24 hr.

DOSE ADJUSTMENTS

Reduce dose by one-half or increase the dosing interval to 36 to 48 hours in patients with moderate or severe renal dysfunction (CrCl less than 50 ml/min). Adjust based on patient response. Half-life may exceed 20 hours if CrCl less than 10 ml/min.

DILUTION

IV injection: Each 20 mg must be diluted with 5 to 10 ml of NS or other compatible infusion solutions for injection (e.g., D5W, D10W, LR, SW. Available premixed 20 mg in 50 ml diluent.

Intermittent infusion: Each 20 mg may be diluted in 100 ml of D5W or other compatible infusion solution and given piggyback.

Storage: Refrigerate vials before dilution. Use diluted solution within 48 hours. Store premixed Galaxy containers at CRT; avoid excessive heat.

INCOMPATIBLE WITH

May form a precipitate with sodium bicarbonate in concentrations greater than 0.2 mg/ml.

COMPATIBLE WITH

(Underline Indicates Conflicting Compatibility Information)

Consult pharmacist; specific conditions may apply; see Compatibilities, p. xvi.

Solutions: Selected TNA and TPN solutions.

Additive: Cefazolin (Kefzol), flumazenil (Romazicon), vancomycin (Vancocin).

Y-site: Acyclovir (Zovirax), allopurinol (Aloprim, Zyloprim), amifostine (Ethyol), aminophylline, ampicillin, ampicillin/sulbactam (Unasyn), atropine, aztreonam (Azactam), bretylium (Bretylate), calcium gluconate, cefazolin (Kefzol), cefoperazone (Cefobid), cefotaxime (Claforan), cefotetan (Cefotan), cefoxitin (Mefoxin), ceftazidime (Fortaz), ceftizoxime (Cefizox), ceftriaxone (Rocephin), cefuroxime (Zinacef), chlorpromazine (Thorazine), cisatracurium (Nimbex), cisplatin (Platinol), cladribine (Leustatin), cyclophosphamide (Cytoxan), cytarabine (ARA-C), dexamethasone (Decadron), dextran 40, digoxin (Lanoxin), diphenhydramine (Benadryl), dobutamine (Dobutrex), docetaxel (Taxotere), dopamine (Intropin), doxorubicin (Adriamycin), doxorubicin liposome (Doxil), droperidol (Inapsine), enalaprilat (Vasotec IV), epinephrine (Adrenalin), erythromycin lactobionate (Erythrocin), esmolol (Brevibloc), etoposide phosphate (Etopophos), filgrastim (Neupogen), fluconazole (Diflucan), fludarabine (Fludara), folic acid (Folvite), furosemide (Lasix), gatifloxacin (Tequin), gemcitabine (Gemzar), gentamicin (Garamycin), granisetron (Kytril), haloperidol (Haldol), heparin, hetastarch in electrolytes (Hextend), hydrocortisone sodium succinate (Solu-Cortef), hydromorphone (Dilaudid), imipenem-cilastatin (Primaxin), inamrinone (Inocor), insulin (regular), isoproterenol (Isuprel), labetalol (Normodyne), lidocaine, linezolid (Zyvox), lorazepam (Ativan), magnesium sulfate, melphalan (Alkeran), meperidine (Demerol), methotrexate (Folex), methylprednisolone (Solu-Medrol), metoclopramide (Reglan), midazolam (Versed), morphine, nafcillin (Nafcil), nitroglycerin (Nitro-Bid IV), nitroprusside sodium, norepinephrine (Levophed), ondansetron (Zofran), oxacillin (Bactocill), paclitaxel (Taxol), perphenazine (Trilafon), phenylephrine (Neo-Synephrine), phenytoin (Dilantin), phytonadione (Aquamephyton), piperacillin (Pipracil), potassium chloride (KCl), potassium phosphates, procainamide (Pronestyl), propofol (Diprivan), remifentanil (Ultiva), sargramostim (Leukine), sodium bicarbonate, teniposide (Vumon), theophylline, thiotepa (Thioplex), ticarcillin (Ticar), ticarcillin/clavulanate (Timentin), tirofiban (Aggrastat), verapamil (Isoptin), vinorelbine (Navelbine).

RATE OF ADMINISTRATION

IV injection: Each 20 mg or fraction thereof over at least 2 minutes.

Intermittent infusion: Each 20-mg dose over 15 to 30 minutes.

ACTIONS

A histamine H_2 antagonist, it inhibits both daytime and nocturnal basal gastric acid secretion. It also inhibits gastric acid secretion stimulated by food and pentagastrin. Onset of action occurs within 30 minutes and lasts for 10 to 12 hours. No cumulative effect with repeated doses. 30 to 60 times more potent than cimetidine. Eliminated by renal and other metabolic routes. Crosses placental barrier. Secreted in breast milk.

INDICATIONS AND USES

Short-term treatment of active duodenal ulcers, benign gastric ulcers, and pathologic hypersecretory conditions in hospitalized patients or in patients unable to take oral medication. ■ Used orally for short-term treatment of gastroesophageal reflux disease (GERD) including erosive or ulcerative esophagitis. IV dose recommendations not yet available.

Unlabeled uses: GI bleeding. ■ Stress ulcer prophylaxis.

CONTRAINDICATIONS

Known hypersensitivity to H_2 receptor antagonists (e.g., cimetidine [Tagamet], famotidine [Pepcid IV], ranitidine [Zantac]) or their components; cross-sensitivity has occurred.

PRECAUTIONS

Use with caution in patients with moderate or severe renal dysfunction; see Dose Adjustments. ■ CNS adverse effects have been reported in patients with impaired renal function. ■ Gastric malignancy may be present even though patient is asymptomatic. ■ Effects maintained with oral dosage. Total treatment usually discontinued after 4 to 8 weeks.

Monitor: Use antacids concomitantly to relieve pain. ■ See Precautions.

Patient Education: Stop smoking or at least avoid smoking after last dose of the day. ■ Gastric pain and ulceration may recur after medication stopped.

Maternal/Child: Category B: use during pregnancy only when clearly needed. ■ Advisable to discontinue breast-feeding. ■ Plasma clearance is reduced and half-life is increased in pediatric patients less than 3 months of age compared to older pediatric patients with pharmacokinetic parameters similar to adults.

Elderly: Response similar to that seen in younger patients; however, greater sensitivity in the elderly cannot be ruled out. ■ Consider risk of renal dysfunction; reduced doses and monitoring of renal function may be indicated; see Dose Adjustments.

DRUG/LAB INTERACTIONS

May inhibit gastric absorption of ketoconazole (Nizoral). ■ May decrease cyclosporine serum levels when famotidine is given concurrently with ketoconazole and cyclosporine.

SIDE EFFECTS

Constipation, diarrhea, dizziness, and headache are the most common side effects. Allergic reactions (bronchospasm, fever, pruritus, rash, eosinophilia) can occur. Abdominal discomfort, agitation, alopecia, anorexia, anxiety, arthralgias, confusion, decreased libido, depression, dry mouth, dry skin, elevated ALT (SGPT), flushing, grand mal seizure, hallucinations, insomnia, malaise, muscular pain, nausea and vomiting, orbital edema, palpitations, paresthesias, somnolence, taste disorder, thrombocytopenia, and tinnitus have been reported.

ANTIDOTE

Notify physician of all side effects. May be treated symptomatically or may respond to decrease in frequency of dosage. Resuscitate as necessary for overdosage.

FAT EMULSION, INTRAVENOUS

Nutritional supplement (fatty acid)

Intralipid 10%, 20% & 30%, Liposyn II 10% & 20%, Liposyn III 10% 20% & 30%

pH 6 to 9

USUAL DOSE

Some solutions may contain aluminum; see Precautions.

Total parenteral nutrition component: 500 ml of 10% or 250 ml of 20% on the first day. Increase dose gradually each day. Do not exceed 60% of the patient's total caloric intake or 2.5 to 3 Gm/kg of body weight.

Fatty acid deficiency: Supply 8% to 10% of the total caloric intake each 24 hours.

PEDIATRIC DOSE

Some solutions may contain aluminum; see Precautions.

Total parenteral nutrition component: Up to 1 Gm/kg of body weight. Increase dose gradually each day. Do not exceed 60% of total caloric intake or 3 to 4 Gm/kg.

Premature infants: Begin with 0.5 Gm fat/kg/24 hr. See comments under Pediatric Dose.

DOSE ADJUSTMENTS

Normal renal function required. Reduced dose may be indicated.

DILUTION

Must be given as prepared by manufacturer; check labels for aluminum content; see Precautions. Use only freshly opened solutions; discard remainder of partial dose. Do not use if there appears to be an oiling out of the emulsion. **Intralipid 30% is not to be given by direct IV infusion.** Packaged for bulk use in a pharmacy admixture program. Must be specifically combined with dextrose solutions and amino acids (TPN) so total fat content does not exceed 20%. Prepared for an individual patient in the pharmacy. Lipids may extract phthalates from phthalate-plasticized PVC. Non-phthalate infusion sets recommended; available with most commercial products.

Storage: Must be stored at temperatures not exceeding 25° C (77° F) or refrigerated. Specific storage conditions required (see literature). Do not freeze. Manufacturer recommends admixtures (3 in 1) be refrigerated for no more than 24 hours after mixing. In actual practice a 7-day supply in individual containers for daily adminstration is frequently prepared and refrigerated for home use.

INCOMPATIBLE WITH

Manufacturer recommends not mixing with any electrolyte or other nutrient solution. Infuse separately; do not disturb emulsion; no additives or medications are to be placed in bottle or tubing with the exception of heparin 1 to 2 units/ml (may be added before administration [activates lipoprotein lipase]). In actual practice, carbohydrates, amino acids, and fat emulsion are mixed in specific percentages and in a specific order to meet individual total parenteral nutritional needs but should be prepared in the pharmacy. Any addition of supplemental vitamins, minerals, or electrolytes (e.g., calcium, magnesium, phosphates) may cause a precipitate unless a specific order is followed. Precipitates are difficult to detect in lipids.

COMPATIBLE WITH **(Underline Indicates Conflicting Compatibility Information)**

Consult pharmacist; specific conditions may apply; see Incompatible With and Compatibilities, p. xvi.

Additive: ***See Incompatible With;*** however, some sources suggest that selected additives may be compatible.

Y-site: Specific TNA solutions may be compatible at Y-site with specific concentrations of aldesleukin (Interleukin-2), <u>amikacin (Amikin)</u>, aminophylline, ampicillin, ampicillin/sulbactam (Unasyn), aztreonam (Azactam), bumetanide (Bumex), buprenorphine (Buprenex), butorphanol (Stadol), calcium gluconate, carboplatin (Paraplatin), cefamandole (Mandol), cefazolin (Kefzol), cefoperazone (Cefobid), cefotaxime (Claforan), cefotetan (Cefotan), cefoxitin (Mefoxin), ceftazidime (Fortaz), ceftizoxime (Cefizox), ceftriaxone (Rocephin), cefuroxime (Zinacef), chlorpromazine (Thorazine), cimetidine (Tagamet), ciprofloxacin (Cipro IV), cisplatin (Platinol), clindamycin (Cleocin), cyclophosphamide (Cytoxan), <u>cyclosporine (Sandimmune)</u>, cytarabine (ARA-C), dexamethasone (Decadron), digoxin, diphenhydramine (Benadryl), dobutamine (Dobutrex), <u>dopamine (Intropin)</u>, enalaprilat (Vasotec IV), erythromycin lactobionate (Erythrocin), famotidine (Pepcid IV), fentanyl (Sublimaze), fluconazole (Diflucan), <u>fluorouracil (5-FU)</u>, furosemide (Lasix), gentamicin (Garamycin), granisetron (Kytril), hydrocortisone (Hydrocortone, Solu-Cortef), <u>hydromorphone (Dilaudid)</u>, ifosfamide (Ifex), imipenem-cilastatin (Primaxin), insulin (regular), isoproterenol (Isuprel), kanamycin (Kantrex), leucovorin calcium, lidocaine, magnesium sulfate, mannitol, meperidine (Demerol), meropenem (Merrem IV), mesna (Mesnex), methotrexate (Folex), methyldopate (Aldomet), methylprednisolone (Solu-Medrol), metoclopramide (Reglan), metronidazole (Flagyl IV), mitoxantrone (Novantrone), morphine, nafcillin (Nafcil), nitroglycerin (Nitro-Bid IV), nitroprusside sodium, norepinephrine (Levophed), octreotide (Sandostatin), ofloxacin (Floxin IV), oxacillin (Bactocill), paclitaxel (Taxol), penicillin G potassium, piperacillin (Pipracil), piperacillin/tazobactam (Zosyn), potassium chloride (KCl), prochlorperazine (Compazine), promethazine (Phenergan), ranitidine (Zantac), sodium bicarbonate, sulfamethoxazole-trimethoprim (Bactrim), tacrolimus (Prograf), ticarcillin (Ticar), ticarcillin/clavulanate (Timentin), tobramycin (Nebcin), vancomycin (Vancocin), zidovudine (AZT, Retrovir).

RATE OF ADMINISTRATION

May be administered via a Y-tube or three-way stopcock near the infusion site. Rates of both solutions (fat emulsion and amino acid products) should be controlled by infusion pumps. Keep fat emulsion line higher than all other lines (has low specific gravity and could run up into other lines). Do not use filters; will disturb emulsion. FDA suggests use of at least a 1.2-micron filter for admixtures containing lipids (e.g., 3 in 1); precipitates difficult to detect in lipids.

Adult: ***10%:*** 1 ml/min or 0.1 Gm fat/min for the first 15 to 30 minutes. If no untoward effects, increase rate to administer 500 ml equally distributed over 4 to 6 hours or 0.2 Gm fat/min.

20%: 0.5 ml/min or 0.1 Gm fat/min for the first 15 to 30 minutes. If no untoward effects, increase rate to administer 250 ml equally distributed over 4 to 6 hours or 0.2 Gm fat/min.

Pediatric: ***10%:*** 0.1 ml/min for the first 10 to 15 minutes. Reduce initial rate to 0.05 ml/min for a ***20%*** solution. If no untoward effects, increase rate to administer 1 Gm/kg of body weight (total usual dose) equally distributed over 4 hours. An infusion pump is recommended. Do not exceed a rate of 50 ml/hr (20%) or 100 ml/hr (10%).

ACTIONS

An isotonic nutrient. Contains emulsified fat particles about 0.4 to 0.5 micron in size. Total caloric value (fat, phospholipid, and glycerol) is 1.1 cal/ml for the 10% emulsion and 2 cal/ml for the 20% emulsion. Metabolized and used as a source of energy. Increases heat production and oxygen consumption. Decreases respiratory quotient. Cleared from the bloodstream by a process not fully understood.

INDICATIONS AND USES

To provide additional calories and essential fatty acids for patients requiring parenteral nutrition whose caloric requirements cannot be met by glucose or who will be receiving parenteral nutrition over extended periods (over 5 days usually). ■ Prevent essential fatty acid deficiency.

CONTRAINDICATIONS

Any condition that disturbs normal fat metabolism, such as pathologic hyperlipemia, lipoid nephrosis, and acute pancreatitis with hyperlipemia; severe egg allergies.

PRECAUTIONS

Isotonic; may be administered by a peripheral vein or central venous infusion. ■ Fatty acids displace bilirubin bound to albumin. Use caution in jaundiced or premature infants. ■ Use caution in pulmonary disease, liver disease, anemia, or blood coagulation disorders, or when there is any danger of fat embolism. ■ Some solutions of potassium acetate contain aluminum. In impaired kidney function, aluminum may reach toxic levels. Premature neonates are particularly at risk because of their immature kidneys and requirement for calcium and phosphate, which also contain aluminum. Research indicates that patients with impaired renal function who receive more than 4 to 5 mcg/kg/day of parenteral aluminum are at risk for developing CNS or bone toxicity associated with aluminum accumulation. ■ See Maternal/Child.

Monitor: Monitor lipids before each infusion; lipemia should clear daily. ■ Monitor hemogram, blood coagulation, liver function tests, plasma lipid profile, and platelet count, especially in neonates. Discontinue use for significant abnormality.

Maternal/Child: Category C: use in pregnancy only when clearly needed; safety not established. ■ Use caution if emulsion is administered to a woman who is breast-feeding. ■ Use extreme caution in neonates; death from intravascular fat accumulation in the lungs has occurred. Frequent, even daily, platelet counts are recommended in neonatal patients receiving TPN with IV fat emulsion.

DRUG/LAB INTERACTIONS

No specific information available; see Dilution.

SIDE EFFECTS

Anaphylaxis, back pain, chest pain, cyanosis, dizziness, dyspnea, elevated temperature, flushing, headache, hypercoagulability, hyperlipemia, nausea and vomiting, pressure over eyes, sepsis (from contamination of IV catheter), sleepiness, sweating, thrombophlebitis (from concurrent hyperalimentation fluids), a delayed overloading syndrome (focal seizures, fever, leukocytosis, splenomegaly, shock), and many others.

ANTIDOTE

Notify physician of all side effects. Many will be treated symptomatically. Treat allergic reaction promptly and resuscitate as necessary. For accidental overdose, stop the infusion. Obtain blood sample for inspection of plasma, triglyceride concentration, and measurement of plasma light-scattering activity by nephelometry. Repeat blood samples until the lipid has cleared. Stop infusion immediately for any signs of acute respiratory distress. May represent pulmonary embolus or interstitial pneumonitis, which may be caused by an unseen precipitate of electrolytes (e.g., calcium and phosphates) in the solution.

FENOLDOPAM MESYLATE

(fhe-knowl′doh-pam mes′uh-lat)

Antihypertensive
Vasodilator

Corlopam

USUAL DOSE

Must be given as a continuous infusion. Avoid hypotension and rapid decreases in BP. Doses ranging from 0.01 to 1.6 mcg/kg/min were studied in clinical trials. Most references suggest an initial dose of 0.1 mcg/kg/min. Doses below 0.1 mcg/kg/min have modest effects and may have minimal use. Initial doses of 0.03 to 0.1 mcg/kg/min have been associated with less reflex tachycardia than initial doses of more than 0.3 mcg/kg/min. As the dose increases, there is a greater and more rapid reduction in BP. Maximum recommended dose is 1.7 mcg/kg/min. To achieve the desired reduction in BP, titrate initial dose upward or downward in increments of 0.05 to 0.1 mcg/kg/min, no more frequently than every 15 minutes. Extend duration of intervals as desired BP goal is approached. Maximum effect of each range usually attained within 15 minutes. When the desired response is achieved, fenoldopam may be discontinued gradually or abruptly; rebound elevation of BP has not been observed. See Precautions and Drug/Lab Interactions.

See product insert for doses used in clinical trials for mild to moderate hypertension and hypertensive emergency. Manufacturer provides extensive charts documenting effects of a wide range of doses but does not suggest a standard initial dose. The manufacturer states that the initial dose may be chosen from the appropriate table and suggests selecting a dose that corresponds to the desired magnitude and rate of BP reduction.

PEDIATRIC DOSE

Safety and effectiveness for use in children not established.

DOSE ADJUSTMENTS

Dose adjustment is not required in end-stage renal disease; in patients on continuous ambulatory peritoneal dialysis (CAPD); in severe hepatic failure; or by age, gender, or race. Effects of hemodialysis have not been evaluated.

DILUTION

To facilitate administration through an infusion pump (e.g., IVAC), each 10 mg (1 ml) must be diluted with 250 ml of NS or D5W and given as a continuous infusion. (10 mg in 250 ml, 20 mg in 500 ml, or 40 mg in 1,000 ml all yield 40 mcg/ml.) For fluid-restricted patients, concentrations of 100 mcg/ml administered through a syringe pump have been used. 10 mg in 100 ml NS or D5W yields 100 mcg/ml.

Storage: Diluted solution is stable at CRT and normal light conditions for 24 hours. Discard any solution not used within 24 hours of preparation.

COMPATIBILITY

Specific information not available. Consider specific use and need for continuous adjustment. Consult pharmacist.

RATE OF ADMINISTRATION

Do not give as a bolus injection; must be given as an infusion. Use of a calibrated, mechanical infusion pump is recommended for accurate, reliable delivery of desired infusion rate. Avoid hypotension and rapid decreases in BP. Infusion may be abruptly discontinued or gradually tapered as indicated by patient condition and/or use of other antihypertensive agents. See chart below for desired infusion rates:

Fenoldopam Infusion Rate Guidelines (40 mcg/ml dilution)					
	Desired Fenoldopam Dose				
Body Weight (kg)	0.025 mcg/kg/min	0.05 mcg/kg/min	0.1 mcg/kg/min	0.2 mcg/kg/min	0.3 mcg/kg/min
	Infusion Rates (ml/min)				
40	0.025	0.05	0.1	0.2	0.3
50	0.031	0.06	0.13	0.25	0.38
60	0.038	0.08	0.15	0.3	0.45
70	0.044	0.09	0.18	0.35	0.53
80	0.05	0.1	0.2	0.4	0.6
90	0.056	0.11	0.23	0.45	0.68
100	0.063	0.13	0.25	0.5	0.75
110	0.069	0.14	0.28	0.55	0.83
120	0.075	0.15	0.3	0.6	0.9
130	0.081	0.16	0.33	0.65	0.98
140	0.088	0.18	0.35	0.7	1.05
150	0.094	0.19	0.38	0.75	1.13

ACTIONS

A peripherally acting rapid-acting vasodilator. Is an agonist at the D_1 receptor and binds with moderate affinity to the $alpha_2$ adrenoreceptor. Causes a dose-dependent fall in systolic and diastolic BP. May cause a reflex increase in HR. Onset of action begins within 5 minutes, and with continuous infusion, steady state concentrations (peak effects) are reached in 15 to 20 minutes. Increases renal blood flow by dilating both afferent and efferent arterioles. Maintains or increases glomerular filtration rate (GFR) in normotensive or hypertensive patients with or without renal insufficiency. Beneficial effects have not been seen in patients with heart failure, hepatic disease, or severe renal disease. Increases sodium excretion and decreases sodium reabsorption. Increases potassium, calcium, and phosphate excretion, with or without an increase in GFR. Elimination half-life is about 5 minutes. Metabolized in the liver primarily by conjugation (without cytochrome P_{450} enzymes). Primarily eliminated in urine; some excretion in feces.

INDICATIONS AND USES

In-hospital, short-term (up to 48 hours) management of severe hypertension when rapid, but quickly reversible, emergency reduction of BP is indicated, including malignant hypertension with deteriorating end-organ function.

Unlabeled uses: Renal protection before study with contrast dye.

CONTRAINDICATIONS

Manufacturer states, "None known."

PRECAUTIONS

Use limited to the hospital. Adequate personnel and appropriate equipment must be available for continuous monitoring. ▪ Use extreme caution in patients with glaucoma or intraocular hypertension. Has caused a dose-dependent increase in intraocular pressure. ▪ Causes a dose-related tachycardia with infusion rates above 0.1 mcg/kg. May diminish over time but is consistent at higher doses. Has not been reported, but could lead to ischemic cardiac events or worsened heart failure. ▪ Although hypotension should be avoided in all patients, use extreme caution in patients with an acute cerebral infarction or hemorrhage. ▪ Rapidly decreases serum potassium leading to hypokalemia; see Monitor. ▪ Use caution; contains sulfites. Sulfite sensitivity is seen more frequently in asthmatic than nonasthmatic individuals. ▪ See Drug/Lab Interactions.

Monitor: Determine patency of vein; avoid extravasation. Monitor BP and HR at least every 15 minutes. Avoid hypotension. More frequent monitoring may be required, but intraarterial BP monitoring has not been required. ▪ Monitor serum electrolytes frequently; monitoring of serum potassium is recommended every 6 hours. Has reduced serum potassium values less than 3 mEq/L in less than 6 hours. Oral or intravenous supplements are required. ▪ Transfer to oral antihypertensive agents when BP is stable. May be added during fenoldopam infusion or following its discontinuation; monitor effects carefully. ▪ See Precautions and Drug/Lab Interactions.

Patient Education: Report IV site burning or stinging promptly. ▪ Request assistance to ambulate.

Maternal/Child: Category B: use only if clearly needed. ▪ Use caution during breast-feeding; not known if fenoldopam is secreted in breast milk (is secreted in milk of rats). ▪ Safety and effectiveness for use in children not established.

Elderly: Reponse similar to other age-groups.

DRUG/LAB INTERACTIONS

No specific drug interaction studies have been conducted. ▪ Concurrent use not recommended with beta-adrenergic blocking agents (e.g., atenolol [Tenormin], esmolol [Brevibloc], metoprolol [Lopressor], propranolol [Inderal]). May cause unexpected hypotension from beta-blocker inhibition of the reflex response to fenoldopam (e.g., tachycardia). ▪ Has been given safely with digitalis and sublingual nitroglycerin. ▪ Limited experience with concomitant use of other antihypertensive agents (e.g., ACE inhibitors [e.g., enalaprilat (Vasotec)], calcium channel blockers [e.g., diltiazem (Cardizem), verapamil (Isoptin)], or thiazide or loop diuretics [e.g., chlorothiazide (Diuril), furosemide (Lasix), torsemide (Demadex)]).

SIDE EFFECTS

Abdominal pain or fullness, anxiety, back pain, constipation, diaphoresis, diarrhea, dizziness, flushing, headache, increased SrCr, injection site reaction, insomnia, nasal congestion, nausea, postural hypotension, urinary infection, and vomiting occurred in up to 5% of patients. Additional side effects have been reported in 0.5% to 5% of patients (see literature).

Major: Cardiac arrhythmias (e.g., bradycardia, extrasystoles, ST-T wave abnormalities, tachycardia), hypotension, hypokalemia, and myocardial infarction can occur with average doses.

ANTIDOTE

Keep physician informed of all side effects. Most will be treated symptomatically. Use oral and/or intravenous potassium to treat hypokalemia. Reduce dose gradually as desired BP is reached. Discontinue fenoldopam immediately for excessive hypotension. Half-life is short. Recovery should begin within 5 to 15 minutes; support patient as indicated (e.g., Trendelenburg position, IV fluids if appropriate). With short half-life the need for vasopressors is unlikely. Discontinue fenoldopam and treat life-threatening arrhythmias as indicated.

FENTANYL CITRATE

(fen′ta-nill sit′rat)

Narcotic analgesic (agonist)
Anesthesia adjunct

Fentanyl, Fentanyl Citrate PF, Sublimaze

pH 4 to 7.5

USUAL DOSE

Adjunct to regional anesthesia: 50 to 100 mcg (0.05 to 0.1 mg).
Adjunct to general anesthesia: ***Low dose:*** 2 mcg/kg of body weight.
Moderate dose: 2 to 20 mcg/kg of body weight. Additional doses of 25 to 100 mcg may be administered as needed.
High dose: 20 to 50 mcg/kg of body weight. Additional doses of 25 mcg to one half the initial loading dose may be administered as needed.
General anesthetic: 50 to 100 mcg/kg of body weight administered with oxygen and a muscle relaxant.
In all situations, use smallest effective dose at maximum intervals.

PEDIATRIC DOSE

Adjunct to general anesthesia in children over 2 years of age: 1 to 3 mcg/kg/dose over 3 to 5 minutes. May repeat in 30 to 60 minutes. To give as an infusion, begin with 1 mcg/kg/hr and titrate to effect. Maximum dose is 3 mcg/kg/hr. See Maternal/Child.

DOSE ADJUSTMENTS

Reduce dose in patients receiving other CNS depressants, such as general anesthetics, alcohol, anticholinergics, antihistamines, barbiturates, cimetidine (Tagamet), hypnotics, sedatives, psychotropic agents, and narcotic analgesics. When administered with narcotics, reduce initial narcotic dose to one fourth to one third of normal. ■ Reduce dose or increase intervals for elderly, debilitated, and poor-risk patients or those with impaired pulmonary, hepatic, or renal function. ■ See Drug/Lab Interactions.

DILUTION

Small volumes may be given undiluted (usually by the anesthesiologist). Further dilution with at least 5 ml of SW or NS for injection to facilitate titration is appropriate. Other IV solutions may be used. May be given through Y-tube or three-way stopcock of infusion set.
Storage: Store at room temperature and protect from light before dilution. Use promptly.

COMPATIBLE WITH (Underline Indicates Conflicting Compatibility Information)

Consult pharmacist; specific conditions may apply; see Compatibilities, p. xvi.

Syringe: Atracurium (Tracrium), atropine, butorphanol (Stadol), chlorpromazine (Thorazine), cimetidine (Tagamet), dimenhydrinate (Dinate), diphenhydramine (Benadryl), droperidol (Inapsine), heparin, hydromorphone (Dilaudid), meperidine (Demerol), metoclopramide (Reglan), midazolam (Versed), morphine, ondansetron (Zofran), pentazocine (Talwin), perphenazine (Trilafon), prochlorperazine (Compazine), promethazine (Phenergan), ranitidine (Zantac), scopolamine.

Y-site: Alatrofloxacin (Trovan IV), amphotericin B cholesteryl (Amphotec), atracurium (Tracrium), cisatracurium (Nimbex), dexamethasone (Decadron), diazepam (Valium), diltiazem (Cardizem), diphenhydramine (Benadryl), dobutamine (Dobutrex), dopamine (Intropin), enalaprilat (Vasotec IV), epinephrine (Adrenalin), esmolol (Brevibloc), etomidate (Amidate), furosemide (Lasix), gatifloxacin (Tequin), haloperidol (Haldol), heparin, hetastarch in electrolytes (Hextend), hydrocortisone sodium succinate (Solu-Cortef), hydromorphone (Dilaudid), ketorolac (Toradol), labetalol (Normodyne), levofloxacin (Levaquin), linezolid (Zyvox), lorazepam (Ativan), metoclopramide (Reglan), midazolam (Versed), milrinone (Primacor), morphine, nafcillin (Nafcil), nicardipine (Cardene IV), nitroglycerin (Nitro-Bid IV), norepinephrine (Levophed), pancuronium (Pavulon), phenobarbital (Luminal), potassium chloride (KCl), propofol (Diprivan), ranitidine (Zantac), remifentanil (Ultiva), sargramostim (Leukine), scopolamine, thiopental (Pentothal), vecuronium (Norcuron).

RATE OF ADMINISTRATION

Administer over a minimum of 3 to 5 minutes. Rapid administration may result in apnea or respiratory paralysis. Rate must be titrated by desired dose and patient response.

ACTIONS

An opium derivative, narcotic analgesic, which is a descending CNS depressant. Approximately 100 times more potent than morphine milligram for milligram. It has definite respiratory-depressant actions that outlast its analgesic effect. In healthy individuals, respiratory rate returns to normal more quickly than with other opiates. Effective within one circulation time and lasts about 30 minutes. Effects are cumulative with repeat doses. Has little hypnotic activity, and histamine release rarely occurs. Cardiovascular system remains stable. Depresses many other senses or reflexes. Metabolized in the liver and excreted in the urine. Crosses the placental barrier. May be secreted in breast milk.

INDICATIONS AND USES

Adjunct to general and regional anesthesia. ■ Short-term analgesia during perioperative period. ■ Useful in short-duration minor surgery in outpatients and in diagnostic procedures or treatments that require the patient to be awake or very lightly anesthetized (e.g., bronchoscopy, radiologic studies, burn dressings, cystoscopy). ■ For administration with a neuroleptic such as droperidol as an anesthetic premedication, for the induction of anesthesia, and as an adjunct in the maintenance of general and regional anesthesia. ■ For use as an anesthetic agent with oxygen in selected high-risk patients, such as those undergoing open heart surgery or certain complicated neurologic or orthopedic procedures.

CONTRAINDICATIONS

Patients with known intolerance to fentanyl. In general, narcotic analgesics are also contraindicated in acute or severe bronchial asthma and if an upper airway obstruction or significant respiratory depression is present. Fentanyl is not recommended for use in labor and delivery.

PRECAUTIONS

Primarily used by or under the direct observation of the anesthesiologist. ■ Use caution in the elderly, in patients with impaired hepatic or renal function, and in patients with pulmonary disease; reduced dose may be indicated. ■ Use extreme caution in craniotomy, head injury, and increased intracranial pressure. ■ Respiratory depression may cause an increased P_{CO_2}, cerebral vasodilation, and increased intracranial pressure. Clinical course of head injury may be obscured. ■ Symptoms of acute abdominal conditions may be masked. ■ Use caution in patients with bradyarrhythmias. ■ Cough reflex is suppressed. ■ Use caution in patients with benign prostatic hypertrophy, diarrhea resulting from poisoning until toxic material is eliminated, hypersensitivity to opiates, and in premature infants or labor and delivery of premature infants.

Monitor: Oxygen, controlled respiratory equipment, naloxone (Narcan), or nalmefene (Revex), and neuromuscular blocking agents (e.g., succinylcholine) must always be available. May cause rigidity of respiratory muscles; may require a muscle relaxant to permit artificial ventilation. ■ Observe patient frequently, monitor vital signs and oxygenation. Patient will appear to be asleep and may forget to breathe unless commanded to do so. ■ Keep patient supine; orthostatic hypotension and fainting may occur. ■ See Precautions.

Patient Education: Avoid alcohol or other CNS depressants (e.g., antihistamines, diazepam [Valium]). ■ Blurred vision, dizziness, drowsiness, or lightheadedness may occur; request assistance with ambulation. ■ Review all medications for interactions.

Maternal/Child: Category C: safety for use in pregnancy not established; has impaired fertility and had embryocidal effects in rats. ■ Postpone breast-feeding for at least 4 to 6 hours after use of fentanyl. ■ Safety for use in children under 2 years not established; has caused chest wall rigidity in neonates and may be associated with methemoglobinemia and hypotension in premature neonates; see Precautions.

Elderly: See Dose Adjustments and Precautions. ■ May markedly decrease pulmonary ventilation. ■ May be more sensitive to effects (e.g., respiratory depression, urinary retention, constipation). ■ Analgesia should be effective with lower doses. ■ Consider age-related organ impairment; may delay postop recovery.

DRUG/LAB INTERACTIONS

Concurrent use of diazepam (Valium) with higher doses of fentanyl may produce vasodilation, prolonged hypotension, and result in delayed recovery. ■ CNS toxicity increased by antidepressants (e.g., amitriptyline [Elavil], nortriptyline [Aventyl]), phenothiazines (e.g., chlorpromazine [Thorazine]); MAO inhibitors (e.g., selegiline [Eldepryl]); neuromuscular blocking agents (e.g., tubocurarine) and beta-adrenergic blocking agents (e.g., propranolol [Inderal]). Reduced dose of both drugs may be indicated. ■ Cardiovascular depression may result from concurrent use of nitrous oxide and high-dose fentanyl. ■ Monitor closely for S/S of respiratory depression and CNS depression with concurrent use of protease inhibitors (e.g., saquinavir [Invirase], ritonavir [Norvir]). ■ Concurrent use with droperidol (Inapsine) may cause hypotension and decrease pulmonary arterial pressure.

SIDE EFFECTS

Bradycardia, diaphoresis, hypersensitivity reactions, hypertension, hypotension, hypothermia, increased intracranial pressure, nausea, orthostatic hypotension, respiratory depression (slight), respiratory muscle rigidity, urinary retention, vomiting.

Overdose: Anaphylaxis, apnea, cardiac arrest, circulatory collapse, coma, excitation, hypotension (severe), inverted T wave on ECG, myocardial depression (severe), pinpoint pupils, respiratory depression (severe), tachycardia, death.

ANTIDOTE

Buprenorphine is sometimes used before the end of surgery to reverse fentanyl-induced anesthesia. With increasing severity of any side effect or onset of symptoms of overdose, discontinue the drug and notify the physician. Naloxone (Narcan) or nalmefene (Revex) will reverse serious respiratory depression. A patent airway, artificial ventilation, oxygen therapy, and other symptomatic treatment must be instituted promptly. A fast-acting muscle relaxant (e.g., succinylcholine) may be required to facilitate ventilation. Use atropine to treat bradycardia. Muscle rigidity during anesthesia induction or surgery must be controlled with neuromuscular blocking agents (e.g., atracurium [Tracrium], vecuronium [Norcuron]) and controlled ventilation with oxygen. Use a neuromuscular blocking agent prophylactically to prevent muscle rigidity or to induce muscle relaxation after rigidity occurs. Resuscitate as necessary.

FILGRASTIM

(fill-grass′stim)

Colony-stimulating factor
Antineutropenic

G-CSF, Human Granulocyte Colony-Stimulating Factor, Neupogen

pH 4

USUAL DOSE

Should not be used 24 hours before to 24 hours after the administration of cytotoxic chemotherapy and/or 12 hours before or after radiotherapy because of the potential sensitivity of rapidly dividing myeloid cells to cytotoxic chemotherapy.

Cancer patients receiving myelosuppressive chemotherapy: 5 mcg/kg/24 hr as a single daily dose for 2 to 4 weeks based on specific chemotherapy protocol and post-nadir absolute neutrophil count (ANC). May be given IV by intermittent or continuous infusion, by SC injection, or as a 24-hour SC infusion. May be increased by 5 mcg/kg/24 hr increments for each chemotherapy cycle. Expect a transient increase in neutrophil counts in the first several days after initiation of therapy. Neutrophil response may not be adequate and dose increases as outlined may be required in heavily pretreated patients, those who have received prior radiation therapy to a significant portion of their medullary bone marrow (e.g., pelvis), bone marrow transplant patients, and/or those receiving dose-intensified chemotherapy. Maximum tolerated dose not identified. Up to 115 mcg/kg/24 hr has been used. For a sustained therapeutic response, therapy must be continued until the post-nadir ANC is 10,000/mm^3 after the expected chemotherapy nadir (lowest point) has passed. Usually discontinued when this point is reached. (Average is 2 weeks or less.) In patients receiving dose-intensified chemotherapy, continue filgrastim until 2 consecutive ANCs equal to or greater than 10,000 cells/mm^3 are documented. (Range is 6 to 28 days.) See Monitor.

Patients with acute myeloid leukemia (AML) receiving induction or consolidation chemotherapy: Suggested dose is based on clinical studies: 5 mcg/kg/24 hr. Begin 24 hours after completion of induction or consolidation chemotherapy and continue daily until the ANC is equal to or greater than 1,000/mm^3 for 3 consecutive days. May be given IV by intermittent or continuous infusion, by SC injection, or as a 24-hour SC infusion.

Bone marrow transplant (BMT): 10 mcg/kg/24 hr as an IV infusion over 4 to 24 hours or as a continuous 24-hour SC infusion. Give the first dose at least 24 hours after cytotoxic chemotherapy and 24 hours after bone marrow infusion.

DOSE ADJUSTMENTS

Reduce dose or discontinue filgrastim if ANC greater than 10,000/mm^3 for 3 days. ■ During neutrophil recovery after BMT titrate the daily dose as follows based on daily or three consecutive-day evaluations:

Guidelines for Filgrastim Dose Adjustments

Absolute Neutrophil Count (ANC)	Filgrastim Dose
ANC >1,000/mm^3 × 3 days	↓ to 5 mcg/kg/24 hr
ANC remains >1,000/mm^3 × 3 more days on 5 mcg/kg/24 hr	DC filgrastim
ANC <1,000/mm^3	Resume at 5 mcg/kg/24 hr
ANC <1,000/mm^3 on 5 mcg/kg/24 hr	↑ to 10 mcg/kg/24 hr

DILUTION

Available as a single-dose vial with either 300 mcg/ml or 480 mcg/1.6 ml. Remove from refrigerator to allow to warm to room temperature (never longer than 24 hours). Confirm expiration date to ensure valid product. Avoid shaking. Contains no preservatives; use sterile technique, entering vial only once to withdraw a single dose. Dilute with 10 to 50 ml D5W to concentrations of 15 mcg/ml or greater. With concentrations from 5 to 15 mcg/ml, the addition of 2 ml of 5% albumin to each 50 ml D5W is required before adding filgrastim. Protects from adsorption to plastics and glass. Discard any unused portion. Should be clear and colorless. Do not dilute to less than 5 mcg/ml.

Storage: Store in refrigerator before use. Do not allow to freeze. Do not expose to direct sunlight. Stable undiluted in a syringe for 24 hours at CRT or up to 7 days if refrigerated. Refrigerate diluted solutions and use within 24 hours.

INCOMPATIBLE WITH

Manufacturer states, "Do not dilute with saline at any time; product may precipitate."

COMPATIBLE WITH (Underline Indicates Conflicting Compatibility Information)

Consult pharmacist; specific conditions may apply; see Compatibilities, p. xvi.

Solution: Diluted in D5W or D5W plus Albumin (human), filgrastim is compatible with glass bottles, PVC and polyolefin IV bags, and polypropylene syringes; see Dilution.

Y-site: Acyclovir (Zovirax), allopurinol (Aloprim, Zyloprim), amikacin (Amikin), aminophylline, ampicillin, ampicillin/sulbactam (Unasyn), aztreonam (Azactam), bleomycin (Blenoxane), bumetanide (Bumex), buprenorphine (Buprenex), butorphanol (Stadol), calcium gluconate, carboplatin (Paraplatin), carmustine (BiCNU), cefazolin (Kefzol), cefotetan (Cefotan), ceftazidime (Fortaz), chlorpromazine (Thorazine), cimetidine (Tagamet), cisplatin (Platinol), cyclophosphamide (Cytoxan), cytarabine (ARA-C), dacarbazine (DTIC), daunorubicin (Cerubidine), dexamethasone (Decadron), diphenhydramine (Benadryl), doxorubicin (Adriamycin), doxycycline (Vibramycin), droperidol (Inapsine), enalaprilat (Vasotec IV), famotidine (Pepcid IV), fluconazole (Diflucan), fludarabine (Fludara), ganciclovir (Cytovene), gentamicin (Garamycin), granisetron (Kytril), haloperidol (Haldol), hydrocortisone (Hydrocortone, Solu-Cortef), hydromorphone (Dilaudid), idarubicin (Idamycin), ifosfamide (Ifex), imipenem-cilastatin (Primaxin), leucovorin calcium, lorazepam (Ativan), mechlorethamine (nitrogen mustard), melphalan (Alkeran), meperidine (Demerol), mesna (Mesnex), methotrexate (Folex), metoclopramide (Reglan), minocycline (Minocin), mitoxantrone (Novantrone), morphine, nalbuphine (Nubain), ondansetron (Zofran), plicamycin (Mithracin), potassium chloride (KCl), promethazine (Phenergan), ranitidine (Zantac), sodium bicarbonate, streptozocin (Zanosar), sulfamethoxazole-trimethoprim (Bactrim), ticarcillin (Ticar), ticarcillin/clavulanate (Timentin), tobramycin (Nebcin), vancomycin (Vancocin), vinblastine (Velban), vincristine (Oncovin), vinorelbine (Navelbine), zidovudine (AZT, Retrovir).

RATE OF ADMINISTRATION

Recent studies suggest that an extended infusion time (intermittent or continuous) promotes increased recovery of neutrophils.

Intermittent infusion: A single dose over 15 to 30 minutes.

Continuous infusion: A single dose over 4 to 24 hours. In all situations flush IV line with D5W before and after administration.

ACTIONS

Colony-stimulating factors are glycoproteins that bind to specific hematopoietic cell surface receptors and stimulate proliferation, differentiation commitment, and some end-cell functional activation. Endogenous granulocyte colony-stimulating factors are produced by monocytes, fibroblasts, and endothelial cells. They are lineage-specific with selectivity for the neutrophil lineage. With recombinant DNA technology, filgrastim is produced by specifically prepared *Escherichia coli* bacteria inserted with the human G-CSF gene. It regulates the production of neutrophils within the bone marrow. Although not species specific, it mimics the actions of endogenous glycoprotein. By accelerating the recovery of neutrophil counts following a variety of chemotherapy regimens, it decreases infections manifested by febrile neutropenia, need for hospitalization, and IV antibiotic usage. May also cause some increase in lymphocyte counts.

Increase in circulating neutrophils is dose-dependent, and a return to baseline occurs shortly after discontinuation (50% of baseline in 1 to 2 days and to pretreatment levels in 1 to 7 days).

INDICATIONS AND USES

Decrease the incidence of infection (febrile neutropenia) in patients with nonmyeloid malignancies receiving myelosuppressive anticancer drugs associated with a significant incidence of severe neutropenia with fever. ■ Reduce the time to neutrophil recovery and the duration of fever, following induction or consolidation chemotherapy treatment of adults with AML. ■ Decrease duration of neutropenia and related clinical problems (e.g., febrile neutropenia) in patients with nonmyeloid malignancies receiving myeloablative chemotherapy followed by BMT. ■ Used SC to treat severe chronic neutropenia (e.g., congenital, cyclic, or idiopathic) after all diseases associated with neutropenia have been ruled out. ■ Used SC or as a 24-hour SC infusion to mobilize hematopoietic progenitor cells into the peripheral blood for collection by leukapheresis with transplantation after myeloablative chemotherapy.

Unlabeled uses: Filgrastim-mobilized peripheral blood progenitor cells (PBPCs) are being used in place of BMT because they provide more rapid recovery of the patient's WBCs (neutrophils), RBCs, and platelets. ■ Increase neutrophil count in adults with myelodysplastic syndrome (MDS). May accelerate progression to usually fatal acute myelogenous leukemia (AML); relationship unclear. ■ Increase neutrophil count in aplastic anemia. ■ Increase neutrophil count in hairy cell leukemia and acute leukemias. ■ Treat granulocytopenia in HIV-infected patients receiving zidovudine. May be used concomitantly with epoetin alfa.

CONTRAINDICATIONS

Hypersensitivity to *E. coli*–derived proteins.

PRECAUTIONS

Should be administered under the direction of a physician knowledgeable about appropriate use for each indication (e.g., expert in bone marrow transplantation). ■ Frequently given by SC injection or SC continuous infusion. ■ Effective in patients receiving chemotherapy with protocols containing cisplatin, cyclophosphamide, doxorubicin, etoposide, ifosfamide, mesna, methotrexate, vinblastine, and similar antineoplastic agents. ■ Effectiveness has not been evaluated in patients receiving chemotherapy associated with delayed myelosuppression (e.g., nitrosoureas [carmustine]), with mitomycin C, or with myelosuppressive doses of antimetabolites (e.g., fluorouracil or cytosine arabinoside). ■ Use extreme caution in any malignancy with myeloid characteristics; can act as a growth factor for any tumor type, particularly myeloid malignancies. ■ Adult respiratory distress syndrome may occur in septic patients. ■ Use caution in patients with pre-existing cardiac disease; cardiac events (e.g., myocardial infarction) have occurred, but the relationship to filgrastim is unclear. ■ Chronic use at varying doses over several years may cause subclinical splenomegaly in adults and children.

Monitor: Obtain a CBC and platelet count before chemotherapy begins and twice weekly thereafter to monitor the neutrophil count and to avoid leukocytosis. Following cytotoxic chemotherapy, the neutrophil nadir occurs earlier during cycles when filgrastim is used, duration of severe neutropenia is reduced, and WBC differentials may have a left shift. ■ Increase monitoring of CBC and platelet count to 3 times a week after bone marrow infusion. ■ Because higher doses of chemotherapy may be tolerated, side effects associated with the chemotherapeutic drug may be more pronounced; observe carefully. ■ Use caution with any additional drugs known to lower the platelet count. ■ See Precautions.

Patient Education: Promptly report any symptoms of infection (e.g., fever) or allergic reaction (itching, redness, swelling at the injection site). ■ May be self-injected SC by the patient at home; requires instruction. Literature includes a patient handout.

Maternal/Child: Category C: safety for use during pregnancy not established. Very large doses have caused fetal damage and death in rabbits. Use only if benefit justifies the potential risk to the fetus. ■ Secretion through breast milk not established; use caution during breast-feeding. ■ Has been used in over 100 children from 3 months to 18 years of age with similar experience to the adult population, even though literature says safety not established. May cause bone pain, fever, or rash.

DRUG/LAB INTERACTIONS

Interaction with other drugs has not been evaluated. ■ Use with caution any drug that may potentiate the release of neutrophils (e.g., lithium). Concurrent use with vincristine (Oncovin) may cause a severe atypical neuropathy (foot pain, severe motor weakness).

SIDE EFFECTS

No serious adverse reactions that would limit the use of the product have been reported. Allergic reactions (itching, redness, swelling at the injection site) have occurred; anaphylaxis has not occurred but is possible. Complaints of dose-related bone pain are common and may require analgesics. With doses above 5 mcg/kg/day, leukocytosis (WBC counts greater than 100,000/mm^3) has occurred in 5% of patients with no adverse effects reported. Cutaneous vasculitis has occurred in a few patients. Reduced dose may be indicated with subsequent treatment.

ANTIDOTE

Notify physician promptly if any signs of infection (fever) or other potential side effects occur. Monitor potential leukocytosis with twice-weekly CBCs. Discontinue therapy after ANC surpasses 10,000/mm^3 and the chemotherapy nadir has occurred. Discontinue filgrastim and notify physician immediately if a generalized allergic reaction should occur. Treat allergic reactions as indicated.

FLUCONAZOLE

(floo-con′a-zole)

Antifungal

Diflucan

pH 4 to 8

USUAL DOSE

IV dose has been used for a maximum of 14 days. Plasma levels are similar with IV or oral, so oral dose can replace IV dose at any time. See Monitor.

Oropharyngeal candidiasis: Initial dose of 200 mg followed by 100 mg daily for a minimum of 14 days. PO maintenance therapy usually required in patients with AIDS to prevent relapse.

Esophageal candidiasis: Initial dose of 200 mg followed by 100 mg daily for a minimum of 21 days and for at least 2 weeks after symptoms subside. Up to 400 mg/24 hr may be used.

Urinary tract or peritoneal candidiasis: 50 to 200 mg daily has been used.

Systemic (disseminated) candidiasis: Initial dose of 400 mg followed by 200 mg daily for a minimum of 28 days and for at least 2 weeks after symptoms subside. Another source suggests optimal dose and duration of therapy not established. Doses up to 400 mg daily have been used.

Treatment of acute cryptococcal meningitis: Initial dose of 400 mg followed by 200 mg daily for a minimum of 10 to 12 weeks after CSF culture becomes negative. Another source suggests a loading dose of 400 mg twice a day for 2 days followed by 400 mg daily for the same duration.

Suppression of cryptococcal meningitis: 200 mg daily. Usually required in patients with AIDS to prevent relapse.

Prevention of candidiasis in bone marrow transplant: 400 mg once daily. If severe neutropenia (less than $500/mm^3$) is expected, begin fluconazole prophylaxis several days ahead of expected neutropenia. Continue for 7 days after neutrophils reach $1{,}000/mm^3$.

PEDIATRIC DOSE

Ages 6 months to 13 years: 10 mg/kg as a loading dose. Maintain with 3 to 6 mg/kg of body weight daily. Begin 24 hours after loading dose. Do not exceed adult dose. Experience with children is limited; see Maternal/Child. A second source recommends the dosing guidelines specific for each indication as follows:

Oropharyngeal candidiasis: Initial dose of 6 mg/kg of body weight followed by 3 mg/kg daily for a minimum of 14 days.

Esophageal candidiasis: Initial dose of 6 mg/kg of body weight followed by 3 mg/kg daily for a minimum of 21 days and for at least 2 weeks after symptoms subside. Up to 12 mg/kg has been used.

Systemic candidiasis: 6 to 12 mg/kg of body weight daily for a minimum of 28 days and for at least 2 weeks after symptoms subside.

Treatment of acute cryptococcal meningitis: Initial dose of 12 mg/kg of body weight followed by 6 mg/kg daily for a minimum of 10 to 12 weeks after CSF culture becomes negative. Up to 12 mg/kg/day has been used.

Suppression of cryptococcal meningitis: 6 mg/kg daily.

NEONATAL DOSE

2 weeks to 3 months of age with meningitis or septicemia: 5 to 6 mg/kg daily PO or by IV infusion over 1 hour, or 10 mg/kg as a ***loading dose*** followed by 5 mg/kg.

Birth to 2 weeks of age with meningitis or septicemia: One source suggests using pediatric doses and extending the intervals to once every 72 hours. Another source suggests 6 mg/kg daily with a reduction to 3 mg/kg in neonates with reduced renal function. A third source suggests a ***loading dose*** of 6 to 12 mg/kg and breaks ***maintenance doses*** down to postconceptual or postnatal age and adjusts both dose and intervals. The younger the neonate, the higher the maintenance dose and the longer the interval. Premature infants younger than 29 weeks postconception receive 5 to 6 mg/kg every 48 to 72 hours. Beginning at 30 weeks postconception, neonates receive a maintenance dose of 3 to 6 mg/kg at intervals of 24 to 48 hours (48-hour interval is for neonates 30 to 36 weeks postconception and full-term infants less than 1 week of age). See Maternal/Child.

Continued

DOSE ADJUSTMENTS

In all adult situations the infecting organism and response to therapy may justify increased doses up to 400 mg daily. ■ Reduce each dose by 50% in patients with a CrCl at or less than 50 ml/min. ■ Give one recommended dose after each dialysis in patients receiving regular dialysis. ■ See Drug/Lab Interactions.

DILUTION

Packaged prediluted and ready for use as an iso-osmotic solution containing 2 mg/ml in both glass bottles and Viaflex Plus plastic containers. Do not remove moisture barrier overwrap of plastic container until ready for use. Tear overwrap down side at slit to open, and remove sterile inner bag. Plastic may appear somewhat opaque due to sterilization process but will clear. Squeeze inner bag firmly to check for leaks. Discard if leakage noted; sterility is impaired. Do not use if cloudy or precipitated.

Storage: Store glass bottles between 5° C (41° F) and 30° C (86° F); store plastic containers between 5° C (41° F) and 25° C (77° F). Protect both from freezing.

INCOMPATIBLE WITH

Manufacturer states, "Do not add supplementary medication."

COMPATIBLE WITH **(Underline Indicates Conflicting Compatibility Information)**

Consult pharmacist; specific conditions may apply; see Compatibilities, p. xvi.

Additive: ***See Incompatible With.*** Another source suggests additive compatibility with acyclovir (Zovirax), amikacin (Amikin), amphotericin B (Fungizone), cefazolin (Kefzol), ceftazidime (Fortaz), clindamycin (Cleocin), gentamicin (Garamycin), heparin, meropenem (Merrem IV), metronidazole (Flagyl IV), morphine, piperacillin (Pipracil), potassium chloride (KCl), theophylline.

Y-site: Acyclovir (Zovirax), aldesleukin (Proleukin), allopurinol (Aloprim, Zyloprim), amifostine (Ethyol), amikacin (Amikin), aminophylline, ampicillin/sulbactam (Unasyn), aztreonam (Azactam), benztropine (Cogentin), cefazolin (Kefzol), cefepime (Maxipime), cefotetan (Cefotan), cefoxitin (Mefoxin), chlorpromazine (Thorazine), cimetidine (Tagamet), cisatracurium (Nimbex), dexamethasone (Decadron), diltiazem (Cardizem), diphenhydramine (Benadryl), dobutamine (Dobutrex), docetaxel (Taxotere), dopamine (Intropin), doxorubicin liposome (Doxil), droperidol (Inapsine), etoposide phosphate (Etopophos), famotidine (Pepcid IV), filgrastim (Neupogen), fludarabine (Fludara), foscarnet (Foscavir), ganciclovir (Cytovene) gatifloxacin (Tequin), gemcitabine (Gemzar), gentamicin (Garamycin), granisetron (Kytril), heparin, hetastarch in electrolytes (Hextend), hydrocortisone sodium phosphate (Hydrocortone), immune globulin intravenous (IGIV), leucovorin calcium, linezolid (Zyvox), lorazepam (Ativan), melphalan (Alkeran), meperidine (Demerol), meropenem (Merrem IV), metoclopramide (Reglan), metronidazole (Flagyl IV), midazolam (Versed), morphine, nafcillin (Nafcil), nitroglycerin (Nitro-Bid IV), ondansetron (Zofran), oxacillin (Bactocill), paclitaxel (Taxol), pancuronium (Pavulon), penicillin G potassium, <u>phenytoin (Dilantin)</u>, piperacillin/tazobactam (Zosyn), prochlorperazine (Compazine), promethazine (Phenergan), propofol (Diprivan), ranitidine (Zantac), remifentanil (Ultiva), sargramostim (Leukine), tacrolimus (Prograf), teniposide (Vumon), theophylline, thiotepa (Thioplex), ticarcillin-clavulanate

(Timentin), tobramycin (Nebcin), vancomycin (Vancocin), vecuronium (Norcuron), vinorelbine (Navelbine), zidovudine (AZT, Retrovir).

RATE OF ADMINISTRATION

A single dose as a continuous infusion at a rate not to exceed 200 mg/hr. Do not use plastic containers in series connections; air embolism could result.

ACTIONS

A synthetic, broad-spectrum, bis-Triazole antifungal agent. Inhibits fungal growth of *Candida* and *Cryptococcus neoformans* by acting on a key enzyme and depriving the fungus of ergosterol; the cell membrane becomes unstable and can no longer function normally. Human sterol synthesis is not affected. Has shown some effectiveness against *Aspergillus flavus, Aspergillus fumigatus, Blastomyces dermatitidis,* and *Coccidioides immitis* in laboratory mice. Peak action achieved in 1 to 2 hours; half-life extends for 30 hours. Initial double dose results in steady-state plasma concentration by day 2 when given IV or orally. Penetrates into all body fluids in similar and effective concentrations and remains constant with daily single-dose administration. 80% excreted as unchanged drug through the kidneys. Secreted in breast milk.

INDICATIONS AND USES

Oropharyngeal and esophageal candidiasis. ■ Serious systemic candidal infections, including GU tract infections, peritonitis, and pneumonia. May be an appropriate and less toxic alternative to amphotericin B. ■ Cryptococcal meningitis, including suppressive therapy to prevent relapse. ■ Prevention of candidiasis in bone marrow transplant patients. ■ Used orally for additional indications (e.g., candidiasis prophylaxis).

Unlabeled uses: Has been used in many other fungal or parasitic infections.

CONTRAINDICATIONS

Concurrent use with cisapride (Propulsid), hypersensitivity to fluconazole or any of its components. Use caution in patients hypersensitive to other azoles (e.g., ketoconazole).

PRECAUTIONS

For IV use only; do not give IM. ■ Use caution in patients with preexisting liver disease.

Monitor: Specimens for fungal culture, serology, and histopathology should be obtained before therapy to isolate and identify causative organisms. Therapy may begin as soon as all specimens are obtained and before results are known. ■ Inadequate treatment may lead to recurrence of active infection; continue treatment until clinical parameters or laboratory tests indicate that active fungal infection has subsided. See specific recommendations in Usual Dose. ■ Serious hepatotoxicity may occur. Causal relationship uncertain, but many patients are taking hepatotoxic drugs for treatment of malignancies and AIDS. Note any increase in liver function tests (e.g., AST [SGOT]). If any clinical signs and symptoms that are consistent with liver disease develop, discontinue drug. Has caused deaths. ■ Exfoliative skin disorders have been reported. ■ See Drug/Lab Interactions.

Patient Education: Review prescription and nonprescription drugs with physician or pharmacist.

Maternal/Child: Category C: safety for use in pregnancy and breast-feeding not established. Use in pregnancy only if potential benefits outweigh risk to fetus. ■ Use in nursing mothers is not recommended. ■ Use in children as young as 6 months of age is supported by clinical studies. ■ Has been used in neonates (unlabeled).

Elderly: Use caution, consider decreased cardiac, hepatic, or renal function and effects of concomitant disease or other drug therapy.

DRUG/LAB INTERACTIONS

Hepatoxicity increased if used concurrently with ketoconazole (Nizoral). ■ Potentiated by hydrochlorothiazide (HydroDIURIL); decreases renal clearance of fluconazole. ■ Inhibits metabolism and increases serum levels of cyclosporine, phenytoin, tacrolimus (Prograf), and theophyllines; careful monitoring of their plasma levels is required; nephrotoxicity has been reported with tacrolimus. ■ Potentiates coumarin-type anticoagulants (e.g., warfarin); monitor PT. ■ Potentiates oral hypoglycemic agents (e.g., glipizide [Glucotrol XL], glyburide [DiaBeta], tolbutamide [Orinase]); monitor blood glucose levels. In all of these situations dose reductions of the above drugs may be indicated. ■ Rifampin increases metabolism; fluconazole dose may need to be increased. One source recommends avoiding concurrent use. ■ Increases serum levels of zidovudine (Retrovir, AZT). ■ Increases serum levels of rifabutin (Mycobutin); uveitis may occur with concurrent use. ■ Studies have not been completed on interactions with pentamidine. ■ Risk of cardiac arrhythmias increased with cisapride (Propulsid), pimozide (Orap), and quinidine, concurrent use not recommended; see Contraindications. ■ Fluconazole plasma concentrations and effectiveness may be decreased by anticonvulsants (e.g., phenytoin [Dilantin], carbamazepine [Tegretol]), and antimycobacterial agents (e.g., isoniazid [INH], rifampin [Rifadin]), may result in treatment failure. ■ May decrease metabolism and increase serum concentrations of celecoxib (Celebrex). ■ May increase serum concentrations and adverse effects of alfentanil (Alfenta), benzodiazepines (e.g., Midazolam [Versed]), buspirone (BuSpar), corticosteroids, glimepiride (Amaryl), losartan (Cozaar), nisoldipine (Sular), tricyclic antidepressants (e.g., amitriptyline [Elavil]), vinca alkaloids (e.g., vincristine [Oncovin]), zolpidem (Ambien). ■ May elevate liver function tests (e.g., ALT [SGPT], AST [SGOT], alkaline phosphatase, and bilirubin).

SIDE EFFECTS

More frequent in HIV-infected patients.

Abdominal pain, agranulocytosis, allergic reactions, diarrhea, dizziness, dry mouth, exfoliative skin disorders, headache, hepatic reactions, increased appetite, increased sweating, nausea, pallor, rash, taste perversion, thrombocytopenia, tremor, vomiting.

Overdose: Cyanosis, decreased motility, decreased respirations, lacrimation, loss of balance, salivation, urinary incontinence. Clonic convulsions preceded death in experimental animals.

ANTIDOTE

Notify physician of all side effects; most will be treated symptomatically. Discontinue drug and notify physician of abnormal liver function tests progressing to clinical signs and symptoms of liver disease. Rash may be the first sign of an exfoliative skin disorder in immunocompromised patients; discontinue drug and notify physician. In overdose a 3-hour dialysis session will decrease plasma levels by 50%. Treat anaphylaxis or resuscitate if indicated.

FLUDARABINE PHOSPHATE

(floo-dar'a-been fos'fat)

Antineoplastic (antimetabolite)

Fludara

pH 7.2 to 8.2

USUAL DOSE

25 mg/M^2 daily for 5 consecutive days. Repeat every 4 weeks. Optimum duration of treatment not established. If there is no major toxicity, treat until maximum response achieved, then administer three additional complete cycles.

DOSE ADJUSTMENTS

Decreased or delayed based on evidence of hematologic or nonhematologic toxicity. Increased toxicity may occur in the elderly and in patients with renal insufficiency or bone marrow impairment. ▪ Reduce dose to 20 mg/M^2 (a 20% reduction) in patients with moderate renal impairment (a CrCl from 30 to 70 ml/min/1.73 M^2); not recommended for use in patients with severe renal impairment (a CrCl less than 30 ml/min/1.73 M^2).

DILUTION

Specific techniques required; see Precautions. Each 50 mg must be initially diluted with 2 ml of SW for injection (25 mg/ml). Should dissolve within 15 seconds. Further dilute a single dose in 100 to 125 ml of NS or D5W and give as an infusion.

Storage: Refrigerate between 2° and 8° C (36° to 46° F) before dilution. No preservative; use within 8 hours of dilution.

COMPATIBLE WITH

Consult pharmacist; specific conditions may apply; see Compatibilities, p. xvi.

Y-site: Allopurinol (Aloprim, Zyloprim), amifostine (Ethyol), amikacin (Amikin), aminophylline, ampicillin, ampicillin/sulbactam (Unasyn), aztreonam (Azactam), bleomycin (Blenoxane), butorphanol (Stadol), carboplatin (Paraplatin), carmustine (BiCNU), cefazolin (Kefzol), cefepime (Maxipime), cefoperazone (Cefobid), cefotaxime (Claforan), cefotetan (Cefotan), ceftazidime (Fortaz), ceftizoxime (Cefizox), ceftriaxone (Rocephin), cefuroxime (Zinacef), cimetidine (Tagamet), cisplatin (Platinol), clindamycin (Cleocin), cyclophosphamide (Cytoxan), cytarabine (ARA-C), dacarbazine (DTIC), dactinomycin (Cosmegen), dexamethasone (Decadron), diphenhydramine (Benadryl), doxorubicin (Adriamycin), doxycycline (Vibramycin), droperidol (Inapsine), etoposide (VePesid), etoposide phosphate (Etopophos), famotidine (Pepcid IV), filgrastim (Neupogen), fluconazole (Diflucan), fluorouracil (5-FU), furosemide (Lasix), gemcitabine (Gemzar), gentamicin (Garamycin), granisetron (Kytril), haloperidol (Haldol), heparin, hydrocortisone (Hydrocortone, Solu-Cortef), hydromorphone (Dilaudid), ifosfamide (Ifex), imipenem-cilastatin (Primaxin), lorazepam (Ativan), magnesium sulfate, mannitol, mechlorethamine (nitrogen mustard), melphalan (Alkeran), meperidine (Demerol), mesna (Mesnex), methotrexate (Folex), methylprednisolone (Solu-Medrol), metoclopramide (Reglan), minocycline (Minocin), mitoxantrone (Novantrone), morphine, multivitamins (MVI), nalbuphine (Nubain), ondansetron (Zofran), pentostatin (Nipent), piperacillin (Pipracil), piperacillin/tazobactam (Zosyn), potassium chloride

(KCl), promethazine (Phenergan), ranitidine (Zantac), sodium bicarbonate, sulfamethoxazole-trimethoprim (Bactrim), teniposide (Vumon), thiotepa (Thioplex), ticarcillin (Ticar), ticarcillin/clavulanate (Timentin), tobramycin (Nebcin), vancomycin (Vancocin), vinblastine (Velban), vincristine (Oncovin), vinorelbine (Navelbine), zidovudine (AZT, Retrovir).

RATE OF ADMINISTRATION

Single daily dose properly diluted for infusion over 30 minutes.

ACTIONS

A potent antineoplastic agent. A fluorinated nucleotide analog of the antiviral agent vidarabine. Rapidly converts to the active metabolite 2-fluoro-ara-ATP and interferes with the synthesis of DNA. Actual mechanism of action unknown and may be multifaceted. Median time to response in studies of patients with refractory chronic lymphocytic leukemia (CLL) was 7 to 21 weeks (range 1 to 68 weeks). Elimination half-life is 9 to 10 hours. Probably excreted in urine.

INDICATIONS AND USES

Treatment of patients with B-cell CLL who have not responded to or progressed during treatment with at least one standard alkylating-agent-containing regimen.

Unlabeled uses: Treatment of non-Hodgkin's lymphoma, macroglobulinemic lymphoma, prolymphocytic leukemia or prolymphocytoid variant of CLL, mycosis fungoides, hairy-cell leukemia, and Hodgkin's disease. Dose and/or efficacy not established.

CONTRAINDICATIONS

Hypersensitivity to fludarabine or its components (e.g., mannitol and sodium hydroxide). Not recommended for use in patients with severely impaired renal function (CrCl less than 30 ml/min/1.73 M^2).

PRECAUTIONS

Follow guidelines for handling cytotoxic agents. See Appendix A, p. 1142. ■ Administered by or under the direction of the physician specialist. ■ Use with caution in advanced age, renal insufficiency, or bone marrow impairment. ■ Most patients have hematologic impairment at baseline because of disease or prior myelosuppressive therapy. Myelosuppression may be severe and cumulative. ■ Use of irradiated blood product has been suggested for patients requiring transfusions during fludarabine therapy because transfusion-associated graft-versus-host disease has been reported. ■ Response can occur within 1 week. Use caution in patients with large tumor burdens; may cause tumor lysis syndrome. ■ Several instances of bone marrow hypoplasia or aplasia resulting in pancytopenia, sometimes resulting in death, have been reported. Clinically significant cytopenias lasted from 2 months to 1 year and occurred in untreated and previously treated patients.

Monitor: Observe closely for signs of toxicity, both hematologic and nonhematologic. ■ Obtain baseline CBC, including differential and platelet count. Repeat regularly to monitor hematopoietic suppression (especially neutrophils and platelets). ■ Observe closely for all signs of infection and any fever of unknown origin. ■ Prophylactic antibiotics may be indicated pending results of C/S in a febrile neutropenic patient. ■ Nausea and vomiting usually less severe than many antineoplastics; prophylactic administration of antiemetics may be indicated. ■ Prevention and treatment of hyperuricemia due to tumor lysis syndrome may be accomplished with adequate hydration and, if necessary, allopurinol (Aloprim, Zyloprim) and alkalinization of urine. ■ Monitor for thrombocytopenia (platelet count less than 50,000/mm^3). Initiate precautions to prevent excessive bleeding (e.g., inspect IV sites, skin, and mucous membranes; use extreme care during invasive procedures; test urine, emesis, stool, and secretions for occult blood).

Patient Education: Nonhormonal birth control recommended. ■ See Appendix D, p. 1148.

Maternal/Child: Category D: avoid pregnancy; may cause fetal harm. ■ Discontinue breast-feeding. ■ Safety for use in children not established.

Elderly: See Precautions and Dose Adjustments.

DRUG/LAB INTERACTIONS

Do not use with pentostatin (Nipent); may increase risk of fatal pulmonary toxicity.

SIDE EFFECTS

Are frequent, may be dose limiting, and may cause death. Agitation, anorexia, bone marrow aplasia or hypoplasia (may result in pancytopenia), bone marrow suppression (may affect multiple cell lines [e.g., anemia, neutropenia, thrombocytopenia]), chills, coma, confusion, diarrhea, edema, GI bleeding, infection (both opportunistic and pneumonia), fatigue, fever, malaise, nausea and vomiting, pain, peripheral neuropathy, pulmonary toxicity (ARDS, dyspnea, interstitial pulmonary infiltrate, pulmonary fibrosis, pulmonary hemorrhage, respiratory distress and failure), rashes, stomatitis, visual disturbances, weakness. Onset of flank pain and hematuria may indicate tumor lysis syndrome (hyperkalemia, hyperphosphatemia, hyperuricemia, hypocalcemia, metabolic acidosis, urate crystalluria, and renal failure); one reported.

Overdose: Severe bone marrow suppression (neutropenia and thrombocytopenia). Severe neurologic toxicity including delayed blindness, coma, and death occurred from 21 to 60 days after the last dose in 36% of patients treated with doses only 4 times greater than the recommended dose. Has occurred (0.2%) with average doses.

ANTIDOTE

Notify physician of all side effects. Most will be treated symptomatically. Some toxicity is necessary to produce remission. Delay or discontinue the drug for serious hematologic depression. Administration of whole blood products (e.g., packed RBCs, platelets, leukocytes) and/or blood modifiers (e.g., darbepoetin alfa [Aranesp], epoetin alfa [Epogen, Procrit], filgrastim [Neupogen], pegfilgrastim [Neulasta], sargramostim [Leukine], oprelvekin [Neumega]) may be indicated to treat bone marrow toxicity. Restart as soon as signs of bone marrow recovery occur. Delay or discontinue if neurotoxicity occurs. There is no specific antidote; supportive therapy as indicated will help sustain the patient in toxicity. Symptoms of pulmonary toxicity may improve with the use of corticosteroids; rule out an infectious origin before use.

FLUMAZENIL

(floo-maz′en-ill)

Romazicon

Benzodiazepine antagonist
Antidote

pH 4

USUAL DOSE

Reversal of conscious sedation or in general anesthesia: 0.2 mg (2 ml) as an initial dose. Assess level of consciousness. May be repeated at 1-minute intervals, assessing level of consciousness between each dose, until desired level of consciousness achieved or a total cumulative dose of 1 mg (10 ml) has been given (average dose to awakening is 0.6 mg to 1 mg). If resedation occurs (may occur if flumazenil wears off before the benzodiazepine) the above process may be repeated at 20-minute intervals as indicated. Do not give more than a cumulative dose of 1 mg in a 20-minute period or 3 mg in any 1 hour.

Management of suspected benzodiazepine overdose: 0.2 mg (2 ml) as an initial dose. Assess level of consciousness. If results inadequate, give an additional dose of 0.3 mg (3 ml) in 1 minute. If results are still inadequate, 0.5 mg (5 ml) may be repeated at 1-minute intervals. Assess level of consciousness between each dose until desired level of consciousness achieved or a total cumulative dose of 3 mg (30 ml) has been given (average dose to awakening is 1 mg to 3 mg). If a partial response is achieved with 3 mg, continue dosing in 0.5-mg increments until awakening or a cumulative dose of 5 mg is reached (rarely required). If patient has not responded to a cumulative dose of 5 mg within 5 minutes, benzodiazepines are not the major cause of sedation; discontinue use. If desired results are achieved and resedation occurs (expected), no more than 1 mg given in 0.5-mg increments may be given in any 20-minute period and no more than a cumulative total dose of 3 mg in any 1 hour.

PEDIATRIC DOSE

Reversal of conscious sedation: 0.01 mg/kg (up to 0.2 mg). Assess level of consciousness. May repeat at 1 minute intervals, assessing level of consciousness between each dose until desired level of consciousness achieved or a maximum total dose of 0.05 mg/kg (or 1 mg) has been given. Mean total dose administered in trials was 0.65 mg. See Maternal/Child. Another source suggests from 10 mcg (0.01 mg)/kg for reversing sedation to 100 mcg (0.1 mg)/kg in a life-threatening overdose to a maximum cumulative dose of 1 mg. Has been given as an infusion at 5 to 10 mcg (0.005 to 0.01 mg)/kg/hr.

DOSE ADJUSTMENTS

Not required for the elderly. ■ Reduce dose and extend intervals after the initial dose in impaired liver function. ■ In high-risk patients, administer the smallest amount that is effective and wait for peak effect (6 to 10 minutes). Slower titration rates and lower total doses may be especially important in these patients (see Precautions) to reduce emergent confusion and agitation and evaluate effect.

DILUTION

May be given undiluted through a free-flowing IV into a large vein (to minimize pain at injection site). Compatible with D5W, D2½W, LR, ½NS, and NS if further dilution required by a specific situation. Discard in 24 hours if drawn undiluted into a syringe or diluted in any solution.

COMPATIBLE WITH

Consult pharmacist; specific conditions may apply; see Compatibilities, p. xvi.

Additive: Aminophylline, cimetidine (Tagamet), dobutamine (Dobutrex), dopamine (Intropin), famotidine (Pepcid IV), heparin, lidocaine, procainamide (Pronestyl), ranitidine (Zantac).

RATE OF ADMINISTRATION

Series of small injections allows control of the reversal of sedation to desired endpoint, avoids abrupt awakening, and minimizes the possibility of adverse effects.

Reversal of conscious sedation or in general anesthesia: Each single dose over 15 seconds.

Management of suspected benzodiazepine overdose: Each single dose (0.2 mg [2 ml], 0.3 mg [3 ml], or 0.5 mg [5 ml] respectively) over 30 seconds.

ACTIONS

A benzodiazepine antagonist. Competes with benzodiazepines, inhibiting their effect at benzodiazepine receptor sites. Action is very specific and reverses the sedative effects of benzodiazepines only. Duration and degree of reversal are dose- and plasma content–related (both for amount of benzodiazepine and amount of flumazenil). Onset of action usually occurs within 1 to 2 minutes of reaching the appropriate dose, with peak effect at 6 to 10 minutes. Enables the physician to control the duration of action of benzodiazepines, helps to evaluate the patient's postoperative condition much earlier than waiting for effect to wear off on its own, and may facilitate the postprocedural course. In overdose, it allows the physician to communicate sooner with patients who have taken an excessive dose. Extensively metabolized in the liver. Excreted in changed form in urine.

INDICATIONS AND USES

Adults: Complete or partial reversal of the effects of general anesthesia induced and/or maintained with benzodiazepines (e.g., diazepam [Valium], midazolam [Versed]). ■ Complete or partial reversal of the sedative effects of benzodiazepines used to produce and/or maintain conscious sedation (e.g., diagnostic and therapeutic procedures). ■ Adjunct to conventional treatment in managing benzodiazepine overdose (e.g., chlordiazepoxide [Librium], diazepam [Valium], lorazepam [Ativan], midazolam [Versed]).

Pediatric patients 1 to 17 years of age: Reversal of conscious sedation induced with benzodiazepines; see Maternal/Child. ■ Not approved for other indications but has been used at doses similar to those used for reversal of conscious sedation; see Maternal/Child.

CONTRAINDICATIONS

Known hypersensitivity to flumazenil or any benzodiazepine, patients who are on benzodiazepine therapy for control of potentially life-threatening conditions (e.g., control of intracranial pressure, status epilepticus), and patients showing signs of serious cyclic antidepressant overdose. ■ Use in treatment of benzodiazepine dependence is not recommended.

PRECAUTIONS

Excess administration increases risk of side effects and decreases desired therapeutics of benzodiazepines. ■ Will not reverse the central nervous system (CNS) effects of drugs such as alcohol, analgesics, antidepressants, barbiturates, and narcotics. In overdose, will bring the patient to a conscious state only if a benzodiazepine is responsible for the sedation. Has reversed benzodiazepine-induced hypotension and bradycardia unresponsive to other measures (e.g., IV fluids, atropine, dopamine). ■ Convulsions may occur, especially in patients who rely on benzodiazepines to control seizures or are physically dependent on benzodiazepines for long-term sedation, in overdose cases where large doses of other drugs have been ingested, in patients showing signs of serious cyclic antidepressant overdose (some clinicians recommend a diagnostic ECG or quantitative analytical testing before use—see Contraindications), or in ICU patients who may have an unrecognized dependence on benzodiazepines because of frequent use as a sedative (can occur with only 3 to 5 days of benzodiazepine administration). Intubation with ventilatory and circulatory support may be the treatment of choice for these high-risk patients; see Dose Adjustments. ■ Risk of adverse reactions increased in patients with a history of alcohol, benzodiazepine, or sedative use (increased frequency of benzodiazepine tolerance and dependence). Can precipitate benzodiazepine withdrawal (also high-risk; see Dose Adjustments). ■ Use extreme caution in head injury (may alter cerebral blood flow or cause convulsions). ■ Do not use until effects of neuromuscular blockade have been fully reversed. ■ May cause panic attacks in patients with a history of panic disorder. ■ Additional ventilatory support may be required in patients with serious lung disease. ■ Half-life prolonged based on amount of hepatic impairment. ■ Ingestion of food increases clearance of flumazenil.

Monitor: Secure airway, ventilation, and IV access before administration. ■ Monitor BP, HR, and respirations closely. ECG monitoring and oxygenation determination by pulse oximetry is recommended. ■ Emergency equipment and supplies, including drugs for seizure control (see Antidote), must always be available. ■ Observe continuously for resedation, respiratory depression, preseizure activity, or other residual benzodiazepine effects for an appropriate period (2 or more hours). ■ Extend observation time for larger doses, in presence of long-acting benzodiazepines (e.g., diazepam [Valium]), or large doses of short-acting benzodiazepines (e.g., more than 10 mg of midazolam [Versed]). ■ Observe ambulatory patients for a minimum of 2 hours after a 1-mg dose; resedation after 2 hours is unlikely. Extend observation time as above. ■ Awake patients may require pain medication sooner than those without benzodiazepine reversal. ■ All postprocedural instructions must be given to the patient verbally and in writing; does not reverse benzodiazepine amnesia. ■ See Drug/Lab Interactions.

Patient Education: Effects of benzodiazepines may recur; for 24 to 48 hours memory and judgment may be impaired. ■ All instructions should be in writing. ■ Do not drive, operate hazardous machinery, or engage in activities that require alertness. ■ Do not take alcohol, other CNS depressants (e.g., antihistamines, barbiturates), or nonprescription drugs for 24 hours.

Maternal/Child: Category C: use only if benefit justifies risk. ■ Not recommended during labor and delivery because effect on newborn unknown. ■ Safety for use in breast-feeding not established. ■ Safety and effectiveness for reversal of conscious sedation induced with benzodiazepines have been established in pediatric patients 1 to 17 years of age. Resedation may occur, especially in children 1 to 5 years of age. Safety and effectiveness of repeated flumazenil doses in children experiencing resedation have not been established. ■ Safety and effectiveness for other uses listed under adult indications have not been established. However, published anecdotal reports have cited safety profiles and dosing guidelines similar to those used in reversal of conscious sedation. ■ Half-life appears to be shorter and more variable in pediatric patients.

Elderly: See Dose Adjustments. Age-related differences in safety and effectiveness have not been observed; however, a greater sensitivity of some older patients cannot be ruled out. ■ Monitor carefully; benzodiazepine-induced sedation may be deeper and more prolonged.

DRUG/LAB INTERACTIONS

May cause cardiac arrhythmias or convulsions in cases of mixed drug overdose. These toxic effects may emerge (especially with cyclic antidepressants [e.g., amitriptyline (Elavil), imipramine (Tofranil)]) with reversal of benzodiazepine effect; see Precautions. May reverse sedative and anticonvulsant effects. ■ May precipitate withdrawal symptoms if given to chronic benzodiazepine users. ■ No specific deleterious interactions noted when flumazenil administered after narcotics, inhalational anesthetics, muscle relaxants, and muscle relaxant antagonists administered in conjunction with sedation or anesthesia. ■ Lab test interactions have not been evaluated.

SIDE EFFECTS

Most common at doses above 1 mg and/or with abrupt reversal.

Abnormal vision, agitation, anxiety, dizziness, dry mouth, dyspnea, emotional lability, fatigue, flushing, headache, hot flashes, hypertension, hyperventilation, insomnia, involuntary movements, irritability, muscle tension, nausea, pain or reaction (rash, thrombophlebitis) at the injection site, palpitations, panic, paresthesia, sweating, tachycardia, tinnitus, tremors, and vomiting. Convulsions may occur; see Precautions.

Overdose: Agitation, anxiety, arrhythmias, convulsions, hyperesthesia, increased muscle tone.

ANTIDOTE

Notify the physician of any side effect. Treat symptoms of benzodiazepine withdrawal (agitation, confusion, dizziness, emotional lability, or sensory distortions) with a barbiturate, benzodiazepine, or other sedative. Larger doses may be required because of presence of flumazenil. Treat convulsions from overdose with barbiturates, benzodiazepines, and phenytoin (Dilantin). Maintain an adequate airway, adequate ventilation, and IV access at all times. Hemodialysis not effective in overdose if 1 hour has passed since administration.

FLUOROURACIL

(flure-oh-yoor′a-sill)

Antineoplastic (antimetabolite)

Adrucil, 5-Fluorouracil, 5-FU

pH 9.2

USUAL DOSE

12 mg/kg of body weight/24 hr for 4 days. Total dose should not exceed 800 mg/24 hr. If no toxicity is observed, one half dose (6 mg/kg) is given on days 6, 8, 10, and 12 unless toxicity occurs. No medication is given on days 5, 7, 9, or 11. Discontinue therapy on day 12, even if no toxicity is apparent. See Precautions/Monitor. The most common form of maintenance therapy is to repeat the entire course of therapy beginning 30 days after the previous course is completed and any toxicity has subsided or to give a single dose of 10 to 15 mg/kg/week, not to exceed 1 Gm. Dose adjustments of subsequent doses are made depending on side effects and tolerance. Other dose regimens are in use.

Advanced colorectal cancer: Various protocols have been used. Examples are leucovorin calcium 20 mg/M^2 followed by fluorouracil 425 mg/M^2, or leucovorin calcium 200 mg/M^2 followed by fluorouracil 370 mg/M^2 daily for 5 days. Repeat at 4-week intervals twice, then repeat every 28 to 35 days based on complete recovery from toxic effects. Do not initiate or continue in any patient with GI toxicity until completely subsided. Reduce fluorouracil dose based on tolerance to previous course; reduce 20% for moderate hematologic or GI toxicity, 30% for severe toxicity. Increase fluorouracil dose 10% if no toxicity. Leucovorin calcium dose is not adjusted. Fluorouracil and leucovorin calcium are also used in combination with irinotecan (Camptosar); see irinotecan monograph.

Breast cancer: Various protocols have been used. An example is fluorouracil 600 mg/M^2 on days 1 and 8 of each cycle combined with cyclophosphamide (Cytoxan) 100 mg/M^2 on days 1 through 14 of each cycle and methotrexate 40 mg/M^2 on days 1 and 8 of each cycle. Repeat cycles monthly (allowing a 2-week rest between cycles). Repeat for 6 to 12 cycles (6 to 12 months). Doxorubicin (Adriamycin) has also been included in this regimen. In patients older than 60 years, reduce the fluorouracil dose to 400 mg/M^2 and the initial methotrexate dose to 30 mg/M^2.

DOSE ADJUSTMENTS

For poor-risk patients or those in a poor nutritional state, either reduce dose by one half or more throughout a course of therapy or give 6 mg/kg/day for 3 days. If no toxicity observed, give 3 mg/kg on days 5, 7, and 9. Give nothing on day 4, 6, or 8. Do not exceed 400 mg/day. ■ Dose based on ideal body weight in presence of edema, ascites, or obesity. ■ Reduce dose in patients who have received high-dose pelvic irradiation or other cytotoxic drug therapy with alkylating agents (e.g., cisplatin, ifosfamide [Ifex]). ■ One source recommends a dose adjustment in patients with impaired hepatic function. Give the full dose if the bilirubin is 5 or less on the day of administration; omit the dose if the bilirubin is greater than 5. ■ Used with other antineoplastic drugs in reduced doses to achieve tumor remission. ■ See Usual Dose.

DILUTION

Specific techniques required; see Precautions. May be slightly discolored without affecting safety and potency. Dissolve any precipitate by heating to 60° C (140° F) and shaking vigorously. Cool to body temperature before using.

IV injection: May be given undiluted. May inject through Y-tube or three-way stopcock of a free-flowing infusion.

Infusion: May be further diluted with D5W or NS and given as an infusion. Doses up to 2 Gm are being given with extreme caution under the specific supervision of experienced specialists. Leucovorin calcium has been mixed into the solution with fluorouracil.

Storage: Store at room temperature; protect from light.

COMPATIBLE WITH (Underline Indicates Conflicting Compatibility Information)

Consult pharmacist; specific conditions may apply; see Compatibilities, p. xvi.

Additive: Bleomycin (Blenoxane), cyclophosphamide (Cytoxan), etoposide (VePesid), heparin, hydromorphone (Dilaudid), ifosfamide (Ifex), leucovorin calcium, magnesium sulfate, methotrexate (Folex), mitoxantrone (Novantrone), potassium chloride (KCl), vincristine (Oncovin).

Syringe: Bleomycin (Blenoxane), cisplatin (Platinol), cyclophosphamide (Cytoxan), doxorubicin (Adriamycin), furosemide (Lasix), heparin, leucovorin calcium, methotrexate (Folex), metoclopramide (Reglan), mitomycin (Mutamycin), vinblastine (Velban), vincristine (Oncovin).

Y-site: Allopurinol (Aloprim, Zyloprim), amifostine (Ethyol), aztreonam (Azactam), bleomycin (Blenoxane), cefepime (Maxipime), cisplatin (Platinol), cyclophosphamide (Cytoxan), doxorubicin (Adriamycin), doxorubicin liposome (Doxil), etoposide phosphate (Etopophos), fludarabine (Fludara), furosemide (Lasix), gatifloxacin (Tequin), gemcitabine (Gemzar), granisetron (Kytril), heparin, hydrocortisone sodium succinate (Solu-Cortef), leucovorin calcium, linezolid (Zyvox), mannitol, melphalan (Alkeran), methotrexate (Folex), metoclopramide (Reglan), mitomycin (Mutamycin), ondansetron (Zofran), paclitaxel (Taxol), piperacillin/tazobactam (Zosyn), potassium chloride (KCl), propofol (Diprivan), sargramostim (Leukine), teniposide (Vumon), thiotepa (Thioplex), vinblastine (Velban), vincristine (Oncovin).

RATE OF ADMINISTRATION

IV injection: A single dose over 1 to 3 minutes.

Infusion: A single dose is usually administered over 24 hours. Toxicity may be lessened by extended administration.

ACTIONS

An antimetabolite. A fluorinated pyrimidine antagonist, cell cycle specific, that interferes with the synthesis of DNA and RNA. Through various chemical processes this deprivation acts more quickly on rapidly growing cells and causes their death. Distributes into tumors, intestinal mucosa, bone marrow, liver, and readily crosses the blood-brain barrier into cerebrospinal fluid and brain tissue. Metabolized by the liver within 3 hours. Half-life is approximately 16 minutes. Excretion is through the urine and as respiratory CO_2.

INDICATIONS AND USES

To suppress or slow neoplastic growth. Palliative treatment of cancers of the breast, colon, pancreas, rectum, and stomach. May be used alone or in combination with other agents.

Unlabeled uses: Has been used for the treatment of bladder, cervical, endometrial, esophageal, head and neck, ovarian, prostatic, skin (topical), and other cancers.

CONTRAINDICATIONS

Potentially serious infections, depressed bone marrow function, poor nutritional state, hypersensitivity, major surgery within the previous month.

PRECAUTIONS

Follow guidelines for handling cytotoxic agents. See Appendix A, p. 1142. ■ Administered by or under the direction of the physician specialist with facilities for monitoring the patient and responding to any medical emergency. ■ Use caution in patients who have had high-dose pelvic irradiation, previous alkylating agents (e.g., cisplatin), other antimetabolic drugs (e.g., methotrexate), metastatic tumor involvement of the bone marrow, impaired hepatic or renal function, or dihydropyrimidine dehydrogenase deficiency. ■ Pseudomembranous colitis has been reported. May range from mild to life-threatening. Consider in patients that present with diarrhea during or after treatment with fluorouracil.

Monitor: Confirm patency of vein. Avoid extravasation. Change peripheral injection site every 48 hours. ■ Obtain a CBC with differential and platelet count before each dose. When given with leucovorin calcium, repeat weekly the first two courses and then at the time of anticipated WBC nadir in following courses. Electrolytes and liver function tests should be done before the first three courses, then every other course. ■ Be alert for signs of bone marrow depression or infection. Prophylactic antibiotics may be indicated pending results of C/S in a febrile neutropenic patient. ■ Examine mouth and lips daily for sores or other signs of stomatitis. ■ Prophylactic antiemetics may reduce nausea and vomiting and increase patient comfort. ■ Toxicity increased by any form of therapy that adds to stress, poor nutrition, and bone marrow depression. ■ Monitor for thrombocytopenia (platelet count less than 50,000/mm^3). Initiate precautions to prevent excessive bleeding (e.g., inspect IV sites, skin, and mucous membranes; use extreme care during invasive procedures; test urine, emesis, stool, and secretions for occult blood). ■ See Drug/Lab Interactions.

Patient Education: Nonhormonal birth control recommended. ■ See Appendix D, p. 1148. ■ Report IV site burning and stinging promptly. ■ Drink at least 2 liters of fluid each day.

Maternal/Child: Category D: avoid pregnancy; can cause fetal harm. ■ Discontinue breast-feeding. ■ Safety for use in children not established.

Elderly: May be more sensitive to toxic effects of the drug. Consider age-related organ impairment. ■ See Dose Adjustments.

DRUG/LAB INTERACTIONS

Potentiates anticoagulants. ■ Do not administer live vaccines to patients receiving antineoplastic drugs. ■ Cimetidine (Tagamet), interferon alfa, and leucovorin calcium may increase toxicity. ■ Additive bone marrow depression may occur with radiation therapy, other bone marrow–depressing agents (e.g., azathioprine [Imuran], chloramphenicol, irinotecan [Camptosar], melphalan [Alkeran], vinorelbine [Navelbine]), and/or agents that cause blood dyscrasias (e.g., metronidazole [Flagyl IV]). ■ Thiazide diuretics (e.g., chlorothiazide [Diuril]) may prolong antineoplastic-induced leukopenia. ■ May decrease metabolism and increase serum levels of phenytoin (Dilantin).

SIDE EFFECTS

Abnormal bromsulphalein (BSP), prothrombin, total protein, sed rate; alopecia (reversible), anaphylaxis, bleeding, bone marrow depression (agranulocytosis, anemia, leukopenia, pancytopenia, thrombocytopenia), cerebellar syndrome, cramps, dermatitis, diarrhea, disorientation, dry lips, erythema, esophagopharyngitis and stomatitis (may lead to sloughing and ulceration), euphoria, frequent stools, GI ulceration and bleeding, headache, hemorrhage from any site, increased skin pigmentation, infection, lacrimal duct stenosis, mouth soreness and ulceration, myocardial ischemia, nail changes, nausea, palmar-plantar erythrodysesthesia syndrome (tingling of hands and feet followed by pain, redness, and swelling), photophobia, photosensitivity, pneumopathy (cough, shortness of breath), thrombophlebitis, visual changes, vomiting (intractable). Diarrhea and stomatitis are most common and may be more severe with a prolonged duration in patients on combination therapy. Pseudomembranous colitis has been reported.

ANTIDOTE

Keep physician informed of any side effects. Discontinue the drug and notify physician promptly at the first sign of toxicity (e.g., bleeding, diarrhea, esophagopharyngitis, gastritis, intractable vomiting, rapidly falling white count, sores in or around the lips or mouth, stomatitis). Nadir of leukocyte count occurs around days 9 to 14. Recovery should be by day 30. Discontinue the drug if the WBC count is less than 3,500/mm^3 or platelets are less than 100,000/mm^3; should reach 4,000/mm^3 and 130,000/mm^3 respectively in 2 weeks; if they do not, discontinue treatment. Administration of whole blood products (e.g., packed RBCs, platelets, leukocytes, and/or blood modifiers (e.g., darbepoetin alfa [Aranesp], epoetin alfa [Epogen, Procrit], filgrastim [Neupogen], pegfilgrastim [Neulasta], sargramostim [Leukine], oprelvekin [Neumega]) may be indicated to treat bone marrow toxicity. Continue to monitor for 4 weeks. Palmar-plantar erythrodysesthesia syndrome has been treated with oral pyridoxine (100 to 150 mg daily). Death may occur from the progression of many side effects. There is no specific antidote; supportive therapy as indicated will help sustain the patient in toxicity.

FOLIC ACID
(foe′lik as′id)

Folvite

Nutritional supplement (vitamin)
Antianemic

pH 8 to 11

USUAL DOSE

Therapeutic dose: 0.25 to 1 mg daily. Larger doses may be required.
Maintenance dose: 0.4 mg daily. ***Pregnant or lactating females:*** 0.8 mg daily.

PEDIATRIC DOSE

Therapeutic dose: 0.25 to 1 mg daily.
Maintenance dose: ***Infants:*** 0.1 mg daily. ***Under 4 years:*** Up to 0.3 mg daily. ***Over 4 years:*** Same as adult.

DOSE ADJUSTMENTS

Increased initial and maintenance doses may be required in alcoholism, hemolytic, anemia, anticonvulsant therapy, or chronic infection.

DILUTION

Each dose (up to 5 mg) should be diluted in at least 50 ml of SW, D5W, or NS. May be added to most IV solutions and given as an infusion.
Storage: Protect from light and freezing.

INCOMPATIBLE WITH

Calcium gluconate (even though a precipitate cannot be seen), doxapram (Dopram), heavy metal ions, iron sulfate, oxidizing agents, reducing agents, solutions with a pH less than 5.

COMPATIBLE WITH

Consult pharmacist; specific conditions may apply; see Compatibilities, p. xvi.
Y-site: Famotidine (Pepcid IV).

RATE OF ADMINISTRATION

5 mg or fraction thereof over a minimum of 1 minute; usually given over 30 minutes or more in an infusion.

ACTIONS

Folic acid (pteroylglutamic acid) is part of the vitamin B complex. In humans, exogenous folate is required for nucleoprotein synthesis and the maintenance of normal erythropoiesis. It is the precursor of tetrahydrofolic acid, an important cofactor involved in the synthesis of amino acids and DNA. Stimulates the production of RBCs, WBCs, and platelets. Metabolized in the liver and excreted in the urine. Crosses the placental barrier. Secreted in breast milk.

INDICATIONS AND USES

For prevention and treatment of folic acid deficiency. Megaloblastic anemias resulting from folic acid deficiency may be seen in sprue, anemias of malnutrition, pregnancy, infancy, and childhood, developmental or surgical anomalies of the GI tract, as well as other conditions.

CONTRAINDICATIONS

Pernicious anemia unless used in combination with diagnostic testing.

PRECAUTIONS

Folic acid is not commonly administered by the IV route. Oral or IM administration provides adequate absorption in most cases. ■ Obscures the peripheral blood picture and prevents the diagnosis of pernicious anemia. May actually aggravate the neurologic symptoms.

Monitor: Obtain CBC before and during therapy.

Maternal/Child: Category A: an important vitamin before and during pregnancy. Folate-deficient mothers have a higher incidence of fetal anomalies and complications of pregnancy. ■ Safe for use during breast-feeding; infant may require supplementation if mother is folate deficient. ■ Some products contain benzyl alcohol as a preservative. Avoid use in neonates.

Elderly: More likely to have folate deficiency.

DRUG/LAB INTERACTIONS

Toxic effects of antineoplastic folic acid antagonists are blocked by folinic acid (leucovorin calcium) but not by folic acid IV. ■ Increases hydantoin metabolism (e.g., phenytoin [Dilantin]); seizures may result. ■ Inhibited by dihydrofolate reductase inhibitors (e.g., methotrexate, trimethoprim), pyrimethamine, and triamterene and by depressed hematopoiesis, alcoholism, and deficiencies of vitamins B_6, B_{12}, C, and E. ■ Aminosalicylic acid (Pamisyl) or sulfasalazine (Azulfidine) may decrease serum folate levels. ■ Oral contraceptives may inhibit folate metabolism.

SIDE EFFECTS

Almost nonexistent. Some slight flushing or feeling of warmth; anaphylaxis can occur.

ANTIDOTE

If anaphylaxis occurs, discontinue drug, treat anaphylaxis, and notify physician. Resuscitate as necessary.

FOMEPIZOLE INJECTION

(foe-mep'i-zoll in-jek'shun)

Antidote

Antizol

USUAL DOSE

Ethylene glycol is the main component of antifreeze and coolants. Methanol is the main component of windshield washer fluid and a component of products such as Sternol (for fondue pots), Heet (gasoline antifreeze), and various paint products. Begin fomepizole treatment immediately upon suspicion of ethylene glycol or methanol ingestion based on patient history and/or anion gap metabolic acidosis, increased osmolar gap, visual disturbances, or oxalate crystals in the urine, or a documented serum ethylene glycol or methanol concentration greater than 20 mg/dl.

Adults with blood concentrations over 20 mg/dl but less than 50 mg/dl: Administer a loading dose of 15 mg/kg as a slow intravenous infusion. Follow with 10 mg/kg every 12 hours times 4 doses, then 15 mg/kg every 12 hours until ethylene glycol or methanol concentrations are undetectable or have been reduced below 20 mg/dl, and the patient is asymptomatic with normal pH.

Adults with blood concentrations of 50 mg/dl or higher, renal failure, or significant or worsening metabolic acidosis: In addition to dosing as above, dialysis should be considered to correct metabolic abnormalities and to lower the ethylene glycol or methanol concentrations below 50 mg/dl.

Dosage with renal dialysis: Amount of loading dose and following doses (mg/kg) remains the same, but fomepizole is dialyzable and the frequency of dosing should be increased to every 4 hours during hemodialysis. Base frequency on the following chart:

Fomepizole Dosing in Patients Requiring Dialysis	
DOSE AT THE BEGINNING OF HEMODIALYSIS	
If <6 hours since last fomepizole dose Do not administer dose	If ≥6 hours since last fomepizole dose Administer next scheduled dose
DOSING DURING HEMODIALYSIS	
Dose every 4 hours	
DOSING AT THE TIME HEMODIALYSIS IS COMPLETED	
Time between last dose and the end of the hemodialysis	
<1 hour	Do not administer dose at the end of hemodialysis
1-3 hours	Administer ½ of next scheduled dose
>3 hours	Administer next scheduled dose
MAINTENANCE DOSING OFF HEMODIALYSIS	
Give next scheduled dose 12 hours from last dose administered	

PEDIATRIC DOSE

Safety and effectiveness for use in pediatric patients has not been established.

DOSE ADJUSTMENTS

Fomepizole has not been studied sufficiently to determine whether the pharmacokinetics differ for the elderly (see Elderly), children, between genders, in renal insufficiency (excreted renally), or in hepatic insufficiency (metabolized by the liver).

DILUTION

Fomepizole solidifies at temperatures less than 25° C (77° F). If it is solidified, liquefy by running the vial under warm water or by holding in the hand. Solidification does not affect the efficacy, safety, or stability. Withdraw the appropriate dose. Each single dose must be diluted in at least 100 ml of NS or D5W and given as an infusion. Mix well.

Storage: Store vials at CRT 20° to 25° C (68° to 77° F). Diluted solutions are stable refrigerated or at CRT for 48 hours; however, manufacturer states should be used within 24 hours of dilution.

COMPATIBILITY

Specific information not available. Consider specific use; consult pharmacist.

RATE OF ADMINISTRATION

Each single dose must be given as a slow intravenous infusion equally distributed over 30 minutes. ***Do not give undiluted or by bolus injection;*** has caused serious venous irritation and phlebosclerosis.

ACTIONS

A synthetic competitive alcohol dehydrogenase inhibitor. Effectively blocks formation of toxic metabolites (glycolic and oxalic acids [ethylene glycol]) and (formic acid [methanol]). These toxins can induce metabolic acidosis, nausea and vomiting, seizures, stupor, coma, calcium oxaluria, acute tubular necrosis, blindness, and death. Has shown minimal CNS depressant effects. Plasma half-life varies with dose and has not been calculated. Rapidly distributes into total body water. Metabolized in the liver by the P_{450} mixed-function oxidase system. Significant increases in the elimination rate occur after 30 to 40 hours. Excreted in urine.

INDICATIONS AND USES

An antidote for ethylene glycol (antifreeze) or methanol (windshield wiper fluid) poisoning, or for use in suspected ethylene glycol or methanol ingestion either alone or in combination with hemodialysis.

CONTRAINDICATIONS

Known serious hypersensitivity to fomepizole or other pyrazoles (e.g., sulfinpyrazone [Anturane]).

PRECAUTIONS

Acute ethylene glycol or methanol poisoning is a medical emergency that is characterized by a syndrome that can include CNS depression, severe metabolic acidosis, renal failure, and coma. Can be lethal if left untreated or when treatment is delayed due to delayed diagnosis. The lethal dose of ethylene glycol is approximately 1.4 ml/kg. The lethal dose of methanol is approximately 1.2 ml/kg. ■ If ethylene glycol or methanol poisoning is left untreated, the natural progression of the poisoning leads to accumulation of toxic metabolites, including glycolic and oxalic acids (ethylene glycol) and formic acid (methanol). These metabolites can induce metabolic acidosis, nausea and vomiting, seizures, stupor, coma, calcium oxaluria, acute tubular necrosis, and death. ■ The diagnosis of these poisonings may be difficult because ethylene glycol and methanol levels diminish in the blood as they are metabolized. ■ The ethylene glycol or methanol concentrations and the acid-base balance, as determined by serum electrolyte (anion gap) and/or arterial blood gas analysis, should be frequently monitored and used to guide treatment. ■ Fomepizole has caused minor allergic reactions (mild rash, eosinophilia).

Monitor: Maintain a patent airway and support ventilation as indicated; CNS and respiratory distress may occur suddenly. ■ Gastric lavage may be indicated if performed soon after ingestion or in patients who are comatose or at risk for seizures. ■ Patients must be managed for metabolic acidosis, acute renal failure (ethylene glycol), adult respiratory distress syndrome, visual disturbances (methanol), and hypocalcemia which may result in tetany. Sodium bicarbonate may be required to treat metabolic acidosis. Correct electrolyte imbalance and maintain adequate urine output with IV fluids. A decrease in the amount of fluids will be required in impending renal failure to prevent fluid overload; monitor closely. ■ Potassium supplementation and oxygen administration are usually necessary. ■ Administer IV calcium to patients with seizures or tetany that may be caused by decreased calcium, but do not attempt to correct hypocalcemia itself (may increase precipitation of calcium oxalate crystals in the tissues). ■ Hemodialysis is necessary in the anuric patient and should be considered in patients with severe metabolic acidosis or azotemia and in any patient with high ethylene glycol or methanol concentrations (equal to or greater than 50 mg/dl). ■ ECG should be continuous to monitor for cardiac irregularities. ■ EEG may be required in the comatose patient. ■ The effective inhibition of alcohol dehydrogenase requires fomepizole plasma concentrations in the range of 100 to 300 micromol/L (8.6 to 24.6 mg/L). ■ To assess treatment success, obtain baseline and frequently monitor measurements of blood gases, pH, electrolytes, BUN, creatinine, and urinalysis in addition to other laboratory tests as indicated by each patient's condition. ■ To assess the status of ethylene glycol or methanol and their respective metabolite clearance, obtain baseline ethylene glycol or methanol plasma and urine concentrations and presence of urinary oxalate crystals (ethylene glycol) and monitor frequently. ■ Obtain baseline and monitor hepatic enzymes and WBC counts during treatment; transient increases in serum transaminase levels and eosinophilia have been noted with repeated fomepizole dosing. ■ Monitor for signs of allergic reactions; see Precautions.

Patient Education: Monitoring of urine output imperative. ■ Cooperation with adequate hydration and frequent laboratory analysis required. ■ Request assistance with ambulation.

Maternal/Child: Category C: use during pregnancy only if clearly needed. ■ Decreased testicular mass in rats. ■ Use caution during breast-feeding; not known if fomepizole is secreted in breast milk.

Elderly: Risk of toxic reactions may be greater in patients with impaired renal function; consider age-related renal impairment.

DRUG/LAB INTERACTIONS

Has not been studied, but reciprocal interactions (increasing or decreasing clearance, effects, or toxicity) may occur with concomitant use of drugs that induce or inhibit the cytochrome P_{450} system (e.g., carbamazepine

[Tegretol], cimetidine [Tagamet], ketoconazole [Nizoral], phenytoin [Dilantin]). Oral fomepizole significantly reduced the rate of elimination of ethanol (by 40%) in healthy subjects. Ethanol decreased the rate of elimination of fomepizole (by 50%).

SIDE EFFECTS

Most common side effects are dizziness, headache, and nausea. Abdominal pain, abnormal smell, allergic reactions (e.g., mild rash, eosinophilia), anemia, anorexia, arrhythmias (bradycardia, tachycardia), back pain (lower), blurred vision, decreased awareness of surroundings, diarrhea, DIC, feeling of drunkenness, fever, hangover, heartburn, hiccups, hypotension, injection site reaction, lightheadedness, lymphangitis, multisystem organ failure, nystagmus, pharyngitis, phlebitis, phlebosclerosis, seizure, shock, slurred speech, somnolence, taste changes (bad or metallic), vertigo, visual problems, vomiting occurred in up to 6% of patients. **Overdose:** Dizziness, nausea, and vertigo occurred in healthy volunteers given 3 to 6 times the recommended dose.

ANTIDOTE

Keep physician informed of all side effects, laboratory results, and concurrent medical problems. Dialysis may be indicated for changes in patient condition (e.g., renal failure, significant or worsening metabolic acidosis, or a measured ethylene glycol or methanol concentration of greater than 50 mg/dl) or in the treatment of overdose. Treat side effects symptomatically as indicated. Resuscitate as necessary.

FOSCARNET SODIUM

(foss-car′net so′de-um)

Antiviral

Foscavir

pH 7.4

USUAL DOSE

Adequate hydration and specific testing required; see Monitor.

CMV retinitis: 90 mg/kg every 12 hours or 60 mg/kg every 8 hours for 14 to 21 days. Length of induction treatment based on clinical response. Begin a maintenance dose of 90 mg/kg/day the next day (day 15 to 22). If retinitis progresses during the maintenance regimen, re-treat with the induction and maintenance regimens. Maintenance dose may be increased to 120 mg/kg/day in patients who show excellent tolerance to foscarnet or those who require early reinduction because of retinitis progression. Normal renal function required.

CMV retinitis combination therapy (foscarnet and ganciclovir) for patients who have relapsed after induction and reinduction monotherapy with either drug (unlabeled): In patients who have received foscarnet induction with 90 mg/kg every 12 hours followed by 120 mg/kg/day maintenance, continue their present therapy (e.g., foscarnet 120 mg/kg/day) and begin ganciclovir induction with 5 mg/kg every 12 hours for 14 to 21 days followed immediately by maintenance doses of foscarnet 90 mg/kg/day and ganciclovir 5 mg/kg/day (see ganciclovir monograph). Monitor renal function very closely with this combination regimen. Information on this combination regimen is available from Roche.

Acyclovir-resistant HSV patients: 40 mg/kg every 8 or 12 hours for 2 to 3 weeks or until healed.

DOSE ADJUSTMENTS

Must be reduced and individualized according to patient's renal function. May be required during treatment even if patient had normal renal function initially. Specific calculation and testing required for both induction and maintenance dose; see the following charts.

Foscarnet Dose Adjustment Guide for Induction				
	Acyclovir-Resistant HSV		CMV Retinitis	
CrCl (ml/min/kg)	Dose of 40 mg/kg q 12 hr	Dose of 40 mg/kg q 8 hr	Dose of 60 mg/kg q 8 hr	Dose of 90 mg/kg q 12 hr
>1.4	40 mg/kg q 12 hr	40 mg/kg q 8 hr	60 mg/kg q 8 hr	90 mg/kg q 12 hr
>1-1.4	30 mg/kg q 12 hr	30 mg/kg q 8 hr	45 mg/kg q 8 hr	70 mg/kg q 12 hr
>0.8-1	20 mg/kg q 12 hr	35 mg/kg q 12 hr	50 mg/kg q 12 hr	50 mg/kg q 12 hr
>0.6-0.8	35 mg/kg q 24 hr	25 mg/kg q 12 hr	40 mg/kg q 12 hr	80 mg/kg q 24 hr

Continued

Foscarnet Dose Adjustment Guide for Induction—cont'd				
	Acyclovir-Resistant HSV		CMV Retinitis	
CrCl (ml/min/kg)	Dose of 40 mg/kg q 12 hr	Dose of 40 mg/kg q 8 hr	Dose of 60 mg/kg q 8 hr	Dose of 90 mg/kg q 12 hr
>0.5-0.6	25 mg/kg q 24 hr	40 mg/kg q 24 hr	60 mg/kg q 24 hr	60 mg/kg q 24 hr
≥0.4-0.5	20 mg/kg q 24 hr	35 mg/kg q 24 hr	50 mg/kg q 24 hr	50 mg/kg q 24 hr
<0.4	Not recommended	Not recommended	Not recommended	Not recommended

Foscarnet Dose Adjustment Guide for Maintenance in CMV Retinitis		
CrCl (ml/min/kg)	90 mg/kg/day (once daily)	120 mg/kg/day (once daily)
>1.4	90 mg/kg q 24 hr	120 mg/kg q 24 hr
>1-1.4	70 mg/kg q 24 hr	90 mg/kg q 24 hr
>0.8-1	50 mg/kg q 24 hr	65 mg/kg q 24 hr
>0.6-0.8	80 mg/kg q 48 hr	105 mg/kg q 48 hr
>0.5-0.6	60 mg/kg q 48 hr	80 mg/kg q 48 hr
≥0.4-0.5	50 mg/kg q 48 hr	65 mg/kg q 48 hr
<0.4	Not recommended	Not recommended

DILUTION

Central venous catheter: Standard 24-mg/ml solution may be given undiluted.

Peripheral vein: Each 1 ml of a calculated dose must be diluted with 1 ml of D5W or NS (yields a 12-mg/ml solution). To avoid any possibility of overdose in either situation, only the calculated dose should be in the infusion bottle. Discard any excess before administration.

INCOMPATIBLE WITH

Manufacturer states, "Administer only with NS or D5W solutions; no other drug or supplement should be administered concurrently via the same catheter." Because of chelating properties, a precipitate can occur. Manufacturer specifically lists as incompatible with 30% dextrose, solutions containing calcium (e.g., LR, TPN), acyclovir (Zovirax), amphotericin B (Fungizone), diazepam (Valium), digoxin (Lanoxin), ***ganciclovir (Cytovene),*** leucovorin calcium, midazolam (Versed), pentamidine, phenytoin (Dilantin), prochlorperazine (Compazine), sulfamethoxazole-trimethoprim (Bactrim), trimetrexate glucuronate, vancomycin (Vancocin). Other sources add diphenhydramine (Benadryl), dobutamine (Dobutrex), droperidol (Inapsine), haloperidol (Haldol), promethazine (Phenergan).

COMPATIBLE WITH (Underline Indicates Conflicting Compatibility Information)

See Incompatible With. Consult pharmacist; specific conditions may apply; see Compatibilities, p. xvi.

Additive: ***Not recommended by manufacturer.*** Potassium chloride (KCl).

Y-site: Aldesleukin (Proleukin), amikacin (Amikin), aminophylline, ampicillin, aztreonam (Azactam), cefazolin (Kefzol), cefoperazone (Cefobid), cefoxitin (Mefoxin), ceftazidime (Fortaz), ceftizoxime (Cefizox), ceftriaxone (Rocephin), cefuroxime (Zinacef), chloramphenicol (Chloromycetin), cimetidine (Tagamet), clindamycin (Cleocin), dexamethasone (Decadron), dopamine (Intropin), erythromycin lactobionate (Erythrocin), fluconazole (Diflucan), furosemide (Lasix), gentamicin (Garamycin), heparin, hydrocortisone sodium succinate (Solu-Cortef), hydromorphone (Dilaudid), imipenem-cilastatin (Primaxin), lorazepam (Ativan), metoclopramide (Reglan), metronidazole (Flagyl IV), morphine, nafcillin (Nafcil), oxacillin (Bactocill), penicillin G potassium, phenytoin (Dilantin), piperacillin (Pipracil), ranitidine (Zantac), sulfamethoxazole-trimethoprim (Bactrim), ticarcillin/clavulanate (Timentin), tobramycin (Nebcin), vancomycin (Vancocin).

RATE OF ADMINISTRATION

Infusion pump required to deliver accurate dose evenly distributed over specific time frame. Excessive plasma levels and toxicity (including hypocalcemia) will occur with too-rapid rate of infusion. Advisable to clear tubing with NS if possible before and after administration through Y-tube or three-way stopcock. Never exceed 1 mg/kg/min.

CMV Retinitis: ***Induction doses:*** Each 60-mg dose equally distributed over a minimum of 1 hour. Increase to 1½ to 2 hours for 90-mg dose.

Maintenance dose: Each dose equally distributed over a minimum of 2 hours.

Acyclovir-resistant HSV: Each dose equally distributed over a minimum of 1 hour.

ACTIONS

An antiviral agent capable of inhibiting replication of all known herpesviruses, including cytomegalovirus (CMV), herpes simplex virus types 1 and 2 (HSV-1, HSV-2), human herpesvirus 6 (HHV-6), Epstein-Barr (EBV), and varicella-zoster virus (VZV). Does not destroy existing viruses but stops them from reproducing and invading healthy cells. Also capable of chelating metal ions (e.g., calcium, magnesium). CMV strains resistant to ganciclovir may be sensitive to foscarnet. Half-life averages 3 hours and increases markedly with renal impairment. Some penetration into bone and cerebrospinal fluid. Probably secreted in breast milk. Excreted unchanged in urine.

INDICATIONS AND USES

Treatment of CMV retinitis in patients with AIDS. Most frequently used in patients who do not tolerate or are resistant to ganciclovir. ■ Combination therapy (foscarnet and ganciclovir) may be indicated with progressive retinitis refractory to single therapy. ■ Treatment of acyclovir-resistant mucocutaneous HSV infections in immunocompromised patients.

CONTRAINDICATIONS

Hypersensitivity to foscarnet.

PRECAUTIONS

For IV use only. ■ May cause potentially life-threatening changes in renal function with cumulative exposure. Careful monitoring of renal function and dose adjustment is imperative. Changes can occur at any time, most likely during second week of therapy. ■ Confirm diagnosis of CMV retinitis by indirect ophthalmoscopy. Diagnosis may be supported by cultures of CMV from urine, blood, throat, etc.; negative culture does not rule out CMV retinitis. ■ Use caution in patients with a history of impaired renal function, altered calcium or other electrolyte levels, neurologic or cardiac abnormalities, a low baseline absolute neutrophil count (ANC), and those receiving other drugs known to influence minerals and electrolytes; see Drug/Lab Interactions. Has caused hyperphosphatemia, hypocalcemia, hypokalemia, hypomagnesemia, and hypophosphatemia, resulting in cardiac disturbances, seizures, and tetany. ■ Foscarnet superior to vidarabine (ARA-A) for treatment of acyclovir-resistant HSV. ■ Resistance has been reported to develop. May be higher in patients treated for a prolonged period. ■ Sensitivity testing for viral isolate is recommended before repeat treatment and/or to evaluate sensitivity versus development of resistance. Cidofovir is a newly approved agent for treatment of CMV retinitis.

Monitor: Baseline 24-hour CrCl verified by creatinine index; baseline SrCr, calcium, magnesium, potassium, phosphorus, and electrolytes required before treatment begins. Correct any deficiencies. ■ Repeat entire testing process 2 to 3 times a week during induction therapy and a minimum of every 2 weeks during maintenance therapy. Foscarnet dose must be adjusted as indicated by test results. More frequent testing may be indicated in specific patients. Supplementation of minerals and electrolytes may be required during treatment. ■ To minimize renal toxicity, hydration adequate to establish diuresis is recommended before and during treatment unless contraindicated. Give 750 to 1,000 ml NS or D5W before the first foscarnet infusion to establish diuresis. With subsequent infusions, give 750 to 1,000 ml concurrently with 90 to 120 mg/kg foscarnet and a minimum of 500 ml concurrently with 40 to 60 mg/kg. ■ Discontinue foscarnet if CrCl drops below 0.4 ml/min/kg or serum creatinine is greater than 2.8 mg/100 ml (1 dl). Monitor patient daily until resolution of renal impairment is ensured. Safety for use in these patients has not been studied. ■ Anemia may be severe enough to require transfusion. ■ Phlebitis or pain may occur at site of infusion; confirm patency of vein and use large veins to ensure adequate blood flow for rapid dilution and distribution. ■ See Drug/Lab Interactions.

Patient Education: Not a cure. Retinitis may recur during maintenance or after treatment; regular ophthalmologic exams imperative. ■ Complete healing of HSV infections may occur, but most relapse. ■ Perioral tingling, numbness in the extremities or paresthesias indicate electrolyte abnormalities; report immediately. ■ Adequate hydration and increased personal hygiene may minimize some side effects. ■ Dose modification or discontinuation may be required for major side effects.

Maternal/Child: Category C: use only if clearly needed; has caused skeletal anomalies in animals. ■ Excreted at three times maternal blood concentrations in lactating rats; human data not available. ■ Safety for use in children not established; deposited in teeth and bones, and deposition greater in young animals. Use only if benefits outweigh risks.

Elderly: Safety and effectiveness not established, however, foscarnet has been used in patients over 65 years of age. Side effects seen are similar to other age-groups. Consider age-related renal impairment in dose selection and monitor renal function; see Dose Adjustments.

DRUG/LAB INTERACTIONS

Because of physical incompatibilities, foscarnet sodium and ganciclovir sodium must never be mixed. ■ Coadministration with any other drugs could theoretically alter its antiviral activity, toxicity, or pharmacokinetics. ■ Has caused hypocalcemia with parenteral pentamidine. ■ Capable of causing calcium or electrolyte disorders. Use caution when administering any drug known to influence minerals or electrolytes (e.g., hypocalcemic agents [gallium nitrate (Ganite)], diuretics [furosemide (Lasix), mannitol], adrenocortical steroids). ■ Elimination of foscarnet may be impaired and toxicity increased by drugs that inhibit renal tubular secretion (e.g., probenecid). ■ Avoid concomitant use with other nephrotoxic drugs (e.g., aminoglycosides [e.g., gentamicin (Garamycin)], amphotericin B [Fungizone], cyclosporine [Sandimmune], pentamidine) unless benefits outweigh risks. ■ Anemia may be additive with zidovudine (AZT). ■ Use with ciprofloxacin (Cipro IV) may cause seizures; monitor patient carefully. ■ Abnormal renal function has been reported in patients receiving foscarnet and ritonavir (Norvir) or foscarnet and ritonavir and saquinavir (Invirase).

SIDE EFFECTS

Impaired renal function, alterations in plasma minerals and electrolytes, and seizures are major side effects and are dose limiting. Abnormal renal function, including acute renal failure, decreased CrCl and increased SrCr (27%); anemia (33%); bone marrow suppression (10%); diarrhea (30%); fever (65%); headache (26%); hyperphosphatemia; hypocalcemia (perioral tingling, numbness in extremities, paresthesias, tetany); hypokalemia; hypomagnesemia; hypophosphatemia; irritation at injection site; irritation and ulcerations of penile and vaginal epithelium; nausea (47%); seizure (10%); vomiting (26%); and death (14%) have occurred. All deaths could not be directly related to foscarnet. Abdominal pain, anorexia, anxiety, asthenia, confusion, coughing, depression, dizziness, dyspnea, granulocytopenia, hypoesthesia, infection, involuntary muscle contractions, leukopenia, malaise, neuropathy, pain, rash, sweating, and vision abnormalities have occurred in 5% of patients. Numerous other side effects have occurred in less than 5% of patients.

ANTIDOTE

There is no specific antidote. Keep physician informed. Adequate hydration and careful monitoring will help reduce potential for renal impairment and may minimize other side effects. Elevations in SrCr are usually reversible (within 1 week) with dose adjustment or discontinuation but have caused death. Discontinue foscarnet if CrCl falls below 0.4 ml/min/kg or SrCr is greater than 2.8 mg/100 ml. Monitor daily until resolution of renal impairment is ensured. Discontinue foscarnet if perioral tingling, numbness in the extremities, or paresthesias occur during or after infusion; evaluate calcium and electrolyte levels (decrease in ionized serum calcium may not be reflected in total serum calcium); notify physician. Administration of foscarnet can be resumed following seizures or cardiac disturbances after treatment of underlying disease, electrolyte disturbance, or after dose adjustment. Overdose can occur with too-rapid rate of infusion. Hemodialysis and hydration are useful in overdose. Treat anaphylaxis and resuscitate as indicated.

FOSPHENYTOIN SODIUM

(foss-fen′i-toy-in so′de-um)

Anticonvulsant (hydantoin)

Cerebyx

pH 8.6 to 9

USUAL DOSE

In all situations, dose of fosphenytoin is expressed as phenytoin sodium equivalents (PE).

Status epilepticus: ***Adult loading dose:*** 15 to 20 mg PE/kg. Full effect is not immediate; concomitant administration of an IV benzodiazepine (e.g., diazepam [Valium]) is usually necessary to control status epilepticus. If seizures are not controlled, consider other anticonvulsants and other measures as needed (e.g., barbiturates or anesthesia). ***Maintenance dose:*** 4 to 6 mg PE/kg/24 hr. ***Elderly loading dose:*** 14 mg PE/kg. See all comments under Usual Dose. See Elderly.

Nonemergent indications: ***Loading dose:*** 10 to 20 mg PE/kg. ***Maintenance dose:*** 4 to 6 mg PE/kg/24 hr. ***Substitute for oral phenytoin:*** May be substituted at the same total daily dose (due to a 10% increase in bioavailability [IV/IM to oral], plasma levels with the IV/IM product may be increased slightly).

PEDIATRIC DOSE

Status epilepticus: 15 to 20 mg PE/kg at a rate of up to 3 mg PE/kg/min. Safety for use in children not established. Limited data available; no significant differences apparent to this date.

DOSE ADJUSTMENTS

Reduced doses may be required in the elderly (see Usual Dose), in impaired renal or hepatic function, or in patients with hypoalbuminemia. ■ See Precautions, Monitor, Drug/Lab Interactions, and Antidote.

DILUTION

Use only clear solutions. Should be diluted in D5W or NS to a concentration of 1.5 to 25 mg PE/ml. Supplied solution is 50 mg PE/ml. Dilute each milliliter of fosphenytoin with 1 ml of diluent to equal 25 mg PE/ml. Dilute a 1,000-mg PE dose in 100 ml diluent to equal 10 mg PE/ml.

Storage: Keep refrigerated; do not store at room temperature for more than 48 hours. After dilution, solutions are stable at room temperature for 8 hours and for 24 hours if refrigerated.

COMPATIBLE WITH

Consult pharmacist; specific conditions may apply; see Compatibilities, p. xvi.

Additive: Potassium chloride (KCl).

Y-site: Lorazepam (Ativan), phenobarbital (Luminal).

RATE OF ADMINISTRATION

Each 100 to 150 mg PE or fraction thereof over a minimum of 1 minute. Risk of hypotension increased if this rate is exceeded. Slow or temporarily stop rate of infusion for burning, itching, numbness, or pain along injection site.

Pediatric rate: Manufacturer recommends 1 to 3 mg PE/kg/min for pediatric patients. Another source suggests a rate of 1.6 mg PE/kg/min.

ACTIONS

A water-soluble prodrug of phenytoin. Converts to phenytoin, phosphate, and formate within 15 minutes of IV/IM administration. An anticonvulsant, chemically related to barbiturates. Selectively stabilizes seizure threshold and depresses seizure activity in the motor cortex. Also exerts a depressant effect on the myocardium by selectively elevating the excitability threshold of the cell, reducing the cell's response to stimuli. Peak levels of fosphenytoin are achieved by the end of an infusion, but conversion to therapeutic serum levels of phenytoin takes longer. Extensively bound to protein, fosphenytoin displaces phenytoin from protein binding sites and increases free phenytoin (dose and rate dependent). Phenytoin is metabolized in the liver by hepatic cytochrome P_{450} enzymes and excreted in urine. Crosses the placental barrier. Secreted in breast milk. Advantages of fosphenytoin over present phenytoin products include solubility in IV solutions, improved infusion site tolerance, more rapid rate of injection, and well-tolerated IM option.

INDICATIONS AND USES

Treatment and control of generalized convulsive status epilepticus. ■ Treatment or prophylaxis of seizures in neurosurgical patients. ■ Substitute for oral phenytoin when oral administration is not feasible or prompt increases in antiepileptic drug levels are needed.

CONTRAINDICATIONS

Hypersensitivity to fosphenytoin, any of its components, phenytoin, or other hydantoins. ■ Sinus bradycardia, sinoatrial block, second- and third-degree AV block, and Adams-Stokes syndrome.

PRECAUTIONS

Doses of fosphenytoin are expressed as phenytoin equivalents; no adjustment required when substituting fosphenytoin or vice versa. Labeling of fosphenytoin has been updated by the manufacturer to reduce the incidence of dosing errors. To ensure accuracy, confirm actual dose, dilution, and amount of injection with pharmacist or another RN. ■ IV route indicated in emergency situations (e.g., status epilepticus). May be given IM in nonemergency situations. ■ Intended for short-term parenteral use (up to 5 days). ■ Transfer to oral phenytoin therapy as soon as feasible. ■ Abrupt withdrawal may cause increased seizure activity. Gradually reduce dose, discontinue, or substitute alternative antiepileptic agents. ■ Discontinue immediately for hypersensitivity reactions; with caution substitute a nonhydantoin anticonvulsant (e.g., phenobarbital [Luminal], valproate sodium [Depacon]). ■ May cause severe cardiovascular depression (e.g., bradycardia, various degrees of AV block, ventricular fibrillation [VF]); use extreme caution in elderly or seriously ill patients. ■ Use with caution in patients with hypotension or severe myocardial insufficiency. ■ May exacerbate porphyria. ■ May cause acute phenytoin hepatotoxicity (e.g., elevated liver function tests, fever, jaundice, lymphadenopathy, skin eruptions). Discontinue immediately and substitute alternate anticonvulsant therapy. ■ Has caused lymphadenopathy and hemopoietic complications (e.g., agranulocytosis, granulocytopenia, leukopenia, thrombocytopenia, or pancytopenia with or without bone marrow suppression). If lymphadenopathy occurs with or without signs of serum sickness (e.g., fever, rash, hepatotoxicity), substitute alternate anticonvulsant therapy. ■ Use caution with low serum albumin levels, and adjust dose as indicated. Phenytoin is highly bound to serum protein, and a reduced albumin causes an increase in free drug availability and may increase toxicity. ■ Not effective for petit mal seizures; combined therapy required if both conditions present. ■ Inhibits insulin release and may increase serum glucose; monitoring indicated in diabetics. ■ May lower serum folate levels.

Monitor: Monitor ECG, BP, and respirations continuously during loading dose and for at least 30 minutes after infusion complete. ■ Allow fosphenytoin time to convert to phenytoin; accurate serum levels are not available until 2 hours after the end of an IV infusion or 4 hours after IM injection. Narrow margin of error between therapeutic and toxic dose. Plasma levels above 10 mcg/ml usually control seizure activity. The acceptable range is 5 to 20 mcg/ml. Toxicity begins with nystagmus at levels exceeding 20 mcg/ml. ■ Observe for rash and discontinue if one appears. If rash is mild, fosphenytoin may be resumed when the rash has completely disappeared. If the mild rash occurs again or the initial rash is serious in nature (e.g., exfoliative, purpuric, bullous) or lupus erythematous, Stevens-Johnson syndrome, or toxic epidermal necrolysis is suspected, discontinue fosphenytoin. Do not resume; consider alternative therapy. ■ Contains phosphates; monitor in patients who require phosphate restriction (e.g., renal impairment). ■ Monitor closely patients who are gravely ill, have impaired liver function, or are elderly. May show early signs of toxicity. ■ Determine absolute patency of vein; avoid extravasation. Not as alkaline as phenytoin.

Patient Education: Report burning, itching, numbness, pain, or rash. ■ Consider birth control options; nonhormonal birth control recommended.

Maternal/Child: Category D: avoid pregnancy. Risk of serious congenital malformations triple that of the general population. ■ An increase in seizure frequency may occur during pregnancy; monitoring of plasma phenytoin levels may be helpful. ■ Newborns whose mothers received phenytoin during pregnancy may develop a life-threatening bleeding disorder that can be prevented by giving vitamin K to the mother before delivery and to the neonate after birth. ■ Discontinue breast-feeding.

Elderly: See Dose Adjustments. ■ Sensitivity and/or toxicity may be increased because serum concentrations may be elevated due to reduced clearance, or low serum albumin may cause a decrease in protein binding and an increase in free phenytoin.

DRUG/LAB INTERACTIONS

No drugs are known to interfere with the conversion of fosphenytoin to phenytoin, although phosphatase activity may have an impact. ■ Capable of innumerable catastrophic drug interactions; review of drug profile by pharmacist imperative. In all situations, monitoring of phenytoin serum levels may be indicated. ■ Serum levels and toxicity of phenytoin may be increased by alcohol (acute intake), amiodarone (Cordarone), anticonvulsants (e.g., succinimides [ethosuximide (Zarontin)]), antidepressants (e.g., fluoxetine [Prozac], trazodone [Deseryl]), antifungal agents (e.g., fluconazole, miconazole, ketoconazole), chloramphenicol, chlordiazepoxide (Librium), H_2 antagonists (e.g., cimetidine [Tagamet]), diazepam (Valium), dicumarol, disulfiram (Antabuse), estrogens, fluorouracil, halothane, isoniazid (Nydrazid), methylphenidate (Ritalin), phenothiazines (e.g., prochlorperazine [Compazine]), phenylbutazone (Butazolidin), salicylates (aspirin), sulfonamides (e.g., sulfisoxazole), tolbutamide (Orinase). ■ Serum levels and effectiveness of phenytoin may be decreased by carbamazepine (Tegretol), chronic alcohol abuse, doxorubicin (with cisplatin), leucovorin calcium, and reserpine (Serpasil). ■ Serum levels of phenytoin may be increased or decreased by phenobarbital (Luminal), valproate sodium (Depacon), valproic acid (Depakene). ■ Tricyclic antidepressants (e.g., amitriptyline [Elavil]) may precipitate seizures in susceptible patients or phenytoin may increase metabolism of antidepressants. Dose adjustment may be indicated for either or both drugs. ■ Phenytoin will inhibit effects of anticoagulants (e.g., warfarin [Coumadin]), corticosteroids, cardiac glycosides (e.g., digoxin), doxycycline, estrogens, furosemide (Lasix), itraconazole (Sporanox), oral contraceptives, rifampin (Rifadin), quinidine, theophylline, vitamin D. ■ In one case report, a patient stabilized on phenytoin and valproic acid experienced seizures and a reduction in antiepileptic drug serum concentration when acyclovir was added to the regimen. ■ Alters some clinical laboratory tests (e.g., may decrease T_4, increase glucose, alkaline phosphatase, and GGT may produce low results in dexamethasone or metyrapone tests).

SIDE EFFECTS

Transient ataxia, dizziness, headache, nystagmus, paresthesia, pruritus, and somnolence are the most common side effects; are dose and rate related; occur within several minutes of the start of the infusion; and usually resolve within 10 minutes of completion. Risks of side effects increased with upper-end doses given at upper-end rates. Coma, hyperreflexia, hypotension, lethargy, nausea, slurred speech, tremor, and vomiting are also signs of increased toxicity. Fosphenytoin breaks down into formate and phosphate metabolites that may cause formate toxicity (hypocalcemia, metabolic acidosis, muscle spasms, paresthesia, and seizures). **Major/overdose:** Arrhythmias (e.g., bradycardia, cardiac arrest, heart block, tachycardia, ventricular fibrillation), coma, hyperreflexia, hypotension, lethargy, nausea, respiratory arrest, slurred speech, syncope, tonic seizures, tremor, and vomiting. Deaths have been reported.

ANTIDOTE

Notify physician of any side effects. Obtain serum plasma levels at first signs of toxicity; reduce dose. If symptoms persist or major side effects appear, discontinue fosphenytoin and notify physician. Treat symptomatically, maintain a patent airway, and resuscitate as necessary. Symptoms of bradycardia or heart block may be reversed with IV atropine. Epinephrine may also be useful. One source says hemodialysis may be helpful in overdose. Another source says hemodialysis, peritoneal dialysis, forced fluid diuresis, exchange transfusions, and plasmapheresis are ineffective. In overdose, measure ionized free calcium levels to guide treatment in phosphate toxicity.

FUROSEMIDE

(fur-oh′se-mide)

Diuretic (loop)
Antihypertensive
Antihypercalcemic

Lasix, ✱Uritol

pH 8 to 9.3

USUAL DOSE

Edema/congestive heart failure: 20 to 40 mg. May be repeated in 1 to 2 hours. If necessary, increase dosage by 20-mg increments (under close medical supervision and no sooner than 2 hours after previous dose) until desired diuresis is obtained. IV bolus dose should not exceed 1 Gm/day. If larger doses are required, give as an infusion. In severe refractory congestive heart failure, doses up to 4 Gm/24 hr have been given with extreme caution. After the initial diuresis the minimum effective dose may be given once or twice every 24 hours as required for maintenance.

Hypertension: Up to 40 mg twice daily. If this dose does not reduce hypertension, the addition of other antihypertensive agents is recommended instead of larger doses of furosemide.

Hypertensive crisis: 40 to 80 mg concomitantly with other antihypertensive agents. AHA guidelines recommend 0.5 to 1 mg/kg over 1 to 2 minutes. If no response, increase dose to 2 mg/kg.

Hypertensive crisis with pulmonary edema or acute renal failure: 100 to 200 mg.

Acute pulmonary edema or post–cardiac arrest cerebral edema: 40 mg. If no response in 1 hour, increase to 80 mg. AHA guidelines recommend 0.5 to 1 mg/kg over 1 to 2 minutes. If no response, increase dose to 2 mg/kg.

Acute or chronic renal failure: Initial dose required can range from 100 mg to 2 Gm. Higher doses are well tolerated in these patients. Increase dose as needed to achieve desired effect. IV bolus dose should not exceed 1 Gm/day. If larger doses are required, give as an infusion. Has been doubled at 2- to 24-hour intervals in some studies. One protocol calls for an infusion of 250 mg over 1 hour. If urine output insufficient in 1 hour, increase to 500 mg infused over 2 hours. If urine output still insufficient after the first hour, increase to 1 Gm over 4 hours. For high-dose infusions, individualize dose and titrate to maximum therapeutic effect from the lowest dose. Highest total IV dose was 6 g.

Hypercalcemia: 80 to 100 mg at 1- to 2-hour intervals. Given concomitantly with NS. Total IV dose required has ranged from 160 mg to 3.2 g.

Diagnostic aid (renal imaging adjunct [unlabeled]): 0.3 to 0.5 mg/kg to maximum dose of 40 mg.

PEDIATRIC DOSE

See Maternal/Child.

Diuretic: 1 mg/kg of body weight. After 2 hours increase by 1-mg/kg increments to effect desired response. Effective dose may be given every 6 to 12 hours. Another source suggests 0.5 to 2 mg/kg/dose every 6 to 12 hours. Do not exceed 6 mg/kg/dose.

Hypercalcemia: 25 to 50 mg. Repeat every 4 hours to desired response. Do not exceed 6 mg/kg/dose.

NEONATAL DOSE

Diuretic: 0.5 to 1 mg/kg/dose every 8 to 24 hours. Maximum dose is 2 mg/kg/dose. See Maternal/Child.

DOSE ADJUSTMENTS

Higher doses may be required in renal insufficiency and acute or chronic renal failure. ■ Reduced dose or extended intervals may be appropriate in the elderly. ■ Extend dosing intervals in neonates because half-life is prolonged. ■ See Drug/Lab Interactions.

DILUTION

May be given undiluted. May be given through Y-tube or three-way stopcock of infusion set. Not usually added to IV solutions, but large doses may be added to NS, LR, D5W, D5NS and given as an infusion. pH of solution must be over 5.5. If obtaining large doses from ampules, use of a filter is recommended to eliminate possible pieces of glass. Some sources recommend protecting diluted solutions from light to prevent photodegradation (minimized at pH 7).

Storage: If diluted for infusion, discard after 24 hours.

COMPATIBLE WITH **(Underline Indicates Conflicting Compatibility Information)**

Consult pharmacist; specific conditions may apply; see Compatibilities, p. xvi.

Additive: Amikacin (Amikin), aminophylline, amiodarone (Cordarone), ampicillin, atropine, bumetanide (Bumex), calcium gluconate, cefamandole (Mandol), cefoperazone (Cefobid), cefuroxime (Zinacef), cimetidine (Tagamet), dexamethasone (Decadron), digoxin (Lanoxin), epinephrine (Adrenalin), gentamicin (Garamycin), heparin, hydrocortisone sodium succinate (Solu-Cortef), kanamycin (Kantrex), lidocaine, meropenem (Merrem IV), morphine, nitroglycerin (Nitro-Bid IV), penicillin G potassium, potassium chloride (KCl), ranitidine (Zantac), scopolamine, sodium bicarbonate, theophylline, tobramycin (Nebcin), verapamil (Isoptin).

Syringe: Bleomycin (Blenoxane), cisplatin (Platinol), cyclophosphamide (Cytoxan), fluorouracil (5-FU), heparin, leucovorin calcium, methotrexate (Folex), mitomycin (Mutamycin).

Y-site: Allopurinol (Aloprim, Zyloprim), amifostine (Ethyol), amikacin (Amikin), amphotericin B cholesteryl (Amphotec), aztreonam (Azactam), bleomycin (Blenoxane), cefepime (Maxipime), cisatracurium (Nimbex), cisplatin (Platinol), cladribine (Leustatin), cyclophosphamide (Cytoxan), cytarabine (ARA-C), dobutamine (Dobutrex), docetaxel (Taxotere), dopamine (Intropin), doxorubicin (Adriamycin), doxorubicin liposome (Doxil), epinephrine (Adrenalin), etoposide phosphate (Etopophos), famotidine (Pepcid IV), fentanyl (Sublimaze), fludarabine (Fludara), fluorouracil (5-FU), foscarnet (Foscavir), granisetron (Kytril), heparin, hetastarch in electrolytes (Hextend), hydrocortisone sodium succinate (Solu-Cortef), hydromorphone (Dilaudid), indomethacin (Indocin), kanamycin (Kantrex), labetalol (Normodyne), leucovorin calcium, linezolid (Zyvox), lorazepam (Ativan), melphalan (Alkeran), meperidine (Demerol), meropenem (Merrem IV), methotrexate (Folex), mitomycin (Mutamycin), morphine, nitroglycerin (Nitro-Bid IV), norepinephrine (Levophed), paclitaxel (Taxol), piperacillin/tazobactam (Zosyn), potassium chloride (KCl), propofol (Diprivan), ranitidine (Zantac), remifentanil (Ultiva), sargramostim (Leukine), tacrolimus (Prograf), teniposide (Vumon), thiotepa (Thioplex), tobramycin (Nebcin).

RATE OF ADMINISTRATION

IV injection: Each 40 mg or fraction thereof should be given over 1 to 2 minutes. A 1-Gm bolus must be given over at least 30 minutes; up to 3 hours is preferred. In oliguric or anuric patients the total dose (undiluted) should be infused at a rate of 4 mg/min. Constant rate infusion pump required.

Infusion: ***Adults and children:*** 0.05 mg/kg/hr. Titrate to effect. High-dose therapy in an infusion should not exceed a rate of 4 mg/min. A 1-Gm dose should take at least 3 hours to prevent ototoxicity.

ACTIONS

A sulfonamide-type diuretic, related to the thiazides. Extremely potent and has a rapid onset of action. Effectiveness is noted within 5 minutes and may last for 2 hours. Apparently acts on the proximal and distal ends of the tubule and the ascending limb of the loop of Henle to excrete water, sodium, chlorides, and potassium. Will produce diuresis in alkalosis or acidosis. Highly protein bound. Metabolized and excreted in the urine. Crosses the placental barrier. Secreted in breast milk.

INDICATIONS AND USES

Edema associated with congestive heart failure, cirrhosis of the liver with ascites, and renal disease including the nephrotic syndrome. ■ Acute pulmonary edema. ■ Edema unresponsive to other diuretic agents. ■ Hypercalcemia. ■ Hypertension. ■ Post–cardiac arrest cerebral edema. **Unlabeled uses:** Renal imaging radionuclide adjunct to increase urine flow and aid in differentiation of mechanical obstruction versus nonobstructive dilatation in patients with hydroureteronephrosis.

CONTRAINDICATIONS

Anuria, severe progressive renal disease with increasing azotemia and oliguria; rarely used in children, pregnancy, and breast-feeding.

PRECAUTIONS

May be used concurrently with aldosterone antagonists (e.g., spironolactone [Aldactone]) for more effective diuresis and to prevent excessive potassium loss. ■ Use caution and improve basic condition first in hepatic coma, electrolyte depletion, and advanced cirrhosis of the liver. ■ May increase risk of gastric hemorrhage during corticosteroid therapy. ■ Use extreme caution in known sulfonamide sensitivity. ■ Risk of ototoxicity increases with higher doses, rapid injection, decreased renal function, or concurrent use with other ototoxic drugs; see Drug/Lab Interactions. ■ May activate or exacerbate systemic lupus erythematosus.

Monitor: Discontinue at least 2 days before elective surgery. ■ Monitor BP frequently, especially during initial therapy. ■ May precipitate excessive diuresis with water and electrolyte depletion. Routine checks on electrolyte panel, CO_2, and BUN are necessary during therapy. Potassium chloride replacement may be required. ■ May increase blood glucose and has precipitated diabetes mellitus. ■ May lower serum calcium level; may cause tetany. ■ Rarely precipitates an acute attack of gout. ■ See Drug/Lab Interactions.

Patient Education: Hypotension may cause dizziness; request assistance with ambulation. ■ Report cramps, dizziness, muscle weakness, or nausea promptly. ■ May cause a decrease in potassium levels and require a supplement. ■ Skin may become photosensitive; avoid unprotected exposure to sun.

Maternal/Child: Category C: use during pregnancy only when clearly needed and benefits outweigh potential risks to fetus. ■ Discontinue breast-feeding. ■ Safety for use in children not established. ■ Prolonged use in premature infants may result in nephrocalcinosis. ■ May increase risk of patent ductus arteriosus in pre-term infants with respiratory distress syndrome; use with caution before delivery. ■ See Contraindications.

Elderly: Consider increased sensitivity to hypotensive and electrolyte effects. ■ May be more susceptible to dehydration; observe carefully. ■ Avoid rapid contraction of plasma volume and hemoconcentration. May cause thromboembolic episodes (e.g., CVA, pulmonary emboli).

DRUG/LAB INTERACTIONS

Causes excessive potassium depletion with corticosteroids, thiazide diuretics (e.g., hydrochlorothiazide [HydroDIURIL]), amphotericin B (all formulations). ■ Potentiates antihypertensive drugs (e.g., nitroglycerin, nitroprusside sodium); reduced dose of the antihypertensive agent or both drugs may be indicated. ■ May cause transient or permanent deafness with doses exceeding the usual or when given in conjunction with other ototoxic drugs (e.g., aminoglycosides [e.g., gentamicin], cisplatin). ■ Amphotericin B (all formulations) may increase potential for ototoxicity and nephrotoxicity, avoid concurrent use. ■ Nephrotoxicity increased by other nephrotoxic agents (e.g., acyclovir [Zovirax], aminoglycosides, ciprofloxacin [Cipro IV], cyclosporine [Sandimmune], vancomycin [Vancocin]), avoid concurrent use. ■ May increase activity of anticoagulants (e.g., warfarin [Coumadin], heparin, streptokinase); monitor PT. ■ May increase serum levels of beta blockers (e.g., propranolol [Inderal]) and of lithium (may cause toxicity). ■ May cause cardiac arrhythmias with amiodarone (Cordarone) or digitalis (potassium depletion). ■ Risk of cardiotoxicity increased with pimozide (Orap) and sparfloxacin (Zagam); concurrent use not recommended. ■ May enhance or inhibit actions of nondepolarizing muscle relaxant (e.g., mivacurium [Mivacron]) or theophyllines. ■ May cause hyperglycemia with insulin or sulfonylureas (e.g., tolbutamide) by decreasing glucose tolerance. ■ Effects may be inhibited by ACE inhibitors (e.g., captopril [Capoten]), NSAIDs (e.g., ibuprofen [Motrin]), probenecid, or in patients with cirrhosis and ascites on salicylates. ■ May cause profound diuresis and serious electrolyte abnormalities with thiazide diuretics (e.g., chlorothiazide [Diuril]) because of synergistic effects. ■ Clofibrate (Atromid-S) may cause increased diuresis. ■ May be inhibited by phenytoin (Dilantin). ■ Do not use concomitantly with ethacrynic acid (Edecrin); risk of ototoxicity markedly increased. ■ Smoking may increase secretion of ADH-decreasing diuretic effects and cardiac output. ■ See Precautions.

SIDE EFFECTS

Usually occur in prolonged therapy, seriously ill patients, or following large doses.

Anemia, anorexia, blurring of vision, deafness (reversible), diarrhea, dizziness, hyperglycemia, hyperuricemia, hypokalemia, leg cramps, lethargy, leukopenia, mental confusion, paresthesia, postural hypotension, pruritus, tinnitus, urinary frequency, urticaria, vomiting, weakness.

Major: Anaphylactic shock, blood volume reduction, circulatory collapse, dehydration, excessive diuresis, hypokalemia, metabolic acidosis, vascular thrombosis, and embolism.

ANTIDOTE

If minor side effects are noted, discontinue the drug and notify the physician, who may treat the side effects symptomatically and continue the drug. If side effects are progressive or any major side effect occurs, discontinue the drug immediately and notify the physician. Treatment of major side effects is symptomatic and aggressive. Resuscitate as necessary.

GALLIUM NITRATE

Antihypercalcemic

(gal′ee-yum ni′trat)

Ganite

pH 6 to 7

USUAL DOSE

Adequate hydration and specific testing required; see Monitor.

200 mg/M^2 daily for 5 consecutive days. Must be administered as an IV infusion. Discontinue treatment at any time the serum calcium levels are lowered into the normal range (8.5 to 10.5 mg/100 ml, corrected for serum albumin). Safety and effectiveness of retreatment not established. See Precautions.

DOSE ADJUSTMENTS

Consider reduction to 100 mg/M^2/day for 5 days in patients with mild hypercalcemia (12 mg/100 ml range corrected for serum albumin) and few symptoms. ■ Reduced dose may be required in impaired renal function based on CrCl (2 to 2.5 mg/100 ml). See Contraindications.

DILUTION

A single daily dose must be diluted in 1,000 ml NS (preferred) or D5W. Less diluent may be used if absolutely necessary in patients with compromised cardiovascular status.

Storage: Store at CRT before dilution. Stable after dilution for 48 hours at CRT and for 7 days if refrigerated.

COMPATIBILITY

Specific information not available. Consider specific use and controlled rate of infusion; consult pharmacist.

RATE OF ADMINISTRATION

A single daily dose equally distributed over 24 hours as an IV infusion. Use of a microdrip (60 gtt/ml) or an infusion pump recommended for even distribution. Too-rapid injection may lead to overdose.

ACTIONS

A hypocalcemic agent that inhibits calcium resorption from bone. Thought to act by reducing increased bone turnover. Does not have cytotoxic effects on bone cells. Plasma levels achieve a steady state 24 to 48 hours after infusion initiated. In one study it normalized serum calcium in 75% of patients who began treatment with a serum calcium corrected for albumin greater than 12 mg/100 ml. Maintains duration of normocalcemia/hypocalcemia longer than calcitonin. Route of metabolism is unknown. Significant excretion occurs through the kidneys.

INDICATIONS AND USES

Treatment of clearly symptomatic cancer-related hypercalcemia that has not responded to adequate hydration. Serum calcium above 12 mg/100 ml corrected for serum albumin. Symptoms may include anorexia, cardiac arrest, coma, confusion, constipation, dehydration, depression, fatigue, muscle weakness, nausea and vomiting.

CONTRAINDICATIONS

Severe renal impairment (SrCr greater than 2.5 mg/100 ml).

PRECAUTIONS

In patients with cancer-related hypercalcemia, the risk of developing severe renal insufficiency is increased with concurrent use of other potentially nephrotoxic drugs (e.g., aminoglycosides [e.g., gentamicin], amphotericin B). If use of these drugs is necessary, discontinue gallium nitrate. Continue hydration for several days after administration of nephrotoxic drugs and closely monitor serum creatinine and urine output during and after their administration. ■ Calcium is bound to serum protein; concentration fluctuates with changes in blood volume. Changes in serum calcium (especially during rehydration) may not reflect true plasma levels. All calcium measurement should be corrected for albumin to establish a basis for treatment and evaluation of treatment. ■ Mild or asymptomatic hypercalcemia will be treated with conservative measures (e.g., saline hydration, with or without diuretics). Consider patient's cardiovascular status. Corticosteroids may be indicated if the underlying cancer is sensitive (e.g., hematologic cancers).

Monitor: Baseline measurements of serum calcium corrected for serum albumin, serum phosphorus, electrolytes, plasma pH, SrCr, and BUN are required. Monitor calcium daily, phosphorus twice weekly, and electrolytes, plasma pH, creatinine, and BUN closely as indicated by baseline results (may be daily). ■ Patients with cancer-related hypercalcemia are frequently dehydrated. Must be adequately hydrated orally and/or intravenously before treatment is initiated. Hydration with saline is preferred to facilitate renal excretion of calcium and correct dehydration. A pretreatment urine output of 2 L/day is recommended. ■ Avoid overhydration in patients with compromised cardiovascular status. Observe frequently for signs of fluid overload. Correct hypovolemia before using diuretics. ■ Maintain adequate hydration and urine output throughout treatment. ■ See Precautions.

Patient Education: Regular visits and assessments of lab tests imperative. ■ Restriction of dietary calcium and vitamin D may be required. ■ Take only prescribed medications. ■ Report abdominal cramps, chills, confusion, fever, muscle spasms, sore throat, and/or any new medical problem promptly.

Maternal/Child: Category C: use in pregnancy has not been studied; use only if clearly needed. ■ Discontinue nursing or do not use gallium nitrate. Consider importance of drug to mother. ■ Safety for use in children not established.

DRUG/LAB INTERACTIONS

Nephrotoxicity may be increased with other nephrotoxic drugs (e.g., aminoglycosides [gentamicin], amphotericin B [Fungizone], Edecrin); see Precautions.

SIDE EFFECTS

Acute renal failure, anemia, asymptomatic decrease in BP, fluid overload, hearing loss, optic neuritis (acute), respiratory alkalosis, tinnitus. Many other side effects, possibly from underlying disease, have occurred in less than 1% of patients.

Overdose: Acute renal failure, anemia, hypocalcemia, hypophosphatemia, nausea, vomiting.

ANTIDOTE

Discontinue drug if CrCl reaches 2.5 mg/100 ml at any time during treatment or if concurrent use of nephrotoxic drugs is indicated. Discontinue drug for any symptoms of overdose. Monitor serum calcium; use vigorous IV hydration, with or without diuretics, for 2 to 3 days. Monitor intake and output to ensure adequacy and balance. For asymptomatic or mild to moderate hypocalcemia (6.5 to 8 mg/100 ml corrected for serum albumin), short-term calcium therapy may be indicated. Oral phosphorus may be required for hypophosphatemia. RBC transfusions may be required in anemia. Keep physician informed. Some side effects may respond to symptomatic treatment. Treat anaphylaxis and resuscitate as indicated.

GANCICLOVIR SODIUM

Antiviral

(gan-sy′clo-ver so′de-um)

Cytovene IV, DHPG

pH 9 to 11

USUAL DOSE

Adequate hydration and specific testing required; see Monitor.

CMV retinitis in adults and children over 3 months: 5 mg/kg of body weight every 12 hours or 2 to 5 mg/kg every 8 hours for 14 to 21 days (has been continued for longer periods). Begin a maintenance dose the next day (day 15 to 22) of 5 mg/kg daily for 7 days each week or 6 mg/kg daily for 5 days each week. See Precautions/Monitor. After IV induction and when retinitis is stable, Cytovene capsules may be used for maintenance therapy; see Precautions. If retinitis progresses during the maintenance regimen, initiate the twice-daily program again. During studies, high-dose induction (unlabeled) of 7.5 mg/kg every 12 hours for 2 weeks was used for reinduction therapy failures. Follow with a maintenance dose of 10 mg daily. A switch to foscarnet was indicated if 2 consecutive relapses occurred in a 10-week period. Treatment continues as long as the patient is immunocompromised, perhaps months or years. Do not exceed recommended dosage or frequency.

CMV retinitis combination therapy (ganciclovir and foscarnet) for patients who have relapsed after induction and reinduction monotherapy with either drug (unlabeled): In patients who have received ganciclovir induction with 5 mg/kg every 12 hours followed by 5 mg/kg/day maintenance, continue their present therapy (e.g., ganciclovir 5 mg/kg/day) and begin foscarnet induction with 90 mg/kg every 12 hours for 14 to 21 days, followed immediately by maintenance doses of ganciclovir 5 mg/kg/day and foscarnet 90 mg/kg/day (see foscarnet monograph). Monitor renal function very closely with this combination regimen. Information on this combination regimen is available from Roche.

Prevention of CMV disease in transplant recipients: 5 mg/kg every 12 hours for 7 to 14 days. Use recommended for 14 days after heart, liver, lung, and pancreas transplants. Follow with maintenance regimen as outlined in CMV retinitis. Length of treatment based on immunosuppression degree and duration; 3 to 4 months or longer is common. CMV disease may occur if treatment stopped prematurely.

PEDIATRIC DOSE

Safety for use in children not established; see Maternal/Child.

7.5 to 10 mg/kg of body weight equally divided and given every 8 or 12 hours for induction has been used, followed by maintenance doses of 2.5 to 5 mg/kg/day.

DOSE ADJUSTMENTS

Dose selection should be cautious in the elderly. Reduced doses may be indicated based on the potential for decreased organ function and concomitant disease or drug therapy. Assess renal function before administration to elderly patients and adjust dose appropriately; see Elderly. ■ Withhold dose if absolute neutrophil count (ANC) less than 500 cells/mm^3 or platelets less than 25,000 cells/mm^3. ■ See Drug/Lab Interactions. ■

With impaired renal function, reduce dose according to the following chart.

Ganciclovir Induction and Maintenance Dose Guidelines in Impaired Renal Function				
Creatinine Clearance (ml/min)	Ganciclovir IV Induction Dose (mg/kg)	Dosing Interval (hours)	Ganciclovir Maintenance Dose (mg/kg)	Dosing Interval (hours)
≥70	5	12	5	24
50-69	2.5	12	2.5	24
25-49	2.5	24	1.25	24
10-24	1.25	24	0.625	24
<10	1.25	3 times per week following hemodialysis	0.625	3 times per week following hemodialysis

DILUTION

Specific techniques required; see Precautions. Initially dissolve the 500-mg vial with 10 ml SW (50 mg/ml). Do not use bacteriostatic water containing parabens; will cause precipitation. Shake well to dissolve completely. Discard if particulate matter or discoloration observed. Withdraw desired dose and further dilute with NS, D5W, Ringer's, or LR to provide a concentration less than 10 mg/ml (70-kg adult at 5 mg/kg equals 350 mg; dissolved in 100 ml of solution equals 3.5 mg/ml).

Storage: Use reconstituted solution within 12 hours. Do not refrigerate. Solution fully diluted for administration must be refrigerated and used within 24 hours to reduce incidence of bacterial contamination.

INCOMPATIBLE WITH

Because of physical incompatibilities, ganciclovir sodium and ***foscarnet sodium*** must never be mixed.

COMPATIBLE WITH

(Underline Indicates Conflicting Compatibility Information)

Consult pharmacist; specific conditions may apply; see Compatibilities, p. xvi.

Y-site: Allopurinol (Zyloprim), amphotericin B cholesteryl (Amphotec), cisatracurium (Nimbex), cisplatin (Platinol), cyclophosphamide (Cytoxan), docetaxel (Taxotere), doxorubicin liposome (Doxil), enalaprilat (Vasotec IV), etoposide phosphate (Etopophos), filgrastim (Neupogen), fluconazole (Diflucan), gatifloxacin (Tequin), granisetron (Kytril), linezolid (Zyvox), melphalan (Alkeran), methotrexate (Folex), paclitaxel (Taxol), propofol (Diprivan), remifentanil (Ultiva), tacrolimus (Prograf), teniposide (Vumon), thiotepa (Thioplex).

RATE OF ADMINISTRATION

A single dose must be administered at a constant rate over 1 hour as an infusion. Use of an infusion pump or microdrip (60 gtt/ml) recommended. ***Do not give by rapid or bolus IV injection.*** Excessive plasma levels and toxicity will occur with too-rapid rate of injection. Advisable to clear tubing with NS before and after administration through Y-tube or three-way stopcock.

ACTIONS

An antiviral agent that inhibits DNA synthesis and stops cytomegalovirus (CMV) from multiplying. Does not destroy existing viruses but stops them from reproducing and invading healthy cells. May allow a weakened immune system to defend the body against the CMV infection. May also be inhibitory against herpes simplex virus 1 and 2, Epstein-Barr virus, and varicella zoster virus, but clinical studies have not been done. Onset of action is prompt, and therapeutic levels are maintained for 3 to 6 hours with some drug remaining 11 hours after infusion. Widely distributed in tissues and body fluids. Half-life is 2.5 to 3.6 hours. Probably crosses the placental barrier. Suspected to be secreted in breast milk. Over 90% excreted unchanged in urine by glomerular filtration in patients with normal renal function.

INDICATIONS AND USES

Treatment of CMV retinitis in immunocompromised individuals, including patients with AIDS. ▪ Combination therapy (ganciclovir and foscarnet) may be indicated with progressive retinitis refractory to single therapy. ▪ CMV disease prevention in at-risk transplant patients. ▪ Now available as an ophthalmic surgical aid (intravitreal implant) to treat CMV retinitis. ▪ Capsules are used for prevention of CMV retinitis in at-risk patients with advanced HIV infection and in the prevention of CMV disease in solid-organ transplant recipients; see Precautions. Valganciclovir (Valcyte) is an oral drug recently approved for the treatment of CMV retinitis, and it is also being used for maintenance.

Unlabeled uses: Treatment of other CMV infections (e.g., gastroenteritis, hepatitis, pneumonitis) in immunocompromised patients. ▪ Treatment of polyradiculopathy caused by CMV infections.

CONTRAINDICATIONS

Hypersensitivity to ganciclovir or acyclovir; patients with a neutrophil count less than 500 cells/mm^3 or a platelet count less than 25,000 cells/mm^3; patients receiving zidovudine (Retrovir), since both drugs cause granulocytopenia.

PRECAUTIONS

A nucleoside analog; follow guidelines for handling and disposal of cytotoxic agents. See Appendix A, p. 1142. ▪ For IV use only; IM or SC administration will cause severe tissue irritation. ▪ Hematologic toxicity (anemia, granulocytopenia, thrombocytopenia) common; see Monitor. ▪ Use with caution in patients with pre-existing cytopenias or a history of cytopenic reactions to other drugs, chemicals, or irradiation. ▪ Resistance has been reported to develop. May be higher in patients treated for a prolonged period. ▪ Cidofovir is also an agent for treatment of CMV retinitis. ▪ Risk of a more rapid rate of disease progression is increased with oral ganciclovir. Use in maintenance recommended only if benefits of avoiding daily IV infusions outweigh risk.

Monitor: Confirm diagnosis of CMV retinitis by indirect ophthalmoscopy. Diagnosis may be supported by cultures of CMV from urine, blood, throat, etc.; negative culture does not rule out CMV retinitis. ▪ CBC with differential and platelet counts, SrCr, and CrCl are required before treatment initiated. Monitor neutrophil and platelet counts every 2 days during twice-daily dosing and weekly thereafter. Monitor daily in patients with previous leukopenia from nucleoside analogs or those with neutrophils less than 1,000 cells/mm^3 at beginning of treatment. Withhold dose if absolute neutrophil count (ANC) less than 500 cells/mm^3 or platelets less than 25,000 cells/mm^3. Monitor SrCr or CrCl every 2 weeks. ▪ Maintain adequate hydration and urine flow before and during infusion. ▪ Phlebitis or pain may occur at site of infusion; confirm patency of vein and use small needles and large veins to ensure adequate blood flow for rapid dilution and distribution. ■ Consider the possibility of viral resistance if retinitis does not show significant improvement with treatment. ■ See Drug/Lab Interactions.

Patient Education: Must use effective birth control throughout treatment. Men should continue barrier contraception for at least 90 days. ■ Not a cure; retinitis may still progress. Frequent ophthalmoscopic examinations important. ■ Cooperation for close monitoring of blood cell counts is imperative to control side effects. ■ Patients with AIDS receiving zidovudine (Retrovir) may not tolerate ganciclovir. ■ High frequency of impaired renal function increased with concomitant use of nephrotoxic agents (e.g., cyclosporine, amphotericin); high risk for transplant recipients.

Maternal/Child: Category C: avoid pregnancy. A potential carcinogen. Teratogenic and embryotoxic; will cause birth defects. Do not use during pregnancy unless risk is justified. May cause temporary or permanent infertility in men and women. ■ Discontinue nursing during treatment; do not resume until at least 72 hours after final dose of ganciclovir. ■ Use extreme caution in children under 12 years of age. Long-term carcinogenicity and reproductive toxicity are probable.

Elderly: Dose selection should be cautious; see Dose Adjustments. Monitor renal function during therapy and adjust dose as indicated.

DRUG/LAB INTERACTIONS

Because of physical incompatibilities, ganciclovir and foscarnet must never be mixed. ■ Additive toxicity may occur with concomitant use of other drugs that inhibit replication of rapidly dividing cell populations (e.g., dapsone, pentamidine, flucytosine [Ancobon], vincristine [Oncovin], vinblastine [Velban], doxorubicin [Adriamycin], amphotericin B [Fungizone], trimethoprim/sulfamethoxazole [Bactrim]). ■ May cause severe granulocytopenia with zidovudine (Retrovir). Combination used in patients with AIDS is rarely tolerated. ■ Concurrent treatment with didanosine (Videx) may cause increased didanosine levels. ■ May cause seizures with imipenem-cilastatin (Primaxin). ■ Potentiated by probenecid and other drugs that may reduce renal clearance; will increase toxicity. ■ Impaired renal function may be markedly increased with other nephrotoxic agents (e.g., cyclosporine, amphotericin B). ■ Concurrent or consecutive use with other bone marrow depressants (e.g., antineoplastics, amphotericin B, zidovudine and/or radiation therapy) may produce additive bone marrow depression. ■ See Contraindications.

SIDE EFFECTS

Granulocytopenia and thrombocytopenia are the most common and are generally reversible if treatment discontinued. Anemia, fever, infection, pain at injection site, phlebitis, rash, and abnormal liver function tests occur in some patients. Fewer than 1% of patients experienced abdominal pain, alopecia, ataxia, chills, coma, confusion, day dreaming, diarrhea, dizziness, dreams, dyspnea, dysrhythmias, edema, eosinophilia, headache, hematuria, hemorrhage, hypersensitivity reactions, hypertension, hypoglycemia, hypotension, increased BUN and CrCl, malaise, nausea, nervousness, paresthesia, pruritus, psychosis, retinal detachment, somnolence, tremor, and urticaria.

Overdose: Anorexia, bloody diarrhea, cytopenia, hypersalivation, increased BUN and liver function tests, testicular atrophy, vomiting, death.

ANTIDOTE

Notify physician of all side effects; most will be treated symptomatically. Filgrastim (Neupogen) 1 to 10 mcg/kg/day has been used to maintain the neutrophil count. Discontinue drug if neutrophils fall below 500 cells/mm^3 or platelets fall below 25,000 cells/mm^3. Hydration and hemodialysis (up to 50% removal) are useful in overdose. Treat anaphylaxis and resuscitate as necessary.

GATIFLOXACIN

(gah-tee-floks'a-sin)

Tequin

Antibacterial (fluoroquinolone)

pH 3.5 to 5.5

USUAL DOSE

200 to 400 mg once every 24 hours. Dose and duration of therapy are based on diagnosis as listed in the following chart. Dose and serum levels similar by oral or IV route. No dose adjustment necessary. Transfer to oral therapy as soon as practical.

Dosage Guidelines for Gatifloxacin

Infection*	Daily Dose†	Duration
Acute bacterial exacerbation of chronic bronchitis	400 mg	5 days
Acute sinusitis	400 mg	10 days
Community–acquired pneumonia	400 mg	7-14 days
Uncomplicated skin and skin structure	400 mg	7-10 days
Uncomplicated urinary tract infections (cystitis)	400 mg or 200 mg	Single dose 3 days
Complicated urinary tract infections	400 mg	7-10 days
Acute pyelonephritis	400 mg	7-10 days
Uncomplicated urethral gonorrhea in men; endocervical and rectal gonorrhea in women	400 mg	Single dose

*Due to the designated pathogens.
†For either the oral or intravenous routes of administration.

DOSE ADJUSTMENTS

No dose adjustment required in impaired hepatic function. Clearance is decreased in patients with impaired renal function. Dose reduction is recommended as outlined in the following chart.

Recommended Dosage of Gatifloxacin in Adult Patients with Renal Impairment		
Creatinine Clearance	**Initial Dose**	**Subsequent Dose***
≥40 ml/min	400 mg	400 mg every day
<40 ml/min	400 mg	200 mg every day
Hemodialysis	400 mg	200 mg every day
Continuous peritoneal dialysis	400 mg	200 mg every day

*Start subsequent dose on Day 2 of dosing.

Give dose after dialysis session in patients receiving hemodialysis. Dose reduction is not required in patients with impaired renal function who are receiving the 400-mg single dose used for treatment of uncomplicated urinary tract infections and gonorrhea or in patients receiving the three-day 200-mg dose used for treatment of uncomplicated urinary tract infections.

DILUTION

Available in 200 mg/20 ml or 400 mg/40 ml single-use vials and as prediluted ready-to-use infusions.

Single-use vials: Must be further diluted to a final concentration of 2 mg/ml with D5W, NS, D5NS, D5LR, 5% sodium bicarbonate, D5 Plasma-Lyte 56, sodium lactate ⅙ M, or D5/½NS with KCl 20 mEq/L (e.g., add 200 mg to 100 ml or 400 mg to 200 ml of one of solutions listed above). No preservatives; enter vial only once. Do not use SW; results in a hypotonic solution.

Premix flexible containers: No further dilution necessary. Available as 200 mg in 100 ml or 400 mg in 200 ml D5W. Instructions for access to and use of premix flexible containers are available from manufacturer. Do not use flexible containers in series connections.

Storage: Store vials and premix bags at CRT. Do not freeze premix bags. Solutions prepared from vials are stable for 14 days at CRT or refrigerated. When diluted to 2 mg/ml with a compatible IV solution except for 5% sodium bicarbonate, may be stored for up to 6 months at –25° to 10° C. Frozen solutions may be thawed at CRT. Solutions that have been thawed are stable for 14 days after removal from the freezer when stored at CRT or in the refrigerator. Discard any unused portion of premixed solutions or opened vials.

INCOMPATIBLE WITH

Manufacturer states, "Limited compatibility information available; other intravenous substances, additives, or other medications should not be added to gatifloxacin or infused simultaneously through the same intravenous line." Flush line with a compatible solution before and after administration of gatifloxacin and/or any other drug through the same IV line.

COMPATIBLE WITH

See Incompatible With. Consult pharmacist; specific conditions may apply; see Compatibilities, p. xvi.

Additive: Manufacturer states, "2 mg/ml concentration compatible with 20 mEq/L KCl in D5/½NS."

Y-site: Acyclovir (Zovirax), alfentanil (Alfenta), amikacin (Amikin), aminophylline, ampicillin, ampicillin/sulbactam (Unasyn), aztreonam (Azactam), bretylium (Bretylate), buprenorphine (Buprenex), butorphanol (Stadol), calcium chloride, calcium gluconate, carboplatin (Paraplatin), cefazolin (Kefzol), cefotetan (Cefotan), ceftazidime (Fortaz), ceftizoxime (Cefizox), ceftriaxone (Rocephin), chlorpromazine (Thorazine), cimetidine (Tagamet), cisatracurium (Nimbex), cisplatin (Platinol), clindamycin (Cleocin), cyclophosphamide (Cytoxan), cyclosporine (Sandimmune), cytarabine (ARA-C), dexamethasone (Decadron), digoxin (Lanoxin), diphenhydramine (Benadryl), dobutamine (Dobutrex), dopamine (Intropin), doxorubicin (Adriamycin), droperidol (Inapsine), enalaprilat (Vasotec IV), esmolol (Brevibloc), etoposide phosphate (Etopophos), famotidine (Pepcid IV), fentanyl (Sublimaze), fluconazole (Diflucan), fluorouracil (5-FU), ganciclovir (Cytovene), gemcitabine (Gemzar), gentamicin (Garamycin), granisetron (Kytril), haloperidol (Haldol), hydrocortisone sodium succinate (Solu-Cortef), hydromorphone (Dilaudid), ifosfamide (Ifex), imipenem-cilastatin (Primaxin), labetalol (Normodyne), leucovorin calcium, lidocaine, lorazepam (Ativan), magnesium sulfate, mannitol, meperidine (Demerol), mesna (Mesnex), methotrexate (Folex), methylprednisolone (Solu-Medrol), metoclopramide (Reglan), metronidazole (Flagyl IV), midazolam (Versed), mitoxantrone (Novantrone), morphine, nalbuphine (Nubain), naloxone (Narcan), nicardipine (Cardene IV), nitroglycerin (Nitro-Bid IV), ondansetron (Zofran), paclitaxel (Taxol), pentamidine, pentobarbital (Nembutal), phenobarbital (Luminal), potassium chloride (KCl), prochlorperazine (Compazine), promethazine (Phenergan), propranolol (Inderal), ranitidine (Zantac), remifentanil (Ultiva), sodium bicarbonate, sodium phosphates, sufentanil (Sufenta), sulfamethoxazole-trimethoprim (Bactrim), theophylline, ticarcillin (Ticar), ticarcillin/clavulanate (Timentin), tobramycin (Nebcin), vecuronium (Norcuron), verapamil (Isoptin), vinblastine (Velban), vincristine (Oncovin), vinorelbine (Navelbine), zidovudine (AZT, Retrovir).

RATE OF ADMINISTRATION

Rapid or bolus intravenous infusion should be avoided. Flush tubing before and after gatifloxacin with a compatible solution. See Precautions. A single dose equally distributed over 60 minutes as an infusion.

ACTIONS

A broad-spectrum methoxyfluoroquinolone antibacterial agent. Active against a wide range of microorganisms including aerobic gram-negative, aerobic gram-positive, and atypical microorganisms (see literature). Inhibits two essential enzymes involved in the replication, transcription, and repair of bacterial DNA. Mechanism of action differs from that of penicillins, cephalosporins, macrolides, aminoglycosides, and tetracyclines. Because of this, may be active against pathogens that are resistant to these antibiotics. There is no cross-resistance between gatifloxacin and the aforementioned antibiotics. Widely distributed throughout the body into many body tissues and fluids. Concentrations in most target tissues are higher than those found in serum. Undergoes limited biotransformation. Undergoes both glomerular filtration and tubular secretion. Excreted as unchanged drug primarily by the kidney. Approximately 5% excreted in feces as unchanged drug. Elimination half-life is 7 to 14 hours.

INDICATIONS AND USES

Treatment of adults with infections caused by susceptible strains of microorganisms in conditions including acute bacterial exacerbation of chronic bronchitis, acute sinusitis, community-acquired pneumonia, uncomplicated skin and skin structure infections, uncomplicated urinary tract infections (cystitis), complicated urinary tract infections, pyelonephritis, uncomplicated urethral and cervical gonorrhea, and acute, uncomplicated rectal infections in women.

Unlabeled uses: Given orally to treat atypical pneumonia, uncomplicated skin and soft tissue infections, and chronic prostatitis.

CONTRAINDICATIONS

History of hypersensitivity to gatifloxacin or any member of the quinolone class of antibiotics (e.g., alatrofloxacin [Trovan], ciprofloxacin [Cipro], levofloxacin [Levaquin], norfloxacin [Noroxin], ofloxacin [Floxin IV]).

PRECAUTIONS

For IV use only. ■ Culture and sensitivity studies indicated to determine susceptibility of the causative organism to gatifloxacin. ■ Cross-resistance has been observed between gatifloxacin and other fluoroquinolones, but some microorganisms resistant to other fluoroquinolones may be susceptible to gatifloxacin. ■ Has the potential to prolong the QTc interval of the electrocardiogram in some patients, increasing the risk for ventricular arrhythmias. Avoid in patients with known prolongation of the QTc interval, patients with uncorrected hypokalemia, and patients receiving class IA (e.g., quinidine [Quinidex], procainamide [Procanbid, Procan SR]) and Class III (amiodarone [Cordarone], sotalol [Betapace]) antiarrhythmic agents. ■ Use with caution in patients receiving drugs that prolong the QTc interval (e.g., antipsychotics, cisapride [Propulsid], erythromycin, and tricyclic antidepressants or in patients with ongoing proarrhythmic conditions (e.g., bradycardia or acute myocardial ischemia). The magnitude of the QTc prolongation increases with increasing concentrations of the drug. Do not exceed recommended dose or rate of infusion. ■ Use with caution in patients with known or suspected CNS disorders, such as severe cerebral atherosclerosis, epilepsy, or other factors that may predispose to seizures. Convulsions, increased intracranial pressure, psychosis, and CNS stimulation have been reported; see Side Effects. ■ Use with caution in patients with impaired renal function; see Dose Adjustments. ■ Ruptures of the shoulder, hand, and Achilles tendons that required surgical repair or resulted in prolonged disability have been reported in patients receiving quinolones. May occur during or after completion of therapy. ■ Pseudomembranous colitis has been reported and may range in severity from mild to life-threatening. Consider this diagnosis in patients that present with diarrhea during or after treatment with gatifloxacin. ■ Gatifloxacin has not been shown to be effective in treatment of syphilis. When used for the treatment of gonorrhea, it may mask or delay the symptoms of incubating syphilis. Patients being treated for gonorrhea should have a serologic test for syphilis.

Monitor: Serious and occasionally fatal hypersensitivity reactions have been reported in patients receiving quinolone therapy. May be seen with first or subsequent doses. Emergency equipment must be readily available; see Side Effects. ■ Obtain baseline and periodic CBC with differential and SrCr. ■ Disturbances in blood glucose, including symptomatic hyperglycemia and hypoglycemia have been reported, usually in diabetic patients or in patients at risk for hyperglycemia. Hypoglycemic episodes, in some cases severe, have been reported in diabetic patients being treated with either sulfonylurea or non-sulfonylurea oral hypoglycemic medications. Episodes usually occur within the first 3 days of treatment but may occur from the fourth to the tenth day of treatment. Monitor blood glucose carefully; see Side Effects and Antidote. ■ Maintain adequate hydration to prevent concentrated urine throughout treatment. Other quinolones have formed crystals. ■ See Drug/Lab Interactions and Antidote.

Patient Education: Drink fluids liberally. ■ Report skin rash or any other hypersensitivity reaction promptly. Report fainting spells or palpitations promptly. ■ Photosensitivity has occurred in patients receiving other quinolones. It is best to avoid excessive sunlight or artificial ultraviolet light. May cause severe sunburn. Use sunscreen and wear dark glasses outdoors. ■ Dizziness or lightheadedness may interfere with ambulation or motor coordination. Use caution in tasks that require alertness. ■ Report tendon pain or inflammation promptly. ■ May produce changes in ECG. ■ Review medicines and disease states with physician or pharmacist before initiating therapy. ■ Monitor blood glucose carefully if diabetic. ■ See Precautions, Monitor, Drug/Lab Interactions, Side Effects, and Antidote.

Maternal/Child: Category C: safety for use in pregnancy and breast-feeding not established. Benefit must outweigh risk to fetus or breast-feeding infant. ■ Safety for use in children and adolescents under 18 years of age not established. Quinolones have caused arthropathy and osteochondrotoxicity in juvenile animals.

Elderly: No overall differences in safety or effectiveness observed. May be at increased risk of toxicity (e.g., QTc prolongation, disturbance in glucose homeostasis) due to potential for decreased organ function, concomitant disease, or drug therapy. ■ Consider age-related renal impairment; monitoring of renal function suggested. See Dose Adjustments.

DRUG/LAB INTERACTIONS

May increase digoxin serum concentrations. Monitor patients for signs and symptoms of digoxin toxicity. ■ Probenecid and cimetidine (Tagamet) decrease clearance and increase gatifloxacin serum concentrations. ■ Effects of warfarin may be enhanced by some quinolones. Although this has not been reported with gatifloxacin, PT or INR should be monitored closely if gatifloxacin is administered with warfarin or one of its derivatives. ■ Concomitant administration of an NSAID (e.g., ibuprofen [Advil, Motrin], naproxen [Aleve, Naprosyn]) and a quinolone may increase the risks of CNS stimulation and convulsions (has not been documented with gatifloxacin to date). ■ Potential for pharmacodynamic interaction between Class IA (e.g., quinidine [Quinidex], procainamide [Procanbid, Procan SR]) and Class III (e.g., amiodarone [Cordarone], sotalol [Betapace]) antiarrhythmic agents. Avoid coadministration. See Precautions. ■ May cause a false-positive when testing for opiates.

SIDE EFFECTS

Most commonly reported side effects were diarrhea (4%), dizziness (3%), headache (3%), injection site reaction (5%), nausea (8%), and vaginitis (8%). Less frequently reported side effects included abdominal pain, abnormal vision, abnormal dreams, allergic reactions, back pain, chest pain, chills, constipation, dyspepsia, dyspnea, dysuria, fever, glossitis, hematuria, insomnia, mouth ulcer, oral moniliasis, palpitation, paresthesia, peripheral edema, pharyngitis, rash, stomatitis, sweating, taste perversion, thrombocytopenia, tinnitus, tremor, vasodilatation, vertigo, and vomiting. Many other rare side effects listed; see literature. Laboratory abnormalities that may have been caused by gatifloxacin and/or the underlying condition being treated included electrolyte abnormalities; increased ALT or AST levels; increased alkaline phosphatase, bilirubin, serum amylase; increased INR/PT levels; and neutropenia.

Major: Allergic reactions (may include or be accompanied by airway obstruction [including bronchospasm, shortness of breath, and acute respiratory distress], anaphylaxis, angioedema [including tongue, laryngeal, throat, or facial edema/swelling], cardiovascular collapse, dyspnea, hypotension/shock, itching, loss of consciousness, seizure, serious skin reactions, tingling, and urticaria); CNS stimulation (e.g., agitation, anxiety, convulsions, depression, hallucinations, insomnia, lightheadedness, nervousness, nightmares, paranoia, or restlessness); hepatitis; hyperglycemia (severe, including hyperosmolar nonketotic hyperglycemia); hypoglycemia (severe); increased intracranial pressure; prolongation of the QTc interval of the electrocardiogram; pseudomembranous colitis; psychosis; rupture of the shoulder, hand, or Achilles tendons; and torsades de pointes.

Overdose: Convulsions, decreased activity and respiratory rate, tremors, and vomiting.

ANTIDOTE

Keep physician informed of all side effects. Most minor side effects will be treated symptomatically; monitor closely. Discontinue gatifloxacin at the first sign of any major side effect (e.g., hypersensitivity, CNS symptoms, dermatologic reaction, symptomatic hyperglycemia or hypoglycemia, tendon rupture) or phototoxicity. Treat allergic reaction as indicated with epinephrine, airway management, oxygen, IV fluids, antihistamines (e.g., diphenhydramine [Benadryl]), corticosteroids (e.g., hydrocortisone [Solu-Cortef]), and pressor amines (e.g., dopamine [Intropin]). Treat CNS symptoms as indicated; may require diazepam (Valium) for seizures. Mild cases of colitis may respond to discontinuation of gatifloxacin. Oral vancomycin (Vancocin) or metronidazole (Flagyl) is treatment of choice for antibiotic-related pseudomembranous colitis. Adequate hydration and supplementation of electrolytes and proteins may be required. Complete rest is indicated for an affected tendon until definitive diagnosis and treatment are available. Maintain hydration in overdose. There is no specific antidote. Monitor patient closely (including ECG monitoring) and provide symptomatic and supportive care as indicated. Not removed by hemodialysis or peritoneal dialysis. Resuscitate as necessary.

GEMCITABINE HYDROCHLORIDE

(gem-sit'a-been hi-droe-klor'id)

Antineoplastic (miscellaneous)

Gemzar

pH 2.7 to 3.3

USUAL DOSE

Pancreatic cancer: 1,000 mg/M^2 once each week for up to 7 weeks (or until toxicity necessitates reducing or holding a dose). Follow with a week of rest. In subsequent cycles, 1,000 mg/M^2 or appropriate reduced or increased dose once each week for 3 consecutive weeks. Follow with a week of rest.

Non–small-cell lung cancer: 1,000 mg/M^2 as an infusion on days 1, 8, and 15 of each 28-day cycle. Given in combination with cisplatin (Platinol). Administer cisplatin 100 mg/M^2 IV on day 1 after the infusion of gemcitabine. An alternate schedule is gemcitabine 1,250 mg/M^2 on days 1 and 8 of each 21-day cycle. Administer cisplatin 100 mg/M^2 IV on day 1 after the infusion of gemcitabine. See cisplatin monograph for administration and hydration guidelines.

Bladder cancer (unlabeled): 1,000 to 1,200 mg/M^2 once each week for 3 weeks. Follow with a week of rest.

Breast cancer (unlabeled): 600 mg/M^2 once each week. Given in combination with cisplatin. An alternate regimen is 800 to 1,250 mg/M^2 as a single agent once each week. With either dose regimen, repeat for 2 or 3 weeks. Follow with a 1-week rest period.

Epithelial ovarian cancer (unlabeled): 800 to 1,250 mg/M^2 as a single agent once each week for 2 to 3 weeks. Follow with a 1-week rest period.

Hodgkin's or non-Hodgkin's lymphoma (unlabeled): 1,000 to 1,250 mg/M^2 on days 1, 8, and 15 of a 28-day cycle. Doses up to 1,500 mg/M^2 have been used.

DOSE ADJUSTMENTS

In all situations, reduce dose based on the degree of hematologic toxicity. See chart below:

Gemcitabine Dosage Reduction Guidelines			
Absolute Granulocyte Count		**Platelet Count**	**% of Full Dose**
≥1,000/mm^3	and	≥100,000/mm^3	100
500-999/mm^3	or	50,000-99,000/mm^3	75
<500/mm^3	or	<50,000/mm^3	Hold

Dose may be increased by 25% (to 1,250 mg/M^2) in patients who complete an entire 7-week initial cycle or a subsequent 3-week cycle at a dose of 1,000 mg/M^2. Absolute granulocyte count nadir must exceed 1,500/mm^3 and platelet nadir must exceed 100,000/mm^3. Nonhematologic toxicity should not be greater than WHO Grade 1 (some examples are: able to eat, reasonable intake, no more than one emesis in 24 hours, asymptomatic heart and lungs, mild paresthesia). If this cycle is tolerated, dose for the next cycle may be increased to 1,500 mg/M^2 providing the same criteria have been met (e.g., granulocyte nadir, platelet nadir, nonhematologic toxicity). ■ Treatment with gemcitabine and cisplatin should be held or decreased by 50% when grade 3 or 4 non-hematologic toxicity occurs.

DILUTION

Specific techniques required; see Precautions. Each 200 mg must be reconstituted with 5 ml NS without preservatives (25 ml NS for 1 Gm). Yields 38 mg/ml. Shake to dissolve. Do not use less solution to reconstitute; dissolution will be incomplete. The appropriate dose may be given without further dilution or may be further diluted with NS to concentrations as low as 0.1 mg/ml. 1,500 mg diluted in 250 ml yields 6 mg/ml. 750 mg in 100 ml yields 7.5 mg/ml.

Storage: Store unopened vials at CRT. Reconstituted or diluted solutions are stable at CRT for 24 hours. Do not refrigerate in any form; may crystallize. Discard unused portion.

COMPATIBLE WITH

Consult pharmacist; specific conditions may apply; see Compatibilities, p. xvi.

Solution: Manufacturer states, "No incompatibilities observed with IV bottles or PVC bags and administration sets."

Y-site: Amifostine (Ethyol), amikacin (Amikin), aminophylline, ampicillin, ampicillin/sulbactam (Unasyn), aztreonam (Azactam), bleomycin (Blenoxane), bumetanide (Bumex), buprenorphine (Buprenex), butorphanol (Stadol), calcium gluconate, carboplatin (Paraplatin), carmustine (BiCNU), cefazolin (Kefzol), cefotetan (Cefotan), cefoxitin (Mefoxin), ceftazidime (Fortaz), ceftizoxime (Cefizox), ceftriaxone (Rocephin), cefuroxime (Zinacef), chlorpromazine (Thorazine), cimetidine (Tagamet), ciprofloxacin (Cipro IV), cisplatin (Platinol), clindamycin (Cleocin), cyclophosphamide (Cytoxan), cytarabine (ARA-C), dactinomycin (Cosmegen), daunorubicin (Cerubidine), dexamethasone (Decadron), dexrazoxane (Zinecard), diphenhydramine (Benadryl), dobutamine (Dobutrex), docetaxel (Taxotere), dopamine (Intropin), doxorubicin (Adriamycin), doxycycline (Vibramycin), droperidol (Inapsine), enalaprilat (Vasotec IV), etoposide (Etopophos, VePesid), famotidine (Pepcid IV), fluconazole (Diflucan), fludarabine (Fludara), fluorouracil (5-FU), gatifloxacin (Tequin), gentamicin (Garamycin), granisetron (Kytril), haloperidol (Haldol), heparin, hydrocortisone (Hydrocortone, Solu-Cortef), hydromorphone (Dilaudid), idarubicin (Idamycin), ifosfamide (Ifex), leucovorin calcium, linezolid (Zyvox), lorazepam (Ativan), mannitol, meperidine (Demerol), mesna (Mesnex), metoclopramide (Reglan), metronidazole (Flagyl IV), minocycline (Minocin), mitoxantrone (Novantrone), morphine, nalbuphine (Nubain), ofloxacin (Floxin IV), ondansetron (Zofran), paclitaxel (Taxol), plicamycin (Mithracin), potassium chloride (KCl), promethazine (Phenergan), ranitidine (Zantac), sodium bicarbonate, streptozocin (Zanosar), sulfamethoxazole-trimethoprim (Bactrim), teniposide (Vumon), thiotepa (Thioplex), ticarcillin (Ticar), ticarcillin/clavulanate (Timentin), tobramycin (Nebcin), topotecan (Hycamtin), vancomycin (Vancocin), vinblastine (Velban), vincristine (Oncovin), vinorelbine (Navelbine), zidovudine (AZT, Retrovir).

RATE OF ADMINISTRATION

A single dose as an infusion equally distributed over 30 minutes. Do not extend infusion time beyond 60 minutes; will increase toxicity.

ACTIONS

A nucleoside analog with antineoplastic activity. Metabolized intracellularly to two active nucleosides. Cell phase specific, these nucleosides induce internucleosomal DNA fragmentation, primarily killing cells undergoing DNA synthesis (S-phase) and also blocking the progression of cells through the G_1/S-phase boundary. Very little is bound to plasma protein. Volume of distribution is increased by infusion length. Half-life is shorter (32 to 94 minutes) with a short infusion (less than 70 minutes), and longer (245 to 638 minutes) with a long infusion (more than 70 minutes). Half-life is slightly longer and rate of clearance is lower in women and in the elderly, resulting in higher concentrations for any given dose. Primarily excreted in urine.

INDICATIONS AND USES

First-line treatment for patients with nonresectable or metastatic cancer of the pancreas and for patients previously treated for cancer of the pancreas with fluorouracil. ■ As a single agent or in combination with cisplatin for the palliative treatment of locally advanced or metastatic non–small-cell lung cancer.

Unlabeled uses: Treatment of metastatic bladder cancer, breast cancer, and epithelial ovarian cancer. ■ Treatment of Hodgkin's and non-Hodgkin's lymphomas.

CONTRAINDICATIONS

Hypersensitivity to gemcitabine or any of its components.

PRECAUTIONS

Follow guidelines for handling cytotoxic agents. See Appendix A, p. 1142. ■ Administered by or under the direction of the physician specialist. ■ Adequate diagnostic and treatment facilities must be available. ■ For IV use only. ■ Prolongation of the infusion time beyond 60 minutes and more frequent than weekly dosing have been shown to increase toxicity. ■ Clearance in women and the elderly is reduced; women, especially older women, were more likely not to proceed to a subsequent cycle and to experience grade 3 or 4 neutropenia and thrombocytopenia. No age or gender dose adjustments recommended. ■ Use with caution in impaired renal or hepatic function. ■ Gemcitabine is a potent radiosensitizer. Depending on the site being radiated, concurrent use with gemcitabine may cause severe, life-threatening esophagitis and pneumonitis. ■ If gemcitabine-induced pneumonitis is confirmed or suspected, discontinue permanently. ■ Use caution in patients who have had previous cytotoxic chemotherapy or radiation therapy.

Monitor: Use caution to prevent bone marrow depression; myelosuppression is the dose-limiting toxicity. See Dose Adjustments. ■ Obtain a CBC, including differential and platelet count, before each dose. ■ Obtain baseline renal function (e.g., SrCr) and liver function tests (e.g., AST [SGOT], ALT [SGPT]) and repeat periodically. ■ Monitor serum calcium, magnesium, potassium, and SrCr during combination therapy with cisplatin. ■ Monitor vital signs. ■ Maintain adequate hydration. ■ Nausea and vomiting are frequent and were severe in 15% of patients; prophylactic administration of antiemetics will increase patient comfort. ■ Observe closely for S/S of infection. May cause fever in the absence of infection or prophylactic antibiotics may be indicated pending results of C/S in a febrile or nonfebrile patient. ■ Monitor for thrombocytopenia (platelet count less than 50,000/mm^3). Initiate precautions to prevent excessive bleeding (e.g., inspect IV sites, skin, and mucous membranes; use extreme care during invasive procedures; test urine, emesis, stool, and secretions for occult blood). ■ Not a vesicant, but monitor injection site for inflammation an/or extravasation.

Patient Education: Nonhormonal birth control recommended. ■ See Appendix D, p. 1148. ■ Report any unusual or unexpected symptoms or side effects (e.g., shortness of breath, blood in stool or urine, S/S of infection, unusual bruising or bleeding) as soon as possible.

Maternal/Child: Category D: avoid pregnancy. May cause fetal harm. ■ Discontinue breast-feeding. ■ Safety and effectiveness for use in children not established.

Elderly: Clearance reduced in the elderly; hematologic toxicity requiring reduction, delay, or omission of subsequent doses is higher than in younger adults; however, incidence of nonhematologic toxicity is similar. Elderly men and women are more likely to experience grade 3 or 4 thrombocytopenia. Elderly women are also more likely to experience grade 3 or 4 neutropenia. Usual dose adjustments based on toxicity are considered appropriate. Age-related impaired renal function may further reduce clearance and increase toxicity.

DRUG/LAB INTERACTIONS

Interaction of gemcitabine with other drugs has not been adequately studied. ■ Additive bone marrow depression may occur with radiation therapy, other bone marrow–depressing agents (e.g., amphotericin B [traditional and lipid], azathioprine [Imuran], chloramphenicol, melphelan [Alkeran]), and/or immunosuppressants (e.g., chlorambucil [Leukeran], cyclophosphamide [Cytoxan], cyclosporine [Sandimmune], glucocorticoid corticosteroids [e.g., dexamethasone], muromonab-CD3 [Orthoclone], tacrolimus [Prograf]); dose reduction may be required. ■ Do not administer live vaccines to patients receiving antineoplastic agents.

SIDE EFFECTS

Alopecia, arrhythmias, bone marrow toxicity (e.g., anemia, leukopenia, neutropenia, thrombocytopenia), bronchospasm, cerebrovascular accident, constipation, diarrhea, dyspnea, edema, elevated lab tests (e.g., alkaline phosphatase, bilirubin, BUN, creatinine, hematuria, proteinuria), fever, flu syndrome (e.g., anorexia, chills, cough, headache, myalgia, weakness), hemorrhage, infection, myocardial infarction, nausea and vomiting (69%), pain, paresthesias, pruritus, pulmonary effects (including pulmonary edema, interstitial pneumonitis, ARDS), rash, somnolence, stomatitis, transient increases in AST (SGOT), ALT (SGPT). Anaphylaxis and hemolytic uremic syndrome (characterized by anemia with evidence of microangiopathic hemolysis, elevation of bilirubin or LDH, reticulocytosis, severe thrombocytopenia and/or evidence of renal failure (elevation of SrCr or BUN) have been reported.

ANTIDOTE

Keep physician informed of all side effects. Symptomatic and supportive treatment is indicated. Reduce dose or withhold gemcitabine until myelosuppression improves to specific criteria; see Dose Adjustments. If gemcitabine-induced pneumonitis or esophagitis is confirmed or suspected, discontinue permanently (in one study severe stomatitis and pharyngeal damage required patients to be fed by feeding tube for up to 12 months after receiving doses of 300 mg/M^2 [25% of the usual dose]). Anemia may require RBC transfusions. Other whole blood products (e.g., platelets, leukocytes) and/or blood modifiers (e.g., darbepoetin alfa [Aranesp], epoetin alfa [Epogen, Procrit], filgrastim [Neupogen], pegfilgrastim [Neulasta], sargramostim [Leukine], oprelvekin [Neumega]) may be indicated to treat bone marrow toxicity. Most side effects are reversible with dose reduction or temporary withholding of gemcitabine. No known antidote for overdose. If hemolytic uremic syndrome occurs, renal failure may not be reversible even with discontinuation of therapy and dialysis may be required. Treat allergic reactions with oxygen, epinephrine, corticosteroids, and antihistamines.

GEMTUZUMAB OZOGAMICIN

(gem-too′zeh-mab oh-zoh-gam′ih-sin)

Mylotarg

Antineoplastic
Monoclonal antibody

USUAL DOSE

Specific procedures may be indicated to prepare patient for therapy; see Precautions and Monitor.

Premedication: To decrease acute transfusion-related symptoms give diphenhydramine (Benadryl) 50 mg PO and acetaminophen (Tylenol) 650 to 1000 mg PO 1 hour before administration of gemtuzumab. Repeat acetaminophen dose every 4 hours for two additional doses.

CD33 positive acute myeloid leukemia: 9 mg/M^2. Repeat dose of 9 mg/M^2 in 14 days. Full recovery from hematologic toxicities is not required for administration of the second dose. 9 mg/M^2 dose expected to saturate all CD33 sites regardless of tumor burden.

PEDIATRIC DOSE

Safety and effectiveness for use in pediatric patients not established.

DOSE ADJUSTMENTS

No dose adjustments recommended. Has not been studied in patients with renal or hepatic impairment.

DILUTION

Specific techniques required; see Precautions. In addition, this product is light-sensitive and must be protected from direct and indirect sunlight and unshielded fluorescent light during preparation and administration. ***All preparation should take place in a biologic safety hood with the fluorescent light off.*** Before reconstitution, allow the vials to come to room temperature. Reconstitute each 5 mg vial with 5 ml of SW to produce a solution with a final concentration of 1 mg/ml. Gently swirl each vial. Withdraw the required volume from each vial and inject into a 100-ml bag of NS. Place finished product in UV protectant bag.

Storage: Refrigerate vials at 2° to 8° C (36° to 46° F) and protect from light. Reconstituted solution may be stored refrigerated and protected from light for up to 8 hours. Use the 100-ml infusion solution immediately after preparation.

COMPATIBILITY

Manufacturer states, "A separate IV line equipped with a low-protein terminal filter must be used for administration." Specific information not available; consult pharmacist.

RATE OF ADMINISTRATION

A single dose must be given as an infusion over 2 hours. ***Do not administer as an IV push or bolus.*** May be given through a peripheral or central line.

Administer through a separate line equipped with a low protein-binding 1.2 micron terminal filter.

ACTIONS

An antineoplastic agent and a humanized IgG_4, kappa recombinant monoclonal antibody linked to a cytotoxic antitumor antibiotic, calicheamicin. Produced by recombinant DNA technology and purified under conditions that remove or inactivate viruses. The antibody portion of the drug binds specifically to the CD33 antigen expressed on the surface of leukemic myeloblasts and immature normal cells of myelomonocytic lineage. The CD33 antigen is not expressed on normal pluripotent hematopoietic stem cells or on nonhematopoietic cells. Binding of the anti-CD33 antibody portion of gemtuzumab ozogamicin with the CD33 antigen results in formation of a complex that has been internalized. Once internalized, the calicheamicin derivative is released and binds to DNA. The end result is DNA double strand breakage and cell death. The cytotoxic effect on normal myeloid precursors leads to substantial myelosuppression, but this is reversible because pluripotent hematopoietic stem cells are spared. Elimination half-lives of total and unconjugated calicheamicin were 45 and 100 hours, respectively after the first dose. After the second dose, the half-life of total calicheamicin was increased to about 60 hours. The half-life of unconjugated calicheamicin remained the same. Crosses the placental barrier.

INDICATIONS AND USES

Treatment of patients with CD33 positive acute myeloid leukemia (AML) in first relapse who are 60 years of age or older and who are not considered candidates for other cytotoxic chemotherapy. Safety and efficacy in patients with poor performance status and organ dysfunction has not been established.

CONTRAINDICATIONS

Known hypersensitivity to gemtuzumab ozogamicin, murine derivatives, or any of its components: anti-CD33 antibody, calicheamicin derivatives, or inactive ingredients.

PRECAUTIONS

Follow guidelines for handling cytotoxic agents. See Appendix A, p. 1142. See Dilution. ■ Administered by or under the supervision of a physician experienced in the treatment of acute leukemia and in facilities equipped to monitor the patient and respond to any medical emergency. ■ Should be used only as single-agent chemotherapy. Should not be used in combination chemotherapy regimens outside clinical trials. ■ Patients with high peripheral blast counts may be at greater risk for pulmonary events and tumor lysis syndrome (TLS), physicians should consider leukoreduction with hydroxyurea or leukophoresis to reduce the peripheral white blood count to less than $30{,}000/mm^3$ before administration of gemtuzumab. Appropriate measures (e.g., hydration and allopurinol), should be taken to prevent hyperuricemia. ■ Severe myelosuppression will occur in all patients given the recommended dose of this agent. ■ Use caution in patients with hepatic impairment. Hepatotoxicity, including hepatic veno-occlusive disease (VOD), has been reported; see Elderly. Patients who receive gemtuzumab before or after hematopoietic stem-cell transplant, patients with underlying hepatic disease or abnormal liver function, and patients receiving gemtuzumab in combination with other chemotherapy may be at increased risk for severe VOD. Deaths from liver failure and VOD have been reported. ■ Use caution in patients with impaired renal function. Renal failure secondary to TLS has been reported. ■ May produce a post-infusion symptom complex of fever and chills, and less commonly hypotension and dyspnea that may occur during the first 24 hours after administration. Premedication may lessen the severity of these reactions. See Usual Dose and Monitor. ■ Can cause severe hypersensitivity reactions, including anaphylaxis and severe pulmonary events (e.g., dyspnea, pulmonary infiltrates, pleural effusions, non-cardiogenic pulmonary edema, pulmonary insufficiency and hypoxia, and acute respiratory distress syndrome). Fatalities have occurred. Patients with WBC counts greater than 30,000 mm^3 may be at increased risk. Strongly consider discontinuing treatment with gemtuzumab in patients who develop anaphylaxis, pulmonary edema, or acute respiratory distress syndrome.

Monitor: Obtain baseline CBC including differential and platelet counts; repeat at regular intervals. In clinical studies, responding patients recovered ANCs to 500/mm^3 by a median of 40.5 days and platelet counts to 25,000/mm^3 by a median of 39 days. ■ Monitor vital signs during the infusion and for four hours following the infusion. ■ Acute infusion-related events may occur after the end of the 2-hour infusion and usually resolve after 2 to 4 hours with a supportive therapy of acetaminophen, diphenhydramine, and IV fluids. See Usual Dose. Fewer infusion-related events were observed after the second dose. ■ Electrolytes, renal and hepatic function, and uric acid levels should be monitored during therapy. ■ Monitor for hepatotoxicity, particularly VOD. Symptoms may include ascites, elevations in bilirubin and/or liver enzymes, hepatomegaly, rapid weight gain, and right upper quadrant pain. ■ TLS may occur. May increase blood uric acid levels, increased doses of antigout agents may be necessary. Allopurinol (Alloprim, Zyloprim) preferred to reduce risk of uric acid nephropathy associated with uricosuric antigout agents. ■ Observe closely for signs of infection, including opportunistic infection. Prophylactic antibiotics may be indicated pending results of C/S in a febrile neutropenic patient. ■ Antiemetics may be administered to increase patient comfort. ■ Monitor for thrombocytopenia (platelet count less than 50,000/mm^3). Initiate precautions to prevent excessive bleeding (e.g., inspect IV sites, skin, and mucous membranes; use extreme care during invasive procedures; test urine, emesis, stool, and secretions for occult blood). ■ See Precautions and Antidote.

Patient Education: Avoid pregnancy. Nonhormonal birth control recommended. See Maternal/Child. ■ Report infusion-related symptoms (chills, dyspnea, fever) and other unusual or unexpected symptoms or side effects promptly. ■ See Appendix D, p. 1148.

Maternal/Child: Category D: may cause fetal harm. Women of childbearing age should use birth control during treatment. ■ Discontinue breast-feeding.

Elderly: Incidence of most adverse effects similar in patients regardless of age. ■ Laboratory parameters associated with hepatic dysfunction (e.g., elevated levels of bilirubin, AST, and ALT) were more consistently observed in patients 60 years of age or older.

DRUG/LAB INTERACTIONS

Formal drug interaction studies have not been performed. ■ Additive bone marrow depression may occur when given with other bone marrow depressants (e.g., other antineoplastics or radiation therapy). ■ Do not administer live-virus vaccines to patients receiving antineoplastic therapy.

SIDE EFFECTS

Acute infusion-related events (e.g., chills, dyspnea, fever, headache, hyperglycemia, hypertension, hypoxia, hypotension, nausea, vomiting), anaphylaxis, antibody formation (rare), asthenia, cerebral hemorrhage, disseminated intravascular coagulation, elevated lactic dehydrogenase (LDH), epistaxis, hematuria, hepatotoxicity (e.g., hyperbilirubinemia, abnormal ALT, AST, or transaminases, jaundice and hepatosplenomegaly, hepatic veno-occlusive disease [has been fatal]), hypokalemia, hypomagnesemia, infection (including Herpes simplex, opportunistic infections pneumonia, and sepsis), intracranial hemorrhage, mucositis, myelosuppression (e.g., severe anemia, neutropenia, thrombocytopenia), peripheral edema, pulmonary events (e.g., dyspnea, pulmonary infiltrates, pleural effusions, non-cardiogenic pulmonary edema, pulmonary insufficiency and hypoxia, and acute respiratory distress syndrome), rash, renal failure secondary to TLS, stomatitis.

ANTIDOTE

Keep physician informed of all side effects. Most will be treated symptomatically. Infusion-related reactions may be attenuated by premedication with acetaminophen and diphenhydramine and with IV hydration. Discontinue infusion if dyspnea or clinically significant hypotension occurs. Monitor until S/S completely resolve. Strongly consider discontinuing treatment with gemtuzumab in patients who develop anaphylaxis, pulmonary edema, or acute respiratory distress syndrome. Monitor V/S and blood counts carefully. Platelet or RBC transfusions and/or blood modifiers (e.g., darbepoetin alfa [Aranesp], epoetin-alfa [Epogen, Procrit], filgrastim [Neupogen], pegfilgrastim [Neulasta], sargramostim [Leukine], oprelvekin [Neumega]) may be indicated. Gemtuzumab is not removed by dialysis. Resuscitate as necessary.

GENTAMICIN SULFATE

(jen-ta-mye′sin sul′fat)

Antibacterial (aminoglycoside)

✤Cidomycin, Garamycin

pH 3 to 5.5

USUAL DOSE

3 mg/kg of body weight/24 hr equally divided into 3 or 4 doses. Up to 5 mg/kg/24 hr may be given if indicated. Reduce to usual dose as soon as feasible. A loading dose of 1 to 2 mg/kg is commonly used. Dosage based on ideal body weight. Recent studies suggest that a single daily dose of 5 to 7 mg/kg (instead of divided into 2 to 3 doses) may provide higher peak levels and enhance drug effectiveness while actually reducing or having no adverse effects on risk of toxicity. Various procedures for monitoring blood levels are in use. Some health facilities are monitoring with trough levels; others may draw levels at predetermined times and plot the concentration on nomograms. Depending on the protocol in place, doses or intervals may be adjusted. See Precautions/Monitor.

Prevention of bacterial endocarditis in dental, respiratory tract, GI or GU tract surgery or instrumentation: 1.5 mg/kg 30 minutes before procedure. Do not exceed 80 mg. Repeat in 8 hours. Given concurrently with ampicillin, vancomycin, or amoxicillin.

Pelvic inflammatory disease: 2 mg/kg as an initial dose. Follow with 1.5 mg/kg every 8 hours for 4 days or 48 hours after patient improves. Given concurrently with clindamycin.

PEDIATRIC DOSE

6 to 7.5 mg/kg of body weight/24 hr (2 to 2.5 mg/kg every 8 hours). A single daily dose is also being used in children. See comments under Usual Dose. 10 mg/ml product available for pediatric use.

Prevention of bacterial endocarditis in dental, respiratory tract, GI or GU tract surgery or instrumentation: 2 mg/kg. See Adult Dose for instructions.

NEONATAL DOSE

2.5 mg/kg. Intervals adjusted based on age as follows:

- **0 to 7 days of age; less than 28 weeks' gestation:** Every 24 hours.
  - **28 to 34 weeks' gestation:** Every 18 hours.
  - **Over 34 weeks' gestation:** Every 12 hours.
- **Over 7 days of age; less than 28 weeks' gestation:** Every 18 hours.
  - **28 to 34 weeks' gestation:** Every 12 hours.
  - **Over 34 weeks' gestation:** Every 8 hours.

Another source suggests that higher doses (4 to 5 mg/kg/dose) at extended intervals (24 to 48 hours) may be used.

DOSE ADJUSTMENTS

Reduce daily dose commensurate with amount of renal impairment and/or increase intervals between injections. ■ Reduced dose or extended intervals may be indicated in the elderly. ■ See Monitor and Drug/Lab Interactions.

DILUTION

Available premixed in several concentrations. Vials equal 10 or 40 mg/ml. Further dilute each single dose in 50 to 200 ml of IV NS or D5W. Decrease volume of diluent for children. Commercially diluted solutions available.

Also available in ADD-Vantage vials for use with ADD-Vantage infusion containers.

INCOMPATIBLE WITH

Manufactuer states, "Do not physically premix with other drugs; administer separately." Inactivated in solution with beta-lactam antibiotics (e.g., cephalosporins, penicillins) and vancomycin. Do not mix in the same solution. Appropriate spacing required because of physical incompatibilities. See Drug/Lab Interactions.

COMPATIBLE WITH (Underline Indicates Conflicting Compatibility Information)

See Incompatible With. Consult pharmacist; specific conditions may apply; see Compatibilities, p. xvi.

Additive: ***Not recommended by manufacturer.*** Atracurium (Tracrium), aztreonam (Azactam), bleomycin (Blenoxane), cefoxitin (Mefoxin), cefuroxime (Zinacef), cimetidine (Tagamet), ciprofloxacin (Cipro IV), clindamycin (Cleocin), cytarabine (ARA-C), dopamine (Intropin), fluconazole (Diflucan), furosemide (Lasix), linezolid (Zyvox), meropenem (Merrem IV), metronidazole (Flagyl IV), ofloxacin (Floxin IV), penicillin G sodium, ranitidine (Zantac), verapamil (Isoptin).

Syringe: ***Not recommended by manufacturer.*** Clindamycin (Cleocin), penicillin G sodium.

Y-site: Acyclovir (Zovirax), alatrofloxacin (Trovan IV), aldesleukin (Proleukin, IL-2), amifostine (Ethyol), amiodarone (Cordarone), atracurium (Tracrium), aztreonam (Azactam), ciprofloxacin (Cipro IV), cisatracurium (Nimbex), cyclophosphamide (Cytoxan), cytarabine (ARA-C), diltiazem (Cardizem), docetaxel (Taxotere), doxorubicin liposome (Doxil), enalaprilat (Vasotec IV), esmolol (Brevibloc), etoposide phosphate (Etopophos), famotidine (Pepcid IV), filgrastim (Neupogen), fluconazole (Diflucan), fludarabine (Fludara), foscarnet (Foscavir), gatifloxacin (Tequin), gemcitabine (Gemzar), granisetron (Kytril), hetastarch in electrolytes (Hextend), hydromorphone (Dilaudid), insulin (regular), labetalol (Normodyne), levofloxacin (Levaquin), linezolid (Zyvox), lorazepam (Ativan), magnesium sulfate, melphalan (Alkeran), meperidine (Demerol), meropenem (Merrem IV), midazolam (Versed), morphine, multivitamins (M.V.I.), ondansetron (Zofran), paclitaxel (Taxol), pancuronium (Pavulon), perphenazine (Trilafon), remifentanil (Ultiva), sargramostim (Leukine), tacrolimus (Prograf), teniposide (Vumon), theophylline, thiotepa (Thioplex), vecuronium (Norcuron), vinorelbine (Navelbine), zidovudine (AZT, Retrovir).

RATE OF ADMINISTRATION

Each single dose, properly diluted, over 30 to 60 minutes, up to 2 hours in children. Recent studies suggest bolus dosing (versus infusion over 30 minutes) may produce an earlier bactericidal effect, which is sustained. No dose, dilution, or rate recommendations are available at this time.

ACTIONS

An aminoglycoside antibiotic with neuromuscular blocking action. Bactericidal against specific gram-negative bacilli, including *Escherichia coli*, *Klebsiella*, *Proteus*, and *Pseudomonas*. Not effective for fungi or viral infections. Well distributed throughout all body fluids; serum and urine levels remain adequate for 6 to 12 hours. Usual half-life is 2 hours. Half-life is prolonged in infants, postpartum females, fever, liver disease and ascites, spinal cord injury, cystic fibrosis, and the elderly; shorter in severe burns. Crosses the placental barrier. Excreted through the kidneys.

INDICATIONS AND USES

Treatment of serious infections of the GI (peritonitis), respiratory, and urinary tracts; CNS (meningitis); skin; bone; soft tissue (burns); septicemia; and bacterial neonatal sepsis. ■ Primarily used when penicillin and other less toxic antibiotics are ineffective or contraindicated. ■ Prevention of bacterial endocarditis in dental, respiratory tract, GI, or GU surgery or instrumentation. ■ Used concurrently with clindamycin to treat pelvic inflammatory disease. ■ Considered initial therapy after culture and sensitivity is drawn in suspected or confirmed gram-negative infections or other serious infections. ■ Treat suspected infection in the immunosuppressed patient. ■ May be used synergistically in gram-positive infections. ■ Used concurrently with penicillin for endocarditis and neonatal sepsis.

CONTRAINDICATIONS

Known gentamicin or aminoglycoside sensitivity, renal failure. Sulfite sensitivity may be a contraindication.

PRECAUTIONS

Sensitivity studies indicated to determine susceptibility of the causative organism to gentamicin. ■ Use extreme caution if therapy is required over 7 to 10 days. ■ Superinfection may occur from overgrowth of nonsusceptible organisms. ■ Use caution in infants, children, and the elderly. ■ May contain sulfites; use caution in patients with asthma. ■ Use extreme caution in patients with end-stage renal disease. ■ Single daily dosing has been used effectively in abdominal, pelvic inflammatory, and GU infections in patients with normal renal function. Not recommended in bacteremia caused by *Pseudomonas aeruginosa,* endocarditis, meningitis, during pregnancy, or in patients less than 6 weeks postpartum. Limited data available for use in all other situations (e.g., burns, cystic fibrosis, elderly, pediatrics, renal impairment). ■ Risk of neurotoxicity (e.g., auditory and vestibular ototoxicity) increased in patients with pre-existing renal damage or in normal renal function with prolonged use. Partial or total irreversible deafness may continue to develop after gentamicin discontinued. ■ Pseudomembranous colitis has been reported. May range from mild to life-threatening. Consider in patients that present with diarrhea during or after treatment with gentamicin.

Monitor: Narrow range between toxic and therapeutic levels. Periodically monitor peak and trough concentrations. Therapeutic level is between 4 and 8 mcg/ml. Monitor frequently in patients with impaired renal function. ■ Watch for decrease in urine output and rising BUN and SrCr. May require decreased dose. ■ Routine serum levels and evaluation of hearing are recommended. ■ Maintain good hydration. ■ Monitor serum calcium, magnesium, sodium, and potassium; levels may decline. Depressed levels have caused mental confusion, paresthesia, positive Chvostek and Trousseau signs (provoked spasm of facial muscles and other muscles; occurs in tetany), and tetany in adults; muscle weakness and tetany in infants. ■ Closely monitor patients with impaired renal function for nephrotoxicity and neurotoxicity (e.g., auditory and vestibular ototoxicity); nephrotoxicity may be reversible. ■ In extended treatment, monitoring of serum levels, electrolytes, renal, auditory, and vestibular functions is recommended daily. ■ See Drug/Lab Interactions.

Patient Education: Report promptly: dizziness, hearing loss, weakness, or any changes in balance. ■ Consider birth control options.

Maternal/Child: Category D: avoid pregnancy. Potential hazard to fetus. ■ Safety for use during breast-feeding not established; use extreme caution. ■ Peak concentrations are generally lower in infants and young children.

Elderly: Consider less toxic alternatives. Half-life prolonged. Longer intervals between doses may be more important than reduced doses. ■ Monitor renal function and drug levels carefully. Measurement of CrCl more useful than BUN or SrCr to assess renal function. ■ See Precautions.

DRUG/LAB INTERACTIONS

Inactivated in solution with penicillins but is synergistic when used in combination with beta-lactam antibiotics (e.g., sulbactam sodium, clavulanate potassium, cephalosporins, penicillins) and vancomycin. Do not mix in the same solution. Dose adjustment and appropriate spacing required because of physical incompatibilities and interactions. Synergism may be inconsistent; measure aminoglycoside levels. ■ Concurrent use topically or systemically with any other ototoxic or nephrotoxic agents should be avoided. May have dangerous additive effects with anesthetics (e.g., enflurane), other neuromuscular blocking antibiotics (e.g., kanamycin, streptomycin), beta-lactam antibiotics (e.g., cephalosporins), diuretics (e.g., furosemide [Lasix]), vancomycin, and many others. ■ Neuromuscular blocking muscle relaxants (e.g., doxacurium [Nuromax], succinylcholine) are potentiated by aminoglycosides. ***Apnea can occur.*** ■ Aminoglycosides are also potentiated by anticholinesterases (e.g., edrophonium), antineoplastics (e.g., nitrogen mustard, cisplatin). ■ May be antagonized by bacteriostatic antibiotics (e.g., chloramphenicol, erythromycin, tetracyclines); bactericidal action may be impacted.

SIDE EFFECTS

Occur more frequently with impaired renal function, higher doses, or prolonged administration, in dehydrated or elderly patients, and in patients receiving other ototoxic or nephrotoxic drugs.

Anorexia, burning, dizziness, fever, headache, hypertension, hypotension, itching, lethargy, muscle twitching, nausea, numbness, rash, roaring in ears, seizures, tingling sensation, tinnitus, urticaria, vomiting, weight loss.

Major: Acute organic brain syndrome; blood dyscrasias; convulsions; elevated bilirubin, BUN, SrCr, AST (SGOT), and ALT (SGPT); hearing loss, laryngeal edema; neuromuscular blockade; oliguria; pseudomembranous colitis; respiratory depression or arrest.

ANTIDOTE

Notify the physician of all side effects. If minor side effects persist or any major symptom appears, discontinue the drug and notify the physician. Treatment is symptomatic. In overdose, hemodialysis may be indicated. Monitor fluid balance, CrCl, and plasma levels carefully. Complexation with ticarcillin may be as effective as hemodialysis. Consider exchange transfusion in the newborn. Calcium salts or neostigmine may reverse neuromuscular blockade. Resuscitate as necessary.

GLUCAGON (rDNA ORIGIN)

(gloo′ka-gon)

Antihypoglycemic
Diagnostic agent
Antidote

GlucaGen, Glucagon for Injection

pH 2.5 to 3

USUAL DOSE

Hypoglycemia in adults and children weighing more than 20 kg (Glucagon [44 lbs]) to 25 kg (GlucaGen [55 lbs]): 1 mg. May be given IV, IM, or SC. Usually awakens an unconscious patient within 15 minutes. May be repeated in 20 minutes. For severe hypoglycemia or when patient fails to respond to glucagon, IV dextrose should be administered. Up to 2 mg of glucagon has been given as initial dose.

Diagnostic aid: stomach, duodenum, and small bowel: 0.5 mg IV 1 minute before procedure begins or 2 mg IM 10 minutes before procedure begins. When diagnostic procedure is over, administer oral carbohydrates; see Monitor.

Diagnostic aid: colon: 2 mg IM 10 minutes before procedure begins. Other sources suggest 0.25 to 1 mg and do not differentiate specific procedures. When diagnostic procedure is over, administer oral carbohydrates; see Monitor.

Reverse effects of beta blockade (unlabeled): 3 to 10 mg or 50 to 150 mcg/kg of body weight. Follow either dose regimen with a continuous infusion of 1 to 5 mg/hr. Specific process required; see Dilution.

PEDIATRIC DOSE

Hypoglycemia in infants and children weighing less than 20 kg (Glucagon [44 lbs]) to 25 kg (GlucaGen [55 lbs]): 20 to 30 mcg/kg or 0.5 mg. See comments under Usual Dose.

DILUTION

Dilute 1 unit (1 mg) with 1 ml SW (supplied). Roll vial gently until completely dissolved. Concentrations greater than 1 mg/ml are not recommended. Do not add to IV solutions. May be given through Y-tube or three-way stopcock of infusion set if a dextrose solution is infusing. A 2-mg dose may be diluted with an equal amount of SW for injection.

Reverse effects of beta blockade: Reconstitute each 1 unit (1 mg) with 1 ml SW. For ***continuous infusion*** this reconstituted solution may be further diluted in D5W to deliver 1 to 5 mg/hr.

Storage: Use immediately after reconstitution. Discard any unused portion. Store ***Glucagon for injection*** at CRT before reconstitution. Refrigerate ***GlucaGen*** before reconstitution, or may be stored at CRT for up to 12 months.

COMPATIBILITY

May form a precipitate with saline solutions and solutions with a pH of 3 to 9.5. Specific information not available. Consider specific use; consult pharmacist.

RATE OF ADMINISTRATION

Too-rapid rate of injection may increase incidence of side effects. 1 unit (1 mg) or fraction thereof over 1 minute.

Reverse effects of beta blockade: A single dose (10 mg) over 1 minute. Follow with an infusion of 1 to 5 mg/hr. Titrate to patient response.

ACTIONS

A polypeptide hormone identical to naturally occurring human glucagon produced by recombinant DNA technology. Induces liver glycogen breakdown, releasing glucose from the liver. Blood glucose is raised within 10 minutes. Glucagon acts only on liver glycogen; hepatic stores of glycogen are necessary for glucagon to produce an antihypoglycemic effect. Extrahepatic effect produces relaxation of the smooth muscle of the stomach, duodenum, small bowel, and colon. Duration of antihypoglycemic effect is 60 to 90 minutes. Duration of smooth muscle relaxation is dose-dependent and ranges from 9 to 25 minutes. Has a half-life of 8 to 18 minutes. Degraded in the liver, kidney, and plasma.

INDICATIONS AND USES

Treatment of severe hypoglycemia (e.g., during insulin therapy in the management of diabetes mellitus and in induced insulin shock during psychiatric therapy). ■ As a diagnostic aid in the radiologic examination of the stomach, duodenum, small bowel, and colon when diminished intestinal motility would be advantageous.

Unlabeled uses: May be helpful in reversing adverse beta-blockade of beta-adrenergic blocking agents (e.g., propranolol [Inderal]) and calcium channel blockers (e.g., diltiazem [Cardizem], verapamil [Isoptin]), or may be used to enhance digitalis effects in heart failure.

CONTRAINDICATIONS

Glucagon for injection: Known hypersensitivity to glucagon or its components, patients with known pheochromocytoma. **GlucaGen:** Known hypersensitivity to GlucaGen or any of its components, patients with pheochromocytoma or insulinoma.

PRECAUTIONS

Easily absorbed IM or SC. ■ If glucagon and glucose do not awaken the patient, coma is probably caused by a condition other than hypoglycemia. ■ Use caution in patients with a history suggestive of insulinoma and/or pheochromocytoma; secondary hypoglycemia may occur. Treat with adequate carbohydrate intake. ■ Evaluation by a physician is recommended for all patients who experience severe hypoglycemia. ■ Use caution in patients with conditions that result in low levels of releasable glucose (e.g., adrenal insufficiency, chronic hypoglycemia, prolonged fasting, starvation). Will result in an inadequate reversal of hypoglycemia. Use of dextrose recommended for treatment of these patients. ■ Use caution; allergic reactions have occurred, usually in association with endoscopic examination during which other agents are administered (e.g., contrast media, local anesthetics). ■ As a smooth muscle relaxant, it is as effective as anticholinergic drugs and has fewer side effects. ■ When used to inhibit gastrointestinal motility, use caution in diabetic patients or in the elderly with known cardiac disease.

Monitor: Should awaken the patient in 5 to 20 minutes. Prolonged hypoglycemic reactions may result in severe cortical damage. ■ Dose may be repeated if necessary. Supplement with IV dextrose (50%) to precipitate awakening and to avoid complications of cerebral hypoglycemia. ■ Blood glucose measurements may be used to monitor patient response. ■ Emesis on awakening is common. Prevent aspiration by turning the patient face down. ■ Depletes glycogen stores especially in children and adolescents; supplement with oral carbohydrates on awakening, to prevent secondary hypoglycemia.

Patient Education: Eat some form of sugar if hypoglycemia recurs. ■ Report episodes of hypoglycemia and glucagon use at home. ■ Teach patient and family proper storage and preparation of glucagon from kits. Include signs of hypoglycemia and procedures to be followed after administration to an unconscious patient.

Maternal/Child: Category B: use during pregnancy only if clearly needed. Use caution during breast-feeding. Not absorbed through the GI tract; it would be unlikely to have any effect on the infant. ■ Safety and effectiveness for use in children as a diagnostic aid not established.

Elderly: If used to inhibit gastrointestinal motility, use caution in elderly patients with known cardiac disease.

DRUG/LAB INTERACTIONS

Potentiates oral anticoagulants.

SIDE EFFECTS

Rare in recommended doses: hyperglycemia (excessive dosage), hypersensitivity reactions (e.g., anaphylaxis, dyspnea, hypotension, rash), increased BP, increased HR, nausea, vomiting. Increases in BP and HR may be greater in patients taking beta-blockers.

Overdose: Nausea and vomiting, increase in BP and HR, inhibition of GI tract motility, hypokalemia.

ANTIDOTE

Nausea and vomiting are tolerable and do occur in hypoglycemia. Antiemetics are indicated when larger doses are given. Increased BP and HR may require treatment in patients with coronary heart disease or pheochromocytoma. Treat sudden increases in BP with phentolamine 5 to 10 mg IV. For any other side effects, discontinue the drug and notify the physician. Treat allergic reactions and resuscitate as necessary. Insulin administration may be indicated in acute overdose.

GLYCOPYRROLATE

(glye-koe-pye′roe-late)

Anticholinergic
Antidote

pH 2 to 3

USUAL DOSE

Peptic ulcer: 0.1 to 0.2 mg at 4-hour intervals 3 to 4 times/day.

Reversal of neuromuscular blockade: 0.2 mg for each 1 mg neostigmine or 5 mg of pyridostigmine. Administer IV simultaneously. May be mixed in the same syringe.

Intraoperative medication: 0.1 mg as needed; may repeat every 2 to 3 minutes. Maximum dose 0.8 mg/24 hr.

Respiratory antisecretory: 0.1 to 0.2 mg every 4 to 8 hours. Maximum single dose 0.2 mg. Maximum in 24 hours is 0.8 mg.

PEDIATRIC DOSE

Intraoperative medication: 0.004 mg/kg of body weight. Do not exceed 0.1 mg as a single dose. May repeat every 2 to 3 minutes. Maximum dose 0.8 mg/24 hr.

Reversal of neuromuscular blockade: Same as adult dose.

Respiratory antisecretory: 0.004 to 0.01 mg/kg every 4 to 8 hours. Do not exceed adult dose.

DOSE ADJUSTMENTS

See Drug/Lab Interactions.

DILUTION

May be given undiluted. Administer through Y-tube or three-way stopcock of infusion tubing containing D5 or D10 in water or saline, NS, or LR. May be further diluted with D5 or D10 in water or saline.

INCOMPATIBLE WITH

Manufacturer states, "Stability is questionable above a pH of 6. May form a precipitate or a gas with chloramphenicol (Chloromycetin), diazepam (Valium), dimenhydrinate (Dinate), methohexitol (Brevital), pentobarbital (Nembutal), sodium bicarbonate, thiopental (Pentothal); do not combine in the same syringe." Dexamethasone (Decadron) or a buffered solution of LR will result in a pH above 6.

COMPATIBLE WITH (Underline Indicates Conflicting Compatibility Information)

Consult pharmacist; specific conditions may apply; see Compatibilities, p. xvi.

Syringe: Manufacturer lists atropine, butorphanol (Stadol), diphenhydramine (Benadryl), droperidol (Inapsine), droperidol and fentanyl (Innovar), fentanyl (Sublimaze), hydromorphone (Dilaudid), levorphanol (Levo-Dromoran), lidocaine, meperidine (Demerol), meperidine and promethazine (Mepergan), morphine, nalbuphine (Nubain), neostigmine (Prostigmin), oxymorphone (Numorphan), pentazocine (Talwin), physostigmine (Antilirium), promethazine (Phenergan), pyridostigmine (Mestinon), scopolamine. Other sources add chlorpromazine (Thorazine), cimetidine (Tagamet), midazolam (Versed), ondansetron (Zofran), prochlorperazine (Compazine), ranitidine (Zantac).

Y-site: Dexmedetomidine (Precedex), propofol (Diprivan).

RATE OF ADMINISTRATION

0.2 mg or fraction thereof over 1 to 2 minutes.

ACTIONS

A synthetic anticholinergic agent. It inhibits the action of acetylcholine. It reduces the volume and free acidity of gastric secretions and controls excessive pharyngeal, tracheal, and bronchial secretions. Antagonizes cholinergic drugs. Onset of action is within 1 minute. Some effects last 2 to 3 hours.

INDICATIONS AND USES

Adjunctive therapy in peptic ulcer. ■ Reversal of neuromuscular blockade (usually intraoperatively). ■ Reduction of salivary, tracheobronchial, and pharyngeal secretions preoperatively. ■ Reduction of volume and free acidity of gastric secretions. ■ Other intraoperative uses controlled by the anesthesiologist (counteract drug-induced or vagal traction reflexes and associated arrhythmias, prevent aspiration pneumonitis).

CONTRAINDICATIONS

Known hypersensitivity to glycopyrrolate. May be contraindicated in patients with glaucoma, obstructive uropathy, obstructive disease of the GI tract, paralytic ileus, unstable cardiovascular status in acute hemorrhage, severe ulcerative colitis, megacolon, and myasthenia gravis, when used for treatment of peptic ulcer disease because of long duration of therapy. ■ Do not use in neonates.

PRECAUTIONS

Use IV only when immediate drug effect is essential. ■ Not recommended for peptic ulcer therapy in children under 12 years of age. ■ Use extreme caution in autonomic neuropathy, asthma, glaucoma, pregnancy, breast-feeding, cardiac arrhythmias, congestive heart failure, coronary artery disease, hepatic or renal disease, hiatal hernia, hypertension, hyperthyroidism, and ulcerative colitis.

Monitor: Urinary retention can be avoided if the patient voids just before each dose. ■ See Drug/Lab Interactions.

Patient Education: Use caution if a task requires alertness; may cause blurred vision, dizziness, or drowsiness. ■ Report constipation, difficulty urinating, dry mouth, flushing, increased light sensitivity, or skin rash promptly.

Maternal/Child: Category B: safety for use in pregnancy not established. ■ It is not known whether this drug is secreted in breast milk; use caution.

Elderly: May produce excitement, agitation, confusion, or drowsiness in the elderly. ■ May precipitate undiagnosed glaucoma. ■ Risk of urinary retention and constipation increased. ■ May increase memory impairment.

DRUG/LAB INTERACTIONS

Potentiated by other drugs with anticholinergic activity (e.g., amantadine [Symmetrel], atropine, phenothiazines [e.g., prochlorperazine (Compazine)], tricyclic antidepressants [e.g., amitriptyline (Elavil)]). Reduced dose of either or both drugs may be indicated. ■ May decrease antipsychotic effects of phenothiazines. Dose adjustment may be required. ■ Risk of ventricular arrhythmias increased when given in presence of cyclopropane. Risk is less than with atropine and when given in doses of 0.1 mg or less. ■ Potentiates atenolol (Tenormin) and digoxin.

SIDE EFFECTS

Anaphylaxis, anticholinergic psychosis, blurred vision, constipation, decreased sweating, dizziness, drowsiness, dry mouth, heat prostration, impotence, increased ocular tension, loss of taste, muscular weakness, nervousness, paralysis, tachycardia, urinary hesitancy and retention.

ANTIDOTE

Notify physician of all side effects. May be treated symptomatically or drug may be discontinued. Neostigmine, in 0.25-mg increments, may be used to counteract peripheral anticholinergic effects. May repeat every 5 to 10 minutes to a maximum dose of 2.5 mg. Physostigmine, in increments of 0.5 to 2 mg, may be used to counteract CNS effects. May repeat as needed to a maximum dose of 5 mg. Proportionately smaller doses should be used in children. Resuscitate as necessary.

GRANISETRON HYDROCHLORIDE

(gra-ni′se-tron hi-droe-klor′id)

Antiemetic
($5HT_3$ receptor antagonist)

Kytril

pH 4.7 to 7.3

USUAL DOSE

Chemotherapy-induced nausea and vomiting (prophylaxis): A single dose of 10 mcg/kg of body weight as an injection or as an infusion. Begin within 30 minutes before giving emetogenic cancer chemotherapy (e.g., cisplatin, carboplatin) and only on the day(s) chemotherapy is given. Clinical trials used doses up to 40 mcg/kg with effects similar to the recommended 10-mcg/kg dose. Recent studies question the effectiveness of a 10-mcg/kg dose. Repeat doses are frequently required to prevent nausea with chemotherapy. Oral granisetron is now available.

Radiation-induced nausea and vomiting (unlabeled, prophylaxis): A single dose of 10 mcg/kg as an injection or as an infusion. Begin within 30 minutes of radiotherapy.

Prevention and treatment of postoperative nausea and vomiting: 1 mg before induction of anesthesia, immediately before reversal of anesthesia, or postoperatively.

PEDIATRIC DOSE

Chemotherapy-induced nausea and vomiting (prophylaxis) in children 2 to 16 years of age: Identical to adult dose.

DOSE ADJUSTMENTS

No dose adjustment required for the elderly or in renal failure or impaired hepatic function.

DILUTION

A single dose may be given undiluted by IV injection or further diluted to a total volume of 20 to 50 ml with NS or D5W and given as an infusion.

Storage: Store vials at CRT or below. Do not freeze; protect from light. Should be administered after dilution (preservative free) but is stable up to 24 hours at room temperature.

INCOMPATIBLE WITH

Manufacturer recommends not mixing in solution with other drugs as a general precaution.

COMPATIBLE WITH

Consult pharmacist; specific conditions may apply; see Compatibilities, p. xvi.

Additive: ***Not recommended by manufacturer.*** Dexamethasone (Decadron), methylprednisolone (Solu-Medrol).

Syringe: ***Not recommended by manufacturer.*** Dexamethasone (Decadron), methylprednisolone (Solu-Medrol).

Y-site: Acyclovir (Zovirax), allopurinol (Aloprim, Zyloprim), amifostine (Ethyol), amikacin (Amikin), aminophylline, amphotericin B cholesteryl (Amphotec), ampicillin, ampicillin/sulbactam (Unasyn), aztreonam (Azactam), bleomycin (Blenoxane), bumetanide (Bumex), buprenorphine (Buprenex), butorphanol (Stadol), calcium gluconate, carboplatin (Paraplatin), carmustine (BiCNU), cefazolin (Kefzol), cefepime (Maxipime), cefoperazone (Cefobid), cefotaxime (Claforan), cefotetan (Cefotan), cefoxitin (Mefoxin), ceftazidime (Fortaz), ceftizoxime (Cefizox), ceftriaxone (Rocephin), cefuroxime (Zinacef), chlorpromazine (Thorazine), cimetidine (Tagamet), ciprofloxacin (Cipro IV), cisplatin (Platinol), cladribine (Leustatin), clindamycin (Cleocin), cyclophosphamide (Cytoxan), cytarabine (ARA-C), dacarbazine (DTIC), dactinomycin (Cosmegen), daunorubicin (Cerubidine), dexamethasone (Decadron), diphenhydramine (Benadryl), dobutamine (Dobutrex), docetaxel (Taxotere), dopamine (Intropin), doxorubicin (Adriamycin), doxorubicin liposome (Doxil), doxycycline (Vibramycin), droperidol (Inapsine), enalaprilat (Vasotec IV), etoposide (Etopophos, VePesid), famotidine (Pepcid IV), filgrastim (Neupogen), fluconazole (Diflucan), fludarabine (Fludara), fluorouracil (5-FU), furosemide (Lasix), ganciclovir (Cytovene), gatifloxacin (Tequin), gemcitabine (Gemzar), gentamicin (Garamycin), haloperidol (Haldol), heparin, hetastarch in electrolytes (Hextend), hydrocortisone (Hydrocortone, Solu-Cortef), hydromorphone (Dilaudid), idarubicin (Idamycin), ifosfamide (Ifex), imipenem-cilastatin (Primaxin), leucovorin calcium, linezolid (Zyvox), lorazepam (Ativan), magnesium sulfate, mechlorethamine (nitrogen mustard), melphalan (Alkeran), meperidine (Demerol), mesna (Mesnex), methotrexate (Folex), methylprednisolone (Solu-Medrol), metoclopramide (Reglan), metronidazole (Flagyl IV), minocycline (Minocin), mitomycin (Mutamycin), mitoxantrone (Novantrone), morphine, nalbuphine (Nubain), ofloxacin (Floxin IV), paclitaxel (Taxol), piperacillin (Pipracil), piperacillin-tazobactam (Zosyn), plicamycin (Mithracin), potassium chloride (KCl), prochlorperazine (Compazine), promethazine (Phenergan), propofol (Diprivan), ranitidine (Zantac), sargramostim (Leukine), sodium bicarbonate, streptozocin (Zanosar), sulfamethoxazole-trimethoprim (Bactrim), teniposide (Vumon), thiotepa (Thioplex), ticarcillin (Ticar), ticarcillin/clavulanate (Timentin), tobramycin (Nebcin), topotecan (Hycamtin), vancomycin (Vancocin), vinblastine (Velban), vincristine (Oncovin), vinorelbine (Navelbine), zidovudine (AZT, Retrovir).

RATE OF ADMINISTRATION

IV injection: A single dose over 30 seconds.

Intermittent infusion: A single dose equally distributed over 5 minutes.

ACTIONS

An antinauseant and antiemetic agent. A selective antagonist of specific serotonin ($5HT_3$) receptors. Chemotherapeutic agents such as cisplatin increase the release of serotonin from specific cells in the GI tract, causing emesis. By antagonizing these receptors, chemotherapy-induced nausea and vomiting are prevented. Has little effect on BP, HR, ECG, plasma prolactin, or aldosterone concentrations. Moderately bound to protein (65%). Distributes freely between plasma and RBCs. Does not induce extrapyramidal side effects. Metabolized in the liver by hepatic cytochrome P_{450} enzymes. Excreted in urine and feces.

INDICATIONS AND USES

Prevention of nausea and vomiting associated with initial and repeat courses of emetogenic cancer therapy, including high-dose cisplatin. Has been shown to be effective with most emetogenic antineoplastic agents. ■ Prevention and treatment of postoperative nausea and vomiting.

Unlabeled uses: Prevention of nausea and vomiting associated with total body radiation or fractional abdominal radiation.

CONTRAINDICATIONS

Known hypersensitivity to granisetron.

PRECAUTIONS

Sterile technique imperative when withdrawing a single dose from the new multidose vial. ■ Stool softeners or laxatives may be required to prevent constipation. ■ See Drug/Lab Interactions. ■ Related to an increased incidence of hepatocellular carcinomas and adenomas in rat studies with large doses. Exceeding maximum suggested dose is not recommended. ■ Cross-sensitivity has been reported between dolasetron (Anzemet) and other $5HT_3$ receptor antagonists (e.g., granisetron, ondansetron).

Monitor: Ambulate slowly to avoid orthostatic hypotension.

Patient Education: Request assistance for ambulation. ■ Report promptly if nausea persists for more than 10 minutes. ■ Maintain adequate hydration. ■ Stool softeners may be required to avoid constipation.

Maternal/Child: Category B: no evidence of impaired fertility or harm to fetus. Use during pregnancy only if benefits justify risks. ■ Use caution if required during breast-feeding. ■ Safety and effectiveness for use in children under 2 years of age have not been established. ■ Response rates seem somewhat less effective in children when compared with those in adults.

Elderly: Response similar to other age groups. ■ Clearance lower and half-life prolonged but has no clinical significance.

DRUG/LAB INTERACTIONS

Metabolism may be inhibited by ketoconazole (Nizoral). ■ Does not induce or inhibit the cytochrome P_{450} drug metabolizing system, but definitive interaction studies have not been done. Its clearance and half-life may be affected by inducers of these enzymes such as anticonvulsants (e.g., carbamazepine [Tegretol], phenytoin [Dilantin]), rifampin (Rifadin) or inhibitors of these enzymes (e.g., cimetidine [Tagamet], calcium channel blockers [e.g., diltiazem (Cardizem), verapamil (Isoptin)], antiviral agents [e.g., indinavir (Crixivan), ritonavir [Norvir], saquinavir [Invirase]). ■ Has been safely administered with benzodiazepines (e.g., lorazepam [Ativan], midazolam [Versed]), neuroleptics (e.g., chlordiazepoxide [Librium]), and antiulcer drugs (e.g., ranitidine [Zantac]) commonly prescribed with antiemetic treatment. ■ Does not appear to interact with emetogenic cancer chemotherapies.

SIDE EFFECTS

Constipation (3%), diarrhea (4%), headache (14%), somnolence (4%), and weakness (5%) occur most frequently. Allergic reactions, including anaphylaxis (rare), have occurred. Transient elevation of AST (SGOT) or ALT (SGPT) may occur. Other side effects have occurred in fewer than 2% of patients but could not be clearly associated with granisetron.

ANTIDOTE

Most side effects will be treated symptomatically. Keep physician informed as indicated. Overdose of up to 38.5 mg has not caused significant problems. There is no specific antidote. Treat anaphylaxis and resuscitate as necessary.

HALOPERIDOL LACTATE

(ha-loe-per′idole lak′tat)

Haldol

Antipsychotic
Sedative/tranquilizer
Antiemetic

pH 3 to 3.6

USUAL DOSE

All IV doses are unlabeled. In all situations observe for effectiveness.

Treatment of agitation and delirium: Initial dose based on degree of agitation. 2 to 5 mg is average. Range is 0.5 to 10 mg.

Acute psychosis: 2 to 50 mg.

Several sources suggest repeating the initial dose as needed every 30 to 60 minutes and extending intervals to 4 to 8 hours as symptoms are controlled. Another source suggests the following regimen: If agitation persists in 20 to 30 minutes, either repeat the first dose one time or give a second dose double the size of the first dose because repeat administration of a dose that does not sedate is ineffective. Continue doubling the dose every 20 to 30 minutes until the patient begins to calm down. The dose given when calming begins is the appropriate dose for that particular patient and may be repeated every hour if necessary. Titrate repeat doses to beginning signs of agitation, observe carefully, and give repeat doses at regular intervals to prevent recurrence of agitation.

Maintenance dose: On succeeding days the total required daily dose is divided and given at specific intervals for that patient (300 mg in 24 hours may be 12.5 mg every 1 hour or 50 mg every 4 hours). IV dosing has been used for up to several days until the source of agitation subsides or is removed. Most patients can then be treated with lower doses of oral haloperidol at less frequent intervals.

Treatment of pain and agitation in cancer patients: 100 to 480 mg/24 hr of haloperidol concurrently with 36 to 480 mg/24 hr of lorazepam has been used in critically ill cancer patients. May be given as a continuous infusion.

Control agitation in critically ill patients requiring mechanical ventilation: 3 to 25 mg/hr as a continuous infusion.

Antiemetic or treatment of intractable hiccups: 2 to 5 mg every 2 hours for 5 to 7 doses. May be used in an antiemetic regimen with dexamethasone in chemotherapy.

DOSE ADJUSTMENTS

Lower initial doses and more gradual adjustments are recommended in children, the elderly, or the debilitated. ■ When a satisfactory response is achieved, gradually reduce dose to the lowest effective maintenance level.

DILUTION

Check vial carefully; only haloperidol lactate can be used IV. May be given undiluted. Give through Y-tube or three-way stopcock of the infusion set. Flush with at least 2 ml of NS before and after administration of haloperidol. A single dose may be added to 30 to 50 ml of D5W and given as an infusion.

Storage: Store below 40° C; protect from light. Do not freeze.

INCOMPATIBLE WITH

One manufacturer recommends that haloperidol not be mixed in syringe or solution with any other drug. May form a precipitate with heparin. Flush line or heparin lock before and after haloperidol administration.

COMPATIBLE WITH (Underline Indicates Conflicting Compatibility Information)

Consult pharmacist; specific conditions may apply; see Compatibilities, p. xvi.

Additive: Buprenorphine (Buprenex).

Syringe: Benztropine (Cogentin), hydromorphone (Dilaudid), lorazepam (Ativan), sufentanil (Sufenta).

Y-site: Amifostine (Ethyol), aztreonam (Azactam), cimetidine (Tagamet), cisatracurium (Nimbex), cladribine (Leustatin), dobutamine (Dobutrex), docetaxel (Taxotere), dopamine (Intropin), doxorubicin liposome (Doxil), etoposide phosphate (Etopophos), famotidine (Pepcid IV), fentanyl (Sublimaze), filgrastim (Neupogen), fludarabine (Fludara), gatifloxacin (Tequin), gemcitabine (Gemzar), granisetron (Kytril), hetastarch in electrolytes (Hextend), hydromorphone (Dilaudid), lidocaine, linezolid (Zyvox), lorazepam (Ativan), melphalan (Alkeran), midazolam (Versed), morphine, nitroglycerin (Nitro-Bid IV), nitroprusside sodium, norepinephrine (Levophed), ondansetron (Zofran), paclitaxel (Taxol), phenylephrine (Neo-Synephrine), propofol (Diprivan), remifentanil (Ultiva), sufentanil (Sufenta), tacrolimus (Prograf), teniposide (Vumon), theophylline, thiotepa (Thioplex), vinorelbine (Navelbine).

RATE OF ADMINISTRATION

IV injection: 5 mg/min. When using multiple drugs, each individual drug should be given at correct rate. (Review text of each drug before administration.)

Intermittent IV: A single dose over 30 minutes.

Infusion: Up to 25 mg/hr has been used. Must be titrated by desired dose and patient response.

ACTIONS

An antipsychotic agent structurally similar to the neuroleptic droperidol with effects similar to selected phenothiazines (e.g., prochlorperazine [Compazine], perphenazine [Trilafon]). A potent dopamine blocker, it produces marked tranquilization and sedation and has a potent antiemetic action. Has minimum effect on cardiac, pulmonary, renal, hepatic, or hematopoietic functions. Peak plasma concentrations occur within 10 to 20 minutes. Half-life is 14 hours. Metabolized in the liver and excreted in urine and feces.

INDICATIONS AND USES

All IV uses are unlabeled. Control acute delirium, especially in emergency situations involving psychotic patients. ▪ Control of agitation or acute delirium interfering with appropriate treatment of cancer, cardiac, surgical, respiratory, and medical patients in intensive care units. ▪ May be given concurrently with lorazepam (Ativan) or midazolam (Versed). Both haloperidol and lorazepam have been given concurrently with morphine in agitation or hydromorphone (Dilaudid) in cancer patients. ▪ Antiemetic in cancer chemotherapy and in surgery patients. ▪ Treatment of intractable hiccups.

CONTRAINDICATIONS

Severe toxic CNS depression or comatose states from any cause. ▪ Hypersensitivity to haloperidol. ▪ Patients with Parkinson's disease.

PRECAUTIONS

Not FDA approved for IV use but is being used. ■ Check vial carefully: only haloperidol lactate can be used IV. Haloperidol decanoate contains sesame oil and is for IM use only. ■ Use should be restricted to closely monitored patients. ■ Rule out other possible causes of agitation (e.g., metabolic and systemic abnormalities, drug toxicity, drug withdrawal) before initiating haloperidol. ■ Use caution with known history of seizures or EEG abnormalities; may lower seizure threshold. Maintain adequate anticonvulsant therapy. ■ Use caution in the presence of severe cardiovascular disorders. ■ Risk of torsades de pointes increases with total daily doses greater than 35 to 50 mg. ■ May cause severe neurotoxicity in patients with thyrotoxicosis; use caution. ■ Development of tardive dyskinesia, usually associated with chronic therapy, has been reported after brief treatment periods at low doses. ■ Neuroleptic malignant syndrome, a rare syndrome manifested by hyperpyrexia, muscle rigidity, autonomic instability, and altered mental status, may develop hours to months after drug initiation. ■ Antiemetic effects may obscure signs of toxicity of other drugs or mask symptoms of another disease. ■ May potentiate Parkinson's disease; see Contraindications.

Monitor: A potent drug. Monitor the patient constantly. Resuscitation equipment, a narcotic antagonist (if a narcotic has been used concurrently), IV infusion line, and drugs to manage hypotension, cardiac arrhythmias, and extrapyramidal symptoms must be readily available. ■ Obtain baseline ECG and monitor periodically in patients receiving higher doses.

Maternal/Child: Safety for use in pregnancy, breast-feeding, and children under 12 years not established.

Elderly: See Dose Adjustments. ■ May have increased serum levels. Sensitivity to postural hypotension, anticholinergic, and sedative effects increased. ■ Risk of extrapyramidal side effects (e.g., tardive dyskinesia) increased especially in elderly women.

DRUG/LAB INTERACTIONS

May cause life-threatening hypotension and bradycardia with propranolol (Inderal). ■ Concurrent use with epinephrine may result in severe hypotension and tachycardia. ■ May potentiate CNS depressants (e.g., anesthetics, narcotics, alcohol). CNS and respiratory depression, as well as hypotensive effects, may all be potentiated. ■ May cause increased intraocular pressure with anticholinergic drugs (e.g., atropine), including antiparkinsonian agents. ■ An encephalopathic syndrome characterized by confusion; elevated serum enzymes, BUN, and FBS; extrapyramidal symptoms, fever, lethargy, leukocytosis, tremulousness, and weakness followed by irreversible brain damage has been reported in a few patients receiving haloperidol and lithium. ■ Haloperidol serum levels may be decreased by phenytoin. ■ See Dose Adjustments.

SIDE EFFECTS

Considered to have a good range of safety, even in large total daily doses. Hypotension (mild), muscle twitching, prolongation of corrected QT interval, tremors, tachycardia.

Major: Apnea, cardiac arrest, excessive sedation, extrapyramidal symptoms (rare), hypotension (severe), impaired vision, jaundice, neuroleptic malignant syndrome, respiratory depression. Numerous other side effects common to phenothiazines and neuroleptic drugs are possible but not common with IV use.

ANTIDOTE

Notify the physician of any side effect. If minor side effects progress or major side effects occur, discontinue the drug, support the patient, treat symptomatically, and notify the physician. Rule out hypovolemia, other hypotensive agents, low cardiac output, and sepsis as causes of hypotension. Then, if indicated, treat hypotension with fluid therapy or vasopressors such as phenylephrine (Neo-Synephrine). Epinephrine is contraindicated for hypotension. Further hypotension will occur. Monitor ECG for QT prolongation or torsades de pointes. Treat cardiac arrhythmias as indicated. Dose reduction or discontinuation of haloperidol may be indicated. Treat extrapyramidal symptoms with benztropine mesylate (Cogentin) or diphenhydramine hydrochloride (Benadryl). Dialysis is not effective in overdose. Resuscitate as necessary.

HEMIN

(hee′men)

Panhematin

Porphyrin inhibitor

USUAL DOSE

A single dose of 1 to 4 mg/kg of body weight/24 hr of hematin for 3 to 14 days. This dose could be repeated in 12 hours for severe cases. Never exceed a total dose of 6 mg/kg/24 hr. Length of treatment dependent on severity of symptoms and clinical response. See Precautions.

DILUTION

Each vial containing 313 mg of hemin must be diluted with 43 ml of SW for injection (provides 301 mg of hematin). Shake well for 2 to 3 minutes to ensure dissolution. Each 1 ml contains 7 mg hematin. Each 0.14 ml contains 1 mg hematin. May be given directly from vial as an infusion or through Y-tube or three-way stopcock of infusion set. Use of a 0.45-micron or smaller filter recommended.

Storage: Store in refrigerator at 2° to 8° C. Contains no preservative, decomposes rapidly; discard unused solution.

COMPATIBILITY

Undergoes rapid chemical decomposition in solution. Manufacturer states, "No drug or chemical agent should be added unless its effect on the chemical and physical stability has been determined." Specific information not available; consult pharmacist.

RATE OF ADMINISTRATION

A single dose evenly distributed over 10 to 15 minutes.

ACTIONS

An iron-containing metalloporphyrin enzyme inhibitor extracted from RBCs. Inhibits rate of porphyria/heme biosynthesis in the liver and bone marrow by an unknown mechanism. Induces remission of symptoms only; not curative. Some excretion occurs in urine and feces.

INDICATIONS AND USES

To control symptoms of recurrent attacks of acute intermittent porphyria in selected patients (often related to the menstrual cycle in susceptible women).

CONTRAINDICATIONS

Hypersensitivity to hemin; porphyria cutanea tarda.

PRECAUTIONS

Confirm diagnosis of acute porphyria before use (positive Watson-Schwartz or Hoechst test). ■ Alternate therapy of 400 Gm glucose/24 hr for 1 to 2 days should be tried before use of hemin initiated. ■ Give as early as possible with onset of attack to achieve the most benefit. ■ Must be given before irreversible neuronal damage of porphyria has begun.

Monitor: Use of a large arm vein or central venous catheter recommended to avoid phlebitis. ■ Effectiveness monitored by decrease in urine concentration of S-aminolevulinic acid (ALA), uroporphyrinogen (UPG), or porphobilinogen (PBG).

Maternal/Child: Category C: safety for use during pregnancy, breast-feeding, and in children not established.

DRUG/LAB INTERACTIONS

Action inhibited by estrogens, barbiturates, and steroid metabolites. Avoid concurrent use. ■ Has anticoagulant effects. Avoid concurrent use with anticoagulants (e.g., heparin, warfarin [Coumadin]).

SIDE EFFECTS

Almost nonexistent with usual dosage and appropriate technique; fever, phlebitis. Reversible renal shutdown has been reported with excessive doses.

ANTIDOTE

Discontinue temporarily if known or questionable side effect appears and notify physician. Renal shutdown of overdose has responded to ethacrynic acid (Edecrin) and mannitol. Treat anaphylaxis (antihistamines, epinephrine, corticosteroids) and resuscitate as necessary.

HEPARIN SODIUM

(hep′a-rin so′de-um)

Anticoagulant

✱Hepalean, Heparin Lock-Flush, Heparin Sodium PF, Hep-Flush 10, Hep-Lock, Hep-Lock U/P, Hep-Pak Lock Flush

pH 5 to 8

USUAL DOSE

Intermittent injection: 10,000 units initially. Dosage is repeated every 4 to 6 hours and adjusted according to clotting time. Usually 5,000 to 10,000 units.

IV infusion: 20,000 to 40,000 units/24 hr in NS or other compatible infusion solution. Available premixed, 12,500 units/250 ml or 25,000 units/250 or 500 ml. An initial bolus dose of 5,000 units is required.

Adjuvant therapy in treatment of AMI: AHA guidelines recommend an initial bolus dose of 60 units/kg of body weight (maximum dose 4,000 units). Follow with an infusion of 12 units/kg/hr. The initial maximum recommended infusion rate is 1,000 units/hr for patients over 70 kg. Adjust to maintain aPTT at 1.5 to 2 times control. Other protocols are in use.

Adjuvant therapy during treatment with thrombolytic agents (e.g., alteplase, reteplase, streptokinase) and glycoprotein GP IIb/IIIa receptor antagonists (e.g., abciximab, eptifibitide, tirofiban): See individual monographs for suggested doses.

Open heart surgery: 150 to 400 units/kg of body weight during surgical procedure.

Maintain patency of indwelling venipuncture devices used with a continuous infusion: 1,000 to 1,500 units to each 1,000 ml IV fluid.

Additive to TPN and IV fat emulsion: 1 to 2 units/ml.

Maintain patency of indwelling venipuncture devices (e.g., central venous line, peripheral lines, heparin plugs) intended for intermittent use: 10 to 100 units diluted in sufficient milliliters of NS to reach the tip of the needle, catheter, or implanted port. Use after each medication injection or every 8 to 24 hours. From 100 units up to 500 units may be required in central venous lines. Confirm patency by aspirating before each injection. Flush with SW or NS before and after any medication incompatible with heparin. Re-instill heparin after second flush. If additional medications are not needed, each single dose of heparin will prevent clotting within the lumen of indwelling venipuncture devices for up to 24 hours. Consult device manufacturers instructions for specific requirements regarding its use.

Blood transfusion: 400 to 600 units/100 ml whole blood.

Treatment of ulcerative colitis (unlabeled): 30,000 to 36,000 units IV daily or 10,000 units SC twice daily. Concomitant administration of sulfasalazine (Azulfidine) is recommended (heparin treatment ineffective without sulfasalazine). Maintain with SC heparin. Improvement should be noted in 1 to 16 weeks. Treatment may continue for more than 6 months.

Reduce incidence of thrombophlebitis from TPN infusions in peripheral lines (unlabeled): 1,500 U and hydrocortisone 15 mg as IV additives to TPN solution. A 5-mg nitroglycerin transdermal patch is applied to the catheter insertion site and changed daily.

PEDIATRIC DOSE

Use a preservative-free solution in neonates; see Maternal/Child.

Full-dose continuous IV infusion: A ***loading dose*** of 50 units/kg followed by a ***maintenance dose*** of 25 units/kg/hr or up to 20,000 units/M^2 equally distributed over 24 hours. Another source suggests a ***loading dose*** of 75 to 100 units/kg and a ***maintenance dose*** (to maintain an aPTT of approximately 60 to 85 seconds) based on age as follows:

Less than 1 year of age: 28 units/kg/hr.

Over 1 year of age: 20 units/kg/hr.

Older children: Dose similar to the weight-adjusted dose in adults (18 units/kg/hr) or a ***loading dose*** of 100 units/kg followed by 50 to 100 units/kg every 4 hours (12.5 to 25 units/kg every hour).

Intermittent IV: An initial dose of 50 units/kg of body weight is followed by a maintenance dose of 10 to 25 units/kg/hr as a continuous infusion or an intermittent infusion of 50 to 100 units/kg every 4 hours. All doses should be adjusted to coagulation tests.

Disseminated intravascular coagulation: 6.25 to 12.5 units/kg/hr by continuous IV infusion or 25 to 50 units/kg every 4 hours by IV injection. Discontinue if no improvement after 4 to 8 hours.

Continued

Patency of indwelling venipuncture devices: Safety and effectiveness of the 100-USP units/ml heparin lock flush solution for pediatric patients not established. Patency for peripheral devices used intermittently may be accomplished with as little as 10 units/ml heparin solution; central lines may require a heparin solution up to 500 units/ml.

DOSE ADJUSTMENTS

Reduction of initial dose indicated in low-birth-weight infants and may be indicated in patients 60 years of age and older (especially women). Dose is based on coagulation tests; see Monitor. ■ Increased dose may be required in smokers (half-life shortened and elimination rate increased).

DILUTION

May be given undiluted or diluted in any given amount of NS, dextrose, or Ringer's solution for infusion and given by IV injection, as an intermittent IV, or continuous IV infusion. Invert container a minimum of 6 times to ensure adequate mixing of heparin with solution in all situations. Available premixed for all uses in suitable dilutions and in ADD-Vantage vials for use with ADD-Vantage infusion containers. Unit-dose heparin flush syringes are not for multiple use; discard unused portions.

Blood transfusion: Add 7,500 units heparin to 100 ml NS. Add 6 to 8 ml of this sterile solution to each 100 ml of whole blood.

Storage: Store at CRT. Do not freeze. Do not use if solution is discolored or contains a precipitate.

INCOMPATIBLE WITH

Several sources recommend not mixing or administering through the same IV line with other drugs until compatibility confirmed. To avoid precipitation with heparin, they also caution to flush with SW or NS before and after any acidic or incompatible medication or solution.

COMPATIBLE WITH **(Underline Indicates Conflicting Compatibility Information)**

Consult pharmacist; specific conditions may apply; see Compatibilities, p. xvi.

Additive: Aminophylline, amphotericin B (Fungizone), <u>ampicillin</u>, ascorbic acid (Cenolate), bleomycin (Blenoxane), calcium gluconate, cefepime (Maxipime), chloramphenicol (Chloromycetin), clindamycin (Cleocin), dimenhydrinate (Dinate), <u>dobutamine (Dobutrex)</u>, dopamine (Intropin), enalaprilat (Vasotec IV), esmolol (Brevibloc), fluconazole (Diflucan), flumazenil (Romazicon), furosemide (Lasix), <u>hydrocortisone sodium succinate (Solu-Cortef)</u>, isoproterenol (Isuprel), lidocaine, lincomycin (Lincocin), magnesium sulfate, meropenem (Merrem IV), methyldopate (Aldomet), methylprednisolone (Solu-Medrol), <u>mitomycin (Mutamycin)</u>, nafcillin (Nafcil), norepinephrine (Levophed), octreotide (Sandostatin), <u>penicillin G potassium and sodium</u>, potassium chloride, ranitidine (Zantac), sodium bicarbonate, <u>teicoplanin (Targocid)</u>, <u>vancomycin (Vancocin)</u>, verapamil (Isoptin).

Syringe: Aminophylline, amphotericin B (Fungizone), ampicillin, atropine, bleomycin (Blenoxane), cefamandole (Mandol), cefazolin (Kefzol), cefoperazone (Cefobid), cefotaxime (Claforan), cefoxitin (Mefoxin), chloramphenicol (Chloromycetin), <u>cimetidine (Tagamet)</u>, cisplatin (Platinol), clindamycin (Cleocin), cyclophosphamide (Cytoxan), diazoxide (Hyperstat IV), digoxin (Lanoxin), dimenhydrinate (Dinate), dobutamine (Dobutrex), dopamine (Intropin), epinephrine (Adrenalin), etomidate (Amidate), fentanyl (Sublimaze), fluorouracil (5-FU), furosemide (Lasix), leucovorin calcium, lidocaine, lincomycin (Lincocin), methotrexate (Folex), metoclopramide (Reglan), mitomycin (Mutamycin), <u>morphine</u>, nafcillin (Nafcil), naloxone (Narcan), neostigmine (Prostigmin), nitroglycerin (Nitro-Bid IV), nitroprusside sodium, norepinephrine (Levophed), pancuronium (Pavulon), penicillin G, phenobarbital (Luminal), piperacillin (Pipracil), ranitidine (Zantac), succinylcholine, sulfamethoxazole-trimethoprim (Bactrim), verapamil (Isoptin), vinblastine (Velban), vincristine (Oncovin).

Y-site: Acyclovir (Zovirax), aldesleukin (Proleukin, IL-2), allpurinol (Aloprim, Zyloprim), amifostine (Ethyol), aminophylline, ampicillin, ampicillin/sulbactam (Unasyn), atracurium (Tracrium), atropine, aztreonam (Azactam), bleomycin (Blenoxane), calcium gluconate, cefazolin (Kefzol), cefotetan (Cefotan), ceftazidime (Fortaz), ceftriaxone (Rocephin), chlordiazepoxide (Librium), chlorpromazine (Thorazine), cimetidine (Tagamet), cisatracurium (Nimbex), cisplatin (Platinol), cladribine (Leustatin), clindamycin (Cleocin), cyclophosphamide (Cytoxan), cytarabine (ARA-C), dacarbazine (DTIC), dexamethasone (Decadron), digoxin (Lanoxin), diltiazem (Cardizem), diphenhydramine (Benadryl), dobutamine (Dobutrex), docetaxel (Taxotere), dopamine (Intropin), doxorubicin (Adriamycin), doxorubicin liposome (Doxil), droperidol (Inapsine), edrophonium (Enlon), enalaprilat (Vasotec IV), epinephrine (Adrenalin), erythromycin lactobionate (Erythrocin), esmolol (Brevibloc), estrogens, conjugated (Premarin), ethacrynate sodium (Edecrin), etoposide phosphate (Etopophos), famotidine (Pepcid IV), fentanyl (Sublimaze), fluconazole (Diflucan), fludarabine (Fludara), fluorouracil (5-FU), foscarnet (Foscavir), furosemide (Lasix), gemcitabine (Gemzar), granisetron (Kytril), hetastarch in electrolytes (Hextend), hydralazine, hydrocortisone sodium succinate (Solu-Cortef), hydromorphone (Dilaudid), insulin (regular), isoproterenol (Isuprel), kanamycin (Kantrex), labetalol (Normodyne), leucovorin calcium, lidocaine, linezolid (Zyvox), lorazepam (Ativan), magnesium sulfate, melphalan (Alkeran), meperidine (Demerol), meropenem (Merrem IV), methotrexate (Folex), methoxamine (Vasoxyl), methyldopate, (Aldomet), methylergonovine (Methergine), methylprednisolone (Solu-Medrol), metoclopramide (Reglan), metronidazole (Flagyl IV), midazolam (Versed), milrinone (Primacor), minocycline (Minocin), mitomycin (Mutamycin), morphine, nafcillin (Nafcil), neostigmine (Prostigmin), nitroglycerin (Nitro-Bid IV), nitroprusside sodium, norepinephrine (Levophed), ondansetron (Zofran), oxacillin (Bactocill), oxytocin (Pitocin), paclitaxel (Taxol), pancuronium (Pavulon), penicillin G potassium, pentazocine (Talwin), phytonadione (Aquamephyton), piperacillin (Pipracil), piperacillin/tazobactam (Zosyn), potassium chloride (KCl), procainamide (Pronestyl), prochlorperazine (Compazine), promethazine (Phenergan), propofol (Diprivan), propranolol (Inderal), pyridostigmine (Mestinon), quinidine gluconate, ranitidine (Zantac), remifentanil (Ultiva), sargramostim (Leukine), scopolamine, sodium bicarbonate, streptokinase, succinylcholine, tacrolimus (Prograf), theophylline, thiopental (Pentothal), thiotepa (Thioplex), ticarcillin (Ticar), ticarcillin/clavulanate (Timentin), tirofiban (Aggrastat), vecuronium (Norcuron), vinblastine (Velban), vincristine (Oncovin), vinorelbine (Navelbine), warfarin (Coumadin), zidovudine (AZT, Retrovir).

RATE OF ADMINISTRATION

First 1,000 units or fraction thereof over 1 minute. After this test dose, any single injection (5,000 units or fraction thereof) may be given over 1 minute. A continuous IV infusion may be given over 4 to 24 hours, depending on specific dosage of heparin required, amount of heparin added, and amount of infusion fluid used as a diluent. Continuous IV infusion is the preferred method of administration. Use an infusion pump for accuracy.

Treatment of ulcerative colitis: A daily dose as a continuous infusion over 24 hours.

ACTIONS

An anticoagulant with immediate and predictable effects on the blood. Heparin combines with other factors in the blood to inhibit the conversion of prothrombin to thrombin and fibrinogen to fibrin. Adhesiveness of platelets is reduced. Well-established clots are not dissolved, but growth is prevented and newer clots may be dissolved. Duration of action is short, about 4 to 6 hours. Average half-life is 30 to 180 minutes. The half-life is prolonged by higher doses and in liver or kidney disease and shortened in patients with pulmonary embolism. Does not cross the placental barrier. Metabolized in the liver and excreted by the kidneys. Has a wide margin of safety.

INDICATIONS AND USES

Prevention and/or treatment of all types of thromboses and emboli including deep vein thrombosis (DVT), pulmonary emboli (PE), and embolization associated with atrial fibrillation (AF). ■ Diagnosis and treatment of disseminated intravascular coagulation (DIC). ■ Prevention of clotting in surgery of the heart or blood vessels, during blood transfusion, and hemodialysis. ■ Adjunct in treatment of coronary occlusion with acute myocardial infarction (MI). ■ Prevention of rethrombosis or reocclusion during MI after thrombolytic therapy (e.g., alteplase, reteplase, streptokinase). ■ Adjunct to use of glycoprotein GP IIb/IIIa receptor antagonists in percutaneous coronary intervention (PCI). ■ Maintain patency of indwelling venipuncture devices (e.g., heparin-lock, needle, catheter, or implanted port) during prolonged IV infusion or for intermittent medication injection or vein access. ■ Additive to TPN to decrease incidence of subclavian vein thrombosis and to IV fat emulsion to activate lipoprotein lipase system and improve clearance of emulsion from bloodstream.

Unlabeled uses: Prevention of left ventricular thrombi and cerebrovascular accidents after MI. ■ Continuous infusion for treatment of myocardial ischemia in unstable angina refractory to conventional treatment. ■ Prevention of cerebral thrombosis in the evolving stroke. ■ Treatment of chronic, refractory, symptomatic ulcerative colitis. ■ Reduce incidence of thrombophlebitis with peripheral TPN. Used concurrently with hydrocortisone and NTG transdermal patch.

CONTRAINDICATIONS

Blood dyscrasias (e.g., severe thrombocytopenia), hypersensitivity to heparin (derived from animal protein), inadequate laboratory facilities, uncontrolled bleeding except in DIC.

PRECAUTIONS

Read label carefully. Comes in many strengths. ■ Unit to milligram conversions are not consistent. ■ Use extreme caution in any disease state or clinical condition where risk of hemorrhage may be increased such as subacute bacterial endocarditis; arterial sclerosis; aneurysm; severe hypertension; during or following spinal tap, spinal anesthesia, or major surgery; hemophilia; thrombocytopenia; ulcerative lesions; diverticulitis; ulcerative colitis; continuous tube drainage of the stomach or small intestine; threatened abortion; menstruation; alcohol abuse; tuberculosis; visceral carcinoma; and severe biliary, liver, or renal disease. ■ Resistance to heparin increased in cancer, fever, infections with thrombosing tendencies, MI, postoperative states, thrombophlebitis, and thrombosis. ■ Use caution if administering ACD-converted blood (variable). ■ See Elderly for additional precautions. ■ Repeated flushing of an indwelling venipuncture device with heparin may result in a systemic anticoagulant effect. ■ Heparin-lock flush solution is intended for maintenance of patency of intravenous injection devices only and is not to be used for anticoagulant therapy. ■ See Maternal/Child.

Monitor: Recent studies show a small reduction in phlebitis when longer IV catheters (30 cm) versus short (3 to 4 cm) are used for heparin infusion. ■ Whole blood clotting time (WBCT), activated coagulation time (ACT), or aPTT must be done before initial injection. Often done before each injection on the first day of treatment or every 4 hours with a continuous infusion. Usually repeated daily thereafter during IV therapy and more often if indicated (some sources recommend an aPTT every 6 hours). Depending on the test chosen the desired therapeutic level is approximately 1½ to 3 times greater than the control level. Confirm desired control level with physician. Obtain test just before next dose due in intermittent injection. Notify the physician if aPTT, ACT, or WBCT is above therapeutic level. ■ Decrease dosage gradually. Abrupt withdrawal may precipitate increased coagulability. ■ Monitor platelet count. Discontinue heparin if it falls below 100,000 or a thrombosis forms. Early or delayed thrombocytopenia can occur and may be dose related. May develop white clot syndrome, which may lead to skin necrosis, gangrene, MI, pulmonary embolism, and stroke. ■ Monitor hematocrit and occult blood in stool also. ■ May cause an increase in free fatty acid serum levels. Patients with dysbetalipoproteinemia (familial hyperlipoproteinemia) cannot catabolize lipid fragments; will result in hyperlipidemia. ■ May cause hyperkalemia in patients with diabetes or renal insufficiency. ■ Use extensive precautionary methods to prevent bleeding if patient requires IM injection, arterial puncture, or venipuncture.

Patency of indwelling venipuncture devices: Obtain a baseline aPTT prior to insertion of an indwelling venipuncture device. Repeated heparin injections can alter aPTT. ■ To avoid precipitation, irrigate indwelling venipuncture devices with NS before and after injecting acidic or incompatible solutions. ■ Heparin and/or NS may interfere with blood samples drawn from these devices, especially if drawn on a frequent basis. Clear the heparin flush solution by aspirating and discarding a volume of solution equal to that of the indwelling venipuncture device before the desired blood sample is drawn.

Patient Education: Report all episodes of bleeding and apply local pressure if indicated. ■ Report tarry stools. ■ Compliance with all measures to minimize bleeding is very important (e.g., avoid use of razors, toothbrushes, other sharp items). ■ Use caution while moving to avoid excess bumping.

Maternal/Child: Category C: preferred anticoagulant in pregnancy but must be used with caution. Hemorrhage most likely to occur during the last trimester or postpartum. Has caused stillbirths and prematurity. ■ Not secreted in breast milk. ■ Some preparations may contain benzyl alcohol;

do not use in neonates. ■ Risk of intraventricular hemorrhage four times greater in low-birth-weight infants. ■ Use heparin-lock flush with caution in infants with diseases with an increased risk of hemorrhage. Use of 100 units/ml concentration is not recommended because of the risk of bleeding especialy in low-birth-weight neonates. Use minimal doses, preservative-free preparations, and monitor carefully. ■ See Dose Adjustments and Precautions.

Elderly: Higher plasma levels of heparin and longer aPTTs may occur in patients over 60 years of age. Higher incidence of bleeding in patients 60 years of age and older (especially women). Lower doses of heparin may be indicated; see Dose Adjustments.

DRUG/LAB INTERACTIONS

Nitroglycerin IV may cause heparin resistance; monitor coagulation status and adjust heparin dose if indicated. ■ Increased risk of bleeding with ACD-converted blood, adrenal cortical steroids (especially chronic therapeutic use), some cephalosporins (e.g., cefamandole [Mandol], cefoperazone [Cefobid], cefotetan, moxalactam [Moxam]), dextran, penicillins, platelet inhibitors (e.g., dipyridamole [Persantine], ticlopidine [Ticlid], phenylbutazone [Butazolidine]), hydroxychloroquine (Chloroquine), NSAIDs (e.g., ibuprofen [Motrin], indomethacin [Indocin], ketorolac [Toradol]), plicamycin (Mithracin), salicylates (e.g., aspirin), other thrombolytic agents (e.g., alteplase, anistreplase [Eminase], streptokinase), thyroid agents (e.g., methimazole [Tapazole], propylthiouracil), valproic acid (Depakote), or any drug that may cause hypothrombinemia, thrombocytopenia, GI ulceration, or hemorrhage. ■ Anticoagulant effect may be prolonged by Probenecid. ■ Resistance to heparin anticoagulation may occur following administration of streptokinase as a systemic thrombolytic agent; adjust dose of heparin based on more frequent aPTTs. ■ Half-life may be decreased and elimination increased in smokers, reducing thrombolytic effect. ■ Inhibited by antihistamines, digitalis, nicotine, tetracyclines, and others; may counteract anticoagulant action of heparin. ■ Potentiates oral anticoagulants. ■ See Precautions/Monitor. ■ Use caution when administered after other anticoagulants. Lab data may not provide an accurate baseline. ■ Blood gas sample errors will occur if heparin is 10% or more of sample volume. ■ Numerous lab values (e.g., imaging studies, thyroid, AST [SGOT], ALT [SGPT], free fatty acid, triglycerides, cholesterol) may be altered. Notify lab of heparin use. Diagnostic results may not be attainable. See Monitor.

SIDE EFFECTS

Bruising, epistaxis, hematuria, hemorrhage (10%), prolonged coagulation time (in excess of two to three times the control level), tarry stools or any other signs of bleeding, thrombocytopenia, white clot syndrome (platelet aggregation, arterial clotting). Allergic reactions, including anaphylaxis, do occur. Vasospastic reactions resulting in a painful, ischemic, cyanotic limb may develop. Alopecia, arthralgias, chest pain, cutaneous necrosis, headache, hypertension, itching on the plantar surface of the feet, osteoporosis, priapism (painful penile erection), rebound hyperlipidemia, and suppressed aldosterone synthesis have been reported. Several studies have shown that moderately high doses of heparin can cause excessive internal bleeding that may lead to paralyzing or lethal strokes. Fewer side effects occur with controlled continuous IV infusion as compared to intermittent.

ANTIDOTE

Discontinue the drug and notify the physician of any side effects. Protamine sulfate is a heparin antagonist and specifically indicated in overdose or desired heparin reversal. Each milligram of protamine neutralizes approximately 100 units heparin. No more than 50 mg should be administered, very slowly, in any 10-minute period. Administration of protamine can cause severe hypotension and anaphylactoid reactions. Use with caution and have emergency equipment and mediations readily available. Whole blood transfusion may be indicated. If heparin-induced thrombocytopenia or white clot syndrome occurs, lepirudin (Refludan), which is an anticoagulant and a direct inhibitor of thrombin, may be indicated. Follow up with oral anticoagulation (e.g., warfarin [Coumadin]) may also be indicated.

HETASTARCH

(het′a-starch)

Plasma volume expander

Hespan, Hextend

pH 5.5

USUAL DOSE

HESPAN, HEXTEND

Shock: Variable, depending on amount of fluid loss and resultant hemoconcentration. Age, weight, and clinical condition of the patient are also considered. Usually 500 to 1,000 ml. Total dose usually does not exceed 1,500 ml/24 hr or 20 ml/kg of body weight. Higher doses, usually in conjunction with blood and/or blood products, have been used in postoperative and trauma patients who have had severe blood loss.

HESPAN

Leukapheresis: 250 to 700 ml in continuous flow centrifugation procedures. Do not use Hextend for leukapheresis.

DOSE ADJUSTMENTS

In patients with a CrCl less than 10 ml/min, the initial dose remains as in Usual Dose; however, subsequent doses should be reduced by 25% to 50%.

DILUTION

Hespan: Available as a 6% solution in 500-ml containers properly diluted in NS and ready for use. Calculated osmolarity is approximately 310 mOsm/L.

Hextend: Available as a 6% solution in 500 ml and 1,000 ml containers properly diluted in lactated electrolyte solution and ready for use. Lactated electrolyte solution contains dextrose, normal physiologic levels of calcium and sodium, and slightly lower than normal physiologic levels of potassium and magnesium.

Storage: Store at CRT. Avoid excessive heat. Do not freeze. Do not use if color is a turbid deep brown or a crystalline precipitate is visible. Discard unused portions.

INCOMPATIBLE WITH

HEXTEND

Safety and compatibility of other additives not established. Contains calcium; do not administer simultaneously through the same administration set as blood; coagulation likely.

COMPATIBLE WITH **(Underline Indicates Conflicting Compatibility Information)**

Consult pharmacist; specific conditions may apply; see Compatibilities, p. xvi.

HESPAN

Additive: Fosphenytoin (Cerebyx).

Y-site: Ampicillin, cefazolin (Kefzol), cimetidine (Tagamet), diltiazem (Cardizem), doxycycline (Vibramycin), enalaprilat (Vasotec IV).

HEXTEND

Y-site: Alatrofloxacin (Trovan IV), alfentanil (Alfenta), amikacin (Amikin), aminophylline, amiodarone (Cordarone), ampicillin, ampicillin/sulbactam (Unasyn), atracurium (Tracrium), azithromycin (Zithromax), bumetanide (Bumex), butorphanol (Stadol), calcium gluconate, cefazolin (Kefzol), cefepime (Maxipime), cefoperazone (Cefobid), cefotaxime (Claforan), cefotetan (Cefotan), cefoxitin (Mefoxin), ceftazidime (Fortaz), ceftizoxime (Cefizox), ceftriaxone (Rocephin), cefuroxime (Zinacef), chlorpromazine (Thorazine), cimetidine (Tagamet), ciprofloxacin (Cipro IV), cisatracurium (Nimbex), clindamycin (Cleocin), dexamethasone (Decadron), digoxin (Lanoxin), diltiazem (Cardizem), diphenhydramine (Benadryl), dobutamine (Dobutrex), dolasetron (Anzemet), dopamine (Intropin), doxycycline (Vibramycin), droperidol (Inapsine), enalaprilat (Vasotec IV), ephedrine, epinephrine (Adrenalin), erythromycin lactobionate (Erythrocin), esmolol (Brevibloc), famotidine (Pepcid IV), fentanyl (Sublimaze), fluconazole (Diflucan), furosemide (Lasix), gentamicin (Garamycin), granisetron (Kytril), haloperidol (Haldol), heparin, hydrocortisone sodium succinate (Solu-Cortef), hydromorphone (Dilaudid), inamrinone (Inocor), isoproterenol (Isuprel), ketorolac (Toradol), labetalol (Normodyne), levofloxacin (Levaquin), lidocaine, lorazepam (Ativan), magnesium sulfate, mannitol, meperidine (Demerol), methylprednisolone (Solu-Medrol), metoclopramide (Reglan), metronidazole (Flagyl IV), midazolam (Versed), milrinone (Primacor), mivacurium (Mivacron), morphine, nalbuphine (Nubain), nitroglycerin (Nitro-Bid IV), nitroprusside sodium, norepinephrine (Levophed), ofloxacin (Floxin IV), ondansetron (Zofran), pancuronium (Pavulon), phenylephrine (Neo-Synephrine), piperacillin (Pipracil), piperacillin/tazobactam (Zosyn), potassium chloride (KCl), procainamide (Pronestyl), prochlorperazine (Compazine), promethazine (Phenergan), ranitidine (Zantac), rocuronium (Zemuron), succinylcholine, sufentanil (Sufenta), sulfamethoxazole-trimethoprim (Bactrim), theophylline, thiopental (Pentothal), ticarcillin (Ticar), ticarcillin/clavulanate (Timentin), tobramycin (Nebcin), vancomycin (Vancocin), vecuronium (Norcuron), verapamil (Isoptin).

RATE OF ADMINISTRATION

Variable, depending on indication, present blood volume, and patient response. Initial 500 ml may be given at rates approaching 20 ml/kg of body weight per hour. Reduce rate in burns or septic shock. If additional hydroxyethyl starch is required, reduce flow to lowest rate possible to maintain hemodynamic status. If pressure infusion is used (flexible containers), withdraw all air through medication port before infusing. If a pumping device is used for administration, discontinue pumping action before the container runs dry or air embolism may result.

Leukapheresis: Usually infused at a constant ratio to venous whole blood (i.e., 1:8).

ACTIONS

A synthetic polymer with properties similar to dextran. Approximates colloidal properties of human albumin. Provides hemodynamically significant plasma volume expansion in excess of the amount infused for about 24 hours. Permits retention of intravascular fluid until hetastarch is replaced by blood proteins. Dilutes total serum protein and hematocrit values. May transiently alter the coagulation mechanism due to hemodilution and a mild direct inhibitory action on Factor VIII. Does not usually interfere with blood typing or cross-matching. **Hextend** supports oncotic pressure and provides electrolytes. Its electrolyte content resembles that of normal plasma. **Hespan** increases erythrocyte sedimentation rate. Granulocyte collection by centrifuging becomes more efficient. Both are enzymatically degraded to molecules small enough to be excreted through the kidneys attached to glucose units.

INDICATIONS AND USES

Hespan and Hextend: Treatment of hypovolemia when plasma volume expansion is desired. An adjunct in treatment of shock due to burns, hemorrhage, sepsis, surgery, or trauma. ■ Used when whole blood or blood products are not available or when cross-matching of blood products cannot be accomplished quickly enough.

Hespan: Adjunct in leukapheresis to improve harvesting and increase yield of granulocytes.

CONTRAINDICATIONS

Severe bleeding disorders, severe congestive heart failure, hypersensitivity to hetastarch, renal disease with oliguria or anuria not related to hypovolemia. ■ Contains lactate; not for use in the treatment of lactic acidosis.

PRECAUTIONS

Hespan and Hextend: For IV use only. ■ Not a substitute for whole blood or plasma proteins. ■ Use caution in heart disease, renal shutdown, congestive heart failure, pulmonary edema, and liver disease. ■ Does not interfere with blood typing or cross-matching. ■ Anaphylactic reactions have occurred, even after solutions containing hetastarch have been discontinued. Patients allergic to corn may also be allergic to hetastarch. ■ Use extreme caution in shock not accompanied by hypovolemia; volume overload may result. ■ Contains dextrose; use caution in patients with overt diabetes.

Hextend: Use extreme caution in patients with metabolic or respiratory alkalosis; contains lactate ions. Excessive lactate may result in metabolic alkalosis. ■ Contains electrolytes; sodium or potassium retention may occur. Use caution in patients receiving corticosteroids, and in renal or cardiac disease particularly in digitalized patients.

Monitor: Monitor HR, BP, central venous pressure, and urine output every 5 to 15 minutes for the first hour and hourly thereafter while indicated. ■ Maintain adequate hydration of patient with additional IV fluids. ■ Change IV tubing or flush with NS before imposing blood. ■ May reduce coagulability of the circulating blood. Observe patient for increased bleeding and/or circulatory overload. ■ Hemoglobin, hematocrit, acid-base balance, electrolyte, and serum protein evaluation are necessary during therapy. During leukapheresis also monitor leukocyte and platelet count, leukocyte differential, PT, and PTT. ■ Observe frequent donors carefully; may have a marked decline in platelet count and hemoglobin levels resulting from hemodilution by hetastarch and saline. Temporary declines in total protein, albumin, calcium, and fibrinogen may also be present.

Maternal/Child: Category C: not recommended for use in pregnancy, especially early pregnancy, unless benefit justifies the potential risk to the fetus. Embryocidal to rabbits. ■ Use caution during breast-feeding. ■ Safety and effectiveness for use in children not established, but has been used. Increased prothrombin time noted.

Elderly: Differences in response between elderly and younger patients not identified. Risk of toxic reactions may be greater in patients with impaired renal function. Monitoring of renal function suggested in the elderly.

DRUG/LAB INTERACTIONS

May increase indirect bilirubin levels. Total bilirubin remained normal.

SIDE EFFECTS

Anemia due to hemodilution, chills, circulatory overload, coagulopathies including DIC, congestive heart failure, elevated serum amylase, fever, headache, hypersensitivity reactions including anaphylaxis, increased urine specific gravity, intracranial bleeding, itching, metabolic acidosis, muscle pains, peripheral edema, pulmonary edema, submaxillary and parotid glandular enlargement, urticaria, and vomiting.

ANTIDOTE

Notify the physician of any side effect. Discontinue the drug immediately at the first sign of an allergic reaction, provided other means of sustaining the circulation are available. Antihistamines such as diphenhydramine (Benadryl) are helpful. Epinephrine (Adrenalin) may also be indicated. Not eliminated by dialysis. Many side effects can result in medical emergencies. Treat as indicated and resuscitate as necessary.

HYDRALAZINE HYDROCHLORIDE

(hye-dral'a-zeen hi-droe-klor'id)

Antihypertensive
Vasodilator

pH 3.4 to 4

USUAL DOSE

10 to 40 mg. Begin with a low dose. Increase gradually as indicated. Repeat every 3 to 6 hours as necessary. Maximum dose is 300 to 400 mg/24 hr.

Eclampsia: 5 to 10 mg every 20 minutes. If no effect after a total dose of 20 mg, use another agent.

PEDIATRIC DOSE

0.1 to 0.2 mg/kg every 4 to 6 hours. Do not exceed 20 mg.

DOSE ADJUSTMENTS

Reduced dose may be required with advanced renal disease and in the elderly. ■ See Drug/Lab Interactions.

DILUTION

May be given undiluted. Do not add to IV solutions. May be given through Y-tube or three-way stopcock of infusion set. Color changes occur in most

10% dextrose solutions and after drawing through a metal filter. Use immediately after drawing up solution.

COMPATIBLE WITH **(Underline Indicates Conflicting Compatibility Information)**

Consult pharmacist; specific conditions may apply; see Compatibilities, p. xvi.

Additive: Dobutamine (Dobutrex).

Y-site: Heparin, hydrocortisone sodium succinate (Solu-Cortef), nitroglycerin (Nitro-Bid IV), potassium chloride, verapamil (Isoptin).

RATE OF ADMINISTRATION

A single dose over 1 minute.

ACTIONS

A potent antihypertensive drug. It lowers BP by direct relaxation of smooth muscle of arteries and arterioles. Peripheral vasodilation and decreased peripheral vascular resistance result. HR, cardiac output, and stroke volume are all increased. Renal blood flow increased in some cases, while cerebral blood flow maintained. Onset of action is 10 to 20 minutes. Average duration of action is 2 to 4 hours. Metabolized by the liver and excreted in urine. Crosses placental barrier. Secreted in breast milk.

INDICATIONS AND USES

Severe essential hypertension. ■ Vasodilation in cardiogenic shock. ■ Drug of choice for pregnancy-induced hypertension (eclampsia).

CONTRAINDICATIONS

Hypersensitivity to hydralazine, coronary artery disease, mitral valvular rheumatic heart disease.

PRECAUTIONS

IV use recommended only when the oral route is not feasible. ■ Rarely the drug of choice for hypertension unless used in combination (effectiveness increased and side effects decreased) with spironolactone (Aldactone), reserpine (Serpasil), guanethidine (Ismelin), and thiazide diuretics. ■ Tolerance is easily developed but subsides about 7 days after the drug is discontinued. ■ Use caution in advanced renal disease, cerebrovascular accidents, congestive heart failure, coronary insufficiency, headache, increased intracranial pressure, and tachycardia. ■ Use in pregnancy should be limited to treatment of eclampsia.

Monitor: Check BP every 5 minutes until stabilized at the desired level. Check every 15 minutes thereafter throughout crisis. Average maximum decrease occurs in 10 to 80 minutes. ■ Withdraw drug gradually to avoid rebound hypertension.

Patient Education: Report chest pain, fatigue, fever, joint or muscle pain promptly.

Maternal/Child: Category C: can cause fetal abnormalities; see Indications and Precautions. ■ Safety for use in children not established. ■ May be used in breast-feeding women.

Elderly: Increased risk of hypotension. ■ Consider age-related renal impairment.

DRUG/LAB INTERACTIONS

Sometimes used with a beta-adrenergic blocking drug (e.g., propranolol [Inderal]) or diuretics (e.g., hydrochlorothiazide [Aldactazide]); use caution, may potentiate effects. ■ Potentiated by anesthetics, MAO inhibitors (e.g., selegiline [Eldepryl]), and other antihypertensive agents. ■ Inhibits epinephrine, levarterenol (Levophed). ■ Use with diazoxide (Hyperstat IV) can cause profound hypotension. ■ NSAIDs (e.g., ibuprofen [Motrin]) may decrease antihypotensive effect.

SIDE EFFECTS

May often be minimized by initiating therapy with a small dose and increasing the dose gradually.

Anxiety, depression, dry mouth, flushing, headache, nausea, numbness, palpitations, paresthesia, postural hypotension, tachycardia, tingling, unpleasant taste, vomiting.

Major: Angina, blood dyscrasias, chills, coronary insufficiency, delirium, dependent edema, fever, ileus, lupus erythematosus (simulated), myocardial ischemia and infarction, rheumatoid syndrome (simulated), toxic psychosis.

ANTIDOTE

If minor side effects occur, notify the physician, who will probably treat them symptomatically. Beta-adrenergic blocking agents (e.g., propranolol [Inderal]) will control tachycardia. Pyridoxine will relieve numbness, tingling, and paresthesia. Antihistamines, barbiturates, and salicylates may be required. Treat hypotension with a vasopressor that is least likely to precipitate cardiac arrhythmias (methoxamine [Vasoxyl]). If side effects are progressive or any major side effects occur, discontinue the drug immediately and notify the physician. Treatment is symptomatic. Resuscitate as necessary. Occasionally methyldopa (Aldomet) will be used as a substitute, since it is effective for the same indications but has fewer side effects.

HYDROCORTISONE SODIUM PHOSPHATE ■ HYDROCORTISONE SODIUM SUCCINATE

(hye-dro-kor′ti-sone so′de-um fos′fat ■ hye-dro-kor′ti-sone so′de-um suk′suh-nat)

Hormone (adrenocorticoid glucocorticoid)
Antiinflammatory
Antiemetic

Hydrocortone Phosphate ■ Solu-Cortef — **pH 7.5 to 8.5 ■ 7 to 8**

USUAL DOSE

The IV route is usually used in an emergency situation or when oral dosing is not feasible. Larger doses may be justified by patient condition. Repeat until adequate response, then decrease dose as indicated. Doses must be individualized and are not always reduced for children. High dose treatment is utilized until patient condition stabilizes, usually no longer than 48 to 72 hours.

Hydrocortisone Phosphate

Average dose range is 15 to 240 mg repeated as necessary every 4 to 6 hours. Another source suggests 100 to 500 mg repeated every 2 to 6 hours. Total dose usually does not exceed 1 Gm/24 hr but may be higher in acute disease.

Acute adrenal insufficiency: 1 to 2 mg/kg initially, follow with 25 to 250 mg/24 hr in equally divided doses every 8 to 12 hours. Another source suggests 100 mg initially. Repeat every 8 to 12 hours in IV fluids.

HYDROCORTISONE SODIUM SUCCINATE

Average dose range is 100 to 500 mg repeated as necessary every 2 to 10 hours. For severe shock, doses up to 2 Gm or more every 2 to 4 hours have been given. Maximum dose is 8 Gm/24 hr. Never give less than 25 mg/24 hr.

Acute asthma: 100 to 500 mg every 6 hr.

Life-threatening shock: 50 mg/kg initially. Repeat in 4 hours and/or every 24 hours as needed *or*

0.5 to 2 Gm initially. Repeat every 2 to 6 hours as needed.

Physiologic replacement: 0.25 to 0.35 mg/kg daily (usually given IM).

PEDIATRIC DOSE

HYDROCORTISONE PHOSPHATE

0.16 to 1 mg/kg of body weight/24 hr or 6 to 30 mg/M^2. May be given as a single dose or equally divided and given every 12 hours. Dose varies with disease.

Adrenal insufficiency: 0.19 to 0.28 mg/kg/24 hr equally divided and given every 8 hours.

HYDROCORTISONE SODIUM SUCCINATE

Acute asthma: 1 to 2 mg/kg/dose every 6 hours for 24 hours; then 2 to 4 mg/kg/24 hr in equally divided doses every 6 hours. For status asthmaticus another source suggests a ***loading dose*** of 4 to 8 mg/kg up to a maximum dose of 250 mg. ***Maintenance dose:*** 8 mg/kg/24 hr in equally divided doses every 6 hours.

Anti-inflammatory: 0.8 to 4 mg/kg/24 hr in equally divided doses every 6 hours.

DOSE ADJUSTMENTS

Reduced dose may be required in the elderly. ■ See Drug/Lab Interactions.

DILUTION

Hydrocortisone phosphate: May be given without mixing or dilution. Always use a separate syringe for hydrocortisone. May be added to NS or dextrose solutions and given by IV infusion. Solution must be used within 24 hours of dilution. Sensitive to heat.

Hydrocortisone sodium succinate: Available in Act-O-Vials and Univials, which are reconstituted by removing the protective cap, turning the rubber stopper a quarter turn, and pressing down, allowing the diluent into the lower chamber. Agitate gently. Using sterile techniques, a needle can be easily inserted through the center of the rubber stopper to withdraw the solution. Also available in flip-top vials. For these other preparations, reconstitute each 250 mg or fraction thereof with 2 ml bacteriostatic water for injection. Agitate gently to mix solution. May be given by IV injection, or each 100 mg (250 mg, 500 mg, etc.) may be further diluted in at least 100 ml (250 ml, 500 ml, etc.) but not more than 1,000 ml of D5W, NS, or D5NS. Sensitive to heat and light. Discard unused solutions after 3 days. If fluid restriction is necessary, 100 to 500 mg may be diluted in 50 ml of the above solutions. Stable for 4 hours.

COMPATIBLE WITH (Underline Indicates Conflicting Compatibility Information)

Consult pharmacist; specific conditions may apply; see Compatibilities, p. xvi.

HYDROCORTISONE SODIUM PHOSPHATE

Solution: Fat emulsion 10% IV.

Additive: Amikacin (Amikin), amphotericin B (Fungizone), bleomycin (Blenoxane), dacarbazine (DTIC), <u>mitoxantrone (Novantrone)</u>, sodium bicarbonate, verapamil (Isoptin).

Syringe: Metoclopramide (Reglan).

Y-site: Allopurinol (Aloprim, Zyloprim), amifostine (Ethyol), aztreonam (Azactam), cefepime (Maxipime), cladribine (Leustatin), docetaxel (Taxotere), etoposide phosphate (Etopophos), famotidine (Pepcid IV), filgrastim (Neupogen), fluconazole (Diflucan), fludarabine (Fludara), gemcitabine (Gemzar), granisetron (Kytril), melphalan (Alkeran), ondansetron (Zofran), paclitaxel (Taxol), piperacillin/tazobactam (Zosyn), teniposide (Vumon), thiotepa (Thioplex), vinorelbine (Navelbine).

Hydrocortisone Sodium Succinate

Solution: Most commonly used IV solutions, fat emulsion 10% IV.

Additive: Amikacin (Amikin), aminophylline, amphotericin B (Fungizone), ampicillin, calcium chloride, calcium gluconate, chloramphenicol (Chloromycetin), clindamycin (Cleocin), cytarabine (ARA-C), daunorubicin (Cerubidine), dimenhydrinate (Dinate), diphenhydramine (Benadryl), dopamine (Intropin), erythromycin lactobionate (Erythrocin), furosemide (Lasix), heparin, kanamycin (Kantrex), lidocaine, magnesium sulfate, metronidazole (Flagyl IV), mitomycin (Mutamycin), mitoxantrone (Novantrone), norepinephrine (Levophed), penicillin G potassium and sodium, piperacillin (Pipracil), potassium chloride (KCl), sodium bicarbonate, theophylline, thiopental (Pentothal), vancomycin (Vancocin), verapamil (Isoptin).

Syringe: Metoclopramide (Reglan), thiopental (Pentothal), selected contrast agents used in radiology.

Y-site: Acyclovir (Zovirax), allopurinol (Aloprim, Zyloprim), amifostine (Ethyol), aminophylline, amphotericin B cholesteryl (Amphotec), ampicillin, atracurium (Tracrium), atropine, aztreonam (Azactam), calcium gluconate, cefepime (Maxipime), chlordiazepoxide (Librium), chlorpromazine (Thorazine), cisatracurium (Nimbex), cladribine (Leustatin), cytarabine (ARA-C), dexamethasone (Decadron), digoxin (Lanoxin), diltiazem (Cardizem), diphenhydramine (Benadryl), docetaxel (Taxotere), dopamine (Intropin), doxorubicin liposome (Doxil), droperidol (Inapsine), edrophonium (Enlon), enalaprilat (Vasotec IV), epinephrine (Adrenalin), esmolol (Brevibloc), estrogens, conjugated (Premarin), ethacrynate sodium (Edecrin), etoposide phosphate (Etopophos), famotidine (Pepcid IV), fentanyl (Sublimaze), filgrastim (Neupogen), fludarabine (Fludara), fluorouracil (5-FU), foscarnet (Foscavir), furosemide (Lasix), gatifloxicin (Tequin), gemcitabine (Gemzar), granisetron (Kytril), heparin, hetastarch in electrolytes (Hextend), hydralazine, inamrinone (Inocor), insulin (regular), isoproterenol (Isuprel), kanamycin (Kantrex), lidocaine, linezolid (Zyvox), lorazepam (Ativan), magnesium sulfate, melphalan (Alkeran), meperidine (Demerol), methoxamine (Vasoxyl), methylergonovine (Methergine), methylprednisolone (Solu-Medrol), minocycline (Minocin), morphine, neostigmine (Prostigmin), norepinephrine (Levophed), ondansetron (Zofran), oxacillin (Bactocill), oxytocin (Pitocin), paclitaxel (Taxol), pancuronium (Pavulon), penicillin G potassium, pentazocine (Talwin), phytonadione (Aquamephyton), piperacillin/tazobactam (Zosyn), procainamide (Pronestyl), prochlorperazine (Compazine), promethazine (Phenergan), propofol (Diprivan), propranolol (Inderal), pyridostigmine (Mestinon), remifentanil (Ultiva), scopolamine, sodium bicarbonate, succinylcholine, tacrolimus (Prograf), teniposide (Vumon), theophylline, thiotepa (Thioplex), vecuronium (Norcuron), vinorelbine (Navelbine).

RATE OF ADMINISTRATION

Hydrocortisone phosphate: IV injection: 25 mg or fraction thereof over 1 minute. Decrease rate of injection if any complaints of burning or tingling along injection site.

Hydrocortisone sodium succinate: IV injection: Each 500 mg or fraction thereof over 30 seconds to 1 minute. Extend to 10 minutes for larger doses. IV injection is usually the route of choice and eliminates the possibility of overloading the patient with IV fluids. At the discretion of the physician, a continuous infusion may be given, properly diluted over the specified time desired.

ACTIONS

Both agents contain the principal hormone secreted by the adrenal cortex and have both glucocorticoid and mineralocorticoid properties. Have potent metabolic, anti-inflammatory, and innumerable other effects. Peak plasma levels achieved promptly. Metabolized in the liver and excreted as inactive metabolites in the urine. Crosses placental barrier. Secreted in breast milk.

INDICATIONS AND USES

Agents of choice for adrenocortical insufficiency; total, relative, and operative. ■ Agents of choice for acute exacerbation of disease for patients on steroid therapy. ■ Occasionally used for asthma or shock, but non-mineralocorticoid steroids are preferred (e.g., dexamethasone, methylprednisolone).

Unlabeled uses: Hydrocortisone 15 mg and heparin 1,500 units as additives to TPN to reduce thrombophlebitis in peripheral lines. A 5-mg transdermal patch of NTG is applied to the catheter insertion site and changed daily.

CONTRAINDICATIONS

Absolute contraindications except in life-threatening situations: Hypersensitivity to any product component, including sulfites; systemic fungal infections.

Relative contraindications: Active or latent peptic ulcer, active or healed tuberculosis, acute psychoses, chickenpox, congestive heart failure, diabetes mellitus, diverticulitis, fresh intestinal anastomoses, hypertension, myasthenia gravis, ocular herpes simplex, osteoporosis, pregnancy, psychotic tendencies, renal insufficiency, thromboembolic tendencies, vaccinia.

PRECAUTIONS

To avoid relative adrenocortical insufficiency, do not stop therapy abruptly. Taper off. Patient is observed carefully, especially under stress, for up to 2 years. The exception is very short-term therapy. ■ Prophylactic antacids may prevent peptic ulcer complications.

Monitor: Monitor electrolytes. May cause sodium retention and potassium and calcium excretion. May cause hypertension secondary to fluid and electrolyte disturbances. ■ May mask signs of infection. ■ May increase insulin needs in diabetes. ■ Administer before 9 AM to reduce suppression of individual's own adrenocortical activity. ■ Periodic ophthalmic exams may be necessary with prolonged treatment. ■ See Drug/Lab Interactions.

Patient Education: Report edema, tarry stools, or weight gain promptly. Anorexia, diarrhea, dizziness, fatigue, low blood sugar, nausea, weakness, weight loss, and vomiting may indicate adrenal insufficiency after dose reduction or discontinuing therapy; report any of these symptoms. ■ May mask signs of infection and/or decrease resistance. ■ Diabetics may have an increased requirement for insulin or oral hypoglycemics. ■ Avoid immunization with live vaccines. ■ Carry ID stating steroid dependent if receiving prolonged therapy.

Maternal/Child: Category C: could produce fetal abnormalities. ■ Discontinue breast-feeding. ■ Observe newborn for hypoadrenalism if mother has received large doses. ■ Some preparations contain benzyl alcohol; do not use in neonates. ■ Observe growth and development in long-term use in children.

Elderly: Reduced muscle mass and plasma volume may require a reduced dose. ■ Monitor BP, blood glucose, and electrolytes carefully; increased risk of hypertension. ■ Higher risk of glucocorticoid-induced osteoporosis. ■ Avoid aluminum-based antacids (risk of Alzheimer's disease).

DRUG/LAB INTERACTIONS

Aminoglutethimide (Cytadren) and mitotane (Lysodren) suppress adrenal function of corticosteroids. Monitor carefully if concurrent use is necessary. ■ Metabolism increased and effects reduced by hepatic enzyme–inducing agents (e.g., alcohol, barbiturates [e.g., phenobarbital], hydantoins [e.g., phenytoin (Dilantin)], and rifampin [Rifadin]); dose adjustment may be required when adding or deleting from drug profile. ■ Risk of hypokalemia increased with amphotericin B or potassium-depleting diuretics (e.g., thiazides, furosemide, ethacrynic acid). Monitor potassium levels and cardiac function. Increased risk of digitalis (e.g., digoxin) toxicity secondary to hypokalemia. ■ May also decrease effectiveness of potassium supplements; monitor serum potassium. ■ Diuretics decrease sodium and fluid retention effects of corticosteroids; corticosteroids decrease sodium excretion and diuretic effects of diuretics. ■ May antagonize effects of anticholinesterases (e.g., neostigmine), isoniazid, salicylates, and somatrem; dose adjustments may be required. ■ Clearance decreased and effects increased with estrogens, oral contraceptives, and ketoconazole (Nizoral). ■ May interact with anticoagulants, nondepolarizing muscle relaxants (e.g., doxacurium [Nuromax]), or theophyllines; may inhibit or potentiate action. ■ Monitor patients receiving insulin or thyroid hormones carefully; dose adjustments of either or both agents may be required. ■ Use with ritodrine (Yutopar) has caused pulmonary edema in the mother; discontinue both agents with onset of S/S of pulmonary edema. ■ Do not vaccinate with attenuated-virus vaccines (e.g., smallpox) during therapy. ■ Altered protein-binding capacity will impact effectiveness of this drug. ■ See Dose Adjustments.

SIDE EFFECTS

Do occur but are usually reversible: alteration of glucose metabolism including hyperglycemia and glycosuria; Cushing's syndrome (moon face, fat pads, etc.); electrolyte and calcium imbalance; euphoria or other psychic disturbances; hypersensitivity reactions including anaphylaxis; increased BP; increased intracranial pressure; masking of infection; menstrual irregularities; perforation and hemorrhage from aggravation of peptic ulcer; protein catabolism with negative nitrogen balance; spontaneous fractures; sweating, headache, or weakness; thromboembolism; transitory burning or tingling; and many others.

ANTIDOTE

Notify the physician of any side effect. Will probably treat the side effect if necessary. Resuscitate as necessary for anaphylaxis and notify physician. Keep epinephrine immediately available.

HYDROMORPHONE HYDROCHLORIDE

(hye-droe-mor′fone hye-droe-klor′id)

Dilaudid

Narcotic analgesic (agonist)

pH 4 to 5.5

USUAL DOSE

Older children and adults: ***IV injection:*** 0.5 to 1 mg every 3 hours as needed. May increase up to 4 mg every 4 to 6 hours if pain is severe.

Infusion: Used postoperatively with a patient-controlled analgesic device (PCA) and in selected terminally ill cancer patients hydromorphone may be administered in doses as high as 2 to 9 mg/hr. Must be administered through a controlled infusion device that may be patient activated. The initial loading dose, the continuous background infusion to provide a level of pain relief and maintain patency of the vein, additional patient-activated doses with specific time interval, additional health professional-provided boluses with specific time interval, and the total dose allowed per hour must be determined by the physician specialist and individualized for each patient. When seeking the required dose to achieve pain relief for an individual patient, increases in increments of at least 25% of the previous dose are suggested. May lower slightly if pain is controlled but patient is too drowsy, or lower dose and increase frequency.

PEDIATRIC DOSE

Individualized on the basis of age and weight. One source suggests 0.015 mg/kg/dose every 4 to 6 hours as needed in children; see Contraindications and Maternal/Child.

DOSE ADJUSTMENTS

Dose selection should be cautious in the elderly. Reduced initial doses may be indicated based on the potential for increased sensitivity, decreased organ function, and concomitant disease or drug therapy. ■ Reduced dose or extended intervals may be required in impaired renal or hepatic function and in elderly or debilitated patients. ■ Doses appropriate for the general population may cause serious respiratory depression in vulnerable patients. ■ See Drug/Lab Interactions.

DILUTION

IV injection: May be given undiluted; further dilution with 5 ml SW or NS to facilitate titration is appropriate. May give through Y-tube or three-way stopcock of infusion set.

Infusion: Each 0.1 to 1 mg is usually diluted in 1 ml NS to provide 0.1 to 1 mg/ml for use in a narcotic syringe infusor system. Available in 1-, 2-, 4-, or 10-mg/ml ampules. Use concentrated preparations for larger doses. May be diluted in larger amounts of D5W, D5NS, D5/½NS, or NS (concentration is usually 1 mg/ml) for infusion and given through a standard infusion pump (requires very close titration).

Storage: Store below 40° C and protect from light and freezing.

COMPATIBLE WITH

(Underline Indicates Conflicting Compatibility Information)

Consult pharmacist; specific conditions may apply; see Compatibilities, p. xvi.

Additive: Fluorouracil (5-FU), midazolam (Versed), ondansetron (Zofran), promethazine (Phenergan), verapamil (Isoptin).

Syringe: Atropine, cefazolin (Kefzol), ceftazidime (Fortaz), chlorpromazine (Thorazine), cimetidine (Tagamet), dexamethasone (Decadron), dimenhydrinate (Dinate), diphenhydramine (Benadryl), fentanyl (Sublimaze), glycopyrrolate, haloperidol (Haldol), ketorolac (Toradol), lorazepam (Ativan), midazolam (Versed), pentazocine (Talwin), pentobarbital (Nembutal), prochlorperazine (Compazine), promethazine (Phenergan), ranitidine (Zantac), scopolamine.

Y-site: Acyclovir (Zovirax), allopurinol (Aloprim, Zyloprim), amifostine (Ethyol), amikacin (Amikin), ampicillin, atropine, aztreonam (Azactam), cefamandole (Mandol), cefazolin (Kefzol), cefepime (Maxipime), cefoperazone (Cefobid), cefotaxime (Claforan), cefoxitin (Mefoxin), ceftazidime (Fortaz), ceftizoxime (Cefizox), cefuroxime (Zinacef), chloramphenicol (Chloromycetin), cisatracurium (Nimbex), cisplatin (Platinol), cladribine (Leustatin), clindamycin (Cleocin), cyclophosphamide (Cytoxan), cytarabine (ARA-C), dexamethasone (Decadron), diltiazem (Cardizem), diphenhydramine (Benadryl), dobutamine (Dobutrex), docetaxel (Taxotere), dopamine (Intropin), doxorubicin (Adriamycin), doxorubicin liposome (Doxil), doxycycline (Vibramycin), epinephrine (Adrenalin), erythromycin lactobionate (Erythrocin), etoposide phosphate (Etopophos), famotidine (Pepcid IV), fentanyl (Sublimaze), filgrastim (Neupogen), fludarabine (Fludara), foscarnet (Foscavir), furosemide (Lasix), gatifloxicin (Tequin), gemcitabine (Gemzar), gentamicin (Garamycin), granisetron (Kytril), haloperidol (Haldol), heparin, hetastarch in electrolytes (Hextend), kanamycin (Kantrex), ketorolac (Toradol), labetalol (Normodyne), linezolid (Zyvox), lorazepam (Ativan), magnesium sulfate, melphalan (Alkeran), methotrexate (Folex), metoclopramide (Reglan), metronidazole (Flagyl IV), midazolam (Versed), milrinone (Primacor), morphine, nafcillin (Nafcil), nicardipine (Cardene IV), nitroglycerin (Nitro-Bid IV), norepinephrine (Levophed), ondansetron (Zofran), oxacillin (Bactocill), paclitaxel (Taxol), penicillin G potassium, phenobarbital (Luminal), Piperacillin (Pipracil), piperacillin/tazobactam (Zosyn), propofol (Diprivan), ranitidine (Zantac), remifentanil (Ultiva), scopolamine, sulfamethoxazole-trimethoprim (Bactrim), tacrolimus (Prograf), teniposide (Vumon), thiotepa (Thioplex), ticarcillin (Ticar), tobramycin (Nebcin), vancomycin (Vancocin), vecuronium (Norcuron), vinorelbine (Navelbine).

RATE OF ADMINISTRATION

IV injection: 2 mg or fraction thereof over 2 to 5 minutes. Frequently titrated according to symptom relief and respiratory rate.

Infusion: All parameters (outlined in Usual Dose) should be ordered by the physician. Any dose requiring a controlled infusion device requires accurate titration and close monitoring.

ACTIONS

An opium derivative narcotic analgesic closely related to morphine. Provides potent analgesia without significant hypnotic effects. Six times more potent than morphine milligram for milligram. Onset of action is 10 to 15 minutes and lasts 2 to 3 hours. Hydromorphone is metabolized in the liver and excreted in the urine. Crosses placental barrier. May be secreted in breast milk.

INDICATIONS AND USES

Moderate to severe acute or chronic pain, especially in situations in which a hypnotic effect is not desirable, such as postoperatively or in some malignancies.

CONTRAINDICATIONS

Acute bronchial asthma, diarrhea caused by poisoning until toxic material eliminated, known hypersensitivity to opiates, pulmonary edema caused by chemical respiratory irritant, respiratory depression, status asthmaticus, upper airway obstruction. ■ Not recommended for use during labor and delivery.

PRECAUTIONS

Use caution in the elderly or debilitated and in patients with impaired hepatic or renal function, pulmonary disease, or concurrent anticoagulation therapy. ■ Use extreme caution in craniotomy, head injury, and increased intracranial pressure. Respiratory depression may cause an increased PCO_2, cerebral vasodilation, and increased intracranial pressure. Clinical course of head injury may be obscured. ■ Symptoms of acute abdominal conditions may be masked. ■ Cough reflex may be suppressed. ■ May cause apnea in the asthmatic. ■ Seizures and myoclonus have been reported in patients administered high doses for cancer and severe pain. ■ Tolerance to hydromorphone gradually increases. A marked increase in dose may precipitate seizures. ■ Physical dependence can develop but is not a factor in the presence of chronic pain of malignancy. ■ Some products may use a latex stopper; may cause an allergic reaction in susceptible patients.

Monitor: Oxygen, controlled respiratory equipment, and naloxone (Narcan) or nalmefene (Revex) must be available. ■ Monitor vital signs and observe patient frequently to continuously based on amount of dose. Keep patient supine; orthostatic hypotension and fainting may occur; less likely with continuous low doses, but observe closely during ambulation. ■ Uncontrolled pain causes sleep deprivation, decreases pain threshold, and increases pain. When pain is finally controlled, expect the patient to sleep more until recovery from sleep deprivation. ■ Stool softeners and/or laxatives will be required to avoid constipation and fecal impaction, especially with increased doses and extended use. Maintain adequate hydration. ■ May increase ventricular response rate in presence of supraventricular tachycardias.

Patient Education: Avoid alcohol or other CNS depressants (e.g., barbiturates, benzodiazepines [e.g., diazepam (Valium)]). ■ May cause blurred vision, drowsiness, or dizziness; use caution in tasks that require alertness. ■ Request assistance with ambulation. ■ May be habit forming.

Maternal/Child: Category C: safety for use during pregnancy or breast-feeding not established. Benefits must outweigh risks. ■ See Contraindications. ■ Pediatric patients may be more sensitive to effects (e.g., respiratory depression). ■ May cause paradoxical excitation.

Elderly: See Dose Adjustments and Precautions. ■ May be more susceptible to effects (e.g., respiratory depression, urinary retention, constipation). ■ Analgesia should be effective with lower doses.

DRUG/LAB INTERACTIONS

Potentiated by phenothiazines and other CNS depressants such as narcotic analgesics, alcohol, anticholinergics, antihistamines, barbiturates, hypnotics, sedatives, MAO inhibitors (e.g., selegiline [Eldepryl]), neuromuscular blocking agents (e.g., tubocurarine), and psychotropic agents. Side effects (e.g., CNS depression, constipation, hypotension) may be additive. Reduced dosages of both drugs may be indicated. ■ Plasma amylase and lipase determinations may be unreliable for 24 hours following narcotic administration.

SIDE EFFECTS

Nausea, vomiting, and drowsiness are less frequent than with morphine. Anorexia, constipation, dizziness, skin rash, urinary retention, urticaria. **Major:** Anaphylaxis, hypotension, respiratory depression, somnolence.

ANTIDOTE

Notify the physician of any side effect. If minor side effects progress or any major side effect occurs, discontinue the drug and notify the physician. Treat anaphylaxis as indicated or resuscitate as necessary. Naloxone (Narcan) or nalmefine (Revex) will reverse serious reactions.

IBRITUMOMAB TIUXETAN

(ib-ri-tyoo′mo-mab ty-uks-e-tan)

Radiopharmaceutical
Monoclonal antibody
Antineoplastic

Zevalin

pH 7.1 (Buffer Vial)

USUAL DOSE

A combination therapeutic regimen consisting of rituximab and two radiolabeled agents (Indium-111 [In-111] ibritumomab tiuxetan and Yttrium-90 [Y-90] ibritumomab tiuxetan). Specific timing of the course of treatment based on the availability of the radioactive components is necessary; see Dilution. These two radiolabeled agents should not be used without the rituximab pre-dose. ***It is imperative that the rituximab monograph be consulted; all information in that monograph must be considered.*** (Deaths from infusion reactions have occurred within 24 hours of rituximab infusion.) The rituximab dose in this combination regimen is reduced to 250 mg/M^2 versus 375 mg/M^2 when it is used as a single agent. Premedication to prevent or attenuate severe hypersensitivity reactions should be considered with the 250 mg/M^2 dose.

DAY 1

Premedication: Acetaminophen (Tylenol) and diphenhydramine (Benadryl) before rituximab to prevent or attenuate severe hypersensitivity reactions.
Rituximab: 250 mg/M^2 as an IV infusion.
In-111 ibritumomab tiuxetan (Zevalin): Within 4 hours following completion of the rituximab infusion, give 5 mCi (1.6 mg total antibody dose) In-111 ibritumomab as an IV injection over 10 minutes.
Assess biodistribution:

- **1st image:** 2 to 24 hours after In-111 ibritumomab injection.
- **2nd image:** 48 to 72 hours after In-111 ibritumomab injection.
- **3rd image:** Optional, 90 to 120 hours after In-111 ibritumomab injection.

If biodistribution is not acceptable, stop therapy now. If biodistribution is acceptable, therapy can proceed on either day 7, day 8 or day 9. Date is selected based on the availability of the radioactive component of Y-90 ibritumomab tiuxetan (may also be adjusted within these 3 days for patient convenience after the availability of the radioactive component is considered).

DAY 7, 8 OR 9 (SELECT ONE DATE)

Premedication: Acetaminophen (Tylenol) and diphenhydramine (Benadryl) before rituximab to prevent or attenuate severe hypersensitivity reactions.

Rituximab: 250 mg/M^2 as an IV infusion.

Y-90 ibritumomab tiuxetan (Zevalin): Within 4 hours following the completion of the rituximab infusion, give Y-90 ibritumomab tiuxetan as an IV injection through a free-flowing IV line over 10 minutes based on platelet count as follows:

0.4 mCi/kg (14.8 MBq/kg) for patients with a normal platelet count *or*
0.3 mCi/kg (11.1 MBq/kg) for patients with a platelet count of 100,000-149,000 cells/mm^3

Do not treat patients with a platelet count less than 100,000/mm^3.

Do not exceed the maximum allowable dose of Y-90 ibritumomab tiuxetan (32 mCi [1184 MBq]), regardless of the patient's weight.

PEDIATRIC DOSE

Safety and effectiveness for use in pediatric patients not established.

DOSE ADJUSTMENTS

See Usual Dose.

DILUTION

Specific timing of the course of treatment based on the availability of the radioactive components is necessary. The In-111 chloride sterile solution (the radioactive component of In-111 ibritumomab tiuxetan) is available from several sources. The Y-90 chloride sterile solution (the radioactive component of Y-90 ibritumomab tiuxetan) is available from only one source and can be delivered on only 2 or 3 days of the week. Specific timing of the course of treatment moves backwards from the day of availability of the Y-90 ibritumomab tiuxetan radioactive component. The radioactive component of In-111 ibritumomab tiuxetan is ordered for 7, 8, or 9 days before that availability.

Changing the ratio of any of the reactants in the radiolabeling process may adversely impact therapeutic results.

Rituximab: See rituximab monograph.

In-111 ibritumomab tiuxetan: A specific kit provides the vials required to produce a single dose. The In-111 chloride sterile solution (the radioactive component) must be ordered separately at the same time the kit is ordered. Other supplies (listed in the package insert) are required for preparation of ibritumomab tiuxetan with In-111 and radiolabeling.

Y-90 ibritumomab tiuxetan: A specific kit provides the vials required to produce a single dose. The Y-90 chloride sterile solution (the radioactive component) will be shipped with the kit when ordered. Other supplies (listed in package insert) are required for the preparation of ibritumomab tiuxetan with Y-90 and radiolabeling.

All preparation, calibration, confirmation of radiochemical purity, and administration of these kits will be by personnel authorized to handle radiopharmaceuticals. Each requires a specific order and specific timing of preparation.

Storage:

In-111 ibritumomab tiuxetan: Store at 2° to 8° C (36° to 46° F) until use and administer within 12 hours of radiolabeling.

Y-90 ibritumomab tiuxetan: Store at 2° to 8° C (36° to 46° F) until use and administer within 8 hours of radiolabeling.

COMPATIBILITY

A radiopharmaceutical; use only the supplies provided in each specific kit. All components, including the rituximab, should not be mixed or diluted with other drugs.

RATE OF ADMINISTRATION

Rituximab: See rituximab monograph.

Both radiopharmaceuticals require the use of a 0.22-micron low-protein binding filter and a vial and syringe shield.

In-111 ibritumomab tiuxetan: A single dose as an IV injection over 10 minutes.

Y-90 ibritumomab tiuxetan: A single dose as an IV injection through a free-flowing IV line over 10 minutes; see Monitor.

ACTIONS

A combination therapeutic regimen consisting of rituximab and two radiolabeled agents (Indium-111 [In-111] ibritumomab tiuxetan and Yttrium-90 [Y-90] ibritumomab tiuxetan). Ibritumomab tiuxetan is the immunoconjugate resulting from a stable thiourea covalent bond between the monoclonal antibody ibritumomab and the linker-chelator tiuxetan. This linker-chelator provides a high affinity, specific chelation site for In-111 or Y-90. The antibody (ibritumomab) is a murine IgG, kappa monoclonal antibody directed against the CD20 antigen found on the surface of normal and malignant B lymphocytes. The CD20 antigen is expressed on pre-B and mature B lymphocytes and on more than 90% of B-cell non-Hodgkin's lymphomas (NHL). Like rituximab, ibritumomab induces apoptosis (fragmentation of the cell). The In-111 component improves detection of the known disease sites. The beta emission from Y-90 induces cellular damage by the formation of free radicals in the target and neighboring cells. After calibration, In-111 decays by electron capture, with a physical half-life of 67.3 hours. After calibration, Y-90 decays by the emission of beta particles, with a physical half-life of 64.1 hours. A small amount of all components is excreted in urine. Administration of the prescribed regimen results in sustained depletion of circulating B-cells (median was zero at 4 weeks [range 0 to 1084 cells/mm^3]). B-cell recovery begins approximately 12 weeks post-treatment and usually progresses to normal range (32 to 341 cells/mm^3) by 9 months post-treatment.

INDICATIONS AND USES

Part of a therapeutic regimen indicated for the treatment of patients with relapsed or refractory low-grade, follicular, or transformed B-cell non-Hodgkin's lymphoma, including patients with rituximab refractory follicular non-Hodgkin's lymphoma. Used in combination with rituximab.

CONTRAINDICATIONS

Known hypersensitivity or anaphylactic reactions to murine proteins or any component of this regimen. ■ Do not administer Y-90 ibritumomab tiuxetan to patients with 25% or greater lymphoma marrow involvement and/or impaired bone marrow reserve (e.g., prior myeloablative therapies, platelet count less than 100,000/mm^3, neutrophil count less than 1,500/mm^3, hypocellular bone marrow [equal to or greater than 15% cellularity or marked reduction in bone marrow precursors] or to patients with a history of failed stem cell collection). ■ Do not administer Y-90 ibritumomab tiuxetan to patients with altered biodistribution as determined by imaging with In-111 ibritumomab tiuxetan. ■ Do not treat patients with a platelet count less than 100,000/mm^3.

PRECAUTIONS

Radiopharmaceuticals are administered by or under the direction of the physician specialist whose experience and training in the safe use and handling of radionuclides have been approved by the appropriate government agency. ■ Contents of the kits are not radioactive; however, during and after radiolabeling, care should be taken to minimize radiation exposure to patients and to medical personnel consistent with institutional good radiation safety practices and patient management procedures. Contact the radiation safety officer. ■ If a splash occurs, flush eyes for at least 15 minutes. For skin contact, wash affected areas thoroughly with soap and water and blot dry; do not abrade skin. In both situations, notify the radiation safety officer and continue the process until no more radiation can be detected. ■ Notify the radiation safety officer immediately if any ingestion occurs. ■ Administer in a facility with adequate personnel, equipment, and supplies to monitor the patient and respond to any medical emergency. ■ Y-90 ibritumomab tiuxetan results in severe and prolonged cytopenias; see Contraindications, Monitor, and Antidote. ■ Expected biodistribution of In-111 ibritumomab tiuxetan includes easily detectable uptake in blood pool areas on the first day, decreasing on days 2 and 3 (for specifics, see package insert). Altered biodistribution necessitates the discontinuation of regimen. It is characterized by diffuse uptake in normal lung that is more intense than the cardiac blood pool on the first day image or more intense than the liver on the second or third day image, kidneys with greater intensity than the liver on the posterior view of the second or third day image, or intense areas of uptake throughout the normal bowel comparable to uptake by the liver on the second or third day images; see Contraindication. ■ May cause severe, and potentially fatal, infusion reactions; see Monitor, Side Effects, and rituximab monograph. ■ Use caution; allergic reactions and/or anaphylaxis can occur. As with all proteins, there is a potential for immunogenicity; patients who have received murine proteins should be screened for human anti-mouse antibodies (HAMA); may be at increased risk of hypersensitivity reactions. ■ Safety of ibritumomab tiuxetan for more than a single course of treatment or for use with other therapeutic regimens has not been established. ■ Contains albumin and carries a theoretical risk for transmission of viral diseases or Creutzfeldt-Jakob disease. Effective donor screening and product manufacturing processes make this risk extremely remote. ■ Secondary malignancies have been reported. ■ Ability to generate a primary or anamnestic humoral response to any vaccine has not been studied.

Monitor: Obtain a baseline CBC, including differential and platelet count. Monitor weekly or more frequently if indicated (e.g., cytopenias, concurrent drugs). Continue until levels recover. Cytopenias (e.g., thrombocytopenia and neutropenia) can be severe; see Precautions, Contraindications, and Antidote. Median time to nadir was 7 to 9 weeks, and the median duration of cytopenias was 22 to 35 days. Some cytopenias extended beyond 12 weeks, and some patients died without recovering. ■ Monitor for infusion reactions. Typically occur within 30 to 120 minutes of the first rituximab infusion and may cause interruption of rituximab, In-111 ibritumomab tiuxetan, or Y-90 ibritumomab tiuxetan. S/S may include angioedema, bronchospasm, hypotension, and hypoxia; see Side Effects for additional symptoms. ■ To reduce unnecessary radiation exposure to vital organs (e.g., thyroid, kidneys, bladder), patients should be well hydrated before, during, and for at least 1 day after administration. Encourage fluid intake and frequent voiding. ■ Establish a free-flowing IV line before administration of Y-90 ibritumomab tiuxetan; avoid extravasation. Monitor closely; if any signs of extravasation occur, discontinue immediately and restart in another vein. ■ Hemorrhage, including fatal cerebral hemorrhage, has occurred. Monitor for thrombocytopenia (platelet count less than 50,000/mm^3) for up to 3 months. Initiate precautions to prevent excessive bleeding (e.g., inspect IV sites, skin, and mucous membranes; use extreme care during invasive procedures; test urine, emesis, stool, and secretions for occult blood). ■ Observe closely for signs of infection for up to 3 months. Prophylactic antibiotics may be indicated pending results of C/S in a febrile neutropenic patient. ■ See rituximab monograph; additional monitoring may be required. ■ See Precautions, Drug/Lab Interactions, and Antidote.

Patient Education: Avoid pregnancy; effective birth control recommended for males and females during treatment and for up to 12 months following therapy. Women should report a suspected pregnancy immediately. ■ Explain importance of increased fluid intake and frequent voiding. ■ Promptly report S/S of infection (e.g., fever, sore throat) or S/S of bleeding (e.g., bruising, nose bleed, dark stools).

Maternal/Child: Category D: avoid pregnancy; can cause fetal harm. Women of childbearing potential should avoid becoming pregnant. ■ Could cause toxic effects on testes and ovaries. Effective contraceptive methods recommended for men and women during treatment and for up to 12 months following therapy. ■ Discontinue breast-feeding.

Elderly: Response similar to that found in younger patients; however, the elderly may have a greater sensitivity to its effects.

DRUG/LAB INTERACTIONS

Risk of bleeding may be increased by any medicine that affects blood clotting, including anticoagulants (e.g., heparin, lepirudin [Refludan], warfarin [Coumadin]); glycoprotein GPIIb/IIIa receptor antagonists (e.g., abciximab [ReoPro], eptifibatide [Integrilin], tirofiban [Aggrastat]); any medication that may cause hypoprothrombinemia, thrombocytopenia, or GI ulceration or bleeding (e.g., selected antibiotics such as cefamandole [Mandol], cefoperazone [Cefobid], cefotetan [Cefotan], ticarcillin [Ticar], aspirin, NSAIDs [e.g., ibuprofen (Advil, Motrin), naproxen (Aleve, Naprosyn), phenylbutazone (Butazolidin)]); and/or any other medication that inhibits platelet aggregation (e.g., dipyridamole [Persantine], plicamycin [Mithracin], sulfinpyrazone [Anturane], ticlopidine [Ticlid], valproate [Depacon, Depakene]). ■ Safety of immunization with live viral vaccines has not been studied. ■ Potential for additive effects with previously administered bone marrow–depressing agents and/or radiation therapy has not been studied.

SIDE EFFECTS

Anorexia, anxiety, arthralgias, cytopenias (e.g., anemia, neutropenia, and thrombocytopenia), dizziness, dyspnea, ecchymosis, GI symptoms (e.g., abdominal pain, diarrhea, nausea, vomiting), and increased cough are common. Abdominal enlargement, asthenia, back pain, chills, constipation, fever, flushing, headache, hypotension, insomnia, myalgia, peripheral edema, rhinitis, and throat irritation have also occurred. Non-hematologic toxicities were considered mild in severity.

Major: Cytopenias (e.g., anemia, neutropenia, and thrombocytopenia) can be severe and prolonged (lasting beyond 3 months [deaths have been reported]). Other major side effects include allergic reactions (e.g., anaphylaxis, angioedema, bronchospasm, hypotension, pruritus, rash), hemorrhage while thrombocytopenic (resulting in death), severe or fatal infusion reactions (e.g., ARDS, cardiogenic shock, hypoxia, MI, pulmonary infiltrates, VF), and infections (predominantly bacterial in origin).

ANTIDOTE

Keep physician informed of all side effects. May constitute a medical emergency or will be treated symptomatically as indicated. Hypersensitivity or infusion-related side effects to any component of the regimen may resolve with slowing or interruption of the infusion and with supportive care (IV saline; diphenhydramine; bronchodilators such as albuterol [Ventolin], terbutaline [Brethaire], or aminophylline; and acetaminophen). Discontinue entire regimen (rituximab, In-111 ibritumomab tiuxetan, and Y-90 ibritumomab tiuxetan) in patients who develop severe infusion reactions (usually to rituximab). Treat anaphylaxis with oxygen, antihistamines (diphenhydramine), epinephrine, and corticosteroids. Maintain a patent airway. Autologous stem cell support, administration of whole blood products (e.g., packed RBCs, platelets, leukocytes), and/or blood modifiers (e.g., darbepoetin alfa [Aranesp], epoetin alfa [Epogen, Procrit], filgrastim [Neupogen], pegfilgrastim [Neulasta], sargramostim [Leukine], oprelvekin [Neumega]) may be indicated to treat bone marrow toxicity or to treat moderate to severe bleeding. Control minor bleeding by local pressure. For severe bleeding, discontinue therapy and obtain PT, aPTT, platelet count, and fibrinogen. Draw blood for type and cross-match. Antibiotic therapy is indicated for infections and may be indicated prophylactically. Death may occur from the progression of some side effects. Resuscitate as indicated.

IBUTILIDE FUMARATE

Antiarrhythmic

(eye-byoo′ti-lide fu′mar-at)

Corvert

pH 4.6

USUAL DOSE

Guidelines for Ibutilide Dosing

Patient Weight	Initial Infusion (over 10 minutes)	Second Infusion
60 kg (132 lb) or more	1 mg ibutilide fumarate (one vial [10 ml])	If the arrhythmia does not terminate within 10 minutes after the end of the initial infusion, a second 10-minute infusion of equal strength may be administered 10 minutes after completion of the first infusion.
Less than 60 kg (132 lb)	0.01 mg/kg ibutilide fumarate (0.1 ml/kg)	

Discontinue infusion promptly when the presenting arrhythmia is terminated (desired effect). Must also be discontinued immediately if sustained or nonsustained ventricular tachycardia or marked prolongation of QT or QTc occur (adverse effects). Postconversion treatment with appropriate antiarrhythmics (e.g., digoxin, verapamil [Isoptin], or propranolol [Inderal]) is usually required.

PEDIATRIC DOSE

Safety and effectiveness for use in children under 18 years of age not established.

DOSE ADJUSTMENTS

Dose selection should be cautious in the elderly. Reduced doses may be indicated based on the potential for decreased organ function and concomitant disease or drug therapy. ■ No adjustments required in patients with impaired hepatic or renal function; see Monitor. Lower doses may be indicated in postcardiac surgery patients. In recent studies one or two infusions of 0.5 mg in patients weighing 60 kg or more or 0.005 mg/kg/dose for patients under 60 kg was effective in terminating atrial fibrillation and/or flutter.

DILUTION

May be given undiluted or may be diluted in 50 ml of NS or D5W and given as an infusion. 1 mg (10 ml of a 0.1-mg/ml solution) of ibutilide in 50 ml diluent yields 0.017 mg/ml.

Storage: Store at CRT in carton until use. Stable after dilution for 24 hours at room temperature, 48 hours if refrigerated.

COMPATIBILITY

Manufacturer lists as compatible with NS and D5W packaged in glass, polyvinyl chloride, or polyolefin infusion containers. Additional information not available; consult pharmacist.

RATE OF ADMINISTRATION

A single dose by injection or infusion over 10 minutes.

ACTIONS

A class III antiarrhythmic agent that produces mild slowing of the sinus rate and atrioventricular conduction. Delays repolarization by activation of a slow inward current (sodium) rather than blocking outward potassium currents. Prolonged atrial and ventricular action potential duration and refractoriness result. Produces dose-related prolongation of the QT interval (may result from dose of ibutilide or rate of injection). Conversion of atrial flutter/fibrillation usually occurs within 30 minutes but may take up to 90 minutes after the start of the infusion. Most patients remain in normal sinus rhythm (NSR) for 24 hours. At recommended doses, ibutilide has no clinically significant effects on cardiac output, mean pulmonary arterial pressure, or pulmonary capillary wedge pressure. Rapidly distributed and metabolized. Elimination half-life is 6 hours (range 2 to 12 hours). Primarily excreted in urine (7% as unchanged drug). Excreted in small amounts in feces.

INDICATIONS AND USES

Rapid conversion of recent onset atrial fibrillation or atrial flutter to sinus rhythm. Patients with more recent onset of arrhythmia have a higher rate of conversion. Effectiveness was less in those with a longer-duration arrhythmia.

CONTRAINDICATIONS

Known hypersensitivity to ibutilide or any of its components. ■ Not recommended in patients who have had a previous polymorphic ventricular tachycardia (e.g., torsades de pointes). ■ See Drug/Lab Interactions.

PRECAUTIONS

Usually administered by or under the direction of the physician specialist. ■ Skilled personnel and proper equipment (e.g., cardiac monitors, intracardiac pacing facilities, cardioverter/defibrillator, emergency drugs) must be immediately available. ■ May cause life-threatening arrhythmias (e.g., torsades de pointes) with or without documented QT prolongation. ■ Correct hypokalemia and hypomagnesemia before use; may exaggerate a prolonged QT and cause arrhythmias. ■ Adequate anticoagulation (usually at least 2 weeks) is required for any patient with atrial fibrillation of more than 2 to 3 days' duration. ■ Select patients carefully; benefits (potential for maintaining sinus rhythm) must outweigh risks. Patients with chronic atrial fibrillation are more likely to revert back to atrial fibrillation after conversion to sinus rhythm. Patients with a QTc interval greater than 440 msec or a serum potassium less than 4.0 mEq/L are at very high risk to develop life-threatening arrhythmias. ■ Patients with a history of CHF may be more susceptible to sustained polymorphic VT. ■ Slightly more effective in atrial flutter than atrial fibrillation. ■ See Drug/Lab Interactions.

Monitor: Obtain weight, baseline vital signs, and ECG before administration. Continuous ECG monitoring during and after infusion indicated to observe for arrhythmias. Watch for QT or QTc prolongation; may cause arrhythmia (torsades de pointes) with or without QT prolongation. ■ Monitor BP and HR. Bradycardia, a varying HR, and/or hypokalemia may increase risk of arrhythmia. ■ Arrhythmia occurs most frequently within 40 minutes of completion of infusion but may occur for up to 3 hours after infusion. Monitor ECG for a minimum of 4 hours or until QTc has returned to baseline. Monitor longer if there are any episodes of arrhythmias or if the patient has impaired liver function.

Patient Education: Report promptly any feeling of faintness, difficulty breathing, or pain or stinging along injection site.

Maternal/Child: Category C: benefits must outweigh risks. Caused birth defects and was embryocidal in rats. ■ Temporarily discontinue breast-feeding. ■ Safety and effectiveness for children under 18 years not established.

Elderly: No age-related differences observed. Median age in clinical trials was 65 years. ■ Lower-end initial doses may be indicated; see Dose Adjustments.

DRUG/LAB INTERACTIONS

Should not be given concurrently with Class Ia antiarrhythmics (e.g., disopyramide [Norpace], procainamide [Pronestyl], quinidine) or other Class III antiarrhythmics (e.g., amiodarone [Cordarone], sotalol [Betapace]). Withhold any of these agents for at least 5 half-lives before ibutilide infusion and for 4 hours after. ■ Incidence of arrhythmia may be increased with other drugs that prolong the QT interval (e.g., phenothiazines [e.g., promethazine (Phenergan)], tricyclic antidepressants [e.g., amitriptyline (Elavil)], tetracyclic antidepressants [e.g., maprotiline (Ludiomil)]). ■ Monitor serum digoxin levels to avoid digoxin toxicity. ■ Use with digoxin, beta blockers, or calcium channel blockers does not alter safety or effectiveness of ibutilide. However, sotalol is a beta-blocker, and its use with ibutilide is restricted because it has Class III antiarrhythmic activity; see first sentence above.

SIDE EFFECTS

Sustained polymorphic VT (1.7%) and nonsustained polymorphic VT (2.7%) can deteriorate into ventricular fibrillation and be fatal. May cause many other arrhythmias (e.g., first-, second-, or third-degree AV block [1.5%], bradycardia [1.2%], bundle branch block [1.9%], nonsustained monomorphic VT [4.9%], prolonged QT segment [1.2%], PVCs [5.1%], tachycardia [2.7%]), CHF (0.5%), headache (3.6%), hypertension (1.2%), hypotension (2%), nausea (1.9%), palpitation (1%).

Overdose: Side effects exaggerated with overdose in humans. Acute overdose in animals resulted in CNS depression, rapid gasping breathing, convulsions.

ANTIDOTE

If proarrhythmias occur, discontinue ibutilide; correct electrolyte abnormalities (e.g., potassium and magnesium). Overdrive cardiac pacing, electrical cardioversion, or defibrillation may be required. Infusions of magnesium sulfate may be helpful. Avoid treatment with antiarrhythmic agents. VT that deteriorates to VF will require immediate defibrillation.

IDARUBICIN HYDROCHLORIDE

(eye-dah-roob′ih-sin hye-droe-klor′id)

Antineoplastic (antibiotic)

Idamycin, Idamycin PFS, IDR

pH 5 to 7

USUAL DOSE

Adult acute myeloid leukemia (AML) induction therapy:

Induction: Idarubicin 12 mg/M²/day for 3 days. Used in combination with cytarabine (Ara-C). Cytarabine 100 mg/M²/day may be given as a continuous infusion on days 1 to 7 (daily for 7 days), or alternately the cytarabine may be given as an IV injection of 25 mg/M² followed immediately by a continuous infusion of cytarabine 200 mg/M²/day on days 1 to 5 (daily for 5 days). See Precautions/Monitor. If unequivocal evidence of leukemia remains after the first course, a second course may be given; see Dose Adjustments.

DOSE ADJUSTMENTS

Delay second course until full recovery if mucositis has occurred and reduce dose by 25%. ■ Consider dose reductions in impaired liver and kidney function based on bilirubin and/or creatinine levels above the normal range. Do not administer if bilirubin above 5 mg/dl.

DILUTION

Specific techniques required (see Precautions). Idamycin PFS is a liquid formulation; each 5 mg of powdered idamycin must be reconstituted with 5 ml of nonbacteriostatic NS for injection (1 mg/ml). Use extreme caution inserting the needle; vial contents are under negative pressure. Avoid any possibility of inhalation from aerosol or any skin contamination.

Storage: PFS product must be refrigerated. Reconstituted idamycin is stable for 7 days under refrigeration (2° to 8° C [36° to 46° F]) or 3 days (72 hours) at room temperature (15° to 30° C [59° to 86° F]). Discard unused solution appropriately.

INCOMPATIBLE WITH

Manufacturer states, "Should not be mixed with other drugs unless specific compatibility data are available," and lists as incompatible with heparin. Prolonged contact with solutions of an alkaline pH (e.g., sodium lactate, sodium bicarbonate) will result in degradation of idarubicin.

COMPATIBLE WITH

Consult pharmacist; specific conditions may apply; see Compatibilities, p. xvi.

Y-site: Amifostine (Ethyol), amikacin (Amikin), aztreonam (Azactam), cimetidine (Tagamet), cladribine (Leustatin), cyclophosphamide (Cytoxan), cytarabine (ARA-C), diphenhydramine (Benadryl), droperidol (Inapsine), erythromycin lactobionate (Erythrocin), etoposide phosphate (Etopophos), filgrastim (Neupogen), gemcitabine (Gemzar), granisetron (Kytril), imipenem-cilastatin (Primaxin), magnesium sulfate, mannitol, melphalan (Alkeran), metoclopramide (Reglan), potassium chloride (KCl), ranitidine (Zantac), sargramostim (Leukine), thiotepa (Thioplex), vinorelbine (Navelbine).

RATE OF ADMINISTRATION

A single dose of properly diluted medication over 10 to 15 minutes through Y-tube or three-way stopcock of a free-flowing infusion of D5W or NS.

ACTIONS

A highly toxic, synthetic, antibiotic, antineoplastic agent. An analog of daunorubicin. Rapidly distributed; has an increased rate of cellular uptake compared to other anthracyclines. It inhibits synthesis of DNA and interacts with the enzyme topoisomerase II. Results in a greater number of remissions and longer survival than previous protocols (daunorubicin and cytarabine). Extensive extrahepatic metabolism. It is severely immunosuppressive. Half-life averages 20 to 22 hours. Slowly excreted in bile and urine.

INDICATIONS AND USES

Treatment of acute myeloid leukemia (AML) in adults in combination with other approved antileukemic drugs.

Unlabeled uses: Treatment of acute lymphoblastic leukemia in pediatric patients; see Maternal/Child.

CONTRAINDICATIONS

Not absolute; pre-existing bone marrow suppression, impaired cardiac function, pre-existing infection; see Precautions/Monitor.

PRECAUTIONS

Follow guidelines for handling cytotoxic agents. See Appendix A, p. 1142. ■ Administered by or under the direction of the physician specialist, with facilities for monitoring the patient and responding to any medical emergency. ■ For IV use only. Do not give IM or SC. ■ Use extreme caution in pre-existing drug-induced bone marrow suppression, existing heart disease, previous treatment with other anthracyclines (e.g., daunorubicin), other cardiotoxic agents (e.g., bleomycin), or radiation therapy encompassing the heart. ■ Myocardial toxicity may cause potentially fatal acute congestive heart failure, acute life-threatening arrhythmias, or other cardiomyopathies. ■ Use with caution in patients with hepatic or renal dysfunction. Metabolism and excretion of idarubicin may be impaired; see Dose Adjustments.

Monitor: Determine absolute patency of vein. A stinging or burning sensation indicates extravasation, but extravasation may occur without stinging or burning; severe cellulitis and tissue necrosis will result. Discontinue injection; use another vein. ■ Monitoring of WBCs, RBCs, platelet count, liver function, kidney function, ECG, chest x-ray, echocardiography, and systolic ejection fraction indicated before and during therapy. ■ Severe myelosuppression occurs with effective therapeutic doses. Observe closely for all signs of infection or bleeding. ■ Monitor for thrombocytopenia (platelet count less than $50,000/mm^3$). Initiate precautions to prevent excessive bleeding (e.g., inspect IV sites, skin, and mucous membranes; use extreme care during invasive procedures; test urine, emesis, stool, and secretions for occult blood). ■ Prophylactic antibiotics may be indicated pending results of C/S in a febrile neutropenic patient. ■ Prophylactic antiemetics may reduce nausea and vomiting and increase patient comfort. ■ Monitor uric acid levels; maintain hydration; allopurinol may be indicated. ■ See Precautions.

Patient Education: Nonhormonal birth control recommended. ■ Report IV site burning or stinging promptly. ■ See Appendix D, p. 1148.

Maternal/Child: Category D: avoid pregnancy. May produce teratogenic effects on the fetus. Contraceptive measures indicated during childbearing years. ■ Discontinue breast-feeding before taking idarubicin. ■ Safety and efficacy for use in children not established but has been used; consult literature.

Elderly: Cardiotoxicity or myelotoxicity may be more severe. Patients over 60 years of age who were undergoing induction experienced CHF, serious arrhythmias, chest pain, myocardial infarction, and asymptomatic declines in left ventricular ejection fraction more frequently than younger patients. ■ Monitor renal, hepatic, and hematologic functions closely.

DRUG/LAB INTERACTIONS

Bone marrow toxicity is additive with other chemotherapeutic agents. ■ Risk of cardiotoxicity increased in patients previously treated with maximum cumulative doses of other anthracyclines (e.g., doxorubicin [Adriamycin], mitoxantrone [Novantrone]) and/or radiation encompassing the heart. ■ Leukopenic and/or thrombocytopenic effects may be increased with drugs that cause blood dyscrasias (e.g., anticonvulsants [e.g., carbamazepine (Tegretol), phenytoin (Dilantin)], NSAIDs [e.g., ibuprofen (Advil, Motrin), naproxen (Aleve, Naprosyn)]). Adjust dose based on differential and platelet count. ■ Do not administer live vaccines to patients receiving antineoplastic drugs. ■ See Precautions/Monitor.

SIDE EFFECTS

Acute congestive heart failure, alopecia (reversible), arrhythmias, bone marrow suppression (marked with average doses), cramping, decrease in systolic ejection fraction, depressed QRS voltage, diarrhea, erythema and tissue necrosis (if extravasation occurs), fever, headache, hemorrhage (severe), hepatic function changes, infection, mucositis, myocarditis, nausea, pericarditis, renal function changes, seizures, skin rash, urticaria (local), vomiting.

ANTIDOTE

Most side effects will be tolerated or treated symptomatically. Keep physician informed. Close monitoring of bone marrow, ECG, chest x-ray, echocardiography, and systolic ejection fraction may prevent most serious and potentially fatal side effects. There is no specific antidote, but adequate supportive care including platelet transfusions, antibiotics, and symptomatic treatment of mucositis is required. For extravasation, elevate the extremity and apply intermittent ice packs over the area immediately and 4 times a day for ½ hour. Continue for 3 days. Consider aspiration of as much infiltrated drug as possible, flooding of the site with NS, and injection of hydrocortisone sodium succinate (Solu-Cortef) throughout extravasated tissue. Use a 27- or 25-gauge needle. Site should be observed promptly by a reconstructive surgeon. If ulceration begins or there is severe persistent pain at the site, early wide excision of the involved area will be considered. Hemodialysis or peritoneal dialysis probably not effective in overdose.

IFOSFAMIDE

(eye-fos′fah-myd)

Antineoplastic
(alkylating agent/nitrogen mustard)

Ifex

pH 6

USUAL DOSE

1.2 Gm/M^2/day for 5 consecutive days. Repeat every 3 weeks as hematologic recovery permits. To initiate this protocol, platelets must be above 100,000/mm^3 and WBCs must be above 4,000/mm^3. To prevent hemorrhagic cystitis, a protector such as mesna should be administered with every dose. Ifosfamide dose has been mixed with the initial mesna dose each day in the same solution. Appears to be compatible.

DOSE ADJUSTMENTS

Reduced dose may be required for adrenalectomized patients and in renal or hepatic impairment. Adequate data not available. ■ Severe myelosuppression is frequent, especially when ifosfamide is given with other chemotherapeutic agents. Dose adjustments of all agents may be required.

DILUTION

Specific techniques required; see Precautions. Each 1 Gm must be diluted with 20 ml SW or bacteriostatic water for injection (parabens or benzyl alcohol preserved only). Shake solution to dissolve. May be further diluted with D5W, NS, LR, or SW for injection. 1 Gm in 20 ml equals 50 mg/ml; 1 Gm in 50 ml equals 20 mg/ml; 1 Gm in 200 ml equals 5 mg/ml (additional diluent recommended by some researchers to reduce side effects). Available in a kit containing ifosfamide and mesna.

Storage: Store dry powder at room temperature, never above 40° C (104° F). Diluted solution may be stored at room temperature up to 1 week except for solutions prepared with SW for injection without preservatives. These must be refrigerated and used within 6 hours.

COMPATIBLE WITH

Consult pharmacist; specific conditions may apply; see Compatibilities, p. xvi.

Additive: Carboplatin (Paraplatin), cisplatin (Platinol), epirubicin (Ellence, Pharmorubicin), etoposide (VePesid), fluorouracil (5-FU), mesna (Mesnex).

Syringe: Epirubicin (Ellence, Pharmorubicin), mesna (Mesnex).

Y-site: Allopurinol (Aloprim, Zyloprim), amifostine (Ethyol), amphotericin B cholesteryl (Amphotec), aztreonam (Azactam), doxorubicin liposome (Doxil), etoposide phosphate (Etopophos), filgrastim (Neupogen), fludarabine (Fludara), gatifloxacin (Tequin), gemcitabine (Gemzar), granisetron (Kytril), linezolid (Zyvox), melphalan (Alkeran), ondansetron (Zofran), paclitaxel (Taxol), piperacillin/tazobactam (Zosyn), propofol (Diprivan), sargramostim (Leukine), sodium bicarbonate, teniposide (Vumon), thiotepa (Thioplex), topotecan (Hycamtin), vinorelbine (Navelbine).

RATE OF ADMINISTRATION

A single dose over a minimum of 30 minutes as an infusion. Extend administration time based on amount of diluent and patient condition.

ACTIONS

An alkylating agent. A synthetic analog of cyclophosphamide chemically related to the nitrogen mustard group. An inert compound; metabolic activation by microsomal liver enzymes is required to produce biologically active metabolites. These alkylated metabolites interact with DNA to effect regression in the size of malignant tumors. Elimination half-life for a usual dose is 7 to 15 hours. Larger doses extend half-life. Extensively metabolized (considerable individual variation); this drug or its metabolites are excreted in urine. Secreted in breast milk.

INDICATIONS AND USES

In combination with other specific antineoplastic agents to suppress or retard neoplastic growth in germ cell testicular cancer. Usually used after other chemotherapy protocols have failed.

Unlabeled uses: Lung, breast, ovarian, pancreatic, and gastric cancer; sarcomas; acute leukemias (except acute myelogenous); malignant lymphomas.

CONTRAINDICATIONS

Hypersensitivity to ifosfamide; patients with severely depressed bone marrow function.

PRECAUTIONS

Follow guidelines for handling cytotoxic agents. See Appendix A, p. 1142. ■ Usually administered by or under the direction of the physician specialist. ■ Use caution in impaired renal function; may increase CNS toxicity. Use caution in patients with compromised bone marrow reserve (e.g., leukopenia, granulocytopenia, extensive bone marrow metastases, prior radiation therapy, treatment with other cytotoxic agents) and patients with severe hepatic or renal disease. ■ May interfere with normal wound healing. Consider waiting 5 to 7 days or more after a major surgical procedure before beginning treatment.

Monitor: Urinalysis before each dose recommended. Withhold drug if RBCs in urine exceed 10 per high-powered field. Reinstitute after complete resolution. Mesna given concurrently should prevent hemorrhagic cystitis. ■ Differential WBC, platelet count, and hemoglobin are recommended before each daily dose and as clinically indicated. WBC count must be above 2,000/mm^3 and platelet count above 50,000/mm^3. ■ Observe constantly for signs of infection (e.g., fever, sore throat, tiredness) or unusual bleeding or bruising. ■ Monitor for thrombocytopenia (platelet count less than 50,000/mm^3). Initiate precautions to prevent excessive bleeding (e.g., inspect IV sites, skin, and mucous membranes; use extreme care during invasive procedures; test urine, emesis, stool, and secretions for occult blood). ■ Prophylactic antibiotics may be indicated pending results of C/S in a febrile neutropenic patient. ■ Adequate hydration required; encourage fluid intake (minimum of 2 L/day) and frequent voiding to prevent cystitis. Bladder irrigation with acetylcysteine (2,000 ml/day) has also been used to prevent hematuria. ■ Prophylactic administration of antiemetics recommended.

Patient Education: Nonhormonal birth control recommended. ■ See Appendix D, p. 1148.

Maternal/Child: Category D: avoid pregnancy. Embryotoxic and teratogenic to the fetus. ■ Discontinue breast-feeding. ■ Safety and effectiveness for use in children not established.

Elderly: Monitor renal, hepatic, and hematologic functions closely.

DRUG/LAB INTERACTIONS

See Dose Adjustments. ■ Because it is a synthetic analog of cyclophosphamide, ifosfamide may share similar interactions with numerous drugs, including allopurinol, antidiabetics, barbiturates, chloramphenicol, corticosteroids, succinylcholine, thiazide diuretics, and other alkylating agents to produce potentially serious reactions. ■ Do not administer live vaccine to patients receiving antineoplastic drugs.

SIDE EFFECTS

Hematuria, hemorrhagic cystitis, and bone marrow depression are dose-limiting side effects. Alopecia, anorexia, confusion, constipation, diarrhea, depressive psychosis with hallucinations, nausea, somnolence, and vomiting occur frequently. Allergic reactions, cardiotoxicity, coagulopathy, coma, cranial nerve dysfunction, dermatitis, dizziness, disorientation, fatigue, fever of unknown origin, hematuria, hemorrhagic cystitis, hypertension, hypotension, infection, liver dysfunction, leukopenia, malaise, neutropenia, phlebitis, polyneuropathy, pulmonary symptoms, thrombocytopenia, or seizures may occur.

ANTIDOTE

Minor side effects will be treated symptomatically if necessary. Discontinue ifosfamide and notify physician immediately if hematuria, hemorrhagic cystitis, confusion, coma, WBC below 2,000/mm^3, or platelets below 50,000/mm^3 occur. Administration of whole blood products (e.g., packed RBCs, platelets, leukocytes) and/or blood modifiers (e.g., darbepoetin alfa [Aranesp], epoetin alfa [Epogen, Procrit], filgrastim [Neupogen], pegfilgrastim [Neulasta], sargramostim [Leukine], oprelvekin [Neumega]) may be indicated to treat bone marrow suppression. There is no specific antidote. Supportive therapy as indicated will help sustain the patient in toxicity. May respond to hemodialysis.

IMIGLUCERASE

(em-ee-glue′sir-ace)

Cerezyme

Enzyme replenisher (glucocerebrosidase)

pH 6.1

USUAL DOSE

Adults and children over 2 years of age: Individualized to each patient based on the severity of illness and patient response. Initial doses range from 2.5 units/kg 3 times a week to 60 units/kg every 2 weeks. Imiglucerase should be given at least every 4 weeks or symptoms and condition may relapse to pretreatment status. Patients beginning imiglucerase therapy are usually given higher-range initial doses for a limited time to stabilize their disease. Patients with very severe Gaucher's disease also may require higher-range initial doses and/or increased frequency because they have accumulated more lipid throughout their bodies, requiring more enzyme to remove the excess stored lipid and bring their disease under control. Some clinicians recommend a test dose; see Rate of Administration.

DOSE ADJUSTMENTS

To utilize each bottle fully and reduce waste, a single dose may be increased or decreased slightly as long as the total monthly dose remains unaltered. ■ After patient response is well established (disease symptoms lessen and the accumulated lipid is reduced), the dose may be adjusted downward to achieve the optimal individualized maintenance dose. Usually progressively lowered at 3- to 6-month intervals while response parameters are closely monitored. Optimal goal is to establish the lowest dose that is effective in maintaining control of the disease and preventing recurrence of symptoms for each patient.

DILUTION

Available in 200-unit and 400-unit vials.

Weight in kg × dose/kg desired ÷ 200 or 400 (units/vial) = # of vials required

A 60-kg man requiring 60 units/kg would require 3,600 units. Number of vials required would be 18 vials at 200 units/vial or 9 vials at 400 units/vial.

Adjust number of vials up or down within monthly dose requirement to fully utilize each vial. Manufacturer has a large plasticized dosing chart/kg to determine vials required for various desired doses. After patient is weighed and appropriate dose is calculated, remove sufficient vials from refrigerator and warm to room temperature. Each 200-unit vial must be diluted with 5.1 ml of SW without preservatives. Each 400-unit vial must be diluted with 10.2 ml. Both equal 40 units/ml. Gently swirl to mix the solution. Do not shake. Let stand for several minutes to allow product to dissolve and bubbles to dissipate. Withdraw exactly 5 ml from the 200-unit vial or 10 ml from the 400-unit vial. A total dose must be further diluted with NS to a volume of 100 to 200 ml. Minimum adequate dilution requires at least 1 or more ml diluent to each 1 ml of imiglucerase. Do not use if discolored or opaque or if particulate matter is present. After dilution, slight flocculation (thin translucent fibers) may occur. The diluted solution may be filtered during administration; see Rate of Administration.

Storage: Refrigerate before use. Do not use after expiration date on bottle. Return of unsuitable vials (reconstituted, before reconstitution, or expired) may be authorized; call 1-800-745-4447. Contains no preservative; do not store opened vials for future use. Should be promptly diluted after reconstitution but has been shown to be stable after reconstitution for up to 12 hours at CRT or under refrigeration. Diluted solutions stable for up to 24 hours under refrigeration.

COMPATIBILITY

Specific information not available. Consider specific use; consult pharmacist.

RATE OF ADMINISTRATION

Use of an inline, low–protein binding, 0.2-micron filter is recommended. Use of a microdrip (60 gtt/ml) or an infusion pump helpful. Flush the IV line with NS at the end of the infusion to ensure the total dose is received.

Test dose: Administer at prescribed rate (0.5 to 1 unit/kg/min) for 5 minutes. Take vital signs and assess patient for symptoms of allergic reaction.

Full dose: A single dose equally distributed over 1 to 2 hours.

ACTIONS

An analog of the human enzyme beta-glucocerebrosidase produced by recombinant DNA technology. Gaucher's disease is characterized by a functional deficiency in beta-glucocerebrosidase enzymatic activity and the resultant accumulation of lipid glucocerebroside in tissue macrophages (Gaucher's cells). These cells are found in the liver, spleen, bone marrow, and occasionally in the lung, kidney, and intestine. Imiglucerase acts like glucocerebrosidase to facilitate the release of the lipid glucocerebrosides. Effective in controlling and actually reversing disease symptoms. Increase in appetite and energy level and improvement in hemoglobin are often the first observable effects and may occur in 2 to 4 months. Cachexia and wasting in children are reduced. Within 6 months splenomegaly and hepatomegaly are significantly reduced, and hemoglobin, hematocrit, erythrocyte, and platelet counts improved. Replenishment of bone marrow and improving mineralization of bone may take several years.

INDICATIONS AND USES

Long-term enzyme replacement therapy for patients with confirmed diagnosis of type I Gaucher's disease, with signs and symptons severe enough to result in one or more of the following conditions: moderate-to-severe anemia, thrombocytopenia, bone disease, hepatomegaly, or splenomegaly. Studies are being conducted to see if dose can be lowered without decreasing effectiveness. Treatment costs (more than $150,000/yr) could be markedly reduced with lower doses.

CONTRAINDICATIONS

None known. Reevaluate if there is significant clinical evidence of hypersensitivity to imiglucerase.

PRECAUTIONS

Effective only via IV route. ■ Should be used under the direction of a physician knowledgeable in the management of Gaucher's disease. ■ A recombinant product; risk of transmission of any bacterial, mycoplasmal, fungal, or viral agent is remote. ■ Approximately 15% of patients have developed IgG antibodies. Most patients who develop antibodies to imiglucerase do so within 12 months of treatment. Patients with antibodies to imiglucerase are at increased risk for developing allergic reactions. Monitor periodically for IgG antibody formation during first year of therapy. ■ Use caution in patients who have had hypersensitivity reaction to alglucerase (Ceredase). ■ Anaphylactoid reactions have been reported. Administer further treatment with caution; see Antidote. ■ Pulmonary hypertension has been reported. It is a known complication of Gaucher's disease and has been observed in these patients whether or not they are receiving imiglucerase. Evaluate patients with respiratory symptoms for the presence of pulmonary hypertension.

Monitor: Evaluation of hemoglobin, hematocrit, platelets, WBC, acid phosphatase (AP), plasma glucocerebroside, liver and/or spleen size, and bone changes are required before and during therapy. Frequency determined by patient response; more frequent when determining response to initial dose and when dose is being adjusted (i.e., every 3 to 6 months). Blood tests will be done more frequently, since anemia is the first symptom to improve. ■ Monitor weight before each dose (used to calculate dose) and monitor vital signs. ■ MRI provides the best evaluation of liver and spleen. ■ Standard x-rays provide adequate evaluation of bone changes. ■ Observe patient closely for signs of improvement (e.g., increased energy, reduced bleeding tendency, reduction in size of liver and/or spleen, reduced joint swelling, reduced bone pain). ■ See Precautions.

Patient Education: Treatment required for life. No longer than 1 month should elapse between treatments, or symptoms and condition may relapse to the pretreatment state.

Maternal/Child: Category C: use in pregnancy only if clearly needed. No studies available on fetal harm or reproductive capacity. ■ Safety for use during breast-feeding not established. Not known if imiglucerase is secreted in breast milk. ■ Has been used in children under 2 years of age, but safety and effectiveness have not been established.

Elderly: Specific information not available in product information.

DRUG/LAB INTERACTIONS

None indicated. Specific information not available.

SIDE EFFECTS

Children 2 to 12 years: Coughing, dyspnea, fever, flushing, nausea, and vomiting were most commonly reported.

Adolescents 13 to 16 years and adults: Headache, pruritus, and rash were most commonly reported. In addition, abdominal discomfort, backache, burning, discomfort, and pruritus at injection site, chills, decreased urinary frequency, diarrhea, dizziness, fatigue, fever, hypotension (mild), nausea, peripheral edema (transient), swelling or sterile abscess at venipuncture site, and tachycardia were reported. A protein immune reaction may develop. Side effects may improve with continued therapy because antibody levels decrease. Hypersensitivity reactions (e.g., anaphylaxis, angioedema, chest discomfort, cyanosis, flushing, hypotension, pruritus, rash, respiratory symptoms, urticaria) have occurred.

ANTIDOTE

Keep physician informed of side effects; may be treated symptomatically if indicated. Discontinue imiglucerase for clinical evidence of hypersensitivity. Patients have successfully continued therapy after pretreatment with antihistamines (e.g., diphenhydramine [Benadryl]) and/or corticosteroids (e.g., dexamethasone [Decadron]) and a reduction in rate of administration. Treat anaphylaxis as necessary.

IMIPENEM-CILASTATIN

(em-ee-pen′em sigh-lah-stat′in)

Primaxin

Antibacterial (carbapenem)

pH 6.5 to 8.5

USUAL DOSE

Range is from 250 mg to 1 Gm every 6 to 8 hours. Dose based on severity of disease, susceptibility of pathogens, condition of the patient, age, weight, and CrCl. Adult doses are limited to patients with a CrCl equal to or greater than 71 ml/min/1.73 M^2 and a body weight equal to or greater than 70 kg. Because of high antimicrobial activity, do not exceed the lower of 50 mg/kg of body weight/24 hr or 4 Gm/24 hr in adults or children. Continue for at least 2 days after all symptoms of infection subside.

Imipenem-Cilastatin Dosing Guidelines

Type or Severity of Infection	Fully Susceptible Organisms	Total Daily Dose	Moderately Susceptible Organisms	Total Daily Dose
Mild	250 mg q 6 hr	1 Gm	500 mg q 6 hr	2 Gm
Moderate	500 mg q 8 hr or 500 mg q 6 hr	1.5 Gm 2 Gm	500 mg q 6 hr or 1 Gm q 8 hr	2 Gm 3 Gm
Severe/life-threatening	500 mg q 6 hr	2 Gm	1 Gm q 8 hr or 1 Gm q 6 hr	3 Gm 4 Gm
Uncomplicated UTI	250 mg q 6 hr	1 Gm	250 mg q 6 hr	1 Gm
Complicated UTI	500 mg q 6 hr	2 Gm	500 mg q 6 hr	2 Gm

PEDIATRIC DOSE

Not recommended for use in pediatric patients with CNS infections because of the risk of seizures, or in pediatric patients weighing less than 30 kg with impaired renal function (no data available).

Infants 3 months of age or less, weight over 1,500 Gm: For non-CNS infections:

Less than 1 week of age: 25 mg/kg every 12 hours.

1 to 4 weeks of age: 25 mg/kg every 8 hours.

4 weeks to 3 months of age: 25 mg/kg every 6 hours.

Premature infants weighing from 670 to 1,890 Gm in the first week of life were given 20 mg/kg every 12 hours in one study (see package insert).

Infants and children over 3 months of age: For non-CNS infections: 15 to 25 mg/kg/dose every 6 hours. See statements in Usual Dose. Maximum dose is 2 Gm/day for treatment of infections caused by fully susceptible organisms and 4 Gm/day for moderately susceptible organisms.

Older children with cystic fibrosis and normal renal function: Higher doses up to 90 mg/kg/day have been used.

DOSE ADJUSTMENTS

Dose adjustments are extensive and required for all patients weighing less than 70 kg, as well as all patients with a CrCl less than 71 ml/min/1.73 M^2.

Dose adjustments also vary based on total daily dose required (e.g., 1, 1.5, 2, 3, or 4 Gm). See charts in package insert. ■ Reduced doses may be required in the elderly based on weight and/or decreased renal function. ■ Cleared by hemodialysis; administer after hemodialysis and at 12-hour intervals thereafter. ■ See Precautions/Monitor and Drug/Lab Interactions.

DILUTION

Reconstitute each single dose with 10 ml of compatible infusion solutions (e.g., D5W, D10W, NS [see chart on inside back cover or literature]); also compatible in D5W with 0.15% KCL and mannitol 5% and 10%. Shake well and transfer the resulting suspension to 100 ml of the same infusion solution. Repeat reconstitution process with an additional 10 ml of infusion solution to ensure complete transfer of vial contents to the infusion solution. Agitate until clear. Also available in ADD-Vantage vials for use with ADD-Vantage infusion containers, monovial vials, and in 120-ml infusion bottles for one-step dilution.

Neonatal dilution: Use preservative-free solutions for reconstitution of neonatal doses.

Storage: Store dry powder at CRT. Diluted solutions are stable at room temperature for 4 hours after preparation or 24 hours if refrigerated. Do not freeze.

INCOMPATIBLE WITH

Manufacturer states, "Should not be mixed with or physically added to other antibiotics." See Drug/Lab Interactions.

COMPATIBLE WITH (Underline Indicates Conflicting Compatibility Information)

Consult pharmacist; specific conditions may apply; see Compatibilities, p. xvi.

Y-site: Acyclovir (Zovirax), amifostine (Ethyol), aztreonam (Azactam), cefepime (Maxipime), cisatracurium (Nimbex), diltiazem (Cardizem), docetaxel (Taxotere), famotidine (Pepcid IV), <u>filgrastim (Neupogen)</u>, fludarabine (Fludara), foscarnet (Foscavir), gatifloxacin (Tequin), granisetron (Kytril), idarubicin (Idamycin), insulin (regular), linezolid (Zyvox), melphalan (Alkeran), methotrexate (Folex), ondansetron (Zofran), propofol (Diprivan), remifentanil (Ultiva), tacrolimus (Prograf), teniposide (Vumon), thiotepa (Thioplex), vinorelbine (Navelbine), zidovudine (AZT, Retrovir).

RATE OF ADMINISTRATION

Intermittent IV: Each 500 mg or fraction thereof over 20 to 30 minutes. Doses greater than 500 mg should be infused over 40 to 60 minutes. Slow infusion rate if patient develops nausea and vomiting, dizziness, hypotension, or sweating. May be given through Y-tube or three-way stopcock of infusion set.

ACTIONS

A potent broad-spectrum antibacterial agent. Imipenem is a carbapenem antibiotic, and cilastatin sodium inhibits its renal metabolism. Both components are present in equal amounts. Bactericidal to many gram-negative, gram-positive, and anaerobic organisms. Bactericidal activity results from the inhibition of bacterial wall synthesis. Effective against many otherwise resistant organisms. Has a high dose of stability in the presence of beta-lactamases produced by gram-negative and gram-positive bacteria. Rapidly and widely distributed into many body fluids and tissues. Metabolized by the kidneys. Half-life is approximately 1 hour. Excreted in the urine. May cross the placental barrier.

INDICATIONS AND USES

Treatment of serious lower respiratory tract, urinary tract, skin and skin structure, bone and joint, gynecologic, intraabdominal, and polymicrobic infections; bacterial septicemia, and endocarditis. Most effective against specific organisms (see literature).

Unlabeled uses: Treatment of febrile neutropenia and melioidosis (a rare infection in humans and animals).

CONTRAINDICATIONS

Known sensitivity to any component of this product. ■ See Maternal/Child and Precautions.

PRECAUTIONS

Specific sensitivity studies are indicated to determine susceptibility of the causative organism to imipenem-cilastatin. ■ Use extreme caution in patients with a history of allergic reactions, especially to other beta-lactam antibiotics. Cross sensitivity is possible. ■ Avoid prolonged use of drug; superinfection caused by overgrowth of nonsusceptible organisms may result. ■ CNS adverse effects, including seizures, have been reported. Incidence increases with higher doses, compromised renal function, or pre-existing CNS disorders. ■ For patients on hemodialysis, benefits of use must outweigh risk of seizures. ■ Not recommended in patients with a CrCl less than 5 ml/min/1.73 M^2 unless hemodialysis is instituted within 48 hours. ■ Pseudomembranous colitis has been reported. May range from mild to life-threatening. Consider in patients that present with diarrhea during or after treatment with imipenem-cilastatin. ■ Safety and effectiveness for use in meningitis not established. ■ See Maternal/Child.

Monitor: May cause thrombophlebitis. Use small needles and large veins, and rotate infusion sites. ■ Electrolyte imbalance and cardiac irregularities resulting from sodium content are possible. Contains 3.2 mEq of sodium/Gm. ■ Monitor renal, hepatic, and hemopoietic systems in prolonged therapy. ■ See Drug/Lab Interactions.

Maternal/Child: Category C: use only if absolutely necessary in pregnancy and breast-feeding.

Elderly: Consider weight and age-related renal impairment. See Dose Adjustments. ■ Response similar to that seen in younger patients; however, greater sensitivity in the elderly cannot be ruled out.

DRUG/LAB INTERACTIONS

May be used concomitantly with aminoglycosides and other antibiotics, but these drugs must never be mixed in the same infusion or given concurrently. ■ Use with ganciclovir (Cytovene) may cause generalized seizures. Use only if benefit outweighs risk. ■ Half-life and plasma levels slightly increased by probenecid. Avoid concurrent use. ■ Concurrent use with cyclosporine (Sandimmune) may increase side effects of both drugs.

SIDE EFFECTS

Full scope of allergic reactions including anaphylaxis. Abdominal pain; abnormal clotting time; altered CBC and electrolytes; anuria; burning, discomfort, and pain at injection site; confusion; diarrhea; dizziness; dyspnea; elevated alkaline phosphotase, AST (SGOT), ALT (SGPT), bilirubin, creatinine, BUN, and LDH; fever; gastroenteritis; glossitis; headache; heartburn; hemorrhagic colitis; hyperventilation; hypotension; increased salivation; myoclonus; nausea and vomiting; paresthesia; pharyngeal pain; polyarthralgia; polyuria; positive direct Coombs' test; presence of WBCs or RBCs, protein, casts, bilirubin, or urobilinogen in urine; pseudomembranous colitis; seizures; somnolence; thrombophlebitis; tinnitus; tongue papillar hypertrophy; transient hearing loss in the hearing impaired; vertigo; and many others.

ANTIDOTE

Notify physician of any side effects. Discontinue the drug if indicated. Treat allergic reaction as indicated with epinephrine (Adrenalin); antihistamines (e.g., diphenhydramine [Benadryl]), and/or corticosteroids (e.g., dexamethasone, hydrocortisone). Resuscitate as necessary. Begin anticonvulsants if focal tremors, myoclonus, or seizures occur. If symptoms continue, decrease dose or discontinue the drug. Infusion rate reactions (e.g., dizziness, hypotension, N/V, and sweating) may respond to a decrease in rate of infusion. Mild cases of colitis may respond to discontinuation of drug. Oral vancomycin or metronidazole (Flagyl) are the treatment of choice for antibiotic-related pseudomembranous colitis. Hemodialysis may be useful in overdose.

IMMUNE GLOBULIN INTRAVENOUS

(im-myoun′ gloh′byou-lin IV)

Immunizing agent (passive)
Platelet count stimulator
Antibacterial
Antiviral
Antipolyneuropathy agent

Gamimune N, Gammagard SD, Gammar P-IV, IGIV, Iveegam, Panglobulin, Polygam SD, Sandoglobulin, Venoglobulin-S

pH 4 to 7.2

USUAL DOSE

PRIMARY IMMUNODEFICIENCY DISEASES

Gamimune N: 100 to 200 mg/kg (2 to 4 ml/kg) as a single-dose IV infusion. May be repeated monthly if indicated. If adequate IgG levels in the circulation or clinical response not achieved, may be increased to 400 mg/kg (8 ml/kg), or a lesser dose may be given more frequently.

Gammagard SD, Polygam SD: 200 to 400 mg/kg of body weight as a single-dose IV infusion. Repeat at least 100 mg/kg monthly.

Gammar P-IV: 200 to 400 mg/kg as a single-dose IV infusion every 3 to 4 weeks. Up to 600 mg/kg may be required. High-end doses may be given initially and for several doses at more frequent intervals based on individual patient response and adequate IgG levels. Reduce dose 100 to 200 mg/kg and/or increase interval when therapeutic IgG levels are achieved.

Iveegam: 200 mg/kg/month as a single-dose IV infusion. If adequate IgG levels in the circulation or clinical response are not achieved, may be increased up to 800 mg/kg or intervals shortened. Do not exceed 800 mg/kg/month.

Panglobulin, Sandoglobulin: 200 mg/kg as a single-dose IV infusion. May be repeated monthly if indicated. If adequate IgG levels in the circulation or clinical response are not achieved, may be given more frequently or increased to 300 mg/kg monthly.

Continued

Venoglobulin-S: 200 mg/kg monthly. If adequate IgG levels in the circulation or clinical response are not achieved, increase to 300 to 400 mg/kg monthly, or a lesser dose may be given more frequently.

IDIOPATHIC THROMBOCYTOPENIC PURPURA (ITP)

Gamimune N, Panglobulin, Sandoglobulin: 400 mg/kg for 2 to 5 consecutive days based on platelet count and clinical response. If clinically significant bleeding occurs or the platelet count falls below 30,000/mm^3, a maintenance dose of 400 mg/kg may be given as a single infusion. If response inadequate, increase to 800 to 1,000 mg/kg. May be given intermittently to maintain platelet count. ***Gamimune N*** 1 Gm/kg may be given as an alternate regimen for induction therapy. Do not use in expanded fluid volume or when fluid volume is a concern. May be repeated the next day only if an adequate increase in the platelet count does not occur from the initial dose.

Gammagard SD, Polygam SD: 1 Gm/kg. Up to 3 doses can be given on alternate days based on clinical response and platelet count.

Venoglobulin-S: Total dose of 2 Gm/kg distributed over 5 days. If clinically significant bleeding occurs or the platelet count falls below 30,000/mm^3, a maintenance dose of 1 Gm/kg may be given as needed to maintain platelet count above 20,000/mm^3 in adults and 30,000/mm^3 in children.

B-CELL CHRONIC LYMPHOCYTIC LEUKEMIA (CLL)

Gammagard SD, Polygam SD: 400 mg/kg every 3 to 4 weeks.

PREVENTION OF INFECTION IN BONE MARROW TRANSPLANT PATIENTS

Gamimune-N: Indicated only in transplant patients over 20 years of age. 500 mg/kg of IGIV on day 7 and day 2 pre-transplant (or at time conditioning therapy for transplant is begun). Give the same dose once each week through day 90 post-transplant.

PREVENTION OF BACTERIAL INFECTIONS IN HIV-INFECTED CHILDREN AND ADULTS

Gamimune-N: 400 mg/kg every 28 days.

KAWASAKI SYNDROME

Gammagard SD, Gamimune-N, Polygam SD, Sandoglobulin: 1 Gm/kg as a single dose or 400 mg/kg for 4 consecutive days beginning within 7 days of onset of fever. Concomitantly give aspirin 80 to 100 mg/kg/day equally divided into 4 doses until fever subsides, then 3 to 10 mg/kg/day for 5 weeks or 3 to 5 mg/kg/day for 6 to 8 weeks or longer.

Iveegam, Venoglobulin-S: 2 Gm/kg as a single dose over 10 to 12 hours. If symptoms persist an additional 2 Gm/kg dose may be given over 10 to 12 hours. Alternately ***Iveegam*** may be given at 400 mg/kg/day for 4 days. Initiate within 10 days of onset of disease. Concomitantly give aspirin 80 to 100 mg/kg/day equally divided into 4 doses through the 14th day after the onset of symptoms or until fever subsides, then 3 to 10 mg/kg/day for 5 weeks or 3 to 5 mg/kg/day for 6 to 8 weeks or longer. Same regimen may be repeated if symptoms persist or recur due to active Kawasaki disease.

PEDIATRIC DOSE

See mg/kg or Gm/kg dose recommendations under Usual Dose. With most brands, clinical studies suggested that no difference in dosing is necessary and no special precautions are indicated. According to the manufacturers, infants and neonates were not included in clinical studies for primary immunodeficiency diseases or Kawasaki disease. All age-groups were represented in clinical studies for idiopathic thrombocytopenic purpura.

Another source recommends the following doses, some of which may be unlabeled in the pediatric population:

Primary immunodeficiency disease: 300 to 400 mg/kg monthly. Optimum dose and frequency are determined by monitoring clinical response and IgG trough levels (increases of 300 to 400 mg/dl over initial pretreatment level are considered ideal).

Idiopathic thrombocytopenic purpura (ITP): ***Initial therapy for acute ITP:*** 0.8 to 1 Gm/kg given in 1 or 2 doses. ***Maintenance therapy:*** Individualized for each patient.

Kawasaki disease: 2 Gm/kg as a single dose over 10 to 12 hours or 400 mg/kg daily on four consecutive days. Start within 10 days of illness. Treatment should include aspirin (see Usual Dose).

Pediatric HIV infection: 400 mg/kg every 28 days.

Bone marrow transplantation: 500 mg/kg on day 7 and day 2 pre-transplant. Repeat 500 mg/kg once each week through day 90 post-transplant. May reduce incidence of infection and death; does not decrease graft-versus-host disease.

Low-birth-weight infants (less than 1,500 Gm): Variable. 500 mg/kg has been used each week or three times in the first week of life and then weekly (target IgG around 700 mg/dl). Not recommended for routine use in preterm infants to prevent late-onset infection.

Parvovirus B19 infection: 400 mg/kg/day for 5 consecutive days or 1 Gm/kg/day for 2 consecutive days.

DILUTION

Absolute sterile technique required at all steps of reconstitution process for each formulation. Gently rotate to dissolve completely. Complete dilution may take up to 20 minutes or longer. For most preparations, filtration is required as drawn into a syringe for administration or as administered through IV tubing. Filtration with filters with larger pore sizes may be used for Panglobulin and Sandoglobulin, but the manufacturer indicates that they are not required. Check each brand for specific equipment. If prepared in a sterile laminar air flow hood, may be pooled into plastic IV infusion bags and refrigerated for up to 24 hours. Mark with date and time of reconstitution and pooling.

Gamimune N: Contains maltose. May be given undiluted (a 5% solution) or may be further diluted with a given amount of D5W to facilitate slow and accurate rate of infusion. Available in 10-, 50-, 100-, 200-, and 250-ml single-dose vials as a 5% solution and in 10-, 50-, 100-, and 200-ml vials as a 10% solution. pH 4 to 4.5.

Gammagard SD, Polygam SD: Must be warmed to room temperature before dilution. Diluent (SW for injection), transfer device, administration set with integral airway, and filter provided with each single-use vial. Available in 2.5-, 5-, and 10-Gm single-dose vials with diluent. Use full amount of diluent (50, 96, 192 ml) to prepare a 5% solution (50 mg/ml) or one half the amount of diluent (25, 48, 96 ml) to prepare a 10% solution (100 mg/ml). Must be used within 2 hours of dilution. pH 6.4 to 7.2.

Gammar P-IV: Contains sucrose; see Precautions. Must be warmed to room temperature before dilution. Diluent (SW for injection) is provided. May provide a transfer device (plastic piercing pin to diluent vial; metal needle to product vial), administration set with integral airway, and filter. Available in 1-, 2.5-, 5-, and 10-Gm single-dose vials with diluent (50 mg/ml) and a bulk pack without diluent. Do not shake to dissolve; rotate or agitate vial. Must be used within 3 hours of dilution. pH 6.4 to 7.2.

Iveegam: Diluent (SW for injection), transfer device, administration set with integral airway, and filter provided with each single-use vial. Available in 0.5-, 1-, 2.5-, and 5-Gm vials with 10, 20, 50, or 100 ml diluent providing 50 mg/ml. Do not shake to dissolve; rotate or agitate vial. Use immediately after dilution. May be further diluted with a given amount of D5W or NS.

Panglobulin: Contains sucrose; see Precautions. Must be warmed to room temperature before dilution. Dilute with NS diluent provided. Makes a 3% solution. Invert so that diluent flows into the IV bottle. Available as 1 (3, 6, or 12) Gm.

Sandoglobulin: Contains sucrose; see Precautions. Must be warmed to room temperature before dilution. Dilute with NS diluent provided. Makes a 3% solution. Invert so that diluent flows into the IV bottle. Available as 1 (3, 6, or 12) Gm with 33 (100 or 200) ml diluent. For a 6% solution use one half diluent provided. Package insert has a chart with dilution requirements for 9% and 12% concentrations. pH 6.4 to 6.8.

Venoglobulin-S: Ready for use as 5% or 10% immune globulin IV in 50, 100, and 200 ml with sterile administration set. pH 5.2 to 5.8.

Storage: Store Gammagard SD, Gammar P-IV, Panglobulin, Polygam SD, Sandoglobulin, and Venoglobulin-S 5% at CRT. Refrigerate Gamimune-N, Iveegam, and Venoglobulin-S 10%. Discard partially used vials. Do not use if turbid or has been frozen.

INCOMPATIBLE WITH

Manufacturers recommend administration through a separate IV line without admixture with other drugs and state, "Do not combine one IGIV product with an IGIV product from another manufacturer." Gamimune N is incompatible with NS.

COMPATIBLE WITH

Consult pharmacist; specific conditions may apply; see Compatibilities, p. xvi.

Solution: ***See Incompatible With.*** Most preparations may be infused sequentially into a primary IV of D5W or NS, or the tubing may be flushed with D5W or NS before and after administration.

Y-site: Fluconazole (Diflucan), sargramostim (Leukine).

RATE OF ADMINISTRATION

Too-rapid infusion may cause a precipitous hypotensive reaction. Decrease rate in patients at risk for thrombotic events and/or neuromuscular disorders. Decrease rate of infusion by one half (5% solution) to one quarter (10% solution) in patients at risk for developing renal dysfunction. See Precautions and specific recommendations below for each product. Decrease rate of infusion at onset of patient discomfort or any adverse reactions; see Antidote. Administer via separate IV tubing with filter or filter needle (provided by most manufacturers). Do not mix with other drugs or IV solutions. An infusion pump will facilitate an accurate rate of administration.

Gamimune N: 0.01 to 0.02 ml/kg/min for the first 30 minutes (0.7 to 1.4 ml/min of undiluted drug for a 70-kg individual). If no discomfort or adverse effects, may be increased to a maximum of 0.08 ml/kg/min. In patients at risk for developing renal dysfunction, maximum flow rate should be less than 0.08 ml/kg/min; see comments under Rate of Administration.

Gammagard SD/Polygam SD: 5% solution 0.5 ml/kg/hr. May be gradually increased to 4 ml/kg/hr if no discomfort or adverse effects. If 5% solution well tolerated at 4 ml/kg/hr, a 10% solution can be used. Begin with 0.5 ml/kg/hr. If no adverse effects, gradually increase up to a maximum of 8 ml/kg/hr. In patients at risk for developing renal dysfunction, the recommended flow rate for 5% concentration is less than 0.27ml/kg/min; the recommended flow rate for 10% concentration is less than 0.13 ml/kg/min.

Gammar P-IV: Contains sucrose; see Precautions. 0.01 ml/kg/min. May be increased to 0.02 ml/kg/min after 15 to 30 minutes. May be gradually increased to 0.03 to 0.06 ml/kg/min if no discomfort or adverse effects. To keep the amount of sucrose infused at less than 3 mg/kg/min in patients at risk for developing renal dysfunction, do not exceed a rate of 0.06 ml IgG/kg/min (1 mg/kg/min).

Iveegam: 1 ml/min. May be increased to a maximum of 2 ml/min in the standard 5% solution. Rate may be adjusted proportionately with further dilution. Note rate for single-dose regimen in Kawasaki disease. In patients at risk for developing renal dysfunction, the maximum recommended flow rate is 0.03 ml/kg/min (less than 1.5 mg/kg/min).

Panglobulin, Sandoglobulin: Contain sucrose, see Precautions. 0.5 to 1 ml/min for 15 to 30 minutes. May then be increased to 1.5 to 2.5 ml/min. After the first infusion, the rate may be initiated at 2 to 2.5 ml/min. After the first dose, a 6% solution may be used to facilitate the administration of larger doses. Begin at 1 to 1.5 ml/min and increase in 15 to 30 minutes to 2 to 2.5 ml/min. To keep the amount of sucrose infused at less than 3 mg/kg/min in patients at risk for developing renal dysfunction, the concentration and infusion rate should be the minimum practicable. Do not exceed a rate of 2 mg IgG/kg/min.

Venoglobulin-S: 0.01 to 0.02 ml/kg/min for 30 minutes. The 5% solution may be gradually increased to a maximum of 0.08 ml/kg/min if no discomfort or adverse effects. The 10% solution may be gradually increased to a maximum of 0.05 ml/kg/min. Subsequent infusions may be given at the higher rate. In patients at risk for developing renal dysfunction, see comments under Rate of Administration. Reduced flow rate is indicated.

Pediatric rate of administration: Begin at 0.01 ml/kg/min. Double rate every 15 to 30 minutes up to a maximum of 0.08 ml/kg/min. If side effects occur, discontinue infusion until they subside. Restart at previously tolerated rate.

ACTIONS

An immune serum containing immune globulin. Obtained, purified, and standardized from human serum or plasma. Specific methods (e.g., detergents, solvents) inactivate blood-borne viruses (e.g., hepatitis). Provides antibodies that bind and neutralize pathogenic autoantibodies with immediate antibody levels against bacterial, viral, parasitic, and mycoplasmic antigens. Half-life approximately 3 weeks but may be decreased by fever or infection (increased catabolism or consumption). Distribution into extravascular fluid, tissue, and cells causes a rapid fall in serum IgG in the first week after infusion.

INDICATIONS AND USES

Provide rapid onset, short-term passive immunization. Labeled uses include: ***Primary immunodeficiency diseases:*** Maintenance and treatment of adults, adolescents, and children unable to produce adequate amounts of

IgG antibodies, especially in the following situations: need for immediate increase in intravascular immunoglobulin levels, small muscle mass or bleeding tendencies that contraindicate IM injection, and selected disease states (e.g., congenital agammaglobulinemia, common variable hypogammaglobulinemia, combined immunodeficiency, Wiskott-Aldrich syndrome). ■ ***Treatment of acute and chronic idiopathic thrombocytopenic purpura:*** Temporary increase in platelet counts in patients with idiopathic thrombocytopenic purpura and with thrombocytopenia associated with bone marrow transplant. ■ ***Adjunct in chronic lymphocytic leukemia:*** Gammagard SD/Polygam SD is used to prevent bacterial infections in patients with hypogammaglobulinemia or recurrent bacterial infection associated with B-cell CLL. ■ ***Infection prophylaxis or control*** and to improve immunologic parameters in select patients with symptomatic AIDS or ARC and children with HIV. ■ ***Bone marrow transplant:*** Reduce risk of serious infections and graft-versus-host disease in bone marrow transplant patients. ■ ***Kawasaki syndrome:*** Prevention of coronary artery aneurysms associated with Kawasaki syndrome.

Unlabeled uses: Infection prophylaxis and control in low-birth-weight neonates, patients with iatrogenically induced or disease-associated immunosuppression (major surgery [e.g., bone marrow or cardiac transplants], hematologic malignancies, extensive burns, or collagen-vascular diseases). ■ Treatment of post-transfusion purpura. ■ Treatment of chronic Parvovirus B19 infection in immunodeficient patients. ■ Prevention of recurrent bacterial infections in patients with IgG subclass deficiencies (e.g., allergies, HIV). ■ Treatment or adjunct in the treatment of dermatomyositis, intractable epilepsy, multiple sclerosis, myasthenia gravis, polymyositis, polyneuropathies, rheumatoid arthritis, and other autoimmune disease (e.g., autoimmune neutropenia, children with type 1 diabetes, chronic fatigue syndrome, Guillain-Barré syndrome, hyperimmunoglobulinemia E syndrome, multifocal motor neuropathy, and many others).

CONTRAINDICATIONS

Individuals known to have allergic response to gamma globulin or its components (e.g., thimerosal); patients with isolated IgA deficiency or pre-existing anti-IgA antibodies. Manufacturer of Gammagard SD states, "None known."

PRECAUTIONS

Check label; must state, "for IV use." ■ Do not use IM or SC. Do not skin test. Will cause a localized chemical skin reaction. ■ Use extreme caution in individuals with a history of prior systemic allergic reactions. Incidence of anaphylaxis may be increased, especially with repeated injections. ■ Some packaging of these products may contain latex; use caution in sensitive individuals. ■ IGIV products have been associated with renal dysfunction, acute renal failure, osmotic nephrosis, and death. Use extreme caution in patients with any degree of renal insufficiency; in patients age 65 years and older; in patients with diabetes mellitus, paraproteinemia, sepsis, volume depletion; and/or in patients receiving known nephrotoxic drugs. If used, should be administered at the minimum concentration available and at the minimum rate of infusion practicable. Products containing sucrose as a stabilizer (Gammar P-IV, Panglobulin, Sandoglobulin, and Swiss Red Cross products) have demonstrated an increased risk of renal dysfunction. Consider benefit versus risk before use. ■ May cause aseptic meningitis syndrome (AMS), especially with 2-Gm/kg doses. May begin from 2 hours to 2 days after treatment. Symptoms are drowsiness, fever, headache (severe), nausea and vomiting, nuchal rigidity, painful eye movements, and photophobia. ▪ IGIV products have been associated with thrombotic events; use caution in patients with a history of cardiovascular disease, thrombotic episodes, and patients with thrombotic risk factors (e.g., cerebrovascular disease, coronary artery disease, diabetes, hypertension).

Monitor: Use of larger veins (e.g., antecubital) recommended to reduce infusion-site discomfort, especially with 10% solutions. ▪ Correct volume depletion before administration. ▪ Monitor vital signs and observe patient continuously during infusion. A precipitous drop in BP or anaphylaxis can occur at any time. Emergency equipment and supplies must be at bedside. ▪ Monitor renal function (e.g., BUN, SrCr) and urine output in patients at increased risk for renal failure. Obtain baseline studies, monitor at intervals, and discontinue IGIV if renal function deteriorates. ▪ Minimal serum level of IgG after infusion should exceed 300 mg/dl.

Patient Education: Report a burning sensation in the head, chills, cyanosis, diaphoresis, dyspnea, faintness or lightheadedness, fatigue, fever, tachycardia, wheezing. ▪ Report decreased urine output, fluid retention, edema, shortness of breath, or sudden weight gain.

Maternal/Child: Category C: use with caution in pregnancy; no adverse effects documented, but adequate studies are not available. ▪ Safety for use in breast-feeding not established. ▪ Response in children usually exceeds response in adults. ▪ Gamimune-N contains maltose and may cause osmotic diuresis.

Elderly: Use with extreme caution. Incidence of renal insufficiency and other side effects increased due to age, potential for decreased organ function, and pre-existing medical conditions; see Precautions.

DRUG/LAB INTERACTIONS

Do not administer live-virus vaccines from 2 weeks before to at least 3 months after immune globulin IV. ▪ Provides immediate antibody levels that last for about 3 weeks. In selected patients, may have an immune-modulating effect that may alter their response to corticosteroids or antineoplastic agents. ▪ Concurrent use with nephrotoxic drugs (e.g., aminoglycosides [e.g., gentamicin (Garamycin)], amphotericin B [Amphotec, Fungizone], cidofovir [Vistide], rifampin [Rifadin]) may increase risk of renal insufficiency.

SIDE EFFECTS

Full range of allergic symptoms, including anaphylaxis, is possible. Angioedema, erythema, fever, and urticaria are most frequently observed. Backache, chills, fatigue, flushing, headache, hypertension (slight), increased BUN and SrCr (may occur as soon as 1 to 2 days following infusion), leg cramps, lightheadedness, nausea, rash, and vomiting have been reported. Acute renal failure, acute tubular necrosis, osmotic nephrosis, and proximal tubular nephropathy have been reported; may result in death. Is made from human plasma; process attempts to eliminate risk of hepatitis or HIV infection. A precipitous hypotensive reaction can occur and is most frequently associated with too-rapid rate of injection. Aseptic meningitis syndrome occurs infrequently. See Precautions.

ANTIDOTE

Reduce rate for patient discomfort, any sign of adverse reaction, and in patients at risk for renal insufficiency. Decreasing the volume of subsequent infusions may also prevent or decrease the incidence of adverse reactions. Loop diuretics (e.g., furosemide [Lasix]) may be helpful in the management of fluid overload. Patients who continue to experience adverse reactions, after rate and/or volume have been reduced, may be premedicated with hydrocortisone 1 to 2 mg/kg 30 minutes prior to the immune globulin infusion. Pretreatment with acetaminophen (Tylenol) and diphenhydramine (Benadryl) or trying a different brand of immune globulin may also be useful. Discontinue the drug immediately for any signs of allergic reaction or renal insufficiency. Notify the physician. May be treated symptomatically, and infusion resumed at slower rate if symptoms subside. Treat anaphylaxis immediately. Epinephrine (Adrenalin), diphenhydramine (Benadryl), oxygen, vasopressors (e.g., dopamine [Intropin]), corticosteroids, and ventilation equipment must always be available. Resuscitate as necessary.

INAMRINONE LACTATE

(in-am′rih-nohn lak′tat)

Inotropic agent

Inocor

pH 3.2 to 4

USUAL DOSE

Previously referred to as amrinone. Name was officially changed to prevent confusion with amiodarone.

Adults and children: 0.75 mg/kg of body weight as the initial loading dose (52.5 mg [10.5 ml] for a 70-kg person).

Inamrinone Loading Dose Determination 0.75 mg/kg (Undiluted)

Patient weight in kg	30	40	50	60	70	80	90	100	110	120
ml of undiluted inamrinone	4.5	6	7.5	9	10.5	12	13.5	15	16.5	18

Follow with a maintenance infusion of 5 to 10 mcg/kg/min. AHA guidelines recommend a maintenance infusion of 5 to 15 mcg/kg/min, titrated to clinical effect. The initial dose (0.75 mg/kg) may be repeated once in 30 minutes if indicated. Manufacturer recommends that the total dose, including the loading doses, not exceed 10 mg/kg/24 hr. Doses up to 18 mg/kg/24 hr have been used in a limited number of patients for shortened durations of therapy.

INFANT/NEONATAL DOSE

0.75 mg/kg as the initial loading dose. May be repeated in 30 minutes if necessary. Another source suggests a loading dose of 3 to 4.5 mg/kg given in divided doses to desired effect. AHA guidelines recommend 0.75 to 1 mg/kg as the initial loading dose and state that the loading dose may be repeated twice to a maximum loading dose of 3 mg/kg. Maintain ***infants*** with an infusion of 5 mcg (0.005 mg) to 10 mcg (0.01 mg)/kg/min and ***neonates*** with an infusion of 3 mcg (0.003 mg) to 5 mcg (0.005 mg)/kg/min.

DOSE ADJUSTMENTS

May be required in impaired renal or hepatic function or if thrombocytopenia occurs.

DILUTION

Available in 100 mg/20 ml ampules. May be given undiluted, or diluted with NS or ½NS to a final concentration of 1 to 3 mg/ml. Addition of 60 ml (300 mg) to 60 ml of solution will provide a final concentration of 2.5 mg/ml. May be given through Y-tube or three-way stopcock of IV infusion set. Use diluted solution within 24 hours.

Storage: Store ampules at CRT. Protect from light. Use diluted solution within 24 hours.

INCOMPATIBLE WITH

Manufacturer lists dextrose solutions (direct dilution only). States, "Forms an immediate precipitate with furosemide."

COMPATIBLE WITH (Underline Indicates Conflicting Compatibility Information)

Consult pharmacist; specific conditions may apply; see Compatibilities, p. xvi.

Syringe: Propranolol (Inderal), verapamil (Isoptin).

Y-site: Aminophylline, atropine, bretylium (Bretylate), calcium chloride, cimetidine (Tagamet), cisatracurium (Nimbex), dextrose solutions, digoxin (Lanoxin), dobutamine (Dobutrex), dopamine (Intropin), epinephrine (Adrenalin), famotidine (Pepcid IV), hetastarch in electrolytes (Hextend), hydrocortisone sodium succinate (Solu-Cortef), isoproterenol (Isuprel), lidocaine, methylprednisolone (Solu-Medrol), nitroglycerin (Nitro-Bid IV), nitroprusside sodium, norepinephrine (Levophed), phenylephrine (Neo-Synephrine), potassium chloride (KCl), procainamide (Pronestyl), propofol (Diprivan), propranolol (Inderal), remifentanil (Ultiva), verapamil (Isoptin).

RATE OF ADMINISTRATION

Loading dose: A single dose over 2 to 3 minutes. AHA guidelines recommend a single dose over 10 to 15 minutes.

Infusion: Using a microdrip (60 gtt/ml) or an infusion pump, deliver inamrinone in recommended doses. See dosage chart defining selected dose in mcg/min/body weight in ml/hr.

Inamrinone Infusion Rate (ml/hr)
(2.5 mg/ml Infusion Concentration)*

Patient weight (kg)	30	40	50	60	70	80	90	100	110	120
Dosage 5 mcg/kg/min	4	5	6	7	8	10	11	12	13	14
7.5 mcg/kg/min	5	7	9	11	13	14	16	18	20	22
10 mcg/kg/min	7	10	12	14	17	19	22	24	26	29

*A 70-kg patient receiving 7.5 mcg/kg/min would have a flow rate of 13 ml/hr with a 2.5 mg/ml concentration.

Adjust as indicated by physician's orders and progress in patient's condition. Reduce rate or stop infusion for excessive drop in BP.

ACTIONS

A class of cardiac inotropic agent that differs in chemical structure and mode of action from digitalis glycosides and catecholamines. It has positive inotropic action with vasodilator activity. Reduces afterload and preload by direct relaxant effect on vascular smooth muscle. Cardiac output is increased without measurable increase in myocardial oxygen consumption or changes in arteriovenous oxygen difference. Pulmonary capillary wedge pressure, total peripheral resistance, diastolic BP, and mean arterial pressure are decreased. HR generally remains the same. With a bolus dose, peak effect occurs within 10 minutes. Continuous administration is required to maintain serum levels. Mean half-life is 3.6 hours. In patients with CHF, mean half-life is 5.8 hours (range 3 to 15). Metabolized by the liver. Excreted primarily in urine and to a small extent in feces.

INDICATIONS AND USES

Short-term management of congestive heart failure in patients who have not responded adequately to digitalis, diuretics, or vasodilators. ■ Short-term management of congestive heart failure, pulmonary hypertension, and postop low cardiac output in neonates and infants up to 2 years.

CONTRAINDICATIONS

Hypersensitivity to inamrinone or bisulfites, severe aortic or pulmonic valvular disease when surgical relief of the obstruction is required.

PRECAUTIONS

Experience in controlled trials does not extend beyond 48 hours. Long-term use of cyclic-AMP–dependent inotropes have been associated with increased risk of hospitalization and death. Patients with NYHA class IV symptoms appear to be at particular risk. ■ May increase ventricular response in atrial flutter/fibrillation. Pretreat with digitalis (recommended). ■ May be given to digitalized patients without causing signs of digitalis toxicity. ■ Use caution in impaired renal or liver function; serum levels may increase considerably. ■ Not recommended for use in the acute phase of myocardial infarction due to lack of clinical trials to date. ■ May aggravate outflow tract obstruction in hypertrophic subaortic stenosis. ■ Contains sulfites, use with caution in patients with allergies.

Monitor: Observe patient continuously; monitoring of ECG, cardiac index, pulmonary capillary wedge pressure, central venous pressure, and plasma concentration are recommended (steady state plasma concentrations of approximately 3 mcg/ml suggested). ■ Monitor BP, urine output, and body weight. Observe for orthopnea, dyspnea, and fatigue. ■ Obtain platelet count before and during therapy to monitor onset of thrombocytopenia. ■ Additional fluids and electrolytes may be required to facilitate appropriate response in patients who have been vigorously diuresed and may have insufficient cardiac filling pressure. Use caution. ■ Monitor electrolytes; hypokalemia secondary to improved cardiac output with improved diuresis may cause arrhythmias. ■ Monitoring of liver function tests suggested. For marked increase in hepatic enzymes or S/S of hepatotoxicity, discontinue inamrinone. If increases in hepatic enzymes are less marked and no clinical symptoms of hepatotoxicity are present, continue inamrinone, decrease dose, or discontinue. Weigh risk versus benefit of continued therapy. ■ Monitor IV site; avoid extravasation.

Maternal/Child: Category C: use during pregnancy only if benefits outweigh risks. ■ Safety during breast-feeding not established. ■ Safety for use in children not established but has been used effectively. ■ Pediatric patients have a shorter elimination half-life.

Elderly: No problems documented; consider possible renal impairment; see Dose Adjustments.

DRUG/LAB INTERACTIONS

May cause excessive hypotension with disopyramide (Norpace).

SIDE EFFECTS

Abdominal pain, anorexia, arrhythmias, burning at site of injection, chest pain, fever, hepatotoxicity, hypotension, nausea and vomiting, thrombocytopenia. Hypersensitivity reactions manifested by ascites, myositis with interstitial shadowing on chest x-ray and elevated sedimentation rate, pericarditis, pleuritis, vasculitis with nodular pulmonary densities, hypoxemia, and jaundice have been reported.

ANTIDOTE

Notify the physician of any side effect. Based on degree of severity and condition of the patient, may be treated symptomatically, and dose may remain the same, be decreased, or the inamrinone may be discontinued. Reduce rate or discontinue the drug at the first sign of marked hypotension and notify the physician. May be resolved by these measures alone or vasopressors (e.g., dopamine [Intropin]) may be required. Treat arrhythmias with the appropriate drug. Resuscitate as necessary.

INDOMETHACIN SODIUM TRIHYDRATE

(in-doe-meth′a-sin so′de-um tri-hye′drat)

Prostaglandin inhibitor (patent ductus arteriosus adjunct)

Indocin IV

pH 6 to 7.5

USUAL DOSE

Neonates: Three IV doses, specific to age at first dose, given at 12- to 24-hour intervals constitute a course of therapy.

Less than 48 hours of age: First dose (0.2 mg/kg of body weight), second dose (0.1 mg/kg), third dose (0.1 mg/kg).

2 to 7 days of age: 0.2 mg/kg for each of 3 doses.

Over 7 days of age: First dose (0.2 mg/kg), then 0.25 mg/kg for the next 2 doses. A second course of 1 to 3 doses may be repeated one time at 12- to 24-hour intervals as above if the ductus arteriosus reopens.

DOSE ADJUSTMENTS

If urine output is less than 0.6 ml/hr at any time a dose is to be given, withhold dose until lab studies confirm normal renal function.

DILUTION

Each 1 mg must be diluted with at least 1 ml NS or SW for injection without preservatives (0.1 mg/0.1 ml); may be diluted with 2 ml diluent (0.05 mg/0.1 ml). The preservative benzyl alcohol is toxic in neonates. Prepare a fresh solution for each dose. Discard any unused portion.

INCOMPATIBLE WITH

Manufacturer states, "Prepare only with preservative-free NS or SW; further dilution with IV solutions is not recommended and may precipitate with solutions with a pH below 6.

COMPATIBLE WITH **(Underline Indicates Conflicting Compatibility Information)**

Consult pharmacist; specific conditions may apply; see Compatibilities, p. xvi.

Y-site: <u>Dextrose</u>, furosemide (Lasix), insulin (regular), potassium chloride (KCl), sodium bicarbonate, nitroprusside sodium.

RATE OF ADMINISTRATION

A single dose, properly diluted, by IV injection over 5 to 10 seconds.

ACTIONS

A potent inhibitor of prostaglandin synthesis. Through an unconfirmed method of action (thought to be inhibition of prostaglandin synthesis), it causes closure of a patent ductus arteriosus 75% to 80% of the time, eliminating the need for surgical intervention. Plasma half-life varies inversely with postnatal age and weight and ranges from 12 to 20 hours. Metabolized in the liver and eventually excreted in urine and bile.

INDICATIONS AND USES

Closure of a hemodynamically significant patent ductus arteriosus in premature infants weighing between 500 and 1,750 Gm if usual medical management (e.g., fluid restriction, diuretics, digitalis, respiratory support) has not been effective after 48 hours.

CONTRAINDICATIONS

Bleeding, especially active intracranial hemorrhage or GI bleeding; coagulation defects; necrotizing enterocolitis; infants with congenital heart disease (e.g., pulmonary atresia, severe coarctation of the aorta, severe tetralogy of Fallot) who require patency of the ductus arteriosus for satisfactory pulmonary or systemic blood flow; proven or suspected untreated infection; significant renal impairment; thrombocytopenia.

PRECAUTIONS

Clinical evidence of a hemodynamically significant patent ductus arteriosus (respiratory distress, a continuous murmur, a hyperactive precordium, cardiomegaly and pulmonary plethora on chest x-ray) should be present before use is considered. ■ For use only in a highly supervised setting such as an intensive care nursery. ■ May increase potential for GI or intraventricular bleeding. ■ Use caution in presence of existing controlled infection; may mask signs and symptoms of exacerbation. ■ For IV use only. ■ Surgery is indicated if condition is not responsive to two courses of therapy.

Monitor: Vital signs, oxygenation, acid-base status, fluid and electrolyte balance, and kidney function must be monitored and maintained. ■ Can cause marked reduction in urine output (over 50%), increase BUN and SrCr, and reduce glomerular filtration rate and CrCl. These symptoms usually disappear when therapy completed but may cause acute renal failure, especially in infants with impaired renal function from other causes. ■ Discontinue drug if signs of impaired liver function appear. ■ Confirm absolute patency of vein. Avoid extravasation; will irritate tissue. ■ See Drug/Lab Interactions.

DRUG/LAB INTERACTIONS

May increase serum levels of aminoglycosides (e.g., gentamicin [Garamycin]) and digitalis. ■ Use with furosemide (Lasix) may help to maintain renal function.

SIDE EFFECTS

Abdominal distention; acidosis; alkalosis; apnea; bleeding into the GI tract (gross or microscopic); bradycardia; DIC; elevated BUN or creatinine; exacerbation of pre-existing pulmonary infection; fluid retention; hyperkalemia; hypoglycemia; hyponatremia; intracranial bleeding; necrotizing enterocolitis; oliguria; oozing from needle puncture sites; pulmonary hemorrhage; pulmonary hypertension; reduced urine sodium, chloride, potassium, urine osmolality, free water clearance or glomerular filtration rate; retrolental fibroplasia; transient ileus; uremia; vomiting.

ANTIDOTE

Discontinue the drug and notify the physician of all side effects. Based on severity, side effects may be treated symptomatically or drug will be completely discontinued in favor of surgical intervention. Resuscitate as necessary.

INFLIXIMAB

(in-flicks′ih-mab)

Remicade

Monoclonal antibody
Inflammatory bowel disease agent
Antirheumatic agent

pH 7.2

USUAL DOSE

Preliminary patient evaluation required; see Monitor.

Crohn's disease and fistulizing Crohn's disease: Begin with an initial dose of 5 mg/kg as an infusion. Repeat at 2 and 6 weeks and every 8 weeks thereafter. For patients who respond and then lose their response, a 10 mg/kg dose may be given on day 1, repeated at 2- and 6-week intervals, and then repeated in 8 weeks (a total of 14 weeks elapsed). If there is no response by week 14, response with continued dosing is unlikely; consider discontinuing infliximab. See Precautions.

Rheumatoid arthritis: 3 mg/kg as an infusion. Repeat dose at 2 and 6 weeks, then every 8 weeks thereafter. Given in combination with methotrexate at a minimum dose of 12.5 mg/week (median dose of 15 mg/week). See methotrexate monograph. If response to infliximab is incomplete, dose may be adjusted up to 10 mg/kg and/or interval decreased to every 4 weeks (e.g., infliximab 3 to 10 mg/kg every 4 to 8 weeks).

DOSE ADJUSTMENTS

Dose adjustment not required based on gender, age, weight, or hepatic or renal function. ■ Do not exceed a dose of 5 mg/kg in patients with mild CHF (NYHA class I/II); see Contraindications.

DILUTION

Each vial contains 100 mg of infliximab. When reconstituted as directed below, each milliliter of solution contains 10 mg of infliximab. Calculate the dose and the number of vials required and the total volume of reconstituted infliximab solution required. Reconstitute each 100-mg vial with 10 ml of SW, using a syringe equipped with a 21-gauge or smaller needle. Direct the stream of SW to side of vial. Do not use vial if vacuum is absent. Swirl gently; do not shake. Allow reconstituted solution to stand for 5 minutes. Solution should be colorless to light yellow and opalescent and may develop a few translucent particles as infliximab is a protein. Do not use if opaque particles, discoloration, or other foreign particles are present. The total dose of reconstituted solution must be further diluted with NS to a final volume of 250 ml. (May withdraw a volume of NS equal to the calculated volume of reconstituted infliximab from a 250-ml bottle or bag of NS and slowly add reconstituted solution.) Mix gently. Infusion concentration should range between 0.4 mg/ml and 4 mg/ml. Must be administered through an infusion set with an in-line, sterile, non-pyrogenic, low–protein-binding filter (pore size equal to or less than 1.2 micron). Flush and prime tubing/filter system with NS before administration of infusion.

Storage: Refrigerate unopened vials at 2° to 8° C (36° to 46° F). Do not freeze. Reconstituted solution may be biochemically stable for 24 hours when stored between 2° and 30° C (36° to 86° F). However, because no preservative is present, manufacturer recommends that administration of infusion solution should begin within 3 hours of preparation. Discard any unused portion.

COMPATIBILITY

Manufacturer recommends not infusing concomitantly in the same IV line with other agents until specific compatibility data are available.

RATE OF ADMINISTRATION

Flush tubing/filter system before administration. A single dose should be given over a period of not less than 2 hours. Upon completion of infusion, IV line should be flushed thoroughly with 15 to 20 ml of NS to ensure all active drug is delivered to the patient.

ACTIONS

A chimeric IgG1 monoclonal antibody that binds specifically to human tumor necrosis factor alpha (TNFα). Is composed of human constant and murine variable regions. Neutralizes the biologic activity of TNFα by binding with high affinity to the soluble and transmembrane forms of TNFα and inhibiting binding of TNFα with its receptors. Infliximab does not neutralize TNFβ. Biologic activities attributed to TNFα include induction of pro-inflammatory cytokines such as IL-1 and IL-6, enhancement of leukocyte migration by increasing endothelial layer permeability and expression of adhesion molecules by endothelial cells and leukocytes, activation of neutrophil and eosinophil functional activity, and induction of acute phase and other liver proteins. Elevated concentrations of TNFα have been found in stools of Crohn's disease patients and in the joints of rheumatoid arthritis patients. These elevated concentrations correlate with elevated disease activity. Treatment with infliximab reduces infiltration of inflammatory cells and TNFα production in inflamed areas of the joint and of the intestine and reduces the proportion of mononuclear cells from the lamina propria able to express TNFα and interferon γ. After treatment, patients have decreased levels of serum IL-6 and C-reactive protein compared to baseline. Infliximab is distributed predominantly within the vascular space. Has a prolonged terminal half-life of 9.5 days. Studies suggest median onset of response to be 2 to 4 weeks and median duration of response to be 12 weeks. Produced by a recombinant cell line cultured by continuous perfusion and is purified by a series of steps that include measures to inactivate and remove viruses.

INDICATIONS AND USES

Treatment of moderately to severely active Crohn's disease for the reduction of the signs and symptoms in patients who have an inadequate response to conventional therapy. ■ Treatment of patients with fistulizing Crohn's disease for reduction in the number of draining enterocutaneous fistula(s). ■ Given in combination with methotrexate to improve physical function, inhibit progression of structural damage, and reduce S/S in patients with rheumatoid arthritis who have had an inadequate response to methotrexate.

Unlabeled uses: Treatment of ankylosing spondylitis and psoriasis.

CONTRAINDICATIONS

Known hypersensitivity to murine proteins or other components of the product, patients with moderate to severe (NYHA class III/IV) CHF.

PRECAUTIONS

Tuberculosis (often disseminated or extrapulmonary at clinical presentation), and invasive fungal infections (e.g., histoplasmosis, listeriosis, and pneumocystosis) have been observed in patients receiving infliximab. Some of these infections have been fatal. ▪ A higher incidence of worsening CHF and increased mortality have been seen in patients with moderate to severe CHF. Occurs more frequently in patients receiving a 10 mg/kg dose. Do not use doses greater than 5 mg/kg in patients with CHF. Discontinue if CHF is worsening, and consider discontinuing in patients with CHF who have not had a significant response to infliximab. Use with caution in patients with mild CHF (NYHA Class I/II); monitor closely. ▪ Hypersensitivity reactions characterized by urticaria, dyspnea, and/or hypotension have occurred in association with infliximab infusion. Discontinue infusion if severe reaction occurs. Medications for management of hypersensitivity reaction (e.g., acetaminophen [Tylenol], diphenhydramine [Benadryl], corticosteroids [e.g., hydrocortisone] and/or epinephrine) should be readily available. ▪ Anti-TNF therapy may result in formation of autoimmune antibodies and, rarely, in the development of a lupus-like syndrome. Discontinue therapy if this occurs. In clinical studies, symptoms resolved with discontinuation of therapy. ▪ TNFα mediates inflammation and modulates cellular immune response. Anti-TNF therapies, including infliximab, may affect normal immune responses. Fatal infections have been reported. Not recommended for patients with a clinically important active infection. Use caution in patients with a chronic infection or history of recurrent infection.▪ Patients with long duration of Crohn's disease and chronic exposure to immunosuppressant therapy are more prone to develop lymphomas and infections. The impact of infliximab treatment on these phenomena is unknown. ▪ In studies of extended treatment, systemic accumulation of infliximab did not occur, clinical benefit was maintained, and retreatment was well tolerated. According to the manufacturer, there have been reports of serum-sickness–like reactions.

Monitor: Evaluate patients for latent tuberculosis (TB) with a TB skin test. Initiate treatment of latent TB before therapy with infliximab. ▪ Before therapy with infliximab, evaluate benefit versus risk in patients who have resided in regions where histoplasmosis is endemic. ▪ If treatment is initiated or continued in a patient witih CHF, monitor cardiac status closely; see Precautions. ▪ Patients receiving infliximab may develop human antichimeric antibody (HACA). Patients who are HACA-positive may be more likely to experience an infusion reaction. The incidence of positive HACA is lower among patients receiving immunosuppressant therapies (e.g., 6-mercaptopurine, azathioprine, corticosteroids). ▪ Monitor BP and pulse every 30 minutes during infusion. If patient experiences a significant change in vital signs (e.g., drop in diastolic BP of 15 to 20 mm Hg) or exhibits any symptoms that may indicate hypersensitivity, stop infusion. Evaluate symptoms and treat appropriately. Continue to monitor patient for at least 30 minutes after completion of the infusion. ▪ Monitor for S/S of infection, discontinue if a serious infection occurs; see Precautions.

Patient Education: Tell health professionals of heart conditions, previous or current infections, and recent or past exposure to TB or histoplasmosis. ▪ Promptly report S/S of heart failure (e.g., shortness of breath, swelling feet), infection, numbness, tingling, or visual disturbances.

Maternal/Child: Category B: use during pregnancy only if clearly needed. ■ Has potential for harm to the nursing infant; discontinue breast-feeding. ■ Safety and effectiveness for use in juvenile rheumatoid arthritis and in children with Crohn's disease not established.

Elderly: Specific differences in safety and effectiveness not noted. Because the impact of infliximab on the incidence of infection is unknown and there is a higher incidence of infections in the elderly population in general, caution should be used in treating the elderly. See Precautions.

DRUG/LAB INTERACTIONS

Specific interaction studies have not been performed. ■ The majority of patients in Crohn's disease clinical trials received one or more of the following concomitant medications without evidence of any type of negative drug interaction: antibiotics, antivirals, corticosteroids, 6-mercaptopurine (Purinethol), azathioprine (Imuran), NSAIDs (e.g., ibuprofen [Motrin, Advil], naproxen [Aleve, Naprosyn], methotrexate, sulfasalazine, and aminosalicylates. ■ Patients receiving immunosuppressants (e.g., 6-mercaptopurine, azathioprine, corticosteroids) tended to experience fewer infusion reactions as compared to patients on no immunosuppressants. ■ Corticosteroid use increases the volume of distribution of infliximab. May be due to corticosteroid-mediated changes in fluid and electrolyte balance. ■ Concurrent administration of live vaccines is not recommended.

SIDE EFFECTS

Most common reasons for discontinuation of therapy were infections or infusion-related reactions (e.g., chest pain, chills, dyspnea, fever, hypertension, hypotension, pruritus, or urticaria) occurring during or within 2 hours of infusion. See Precautions. Most commonly reported side effects include abdominal pain, coughing, fatigue, headache, nausea, pharyngitis, upper respiratory tract infections, and vomiting. Other less common side effects include abscess, anemia, anxiety, arthralgia, autoantibodies/lupus-like syndrome, back pain, conjunctivitis, constipation, depression, diarrhea, dizziness, dyspepsia, dysuria, flushing, hot flashes, HACA development, hepatic enzyme increases, insomnia, intestinal obstruction, lymphoproliferative disorders, moniliasis, myalgia, pain, paresthesia, peripheral edema, rash, stomatitis, tachycardia, vertigo, and visual disturbances. See Precautions. TB, invasive fungal infections (e.g., histoplasmosis, listeriosis, and pneumocystosis), worsening CHF, and deaths have been reported.

ANTIDOTE

Notify physician of any side effects; most will be treated symptomatically. Discontinue infliximab if patient experiences significant changes in vital signs, new or worsening S/S of heart failure, a hypersensitivity reaction, a serious infection, or a lupus-like syndrome (fever, pleuritic pain, pleural effusion). Treat with acetaminophen (Tylenol), antihistamines (diphenhydramine [Benadryl]), corticosteroids, dopamine (Intropin), and epinephrine as indicated. If infusion is stopped but the reaction is not severe and does not require treatment with drugs such as epinephrine or corticosteroids, the infusion may be restarted with caution. A physician should be present during initiation of any subsequent infusion for a patient who has had a previous reaction. Lupus-like syndrome usually subsides within 10 days of discontinuing infliximab.

INSULIN INJECTION (REGULAR)

(in′su-lin in-jek′shun)

Hormone
Antidiabetic agent

Humulin R, ✦ Novolin ge Toronto,
Regular Iletin II (pork), Regular Iletin II (purified pork),
Regular Insulin (pork), Regular Insulin (purified pork) **pH 7 to 7.8**

USUAL DOSE

Only regular insulin may be given IV. Confirm by label or package insert that a particular insulin product is for IV use; see Precautions.

Dose varies greatly. Will be dependent on patient's condition and response. It is imperative that dosing is individualized and adjusted based on blood and urine glucose determinations because of the marked loss of insulin from adsorption to glass and plastic infusion containers and tubing; see Precautions.

Low-dose treatment in ketoacidosis or diabetic coma: 0.15 units/kg as an optional loading dose (10.5 units for a 70-kg patient), followed by a continuous infusion of 0.1 units/kg/hr (7 units/hr for a 70-kg patient). Another source recommends 10 to 30 units initially followed by a continuous infusion of 2 to 12 units/hr. See Precautions. Decrease the rate of infusion when plasma glucose reaches 300 mg/dl. Start a separate IV of D5W when plasma glucose reaches 250 mg/dl. Administer an appropriate dose of insulin SC 30 minutes before discontinuing the insulin infusion (intermediate-acting insulin recommended).

Diagnosis of growth hormone deficiency (unlabeled use): 0.05 to 0.15 units/kg of body weight as a rapid, one-time injection.

Myocardial infarction (glucose, insulin, potassium therapy [GIK therapy] unlabeled): Insulin 20 or 50 units/liter in combination with potassium chloride 40 or 80 mEq/liter respectively and a liter of 10% or 25% IV dextrose solution (20 units insulin with 40 mEq KCl in 1 liter of D10W or 50 units insulin with 80 mEq KCl in 1 liter of D25W). Low-dose regimen is infused at 1 ml/kg/hr for 24 hours, high-dose regimen at 1.5 ml/kg/hr for 24 hours. High-dose regimen may be more effective.

PEDIATRIC DOSE

Ketoacidosis: 0.1 unit/kg as an IV bolus. Follow with a continuous infusion of 0.1 unit/kg/hr. Rate of glucose fall should not exceed 80 to 100 mg/dl/hr. Increase insulin to 0.14 to 0.2 unit/kg/hr if glucose falls less than 50 mg/dl/hr. If glucose falls faster than 100 mg/dl/hr, continue insulin infusion (0.1 unit/kg/hr) and add 5% dextrose to IV fluids. As glucose approaches 250 to 300 mg/dl, add 5% dextrose to IV fluids.

DOSE ADJUSTMENTS

A reduced dose of insulin may be indicated when infusions are discontinued and SC administration is indicated. As in Usual Dose, base on blood and urine determinations and patient's response to therapy.

DILUTION

Use only if water clear. May be given undiluted either directly into the vein or through a Y-tube or three-way stopcock. Insulin is compatible with commonly used IV solutions and may be given as an infusion. Usually diluted in NS or ½NS for infusion. Fifty units of insulin added to 500 ml of infusion solution given at a rate of 1 ml/min will deliver 6 units/hr.

Another regimen adds 100 units of insulin (1 ml) to 100 ml of NS. This solution yields 1 unit/ml and is usually given at a rate of 0.1 unit/kg of body weight/hr (70-kg adult would receive 7 units/hr). See Precautions.

Storage: Store unopened vials in refrigerator; vial that is in use may be stored in a cool, dark room. Protect from sunlight and freezing. Discard any open vial not used for several weeks.

COMPATIBLE WITH

(Underline Indicates Conflicting Compatibility Information)

Consult pharmacist; specific conditions may apply; see Compatibilities, p. xvi.

Additive: Bretylium (Bretylate), cimetidine (Tagamet), lidocaine, meropenem (Merrem IV), ranitidine (Zantac), verapamil (Isoptin).

Syringe: Metoclopramide (Reglan).

Y-site: Amiodarone (Cordarone), ampicillin, ampicillin/sulbactam (Unasyn), aztreonam (Azactam), cefazolin (Kefzol), cefotetan (Cefotan), digoxin (Lanoxin), diltiazem (Cardizem), dobutamine (Dobutrex), esmolol (Brevibloc), famotidine (Pepcid IV), gentamicin (Garamycin), heparin, imipenem-cilastatin (Primaxin), indomethacin (Indocin), levofloxacin (Levaquin), magnesium sulfate, meperidine (Demerol), meropenem (Merrem IV), midazolam (Versed), milrinone (Primacor), morphine, nitroglycerin (Nitro-Bid IV), nitroprusside sodium, oxytocin (Pitocin), pentobarbital (Nembutal), potassium chloride (KCl), propofol (Diprivan), sodium bicarbonate, tacrolimus (Prograf), ticarcillin (Ticar), ticarcillin/clavulanate (Timentin), tobramycin (Nebcin), vancomycin (Vancocin).

RATE OF ADMINISTRATION

Each 50 units or fraction thereof over 1 minute. When given in an IV infusion, the rate should be ordered by the physician and will depend on insulin and fluid needs; see Dilution for example. Decrease rate when plasma glucose reaches 300 mg/dl.

ACTIONS

A hormone produced by the pancreas. Responsible for storage, metabolism, and uptake of carbohydrates, proteins, and fat. Stimulates protein and free fatty acid synthesis and promotes conversion of glucose to glycogen. Rapidly and widely distributed. Half-life is 5 to 6 minutes. Eliminated to some extent renally. Does not cross the placenta. Not found in breast milk.

INDICATIONS AND USES

Treatment of diabetes mellitus (Type I, Type II, and gestational). ■ Treatment of complications associated with diabetes (e.g., diabetic coma, ketoacidosis). ■ In combination with glucose to treat hyperkalemia. ■ Add to total parenteral nutrition to control hyperglycemia.

Unlabeled uses: Diagnosis of growth hormone deficiency. ■ Continuous intravenous infusions administered via a special pump have been used to treat severe brittle diabetics who have failed more conventional therapy. ■ Induction of insulin shock for psychotherapy. ■ GIK therapy for metabolic modulation post MI. May have potential beneficial effects on morbidity and mortality. Has been used in combination with thrombolytics or percutaneous coronary intervention (PCI).

CONTRAINDICATIONS

There are no contraindications when insulin is indicated as a life-saving measure.

PRECAUTIONS

Only regular insulin may be given IV. Humulin R is one of the newest products (recombinant DNA origin). All insulin is standardized at 100 units/ml. ■ Insulin potency may be reduced by at least 20% and possibly up to 80%

via the glass or plastic infusion container and plastic IV tubing before it actually reaches the venous system in an infusion. The percentage adsorbed is inversely proportional to the concentration of insulin (the larger the dose, the less adsorption) and takes place within 30 to 60 minutes. Albumin is sometimes added to reduce this adsorption. Other additives (e.g., electrolytes, other drugs, vitamins) may also reduce adsorption. Other methods of compensation for insulin loss include the addition of added insulin to saturate binding sites or the use of a syringe pump (instead of infusion containers) to reduce surface area for adsorption. ■ In low-dose treatment of diabetic coma or ketoacidosis, an initial priming dose of 10 units followed by 2 to 12 units/hr has achieved normal plasma levels of 100 to 200 microunits/ml of blood more quickly than previously used large doses. ■ Circulating levels of insulin may be increased in patients with renal or hepatic failure.

Monitor: Response to insulin measured by blood glucose, blood pH, acetone, BUN, sodium, potassium, chloride, and CO_2 levels. Monitor patient carefully in all situations. Use frequent blood glucose and ketone monitoring. ■ Hypovolemia is a common complication of diabetic acidosis. ■ See Drug/Lab Interactions. ■ Insulin is inactivated at pH above 7.5.

Patient Education: Monitor blood glucose as directed. ■ Adhere to consistent diet and exercise programs. ■ Avoid alcohol.

Maternal/Child: Category B: human insulin is drug of choice for control of diabetes in pregnancy. Additional insulin may be required to control serum glucose and avoid ketoacidosis. Monitor carefully; insulin requirements may drop immediately postpartum. Normal prepregnancy dose should be achieved within 6 weeks. Patients with gestational diabetes usually do not require insulin therapy following childbirth. ■ Breast-feeding may decrease insulin requirements. ■ Inadequately controlled maternal blood glucose late in pregnancy may cause increased insulin production in the fetus. Monitor and treat neonatal hypoglycemia postpartum.

DRUG/LAB INTERACTIONS

Hypoglycemic effect is potentiated by alcohol, anabolic steroids (e.g., nandrolone [Durabolin]), beta-adrenergic blockers (e.g., propranolol [Inderal]), guanethidine, isoniazid, MAO inhibitors (e.g., selegiline [Eldepryl]), pyrazolone compounds (e.g., phenylbutazone [Butazolidin]), salicylates, sulfonamides, tetracyclines, and many others. ■ Inhibited by corticosteroids, thiazide diuretics, dobutamine (Dobutrex), epinephrine (Adrenalin), furosemide (Lasix), oral contraceptives, thyroid preparations, and others. ■ Hypoglycemic effects may be decreased in smokers; dose adjustment may be required. ■ Will affect serum potassium levels; use caution in patients taking digitalis products. ■ Octreotide (Sandostatin) may alter insulin, glucagon, and growth hormone secretion, resulting in hypoglycemia or hyperglycemia. Monitor serum glucose and adjust insulin dose as indicated. ■ Pentamidine is toxic to the beta cells of the pancreas. Patients may develop hypoglycemia initially as insulin is released. This may be followed by hypoinsulinemia and hyperglycemia with continued pentamidine therapy. ■ Octreotide (Sandostatin) markedly increases adsorption of insulin to glass and plastic and reduces availability.

SIDE EFFECTS

Hypoglycemia with overdose. ***Early:*** Ashen color, clammy skin, drowsiness, faintness, fatigue, headache, hunger, nausea, nervousness, sweating, tremors, weakness. ***Advanced:*** Coma, convulsions, disorientation, hypokalemia (with ECG changes), psychic disturbances, unconsciousness, hypersensitivity reactions including anaphylaxis; death is rare.

ANTIDOTE

Discontinue the drug immediately and notify physician. ***Glucagon*** 1 to 2 mg IM is the specific antidote for insulin overdose. It may be supplemented by glucose 50% IV and/or oral carbohydrates such as glucose gel or orange juice. Oral carbohydrates may be sufficient to combat early symptoms of hypoglycemia. Allergic reactions usually respond to symptomatic treatment.

INTERFERON ALFA-2b, RECOMBINANT

(in-ter-feer′on al′fah)

Biologic response modifier
Antineoplastic

Intron A

pH 6.9 to 7.5

USUAL DOSE

Malignant melanoma: ***Induction:*** 20,000,000 IU/M^2 as an infusion each day for 5 consecutive days per week for 4 weeks. Begin therapy within 56 days of surgical resection.

Maintenance: Follow with 10,000,000 IU/M^2 as a SC injection three times each week for 48 weeks.

Total treatment regimen lasts for 1 year and should be completed unless there is progression of disease or the drug is discontinued because of specific side effects.

PEDIATRIC DOSE

Safety for use in children under 18 years of age not established.

DOSE ADJUSTMENTS

Temporarily discontinued for serious adverse reactions, if granulocytes decrease to less than 500/mm^3, or ALT (SGPT)/AST (SGOT) increases to more than 5 times upper limit of normal. When adverse reactions subside or improvement of granulocytes or liver function tests occur, treatment can be restarted at 50% of the previous dose. Discontinue permanently if serious adverse reactions persist, if granulocytes decrease to less than 250/mm^3, or if ALT/AST increases to more than 10 times the upper limit of normal.

DILUTION

Prepare immediately before use. Only the sterile powder is suitable for dilution for IV use. Do not use different brands of interferon in any single treatment regimen; variations exist and may adversely affect dosage and response to treatment. Available in 3, 5, 10, 18, 25, and 50 million IU vials; select one most appropriate for desired dose. Reconstitute with the diluent provided. Withdraw desired dose and inject into 100 ml of NS. Final concentration should be at least 10 million IU/100 ml.

Storage: Unopened vials of powder for injection should be refrigerated; stable at room temperature for up to 7 days. Refrigerate reconstituted solution if not used immediately; stable for 1 month.

COMPATIBILITY

Specific information not available. Consider specific use; consult pharmacist. One source indicates compatibility with NS, LR, and R solutions and incompatibility with dextrose solutions.

RATE OF ADMINISTRATION

A single dose equally distributed over 20 minutes. Administration at bedtime and the use of acetaminophen may prevent or partially reduce common side effects (e.g., fever, headache, "flu-like" symptoms).

ACTIONS

A naturally occurring small protein and glycoprotein of the interferon family produced by recombinant DNA techniques. It binds to specific membrane receptors on the cell surface and initiates a complex sequence of intracellular events (e.g., induction of specific enzymes, suppression of cell proliferation, immunomodulating activities [e.g., enhancement of phagocytic activity of macrophages, augmentation of the specific cytotoxicity of lymphocytes for target cells, inhibition of virus replication in virus-infected cells]). Peak concentration achieved within 30 minutes. Half-life about 2 hours; undetectable 4 hours after infusion. Has produced a significant increase in relapse-free and overall survival in patients with malignant melanoma. The kidney may be the site of interferon catabolism.

INDICATIONS AND USES

Adjuvant to surgical treatment in patients with malignant melanoma who are free of disease but at high risk for systemic recurrence. ■ Used IM or SC to treat hairy cell leukemia, AIDS-related Kaposi's sarcoma, chronic hepatitis non-A, non-B/C, chronic hepatitis B, chronic hepatitis C in patients unresponsive to previous therapy, in combination with recombinant ribavirin to treat chronic hepatitis C in patients with compensated liver disease who have relapsed following interferon alfa therapy, and intralesionally to treat condylomata acuminata.

CONTRAINDICATIONS

Hypersensitivity to interferon alfa or any of its components (benzyl alcohol, glycine, human albumin, and sodium phosphate dibasic and monobasic). Not recommended for patients with a pre-existing psychiatric condition, especially depression or a history of severe psychiatric disorder. Not recommended for patients with pre-existing thyroid abnormalities if they cannot be maintained within the normal range with medication.

PRECAUTIONS

Use cautiously in patients with a history of pulmonary disease (e.g., COPD), diabetes mellitus prone to ketoacidosis, coagulation disorders (e.g., thrombophlebitis, pulmonary embolism) or severe myelosuppression. ■ Use cautiously in patients with a history of cardiovascular disease (e.g., unstable angina, uncontrolled CHF, recent MI, and previous or current arrhythmic disorder). ■ May cause depression and suicidal behavior. ■ May aggravate life-threatening or fatal neuropsychiatric, autoimmune, ischemic, or infectious disorders listed in above precautions. Close monitoring required. Discontinue therapy if S/S of any of the above conditions worsen. Symptoms may resolve. ■ Severe cytopenias, including rare cases of aplastic anemia, have been reported; see Monitor. ■ Use caution in patients with psoriasis; may exacerbate disease. ■ Serum neutralizing antibodies have been detected in some patients; clinical significance unknown.

Monitor: Obtain baseline CBC including differential and platelet count, blood chemistries (electrolytes, liver function tests, and TSH), chest x-ray. Obtain baseline eye exam for patients with diabetes or hypertension. Obtain baseline ECG if there is a history of cardiovascular disease and/or patient is in advanced stages of cancer. Monitor all tests periodically during therapy. ■ Monitor differential WBC and liver function tests weekly during the induction phase and monthly during maintenance. Dose adjustments will be determined by results. Discontinue therapy if neutrophil count drops below 500 cells/mm^3. ■ Closely monitor any patient with a history of cardiovascular disease (see Precautions); arrhythmias including tachycardia, hypotension, and transient reversible cardiomyopathy have occurred. ■ Hypotension may occur during administration or up to 2 days posttherapy; monitor frequently. May require fluid replacement. ■ Maintain adequate hydration, particularly during initial states of treatment. ■ Monitor for signs of depression and/or suicidal behavior. ■ Use of narcotics, hypnotics, or sedatives may be required to manage adverse effects; use with caution and monitor carefully. ■ Monitor for thrombocytopenia (platelet count less than 50,000/mm^3). Discontinue therapy if platelet count drops below 25,000/mm^3. Initiate precautions to prevent excessive bleeding (e.g., inspect IV sites, skin, and mucous membranes; use extreme care during invasive procedures; test urine, emesis, stool, and secretions for occult blood). ■ Monitor thyroid function; abnormalities not normalized by medication may require discontinuing interferon. ■ Determine cause of persistent fever. ■ Repeat chest x-ray if cough, dyspnea, fever, or other respiratory symptoms occur. Monitor closely if pulmonary infiltrates or evidence of pulmonary function impairment is present; may require discontinuing interferon. ■ Obtain an eye exam for any patient who complains of changes in visual acuity, visual fields, or other ophthalmologic symptoms; retinal hemorrhages, cotton-wool spots, and retinal artery or vein obstruction have been observed rarely. ■ See Precautions.

Patient Education: Must use effective birth control throughout treatment; nonhormonal birth control preferred. ■ Cooperation for close monitoring and reporting of side effects is imperative. ■ Manufacturer provides a patient information sheet. ■ Home use may require extensive patient education. ■ See Appendix D, p. 1148. ■ Do not change brands of interferon without medical consultation. ■ Do not drive or operate machinery; mental alertness may be impaired. ■ Administration at bedtime and/or use of acetaminophen may be helpful to prevent the most common "flu-like" side effects. ■ Side effects may decrease in severity as treatment continues. Avoid excessive sunlight or artificial ultraviolet light. Potential for photosensitivity; wear protective clothing, sunscreens, and sunglasses.

Maternal/Child: Category C: has abortifacient effects. Should be used only if benefits justify risks. ■ Discontinue breast-feeding. ■ Safety for use in children under age 18 not established.

Elderly: Incidence of obtundation and coma has occurred, especially at higher doses.

DRUG/LAB INTERACTIONS

Specific information not available. Use caution with any other potentially myelosuppressive agent (e.g., cisplatin [Platinol], zidovudine [AZT]). ■ May increase serum levels of aminophylline; monitoring of aminophylline levels recommended. ■ May have synergistic additive effects with zidovudine (AZT) and increase incidence of neutropenia; monitor WBC closely.

SIDE EFFECTS

Occur in high percentages of patients and may be serious enough to require a decreased dose or discontinuation of drug. Usually rapidly reversible after therapy discontinued, but may require up to 3 weeks to resolve. Alopecia, anemia, anorexia, arrhythmias, bleeding, coughing, depression, diarrhea, dizziness, dyspnea, "flu-like" symptoms (e.g., chills, fatigue, fever, headache, myalgia), granulocytopenia, increased AST and/or ALT, leukopenia, nausea, pain (variable), paresthesia, rash, taste alteration, thrombocytopenia. Many other side effects may occur. Acute serious hypersensitivity reactions (e.g., anaphylaxis, angioedema, bronchoconstriction, urticaria) are rare but have occurred.

ANTIDOTE

Keep physician informed of all side effects. Some will be tolerated or treated symptomatically. Discontinue interferon immediately for any acute serious hypersensitivity reactions and treat as appropriate. Discontinue drug for any patient developing severe depression or other psychiatric disorder, myelosuppression that persists after dose reduction, thyroid abnormalities not normalized by medication, serious liver function abnormalities, serious pulmonary function impairment, or pulmonary infiltrates. Resuscitate as necessary.

IRINOTECAN HYDROCHLORIDE

(eye′rih-noh-tee′kan hye-droe-klor′id)

Antineoplastic (topoisomerase 1 inhibitor)

Camptosar, CPT-II

pH 3 to 3.8

USUAL DOSE

Recent studies conducted with the Saltz regimen (Regimen 1 of the combination therapy for first line treatment of colorectal cancer) were halted because of increased adverse reactions, including deaths. Some investigators have recommended dose reductions and increased monitoring for toxicity. Contact Pharmacia and Upjohn for additional information (1-800-323-4204). Studies documented in the June 21, 2001 issue of *The New England Journal of Medicine.*

Premedication with antiemetics recommended. Dexamethasone 10 mg and a $5HT_3$ blocker (e.g., ondansetron or granisetron) should be given on the day of treatment. Begin at least 30 minutes before giving irinotecan. See Monitor.

First-line treatment of colorectal cancer: The Saltz regimen or Regimen 1 is a combination therapy. It is administered once each week for 4 weeks (days 1, 8, 15, and 22) followed by a 2-week rest period. Premedication as described above is recommended. In addition prophylactic or therapeutic atropine may be indicated in patients experiencing cholinergic symptoms. Initiate regimen with the infusion of irinotecan over 90 minutes. Follow immediately with the infusion of leucovorin calcium (see leucovorin calcium monograph). Follow the leucovorin immediately with the infusion of fluorouracil over 24 hours (see fluorouracil monograph). Doses and modified dosing recommendations are based on the chart Combination-Agent Dosage Regimens & Dose Modifications. Doses of irinotecan and fluorouracil may require modification based on toxicity. See Dose Adjustments, combination therapy and/or package insert.

Regimen 2, called the Douillard or European regimen, is another regimen. Used primarily in Europe, doses are considerably higher, intervals are different, and side effects more pronounced. See chart Combination-Agent Dosage Regimens & Dose Modifications and see Dose Adjustments, combination therapy and/or package insert.

Combination-Agent Dosage Regimens & Dose Modifications[a] (Irinotecan/Fluorouracil [5FU]/Leucovorin Calcium [LV])

Regimen 1 6-wk course with bolus 5-FU/LV (next course begins on day 43)	irinotecan leucovorin 5-FU	125 mg/m^2 IV over 90 min, day 1, 8, 15, 22 20 mg/m^2 IV bolus, day 1, 8, 15, 22 500 mg/m^2 IV bolus, day 1, 8, 15, 22		
		Starting Dose & Modified Dose Levels (mg/m^2)		
		Starting Dose	Dose Level −1	Dose Level −2
	irinotecan	125	100	75
	leucovorin	20	20	20
	5-FU	500	400	300
Regimen 2 6-wk course with infusional 5-FU/LV (next course begins on day 43)	irinotecan leucovorin 5-FU Bolus 5-FU Infusion[b]	180 mg/m^2 IV over 90 min, day 1, 15, 29 200 mg/m^2 IV over 2 hr, day 1, 2, 15, 16, 29, 30 400 mg/m^2 IV bolus, day 1, 2, 15, 16, 29, 30 600 mg/m^2 IV over 22 hr, day 1, 2, 15, 16, 29, 30		
		Starting Dose & Modified Dose Levels (mg/m^2)		
		Starting Dose	Dose Level −1	Dose Level −2
	irinotecan	180	150	120
	leucovorin	200	200	200
	5-FU Bolus	400	320	240
	5-FU Infusion[b]	600	480	360

[a]Dose reductions beyond dose level −2 by decrements of ~20% may be warranted for patients continuing to experience toxicity. Provided intolerable toxicity does not develop, treatment with additional courses may be continued indefinitely as long as patients continue to experience clinical benefit.
[b]Infusion follows bolus administration.

Treatment of colorectal cancer after failure of treatment with fluorouracil: Irinotecan: Administer based on chart Single-Agent Regimens of Irinotecan and Dose Modifications as an infusion once each week for 4 weeks, followed by a 2-week rest period. See Premedication. After adequate recovery, additional doses may be repeated in a similar 6-week cycle and continued indefinitely in patients who attain a response or in those whose disease remains stable.

Continued

Irinotecan Single-Agent Regimens and Dose Modifications			
Weekly Regimen[a]	125 mg/m² IV over 90 min, day 1, 8, 15, 22 then 2-wk rest		
	Starting Dose & Modified Dose Levels[c] (mg/m²)		
	Starting Dose	Dose Level −1	Dose Level −2
	125	100	75
Once-Every-3-Week Regimen[b]	350 mg/m² IV over 90 min, once every 3 wks[c]		
	Starting Dose & Modified Dose Levels (mg/m²)		
	Starting Dose	Dose Level −1	Dose Level −2
	350	300	250

[a]Subsequent doses may be adjusted as high as 150 mg/m² or to as low as 50 mg/m² in 25 to 50 mg/m² decrements depending upon individual patient tolerance.
[b]Subsequent doses may be adjusted as low as 200 mg/m² in 50 mg/m² decrements depending upon individual patient tolerance.
[c]Provided intolerable toxicity does not develop, treatment with additional courses may be continued indefinitely as long as patients continue to experience clinical benefit.

DOSE ADJUSTMENTS

Combination therapy: Decrease dose based on toxicity as described in the following chart, Guidelines for Dose Adjustments in Combination Schedules.

Guidelines for Dose Adjustments in Combination Schedules (Irinotecan Fluorouracil [5-FU]/Leucovorin Calcium [LV])		
Patients should return to pretreatment bowel function without requiring antidiarrhea medications for at least 24 hours before the next chemotherapy administration. A new course of therapy should also not begin until the granulocyte count has recovered to ≥1500/mm³, and the platelet count has recovered to ≥100,000/mm³. Treatment should be delayed 1 to 2 weeks to allow for recovery from treatment-related toxicities. If the patient has not recovered after a 2-week delay, consideration should be given to discontinuing therapy.		
Toxicity NCI CTC Grade[a] (Value)	During a Course of Therapy	At the Start of Subsequent Courses of Therapy[b]
No toxicity	Maintain dose level	Maintain dose level
Neutropenia		
1 (1500 to 1999/mm³)	Maintain dose level	Maintain dose level
2 (1000 to 1499/mm³)	↓1 dose level	Maintain dose level
3 (500 to 999/mm³)	Omit dose, then ↓1 dose level when resolved to ≤grade 2	↓1 dose level
4 (<500/mm³)	Omit dose, then ↓2 dose levels when resolved to ≤grade 2	↓2 dose levels
Neutropenic fever (grade 4 neutropenia and ≥grade 2 fever)	Omit dose, then ↓2 dose levels when resolved	↓2 dose levels
Other hematologic toxicities	Dose modifications for leukopenia or thrombocytopenia during a course of therapy and at the start of subsequent courses of therapy are also based on NCI toxicity criteria and are the same as recommended for neutropenia above.	

Continued

Guidelines for Dose Adjustments in Combination Schedules (Irinotecan Fluorouracil [5-FU]/Leucovorin Calcium [LV])—cont'd		
Patients should return to pretreatment bowel function without requiring antidiarrhea medications for at least 24 hours before the next chemotherapy administration. A new course of therapy should also not begin until the granulocyte count has recovered to ≥1500/mm³, and the platelet count has recovered to ≥100,000/mm³. Treatment should be delayed 1 to 2 weeks to allow for recovery from treatment-related toxicities. If the patient has not recovered after a 2-week delay, consideration should be given to discontinuing therapy.		
Toxicity NCI CTC Grade[a] (Value)	During a Course of Therapy	At the Start of Subsequent Courses of Therapy[b]
Diarrhea		
1 (2-3 stools/day >pretx[c])	Maintain dose level	Maintain dose level
2 (4-6 stools/day >pretx)	↓1 dose level	Maintain dose level
3 (7-9 stools/day >pretx)	Omit dose, then ↓1 dose level when resolved to ≤grade 2	↓1 dose level
4 (≥10 stools/day >pretx)	Omit dose, then ↓2 dose levels when resolved to ≤grade 2	↓2 dose levels
Other nonhematologic toxicities		
1	Maintain dose level	Maintain dose level
2	↓1 dose level	Maintain dose level
3	Omit dose, then ↓1 dose level when resolved to ≤ grade 2	↓1 dose level
4	Omit dose, then ↓2 dose levels when resolved to ≤ grade 2 *For mucositis/stomatitis decrease only 5-FU, not irinotecan*	↓2 dose levels *For mucositis/stomatitis decrease only 5-FU, not irinotecan*

[a]National Cancer Institute Common Toxicity Criteria.
[b]All dose modifications should be based on the worst preceding toxicity.
[c]Pretreatment.

Single agent therapy: Discontinue if neutropenic fever occurs or absolute neutrophil count drops below 500/mm³. ▪ Reduce dose based on toxicity levels in chart, Irinotecan Guidelines for Dose Adjustments in Single-Agent Schedules. Most common reasons for dose reduction are late diarrhea, neutropenia, and leukopenia. ▪ Dose reduction may be required in patients over 65 and 70 years of age (see Elderly) and in patients who have previously received pelvic/abdominal irradiation.

Continued

Irinotecan Guidelines for Dose Adjustments in Single-Agent Schedules[a]

A new course of therapy should not begin until the granulocyte count has recovered to ≥1500/mm³, and the platelet count has recovered to ≥100,000/mm³, and treatment-related diarrhea is fully resolved. Treatment should be delayed 1 to 2 weeks to allow for recovery from treatment-related toxicities. If the patient has not recovered after a 2-week delay, consideration should be given to discontinuing irinotecan.

Worst Toxicity NCI CTC Grade[b] (Value)	During a Course of Therapy	At the Start of the Next Courses of Therapy (After Adequate Recovery). Compared with the Starting Dose in the Previous Course[a]	
	Weekly	Weekly	Once Every 3 Weeks
No toxicity	Maintain dose level	↑25 mg/m² up to a maximum dose of 150 mg/m²	Maintain dose level
Neutropenia			
1 (1500 to 1999/mm³)	Maintain dose level	Maintain dose level	Maintain dose level
2 (1000 to 1499/mm³)	↓25 mg/m²	Maintain dose level	Maintain dose level
3 (500 to 999/mm³)	Omit dose, then ↓25 mg/m² when resolved to ≤grade 2	↓25 mg/m²	↓50 mg/m²
4 (<500/mm³)	Omit dose, then ↓50 mg/m² when resolved to ≤grade 2	↓50 mg/m² dose levels	↓50 mg/m²
Neutropenic fever (grade 4 neutropenia and ≥grade 2 fever)	Omit dose, then ↓50 mg/m² when resolved	↓50 mg/m²	↓50 mg/m²
Other hematologic toxicities	Dose modifications for leukopenia, thrombocytopenia, and anemia during a course of therapy and at the start of subsequent courses of therapy are also based on NCI toxicity criteria and are the same as recommended for neutropenia above.		
Diarrhea			
1 (2-3 stools/day >pretx[c])	Maintain dose level	Maintain dose level	Maintain dose level
2 (4-6 stools/day >pretx)	↓25 mg/m²	Maintain dose level	Maintain dose level
3 (7-9 stools/day >pretx)	Omit dose, then ↓25 mg/m² when resolved to ≤grade 2	↓25 mg/m²	↓50 mg/m²
4 (≥10 stools/day >pretx)	Omit dose, then ↓50 mg/m² when resolved to ≤grade 2	↓50 mg/m²	↓50 mg/m²
Other nonhematologic toxicities			
1	Maintain dose level	Maintain dose level	Maintain dose level
2	↓25 mg/m²	↓25 mg/m²	↓50 mg/m²
3	Omit dose, then ↓25 mg/m² when resolved to ≤grade 2	↓25 mg/m²	↓50 mg/m²
4	Omit dose, then ↓50 mg/m² when resolved to ≤grade 2	↓50 mg/m²	↓50 mg/m²

[a]All dose modifications should be based on the worst preceding toxicity.
[b]National Cancer Institute Common Toxicity Criteria.
[c]Pretreatment.

DILUTION

Specific techniques required; see Precautions. Must be diluted for infusion with D5W (preferred) or NS to concentrations between 0.12 to 2.8 mg/ml. Usually diluted in 250 to 500 ml D5W.

Storage: Packaged in a blister pack to protect against accidental breakage and leakage. Store in carton protected from light at CRT. Do not freeze. If damaged, incinerate the unopened package. Recommended that diluted solution be used within 24 hours if refrigerated, within 6 hours if kept at CRT. However, when mixed with D5W, is stable for 48 hours if refrigerated and 24 hours at CRT. Do not refrigerate if mixed with NS; a precipitate may form. Stable for 24 hours at CRT.

COMPATIBILITY

Manufacturer states, "Other drugs should not be added to the infusion solution." Consider specific use and toxicity; consult pharmacist.

RATE OF ADMINISTRATION

A single dose as an infusion equally distributed over 90 minutes.

ACTIONS

An alkaloid extract from plants such as *Camptotheca acuminata.* A new class of antineoplastic agent that inhibits the enzyme topoisomerase I required for DNA replication. Together with its active metabolite SN-38 it causes cell death by damaging DNA produced during the S-phase of cell synthesis. Maximum plasma SN-38 levels are reached within 1 hour of infusion end. Extensively distributed to body tissues. Terminal half-life of irinotecan is about 6 hours; SN-38 is 10 hours. Irinotecan is moderately bound to plasma proteins (35%), but SN-38 is highly bound (95%). Metabolic conversion of irinotecan to SN-38 primarily occurs in the liver. Approximately 25% to 50% excreted through bile and urine.

INDICATIONS AND USES

First-line therapy for the treatment of metastatic colorectal cancer in combination with fluorouracil and leucovorin calcium. ■ As a single agent in the treatment of metastatic carcinoma of the colon or rectum that has recurred or progressed following treatment with fluorouracil.

CONTRAINDICATIONS

Hypersensitivity to irinotecan or any of its components. ■ Combination therapy is not recommended for use in patients with a bilirubin more than 2 mg/dl.

PRECAUTIONS

Follow guidelines for handling cytotoxic agents. See Appendix A, p. 1142. ■ Administered by or under the direction of the physician specialist. ■ Adequate diagnostic and treatment facilities must be available. ■ Must have normal biliary function. Hepatic dysfunction may impair the metabolism of both irinotecan and SN-38. Patients with a bilirubiin of 1 to 2 mg/dl are at increased risk for developing grade 3 or 4 neutropenia. ■ Use caution in the elderly (may have an increased incidence and severity of diarrhea) and in patients who have had previous cytotoxic therapy or previous pelvic/abdominal irradiation (likely to have an increased incidence and severity of myelosuppression). Monitor closely. ■ Use caution in patients with poor performance status. Patients with a baseline performance status of 2 had higher rates of hospitalization, neutropenic fever, thromboembolism, first-cycle treatment discontinuation, and early deaths than patients with a performance status of 0 or 1. ■ Use caution in patients with a history of allergies. ■ Use caution in patients with pleural effusions and/or with impaired pulmonary function. ■ Colitis complicated by ulceration, ileus, and what was described as toxic megacolon has been reported. ■ Do not use with the Mayo Clinic regimen of 5-FU/LV (administered for 4 to 5 days every 28 days). Regimen has caused increased toxicity and death. ■ See Monitor.

Monitor: Obtain a WBC with differential, hemoglobin, and platelet count before each dose. Expected nadir for platelets is 14 days, and 21 days for hemoglobin, neutrophils, and leukocytes. ■ Prophylactic antiemetics are recommended; see Usual Dose. To reduce nausea and vomiting and increase patient comfort after initial dosing, additional antiemetics should be available (e.g., ondansetron, granisetron). ■ Consider obtaining baseline electrolytes and liver function tests. ■ Not a vesicant, but monitor injection site for inflammation and/or extravasation. ■ Monitor vital signs. ■ Obtain an accurate bowel history to evaluate changes in bowel habits after administration of irinotecan. ■ Monitor for "early" diarrhea. Occurs during or within 24 hours of irinotecan administration and is cholinergic in nature. May be accompanied by other cholinergic symptoms (e.g., diaphoresis, flushing, increased salivation, lacrimation, miosis, rhinitis). Patients who have a cholinergic reaction to irinotecan will probably have similar reactions to subsequent doses. Atropine 0.25 to 1 mg IV or SC may be considered for treatment or for prophylactic use unless clinically contraindicated. ■ Monitor for "late" diarrhea (more than 24 hours after irinotecan administration), which probably results from cytotoxic effects on GI epithelium. May be prolonged; cause dehydration, electrolyte imbalances, or sepsis; and can be life threatening. At first onset give loperamide (Imodium) 4 mg; give 2 mg every 2 hours (4 mg every 4 hours during the night) until diarrhea-free for a minimum of 12 hours. An alternate regimen suggests loperamide 4 mg every 3 hours in combination with diphenhydramine (Benadryl) 25 mg every 6 hours. Monitor carefully; replace fluids and electrolytes as needed. ■ Premedication or prophylaxis with loperamide is not recommended. If grade 3 or 4 late diarrhea develops, hold irinotecan therapy until patient recovers, then decrease subsequent doses; see Dose Adjustments. ■ Use of laxatives is not recommended; however, they may be used in patients requiring them for constipation caused by narcotics. Close supervision is required. ■ Initiate antibiotic therapy in patients who develop ileus, fever, or severe neutropenia. After the first treatment, subsequent weekly chemotherapy treatments should be delayed until the return of pretreatment bowel function for at least 24 hours without the need for antidiarrheal medication. ■ Maintain adequate hydration. Orthostatic hypotension or dizziness may indicate dehydration. Rare cases of renal impairment or acute renal failure have been reported, usually in patients who became dehydrated from vomiting and/or diarrhea. ■ Be alert for signs of bone marrow suppression or infection. Prophylactic antibiotics may be indicated pending results of C/S in a febrile or nonfebrile neutropenic patient. ■ Patients who have a cholinergic reaction to irinotecan will probably have similar reactions to subsequent doses. Atropine may be considered for prophylactic use. No studies available. ■ Monitor for thrombocytopenia (platelet count less than 50,000/mm^3). Initiate precautions to prevent excessive bleeding (e.g., inspect IV sites, skin, and mucous membranes; use extreme care during invasive procedures; test urine, emesis, stool, and secretions for occult blood). ■ See Dose Adjustments.

Patient Education: Manufacturer provides a patient education brochure, "Important Facts About Your Chemotherapy." ■ Report any unusual or unexpected symptoms or side effects as soon as possible. ■ Report black or bloody stools, diarrhea not under control within 24 hours, dry mouth, fever or chills, inability to retain oral fluids due to nausea and vomiting, infections, symptoms of dehydration (e.g., lightheadedness, dizziness, fainting), urine changes, or vomiting immediately; each must be treated promptly. Have loperamide (Imodium) available. ■ Compliance with regimen imperative (e.g., taking temperature, obtaining lab work, adequate rest, nourishment, and fluids). ■ Avoid caffeine and alcohol. May worsen dehydration. ■ Avoid raw fruits and vegetables, bran, fatty foods, or any other food that may aggravate diarrhea. ■ Nonhormonal birth control recommended. ■ Inform healthcare professionals of any problems with previous treatments. ■ See Appendix D, p. 1148.

Maternal/Child: Category D: avoid pregnancy. May cause fetal harm. ■ Discontinue breast-feeding. ■ Safety and effectiveness for use in children not established.

Elderly: Half-life slightly extended. ■ Reduction in starting dose by one dose level may be considered in patients over 65. Reduce starting dose by one dose level to 300 mg/M^2 in patients 70 years and older in the single agent once every 3 week regimen. See Usual Dose and Dose Adjustments. ■ Risk of severe diarrhea increased in the elderly. ■ Monitor carefully; may dehydrate more quickly from diarrhea. Begin loperamide therapy promptly. Avoid laxatives.

DRUG/LAB INTERACTIONS

Interaction of irinotecan with other drugs has not been adequately studied. ■ Additive bone marrow depression may occur with radiation therapy and/or other bone marrow–depressing agents (e.g., azathioprine [Imuran], chloramphenicol, melphalan [Alkeran]). Dose reduction may be required. ■ Concurrent administration with irradiation is not recommended. ■ Dexamethasone for antiemetic prophylaxis may increase lymphocytopenia and may contribute to hyperglycemia in patients with diabetes. ■ Administration of prochlorperazine (Compazine) and irinotecan on the same day may increase the risk of akathisia (inability to sit still, urge to move about constantly). ■ Use caution or withhold diuretics (e.g., furosemide [Lasix]) and laxatives during treatment; may increase risk of dehydration secondary to vomiting and/or diarrhea. ■ St. John's wort may decrease serum levels and effectiveness. ■ Do not administer live vaccines to patients receiving antineoplastic drugs.

SIDE EFFECTS

Myelosuppression (anemia, leukopenia, neutropenia) and diarrhea ("early" [e.g., abdominal cramping or pain, diaphoresis] or "late") occur in patients and are the most common dose-limiting toxicities. Nausea and vomiting occur in most patients and can be severe, may occur early (within 24 hours of administration) or late (more than 24 hours after administration). Abdominal bloating, allergic reactions (including anaphylaxis), alopecia, anorexia, asthenia, back pain, chills, confusion, constipation, coughing, dehydration, dizziness, dyspepsia, dyspnea, edema, exfoliative dermatitis, fever, flatulence, flushing, headache, hypotension, increased alkaline phosphatase and AST (SGOT), increased bilirubin, infection, insomnia, mucositis, myocardial infarction, neutropenic fever, neutropenic infection, pneumonia, pulmonary embolism, rash, rhinitis, somnolence, stomatitis, thrombocytopenia, thrombophlebitis, and weight loss may occur. Death was preceded by cyanosis, tremors, respiratory distress, and convulsions. In addition, ileus without preceding colitis has occurred. Renal impairment or failure has occurred usually in patients who became volume depleted from severe vomiting and/or diarrhea.

ANTIDOTE

Keep physician informed of all side effects and monitor carefully. Adjust or omit dose as indicated for toxicity; see Dose Adjustments. Treat diarrhea immediately; see Monitor. Administration of whole blood products (e.g., packed RBCs, platelets, leukocytes) and/or blood modifiers (e.g., darbepoetin alfa [Aranesp], epoetin alfa [Epogen, Procrit], filgrastim [Neupogen], pegfilgrastim [Neulasta], sargramostim [Leukine], oprelvekin [Neumega]) may be indicated to treat bone marrow toxicity. Death may occur from the progression of many side effects. No known antidote for overdose. Maximum supportive care (e.g., to prevent dehydration due to diarrhea and to treat any infectious complications) will help sustain patient in toxicity. If extravasation occurs, flush site with SW, elevate the extremity, and apply ice.

IRON DEXTRAN INJECTION

(i′ern deks′tran in-jek′shun)

Antianemic
Iron supplement

DexFerrum, ✤DexIron, InFeD, ✤Infufer

pH 5.2 to 6.5

USUAL DOSE

0.5 ml (25 mg) on the first day as a test dose. Wait 1 hour. If no adverse reactions, may be increased gradually to 2 ml (100 mg)/24 hr and repeated daily until results achieved or maximum calculated dosage reached (see dosage tables in literature or formula below). A total calculated dose has been given as an infusion. Though not FDA approved, this method is preferred by some to multiple small-dose infusions or injections.

To calculate the total amount of iron dextran (ml) required to restore hemoglobin and to replenish iron stores in adults and children weighing over 15 kg (lean body weight [LBW]):

$$\text{Dose (ml)} = 0.0442\,(\text{desired Hb} - \text{observed Hb}) \times \text{LBW in kg} + (0.26 \times \text{LBW in kg}).$$

If actual weight is less than LBW or in children between 5 to 15 kg, use actual weight in kg.

PEDIATRIC DOSE

0.5 ml (25 mg) on the first day as a test dose. Wait 1 hour. If no adverse reactions, may give remainder of daily dose. The following daily doses have been recommended by one source: ***less than 5 kg,*** 25 mg; ***5 to 10 kg,*** 50 mg; ***more than 10 kg,*** 100 mg. Repeat daily until results achieved or maximum calculated dosage reached (see dosage tables in literature or formula above).

DILUTION

Check vial carefully; must state, "for IV use." Given undiluted, or up to the total desired dose may be further diluted in 50 to 1,000 ml NS for infusion. D5W may cause additional local pain and phlebitis.

Storage: Store unopened vials at CRT, protect from freezing.

COMPATIBILITY

Manufacturer states, "Do not mix with other medications or add to parenteral nutrition solutions."

RATE OF ADMINISTRATION

IV injection: 1 ml (50 mg) or fraction thereof over 1 minute or more.

Infusion: Test dose of 25 mg over 5 minutes (Dexferrum), over 30 seconds (InFed). If no adverse reactions, infuse remaining dose over 1 to 8 hours (based on amount of dose, amount of diluent, and patient comfort). Another source suggests a test infusion (diluted in 500 ml) of 10 gtts/minute for 10 minutes and infusion over 4 to 5 hours. Discontinue IV infusion solutions during administration of iron dextran injection.

ACTIONS

The iron-dextran complex is separated into smaller molecules by cellular systems in the bone marrow, liver, spleen, etc. By chemical processes usable iron (e.g., ferritin) can then be absorbed into the hemoglobin. Serum ferritin peaks in 7 to 9 days and returns to baseline in 3 weeks. After hemoglobin needs of the blood are met, iron is stored in the body for reserve use. Small amounts of unabsorbed iron are excreted in the urine, feces, and bile. Crosses the placental barrier. Trace amounts of unmetabolized iron dextran are excreted in breast milk.

INDICATIONS AND USES

Iron-deficiency anemia in patients for whom oral administration is unsatisfactory or impossible; identify and treat the cause of the anemia.

Unlabeled uses: Iron supplementation for patients taking epoetin alfa (Epogen, Procrit).

CONTRAINDICATIONS

Manifestation of allergic reaction, any anemia other than iron deficiency.

PRECAUTIONS

Use only when truly indicated to avoid excess storage of iron. One source recommends discontinuing oral iron before administering parental iron. ▪ Increases joint pain and swelling in patients with rheumatoid arthritis. ▪ Fatal anaphylactic reactions have been reported. Facilities for monitoring the patient and responding to any medical emergency must be available. ▪ Use caution with history of asthma or allergies. ▪ Allergic reactions are often delayed, are more frequent with certain batches, and may happen at any time during an infusion even if no reaction from test dose. ▪ Use only if absolutely necessary in liver disease. ▪ Do not use during acute phase of an infectious kidney disease.

Monitor: Keep patient lying down after injection to prevent postural hypotension. ▪ Observe continuously for an allergic reaction during an infusion. Monitor vital signs. ▪ Monitor serum ferritin assays in prolonged therapy. Consider possibility of false results for months after injection caused by delayed utilization.

Maternal/Child: Category C: use only if absolutely necessary in pregnancy, breast-feeding, or childbearing years. Known hazard to fetus. ▪ Not recommended in infants younger than 4 months of age.

DRUG/LAB INTERACTIONS

Inhibited by chloramphenicol. ■ Effectiveness negated by deferoxamine (Desferal), an iron chelating agent. May be affected by other chelating agents (e.g., edetate disodium). Give iron dextran at least 2 hours after a chelating agent. ■ May cause false serum iron values within 1 to 2 weeks of large doses of iron dextran. ■ May cause a false elevated bilirubin, false decreased calcium, or affect numerous other tests or scans. ■ See Monitor.

SIDE EFFECTS

Backache, dizziness, headache, itching, local phlebitis at injection site, malaise, nausea, rash, shivering, transitory paresthesias.

Major: Anaphylaxis (fatalities have occurred); arthritic reactivation; dyspnea; febrile episodes; hypotension; leukocytosis; local phlebitis; lymphadenopathy; peripheral vascular flushing, especially with too-rapid injection; urticaria; tachycardia; shock (severe iron toxicity increases vasodilation and venous pooling and decreases circulating blood volume. Results in decreased cardiac output, hypotension, increased peripheral vascular resistance, and shock).

Overdose: Produces no acute toxicity, may result in hemosiderosis. Excess iron may increase susceptibility to infection.

ANTIDOTE

Discontinue the drug and notify the physician of early symptoms. For severe symptoms, discontinue drug, treat allergic reactions, or resuscitate as necessary, and notify physician. Epinephrine (Adrenalin) and diphenhydramine (Benadryl) should always be available. Deferoxamine is an iron chelating agent and may be useful in iron toxicity or overdose.

IRON SUCROSE
(i'ren soo'kros)

Venofer

Hematinic
Antianemic

pH 10.5 to 11.1

USUAL DOSE

Dose is expressed in terms of mg of elemental iron. Administered during the dialysis session.

Test dose (optional): 50 mg. Test dose is not required, but may be given at the physician's discretion.

Treatment of iron deficiency in hemodialysis patients: 100 mg (5 ml) one to three times a week to a total dose of 1,000 mg in 10 doses. Repeat as needed to maintain target levels of hemoglobin, hematocrit, and laboratory parameters of iron stores within acceptable limits. Frequency of dosing should be no more than three times weekly.

PEDIATRIC DOSE

Safety and effectiveness in children has not been established.

DOSE ADJUSTMENTS

Begin at the low end of the dosing range in elderly patients. ■ Withhold in patients with evidence of tissue iron overload; see Monitor.

DILUTION

Available in vials containing 100 mg/5 ml (20 mg/ml) of elemental iron.

Test dose: 50 mg (2.5 ml) should be diluted in 50 ml of NS.

Therapeutic dose: May be given undiluted or further diluted in a maximum of 100 ml of NS.

Storage: Store unopened vials in original carton at CRT. Do not freeze. Diluted iron infusions should be used immediately after preparation. Discard any unused portion.

COMPATIBILITY

Manufacturer states, "Do not mix with other medications or add to parenteral nutrition solutions."

RATE OF ADMINISTRATION

Administer into the dialysis line during the dialysis session. Too-rapid administration may cause hypotension or symptoms of overdose; see Side Effects.

Test dose: A single dose over 3 to 10 minutes.

Slow IV injection: A single undiluted dose at a rate of 20 mg/min (i.e., 5 minutes for a 100-mg dose).

Infusion: A single dose equally distributed over at least 15 minutes. This method of administration may reduce the risk of hypotensive episodes.

ACTIONS

An aqueous, complex of polynuclear iron (III)-hydroxide in sucrose. Used to replenish the total body iron stores in patients with iron deficiency on chronic hemodialysis. Iron is critical for normal hemoglobin synthesis to maintain oxygen transport and necessary for metabolism and synthesis of DNA and various other processes. Following intravenous administration, iron sucrose is dissociated by the reticuloendothelial system into iron and sucrose. Iron distributes into liver, spleen, and bone marrow. Since iron disappearance from serum depends on the need for iron in the iron stores and iron-utilizing tissues of the body, serum clearance of iron is expected to be more rapid in iron deficient patients as compared to healthy individuals. Half-life of the iron component is 6 hours. The sucrose component is eliminated mainly by urinary excretion. Most iron is stored in the body in hemoglobin, bone marrow, spleen, liver, and ferritin. Small amounts are eliminated in the urine.

INDICATIONS AND USES

Treatment of iron deficiency anemia in patients undergoing chronic hemodialysis who are receiving supplemental erythropoietin therapy.

CONTRAINDICATIONS

Patients with evidence of iron overload, with anemia not caused by iron deficiency, or with known hypersensitivity to iron sucrose or any of its inactive components.

PRECAUTIONS

Use only when truly indicated to avoid excess storage of iron. Not recommended for use in patients with iron overload. ■ Potentially fatal hypersensitivity reactions characterized by anaphylactic shock, loss of consciousness, collapse, hypotension, dyspnea, or convulsions have been reported. Medications and equipment for resuscitation must be readily available. ■ Hypotension has been reported frequently and may be related to rate of administration and/or total dose administered. Follow guidelines for dosing and administration. See Usual Dose and Rate of Administration.

Monitor: Monitor vital signs during and immediately following administration. Recumbent position during and after administration may help to prevent postural hypotension. Hypotensive effects may be additive to transient hypotension during dialysis and/or from too-rapid rate of administration. ■ Periodic monitoring of hematologic and hematinic parameters (hemoglobin, hematocrit, serum ferritin and transferrin saturation) is indicated during parenteral iron replacement therapy. Transferrin saturation values increase rapidly after IV adminstration of iron sucrose; thus serum iron values may be reliably obtained 48 hours after IV dosing. Avoid excess tissue iron; withhold in patients with evidence of tissue iron overload.

Patient Education: Report S/S of allergic reaction promptly.

Maternal/Child: Category B: use in pregnancy only if clearly needed. ■ Safety for use during breast-feeding and in children not established.

Elderly: Differences in response between elderly and younger patients have not been identified. Lower-end initial doses may be appropriate in the elderly based on the potential for decreased organ function and concomitant disease or drug therapy.

DRUG/LAB INTERACTIONS

Drug interactions involving iron sucrose have not been studied. May reduce the absorption of concomitantly administered oral iron preparations, concurrent use not recommended.

SIDE EFFECTS

Frequent: Cramps/leg cramps, diarrhea, headache, hypotension, nausea, and vomiting.

Less frequent: Abdominal pain, asthenia, chest pain, cough, dizziness, dyspnea, elevated liver enzymes, fever, hypersensitivity reactions (e.g., pruritus, rash, anaphylactic shock, loss of consciousness, collapse dyspnea, hypotension, or convulsions), hypertension, hypervolemia, injection site pain, malaise, musculoskeletal pain, pneumonia, pruritus.

Overdose: Abdominal and muscle pain, bleeding in the GI tract and lungs, cardiovascular collapse, diarrhea, edema, headache, hemosiderosis, hypoactivity, hypotension, joint aches, nausea, pale eyes, paresthesia, sedation, vomiting.

ANTIDOTE

Reduce rate of infusion for hypotension or other symptoms. Most symptoms are successfully treated with IV fluids, hydrocortisone (Solu-Cortef), and/or antihistamines (e.g., diphenhydramine [Benadryl]). Volume expanders (e.g., albumin, dextran, hetastarch [Hespan]) may be indicated. Slowing the rate of the infusion may also help alleviate symptoms. Keep physician informed of all side effects. Discontinue drug and treat severe allergic reaction as indicated (e.g., diphenhydramine [Benadryl], corticosteroids [Solu-Cortef], H_2 antagonists [e.g., cimetidine (Tagamet)], dopamine [Intropin], and IV fluids). Resuscitate as needed.

ISOPROTERENOL HYDROCHLORIDE

(eye-soe-proe-ter′e-nole hye-droe-klor′id)

Cardiac stimulant (inotropic/chronotropic)
Bronchodilator
Antiarrhythmic

Isuprel Hydrochloride

pH 3.5 to 4.5

USUAL DOSE

Asthma unresponsive to inhalation therapy: 0.01 to 0.02 mg (0.5 to 1 ml of a 1:50,000 dilution). Repeat as necessary.

Control bronchospasm during anesthesia: 0.01 to 0.02 mg (0.5 to 1 ml of a 1:50,000 dilution). Repeat as necessary.

Atropine-resistant hemodynamically significant bradycardia: 0.02 to 0.06 mg (1 to 3 ml of a 1:50,000 dilution) as an initial dose. Subsequent doses may range from 0.01 to 0.2 mg (0.5 to 10 ml of a 1:50,000 dilution) or may be maintained with an infusion. 5 mcg/min (1.25 ml of a 1:250,000 dilution) is the average initial dose. Range is 2 to 20 mcg/minute. AHA recommendation is 2 to 10 mcg/min if an external pacemaker is not available.

Complete heart block following closure of ventricular septal defects: 0.04 to 0.06 mg (2 to 3 ml of a 1:50,000 dilution) as a bolus injection. May maintain a sinus rhythm with a HR above 90 to 100/min or may relapse into complete heart block again.

Shock: 0.5 to 5 mcg/min as an infusion (0.25 to 2.5 ml of a 1:500,000 dilution [2 mcg/ml]). Titrate to patient response (e.g., HR, central venous pressure, BP, urine output). Up to 30 mcg/min have been used in advanced stages of shock. Administer only for 1 hour or less in patients with septic shock.

Diagnosis of mitral regurgitation: 4 mcg/min as an infusion (1 ml/min of a 1:250,000 dilution).

Diagnosis of coronary artery disease or lesions: 1 to 3 mcg/min as an infusion (0.25 to 0.75 ml/min of a 1:250,000 dilution).

Intracardiac: 0.02 mg (0.1 ml) of a 1:5,000 dilution (rarely used).

Refractory torsades de pointes, bradycardia in heart transplant patients, beta-adrenergic blocker poisoning: AHA recommends 2 to 10 mcg/min (0.5 to 2.5 ml/min of a 1:250,000 dilution [4 mcg/ml]). Titrate to adequate heart rate. In torsades de pointes titrate to increase heart rate until VT is suppressed.

PEDIATRIC DOSE

Safety and effectiveness in pediatric patients not established; see Maternal/Child.

Status asthmaticus: 0.08 to 1.7 mcg/kg/min as an infusion. Begin with 0.1 mcg/kg/min and increase every 5 to 10 minutes by 0.1 mcg/kg/min until desired effect. Reduce rate for tachycardia over 180 or if arrhythmia occurs. Continuous assessment of VS, frequent ECGs, and daily measurement of cardiac enzymes (e.g., CPK, MB) is suggested; see Maternal/Child.

Atropine-resistant hemodynamically significant bradycardia: Begin with 0.1 mcg/kg/min as an infusion. Increase by 0.1 mcg/kg/min until desired effect. Titrate to patient response and monitor cardiac status carefully. Maximum dose is 1 mcg/kg/min.

Complete heart block after closure of ventricular septal defects in infants: 0.01 to 0.03 mg (0.5 to 1.5 ml of a 1:50,000 dilution) as a bolus injection. See comments in Usual Dose.

DOSE ADJUSTMENTS

Lower-end initial doses may be appropriate in the elderly; see Elderly.

DILUTION

IV injection: Available in a 1:50,000 solution or dilute 0.2 mg (1 ml) of a 1:5,000 solution with 9 ml NS for injection (1:50,000 solution).

Infusion: 1 mg (5 ml) of a 1:5,000 solution in 250 ml (2 mg [10 ml] in 500 ml) of D5W. 1 ml equals 4 mcg in this 1:250,000 solution. Dilute 1 mg in 500 ml (1:500,000 solution [2 mcg/ml]) to treat shock. Use an infusion pump or microdrip (60 gtt equals 1 ml) to administer. Less diluent may be used to reduce fluid intake.

Pediatric infusion: 0.6 mg/kg isoproterenol in 100 ml D5W. 1 ml/hr equals 0.1 mcg/kg/min.

Intracardiac: 1:5,000 solution undiluted (rarely used). No longer recommended as an acceptable route for bradycardia or cardiac arrest.

Do not use if pink or brown in color or contains a precipitate.

COMPATIBLE WITH

Consult pharmacist; specific conditions may apply; see Compatibilities, p. xvi.

Additive: Atracurium (Tracrium), calcium chloride, cimetidine (Tagamet), dobutamine (Dobutrex), heparin, magnesium sulfate, multivitamins (M.V.I.), potassium chloride (KCl), ranitidine (Zantac), succinylcholine, verapamil (Isoptin).

Syringe: Ranitidine (Zantac).

Y-site: Amiodarone (Cordarone), atracurium (Tracrium), bretylium (Bretylate), cisatracurium (Nimbex), famotidine (Pepcid IV), heparin, hetastarch in electrolytes (Hextend), hydrocortisone sodium succinate (Solu-Cortef), inamrinone (Inocor), levofloxacin (Levaquin), milrinone (Primacor), pancuronium (Pavulon), potassium chloride (KCl), propofol (Diprivan), remifentanil (Ultiva), tacrolimus (Prograf), vecuronium (Norcuron).

RATE OF ADMINISTRATION

IV injection: Each 1 ml of a 1:50,000 (0.02 mg) solution or fraction thereof over 1 minute. Follow with a 20 ml flush of NS if indicated to ensure distribution to circulation.

Infusion: Titrate to desired dose, HR, and rhythm. Decrease rate of infusion as necessary. Ventricular rate generally should not exceed 110 beats/min.

Isoproterenol (Isuprel) Infusion Rates						
Desired Dose	1 mg in 500 ml D5W (2 mcg/ml)			1 mg in 250 ml D5W 2 mg in 500 ml D5W (4 mcg/ml)		
mcg/min	mcg/hr	ml/min	ml/hr	mcg/hr	ml/min	ml/hr
2	120	1	60	120	0.5	30
5	300	2.5	150	300	1.25	75
10	600	5	300	600	2.5	150

Continued

Isoproterenol (Isuprel) Infusion Rates—cont'd						
Desired Dose	1 mg in 500 ml D5W (2 mcg/ml)			1 mg in 250 ml D5W 2 mg in 500 ml D5W (4 mcg/ml)		
mcg/min	mcg/hr	ml/min	ml/hr	mcg/hr	ml/min	ml/hr
15	900	7.5	450	900	3.75	225
20	1,200	10	600	1,200	5	300
25	1,500	12.5	750	1,500	6.25	375
30	1,800	15	900	1,800	7.5	450

Pediatric infusion: 0.6 mg/kg in 100 ml D5W 1 ml/hr = 0.1 mcg/kg/min.

Intracardiac: Each 0.1 ml of a 1:5,000 solution over 1 second. See note in Dilution for this route.

ACTIONS

A synthetic cardiac beta receptor stimulant (sympathomimetic amine) similar to epinephrine and norepinephrine. Has positive inotropic and chronotropic actions more potent than those of epinephrine. It increases cardiac output, cardiac work, coronary flow, and venous return. Improves atrioventricular conduction. Stimulates only the higher ventricular foci, allowing a more normal cardiac pacemaker to take over, thus suppressing ectopic pacemaker activity. Decreases peripheral vascular resistance by relaxing arterial smooth muscle and is a most effective bronchial smooth muscle relaxant. Onset of action is immediate and lasts 1 to 2 hours. Excreted in the urine.

INDICATIONS AND USES

Atrioventricular (AV) heart block and Stokes-Adams syndrome. ■ Some ventricular arrhythmias due to AV nodal block. ■ Treatment of refractory torsades de pointes until pacemaker implanted. ■ Temporary control of symptomatic bradycardia in denervated hearts of heart transplant patients until pacemaker implanted. ■ Bronchospasm during anesthesia. ■ Management of shock (cardiogenic, CHF, hypoperfusion [low cardiac output], hypovolemic, septic). Adequate fluid and electrolyte replacement required. ■ Pulmonary embolism, to increase pulmonary blood volume and decrease pulmonary arterial pressure and vascular resistance. ■ Cardiac catheterization to simulate exercise. ■ On occasion as an antidote to reverse severe hypotension caused by tricyclic antidepressants (e.g., amitriptyline [Elavil]). ■ AHA recommends cautious use in symptomatic bradycardia if a pacemaker is not available, and use in the treatment of refractory torsades de pointes unresponsive to magnesium sulfate, and poisoning from beta-adrenergic blockers (e.g., metoprolol [Lopressor]).

CONTRAINDICATIONS

Tachyarrhythmias, patients with tachycardia or heart block caused by digitalis intoxication, angina pectoris, ventricular arrhythmias that require inotropic therapy.

PRECAUTIONS

Intracardiac or IV injection in cardiac standstill must be accompanied by cardiac massage to perfuse drug into the myocardium. Current JAMA recommendations do not include isoproterenol in the treatment of cardiac arrest or hypotension. ■ Fourth-line agent for bradycardia; considered possibly helpful but may be harmful. ■ Can cause a severe drop in BP and can be very harmful in bradycardia. ■ Use extreme caution when inhalant anesthetics (e.g., cyclopropane) are being administered and supplementary to digitalis administration. ■ Use caution in coronary insufficiency, diabetes, hyperthyroidism, known sensitivity to sympathomimetic amines, and pre-existing cardiac arrhythmias with tachycardia. ■ Increased cardiac output and work can increase ischemia and worsen arrhythmias. ■ Contains sulfites; use caution in allergic patients.

Monitor: Decrease rate of infusion as necessary. Ventricular rate generally should not exceed 110 beats/min. Maintain adequate blood volume and correct acidosis. ■ Continuous cardiac monitoring, central venous pressure readings, BP, and urine flow measurements are advisable during therapy with isoproterenol. ■ See Drug/Lab Interactions and Maternal/Child.

Maternal/Child: Category C: safety for use in pregnancy or breast-feeding not established. Benefits must outweigh risks. ■ Safety and effectiveness in pediatric patients not established. ■ In asthmatic children, IV infusion of isoproterenol has caused clinical deterioration, myocardial necrosis, CHF, and death. Risks of cardiac toxicity may be increased by other factors such as acidosis, hypoxemia, co-administration of corticosteroids or methylxanthines (e.g., aminophylline). Continuous assessment of VS, frequent ECGs, and daily measurement of cardiac enzymes (e.g., CPK, MB) is suggested if isoproterenol infusion is required.

Elderly: Difference in response from younger patients not known. Elderly patients may be less responsive to beta-adrenergic stimulation than younger patients. Lower-end initial doses may be appropriate based on potential for decreased organ function and concomitant disease or drug therapy; see Dose Adjustments.

DRUG/LAB INTERACTIONS

May be used alternately with epinephrine (Adrenalin), but they may not be used together. Both are direct cardiac stimulants; serious arrhythmias and death may result. An adequate interval between doses must be maintained. ■ Simultaneous use with oxytoxics may cause hypertensive crisis. ■ May cause hypertension with guanethidine (Ismelin). ■ May cause arrhythmia with bretylium. ■ Halogenated hydrocarbon anesthetics (e.g., halothane) may sensitize myocardium and cause serious arrhythmias. ■ Antagonized by propranolol (Inderal). May be used to treat tachycardia caused by isoproterenol, but tachycardia and hypotension secondary to peripheral vasodilation may occur. ■ Potentiated by tricyclic antidepressants. ■ Severe hypotension and bradycardia may occur with hydantoins (e.g., phenytoin [Dilantin]).

SIDE EFFECTS

Anginal pain, cardiac arrhythmias, flushing, headache, nausea, nervousness, palpitations, sweating, tachycardia, vomiting. Cardiac dilation, marked hypotension, pulmonary edema, and death may occur with prolonged use or overdose.

ANTIDOTE

Notify the physician of any side effect. Treatment will probably be symptomatic. For ventricular rate over 110 beats/min, PVCs, or ECG changes, decrease rate of infusion or discontinue drug. For accidental overdose, discontinue drug immediately, resuscitate and sustain patient, and notify physician.

ITRACONAZOLE

(it-ra-con′a-zol)

Sporanox

Antifungal

pH 4.8

USUAL DOSE

Very specific procedures required before administration. See Dilution, Incompatible With, Monitor, and Rate of Administration.

Empiric therapy in febrile, neutropenic patients (ETFN): 200 mg as an infusion. Dedicated infusion line required. Give twice daily for 4 doses, followed by 200 mg daily for up to 14 days. Treatment should continue with itraconazole oral solution twice daily until resolution of clinically significant neutropenia. The safety and efficacy of itraconazole use for more than 28 days in ETFN is not known.

Treatment of fungal infections (blastomycosis, histoplasmosis, aspergillosis): 200 mg as an infusion. Dedicated infusion line required. Give twice daily for 4 doses, then daily thereafter. Another source suggests a loading dose of 200 mg three times a day for the first three days of therapy in life-threatening infections. Follow with oral itraconazole for a minimum of 3 months until clinical parameters and laboratory tests indicate that the active fungal infection has subsided. Safety and effectiveness of IV formulation for longer than 14 days is not known.

PEDIATRIC DOSE

Safety and effectiveness for use in pediatric patients not established; see Maternal/Child.

DOSE ADJUSTMENTS

No dose adjustments required. Not recommended for use in patients with creatinine clearance less than 30 ml/min.

DILUTION

Supplied as a kit containing one 25-ml ampule of itraconazole (10 mg/ml or 250 mg/ampule), 100-ml capacity infusion bag containing 50 ml NS (do not use bacteriostatic NS, see Compatibility), and one filtered infusion set. Withdraw the full contents of the ampule and transfer to the infusion bag of NS. Final concentration will be 3.33 mg/ml. This precise mixing ratio is required to obtain a stable solution. A precipitate will form if the 3.33 mg/ml concentration is not maintained. Mix gently after the transfer is complete. Withdraw and discard 15 ml of the solution; 60 ml (200 mg) will remain.

Storage: Store kits at or below 25° C (77° F). After reconstitution, stable for 48 hours refrigerated (2° to 8° C) or at CRT when protected from direct light.

COMPATIBILITY

Manufacturer states, "Use only the components provided in the kit by the manufacturer. ***Do not substitute.*** Do not dilute in D5W or LR alone or in combination with any other diluent. Do not introduce concomitant medication in the same infusion bag or through the same line as itraconazole." Recommends administering other medications as required after flushing the line/catheter as described under Rate of Administration and removing and replacing the entire infusion line. Alternatively, use another lumen (e.g., as in a multi-lumen catheter).

RATE OF ADMINISTRATION

Using a flow control device, infuse 60 ml (200 mg) of the diluted solution over 60 minutes. Use of a flow control device and an additional extension line required in addition to provisions in kit. Protection from light not required during administration. After administration, flush the infusion set with 15 to 20 ml of NS over 30 seconds to 15 minutes via the two-way stopcock on the extension line (itraconazole line to stopcock turned off to prevent backflow and guarantee flushing of extension line). Discard the entire extension line.

ACTIONS

A synthetic triazole antifungal agent. Inhibits the cytochrome P_{450}-dependent synthesis of ergosterol, which is a vital component of fungal cell membranes. Inhibits azole antifungals endogenous respiration, causes accumulation of phospholipids and unsaturated fatty acids within fungal cells, and disrupts chitin (polysaccharide found in certain fungi) synthesis. Steady-state plasma concentrations reached after the fourth dose during clinical trials. Half-life ranges from 6 to 64.8 hours. Extensively protein bound (99.8%). Metabolized to several metabolites including its major metabolite, hydroxyitraconazole. 40% excreted as inactive metabolites in urine, some excretion in feces. Secreted in breast milk.

INDICATIONS AND USES

Treatment of fungal infections in immunocompromised and non-immunocompromised patients. Approved for treatment of blastomycosis (pulmonary and extrapulmonary), histoplasmosis (including chronic cavitary pulmonary disease and disseminated, non-meningeal histoplasmosis), and aspergillosis (pulmonary and extrapulmonary, in patients who are intolerant of or who are refractory to amphotericin B therapy). ■ Empiric therapy in febrile neutropenic patients with suspected fungal infections. **Unlabeled uses:** Has been used in many other fungal or parasitic infections.

CONTRAINDICATIONS

Hypersensitivity to itraconazole or any of its components. Use caution in patients hypersensitive to other azoles (e.g., fluconazole, ketoconazole); risk of cross-hypersensitivity not known. ■ Coadministration is specifically contraindicated with the following drugs metabolized by the cytochrome P_{450} 3A4 isoenzyme system (CYP3A4): cisapride (Propulsid), dofetilide (Tikosyn), HMG CoA-reductase inhibitors (lovastatin [Mevacor], simvastatin [Zocor]), oral midazolam (Versed), pimozide (Orap), quinidine, and triazolam (Halcion); may result in life-threatening cardiovascular events, including QT prolongation, torsades de pointes, ventricular tachycardia, cardiac arrest, and sudden death. Astemizole and terfenadine would be included in this list but are no longer commercially available. See Drug/Lab Interactions.

PRECAUTIONS

Do not give as an IV bolus; for infusion only. ■ Inadequate treatment may lead to recurrence of active infection. Continue treatment until clinical parameters or laboratory tests indicate that active fungal infection has subsided. ■ Itraconazole has been associated with rare cases of serious hepatotoxicity, including liver failure and death. Some cases developed within the first week of therapy. Pre-existing liver disease was not always present. If clinical S/S consistent with liver disease develop, treatment should be discontinued and liver function monitored. Continuing or reinstituting therapy is strongly discouraged unless benefit outweighs risk; see

Monitor. ■ Use discouraged in patients with pre-existing liver disease or in those who have experienced hepatotoxicity with other drugs, unless there is a serious or life-threatening situation in which the expected benefit exceeds the risk. Monitoring of liver function imperative; see Monitor. ■ Not recommended for use in patients with a creatinine clearance less than 30 ml/min; accumulation of metabolites is seen. ■ Has negative inotropic effects; not recommended for patients with evidence of ventricular dysfunction unless benefit clearly outweighs risk. Evaluate benefit versus risk and use with caution in patients with risk factors for CHF (e.g., ischemic and valvular disease, significant pulmonary disease [e.g., COPD], renal failure, and/or other edematous disorders); see Monitor. ■ Fungal species with decreased susceptibility to itraconazole have been isolated during prolonged therapy. Fungi with reduced susceptibility to one azole antifungal agent may also be less susceptible to other azole derivatives. ■ One of the components of itraconazole injection has produced pancreatic adenocarcinomas in a rat carcinogenicity study; clinical relevance unknown.

Monitor: Specimens for fungal culture, serology, and histopathology should be obtained before therapy to isolate and identify causative organisms. Therapy may begin as soon as all specimens are obtained and before results are known. Reassess after test results are known. ■ Hepatotoxicity has been reported; monitor liver function tests (e.g., AST, ALT) in patients with pre-existing impaired hepatic function and any time S/S suggestive of liver dysfunction develop (e.g., jaundice, lethargy). ■ Cases of CHF, peripheral edema, and pulmonary edema have been reported. Monitor patients with risk factors of CHF carefully for S/S of CHF during treatment (e.g., dry cough, edema, paroxysmal nocturnal dyspnea, shortness of breath, weight gain). If symptoms develop, consider other treatment alternatives; may require discontinuation of itraconazole. ■ See Drug/Lab Interactions.

Patient Education: Promptly report shortness of breath, rapid heart rate, or swelling of extremities. Report any S/S of liver dysfunction (anorexia, fatigue, jaundice, nausea and vomiting, dark urine or pale stools). ■ One of the components of itraconazole has produced pancreatic adenocarcinomas in a rat carcinogenicity study. Findings not observed in a similar mouse carcinogenicity study. Relevance unknown.

Maternal/Child: Category C: use during pregnancy only if benefits outweigh potential risks to fetus. Has been found to be embryotoxic and teratogenic in rats and mice. ■ Secreted in human milk; weigh benefits to mother against potential risk to an infant being breast-fed. CDC advises HIV-infected women not to breast-feed. ■ Safety and effectiveness in children not established. Small numbers of children have been treated with oral itraconazole with no adverse effects. Has caused bone defects in some rat studies. Similar bone toxicity not found in adults, but long-term effects in children unknown.

Elderly: Use caution; consider decreased cardiac, hepatic, or renal function and effects of concomitant disease or other drug therapy.

DRUG/LAB INTERACTIONS

Interactions are numerous and potentially life-threatening. Review of drug profile by pharmacist is imperative. **Contraindicated** with antiarrhythmics **(dofetilide [Tikosyn], quinidine),** antipsychotic **pimozide (Orap),** benzodiazepines **(oral midazolam, triazolam [Halcion]),** GI motility agents **(cisapride [Propulsid]),** HMG CoA-reductase inhibitors **(lovastatin [Mevacor], simvastatin [Zocor]).**

Astemizole and terfenadine would be included in this list but are no longer commercially available. See Contraindications, may result in life-threatening cardiovascular events, including QT prolongation, torsades de pointes, ventricular tachycardia, cardiac arrest, and sudden death. ■ A potent inhibitor of the cytochrome P_{450} enzyme system. Coadministration of itraconazole and drugs primarily metabolized by the cytochrome P_{450} enzyme system may result in increased plasma concentrations of the other drug that could increase or prolong its therapeutic and/or adverse effects. Unless otherwise specified, concomitant medications metabolized by the P_{450} enzyme system should be discontinued as medically indicated. ***In addition to the contraindicated drugs above, plasma levels of the following drugs are predicted to be increased by itraconazole:*** alfentanil (Alfenta), antiarrhythmics (digoxin), anticonvulsants (carbamazepine [Tegretol], phenytoin [Dilantin]), anti-HIV protease inhibitors (e.g., indinavir [Crixivan], ritonavir [Norvir], saquinavir [Invirase, Fortovase]), antimycobacterials (rifabutin [Mycobutin]), antineoplastic agents (e.g., busulfan [Myleran], docetaxel [Taxotere], vinca alkaloids [e.g., vinblastine (Velban), vincristine (Oncovin)]), benzodiazepines (e.g., alprazolam [Xanax], diazepam [Valium], midazolam [Versed]), buspirone (BuSpar), calcium channel blockers (e.g., verapamil [Isoptin], dihydropyridine calcium channel blockers [e.g., nifedipine (Procardia), felodipine (Plendil)]), cholesterol-lowering agents (HMG-CoA-reductase inhibitors [e.g., atorvastatin (Lipitor)]), immunosuppressive agents (e.g., cyclosporine [Sandimmune], sirolimus [Rapamune], tacrolimus [Prograf]), oral hypoglycemics (e.g., glyburide [DiaBeta, Micronase]. Glipizide [Glucotrol]), steroids (e.g., methylprednisone [Solu-Medrol]), trimetrexate (Neutrexin), warfarin [Coumadin]), and others. ■ Metabolism of vinca alkaloids and steroids may be inhibited and toxicity increased with concurrent itraconazole administration. Dose adjustments may be indicated. ■ Hypnotic and sedative effects of benzodiazepines may be prolonged with concurrent use; monitor patient carefully (oral midazolam and triazolam are contraindicated). ■ May cause edema with dihydropyridine calcium channel blockers; dose adjustments may be necessary. In addition calcium channel blockers have a negative inotropic effect which may be additive to the negative inotropic effect caused by itraconazole. ■ Concurrent administration with cholesterol-lowering agents (e.g., HMG-CoA reductase inhibitors) has been associated with skeletal muscle toxicity including rhabdomyolysis; temporarily discontinue during itraconazole therapy. ■ Concurrent use with buspirone may cause increased buspirone plasma levels. Introduce buspirone at lower doses and monitor plasma levels if itraconazole started. ■ Monitor digoxin plasma concentrations during concurrent use. ■ Dose adjustment of immunosuppressive agents may be indicated. ■ May cause hypoglycemia with oral hypoglycemic agents such as glyburide (DiaBeta, Micronase), glipizide (Glucotrol); monitor blood glucose concentrations carefully. ■ May cause tinnitus and ototoxicity in addition to cardiac arrhythmias with quinidine. ■ Itraconazole plasma concentrations and effectiveness may be decreased by anticonvulsants (e.g., carbamazepine [Tegretol], phenobarbital [Luminal], phenytoin [Dilantin]), antimycobacterial agents (e.g., isoniazid [INH], rifampin [Rifadin], rifabutin [Mycobutin]), didanosine (Videx), reverse transcriptase inhibitors (e.g., nevirapine [Viramune], and others. Monitor itraconazole serum levels with concurrent use; increased doses of itraconazole may be indicated. If antimycobacterial agents are indicated, alternate antifungal therapy should be considered. ■ Prior treatment with itraconazole may reduce or inhibit the activity of polyenes (e.g., amphotericin B); clinical significance not defined. ■ Itraconazole plasma concentrations and toxicity may be increased by macrolide antibiotics (e.g., clarithromycin [Biaxin], erythromycin). ■ Plasma concentrations of both drugs may be affected with concurrent administration of itraconazole and anti-HIV protease inhibitors (e.g., ritonavir [Norvir], indinavir [Crixivan]). Studies to date show that plasma levels of the anti-HIV reverse transcriptase inhibitor zidovudine (AZT) are not affected; other agents have not been studied.

SIDE EFFECTS

Incidence difficult to assess because of multiple medical conditions and multiple medications. Abdominal pain, abnormal renal function, albuminuria, alopecia, CHF, diaphoresis, diarrhea, dizziness, edema, headache, hypertriglyceridemia, hypokalemia, hypomagnesemia, increased liver function tests (e.g., alkaline phosphatase, AST, ALT, BUN, NPN), injection site reactions, menstrual disorders, nausea, neutropenia, neuropathy, pain, peripheral edema, pulmonary edema, rash, vomiting. Allergic reactions (e.g., angioedema, pruritus, rash, anaphylaxis, Stevens-Johnson syndrome), idiosyncratic hepatitis (rare), and hepatotoxicity (rare) have been reported.

ANTIDOTE

Notify physician of all side effects; most will be treated symptomatically. Discontinue drug and notify physician of abnormal liver function tests progressing to clinical signs and symptoms of liver disease. Rash may be the first sign of an exfoliative skin disorder in immunocompromised patients; discontinue drug and notify physician. Notify physician of onset of S/S of CHF, may require discontinuation of itraconazole. Not removed by hemodialysis. Treat anaphylaxis or resuscitate if indicated.

KANAMYCIN SULFATE

(kan-a-mye′sin sul′fat)

Antibacterial (aminoglycoside)

Kantrex

pH 4.5

USUAL DOSE

Up to 15 mg/kg of body weight/24 hr equally divided into 2 or 3 doses. Dosage based on ideal body weight. Do not exceed a total adult dose of 1.5 Gm by all routes in 24 hours. Recent studies suggest that a single daily dose of 15 to 20 mg/kg (instead of divided into 2 or 3 doses) may provide higher peak levels and enhance drug effectiveness while actually reducing or having no adverse effects on risk of toxicity. Various procedures for monitoring blood levels are in use. Some health facilities are monitoring with trough levels; others may draw levels at predetermined times and plot the concentration on nomograms. Depending on the protocol in place, doses or intervals may be adjusted. See Precautions.

***Mycobacterium avium* complex:** 11 to 13 mg/kg/24 hr in equally divided doses every 8 to 12 hours (part of a 3- to 5-agent regimen).

Tuberculosis: 15 to 30 mg/kg to maximum dose of 1 Gm daily.

PEDIATRIC DOSE

15 to 30 mg/kg/24 hr in equally divided doses every 12 hours. Maximum dose is 1.5 Gm.

A single daily dose is also being used in children. See comments under Usual Dose.

NEONATAL DOSE

Less than 2,000 Gm; under 7 days of age: 7.5 mg/kg every 12 hours. **Over 7 days of age:** 6.67 mg/kg every 8 hours.

Over 2,000 Gm; under 7 days of age: 10 mg/kg every 12 hours. **Over 7 days of age:** 10 mg/kg every 8 hours.

DOSE ADJUSTMENTS

Reduce daily dose for renal impairment or increase intervals between injections. ■ Reduced dose or extended intervals may be required in the elderly. ■ See Monitor and Drug/Lab Interactions.

DILUTION

Each 500 mg or fraction thereof must be diluted with at least 100 ml of D5W, D5NS, or NS for infusion, or see chart on inside back cover. Discard partially used vials after 48 hours.

INCOMPATIBLE WITH

Manufacturer states, "Do not physically premix with other drugs; administer separately." Inactivated in solution with beta-lactam antibiotics (e.g., cephalosporins, penicillins) and vancomycin. Do not mix in the same solution. Appropriate spacing required because of physical incompatibilities. See Drug/Lab Interactions.

COMPATIBLE WITH **(Underline Indicates Conflicting Compatibility Information)**

See Incompatible With. Consult pharmacist; specific conditions may apply; see Compatibilities, p. xvi.

Additive: ***Not recommended by manufacturer.*** Ascorbic acid (Cenolate), cefoxitin (Mefoxin), chloramphenicol (Chloromycetin), clindamycin (Cleocin), dopamine (Intropin), furosemide (Lasix), hydrocortisone sodium succinate (Solu-Cortef), penicillin G potassium and sodium, sodium bicarbonate.

Syringe: Penicillin G sodium.

Y-site: Cyclophosphamide (Cytoxan), furosemide (Lasix), hydromorphone (Dilaudid), magnesium sulfate, meperidine (Demerol), morphine, perphenazine (Trilafon), potassium chloride (KCl).

RATE OF ADMINISTRATION

Do not exceed a rate of 3 to 4 ml/min diluted solution. Give total dose over 30 to 60 minutes.

ACTIONS

An aminoglycoside antibiotic with neuromuscular blocking action. Bactericidal against many gram-negative organisms resistant to other antibiotics. Well distributed through all body fluids; crosses the placental barrier. Usual half-life is 2 to 3 hours. Half-life is prolonged in infants, postpartum females, fever, liver disease and ascites, spinal cord injury, cystic fibrosis, and the elderly; shorter in severe burns. Excreted in high concentrations through the kidneys. Secreted in breast milk. Cross-allergenicity does occur between aminoglycosides.

INDICATIONS AND USES

Short-term treatment of serious infections caused by susceptible organisms. ■ Concurrent therapy with a penicillin or cephalosporin sometimes indicated. ■ Treatment of tuberculosis. ■ Primarily used when penicillin and other less toxic antibiotics are ineffective or contraindicated. **Unlabeled uses:** Treatment of *Mycobacterium avium* complex, a common infection in AIDS (part of a multiple drug [3 to 5] regimen).

CONTRAINDICATIONS

Known kanamycin or aminoglycoside sensitivity, prior hearing damage by kanamycin or other ototoxic agents unless infection is life threatening. Sulfite sensitivity may be a contraindication.

PRECAUTIONS

Most frequently given IM. ■ Use extreme caution if therapy required over 7 to 10 days. ■ Sensitivity studies necessary to determine susceptibility of causative organism to kanamycin. ■ Superinfection may occur from overgrowth of nonsusceptible organisms. ■ Use caution in children and elderly. ■ May cause "malabsorption syndrome" (increase in fecal fat, decrease in serum carotene and xylose absorption); most common in prolonged therapy. ■ May contain sulfites; use caution in patients with asthma. ■ Single daily dosing has been used effectively in abdominal, pelvic inflammatory, and GU infections in patients with normal renal function. Not recommended in bacteremia caused by *Pseudomonas aeruginosa*, endocarditis, meningitis, during pregnancy, or in patients less than 6 weeks postpartum. Limited data available for use in all other situations (e.g., burns, cystic fibrosis, elderly, pediatrics, renal impairment). ■ Risk of neurotoxicity (e.g., auditory and vestibular ototoxicity) increased in patients with preexisting renal damage or in normal renal function with prolonged use. Partial or total irreversible deafness may continue to develop after kanamycin discontinued. ■ Pseudomembranous colitis has been reported. May range from mild to life-threatening. Consider in patients that present with diarrhea during or after treatment with kanamycin.

Monitor: Routine evaluation of hearing is necessary. Watch for decrease in urine output, rising BUN and SrCr, and declining CrCl levels. Dose may need to be decreased. ■ Narrow range between toxic and therapeutic levels. Periodically monitor peak and trough concentrations to avoid peak serum concentrations above 30 mcg/ml and trough concentrations above 5 mcg/ml. ■ Maintain good hydration. ■ Monitor serum calcium, magnesium, potassium, and sodium; levels may decline. ■ Closely monitor patients with impaired renal function for nephrotoxicity and neurotoxicity (e.g., auditory and vestibular ototoxicity); nephrotoxicity may be reversible. ■ In extended treatment, daily monitoring of serum levels, electrolytes, renal, auditory, and vestibular functions is recommended. ■ See Drug/Lab Interactions.

Patient Education: Report promptly dizziness, hearing loss, weakness, or any changes in balance. ■ Consider birth control options.

Maternal/Child: Category D: avoid pregnancy. Use during pregnancy and breast-feeding only when absolutely necessary. Potential hazard to fetus. ■ Rarely used IV in infants. Use extreme caution in premature infants and neonates; immature kidney function will result in prolonged half-life.

Elderly: Consider less toxic alternatives. ■ Half-life prolonged. ■ Longer intervals between doses may be more important than reduced doses. ■ Monitor renal function and drug levels carefully. Measurement of CrCl more useful than BUN or SrCr to assess renal function. ■ See Precautions.

DRUG/LAB INTERACTIONS

Inactivated in solution with penicillin but is synergistic when used in combination with beta-lactam antibiotics (e.g., sulbactam sodium, clavulanate potassium, cephalosporins, penicillins) and vancomycin. Do not mix in the same solution. Dose adjustment and appropriate spacing required because of physical incompatibilities and interactions. Synergism may be inconsistent; measure aminoglycoside levels. ■ Concurrent use topically or systemically with any other ototoxic or nephrotoxic agents should be avoided. May have dangerous additive effects with anesthetics (e.g., enflurane), other neuromuscular blocking antibiotics (e.g., gentamicin), diuretics (e.g., furosemide [Lasix]), beta-lactam antibiotics (e.g., cephalosporins), vancomycin, and many others. ■ Neuromuscular blocking muscle relaxants (e.g., doxacurium [Nuromax], succinylcholine) are potentiated by aminoglycosides. ***Apnea can occur.*** ■ Aminoglycosides are also potentiated by anticholinesterases (e.g., edrophonium), antineoplastics (e.g., nitrogen mustard, cisplatin). ■ Digoxin dose may need adjustment. ■ May be antagonized by bacteriostatic antibiotics (e.g., chloramphenicol, erythromicin, and tetracyclines); bactericidal action may be impacted.

SIDE EFFECTS

Occur more frequently with impaired renal function, higher doses, prolonged administration, in dehydrated or elderly patients, and in patients receiving other ototoxic or nephrotoxic drugs.

Fever, headache, paresthesias, seizures, skin rash, thrombophlebitis.

Major: Apnea; azotemia; elevated BUN, nonprotein nitrogen, creatinine; granular casts; hearing loss; malabsorption syndrome; neuromuscular blockade; oliguria; proteinuria; pseudomembranous colitis; tinnitus; vertigo.

ANTIDOTE

Notify the physician of all side effects. If minor symptoms persist or any major symptom appears, discontinue the drug and notify the physician. Treatment is symptomatic, or a reduction in dose may be required. In overdose, hemodialysis may be indicated. Monitor fluid balance, CrCl, and plasma levels carefully. Complexation with ticarcillin may be as effective as hemodialysis. Consider exchange transfusion in the newborn. Calcium salts or neostigmine may reverse neuromuscular blockade. Resuscitate as necessary.

KETOROLAC TROMETHAMINE

(kee-toe′role-ak tro-meth′ah-men)

Toradol

Analgesic (NSAID)

pH 6.9 to 7.9

USUAL DOSE

Adults less than 65 years: 30 mg. May repeat every 6 hours. Maximum dose is 120 mg in 24 hours. Do not increase the dose or frequency for breakthrough pain. Consider alternating with low doses of opioids (e.g., morphine or meperidine). Ketorolac oral may be used only as continuation therapy to parenteral dosing. Maximum oral dose is 40 mg/24 hours. Do not administer for longer than 5 days (IV/IM alone or combined use with oral).

Adults over 65 years, impaired renal function, and/or patients under 50 kg (110 lb): 15 mg. May repeat every 6 hours. Maximum dose is 60 mg in 24 hours. Note all restrictions for adults less than 65 years outlined above.

PEDIATRIC DOSE

See Maternal/Child.

Short-term postoperative pain management (unlabeled): 1 mg/kg alone or as an adjunct.

DOSE ADJUSTMENTS

Required for patients under 50 kg (110 lb), over 65 years of age, and those with reduced renal function; see Usual Dose. Further dose reductions may be required with high-dose salicylates; see Drug/Lab Interactions.

DILUTION

Confirm IV use. Some 2 ml tubex syringes are for IM use only. May be given undiluted through Y-tube or three-way stopcock of infusion set. Administration through a free-flowing IV is preferred.

Storage: Store at CRT; protect from light.

INCOMPATIBLE WITH

May form a precipitate if admixed with drugs with a low pH (e.g., meperidine [Demerol], morphine, promethazine [Phenergan]).

COMPATIBLE WITH

(Underline Indicates Conflicting Compatibility Information)

Consult pharmacist; specific conditions may apply; see Compatibilities, p. xvi.

Syringe: Hydromorphone (Dilaudid), sufentanil (Sufenta).

Y-site: Alatrofloxacin (Trovan IV), cisatracurium (Nimbex), fentanyl (Sublimaze), hetastarch in electrolytes (Hextend), hydromorphone (Dilaudid), morphine, remifentanil (Ultiva), sufentanil (Sufenta).

RATE OF ADMINISTRATION

A single dose over a minimum of 15 seconds; evenly distributed over 1 to 2 minutes is preferred.

ACTIONS

A nonsteroidal antiinflammatory drug (NSAID) with peripheral analgesic, antiinflammatory, and antipyretic actions. Inhibits prostaglandin synthesis. 30 to 60 mg produces analgesia similar to morphine 12 mg or Demerol 100 mg. Studies reflect less drowsiness, nausea, and vomiting. Not a narcotic agonist or antagonist. Cardiac and hemodynamic parameters are not altered. Onset of action is 30 to 60 minutes. Half-life varies from 3.8 to 8.6 hours based on age and clinical status. Relief in some patients may last 6 to 8 hours. Excreted primarily in urine. Secreted in breast milk.

INDICATIONS AND USES

Short-term management of moderately severe, acute pain (no longer than 5 days).

Unlabeled uses: Postoperative short-term pain management in children.

CONTRAINDICATIONS

Hypersensitivity to ketorolac or its components, labor and delivery, breast-feeding, preoperative or intraoperative medication, patients currently receiving ASA or NSAIDs (e.g., ibuprofen [Advil, Motrin], naproxen [Aleve, Naprosyn]), active peptic ulcer disease, recent GI bleeding or perforation, patients with a history of peptic ulcer disease or GI bleeding, suspected or confirmed cerebrovascular bleeding, hemorrhagic diathesis, incomplete hemostasis, high risk of bleeding, advanced renal impairment, or patients at risk for renal failure because of volume depletion. Do not use for epidural or intrathecal administration, contains alcohol. See Drug/Lab Interactions.

PRECAUTIONS

Inhibits platelet aggregation and may prolong bleeding time. ■ May cause serious GI ulceration and bleeding without warning. ■ In addition to the usual caution in patients with reduced hepatic or renal function, ketorolac may also cause a dose-dependent reduction in renal prostaglandin formation. Can precipitate renal failure in patients with impaired renal function, heart failure, or liver dysfunction; in the elderly or in patients receiving diuretics. ■ Use caution in patients with cardiac decompensation, hypertension, or similar conditions; may cause fluid retention and edema. ■ Use caution in patients with pre-existing asthma, especially aspirin-sensitive asthma. Severe bronchospasm has been reported.

Monitor: Correct hypovolemia before giving ketorolac and maintain adequate hydration. ■ Observe patient frequently, especially for heartburn or signs and symptoms of GI upset or bleeding, and monitor vital signs. ■ Observe closely during ambulation. ■ Low doses of narcotics may be required to treat breakthrough pain.

Patient Education: Side effects have resulted in extended hospitalization and could be fatal. ■ Discard any remaining oral ketorolac at end of 5-day total cumulative maximum time for use.

Maternal/Child: See Contraindications. ■ Category C: safety for use not established. Use only if other alternatives are not available. ■ Discontinue breast-feeding. ■ Not recommended for use in children under 16 years of age.

Elderly: See Dose Adjustments and Precautions. ■ More sensitive to side effects. ■ Incidence of GI bleeding and acute renal failure increases with age.

DRUG/LAB INTERACTIONS

Probenecid inhibits clearance and may triple plasma levels of ketorolac. Concomitant use is contraindicated. ■ Potentiated by salicylates (especially high-dose regimens). May double plasma levels of ketorolac. Reduce dose of ketorolac by half. ■ May decrease clearance and increase toxicity of methotrexate. ■ Additive if used with other NSAIDs (see Contraindications); side effects may increase markedly. ■ May potentiate lithium levels. ■ May increase risk of bleeding, especially from the GI tract, when given concomitantly with anticoagulants (e.g., warfarin [Coumadin], heparin) or thrombolytic agents (e.g., alteplase [tPA]). ■ May increase risk of bleeding when given with agents that may cause hypoprothrombinema or inhibit platelet aggregation (e.g., cefamandole [Mandol], cefaperazone [Cefobid], valproic acid [Depacon]). ■ Can precipitate renal failure concomitantly with diuretics (e.g., furosemide [Lasix]); see Precautions. ■ Can reduce response to furosemide (Lasix) in normovolemic healthy individuals. ■ May increase risk of renal impairment with ACE inhibitors (e.g., enalapril [Vasotec]). ■ Nephrotoxicity of both agents may be increased with other nephrotoxic agents (e.g., aminoglycosides [e.g., gentamicin], cyclosporine [Sandimmune]). ■ May potentiate nondepolarizing muscle relaxants (e.g., doxacurium [Nuromax]). ■ Has caused seizures in a few patients taking antiepileptics (e.g., phenytoin [Dilantin], carbamazepine [Tegretol]). ■ May cause hallucinations with antipsychotics (e.g., thiothixene [Navane]), antidepressants (e.g., fluoxetine [Prozac]). ■ May cause elevations of liver function tests AST (SGOT), ALT (SGPT).

SIDE EFFECTS

Average dose: Diarrhea, dizziness, dyspepsia, drowsiness, edema, GI bleeding, GI pain, headache, injection site pain, nausea, and sweating are most common. Capable of all side effects of other NSAIDs, especially with extended use: abnormal taste, abnormal vision, asthenia, asthma, confusion, constipation, depression, dry mouth, dypsnea, euphoria, excessive thirst, flatulence, inability to concentrate, insomnia, liver function abnormalities, melena, myalgia, nervousness, oliguria, pallor, paresthesia, peptic ulcer, rectal bleeding, stimulation, stomatitis, pruritus, purpura, urinary frequency, urticaria, vasodilation, vertigo, vomiting.

Overdose: Abdominal pain, diarrhea, labored breathing, metabolic acidosis, pallor, peptic ulcer, rales, vomiting.

ANTIDOTE

With increasing severity of any side effect or onset of symptoms of overdose, discontinue the drug and notify the physician. A patent airway, artificial ventilation, oxygen therapy, and other symptomatic treatment must be instituted promptly if indicated. Treat anaphylaxis with epinephrine (Adrenalin), diphenhydramine (Benadryl), and corticosteroids as indicated. Not significantly cleared by dialysis.

LABETALOL HYDROCHLORIDE

(la-bet′a-lole hye-droe-klor′id)

Alpha/beta-adrenergic blocking agent
Antihypertensive

Normodyne, Trandate

pH 3 to 4

USUAL DOSE

20 mg as an initial dose by IV injection. May repeat with injections of 40 to 80 mg at 10-minute intervals until desired BP is achieved, or may be diluted and given as a continuous infusion. Usually effective with 50 to 200 mg. Do not exceed a total dose of 300 mg. Initiate oral labetalol after desired BP has been achieved and the supine diastolic pressure starts to rise. See literature for dose regimen. AHA recommends 10 mg IV over 1 to 2 minutes. May repeat or double dose every 10 minutes to a maximum dose of 150 mg. Or initial dose may be given by IV injection followed by an infusion of 2 to 8 mg/min. Titrate slowly to achieve desired results without exceeding maximum dose.

DOSE ADJUSTMENTS

See Precautions and Drug/Lab Interactions.

DILUTION

IV injection: May be given undiluted.

Continuous infusion: May be diluted in most commonly used IV solutions (see chart on inside back cover). Addition of 200 mg (40 ml) to 160-ml solution yields 1 mg/ml, 300 mg (60 ml) to 240 ml yields 1 mg/ml, or 200 mg (40 ml) to 250 ml yields 2 mg/3 ml. Amount of solution may be decreased if required by fluid restrictions of the patient.

Storage: Stable after dilution for 24 hours at room temperature.

INCOMPATIBLE WITH

Manufacturer lists 5% sodium bicarbonate.

COMPATIBLE WITH

(Underline Indicates Conflicting Compatibility Information)

Consult pharmacist; specific conditions may apply; see Compatibilities, p. xvi.

Y-site: Amikacin (Amikin), aminophylline, amiodarone (Cordarone), ampicillin, butorphanol (Stadol), calcium gluconate, cefazolin (Kefzol), ceftazidime (Fortaz), ceftizoxime (Cefizox), chloramphenicol (Chloromycetin), cimetidine (Tagamet), clindamycin (Cleocin), diltiazem (Cardizem), dobutamine (Dobutrex), dopamine (Intropin), enalaprilat (Vasotec IV), epinephrine (Adrenalin), erythromycin lactobionate (Erythrocin), esmolol (Brevibloc), famotidine (Pepcid IV), fentanyl (Sublimaze), furosemide (Lasix), gatifloxacin (Tequin), gentamicin (Garamycin), heparin, hetastarch in electrolytes (Hextend), hydromorphone (Dilaudid), insulin (regular), lidocaine, linezolid (Zyvox), lorazepam (Ativan), magnesium sulfate, meperidine (Demerol), metronidazole (Flagyl IV), midazolam (Versed), milrinone (Primacor), morphine, nicardipine (Cardene IV), nitroglycerin (Nitro-Bid IV), nitroprusside sodium, norepinephrine (Levophed), oxacillin (Bactocill), penicillin G potassium, piperacillin (Pipracil), potassium chloride (KCl), potassium phosphates, propofol (Diprivan), ranitidine (Zantac), sodium acetate, sulfamethoxazole-trimethoprim (Bactrim), tobramycin (Nebcin), vancomycin (Vancocin), vecuronium (Norcuron).

RATE OF ADMINISTRATION

IV injection: Each 20 mg or fraction thereof over at least 2 minutes.

Continuous infusion: Begin at 2 mg/min. Adjust according to orders of physician and BP response. Another source suggests 0.5 to 2 mg/min. Use of a microdrip (60 gtt/ml) or an infusion pump may be helpful.

ACTIONS

Labetalol is an alpha-/beta-adrenergic blocking agent. Causes dose-related falls in BP without reflex tachycardia or significant reduction in HR. Maximum effect of each dose is reached in 5 minutes. Half-life is about 5 hours, but some effects last up to 16 hours. Metabolized and excreted as metabolites in urine and through bile to feces. Crosses the placental barrier. Present in small amounts in breast milk.

INDICATIONS AND USES

Control of BP in severe hypertension.

Unlabeled uses: Treatment of clonidine withdrawal hypertension. ■ Decrease BP and relieve symptoms in patients with pheochromocytoma.

CONTRAINDICATIONS

Obstructive airway disease including asthma, cardiogenic shock, greater than first-degree heart block, overt cardiac failure, severe bradycardia, and hypersensitivity to labetalol or its components.

PRECAUTIONS

Use caution in impaired liver function. ■ Use extreme caution in patients with any degree of cardiac failure; may further depress myocardial contractility. Does not alter effectiveness of digitalis on heart muscle. ■ Effective in lowering BP in pheochromocytoma, but may cause a paradoxical hypertensive response. ■ Use with extreme caution in diabetics or patients with a history of hypoglycemia. May mask the symptoms of hypoglycemia. ■ Some authorities recommend that drugs with beta-adrenergic properties be discontinued 48 hours before major surgery (beta blockade interferes with cardiac response to reflex stimuli). ■ See Drug/Lab Interactions.

Monitor: Keep patient supine. Postural hypotension can occur for several hours after administration. Ambulate with care and assistance. ■ Monitor BP before and 5 and 10 minutes after each direct IV injection. Monitor at least every 5 minutes during infusion. Avoid rapid or excessive falls in either systolic or diastolic BP. When severely elevated BP drops too rapidly, catastrophic reactions can occur (e.g., cerebral infarction, optic nerve infarction, angina, ischemic ECG changes). ■ Although rebound angina, myocardial infarction, or ventricular arrhythmias have not been a problem with labetalol, it is recommended that the dose of beta-adrenergic blockers be reduced gradually to avoid these conditions. ■ See Drug/Lab Interactions.

Patient Education: Report cough, dizziness, irregular pulse, or shortness of breath promptly. ■ May cause dizziness or fainting; request assistance with ambulation.

Maternal/Child: Category C: use in pregnancy only when clearly indicated and benefit outweighs risk. Has been used during labor and delivery. ■ Use caution during breast-feeding. ■ Safety for use in children not established.

Elderly: Use with caution in age-related peripheral vascular disease; risk of hypothermia increased. ■ May exacerbate mental impairment.

DRUG/LAB INTERACTIONS

May potentiate tricyclic antidepressants (e.g., imipramine [Tofranil]). ■ Inhibits beta-agonist bronchodilators (e.g., epinephrine); increased doses may be required, especially in asthmatics. ■ Synergistic with halothane anesthesia. Notify anesthesiologist that patient is receiving labetalol. ■ Potentiated by cimetidine (Tagamet). ■ May cause further hypotension with nitroglycerin. The use of labetalol with calcium channel blockers (e.g., diltiazem [Cardizem], verapamil [Isoptin]) may potentiate both drugs and result in severe depression of myocardium, AV conduction, and severe hypotension. ■ May decrease insulin availability; dose of antidiabetics may need to be adjusted. ■ May interfere with lab tests in diagnosis of pheochromocytoma.

SIDE EFFECTS

Diaphoresis, dizziness, flushing, moderate hypotension, numbness, severe postural hypotension, somnolence, tingling of scalp, and ventricular dysrhythmias (e.g., intensified atrioventricular block) occur most frequently.

ANTIDOTE

Notify the physician of all side effects. Decrease rate or discontinue drug if hypotension occurs. Notify physician immediately. Trendelenburg position may be appropriate. May require treatment with IV fluids or vasopressors (e.g., norepinephrine [levarterenol], dopamine [Intropin]). Use atropine for severe bradycardia; digitalis and diuretics for cardiac failure. Unresponsive hypotension and bradycardia may be reversed by glucagon 5 to 10 mg over 30 seconds followed by a continuous infusion of 5 mg/hr. Reduce rate as condition improves. Treat other side effects symptomatically and resuscitate as necessary. Hemodialysis is not effective.

LEPIRUDIN

(leh-peer'u-din)

Refludan

Anticoagulant

pH 7

USUAL DOSE

A baseline aPTT should be determined before initiation of therapy with lepirudin. To avoid a potential overdose, therapy should not be started in patients with a baseline aPTT ratio of 2.5 or more. The aPTT ratio is the aPTT in a given patient at a given time over an aPTT reference value; usually median of the laboratory normal range for aPTT.

Anticoagulation in adult patients with heparin-induced thrombocytopenia (HIT) and associated thromboembolic disease. ***Bolus dose:*** 0.4 mg/kg body weight (up to 110 kg).

Lepirudin Standard Bolus Injection Volumes According to Body Weight for a 5 mg/ml Concentration		
Body Weight (kg)	Injection Volume	
	Dosage 0.4 mg/kg	Dosage 0.2 mg/kg*
50	4 ml	2 ml
60	4.8 ml	2.4 ml
70	5.6 ml	2.8 ml
80	6.4 ml	3.2 ml
90	7.2 ml	3.6 ml
100	8 ml	4 ml
≥110	8.8 ml	4.4 ml

*Dosage recommended for all patients with renal insufficiency.

Maintenance infusion: 0.15 mg/kg body weight (up to 110 kg)/hr for 2 to 10 days or longer as clinically indicated. Adjust rate to maintain an aPTT ratio of 1.5 to 2.5. See Dose Adjustments and Precautions/Monitor.

DOSE ADJUSTMENTS

Normally the initial dose depends on body weight. This is valid up to a body weight of 110 kg. In patients weighing more than 110 kg, the initial dose should not be increased beyond the 110-kg body weight dose (i.e., the initial bolus dose should not exceed 44 mg and the initial infusion rate should not exceed 16.5 mg/hr). ■ If possible, an aPTT ratio outside of the target range (aPTT 1.5 to 2.5) should be confirmed before any dose adjustment. If the confirmed aPTT ratio is above the target range, the infusion should be stopped for 2 hours and then restarted at half the previous infusion rate. If the confirmed aPTT ratio is below the target range, the infusion rate should be increased in 20% increments. ■ Dose reduction is required in patients with renal impairment as measured by a CrCl of less than 60 ml/min or a SrCr of greater than 1.5 mg/dl. Reduce bolus dose to 0.2 mg/kg body weight. Adjust infusion rate as indicated in the following chart.

Reduction of Lepirudin Infusion Ratio in Patients With Renal Impairment			
		Adjusted Infusion Rate	
Creatinine Clearance (ml/min)	Serum Creatinine (mg/dl)	(% of Standard Initial Infusion Rate)	(mg/kg/hr)
45-60	1.6-2	50%	0.075
30-44	2.1-3	30%	0.045
15-29	3.1-6	15%	0.0225
Below 15*	Above 6*	Avoid or STOP infusion*	

*In hemodialysis patients or in case of acute renal failure (CrCl <15 ml/min or SrCr >6 mg/dl). Infusion of lepirudin is to be avoided or stopped. Additional intravenous bolus doses of 0.1 mg/kg body weight should be considered every other day only if the aPTT ratio falls below the lower therapeutic limit of 1.5.

■ There are limited data regarding concomitant use of lepirudin with thrombolytic therapy (e.g., alteplase [tPA, Activase], streptokinase [Streptase], urokinase [Abbokinase]). A dose reduction of 0.2 mg/kg of body weight for the bolus dose and 0.1 mg/kg of body weight/hr for the continuous infusion has been recommended. ■ In patients scheduled to receive a coumarin derivative for oral anticoagulation after lepirudin therapy, the rate should be decreased gradually until an aPTT ratio just above 1.5 is reached. Initiate oral anticoagulant therapy at this point. Coumarin derivatives should be initiated only when platelet counts are normalizing. Do not use a loading dose; administer the intended maintenance dose. Discontinue lepirudin when target INR is reached. May take 4 to 5 days. See package insert. ■ Clearance of lepirudin is lower in women and in the elderly. Dose adjustments may be necessary.

DILUTION

Warm preparation to room temperature before administration.

Bolus: Reconstitute 50-mg vial with 1 ml of SW or NS and shake gently. Transfer the contents of the vial to a sterile syringe and further dilute with NS, SW, or D5W to a total volume of 10 ml. This provides a final concentration of 5 mg/ml, which is suitable for bolus injection. Calculate volume of dilution to be administered. See Usual Dose. Discard any unused solution.

Infusion: Reconstitute 2 vials with 1 ml each of SW or NS. Add the contents of both vials (100 mg) to 250 ml or 500 ml of NS or D5W to obtain a final concentration of 0.4 mg/ml or 0.2 mg/ml, respectively.

Storage: Store unopened vials at 2° to 25° C (36° to 77° F). Once reconstituted, lepirudin should be used immediately. Stable for 24 hours at room temperature (e.g., during infusion).

COMPATIBILITY

Manufacturer states, "Should not be mixed with other drugs except for SW, NS, or D5W."

RATE OF ADMINISTRATION

Bolus: A single dose over 15 to 20 seconds.

Infusion: Administer at the determined rate according to body weight. See Usual Dose, Dose Adjustments, and the following chart. An infusion rate of 0.21 mg/kg/hr should not be exceeded without checking for coagulation abnormalities, which might prevent an appropriate aPTT response.

Lepirudin Standard Infusion Rates According to Body Weight		
	Infusion Rate at 0.15 mg/kg/hr	
Body Weight (kg)	500-ml Infusion Bag (0.2 mg/ml)	250-ml Infusion Bag (0.4 mg/ml)
50	38 ml/hr	19 ml/hr
60	45 ml/hr	23 ml/hr
70	53 ml/hr	26 ml/hr
80	60 ml/hr	30 ml/hr
90	68 ml/hr	34 ml/hr
100	75 ml/hr	38 ml/hr
≥110	83 ml/hr	41 ml/hr

ACTIONS

An anticoagulant that is a highly specific direct inhibitor of thrombin. A recombinant hirudin that is derived from yeast cells. One molecule of lepirudin binds to one molecule of thrombin, thereby blocking the thrombogenic activity of thrombin. Inhibits both free and clot-bound thrombin without requiring endogenous cofactors (i.e., mode of action is independent of antithrombin III and heparin cofactor II and is not inhibited by platelet factor 4). Produces a dose-dependent increase in aPTT. Distribution is restricted primarily to the extracellular space. Excreted almost exclusively by the kidneys. Terminal half-life approximately 1.3 hours.

INDICATIONS AND USES

Anticoagulation in patients with heparin-induced thrombocytopenia (HIT) and associated thromboembolic disease to prevent further thromboembolic complications.

CONTRAINDICATIONS

Known hypersensitivity to hirudins.

PRECAUTIONS

Intracranial bleeding in the absence of concomitant thrombolytic therapy has been reported. Concomitant therapy with thrombolytic agents (e.g., alteplase [tPA, Activase], streptokinase [Streptase], urokinase [Abbokinase]) may increase the risk of bleeding, including life-threatening intracranial bleeding. See Dose Adjustments and Drug/Lab Interactions. ■ Use with extreme caution and weigh risk versus benefit in all patients with an increased risk of bleeding. Conditions of concern include recent significant surgery, anomaly of vessels or organs, bacterial endocarditis, severe uncontrolled hypertension, advanced renal impairment, hemorrhagic diathesis, recent puncture of large vessels, recent CVA, stroke, intracerebral surgery or other neuraxial procedures, recent organ biopsy, and recent major bleeding (e.g., intracranial, gastrointestinal, intraocular, or pulmonary bleeding). ■ Hepatic impairment may enhance the anticoagulant effect of lepirudin due to coagulation defects secondary to reduced generation of vitamin K–dependent coagulation factors. ■ There are limited data regarding reexposure to lepirudin. A case of mild allergic skin reaction upon reexposure has been reported. ■ Antihirudin antibody formation has been reported in about 40% of patients receiving lepirudin. This may increase the drug's anticoagulant effect. To date, there is no evidence that antibody formation may lead to neutralization of lepirudin. ■ Allergic reactions, including anaphylaxis resulting in shock or death, have been reported and have occurred during initial administration and on re-exposure.

Monitor: Monitor renal function. CrCl is preferred method of monitoring. May use SrCr if CrCl is not available. See Dose Adjustments. ■ Determine a baseline aPTT ratio. Infusion rate should be adjusted according to the aPTT ratio. See Dose Adjustments. An aPTT ratio should be determined 4 hours after the start of the infusion and 4 hours after any change in infusion rate. Follow-up aPTT ratios should be determined at least once daily. More frequent monitoring is recommended in patients with renal or hepatic impairment. ■ Obtain baseline and monitor platelet count, hemoglobin, hematocrit, and occult blood in stool. ■ Strict monitoring of aPTT indicated in prolonged therapy to monitor for antihirudin antibodies. ■ See Precautions.

Patient Education: Report all episodes of bleeding. ■ Report tarry stools. ■ Compliance with all measures to minimize bleeding is very important (e.g., avoid use of razors, toothbrushes, other sharp items). ■ Use caution while moving to avoid excess bumping.

Maternal/Child: Category B: safety for use in pregnancy not established. Benefits must outweigh risks. ■ In lactating women, the decision should be made to discontinue breast-feeding or to discontinue the drug, taking into account the importance of the drug to the mother. ■ Safety and efficacy have not been established for children. Was used during trials in two older children without adverse events.

Elderly: Clearance is reduced in the elderly, possibly due to age-related renal impairment. See Dose Adjustments.

DRUG/LAB INTERACTIONS

Concomitant treatment with thrombolytics (e.g., alteplase [tPA, Activase], reteplase [Retavase], streptokinase [Streptase], urokinase [Abbokinase]) may increase the risk of bleeding complications and enhance the effect of lepirudin on aPTT prolongation. See Dose Adjustments. ■ Concomitant treatment with coumarin derivatives (warfarin [Coumadin]) and drugs that affect platelet function such as dipyridamole (Persantine), NSAIDs (e.g., ibuprofen [Advil, Motrin], naproxen [Aleve, Naprosyn]) may also increase the risk of bleeding. ■ Other thrombin-dependent coagulation assays will be changed by lepirudin.

SIDE EFFECTS

Bleeding is the most frequent adverse event.

Abnormal kidney or liver function, allergic reactions (including anaphylaxis), fever, heart failure, infection, intracranial bleeding, multi-organ failure, pericardial effusion, pneumonia, ventricular fibrillation.

ANTIDOTE

No specific antidote is available. If life-threatening bleeding develops and excessive plasma levels of lepirudin are suspected, immediately stop lepirudin infusion. Determine aPTT and hemoglobin and prepare for blood transfusion as appropriate. Follow current guidelines for treatment of shock as indicated (fluid, vasopressors [e.g., dopamine], Trendelenburg position, plasma expanders [e.g., albumin, hetastarch]). Hemodialysis or hemofiltration may be useful in overdose situation; see package insert for specifics.

LEUCOVORIN CALCIUM

(loo-koe-vor′in kal′se-um)

Antidote
Antineoplastic adjunct

Citrovorum Factor, Folinic Acid

pH 6 to 8.1

USUAL DOSE

Delayed excretion or overdose of methotrexate (MTX): 10 mg/M^2 every 6 hours until the serum MTX level is less than 0.05 micromolar. Milligram for milligram or greater than the dose of MTX is common. Administer within the first hour (or as soon as possible) in overdose or within 24 hours of MTX dose if there is delayed excretion. At least every 24 hours, obtain a SrCr and MTX level. If SrCr is more than 50% above pretreatment level, increase the leucovorin dose to 100 mg/M^2 every 3 hours until the serum MTX level is less than 0.05 micromolar.

Leucovorin rescue after high-dose MTX therapy: With high-dose methotrexate (12 to 15 Gm/M^2 as an infusion over 4 hours); begin leucovorin 15 mg (approximately 10 mg/M^2) 24 hours after MTX infusion started. Repeat every 6 hours for 10 doses. If MTX elimination is delayed, extend every-6-hour dosing until MTX level is less than 0.05 micromolar. If there is evidence of acute renal injury, increase leucovorin to 150 mg every 3 hours until MTX level is less than 1 micromolar, then 15 mg every 3 hours until MTX level is less than 0.05 micromolar. In both situations obtain SrCr and MTX level at least every 24 hours. Other protocols are in use. Amount of leucovorin is dependent on MTX dose, MTX serum levels, and SrCr.

Megaloblastic anemia: Up to 1 mg daily.

Advanced colorectal cancer: 200 mg/M^2 followed by fluorouracil (5-FU) 370 mg/M^2 or leucovorin 20 mg/M^2 followed by 5-FU 425 mg/M^2 daily for 5 days. Repeat at 4-week intervals twice, then repeat every 28 to 35 days based on complete recovery from toxic effects. Reduce 5-FU dose based on tolerance to previous course, 20% for moderate hematologic or GI toxicity, 30% for severe. Leucovorin doses remain the same. Increase 5-FU dose 10% if no toxicity. Other protocols are in use. Recently approved for use with irinotecan and 5-FU.

DOSE ADJUSTMENTS

See adjustments in Usual Dose; larger reductions may be required in the elderly based on the potential for decreased renal function, especially in combination with fluorouracil. ■ See Precautions/Monitor.

DILUTION

Each 50-mg, 100-mg, or 350-mg vial should be diluted to a 10 mg to 20 mg/ml solution. For total doses less than 10 mg/M^2, dilute with bacteriostatic water for injection (contains benzyl alcohol as a preservative). Use SW for injection without a preservative for any dose 10 mg/M^2 or greater. May be further diluted in 100 to 500 ml of D5W, D10W, NS, R, or LR. 1-ml (3-mg) ampules may be given undiluted (contain benzyl alcohol).

Storage: If prepared without a preservative, use immediately; stable up to 7 days with a preservative.

INCOMPATIBLE WITH

Several sources cite incompatibility with fluorouracil (5-FU) as an additive.

COMPATIBLE WITH (Underline Indicates Conflicting Compatibility Information)

Consult pharmacist; specific conditions may apply; see Compatibilities, p. xvi.

Additive: Cisplatin (Platinol), methotrexate (Folex).

Syringe: Bleomycin (Blenoxane), cisplatin (Platinol), cyclophosphamide (Cytoxan), doxorubicin (Adriamycin), fluorouracil (5-FU), furosemide (Lasix), heparin, methotrexate (Folex), metoclopramide (Reglan), mitomycin (Mutamycin), vinblastine (Velban), vincristine (Oncovin).

Y-site: Amifostine (Ethyol), aztreonam (Azactam), bleomycin (Blenoxane), cefepime (Maxipime), cisplatin (Platinol), cladribine (Leustatin), cyclophosphamide (Cytoxan), docetaxel (Taxotere), doxorubicin (Adriamycin), doxorubicin liposome (Doxil), etoposide phosphate (Etopophos), filgrastim (Neupogen), fluconazole (Diflucan), fluorouracil (5-FU), furosemide (Lasix), gatifloxacin (Tequin), gemcitabine (Gemzar), granisetron (Kytril), heparin, linezolid (Zyvox), methotrexate (Folex), metoclopramide (Reglan), mitomycin (Mutamycin), piperacillin/tazobactam (Zosyn), tacrolimus (Prograf), teniposide (Vumon), thiotepa (Thioplex), vinblastine (Velban), vincristine (Oncovin).

RATE OF ADMINISTRATION

Because of calcium content, do not exceed a rate of 160 mg/min (16 ml of a 10-mg/ml or 8 ml of a 20-mg/ml solution). May be given more slowly. Large doses may be infused equally distributed over 1 to 6 hours. Never exceed above limits.

ACTIONS

Potent agent for neutralizing immediate toxic effects of methotrexate (and other folic acid antagonists) on the hematopoietic system. Preferentially rescues normal cells without reversing the oncolytic effect of methotrexate. Also enhances the therapeutic and toxic effects of fluoropyrimidines (e.g., fluorouracil [5-FU]).

INDICATIONS AND USES

Treatment of accidental folic acid antagonist (e.g., methotrexate) overdose or delayed excretion of MTX. ■ Folinic acid rescue to prevent or decrease the toxicity of massive MTX doses used to treat resistant neoplasms. ■ Treatment of megaloblastic anemia due to folic acid deficiency when oral therapy not appropriate. ■ In combination with fluorouracil or fluorouracil and irinotecan (Camptosar) to treat colorectal cancer.

Unlabeled uses: Adjunct in the treatment of Ewing's sarcoma, head and neck cancer, non-Hodgkin's lymphomas, and trophoblastic tumors.

CONTRAINDICATIONS

Pernicious anemia and other megaloblastic anemias secondary to lack of vitamin B_{12}. None when used as indicated for other specific uses.

PRECAUTIONS

Usually administered in the hospital by or under the direction of the physician specialist. ■ Permits use of massive doses of methotrexate. ■ Do not discontinue leucovorin calcium until methotrexate serum levels fall below toxic levels. ■ Much less effective in accidental overdose after a 1-hour delay. ■ Delayed MTX excretion may occur from third-space fluid accumulation (ascites, pleural effusion), renal insufficiency, or inadequate hydration. ■ All doses over 25 mg should be given IM or IV (no more than 25 mg can be absorbed orally). ■ IM or IV dosing required in presence of GI toxicity, nausea, or vomiting. ■ Benzyl alcohol associated with gasping syndrome in premature infants.

Monitor: Monitor serum blood levels of MTX and SrCr levels at least daily until level is less than 0.05 micromolar. Death can occur in 5 to 10 days if MTX remains at toxic levels longer than 48 hours. ■ Minimum fluid intake of 3 L/24 hr and alkalinization of urine to a pH of 7 or more with oral sodium bicarbonate recommended. Begin 12 hours before MTX dose and continue for 48 hours after final dose in each sequence. Does not reduce nephrotoxicity of MTX from drug or metabolite precipitation in the kidney. ■ See methotrexate or fluorouracil monograph.

Maternal/Child: Category C: safety for use in pregnancy and breast-feeding not established. Benefits must outweigh risks.

Elderly: Response similar to that seen in younger patients; however, use caution, may have greater sensitivity to its toxic effects (e.g., greater risk for GI toxicity and severe diarrhea in combination with fluorouracil). Monitoring of renal function suggested. ■ See Dose Adjustments.

DRUG/LAB INTERACTIONS

May inhibit phenytoins (e.g., Dilantin), phenobarbital, and primidone; may cause increased frequency of seizures. ■ Is used in combination with fluorouracil, use caution, leucovorin calcium may increase toxic as well as therapeutic effects of fluorouracil. ■ When given with MTX avoid any drug that may interfere with MTX elimination or binding to serum albumin (e.g., NSAIDs [e.g., ibuprofen (Advil, Motrin), indomethacin, ketoprofen, naproxen (Aleve, Naprosyn)], probenecid, procarbazine [Matulane], salicylates, sulfonamides). Consider as possible cause of toxicity. ■ Concurrent use with sulfamethoxazole and trimethoprim (Bactrim) may cause treatment failure and increased morbidity in HIV patients being treated for ***pneumocystis carinii*** pneumonia.

SIDE EFFECTS

Allergic reactions including anaphylaxis have occurred rarely. Methotrexate or fluourouracil may cause many serious and dose-limiting side effects; see individual monographs.

ANTIDOTE

Keep physician informed of patient's condition. Symptomatic treatment indicated.

LEVOCARNITINE

(lee-voh-kar′ne-teen)

Nutritional supplement

L-Carnitine, Carnitor

pH 6 to 6.5

USUAL DOSE

Metabolic secondary carnitine deficiency in adults and children: 50 mg/kg/24 hr in equally divided doses every 3 to 4 hours (preferred). Intervals between administration must never exceed 6 hours. Repeat daily and adjust dose as indicated by clinical response or as therapy may require. In ***severe metabolic crisis*** an initial loading dose of 50 mg/kg may be given followed by an equivalent dose (50 mg/kg) in equally divided doses every 3 to 4 hours over 24 hours. Then give 50 mg/kg/day. Up to 300 mg/kg/24 hr has been given.

Carnitine deficiency in adult and pediatric dialysis patients: 10 to 20 mg/kg of dry body weight into the venous return line after each dialysis session. Initiate therapy if trough (pre-dialysis) plasma levocarnitine concentrations are below a normal of 40 to 50 mcM/L. Do not use oral levocarnitine in patients with end-stage renal disease (ESRD); see Precautions.

Pediatric cardiomyopathy: 50 mg/kg/24 hr in equally divided doses every 3 to 4 hours. Intervals must never exceed 6 hours. Repeat daily; adjust dose as indicated by clinical response. Cardiomyopathy may be part of a carnitine deficiency or be idiopathic. May have a dramatic response; in some cases the heart has returned to normal size within 72 hours.

DOSE ADJUSTMENTS

In dialysis patients, reduce dose based on trough (pre-dialysis) plasma levocarnitine concentrations. Reductions to 5 mg/kg may be indicated as early as the third or fourth week of therapy. ■ See Precautions.

DILUTION

May be given by IV injection or added to NS or LR for infusion.

Storage: Store ampules at CRT in carton to protect from light. Discard any unused portion; contains no preservative. Infusion solutions ranging from 0.5 to 8 mg/ml are stable for 24 hours at CRT.

COMPATIBILITY

Specific information not available; consult pharmacist. Manufacturer lists compatibility with PVC infusion bags.

RATE OF ADMINISTRATION

IV injection: A single dose equally distributed over 2 to 3 minutes.

Infusion: Give at rate ordered for primary infusion. Do not exceed direct IV rate.

ACTIONS

A naturally occurring substance required in energy metabolism. Facilitates entry of long-chain fatty acids into cellular mitochondria, providing substrate for oxidation and subsequent energy production. Fatty acids are used as an energy source in all tissues except the brain. Primary systemic carnitine deficiency is characterized by low concentrations of carnitine in plasma, RBCs and/or tissues. Secondary carnitine deficiency may be caused by inborn errors in metabolism or by iatrogenic factors such as hemodialysis. Levocarnitine promotes the excretion of excess organic or fatty acids in patients with defects in fatty acid metabolism and/or specific organic acidopathies that bioaccumulate acyl CoA esters. Can correct acidosis from these specific causes, which can be life threatening. Clears toxic organic acids by forming acyl carnitine, which is excreted primarily in the urine. Has a short half-life that necessitates dosing at least every 6 hours to maintain desired blood levels.

INDICATIONS AND USES

Acute and chronic treatment of patients (including infants and children) with an inborn error of metabolism that results in secondary carnitine deficiency (e.g., glutaric aciduria II, methyl malonic aciduria, propionic acidemia, medium chain fatty acyl CoA dehydrogenase deficiency). ■ Prevention and treatment of carnitine deficiency in end-stage renal disease patients undergoing dialysis. ■ Treatment of pediatric cardiomyopathy (orphan designation).

Unlabeled uses: Treatment of secondary carnitine deficiency in valproate toxicity. Treatment of zidovudine-induced mitochondrial myopathy.

CONTRAINDICATIONS

None known at this time when used as directed for specific indications.

PRECAUTIONS

Oral dose form used to treat primary carnitine deficiency and when feasible in secondary deficiency. ■ Safety and effectiveness of oral levocarnitine has not been evaluated in patients with renal dysfunction. Chronic administration in patients with severe renal impairment may lead to accumulation of potentially toxic metabolites that are normally excreted in urine. Use only the IV formulation in patients with ESRD, patients receiving dialysis, or patients with severe impaired renal function. ■ See Drug/Lab Interactions.

Monitor: Obtain baseline plasma carnitine levels before treatment and monitor weekly and then monthly based on response (normal range of free carnitine levels is 35 to 60 micromoles/L). ■ Monitor blood chemistries, free fatty acid concentrations, triglycerides, vital signs, and overall clinical condition before treatment, as indicated during acute phase and weekly to monthly thereafter. ■ End Stage Renal Disease (ESRD) patients on maintenance hemodialysis may have low plasma carnitine concentrations and an increased ratio of acylcarnitine/carnitine because of reduced intake of meat and dairy products, reduced renal synthesis and dialytic losses. Certain clinical conditions common in hemodialysis patients such as malaise, muscle weakness, cardiomyopathy, and cardiac arrhythmias may be related to abnormal carnitine metabolism.

Patient Education: Stress importance of follow-up evaluation and treatment.

Maternal/Child: Category B: no adequate studies; use only if clearly needed. ■ Carnitine is a normal component of breast milk. Highly probable that L-carnitine is secreted in breast milk also; discontinue breast-feeding.

DRUG/LAB INTERACTIONS

Vitamin B_T (D, L-carnitine), sold in health food stores, competitively inhibits L-carnitine and can cause a secondary deficiency. ■ Carnitine requirements may be increased in patients taking valproic acid.

SIDE EFFECTS

Abdominal cramps, diarrhea, gastritis, and transient nausea and vomiting may occur; most common with oral dosing. Drug-related body odor (11%). Seizures may occur with or without a history of seizures. An increased incidence of seizures has been reported in patients with a history of seizures.

ANTIDOTE

Keep physician informed. If clinically appropriate, dose reduction may decrease or eliminate body odor and GI symptoms. No reports of toxicity, but treatment would be supportive. Removed by dialysis.

LEVOFLOXACIN

(lee-voh-flox'a-sin)

Levaquin

Antibacterial (fluoroquinolone)

pH 3.8 to 5.8

USUAL DOSE

250 to 750 mg once every 24 hours. Dose and duration of treatment are based on degree of infection and specific diagnosis. CrCl equal to or greater than 50 ml/min is required. Dose and serum levels similar by oral or IV route. Transfer to oral dose as soon as practical.

Levofloxacin Dosing Guidelines

Infection*	Unit Dose	Freq.	Duration	Total Daily Dose
Acute Bacterial Exacerbation of Chronic Bronchitis	500 mg	q24h	7 days	500 mg
Nosocomial Pneumonia	750 mg	q24h	7-14 days	750 mg
Comm. Acquired Pneumonia	500 mg	q24h	7-14 days	500 mg
Acute Maxillary Sinusitis	500 mg	q24h	10-14 days	500 mg
Complicated SSSI[1]	750 mg	q24h	7-14 days	750 mg
Uncomplicated SSSI[1]	500 mg	q24h	7-10 days	500 mg
Complicated UTI[2]	250 mg	q24h	10 days	250 mg
Acute pyelonephritis	250 mg	q24h	10 days	250 mg
Uncomplicated UTI[2]	250 mg	q24h	3 days	250 mg

*DUE TO THE DESIGNATED PATHOGENS (See Indications and Usage.)
[1]Skin and Skin Structure Infections
[2]Urinary Tract Infections

DOSE ADJUSTMENTS

Clearance is reduced and half-life is prolonged in patients with a CrCl equal to or less than 80 ml/min. See chart for dosing guidelines. See Important IV Therapy Facts on p. xxii for formula to convert SrCr to CrCl. ■ Supplemental doses are not required after hemodialysis or peritoneal dialysis. ■ No dose adjustment is required specifically for age, gender, race, or in impaired hepatic function.

Levofloxacin Dosing Guidelines in Impaired Renal Function		
Renal Status	**Initial Dose**	**Subsequent Dose**
Acute Bacterial Exacerbation of Chronic Bronchitis/Comm. Acquired Pneumonia/ Acute Maxillary Sinusitis/Uncomplicated SSSI		
CrCl from 50 to 80 mL/min	No dosage adjustment required	
CrCl from 20 to 49 mL/min	500 mg	250 mg q24h
CrCl from 10 to 19 mL/min	500 mg	250 mg q48h
Hemodialysis	500 mg	250 mg q48h
Peritoneal dialysis	500 mg	250 mg q48h
Complicated SSSI/Nosocomial Pneumonia		
CrCl from 50 to 80 mL/min	No dosage adjustment required	
CrCl from 20 to 49 mL/min	750 mg	750 mg q48h
CrCl from 10 to 19 mL/min	750 mg	500 mg q48h
Hemodialysis	750 mg	500 mg q48h
Peritoneal dialysis	750 mg	500 mg q48h
Complicated UTI/Acute Pyelonephritis		
CrCl ≥20 mL/min	No dosage adjustment required	
CrCl from 10 to 19 mL/min	250 mg	250 mg q48h
Uncomplicated UTI	No dosage adjustment required	

DILUTION

Available in single-use vials and as prediluted, ready-to-use infusions.

Single-use vials: Withdraw desired dose from single-use vial (10 ml for 250 mg, 20 ml for 500 mg, 30 ml for 750 mg). Each 10 ml (250 mg) must be further diluted with a minimum of 40 ml NS, D5W, D5NS, D5LR, D5/plasma-Lyte 56, D5/½NS with 0.15% KCl, or ⅙ M sodium lactate. Desired concentration is 5 mg/ml. No preservatives; enter vial only once. When 500 mg (20 ml) vial is used to prepare two 250-mg doses, withdraw entire contents of vial at once into separate syringes, prepare and store second dose for subsequent use.

Premix flexible containers: No further dilution necessary. Available as 250 mg in 50 ml, 500 mg in 100 ml, or 750 mg in 150 ml D5W. Instructions for access to and use of premix flexible containers are on its storage carton. Do not use flexible containers in series connections.

Storage: Store vials at CRT; protect from light. Store premix at or below 25° C (77° F); protect from freezing, light, and excessive heat. Both are stable to expiration date. Solutions diluted from vials are stable at CRT for 3 days, up to 14 days if refrigerated. May be frozen for up to 6 months. Do not force thaw (e.g., microwave or water bath) and do not refreeze. Discard any unused portion of premixed solutions and/or opened vials.

INCOMPATIBLE WITH

Manufacturer states, "Limited compatibility information available; other intravenous substances, additives, or other medications should not be added to levofloxacin or infused simultaneously through the same intravenous line." Never administer in the same IV or through the same tubing with any solution containing multivalent cations (e.g., calcium, magnesium). Flush line with a compatible solution before and after administration of levofloxacin and/or any other drug through the same IV line.

COMPATIBLE WITH

See Incompatible With. Consult pharmacist; specific conditions may apply; see Compatibilities, p. xvi.

Additive: ***Not recommended by manufacturer.*** Linezolid (Zyvox).

Y-site: Amikacin (Amikin), aminophylline, ampicillin, caffeine citrate, cefotaxime (Claforan), cimetidine (Tagamet), clindamycin (Cleocin), dexamethasone (Decadron), dobutamine (Dobutrex), dopamine (Intropin), epinephrine (Adrenalin), fentanyl (Sublimaze), gentamicin (Garamycin), hetastarch in electrolytes (Hextend), insulin (regular), isoproterenol (Isuprel), lidocaine, linezolid (Zyvox), lorazepam (Ativan), metoclopramide (Reglan), morphine, oxacillin (Bactocill), pancuronium (Pavulon), penicillin G sodium, phenobarbital (Luminal), phenylephrine (Neo-Synephrine), sodium bicarbonate, vancomycin (Vancocin).

RATE OF ADMINISTRATION

Each 250- or 500-mg dose must be equally distributed over 60 minutes as an infusion. A 750-mg dose must be equally distributed over 90 minutes as an infusion. Too-rapid administration may cause hypotension. May be given through a Y-tube or three-way stopcock of infusion set. Temporarily discontinue other solutions infusing at the same site and flush tubing with compatible solutions before and after levofloxacin.

ACTIONS

A synthetic, broad-spectrum, fluoroquinolone antibacterial agent. First once-daily antiinfective indicated to treat all three of the most difficult to treat bacterial respiratory infections in adults. Bactericidal to a wide range of aerobic gram-negative and gram-positive organisms, as well as some anaerobic organisms through interference with an enzyme (topoisomerase II) needed for synthesis of bacterial DNA. May be active against bacteria resistant to aminoglycosides, beta-lactam antibiotics, and macrolides. Onset of action is prompt, and serum levels are dose related. Mean terminal half-life is 6 to 8 hours. Steady state is achieved within 48 hours. Widely distributed into body tissues, including blister fluid and lung tissues. Moderately bound to serum protein (24% to 38%). Metabolism is minimal; primarily excreted as unchanged drug in urine. Very small amounts found in bile and feces. May cross placental barrier. May be secreted in breast milk.

INDICATIONS AND USES

Treatment of adults with mild, moderate, and severe infections caused by susceptible strains of microorganisms in conditions including acute maxillary sinusitis, acute bacterial exacerbation of chronic bronchitis, and community-acquired pneumonia and nosocomial pneumonia. Treatment of pneumonia caused by susceptible strains of *Streptococcus pneumoniae*, including penicillin-resistant strains. ■ Treatment of complicated skin and skin structure infections, mild to moderate uncomplicated skin and skin structure infections, complicated and uncomplicated urinary tract infections, and acute pyelonephritis.

CONTRAINDICATIONS

History of hypersensitivity to levofloxacin, its components, or any other quinolone antimicrobial agents (e.g., ciprofloxacin [Cipro], norfloxacin [Noroxin], ofloxacin [Floxin IV]).

PRECAUTIONS

For IV use only. ■ Culture and sensitivity studies indicated to determine susceptibility of the causative organism to levofloxacin. Tests for sensitivity to ofloxacin may be used until specific tests for levofloxacin are available. ■ *Pseudomonas aeruginosa* may develop resistance during treatment. Ongoing culture and sensitivity studies indicated. ■ Prolonged use may cause superinfection because of overgrowth of nonsusceptible organisms. ■ Use with caution in patients with known CNS disorders that predispose to seizures or alter seizure threshold (e.g., epilepsy, severe cerebral arteriosclerosis, concomitant drug therapy). Convulsions, toxic psychosis, increased intracranial pressure, and CNS stimulation have been reported. ■ Use caution in patients with impaired renal function; see Dose Adjustments. ■ May be used by patients who are allergic to penicillin or intolerant of macrolides (e.g., erythromycin). ■ Cross-resistance may occur with other fluoroquinolones, but some microorganisms resistant to other fluoroquinolones may be susceptible to levofloxacin. ■ Rupture of shoulder, hand, and achilles tendons that required surgical repair or resulted in prolonged disability have been reported in patients receiving quinolones. ■ Prolongation of the QT interval on ECG and infrequent cases of arrhythmia (including torsades de pointes) have been reported. The risk of arrhythmia may be reduced by avoiding use of levofloxacin in the presence of hypokalemia, significant bradycardia, cardiomyopathy, or concurrent treatment with class 1A antiarrhythmic agents (e.g., quinidine [Quinidex], procainamide [Procanbid, Procan SR]) or Class III antiarrhythmic agents (e.g., amiodarone [Cordarone], sotalol [Betapace]). ■ Pseudomembranous colitis has been reported. May range from mild to life-threatening. Consider in patients that present with diarrhea during or after treatment with levofloxacin.

Monitor: Hypersensitivity reactions, including anaphylaxis with the first or succeeding doses, has been reported in patients receiving quinolones, even in those without known hypersensitivity. Emergency equipment must always be available. ■ Obtain baseline CBC with differential, CrCl, and blood glucose. Periodic monitoring of organ systems, including hematopoietic, hepatic, and renal, is recommended. ■ Maintain adequate hydration to prevent concentrated urine throughout treatment. Other quinolones have formed crystals. ■ Monitor infusion site for inflammation and/or extravasation. ■ Symptomatic hyperglycemia or hypoglycemia may occur, usually in diabetic patients receiving oral hypoglycemic agents (e.g., glyburide) or insulin. Monitor blood glucose closely. ■ See Drug/Lab Interactions and Antidote.

Patient Education: Drink fluids liberally. ■ Report skin rash or any other hypersensitivity reaction promptly. ■ Photosensitivity has occurred in a minimal number of patients, but it is best to avoid excessive sunlight or artificial ultraviolet light. May cause severe sunburn; use sunscreen and wear dark glasses outdoors. ■ Dizziness or lightheadedness may interfere with ambulation and motor coordination. Use caution in tasks that require alertness. ■ Effects of caffeine, theophylline preparations, and/or warfarin (Coumadin) may be increased; notify your physician if you take any of these agents. If diabetic and on medication, monitor your blood glucose carefully. If a hypoglycemia reaction occurs, discontinue levofloxacin and consult physician. ■ Report tendon pain or inflammation promptly. ■ See Precautions, Monitor, Drug/Lab Interactions, and Antidote.

Maternal/Child: Category C: safety for use in pregnancy not established; benefits must outweigh risks. ■ Discontinue breast-feeding. ■ Safety for use in children and adolescents under 18 years of age not established. Quinolones have caused arthropathy and osteochondrosis in juvenile animals.

Elderly: Half-life may be slightly extended due to age-related renal impairment. Dose reduction required only in the elderly with a CrCl of 50 ml/min or less. ■ Safety and effectiveness similar to that in younger adults, but monitoring of renal function may be useful. ■ See Dose Adjustments and Precautions.

DRUG/LAB INTERACTIONS

Risk of CNS stimulation and convulsive seizures may be increased with NSAIDs (e.g., ibuprofen [Advil, Motrin], naproxen [Aleve, Naprosyn]). ■ May cause hyperglycemia and hypoglycemia with concurrent administration of antidiabetic agents (e.g., metformin [Glucophage], insulin); monitoring of blood glucose recommended. ■ Concomitant administration with cimetidine or probenecid reduces levofloxacin renal clearance by 24% and 35% respectively, but dose adjustment is not required. ■ Interactions with theophylline that occur with other quinolones have not been noted, but monitoring of theophylline levels is recommended with concomitant use. ■ May enhance effects of warfarin (Coumadin); monitoring of PT or INR is recommended with concomitant use. ■ No dose adjustment required for either drug when levofloxacin is administered concomitantly with cyclosporine or digoxin. ■ See Precautions. ■ May cause false-positive when testing for opiates.

SIDE EFFECTS

Abdominal pain, anorexia, anxiety, constipation, decreased glucose, decreased lymphocytes, diarrhea, dizziness, dyspepsia, dysphonia, edema, fatigue, flatulence, genital moniliasis, headache, increased INR/PT, injection site reaction, insomnia, leukorrhea, malaise, nausea, phototoxicity (sun sensitivity), pruritus, rash, sweating, taste disturbances, tremor, urticaria, vaginitis, vomiting. Capable of numerous other reactions in less than 1% of patients.

Major: Allergic reactions (e.g., anaphylaxis, cardiovascular collapse, death, dyspnea, edema [facial, laryngeal, or pharyngeal]); allergic pneumonitis; arrhythmias (e.g., torsades de pointes), CNS stimulation (e.g., anxiety, confusion, depression, encephalopathy, hallucinations), convulsions, increased intracranial pressure, and toxic psychoses; eosinophilia; fever, rash, and severe dermatologic reactions (e.g., toxic epidermal necrolysis, Stevens-Johnson syndrome); hemolytic anemia; hypoglycemic reactions; multisystem organ failure; pseudomembranous colitis; and pain, inflammation, and ruptures of the shoulder, hand, and Achilles tendons have all been reported in patients receiving quinolones.

ANTIDOTE

Keep physician informed of all side effects. Most minor side effects will be treated symptomatically; monitor closely. Discontinue levofloxacin at the first sign of any major side effect (hypersensitivity, CNS symptoms, dermatologic reactions, hypoglycemic reactions, pseudomembranous colitis, tendon rupture) or phototoxicity. Treat allergic reactions as indicated with epinephrine, airway management, oxygen, IV fluids, antihistamines (e.g., diphenhydramine [Benadryl]), corticosteroids (e.g., Solu-Cortef), and pressor amines (e.g., dopamine [Intropin]). Treat CNS symptoms as indicated; may require diazepam (Valium) for seizures. Mild cases of colitis may respond to discontinuation of levofloxacin. Oral vancomycin (Vancocin) or metronidazole (Flagyl) is the treatment of choice for antibiotic-related pseudomembranous colitis. Adequate hydration and supplementation of electrolytes and proteins usually indicated. Complete rest is indicated for an affected tendon until treatment is available. Maintain hydration in overdose. No specific antidote; not removed by hemodialysis or peritoneal dialysis. Maintain patient until drug is excreted and symptoms subside.

LEVORPHANOL TARTRATE

(lee-vor′fa-nole tahr′trat)

Narcotic analgesic (agonist)
Anesthesia adjunct

Levo-Dromoran

pH 4.3

USUAL DOSE

Up to 1 mg every 3 to 6 hours. Doses as high as 2 to 3 mg may be indicated in severe pain (usually given SC). Titrate to symptom relief and respiratory rate. When seeking the required dose to achieve pain relief for an individual patient, increases in increments of at least 25% of the previous dose are suggested. Allow adequate time (approximately 72 hours) after each dose adjustment for patient to reach new steady-state level. Lower slightly if pain is controlled but patient is too drowsy; or lower dose and increase frequency.

Anesthesia adjunct: Optimum IV dose not established. 1 to 2 mg SC 60 to 90 minutes before surgery has been used.

PEDIATRIC DOSE

Not recommended for use in children under 18 years of age. If used, must be individualized on basis of age and weight; see Maternal/Child.

DOSE ADJUSTMENTS

Reduced dose may be required with hepatic or renal disease. ■ Reduce dose by 50% in patients with conditions affecting respiratory reserve or receiving other drugs that may depress respiration. Titrate subsequent doses to each individual. ■ Doses appropriate for the general population may cause serious respiratory depression in vulnerable patients. ■ See Drug/Lab Interactions.

DILUTION

May be given undiluted; further dilution with 5 ml SW or NS to facilitate titration is appropriate. Do not add to IV solutions. May give through Y-tube or three-way stopcock of infusion set.

Storage: Store at CRT.

INCOMPATIBLE WITH

Manufacturer lists aminophylline, ammonium chloride, chlorothiazide (Diuril), heparin, methicillin (Staphcillin), pentobarbital (Nembutal), perphenazine (Trilafon), phenobarbital (Luminal), phenytoin (Dilantin), sodium bicarbonate, sodium iodide, thiopental (Pentothal).

COMPATIBLE WITH

Consult pharmacist; specific conditions may apply; see Compatibilities, p. xvi.

Syringe: Glycopyrrolate.

Y-site: Propofol (Diprivan).

RATE OF ADMINISTRATION

2 mg or fraction thereof over 4 to 5 minutes. Usually titrated to symptom relief and respiratory rate.

ACTIONS

A synthetic narcotic analgesic and CNS depressant closely related to morphine. Five times more potent than morphine milligram for milligram. Onset of action is immediate and lasts 4 to 5 hours. Levorphanol is metabolized in the liver and excreted in the urine. Crosses the placental barrier. May be secreted in breast milk.

INDICATIONS AND USES

Relief of moderate to severe, acute or chronic pain. ■ Preanesthetic sedation.

CONTRAINDICATIONS

Acute alcoholism, anoxia, bronchial asthma, diarrhea caused by poisoning until toxic material eliminated, increased intracranial pressure, known hypersensitivity to levorphanol, respiratory depression, upper airway obstruction. ■ Not recommended for use during labor and delivery. ■ Not recommended for use in biliary surgery.

PRECAUTIONS

IV is not the route of choice. Usually given SC. ■ Tolerance to levorphanol gradually increases. ■ Use caution in the elderly and in patients with impaired hepatic or renal function, pulmonary disease, and those receiving concurrent anticoagulation therapy. ■ Use extreme caution in craniotomy, head injury, and increased intracranial pressure; respiratory depression and intracranial pressure may be further increased. ■ May cause apnea in the asthmatic. ■ Symptoms of acute abdominal conditions may be masked. ■ May increase ventricular response rate in presence of supraventricular tachycardias. Limit use in acute MI or cardiac patients, other effects on the heart are not known. ■ May cause marked rise in pressure in the common bile duct; see Contraindications. ■ Cough reflex is suppressed.

Monitor: Oxygen, controlled respiratory equipment, and naloxone (Narcan) or nalmefene (Revex) must be available. ■ Observe patient frequently and monitor vital signs. Keep patient supine; orthostatic hypotension and fainting may occur. ■ Uncontrolled pain causes sleep deprivation, decreases pain threshold, and increases pain. When pain is finally controlled, expect the patient to sleep more until recovery from sleep deprivation. ■ See Precautions and Drug/Lab Interactions.

Patient Education: Avoid alcohol or other CNS depressants (e.g., barbiturates, benzodiazepines such as diazepam [Valium]). ▪ May cause blurred vision, dizziness, or drowsiness; use caution in tasks that require alertness. ▪ Request assistance with ambulation. ▪ May be habit forming.

Maternal/Child: Category C: safety for use in pregnancy or breast-feeding not established. Benefits must outweigh risks. ▪ Pediatric patients may be more sensitive to effects (e.g., respiratory depression). ▪ May cause paradoxical excitation.

Elderly: See Precautions. ▪ May be more sensitive to effects (e.g., respiratory depression, constipation, urinary retention). ▪ Analgesia should be effective with lower doses. ▪ Consider age-related organ impairment.

DRUG/LAB INTERACTIONS

CNS toxicity potentiated by phenothiazines (e.g., chlorpromazine [Thorazine]) and other CNS depressants, such as narcotic analgesics, alcohol, anticholinergics, antidepressants (e.g., amitriptyline [Elavil], nortriptyline [Aventyl]), antihistamines, barbiturates, hypnotics, sedatives, MAO inhibitors (e.g., selegiline [Eldepryl]), neuromuscular blocking agents (e.g., tubocurarine), and psychotropic agents. Side effects (e.g., CNS depression, constipation, hypotension) may be additive. Reduced dosage of both drugs may be indicated. ▪ Administration of agonist/antagonist analgesics (e.g., butorphanol [Stadol]) to an opiate-dependent patient receiving a pure opiate may precipitate withdrawal symptoms. ▪ Plasma amylase and lipase determinations may be unreliable for 24 hours following narcotic administration.

SIDE EFFECTS

Nausea, vomiting, and constipation are less frequent than with morphine. Dizziness, skin rash, urinary retention, urticaria.

Major: Anaphylaxis, cardiac arrhythmias, hypotension, respiratory depression.

ANTIDOTE

With increasing severity of any side effect or onset of symptoms of overdose, discontinue the drug and notify the physician. Naloxone (Narcan) or nalmefene (Revex) will reverse serious reactions. A patent airway, artificial ventilation, oxygen therapy, and other symptomatic treatment must be instituted promptly. Resuscitate as necessary.

LEVOTHYROXINE SODIUM

(lee-voe-thye-rox′een so′de-um)

Hormone (thyroid)

Synthroid, T_4, L-Thyroxine

USUAL DOSE

When oral ingestion is not practical, IV dose should be ½ of any previously established oral dose. Adjust in small increments as indicated. Initiate oral treatment as soon as possible. 0.05 to 0.06 mg (50 to 60 mcg) equals approximately 60 mg (gr 1) thyroid hormone.

Hypothyroidism: Usual IV starting dose would be 25 mcg/day. Increase in increments of 12.5 to 25 mcg. Average maintenance dose is 50 to 100 mcg/day.

Myxedema coma: 400 mcg as initial dose. Range is 200 to 500 mcg. 100 to 300 mcg may be repeated the next day unless considerable improvement has occurred, as indicated by patient response or serum protein-bound iodine levels. Maintenance dose ranges from 50 to 200 mcg. See Precautions. Liothyronine (Triostat) is the drug of choice for myxedema coma.

Thyroid suppression therapy: 1.3 mcg/kg/day for 7 to 10 days; usually yields normal serum T_4 and T_3 levels and lack of response to TSH.

PEDIATRIC DOSE

Given orally (may be crushed in food or liquid). See Precautions. Any IV dose should be 75% of oral dose. Size of ***oral*** dose is inversely proportional to age from 8 to 10 mcg/kg/24 hr at 0 to 6 months to 2 to 3 mcg/kg/24 hr for over 12 years.

DOSE ADJUSTMENTS

See Drug/Lab Interactions. Reduce dose in elderly, functional or ECG evidence of cardiovascular disease including angina, long-standing thyroid disease, other endocrinopathies, and severe hypothyroidism.

DILUTION

Each 100 mcg of lyophilized powder is diluted with 1 ml of NS for injection (without preservatives). Shake well to dissolve completely. 1 ml equals 100 mcg. More diluent may be added to Synthroid (5 ml to 200 mcg yields 40 mcg/ml) and bacteriostatic NS may be used. Do not add to IV solutions. May be given through Y-tube or three-way stopcock of infusion set. Must be used immediately after dilution; any remaining solution is discarded.

COMPATIBILITY

Specific information not available. Consider specific use; consult pharmacist.

RATE OF ADMINISTRATION

100 mcg or fraction thereof over 1 minute.

ACTIONS

A synthetic thyroid hormone. Effective replacement for decreased or absent thyroid function. Requires peripheral metabolic conversion to active hormone T_3 to be effective. Process inhibited by illness or stress. Onset of action is slow. Up to 5 or 6 hours is required before any noticeable improvements occur, and 24 hours may be required to note full benefits. Thyroid hormone is essential to many body functions, including rate of metabolism.

INDICATIONS AND USES

Hypothyroid states due to any cause. ■ An emergency measure in myxedema coma. ■ Thyroid suppression therapy.

CONTRAINDICATIONS

Hypersensitivity to levothyroxine, myocardial infarction, thyrotoxicosis.

PRECAUTIONS

Correct adrenocortical insufficiency before administration or acute adrenal crisis and death may result. ■ Corticosteroid therapy is also required concomitantly to prevent acute adrenal insufficiency in myxedema coma or any pre-existing manifestation of adrenal insufficiency. ■ Use caution in diabetes and cardiovascular disease. ■ Larger doses (e.g., 0.3 to 0.4 mg) may cause cardiovascular side effects; use with extreme caution.

Monitor: Observe patient continuously and monitor vital signs. ■ Monitor thyroid function tests (e.g., free T_4 index, TSH).

Maternal/Child: Category A: may be used during pregnancy. ■ Presumed safe in breast-feeding; use caution and observe infant. ■ Avoid excessive dose in children; can cause brain damage in thyrotoxicosis during infancy. Can also accelerate bone age and cause craniosynotosis (premature closing of sutures in the skull).

Elderly: See Dose Adjustments; more sensitive to effects.

DRUG/LAB INTERACTIONS

Increases rate of metabolism and requires dose adjustment for anticoagulants, antidepressants, oral antidiabetics, barbiturates, digitalis, catecholamines (e.g., epinephrine), beta-adrenergic blockers (e.g., propranolol), insulin, estrogens, theophylline, and others. Cardiac arrhythmias, hypoglycemia, and bleeding can occur with unadjusted dose of some of these drugs.

SIDE EFFECTS

Chest pain, diarrhea, heart palpitations, muscle cramps, nervousness, perspiration, tachycardia, vomiting.

ANTIDOTE

Notify the physician of any side effect. A reduction in dose will usually decrease symptoms. In massive overdose control fever, hypoglycemia, and fluid loss. Digitalis may be indicated for CHF; propranolol (Inderal) has been used to treat increased sympathetic activity (1 to 3 mg IV over 10 minutes). Adrenal insufficiency may be unrecognized.

LIDOCAINE HYDROCHLORIDE

Antiarrhythmic

(lye′doe-kane hye-droe-klor′id)

Lidocaine PF, Xylocaine PF, ✤Xylocard

pH 5 to 7

USUAL DOSE

Refractory ventricular fibrillation or ventricular tachycardia: 1 to 1.5 mg/kg of body weight (50 to 100 mg) as a ***loading dose.*** May repeat 0.5 to 1.5 mg/kg every 5 to 10 minutes to desired effect, up to a total of 3 mg/kg. Should not exceed 200 to 300 mg/hr. AHA recommends repeat doses of 0.5 to 0.75 mg/kg.

Maintenance dose: With return of perfusion, initiate an infusion of 1 to 4 mg/min (20 to 50 mcg/kg/min). ***Do not exceed 4 mg/min rate.*** If arrhythmias occur during an infusion, give a small bolus of 0.5 mg/kg to increase plasma concentration.

Prophylactic dose: Initiate a keep-open IV of D5W. Begin with a bolus dose of 0.5 mg/kg. Repeat 0.5 mg/kg bolus every 5 minutes to a total dose of 2 mg/kg if ventricular ectopic activity is present. Not recommended in uncomplicated acute MI or ischemia without PVCs.

Status epilepticus (unlabeled): 1 mg/kg as a loading dose. If seizure does not terminate in 2 minutes, give an additional 0.5 mg/kg to prevent recurrences; a maintenance infusion of 30 mcg/kg/min has been used. Another source suggests a loading dose of 100 mg. Give an additional 50 mg in 20 minutes. Follow with a maintenance infusion of 1 to 3 mg/min. Reduce infusion rate gradually based on patient response; complete withdrawal may take several days.

Cardiac arrest: AHA considers a single dose of 1.5 mg/kg acceptable. 2 to 4 mg/kg may be given intratracheally.

PEDIATRIC DOSE

1 mg/kg IV or intratracheally. May repeat in 10 to 15 minutes times 2 if indicated. Maximum total dose is 3 to 4.5 mg/kg/hr. Follow with an infusion of 20 to 50 mcg/kg/min. AHA recommends 1 mg/kg as an IV injection followed immediately by an infusion of 20 to 50 mcg/kg/min.

DOSE ADJUSTMENTS

Reduce loading dose in digitalis toxicity with AV block. ■ Consider loading dose reduction (not universally recommended) in congestive heart failure, reduced cardiac output and liver disease. ■ Lower-end initial doses may be indicated in the elderly based on potential for decreased organ function and concomitant disease or drug therapy. ■ One source suggests patients over 65 years of age should be dosed cautiously based on body weight. ■ Reduce maintenance dose by one half in presence of decreased cardiac output (e.g., acute MI, congestive heart failure, or shock from any cause), impaired liver function, the elderly (over 65), and in patients receiving drugs that may decrease clearance of lidocaine or decrease liver blood flow (e.g., beta-blockers [propranolol (Inderal), cimetidine (Tagamet)]). ■ Reduce maintenance dose after 24 hours or monitor blood levels; half-life of lidocaine increases with prolonged administration.

DILUTION

Label must state, "for IV use" and be preservative free. Bolus dose may be given undiluted.

Infusion: Add 1 Gm of lidocaine to 500 or 250 ml of D5W (preferred), D5/½NS, D5NS, LR, or other compatible solutions; see chart on inside back cover. Solution gives 2 or 4 mg/ml of lidocaine. Available prediluted (2, 4, or 8 mg/ml). Titrate to desired response.

Pediatric infusion: Add 120 mg of lidocaine to 100 ml of diluent (1,200 mcg/ml). 1 to 2.5 ml/kg/hr will deliver 20 to 50 mcg/kg/min or add 6 mg/kg to 100 ml diluent. 1 ml/hr equals 1 mcg/kg/min.

Storage: Store at CRT. Discard diluted solution after 24 hours.

INCOMPATIBLE WITH

Additives should not be introduced into premixed solutions of lidocaine.

COMPATIBLE WITH **(Underline Indicates Conflicting Compatibility Information)**

Consult pharmacist; specific conditions may apply; see Compatibilities, p. xvi.

Additive: *Physically compatible with numerous drugs. Combination may not be practical because of extensive individualized rate adjustments to achieve desired effects.* Alteplase (Activase, tPA), aminophylline, amiodarone (Cordarone), atracurium (Tracrium), bretylium (Bretylate), calcium chloride, calcium gluconate, chloramphenicol (Chloromycetin), chlorothiazide (Diuril), cimetidine (Tagamet), ciprofloxacin (Cipro IV), dexamethasone (Decadron), digoxin (Lanoxin), diphenhydramine (Benadryl), dobutamine (Dobutrex), dopamine (Intropin), ephedrine sulfate, erythromycin lactobionate (Erythrocin), fentanyl (Sublimaze), flumazenil (Romazicon), furosemide (Lasix), heparin, hydrocortisone sodium succinate (Solu-Cortef), insulin (regular), nafcillin (Nafcil), nitroglycerin (Nitro-Bid IV), penicillin G potassium, pentobarbital (Nembutal), phenylephrine (Neo-Synephrine), potassium chloride (KCl), procainamide (Pronestyl), prochlorperazine (Compazine), ranitidine (Zantac), sodium bicarbonate, sodium lactate, theophylline, verapamil (Isoptin).

Syringe: Ampicillin, ceftriaxone (Rocephin), glycopyrrolate, heparin, metoclopramide (Reglan), milrinone (Primacor), nalbuphine (Nubain), sodium bicarbonate.

Y-site: Alteplase (Activase, tPA), amiodarone (Cordarone), cefazolin (Kefzol), ciprofloxacin (Cipro IV), cisatracurium (Nimbex), diltiazem (Cardizem), dobutamine (Dobutrex), dopamine (Intropin), enalaprilat (Vasotec IV), etomidate (Amidate), famotidine (Pepcid IV), gatifloxacin (Tequin), haloperidol (Haldol), heparin, hetastarch in electrolytes (Hextend), inamrinone (Inocor), labetalol (Normodyne), levofloxacin (Levaquin), linezolid (Zyvox), meperidine (Demerol), morphine, nitroglycerin (Nitro-Bid IV), nitroprusside sodium, potassium chloride (KCl), propofol (Diprivan), remifentanil (Ultiva), streptokinase, theophylline, tirofiban (Aggrastat), warfarin (Coumadin).

RATE OF ADMINISTRATION

Bolus dose: 25 to 50 mg or fraction thereof over 1 minute. Too-rapid injection may cause seizures.

Infusion: Using a microdrip (60 gtt/ml) or an infusion pump delivers lidocaine in recommended doses. Adjust as indicated by progress in patient's condition. See Dose Adjustments.

Lidocaine Infusion Rates						
Desired Dose	1 Gm in 500 ml Diluent (2 mg/ml)			1 Gm in 250 ml Diluent (4 mg/ml)		
mg/min	mg/hr	ml/min	ml/hr	mg/hr	ml/min	ml/hr
1	60	0.5	30	60	0.25	15
2	120	1	60	120	0.5	30
3	180	1.5	90	180	0.75	45
4	240	2	120	240	1	60
Pediatric infusion: 120 mg to 100 ml diluent = 1,200 mcg/ml 1 to 2.5 ml/kg/hr = 20 to 50 mcg/kg/min or 6 mg/kg to 100 ml diluent 1 ml/hr = 1 mcg/kg/min						

ACTIONS

A local anesthetic agent. Exerts an antiarrhythmic effect similar to procainamide but is more potent. Decreases ventricular excitability without depressing the force of ventricular contractions by increasing the stimulation threshold of the ventricle during diastole. Decreases cell membrane permeability and prevents loss of sodium and potassium ions. Onset of action should occur within 2 minutes and last approximately 10 to 20 minutes. Crosses placental barrier. Metabolized in the liver and excreted in the urine.

INDICATIONS AND USES

Drug of choice for treatment of ventricular arrhythmias (e.g., PVCs, ventricular tachycardia [VT], ventricular fibrillation [VF]) occurring during acute myocardial infarction and during cardiac and other surgery. ■ Wide-complex tachycardia of uncertain origin. ■ Wide-complex PSVT. ■ Prophylactic administration to reduce incidence of primary VF in acute MI.

Unlabeled uses: Pediatric cardiac arrest, status epilepticus.

CONTRAINDICATIONS

Known sensitivity to lidocaine or any other local anesthetic of the amide type; Wolff-Parkinson-White syndrome, Stokes-Adams syndrome or any other severe first-, second-, or third-degree heart block without an artificial pacemaker in place.

PRECAUTIONS

Oral antiarrhythmic drugs are preferred for maintenance. ■ Use caution in severe liver or renal disease, hypovolemia, shock, all forms of heart block, and untreated bradycardia. ■ Acceleration of ventricular rate may occur in patients with atrial flutter or fibrillation.

Monitor: Monitor IV flow rate and the patient's ECG continuously. Therapeutic serum levels range from 1.5 to 5 mcg/ml; above 6 mcg/ml is usually toxic. ■ Half-life increases over time. Reduce dose of continuous infusion after 24 hours and monitor blood levels. ■ Keep patient lying down to reduce hypotensive effects. ■ Discontinue lidocaine when patient's cardiac condition is stable or any signs of toxicity become apparent. ■ Keep a bolus dose, 100 mg (5 ml), available at all times for emergency use in myocardial infarction.

Patient Education: May cause dizziness; remain at bed rest; request assistance if ambulation permitted.

Maternal/Child: Category C: safety not established. Benefits must outweigh risks. ■ Safety for use in breast-feeding and children not established.

Elderly: Lower-end initial dosing and/or mg/kg dose may be appropriate. See Dose Adjustments. ■ Decreased lidocaine clearance and increased sensitivity to adverse effects. ■ Consider age-related hepatic impairment.

DRUG/LAB INTERACTIONS

Cross-sensitivity and/or potentiation may occur with other antiarrhythmics (e.g., procainamide or quinidine); may cause conduction abnormalities. ■ Potentiated by amiodarone (Cordarone), beta-adrenergic blockers (e.g., propranolol [Inderal]), and cimetidine (Tagamet); toxicity can occur. Monitor cardiac function. ■ May produce excessive cardiac depression with phenytoin (Dilantin). ■ Potentiates neuromuscular blockade of muscle relaxants (e.g., tubocurarine, succinylcholine) and aminoglycoside antibiotics (e.g., gentamicin [Garamycin]). ■ Effects may be altered by smoking; monitor carefully.

SIDE EFFECTS

Transient because of short duration of action of lidocaine.

Apprehension, blurred vision, confusion, dizziness, "doom" anxiety, drowsiness, edema, euphoria, hallucinations, lightheadedness, mood changes, nervousness, sensations of heat, cold, and numbness, slurred speech, tinnitus, urticaria, vomiting.

Major: Anaphylaxis, bradycardia, cardiac arrest, cardiovascular collapse, convulsions, hypotension, malignant hyperthermia (tachycardia, tachypnea, metabolic acidosis, fever), PR interval prolonged, QRS complex widening, respiratory depression, tremors, twitching, unconsciousness.

ANTIDOTE

Notify the physician of any side effects. For major side effects, discontinue the drug immediately and institute appropriate measures. For anaphylactic shock use epinephrine and corticosteroids, etc. To correct CNS stimulation use diazepam (Valium), rapid ultra-short-acting barbiturates (e.g., thiopental [Pentothal]), or if under anesthesia, muscle relaxants (e.g., succinylcholine). Use vasopresssors (e.g., dopamine [Intropin]) and IV fluids to correct hypotension. Maintain and support patient; resuscitate as necessary.

LINEZOLID

(li-nee′zoh-lid)

Zyvox

Antibacterial (oxazolidinone)

USUAL DOSE

Dose and duration of therapy are based on diagnosis and designated pathogens. May be transferred to oral dosing when appropriate. See Precautions.

Recommended Linezolid Doses in Pediatric and Adult Patients			
	Dosage and Route of Administration		
Infection*	Pediatric Patients† (Birth Through 11 Years of Age)	Adults and Adolescents (12 Years of Age and Older)	Recommended Duration of Treatment (Consecutive Days)
Complicated skin and skin structure infections	10 mg/kg IV or PO‡ q8h	600 mg IV or PO‡ q12h	10 to 14
Community-acquired pneumonia, including concurrent bacteremia			
Nosocomial pneumonia			
Vancomycin-resistant *Enterococcus faecium* infections, including concurrent bacteremia	10 mg/kg IV or PO‡ q8h	600 mg IV or PO‡ q12h	14 to 28
Methicillin-resistant *Staphylococcus aureus* (MRSA) infections	—	600 mg IV or PO‡ q12h	7 to 28
Uncomplicated skin and skin structure infections	Less than 5 years: 10 mg/kg PO‡ q8h 5-11 years: 10 mg/kg PO‡ q12h	Adults: 400 mg PO‡ q12h Adolescents: 600 mg PO‡ q12h	10 to 14

*Due to the designated pathogens (see Indications and Uses and package insert).

†Neonates less than 7 days of age: Most preterm neonates less than 7 days of age (gestational age less than 34 weeks) have lower systemic linezolid clearance values and larger AUC values than many full-term neonates and older infants. These neonates should be initiated with a dosing regimen of 10 mg/kg q12h. Consideration may be given to the use of 10 mg/kg q8h regimen in neonates with a suboptimal clinical response. All neonatal patients should receive 10 mg/kg q8h by 7 days of life.

‡Oral dosing using either linezolid tablets or linezolid for oral suspension.

PEDIATRIC DOSE

See Usual Dose.

DOSE ADJUSTMENTS

Dose adjustment based on age, gender, renal insufficiency, or hepatic insufficiency is not required.

DILUTION

Available in ready-to-use flexible plastic infusion bags in a foil laminate overwrap. Available as a 2 mg/ml solution in 200-, 400-, and 600-mg infusion bags. Prior to use, remove overwrap and check for leaks by squeezing the bag. Do not use flexible containers in series connections. ***Storage:*** Store at CRT. Protect from light and freezing. Keep in overwrap until ready to use. Solution may exhibit a yellow color that can intensify with time. Will not adversely affect potency.

INCOMPATIBLE WITH

Manufacturer states, "Additives should not be added to the infusion bag." If administered through the same tubing as other medications, flush line before and after infusion of linezolid with a solution that is compatible with linezolid and with any medications administered through the common line.

Y-site: Manufacturer lists amphotericin B (Fungizone), ceftriaxone (Rocephin), chlorpromazine (Thorazine), diazepam (Valium), erythromycin lactobionate (Erythrocin), pentamidine, phenytoin (Dilantin), sulfamethoxazole-trimethoprim (Bactrim, Septra).

COMPATIBLE WITH

Consult pharmacist; specific conditions may apply; see Compatibilities, p. xvi.

Additive: ***Not recommended by manufacturer.*** Aztreonam (Azactam), cefazolin (Kefzol), ceftazidime (Fortaz), ciprofloxacin (Cipro IV), gentamicin (Garamycin), levofloxacin (Levaquin), ofloxacin (Floxin IV), piperacillin (Pipracil), tobramycin (Nebcin).

Y-site: Acyclovir (Zovirax), alfentanil (Alfenta), amikacin (Amikin), aminophylline, ampicillin, ampicillin/sulbactam (Unasyn), aztreonam (Azactam), bretylium (Bretylate), buprenorphine (Buprenex), butorphanol (Stadol), calcium gluconate, carboplatin (Paraplatin), cefazolin (Kefzol), cefoperazone (Cefobid), cefotetan (Cefotan), cefoxitin (Mefoxin), ceftazidime (Fortaz), ceftizoxime (Cefizox), ceftriaxone (Rocephin), cefuroxime (Zinacef), cimetidine (Tagamet), ciprofloxacin (Cipro IV), cisatracurium (Nimbex), cisplatin (Platinol), clindamycin (Cleocin), cyclophosphamide (Cytoxan), cyclosporine (Sandimmune), cytarabine (ARA-C), dexamethasone (Decadron), D5/½NS, D5NS, digoxin (Lanoxin), diphenhydramine (Benadryl), dobutamine (Dobutrex), dopamine (Intropin), doxorubicin (Adriamycin), doxycycline (Vibramycin), droperidol (Inapsine), enalaprilat (Vasotec IV), esmolol (Brevibloc), etoposide phosphate (Etopophos), famotidine (Pepcid IV), fentanyl (Sublimaze), fluconazole (Diflucan), fluorouracil (5-FU), furosemide (Lasix), ganciclovir (Cytovene), gemcitabine (Gemzar), gentamicin (Garamycin), granisetron (Kytril), haloperidol (Haldol), heparin, hydrocortisone sodium succinate (Solu-Cortef), hydromorphone (Dilaudid), ifosfamide (Ifex), imipenem-cilastatin (Primaxin), labetalol (Normodyne), leucovorin calcium, levofloxacin (Levaquin), lidocaine, lorazepam (Ativan), magnesium sulfate, mannitol, meperidine (Demerol), meropenem (Merrem IV), mesna (Mesnex), methotrexate (Folex), methylprednisolone (Solu-Medrol), metoclopramide (Reglan), metronidazole (Flagyl IV), midazolam (Versed), minocycline (Minocin), mitoxantrone (Novantrone), morphine, nalbuphine (Nubain), naloxone (Narcan), nicardipine (Cardene IV), nitroglycerin (Nitro-Bid IV), ofloxacin (Floxin IV), ondansetron (Zofran), paclitaxel (Taxol), pentobarbital (Nembutal), phenobarbital (Luminal), piperacillin (Pipracil), piperacillin/tazobactam (Zosyn), potassium chloride (KCl), prochlorperazine (Compazine), promethazine (Phenergan), propranolol (Inderal), ranitidine (Zantac), remifentanil (Ultiva), Ringer's solution, sodium bicarbonate, sufentanil (Sufenta), theophylline, ticarcillin (Ticar), tobramycin (Nebcin), vancomycin (Vancocin), vecuronium (Norcuron), verapamil (Isoptin), vincristine (Oncovin), zidovudine (AZT, Retrovir).

RATE OF ADMINISTRATION

Administer as an infusion over 30 to 120 minutes. Flush line before and after administration if indicated; see Incompatible With.

ACTIONS

A synthetic antibacterial agent. The first agent of a new class of antibiotics, the oxazolidinones. Clinically useful in the treatment of infections caused by aerobic gram-positive bacteria. See Indications and Uses and manufacturer's literature. Inhibits bacterial protein synthesis through a mechanism of action different from that of other antibacterial agents; therefore, cross-resistance between linezolid and other classes of antibiotics is unlikely. Bacteriostatic against enterococci and staphylococci. Bactericidal against most strains of streptococci. Readily distributes into well-perfused tissues. Metabolized to two inactive metabolites. Approximately 30% of a dose is excreted in the urine as linezolid and 50% is excreted as metabolites. Half-life is 4.8 hours.

INDICATIONS AND USES

Treatment of adults, adolescents, and pediatric patients with the following infections caused by susceptible strains of the designated microorganisms: vancomycin-resistant *Enterococcus faecium,* including cases with concurrent bacteremia; nosocomial pneumonia caused by *Staphylococcus aureus* (methicillin-susceptible and methicillin-resistant strains) or *Streptococcus pneumoniae* (penicillin-susceptible strains only); complicated skin and skin-structure infections caused by *Staphylococcus aureus* (methicillin-susceptible and methicillin-resistant strains), *Streptococcus pyogenes*, or *Streptococcus agalactiae;* uncomplicated skin and skin-structure infections caused by *Staphylococcus aureus* (methicillin-susceptible strains only) or *Streptococcus pyogenes*; and community-acquired pneumonia caused by *Streptococcus pneumoniae* (penicillin-susceptible strains only), including cases with concurrent bacteremia, or *Staphylococcus aureus* (methicillin-susceptible strains only). ■ Treatment of diabetic foot and decubitus ulcers not included in clinical studies. ■ Given orally to treat uncomplicated skin and skin-structure infections.

CONTRAINDICATIONS

History of hypersensitivity to linezolid or any of its components.

PRECAUTIONS

Culture and sensitivity studies are indicated to determine susceptibility of the causative organism to linezolid. ■ Due to concerns about inappropriate use of antibiotics leading to an increase in resistant organisms, prescribers should carefully consider alternatives before initiating treatment with linezolid in the outpatient setting. Vancomycin-resistant enterococci (VRE) have been reported in patients taking linezolid. ■ Combination therapy may be clinically indicated in treatment of nosocomial pneumonia or complicated skin and skin-structure infections if the documented or presumptive pathogens include gram-negative organisms. ■ Use with caution in patients with renal failure. Although dose adjustments are not recommended in this patient population, the metabolites may accumulate. The clinical significance of this accumulation is unknown. Dose should be given after hemodialysis. ■ Use with caution in patients with uncontrolled hypertension, severe hepatic insufficiency, pheochromocytoma, carcinoid syndrome, or untreated hyperthyroidism. Use has not been studied in these patient populations. ■ Safety and efficacy of linezolid given for longer than 28 days have not been evaluated. ■ Neuropathy (peripheral and optic) has been reported. May occur in patients treated with linezolid for shorter periods, as well as in patients treated for more than 28 days. ■ Superinfection, caused by the overgrowth of nonsusceptible organisms, may occur with antibiotic use. Treat as indicated. ■ Pseudomembranous colitis has been reported and may range from mild to life-threatening. Consider in patients that present with diarrhea during or after treatment with linezolid. ■ See Monitor and Patient Education.

Monitor: Myelosuppression (including anemia, leukopenia, pancytopenia, and thrombocytopenia) has been reported. CBC with differential and platelet count should be monitored weekly, especially in patients who receive linezolid for longer than 2 weeks; those with pre-existing myelosuppression; those receiving concomitant drugs that produce bone marrow suppression (e.g., antineoplastics [cisplatin (Platinol), gemcitabine (Gemzar)], chloramphenicol, immunosuppressants [e.g., azathioprine (Imuran)]) or affect platelet function (e.g., aspirin, epoprostenol [Flolan], NSAIDs [e.g., ibuprofen (Advil, Motrin), naproxen (Aleve, Naprosyn)], platelet aggregation inhibitors [e.g., abciximab (ReoPro), clopidogrel (Plavix), dipyridamole (Persantine), eptifibatide (Integrilin)], selected antibiotics [e.g., piperacillin (Pipracil), ticarcillin (Ticar)], valproic acid (Depacon, Depakene)]). Discontinuation of therapy should be considered in patients who develop or have worsening myelosuppression. Myelosuppression appears to be reversible following discontinuation of linezolid. ■ Monitor dietary intake of tyramine; see Patient Education. Hypertension may result from excessive tyramine intake (less than 100 mg/day).

Patient Education: Avoid foods or beverages high in tyramine (e.g., aged cheeses, fermented or air-dried meats, sauerkraut, soy sauce, tap beers, red wines). ■ Inform physician of any history of hypertension. See Precautions. ■ Inform physician if taking any medications containing pseudoephedrine or phenylpropanolamine (found in many cold or allergy preparations or diet aids), or if taking serotonin re-uptake inhibitors (e.g., fluoxetine [Prozac], sertraline [Zoloft], paroxetine [Paxil]) or other antidepressants. See Drug Interactions.

Maternal/Child: Category C: safety for use in pregnancy and breast-feeding not established; benefits must outweigh risks. ■ Volume of distribution is similar regardless of age in pediatric patients; however, clearance varies as a function of age. Clearance is most rapid in the youngest age-groups (ranging from less than 1 week old to 11 years of age), resulting in lower single-dose systemic exposure (AUC) and shorter half-life. ■ AUC values in patients from birth to 11 years of age dosed every 8 hours are similar to adolescents and adults dosed every 12 hours.

Elderly: No overall difference in safety or effectiveness has been observed between these patients and younger patients. Pharmacokinetics are not significantly altered in the elderly. See Dose Adjustments.

DRUG/LAB INTERACTIONS

Linezolid is a reversible, nonselective inhibitor of monoamine oxidase and therefore has the potential to interact with adrenergic and serotonergic agents and with tyramine-containing foods. ■ A reversible enhancement of the pressor response to indirect-acting sympathomimetic agents or vasopressor or dopaminergic agents (e.g., pseudoephedrine [Sudafed], phenylpropanolamine, epinephrine [Adrenalin], dopamine [Intropin]) may be seen with concomitant use. Initial doses of adrenergic agents, such as epinephrine or dopamine, should be reduced and titrated to achieve the desired response. ■ In clinical trials, coadministration of linezolid and serotonergic agents (e.g., dextromethorphan [Benylin DM], fluoxetine [Prozac], paroxetine [Paxil], sertraline [Zoloft]) was not associated with serotonin syndrome (e.g., blushing, cognitive dysfunction, confusion, diaphoresis, delirium, hyperpyrexia, restlessness, and tremors). However, experience with co-administration of these agents is limited. Patients receiving both therapies should be monitored for the development of serotonin syndrome. ■ Does not appear to induce or be induced by the cytochrome P_{450} system and should therefore not affect drugs metabolized by this system (e.g., warfarin [Coumadin], phenytoin [Dilantin]). ■ Has been co-administered with aztreonam (Azactam) and gentamicin (Garamycin). When linezolid was co-administered with either one of these agents no alteration of pharmacokinetics occurred in either drug. ■ Severe myelosuppression may occur with bone marrow depressants and other drugs that affect platelet function; see Monitor.

SIDE EFFECTS

Children up to 11 years of age: Most common side effects are diarrhea, neutropenia, increased ALT (SGPT).

Adults and adolescents: Most common side effects are diarrhea, headache, and nausea. Other reported side effects include abdominal pain, constipation, dizziness, dysgeusia (change in sense of taste), dyspepsia, fever, hypertension, insomnia, myelosuppression (anemia, leukopenia, pancytopenia, thrombocytopenia), neuropathy (peripheral and optic), oral moniliasis, pruritus, pseudomembranous colitis, rash, tongue discoloration, vaginal moniliasis, and vomiting.

ANTIDOTE

Keep physician informed of all side effects. Discontinue drug if indicated. Consider discontinuing linezolid in patients who develop or have worsening myelosuppression. Mild cases of colitis may respond to discontinuation of drug. Treat antibiotic-related pseudomembranous colitis with fluid, electrolytes, protein supplements, and oral vancomycin (Vancocin) or metronidazole (Flagyl) as indicated. In the event of an overdose, initiate supportive care and maintain glomerular filtration. Both linezolid and its metabolites are partially removed by hemodialysis.

LIOTHYRONINE SODIUM

(lye-oh-thye′roe-neen so′de-um)

Hormone (thyroid)

T_3, Triostat

pH 9.5 to 11.5

USUAL DOSE

Preadministration testing and adjunctive therapy with corticosteroids required (see Precautions/Monitor).

Initial and subsequent doses must be determined on the basis of continuous monitoring of clinical condition and response to liothyronine therapy. An adequate dose is important in determining clinical outcome.

Myxedema coma: 25 to 50 mcg as an initial dose. At least 4 hours but no more than 12 hours should elapse between doses; allows sufficient time to evaluate response and avoids fluctuation in hormone levels. Myxedematous patients have an increased sensitivity to thyroid hormones. Begin with lower doses and increase gradually. Use caution in adjusting dose to avoid large changes that may precipitate adverse cardiovascular events. A total daily dose of 65 mcg/day in the initial days of treatment has decreased mortality. Experience with doses above 100 mcg/day is limited.

Transfer to oral therapy: Initiate oral therapy as soon as condition is stabilized and patient is able to take oral medications. With oral liothyronine, discontinue IV liothyronine and begin with low doses. Increase gradually based on response. If L-thyroxine (Synthyroid, T_4) is used, discontinue IV therapy gradually to compensate for several-day delay in effectiveness of oral L-thyroxine.

DOSE ADJUSTMENTS

Reduce initial dose to 10 to 20 mcg in known or suspected cardiovascular disease. ■ Begin with lower doses in the elderly based on the potential for decreased organ function and concomitant disease or drug therapy. ■ See Drug/Lab Interactions.

DILUTION

May be given undiluted. Available as 10 mcg/ml in 1-ml vials.

Storage: Must be refrigerated until administration. Discard unused portion.

COMPATIBILITY

Specific references not available. Consider specific use; consult pharmacist.

RATE OF ADMINISTRATION

Each 10 mcg or fraction thereof over 1 minute.

ACTIONS

A synthetic form of the natural thyroid hormone triiodothyronine (T_3). Enters peripheral tissues readily and binds to specific nuclear receptor(s) to initiate hormonal, metabolic effects. Affinity for these receptors is 10-fold higher than prohormone T_4 (levothyroxine) and no additional conversion (T_4 to T_3) is required. Increases metabolic rate and reverses the loss of consciousness, hypothermia, lactic acidosis, and other symptoms of myxedema coma. Thyroid hormones have many beneficial effects on general metabolism and the cardiovascular system. Liothyronine produces a detectable metabolic response in 2 to 4 hours. Achieves maximum therapeutic response within 48 hours. Has a rapid cutoff of activity, permitting quick dose adjustments and/or control of overdose. Metabolized in the liver to an inactive metabolite. Does not readily cross the placental barrier. Minimal secretion in breast milk.

INDICATIONS AND USES

Treatment of myxedema coma and precoma (patient not completely unconscious). ■ May be used in patients allergic to desiccated thyroid or thyroid extract derived from pork or beef.

CONTRAINDICATIONS

Concomitant use with artificial patient rewarming; generally contraindicated in diagnosed but uncorrected adrenal cortical insufficiency or untreated thyroxicosis; hypersensitivity to any components (no documented evidence of true allergic idiosyncratic reactions). Not justified for use in treatment of obesity or male or female infertility without hypothyroidism.

PRECAUTIONS

For IV use only. ■ Myxedema coma is a medical emergency usually precipitated in a hypothyroid patient by illness, sedatives, or anesthetics. Has a 50% to 70% mortality rate even with aggressive therapy. ■ Use with caution in presence of any compromised cardiac function or cardiac disease, particularly of the coronary arteries. ■ May precipitate a hyperthyroid state or may aggravate existing hyperthyroidism. ■ Due to the rarity of myxedema coma and precoma, no systematic studies have been performed with IV liothyronine.

Monitor: Confirm diagnosis with serum TSH (greater than 60 mcU/ml), serum total T_4 and free T_4 (low), and serum total T_3 and free T_3 (normal or low). Repeat as indicated to evaluate response to treatment. ■ ECG, chest x-ray, CBC, AST (SGOT), CPK, LDH, lipids, serum electrolytes, serum cortisol, cerebrospinal fluid examination, and EEG are helpful before dose administration. Monitor progress by repeat evaluations at selected intervals. ■ Correct adrenocortical insufficiency before administration or acute adrenal crisis and death may result. Corticosteroids (e.g., dexamethasone [Decadron], methylprednisolone [Solu-Medrol]) should be administered routinely in the initial emergency treatment of all myxedema coma patients; required before starting liothyronine or simultaneously with administration in pituitary myxedema; recommended in primary myxedema. During therapy metabolism increases at a greater rate than adrenocortical activity; can precipitate adrenocortical insufficiency and shock; corticosteroids may be needed throughout therapy. ■ In any patient with compromised cardiac function, monitoring of cardiac function is required. ■ Assisted or artificial ventilation may be required. ■ Treatment should correct electrolyte disturbances, possible infection, or other illness. ■ IV fluids will be required, but use caution to prevent cardiac decompensation and be alert for water intoxication from inappropriate secretion of ADH. ■ Do not rewarm patient artificially; may further decrease circulation to vital internal organs and increase shock. Normal body temperature can be restored in 24 to 48 hours by preventing heat loss. Keep patient covered with blankets in a warm room. ■ See Drug/Lab Interactions.

Maternal/Child: Category A: clinical experience does not indicate adverse effect on fetus. ■ Observe infant carefully for any adverse symptoms if breast-feeding; minimal amounts secreted in breast milk. ■ Experience with children under 18 is limited; safety and effectiveness not established.

Elderly: Response similar to other age-groups; however, may be more sensitive to effects. Evaluate carefully for any occult cardiac disease; see Precautions/Monitor. ■ Reduced dose may be indicated; see Dose Adjustments.

DRUG/LAB INTERACTIONS

Metabolic requirements are markedly reduced in hypothyroid patients. Concomitant use with vasopressors (e.g., epinephrine, dopamine [Intropin]) may increase risk of coronary insufficiency, arrhythmias, or circulatory collapse. Use lower doses and extreme caution. ■ Observe any patient previously stabilized on anticoagulants carefully; dose reduction may be required. Monitor PT. ■ Increased doses of insulin or oral hypoglycemics may be required. ■ Higher doses of levothyroxine may be required with estrogens or estrogen-containing oral contraceptives in the patient with a nonfunctioning thyroid. ■ May cause transient cardiac arrhythmias with tricylic antidepressants (e.g., imipramine [Tofranil]). ■ May potentiate toxic effects of digitalis, while increased metabolism may require a higher digitalis dose. ■ Hypertension and tachycardia are probable with ketamine anesthesia. Be prepared to treat promptly. ■ Pregnancy, as well as many drugs (e.g., androgens, corticosteroids, estrogens, estrogen oral contraceptives, iodine preparations, salicylates) in combination with thyroid preparations, interfere with accurate interpretation of lab tests. Consult with lab personnel.

SIDE EFFECTS

Average dose: Arrhythmia (6%), cardiopulmonary arrest (2%), hypotension (2%), myocardial infarction (2%), tachycardia (3%). Angina, congestive heart failure, fever, hypertension, phlebitis, and twitching occurred in 1% or less.

Overdose: Acute myocardial infarction, angina pectoris, arrhythmia, congestive heart failure, headache, increased bowel motility, irritability, menstrual irregularities, nervousness, shock, sweating, tachycardia, thyroid storm, tremor.

ANTIDOTE

Keep physician informed of all side effects. If side effects progress or overdose occurs, reduce or temporarily discontinue liothyronine. Restart at lower doses when feasible. Treatment is symptomatic and supportive. Oxygen and artificial ventilation may be required. Treat increased sympathetic activity with beta-adrenergic antagonists (e.g., esmolol [Brevibloc]). Monitor fever, hypoglycemia, and fluid loss and treat as needed. Digoxin (Lanoxin) may be required in congestive heart failure.

LORAZEPAM

(lor-a′ze-pam)

Benzodiazepine
Sedative-hypnotic
Antianxiety agent
Anticonvulsant
Amnestic
Skeletal muscle relaxant
Antiemetic

Ativan

USUAL DOSE

Dose must be individualized, especially when used in conjunction with other medications that may cause CNS depression. See Dose Adjustments, Precautions, and Drug/Lab Interactions.

Antianxiety/amnestic: 2 mg or 0.044 mg/kg of body weight, whichever is smaller, 15 to 20 minutes before procedure. For greater lack of recall 0.05 mg/kg up to 4 mg may be given. 2 mg is usually the maximum dose for patients over 50 years of age.

Sedation: 2 mg as the initial dose (may not be necessary if patient is receiving intermittent benzodiazepines [e.g., diazepam, midazolam]). Follow with an infusion of 0.5 to 1 mg/hr (0.25 to 0.5 mg/hr if less agitated or has cardiorespiratory problems). Titrate to achieve adequate sedation. Increase in 1 mg/hr increments. Up to 5 to 10 mg/hr has been used. When sedation is adequate, reduce to lowest amount needed.

Status epilepticus: 4 mg as the initial dose. May repeat once in 10 to 15 minutes if seizures continue. Experience with further doses is very limited. Additional intervention (e.g., concomitant administration of phenytoin) may be required. Another source suggests 0.05 mg/kg of body weight to a total dose of 4 mg. May repeat once in 10 to 15 min. If still not effective, use another anticonvulsant agent (e.g., phenytoin). Do not exceed a total dose of 8 mg in 12 hours.

High-dose therapy for refractory status epilepticus (unlabeled): With continuous EEG monitoring, begin a continuous infusion of lorazepam at 1 mg/hr. Increase by 1 mg/hr at 15-minute intervals until patient is seizure free. Maintain seizure-free state with lorazepam for 24 hours. Use therapeutic doses of phenytoin and phenobarbital in addition to lorazepam. At the end of 24 hours, begin to reduce the lorazepam by 1 mg/hr at hourly intervals. Observe closely and monitor EEG for signs of recurrent seizures. Repeat process if seizures recur.

Management of emetic-inducing chemotherapy (unlabeled): 2 mg 30 minutes before chemotherapy is begun. Repeat every 4 hours as needed. Another source suggests 1.5 mg/M^2 (up to a maximum of 3 mg/M^2) over 5 minutes. Administer 30 to 45 minutes before administration of antineoplastic agent. May be given in combination with metoclopramide and dexamethasone. Repeat every 4 hours as needed.

Control of acute agitated delirium in combination with haloperidol (unlabeled): Range is from 0.5 to 10 mg lorazepam every hour until agitation subsides. Begin with a small dose and increase gradually until agitation subsides. Repeat successful dose as needed for agitation. Consult haloperidol monograph.

Treatment of pain and agitation in critically ill cancer patients in combination with haloperidol and hydromorphone [Dilaudid] (unlabeled): Range is from 0.5 to 10 mg lorazepam every 20 to 30 minutes. Begin with a small dose and increase gradually until agitation subsides, then discontinue lorazepam. Consult haloperidol monograph and hydromorphone monograph.

PEDIATRIC DOSE

Safety for use in pediatric patients under 12 years of age has not been fully studied, but it has been used for status epilepticus in neonates, infants, and children; see Maternal/Child.

Sedation: 0.05 mg/kg up to a maximum of 2 mg/dose every 4 to 8 hours.

Status epilepticus (unlabeled): ***Neonates, infants, and children:*** 0.05 to 0.1 mg/kg up to a maximum of 4 mg/dose. May repeat 0.05 mg/kg once in 5 to 10 minutes if needed.

Antiemetic, adjunct therapy (unlabeled): 0.04 to 0.08 mg/kg/dose up to a maximum of 4 mg/dose. May repeat every 6 hours as needed.

DOSE ADJUSTMENTS

Start with a small dose in the elderly and increase gradually based on response. Consider the potential for decreased organ function and concomitant disease or drug therapy. ■ Dose adjustments are not required with impaired liver function. ■ Dose adjustments are not required with impaired renal function unless frequent doses are given over a short period of time. ■ Reduced dose may be indicated in the presence of other CNS depressants. ■ Reduce dose by 50% when given concurrently with probenicid (Benemid) or valproate (Depacon). ■ See Drug/Lab Interactions.

DILUTION

IV injection: Dilute immediately before use with an equal volume of SW, D5W, or NS. Do not shake vigorously, will result in air entrapment. Gently invert repeatedly until completely in solution. May be given by IV injection or through Y-tube or three-way stopcock of infusion tubing.

Infusion (unlabeled): Has been further diluted in D5W or NS and given as an infusion. Best solubility is in concentrations of 0.1 mg/ml or 0.2 mg/ml.

Lorazepam Guidelines for Dilution and Infusion				
Base Concentration	**2 mg/ml**		**4 mg/ml**	
Desired Concentration	**0.1 mg/ml**	**0.2 mg/ml**	**0.1 mg/ml**	**0.2 mg/ml**
Volume of diluent required for each 1 ml lorazepam	19 ml	9 ml	39 ml	19 ml

Very viscous; mix well and observe for crystallization. Crystallization does occur and is thought to be due to propylene glycol preservative. May occur more frequently in NS than in D5W and with 4-mg/ml vials of lorazepam base than with 2-mg/ml vials. Prepare only enough to last for 12 hours. If necessary for fluid restriction, a 2-mg/ml vial has been stable for 24 hours when diluted in a 1 mg (lorazepam base) to 1 ml diluent (D5W preferred). Monitor carefully.

Storage: Refrigerate before dilution; protect from light. Use only freshly prepared solutions; discard if discolored or precipitate forms. Infusions stable at room temperature for 12 hours in plastic, 24 hours in glass.

COMPATIBLE WITH (Underline Indicates Conflicting Compatibility Information)

Consult pharmacist; specific conditions may apply; see Compatibilities, p. xvi.

Syringe: Cimetidine (Tagamet), haloperidol (Haldol), hydromorphone (Dilaudid).

Y-site: Acyclovir (Zovirax), alatrofloxacin (Trovan IV), albumin (Albuminar), allopurinol (Aloprim, Zyloprim), amifostine (Ethyol), amikacin (Amikin), amphotericin B cholesteryl (Amphotec), atracurium (Tracrium), bumetanide (Bumex), cefepime (Maxipime), cefotaxime (Claforan), ciprofloxacin (Cipro IV), cisatracurium (Nimbex), cisplatin (Platinol), cladribine (Leustatin), cyclophosphamide (Cytoxan), cytarabine (ARA-C), dexamethasone (Decadron), diltiazem (Cardizem), dobutamine (Dobutrex), docetaxel (Taxotere), dopamine (Intropin), doxorubicin (Adriamycin), doxorubicin liposome (Doxil), epinephrine (Adrenalin), erythromycin lactobionate (Erythrocin), etomidate (Amidate), etoposide phosphate (Etopophos), famotidine (Pepcid IV), fentanyl (Sublimaze), filgrastim (Neupogen), fluconazole (Diflucan), fludarabine (Fludara), <u>foscarnet (Foscavir)</u>, fosphenytoin (Cerebyx), furosemide (Lasix), gatifloxacin (Tequin), gemcitabine (Gemzar), gentamicin (Garamycin), granisetron (Kytril), haloperidol (Haldol), heparin, hetastarch in electrolytes (Hextend), hydrocortisone sodium succinate (Solu-Cortef), hydromorphone (Dilaudid), labetalol (Normodyne), levofloxacin (Levaquin), linezolid (Zyvox), melphalan (Alkeran), methotrexate (Folex), metronidazole (Flagyl IV), midazolam (Versed), milrinone (Primacor), morphine, nicardipine (Cardene IV), nitroglycerin (Nitro-Bid IV), norepinephrine (Levophed), paclitaxel (Taxol), pancuronium (Pavulon), piperacillin (Pipracil), piperacillin/tazobactam (Zosyn), potassium chloride (KCl), propofol (Diprivan), ranitidine (Zantac), remifentanil (Ultiva), sulfamethoxazole-trimethoprim (Bactrim), tacrolimus (Prograf), teniposide (Vumon), <u>thiopental (Pentothal)</u>, thiotepa (Thioplex), vancomycin (Vancocin), vecuronium (Norcuron), vinorelbine (Navelbine), zidovudine (AZT, Retrovir).

RATE OF ADMINISTRATION

IV injection: Each 2 mg or fraction thereof over 2 to 5 minutes.

Infusion: Use a microdrip or infusion pump for accuracy to deliver desired dose and/or titrate to desired level of sedation.

Pediatric rate: 1 mg or fraction thereof over 2 to 5 minutes.

ACTIONS

A benzodiazepine with antianxiety, sedative, and anticonvulsant effects. Inhibits ability to recall events. Interacts with the GABA-benzodiazepine receptor complex in the brain. Effective in 15 to 30 minutes. Effects last an average of 6 to 8 hours, but may last as long as 12 to 24 hours. Half-life is 9.5 to 19.5 hours. Widely distributed in body fluids. Metabolized by the liver to inactive metabolites; some is slowly excreted in urine. Crosses the placental barrier. Excreted in breast milk.

INDICATIONS AND USES

Preanesthetic medication for adult patients. ■ Produce sedation, relieve anxiety, and provide anterograde amnesia. ■ Management of status epilepticus.

Unlabeled uses: Treatment of severe agitation concurrently with haloperidol. ■ Treatment of pain and agitation in critically ill cancer patients concurrently with haloperidol and hydromorphone or morphine sulfate. ■ High-dose therapy for status epilepticus clinically or EEG diagnosed as refractory to high doses of phenytoin and phenobarbital. ■ Management of emetic-inducing chemotherapy. ■ Antipanic agent. ■ Treatment of alcohol withdrawal. ■ Amnestic during endoscopic procedures. ■ Skeletal muscle relaxant adjunct. ■ Treatment of tension headaches.

CONTRAINDICATIONS

Hypersensitivity to benzodiazepines (diazepam [Valium], chlordiazepoxide [Librium], etc.), glycols, or benzyl alcohol. Patients with acute narrow angle glaucoma, sleep apnea syndrome, or severe respiratory insufficiency (except patients requiring relief of anxiety and/or diminished recall of events while being mechanically ventilated). Intraarterial injection.

PRECAUTIONS

Rapidly and completely absorbed IM. ■ When given as a sedative, patient is able to respond to simple instructions. ■ Airway support, emergency drugs, and equipment must be immediately available. ■ Dependence is possible with prolonged use or high dose. ■ Use with extreme caution in the elderly, the very ill, or patients with limited pulmonary reserve; risk of hypoventilation and/or hypoxic cardiac arrest is increased. ■ Use as a premedicant before local or regional anesthesia may cause excessive drowsiness and interfere with assessment of levels of anesthesia. More likely to occur with doses greater than 0.05 mg/kg or when other narcotic agents are used concomitantly. ■ Use with caution in patients with mild to moderate renal or hepatic disease. ■ There have been reports of possible propylene and polyethylene glycol toxicity when lorazepam has been administered at higher than recommended doses. Patients with renal impairment may be at increased risk of developing toxicity. ■ See Antidote (e.g., risk of seizure with flumazenil).

Monitor: Bed rest required for a minimum of 3 hours after IV injection and assistance required for up to 8 hours. ■ To reduce incidence of thrombophlebitis, avoid smaller veins. Extravasation is hazardous; arterial administration may cause arteriospasms and gangrene and/or require amputation. ■ Monitor and maintain patent airway. Respiratory assistance and flumazenil (Romazicon) must be available. ■ Establish an IV and monitor vital signs. ***Status epilepticus:*** In addition to the above, observe for and correct any other possible cause of seizure (e.g., hypoglycemia, hyponatremia, other metabolic disorders). ■ Sedative effects may add to the impairment of consciousness seen in the post-ictal state (e.g., after a seizure). ■ Neurologic consult is suggested for any patient who fails to regain consciousness.

Patient Education: May produce drowsiness or dizziness; request assistance with ambulation and use caution performing tasks that require alertness for 24 to 48 hours or until the effects of the drug have subsided. ■ Avoid use of alcohol or other CNS depressants (e.g., antihistamines, barbiturates) for 24 to 48 hours or until the effects of the drug have subsided. ■ May be habit-forming with long-term use or high-dose therapy. ■ Has amnestic potential; may impair memory. ■ Consider birth control options.

Maternal/Child: Category D: avoid pregnancy. May cause fetal damage. Not recommended during pregnancy, labor and delivery, breast-feeding, or in children under 12 years of age. ■ Has FDA approval for treatment of status epilepticus in adults over 18 years of age. Safety for use in pediatric patients has not been fully studied, but has been used for status epilepticus in neonates, infants, and children. ■ Half-life prolonged in pediatric patients.

Elderly: Dosing should be cautious in the elderly; see Dose Adjustments. ■ More sensitive to therapeutic and adverse effects (e.g., ataxia, dizziness, oversedation). ■ IV injection may be more likely to cause apnea, bradycardia, CNS depression, hypotension, respiratory depression, and cardiac arrest. ■ See Precautions and Drug/Lab Interactions.

DRUG/LAB INTERACTIONS

Concurrent use with other CNS depressants such as alcohol, antihistamines, barbiturates, MAO inhibitors (e.g., selegiline [Eldepryl]), narcotics (e.g., morphine, meperidine [Demerol], fentanyl), phenothiazines (e.g., prochlorperazine [Compazine]), and tricyclic antidepressants (e.g., imipramine [Tofanil-PM]) may result in additive effects for up to 48 hours. Reduced dose may be indicated. ■ Concurrent administration with valproate (Depacon) or probenicid (Benemid) will decrease clearance of lorazepam. Reduce dose of lorazepam by one half in patients receiving concurrent valproate or probenicid. ■ Apnea, arrhythmia, bradycardia, cardiac arrest, and coma have been reported when used concurrently with haloperidol (Haldol). ■ Significant hypotension, respiratory depression, and stupor have been reported (rare) with concomitant use of loxapine (Loxapac). ■ May increase serum concentrations of digoxin and phenytoin (Dilantin); monitor digoxin and phenytoin serum levels. ■ Benzodiazepines may decrease clearance and increase toxicity of zidovudine (AZT). ■ Hypotensive effects of benzodiazepines may be increased by any agent that induces hypotension (e.g., antihypertensives, bretylium, CNS depressants, diuretics, lidocaine, paclitaxel). ■ Use with rifampin (Rifadin) increases clearance and reduces effects of benzodiazepines. ■ Theophyllines (Aminophylline) antagonize sedative effects of benzodiazepines. ■ clozapine (Clozaril) has caused respiratory distress or cardiac arrest in a few patients; use concurrently with extreme caution. ■ Estrogen-containing oral contraceptives increase clearance and decrease effects. ■ Scopolamine increases sedation, hallucinations, and irrational behavior. ■ Inhibits antiparkinson effectiveness of levodopa.

SIDE EFFECTS

Airway obstruction, apnea, blurred vision, confusion, crying, delirium, depression, excessive drowsiness, hallucinations, hypotension, injection site reaction, respiratory depression, restlessness, somnolence.

Overdose: Ataxia, coma, hypotension, hypotonia, hypnosis, and very rarely death.

ANTIDOTE

Notify physician of all symptoms. Reduction of dose may be required. Treat hypotension with dopamine (Intropin) or norepinephrine (Levophed). In overdose, flumazenil (Romazicon) will reverse all sedative effects of benzodiazepines. See flumazenil monograph (risk of seizures). A patent airway, artificial ventilation, oxygen therapy, and other symptomatic and supportive treatment must be instituted promptly. Monitor vital signs and fluid status carefully. Forced diuresis and osmotic diuretics (e.g., mannitol) may increase rate of lorazepam elimination. The value of dialysis has not been adequately determined.

LYMPHOCYTE IMMUNE GLOBULIN

Immunosuppressant

(lim′fo-sit uh-mun′ glob′u-lin)

Anti-Thymocyte Globulin [Equine], Atgam

pH 6.8

USUAL DOSE

Range is 10 to 30 mg/kg of body weight/24 hr. Actual potency and activity may vary from lot to lot. Given concomitantly with other immunosuppressive therapy (antimetabolites such as azathioprine [Imuran] and corticosteroids). Skin test required; see Monitor.

Delay onset of renal allograft rejection: 15 mg/kg/24 hr for 14 days, then every other day for 7 more doses. Initial dose should be given 24 hours before or after the transplant.

Treat allograft rejection: 10 to 15 mg/kg/24 hr for 14 days, then every other day for 7 more doses (optional). Initial dose should be given when first rejection episode is diagnosed.

Aplastic anemia: 10 to 20 mg/kg/24 hr for 8 to 14 days. Additional alternate-day therapy up to a total of 21 doses may be given.

PEDIATRIC DOSE

Range is 5 to 25 mg/kg/24 hr.

DILUTION

Total daily dose must be further diluted with NS, D5/¼NS, or D5/½NS for infusion. Invert solution while injecting drug so contact is not made with air in infusion bottle. Gently rotate diluted solution. Do not shake. Concentration should not exceed 4 mg/ml. May be infused into a vascular shunt, AV fistula, or high-flow central vein. Use of a 0.2- to 1-micron filter recommended.

Storage: Keep refrigerated before and after dilution. Discard diluted solution after 24 hours.

COMPATIBILITY

Manufacturer states lymphocyte immune globulin may precipitate in dextrose solutions and may be unstable with highly acidic solutions.

RATE OF ADMINISTRATION

A total daily dose equally distributed over a minimum of 4 hours.

ACTIONS

A lymphocyte-selective immunosuppressant. Reduces the number of thymus-dependent lymphocytes and contains low concentrations of antibodies against other formed elements in blood. Effective without causing severe lymphopenia. Supports an increase in the frequency of resolution of an acute rejection episode. Has a serum half-life of 5 to 8 days.

INDICATIONS AND USES

Management of allograft rejection in renal transplant patients. ■ Adjunctive to other immunosuppressive therapy to delay onset of initial rejection episode. ■ Treatment of moderate to severe aplastic anemia in patients who are not candidates for bone marrow transplant.

CONTRAINDICATIONS

Systemic hypersensitivity reaction to previous injection of lymphocyte immune globulin or any other equine gamma-globulin preparation.

PRECAUTIONS

Administered only under the direction of a physician experienced in immunosuppressive therapy and management of renal transplant patients in a facility with adequate laboratory and supportive medical resources. ■ Use caution in repeated courses of therapy; observe for signs of allergic reaction.

Monitor: Intradermal skin test required before administration. Use 0.1 ml of a 1:1,000 dilution in NS and a saline control. If a systemic reaction (rash, dyspnea) occurs, do not administer. If a limited reaction (10 mm wheal or erythema) occurs, proceed with extreme caution. Anaphylaxis can occur even if skin test is negative. ■ Will cause chemical phlebitis in peripheral veins. ■ Monitor carefully for signs of infection, leukopenia, or thrombocytopenia. Thrombocytopenia is usually transient in renal transplant patients. Platelet transfusions may be necessary in patients with aplastic anemia. Notify physician immediately so prompt treatment can be instituted and/or drug discontinued. ■ Prophylactic antibiotics may be indicated pending results of C/S in a febrile neutropenic patient. ■ Masked reactions may occur as dose of corticosteroids and antimetabolites is decreased. Observe carefully. ■ Antihistamines (e.g., diphenhydramine [Benadryl]) may be required to control itching. ■ Anaphylaxis can occur at any time. Emergency equipment and supplies must be at bedside.

Patient Education: See Appendix D, p. 1148.

Maternal/Child: Category C: no studies conducted in pregnant patients. Use caution. ■ Safety for use in breast-feeding not established. Limited experience on use in children.

DRUG/LAB INTERACTIONS

See Monitor.

SIDE EFFECTS

Full range of allergic symptoms including anaphylaxis is possible. Arthralgia, back pain, chest pain, chills, clotted AV fistula, diarrhea, dyspnea, fever, headache, hypotension, infusion site pain, leukopenia, nausea, night sweats, pruritus, rash, stomatitis, thrombocytopenia, thrombophlebitis, urticaria, vomiting, wheal and flare.

ANTIDOTE

Notify physician of all side effects. Discontinue if anaphylaxis, severe and unremitting thrombocytopenia, and/or severe and unremitting leukopenia occur; see Monitor. May be discontinued if infection or hemolysis present even if appropriately treated. Clinically significant hemolysis may require erythrocyte transfusion, IV mannitol, furosemide, sodium bicarbonate, and fluids. Prophylactic or therapeutic antihistamines (e.g., diphenhydramine [Benadryl]) or corticosteroids should control chills caused by release of endogenous leukocyte pyrogens. Treat anaphylaxis immediately. Epinephrine (Adrenalin), diphenhydramine (Benadryl), oxygen, vasopressors (e.g., dopamine [Intropin]), corticosteroids, and ventilation equipment must always be available. Resuscitate as necessary.

MAGNESIUM SULFATE
(mag-nee′zee-um sul′fat)

Electrolyte replenisher
Anticonvulsant
Antiarrhythmic
Uterine relaxant

pH 5.5 to 7

USUAL DOSE

Convulsive states: 1 to 4 Gm (8 to 32 mEq [10 to 40 ml of a 10% solution]). Repeat as indicated, observing all necessary precautions. An alternate regimen is 4 Gm diluted in 250 ml of D5W infused at a rate not to exceed 3 ml/min. In severe ***preeclampsia or eclampsia,*** a total dose of 8 to 15 Gm may be required depending on body weight. Repeat doses are frequently given IM or an infusion of 1 to 2 Gm/hr is initiated.

Hypomagnesemia (mild): 1 Gm every 6 hours for 4 doses.

Hypomagnesemia (severe): 5 Gm (40 mEq) in 1,000 ml D5W or NS as an infusion evenly distributed over 3 hours.

Hyperalimentation in adults: 8 to 24 mEq/24 hr (1 to 3 Gm).

Cardiac arrest (hypomagnesemia or torsades de pointes): AHA recommends 1 to 2 Gm (2 to 4 ml of a 50% solution) diluted in 10 ml D5W IV push.

Torsades de pointes (not during cardiac arrest): AHA recommends a loading dose of 1 to 2 Gm in 50 to 100 ml D5W as an infusion over 5 to 60 minutes. Follow with 0.5 to 1 Gm/hr and titrate to control the torsades.

Refractory ventricular tachycardia/ventricular fibrillation: 1 to 2 Gm (8 to 16 mEq) in 100 ml D5W over 1 to 2 min. 2 to 6 Gm has been used with extreme caution over several minutes followed by an infusion of 3 to 20 mg/min for 5 to 48 hours.

Reduce incidence of postinfarction arrhythmias associated with hypomagnesemia: ***Loading dose:*** 1 to 2 Gm (8 to 16 mEq) in 50 to 100 ml D5W over 5 to 60 minutes. Follow with an ***infusion*** of 0.5 to 1 Gm (4 to 8 mEq) per hour for up to 24 hours. Base rate and duration on level of hypomagnesemia. 3 to 4 Gm (30 to 40 ml) of a 10% solution has been used ***with extreme caution over 30 seconds*** in the management of paroxysmal atrial tachycardia.

Barium poisoning: 1 to 2 Gm.

Alternative to thrombolytic therapy post MI (unlabeled): 22 Gm equally distributed over 48 hours. Effectively decreases incidence of arrhythmias in acute MI patients who cannot receive thrombolytic therapy. Does not decrease incidence of CHF or conduction disturbances.

Alleviate bronchospasm in acute asthma (unlabeled): 2 Gm given IV over 20 minutes. Usually given concurrently with inhaled albuterol (Proventil) and IV corticosteroids.

PEDIATRIC DOSE

Hypomagnesemia or hypocalcemia: 25 to 50 mg/kg of body weight. May repeat at 4- to 6-hour intervals for 3 or 4 doses. Maintain with 30 to 60 mg/kg/24 hr (approximately 0.25 to 0.5 mEq/kg/24 hr). Maximum dose is 1 Gm/24 hr. AHA recommends 25 to 50 mg/kg as an infusion over 10 to 20 minutes for ***asthma, suspected hypomagnesemia, ventricular tachycardia, or torsades de pointes.*** Maximum recommended dose is 2 Gm.

Acute nephritis in children: 100 to 200 mg/kg as a 1% to 3% solution (1 Gm in 100 ml = 1% solution, 3 Gm in 100 ml = 3%). One-half dose should be given over 15 to 20 minutes. Complete balance of dose within 1 hour. **Alleviate bronchospasm in acute asthma (unlabeled):** 25 to 40 mg/kg. Given IV over 20 minutes. Do not exceed 2 Gm. Usually given concurrently with inhaled albuterol (Proventil) and IV corticosteroids.

Hyperalimentation: ***Children:*** 0.25 to 1.25 Gm/24 hr (2 to 10 mEq/24 hr). ***Infants:*** 30 to 60 mg/kg/24 hr (0.25 to 0.6 mEq/kg/24 hr) up to a maximum dose of 1 Gm.

DOSE ADJUSTMENTS

Reduce dose of other CNS depressants (e.g., narcotics, barbiturates) when given in conjunction with magnesium sulfate. ■ Reduce dose in impaired renal function and in the elderly.

DILUTION

Must be diluted to a concentration of 20% (200 mg/ml) or less for IV administration. D5W or NS are the most common diluents. Available in vials or syringes as 10% (100 mg/ml), 12.5% (125 mg/ml), 20% (200 mg/ml), and 50% (500 mg/ml); premixed in SW as a 4% solution (40 mg/ml) in 100, 500, or 1,000 ml containers; premixed as an 8% solution (80 mg/ml) in 50 ml; and premixed as a 1% solution (10 mg/ml) in 100 or 1,000 ml D5W or a 2% solution (20 mg/ml) in 500 or 1,000 ml D5W. See Usual Dose for specific dilutions. May be given through Y-tube or three-way stopcock of infusion set.

INCOMPATIBLE WITH

Will form various precipitates with alkali carbonates, alkali hydroxides, arsenates, barium, calcium, lead, phosphates, salicylates, strontium, and tartrates. Use caution; consult pharmacist.

COMPATIBLE WITH **(Underline Indicates Conflicting Compatibility Information)**

See Incompatible With. Consult pharmacist; specific conditions may apply; see Compatibilities, p. xvi.

Additive: <u>Calcium gluconate</u>, chloramphenicol (Chloromycetin), cisplatin (Platinol), heparin, <u>hydrocortisone sodium succinate (Solu-Cortef)</u>, isoproterenol (Isuprel), linezolid (Zyvox), meropenem (Merrem IV), methyldopate (Aldomet), norepinephrine (Levophed), penicillin G potassium, <u>potassium phosphate</u>, verapamil (Isoptin).

Syringe: Metoclopramide (Reglan).

Y-site: Acyclovir (Zovirax), aldesleukin (Proleukin, IL-2), amifostine (Ethyol), amikacin (Amikin), ampicillin, aztreonam (Azactam), cefamandole (Mandol), cefazolin (Kefzol), cefoperazone (Cefobid), cefotaxime (Claforan), cefoxitin (Mefoxin), chloramphenicol (Chloromycetin), <u>ciprofloxacin (Cipro IV)</u>, cisatracurium (Nimbex), <u>clindamycin (Cleocin)</u>, dobutamine (Dobutrex), docetaxel (Taxotere), doxorubicin liposome (Doxil), doxycycline (Vibramycin), enalaprilat (Vasotec IV), erythromycin lactobionate (Erythrocin), esmolol (Brevibloc), etoposide phosphate (Etopophos), famotidine (Pepcid IV), fludarabine (Fludara), gatifloxacin (Tequin), gentamicin (Garamycin), granisetron (Kytril), heparin, hetastarch in electrolytes (Hextend), <u>hydrocortisone sodium succinate (Solu-Cortef)</u>, hydromorphone (Dilaudid), idarubicin (Idamycin), insulin (regular), kanamycin (Kantrex), labetalol (Normodyne), linezolid (Zyvox), meperidine (Demerol), metronidazole (Flagyl IV), milrinone (Primacor), minocycline (Minocin), morphine, nafcillin (Nafcil), ondansetron (Zofran), oxacillin (Bactocill), paclitaxel (Taxol), penicillin G potassium, piperacillin

(Pipracil), piperacillin/tazobactam (Zosyn), potassium chloride (KCl), propofol (Diprivan), remifentanil (Ultiva), sargramostim (Leukine), sulfamethoxazole-trimethoprim (Bactrim), thiotepa (Thioplex), ticarcillin (Ticar), tobramycin (Nebcin), vancomycin (Vancocin).

RATE OF ADMINISTRATION

IV injection: 1.5 ml of a 10% solution or its equivalent over at least 1 minute or as directed in Usual Dose. Too-rapid administration may cause hypotension and asystole.

IV infusion: As directed in Usual Dose.

ACTIONS

A CNS depressant and a depressant of smooth, skeletal, and cardiac muscle. It also possesses a mild diuretic effect and vasodilating effect. Can reverse refractory VF caused by hypomagnesemia and help replenishment of intracellular potassium. Onset of action is immediate and effective for about 30 minutes. Excreted in the urine. Secreted in breast milk. Crosses the placental barrier.

INDICATIONS AND USES

Prevention and control of convulsive states (eclampsia, glomerulonephritis, hypoparathyroidism). ■ Severe hypomagnesemia. ■ Nutritional supplementation in hyperalimentation. ■ Cerebral edema. ■ Uterine tetany, especially after large doses of oxytocin. ■ Treatment of choice in torsades de pointes, recurrent and refractory ventricular tachycardia, and ventricular fibrillation (VT/VF). ■ Reduce the incidence of postinfarction arrhythmias by counteracting postinfarction hypomagnesemia (given on admission to CCU of a patient with suspected myocardial infarction). ■ Counteract muscle-stimulating effects of barium poisoning. ■ Acute nephritis in children to control hypertension, encephalopathy, and convulsions.

Unlabeled uses: Inhibit premature labor. ■ Treatment of alcohol withdrawal. ■ Adjunctive to alleviate bronchospasm in acute asthma. ■ Alternative to thrombolytic therapy in post myocardial infarction patients. ■ Chronic fatigue syndrome. ■ Adjunctive therapy with digoxin in treatment of new-onset atrial fibrillation. ■ Decrease complications during premature labor and/or decrease incidence of cerebral palsy.

CONTRAINDICATIONS

Presence of heart block or myocardial damage; within 2 hours of delivery.

PRECAUTIONS

Do not administer during the 2 hours preceding delivery of the toxemic patient. May cause magnesium toxicity in the newborn requiring assisted ventilation and calcium administration. ■ Each 1 Gm contains 8.12 mEq of magnesium. A normal adult body contains 20 to 30 Gm of magnesium. ■ Use caution in impaired renal function and in patients receiving digitalis. Even in normal renal function, use caution to prevent exceeding renal excretory capacity. ■ Hypomagnesemia can precipitate refractory VF and hinder potassium replacement.

Monitor: Discontinue IV administration when the desired therapeutic effect is obtained. ■ Test knee jerks and observe respirations before each additional dose. If the knee jerk is absent or respirations are less than 16/min, do not give additional magnesium sulfate. ■ Equipment to maintain artificial ventilation must be available at all times. Patient must be continuously observed. Maintain minimum of 100 ml of urine output every 4 hours. ■ Closely monitor patients with suspected or probable MI for hypotension or asystole and measure magnesium levels.

Maternal/Child: See Precautions. ■ Category A: appears to be safe for use during pregnancy except for the last 2 hours before delivery; see Contraindications. ■ A continuous infusion given to control convulsions in toxemic mothers before delivery (especially in the 24 hours preceding) may cause signs of magnesium toxicity in the newborn (e.g., respiratory depression). ■ Some literature indicates possible harm to the fetus during pregnancy if mother is not toxic. ■ Use caution during breast-feeding. ■ Safety for children not established.

Elderly: See Dose Adjustments.

DRUG/LAB INTERACTIONS

See Dose Adjustments and Monitor. ■ Potentiates neuromuscular blocking agents (e.g., tubocurarine [Curare], vecuronium [Norcuron], succinylcholine). ■ May reduce the antibiotic activity of streptomycin, tetracycline, and tobramycin (Nebcin).

SIDE EFFECTS

Usually the result of magnesium intoxication. Absence of knee-jerk reflex; cardiac arrest; circulatory collapse; CNS depression; complete heart block; flaccid paralysis; flushing; hypocalcemia with signs of tetany; hypotension; hypothermia; increased PR interval; increased QRS complex; prolonged QT interval; respiratory depression, paralysis, and failure; stupor; sweating.

ANTIDOTE

Discontinue the drug and notify the physician of the occurrence of any side effect. Calcium gluconate and calcium gluceptate are specific antidotes; 5 to 10 mEq should reverse respiratory depression and heart block. Physostigmine 0.5 to 1 mg SC may be helpful. Treat hypotension with dopamine (Intropin). Employ artificial ventilation as necessary and resuscitate as necessary. Peritoneal dialysis or hemodialysis are effective in overdose. **Newborn resuscitation:** Will require endotracheal intubation, assisted ventilation, and calcium 1 mEq as an antidote.

MANNITOL

(man′nih-tol)

Osmitrol

Diuretic (osmotic)

pH 4.5 to 7

USUAL DOSE

Test dose may be required; see Monitor. 1 to 2 Gm/kg of body weight or 20 to 200 Gm/24 hr. Very flexible. 1 Gm equal to approximately 5.5 mOsm.

Available as:
5% solution (50 Gm/L)
10% solution (50 Gm/500 ml, 100 Gm/L)
15% solution (75 Gm/500 ml)
20% solution (50 Gm/250 ml, 100 Gm/500 ml)
25% solution (12.5 Gm/50 ml)

Prevention of oliguric phase of acute renal failure: 50 to 100 Gm as a 5% to 25% solution.

Treatment of oliguria: 300 to 400 mg/kg of body weight of a 15% to 25% solution or 50 to 100 Gm of a 15% to 25% solution.

Management of intracranial pressure in neurologic emergencies: AHA recommends 0.5 to 1 Gm/kg over 5 to 10 minutes. Repeat 0.25 to 2 Gm/kg every 4 to 6 hours as needed. Another source suggests 0.25 to 2 Gm/kg of body weight as a 15% to 25% solution.

Reduction of intraocular pressure: 0.25 to 2 Gm/kg of body weight as a 15%, 20%, or 25% solution. May be used 60 to 90 minutes before surgery.

Promote diuresis in intoxication: 50 to 200 Gm. Discontinue if no benefit derived from this dose.

Measurement of glomerular filtration rate: 100 ml of a 20% solution (20 Gm) diluted with 180 ml of NS should be infused at a rate of 20 ml/min. Collect urine and plasma samples as ordered.

PEDIATRIC DOSE

Test dose may be required; see Monitor. 0.25 to 2 Gm/kg of body weight or 30 to 60 Gm/M^2 of body surface as a 15% to 20% solution. Start with low dose and increase gradually based on clinical situation.

Promote diuresis in intoxication: 0.25 to 2 Gm/kg or 30 to 60 Gm/M^2 as a 5% or 10% solution.

Anuria/oliguria: 0.5 to 1 Gm/kg as an initial dose. Maintain with 0.25 to 0.5 Gm/kg every 4 to 6 hours.

Cerebral edema: 0.25 Gm/kg. May repeat every 5 minutes as indicated. May give furosemide (Lasix) 1 mg/kg 5 minutes before or concurrently. May gradually increase dose of mannitol to 1 Gm/kg to effect satisfactory response.

Preoperative for neurosurgery: 1.5 to 2 Gm/kg over 30 to 60 min.

DOSE ADJUSTMENTS

Reduce dose by one half for small or debilitated patients. ■ Reduced dose may be required in oliguria or impaired renal function; see Monitor.

DILUTION

No further dilution is necessary; however, if there are any crystals present in the solution, they must be completely dissolved before administration. Warm ampule or bottle in hot water (to 50° C [122° F]) and shake vigorously at intervals. Cool to at least body temperature before administration. Use an in-line filter for 15%, 20%, and 25% solutions. Discard unused portions.

Glomerular filtration rate: See Usual Dose.

Storage: Store below 40° C.

INCOMPATIBLE WITH

Sources list strongly acidic or alkaline solutions. 20% or 25% solutions of mannitol may precipitate with potassium chloride (KCl) or sodium chloride. Concomitant administration of electrolyte-free mannitol solutions with whole blood may cause pseudoagglutination; consult pharmacist.

COMPATIBLE WITH

Consult pharmacist; specific conditions may apply; see Compatibilities, p. xvi.

Additive: Amikacin (Amikin), bretylium (Bretylate), cefamandole (Mandol), cefoxitin (Mefoxin), cimetidine (Tagamet), cisplatin (Platinol), dopamine (Intropin), fosphenytoin (Cerebyx), furosemide (Lasix), gentamicin (Garamycin), metoclopramide (Reglan), ofloxacin (Floxin IV), ondansetron (Zofran), sodium bicarbonate, tobramycin (Nebcin), verapamil (Isoptin).

Y-site: Allopurinol (Aloprim, Zyloprim), amifostine (Ethyol), amphotericin B cholesteryl (Amphotec), aztreonam (Azactam), cisatracurium (Nimbex), cladribine (Leustatin), docetaxel (Taxotere), etoposide phosphate (Etopophos), fludarabine (Fludara), fluorouracil (5-FU), gatifloxacin (Tequin), gemcitabine (Gemzar), hetastarch in electrolytes (Hextend), idarubicin (Idamycin), linezolid (Zyvox), melphalan (Alkeran), ondansetron (Zofran), paclitaxel (Taxol), piperacillin/tazobactam (Zosyn), propofol (Diprivan), remifentanil (Ultiva), sargramostim (Leukine), teniposide (Vumon), thiotepa (Thioplex), vinorelbine (Navelbine).

RATE OF ADMINISTRATION

A single dose should be given over 30 to 90 minutes. Up to 3 Gm/kg have been given over this time span. A test dose (see Monitor) or loading doses may be given over 3 to 5 minutes.

Oliguria: A single dose over 90 minutes to several hours.

Reduction of intracranial pressure and brain mass: A single dose over 30 to 60 minutes.

Treatment of edema or ascites in pediatric patients: A single dose over 2 to 6 hours.

Glomerular filtration rate: See Usual Dose.

ACTIONS

A sugar alcohol and most effective osmotic diuretic. It is a stable, inert, nontoxic solution. Distribution in the body is limited to extracellular compartments. Mannitol is not reabsorbed by the tubules of the kidneys. It is excreted almost completely in the urine along with water, sodium, and chloride. Onset of diuresis is 1 to 3 hours. Reduction in cerebrospinal and intraocular fluid occurs within 15 minutes and lasts 4 to 8 hours. Rebound may occur within 12 hours.

INDICATIONS AND USES

Prophylaxis of acute renal failure (cardiovascular procedures, severe trauma, surgery in presence of jaundice, and hemolytic transfusion reactions). ■ Reduction of intracranial pressure and brain mass before and after surgery. ■ Reduction of extremely high intraocular pressure. ■ Promotion of excretion of toxic substances. ■ Kidney function test (glomerular filtration rate). ■ Reduction of generalized edema and ascites. ■ Oliguric phase of acute renal failure.

CONTRAINDICATIONS

Anuria, edema associated with capillary fragility of membrane permeability, fluid and electrolyte depletion, intracranial bleeding except during craniotomy, some cases of metabolic edema, severe congestive heart failure, severe dehydration, severe pulmonary congestion or frank pulmonary edema, severe renal impairment or progressive renal dysfunction, including increasing azotemia or oliguria.

PRECAUTIONS

Evaluate cardiac status to avoid fulminating congestive heart failure. Use caution in renal failure, fluid overload may result.

Monitor: Test dose should be used in patients with marked oliguria or impaired renal functions. Give 200 mg/kg of body weight over 3 to 5 minutes. 40 ml of urine should be produced in 1 hour. If adequate urine not produced, repeat once. If still ineffective, reevaluate patient. ■ Observe urine output continuously; should exceed 30 to 50 ml/hr. Insert Foley catheter if necessary. ■ Monitor fluid status and osmolality (not to exceed 310 mOsm/kg). ■ Electrolyte depletion may occur. Check with laboratory studies and replace as necessary. ■ Observe infusion site to prevent infiltration. ■ Maintain hydration; may obscure signs of inadequate hydration or hypovolemia. ■ Before attempting to reduce intracranial pressure and brain mass, evaluate circulatory and renal reserve, fluid and electrolyte balance, body weight, and total input and output before and after mannitol infusion. Support with adequate ventilation and oxygenation. Reduced cerebrospinal fluid pressure must be observed within 15 minutes after starting infusion.

Maternal/Child: Category C: safety for use in pregnancy not established. Benefits must outweigh risks. ■ Use caution in breast-feeding. ■ Doses for children under 12 years not established but are used clinically.

DRUG/LAB INTERACTIONS

May increase lithium excretion, thereby decreasing its effectiveness. ■ Mannitol-induced hypokalemia may increase the potential for digoxin toxicity.

SIDE EFFECTS

Rare when used as directed but may include backache, blurred vision, chest pain, chills, convulsions, decreased chloride levels, decreased sodium levels, dehydration, diuresis, dizziness, dryness of mouth, edema, fever, fulminating congestive heart failure, headache, hyperosmolality, hypertension, hypotension, nausea, polyuria then oliguria, pulmonary edema, rhinitis, tachycardia, thirst, thrombophlebitis, and urinary retention.

ANTIDOTE

If minor side effects persist, notify the physician. For all major side effects or if urine output is under 30 to 50 ml/hr, discontinue the drug and notify the physician. Treatment will be supportive to correct fluid and electrolyte imbalances. Hemodialysis may be used to clear mannitol and reduce serum osmolality.

MECHLORETHAMINE HYDROCHLORIDE

(meh-klor-eth′ah-meen hye-droe-klor′id)

Antineoplastic (alkylating agent/nitrogen mustard)

HN_2, Mustargen, Nitrogen Mustard

pH 3 to 5

USUAL DOSE

0.4 mg/kg of body weight as a single dose is preferred, or may be divided into 2 to 4 equal doses and given daily for 2 to 4 days. Allow about 3 to 6 weeks between courses of therapy. Confirm bone marrow recovery. Results with subsequent courses are rarely as satisfactory as the initial course.

Hodgkin's disease: 6 mg/M^2 on days 1 and 8 of a monthly treatment cycle.

DOSE ADJUSTMENTS

Dose based on average weight in presence of ascites or edema. ■ Used in reduced doses with other chemotherapeutic agents to produce tumor remission. ■ See Drug/Lab Interactions.

DILUTION

Specific techniques required; see Precautions. Highly toxic. Both powder and solution must be handled with care. Mix solution immediately before use. Very unstable. Dilute each 10-mg vial with 10 ml of SW or NS. Do not remove needle and syringe. Hold securely and shake vial to dissolve completely. Withdraw desired dose. Contains 1 mg/ml. Do not use if solution is discolored or if droplets of water remain isolated in the vial. May be given by IV injection, but administration through a Y-tube or three-way stopcock of a free-flowing infusion is preferred. Neutralize unused portion with equal volumes of 5% sodium thiosulfate and 5% sodium bicarbonate solution and let stand 45 minutes, then discard appropriately.

INCOMPATIBLE WITH

Rapidly decomposes in IV solutions; addition not recommended.

COMPATIBLE WITH

Consult pharmacist; specific conditions may apply; see Compatibilities, p. xvi.

Y-site: Amifostine (Ethyol), aztreonam (Azactam), filgrastim (Neupogen), fludarabine (Fludara), granisetron (Kytril), melphalan (Alkeran), ondansetron (Zofran), sargramostim (Leukine), teniposide (Vumon), vinorelbine (Navelbine).

RATE OF ADMINISTRATION

Total daily dose equally distributed over 3 to 5 minutes.

ACTIONS

An alkylating agent, cell cycle phase–nonspecific, with antitumor activity. It has a selective cytotoxic effect on rapidly growing cells. Palliative, not curative, in its effects; regression in the size of malignant tumor may occur; pain and fever subside; appetite, strength, and a sense of well-being are increased. Rapidly metabolized. Excreted in changed form in the urine.

INDICATIONS AND USES

To suppress or retard neoplastic growth. Good response is inconsistent but has been experienced in Hodgkin's disease, lymphosarcoma, bronchogenic carcinoma, specific types of chronic leukemia, polycythemia vera, and mycosis fungoides. Used in generalized metastasis and in patients refractory to radiation therapy.

CONTRAINDICATIONS

Not recommended in patients with infectious disease, previous anaphylactic reactions, or in terminal stages of malignancy.

PRECAUTIONS

Follow guidelines for handling cytotoxic agents. See Appendix A, p. 1142. ■ Administered by or under the direction of the physician specialist. ■ Highly toxic; a probable carcinogen. Must not be inhaled or come into contact with skin or any mucous membrane, especially the eyes, at any stage of mixing, administration, or destruction. For accidental contact, copious irrigation with water for at least 15 minutes is indicated. Follow with rinse of 2% sodium thiosulfate and seek medical attention. If accidental eye exposure occurs, irrigate for 15 minutes with water, NS, or a balanced salt ophthalmic irrigating solution and seek ophthalmologic consultation. Contaminated clothing should be removed and destroyed. ■ Use precaution with radiation therapy, other chemotherapy, severe leukopenia, thrombocytopenia, anemia, and bone marrow infiltrated with malignant cells. ■ Specific tissue can be protected from the effects of this agent by temporary interruption of its blood supply during and immediately after injection. ■ In the presence of acute or chronic suppurative inflammation, do not use nitrogen mustard. May cause rapid development of amyloidosis.

Monitor: Extremely narrow margin of safety; dose is individual, and frequent blood examinations are mandatory. ■ Extravasation into surrounding tissue can cause sloughing and possible necrosis. ■ Often given in the late evening with antiemetics and sedatives to promote patient comfort. ■ Maintain adequate hydration. ■ Allopurinol may prevent formation of uric acid crystals. ■ Observe closely for all signs of infection. Prophylactic antibiotics may be indicated pending results of C/S in a febrile neutropenic patient. ■ Monitor for thrombocytopenia (platelet count less than 50,000/mm^3). Initiate precautions to prevent excessive bleeding (e.g., inspect IV sites, skin, and mucous membranes; use extreme care during invasive procedures; test urine, emesis, stool, and secretions for occult blood).

Patient Education: Report IV site burning or stinging promptly ■ Nonhormonal birth control recommended. ■ See Appendix D, p. 1148.

Maternal/Child: Category D: avoid pregnancy. May produce teratogenic effects on the fetus. Has mutagenic potential. ■ Discontinue breastfeeding. ■ Limited use in children; safety not established.

DRUG/LAB INTERACTIONS

Alkylating agents interact with radiation therapy, other antineoplastics, and other bone marrow depressants (e.g., doxorubicin [Adriamycin], vincristine [Oncovin]) to produce serious reaction. ■ Do not administer live vaccines to patients receiving antineoplastic drugs.

SIDE EFFECTS

Alopecia, anaphylaxis, anorexia, bleeding, bone marrow depression, cerebrovascular accidents, delayed catamenia, depression of formed elements in circulating blood, diarrhea, hemolytic anemia, hyperuricemia, jaundice, leukopenia, nausea, petechiae, sloughing, susceptibility to infection, tinnitus, thrombophlebitis, vertigo, vomiting, weakness, death.

ANTIDOTE

For external contact and cleaning purposes, use a 2% sodium thiosulfate solution. ■ To prevent sloughing and necrosis in areas where extravasation has occurred, inject isotonic sodium thiosulfate with a fine hypodermic needle into the indurated area. Apply ice compress for 6 to 12 hours. Elevate extremity. ■ Use chlorpromazine (Thorazine) or other phenothiazines to control nausea and sodium pentobarbital (Nembutal) to produce sedation. ■ Notify physician of any side effect. Discontinue the drug and use supportive therapy as necessary to sustain the patient in toxicity. Administration of whole blood products (e.g., packed RBCs, platelets, leukocytes) and/or blood modifiers (e.g., darbepoetin alfa [Aranesp], epoetin alfa [Epogen, Procrit], filgrastim [Neupogen], pegfilgrastim [Neulasta], sargramostim [Leukine], oprelvekin [Neumega]) may be indicated to treat bone marrow toxicity.

MELPHALAN HYDROCHLORIDE

(mel′fah-lan hye-droe-klor′id)

Antineoplastic (alkylating agent/nitrogen mustard)

Alkeran, L-PAM, Phenylalanine Mustard, L-Sarcolysin

pH 6.5 to 7

USUAL DOSE

16 mg/M^2 every 2 weeks for 4 doses. After recovery from toxicity, repeat a dose every 4 weeks. Prednisone is administered concurrently (0.6 mg/kg daily with dose reductions every 2 weeks). WBC should be above 4,000/mm^3 and platelets above 100,000/mm^3. Other similar regimens are in use. No exact dosage conversion from oral to parenteral or parenteral to oral.

PEDIATRIC DOSE

See Unlabeled uses.

DOSE ADJUSTMENTS

Reduce dose by 50% if BUN greater than 30 mg/dl or SrCr greater than 1.5 mg/dl. ■ Reduce dose based on myelotoxicity; by 25% if WBC between 3,000 to 4,000/mm^3 and platelets between 75,000 to 100,000/mm^3; by 50% if WBC between 2,000 and 3,000/mm^3 and platelets between 50,000 to 75,000/mm^3. Withhold dose for WBC below 2,000/mm^3 and platelets below 50,000/mm^3. ■ Somewhat reduced dose may be appropriate for patients undergoing hemodialysis.

DILUTION

Specific techniques required; see Precautions. Reconstitution to completion of administration must take place within 60 minutes due to instability of melphalan (rapid hydrolysis). Rapidly inject 10 ml of supplied diluent into vial. Shake vigorously until a clear solution results (5 mg/ml). Use only clear solutions. Has been given without further dilution via a central line. Usually further diluted in NS to a concentration of 0.1 to 0.45 mg/ml (45 mg in 100 ml equals 0.45 mg/ml). Must always be further diluted for use in peripheral lines.

Storage: Protect from light and store at room temperature before reconstitution. Reconstituted solution is stable for only 90 minutes maximum.

Stable at a concentration of 0.1 to 0.45 mg/ml for only 60 minutes. Will precipitate if refrigerated.

COMPATIBLE WITH

Consult pharmacist; specific conditions may apply; see Compatibilities, p. xvi.

Y-site: Acyclovir (Zovirax), amikacin (Amikin), aminophylline, ampicillin, aztreonam (Azactam), bleomycin (Blenoxane), bumetanide (Bumex), buprenorphine (Buprenex), butorphanol (Stadol), calcium gluconate, carboplatin (Paraplatin), carmustine (BiCNU), cefazolin (Kefzol), cefepime (Maxipime), cefoperazone (Cefobid), cefotaxime (Claforan), cefotetan (Cefotan), ceftazidime (Fortaz), ceftizoxime (Cefizox), ceftriaxone (Rocephin), cefuroxime (Zinacef), cimetidine (Tagamet), cisplatin (Platinol), clindamycin (Cleocin), cyclophosphamide (Cytoxan), cytarabine (ARA-C), dacarbazine (DTIC), dactinomycin (Cosmegen), daunorubicin (Cerubidine), dexamethasone (Decadron), diphenhydramine (Benadryl), doxorubicin (Adriamycin), doxycycline (Vibramycin), droperidol (Inapsine), enalaprilat (Vasotec IV), etoposide (VePesid), famotidine (Pepcid IV), fluconazole (Diflucan), fludarabine (Fludara), fluorouracil (5-FU), furosemide (Lasix), ganciclovir (Cytovene), gentamicin (Garamycin), granisetron (Kytril), haloperidol (Haldol), heparin, hydrocortisone (Hydrocortone, Solu-Cortef), hydromorphone (Dilaudid), idarubicin (Idamycin), ifosfamide (Ifex), imipenem-cilastatin (Primaxin), lorazepam (Ativan), mannitol, mechlorethamine (nitrogen mustard), meperidine (Demerol), mesna (Mesnex), methotrexate (Folex), methylprednisolone (Solu-Medrol), metoclopramide (Reglan), metronidazole (Flagyl IV), minocycline (Minocin), mitomycin (Mutamycin), mitoxantrone (Novantrone), morphine, nalbuphine (Nubain), ondansetron (Zofran), pentostatin (Nipent), piperacillin (Pipracil), plicamycin (Mithracin), potassium chloride (KCl), prochlorperazine (Compazine), promethazine (Phenergan), ranitidine (Zantac), sodium bicarbonate, streptozocin (Zanosar), sulfamethoxazole-trimethoprim (Bactrim), teniposide (Vumon), thiotepa (Thioplex), ticarcillin (Ticar), ticarcillin/clavulanate (Timentin), tobramycin (Nebcin), vancomycin (Vancocin), vinblastine (Velban), vincristine (Oncovin), vinorelbine (Navelbine), zidovudine (AZT, Retrovir).

RATE OF ADMINISTRATION

IV injection: A single dose less than 23 mg/M^2 over 2 to 5 minutes via a peripheral vein; up to 200 mg/M^2 over 2 to 20 minutes via a central line.

Intravenous infusion: A single dose over 15 minutes.

ACTIONS

A phenylalanine derivative of nitrogen mustard that is a bifunctional alkylating antineoplastic agent. Cytotoxicity is related to the extent of its interstrand cross-linking with DNA. Not dependent on cell cycle phase. Active against both resting and dividing tumor cells. Eliminated from plasma primarily by chemical hydrolysis rather than metabolism. 30% bound to plasma protein. Distribution to terminal half-life is 10 to 75 minutes. About 10% excreted as unchanged drug in urine.

INDICATIONS AND USES

Palliative treatment of patients with multiple myeloma when oral therapy is not appropriate.

Unlabeled uses: Treatment of multiple myeloma in combination with other cytotoxic agents. ■ Treatment of refractory multiple myeloma (high-dose melphalan [100 to 140 mg/M^2] in combination with prednisone [MP], vincristine, doxorubicin [Adriamycin], and dexamethasone [Decadron],

[VAD], and bone marrow support). ▪ Treatment of newly diagnosed aggressive multiple myeloma in combination with other cytotoxic agents and interferon. ▪ High doses (above 100 mg/M^2) with bone marrow reinfusion or colony-stimulating factor (e.g., filgrastim [GCSF]) to treat poor-prognosis Hodgkin's and non-Hodgkin's lymphoma, leukemia, multiple myeloma, and neuroblastoma. ▪ High-dose melphalan (180 to 220 mg/M^2) with bone marrow rescue to treat neuroblastoma, Ewing's sarcoma and soft tissue sarcoma, leukemia, and lymphoma in children over 1 year. May be combined with other cytotoxic agents, surgery, and/or total body irradiation. See Maternal/Child. ▪ Intraarterial injection (hyperthermic isolated limb perfusion) is used with surgery for extremity melanoma and as a palliative treatment with locally advanced, unresectable malignant melanoma of the extremity. ▪ Intraperitoneal route used to treat advanced ovarian cancers.

CONTRAINDICATIONS

Prior resistance to or hypersensitivity to melphalan.

PRECAUTIONS

Follow guidelines for handling cytotoxic agents. See Appendix A, p. 1142. ▪ Administered by or under the direction of the physician specialist, with facilities for monitoring the patient and responding to any medical emergency. ▪ Use extreme caution in patients whose bone marrow is compromised by or recovering from previous radiation or chemotherapy. ▪ Severe myelotoxicity (WBC below 1,000/mm^3 and platelets below 25,000/mm^3) is more common with IV dosing. ▪ Do not abandon treatment prematurely. Improvement may continue slowly over many months with repeated courses. ▪ Patients with an elevated BUN had a greater incidence of severe leukemia.

Monitor: Determine absolute patency of vein. A stinging or burning sensation indicates extravasation; cellulitis and tissue necrosis may result. Discontinue injection; use another vein. ▪ Monitor platelet count, hemoglobin, white blood cell count, and differential frequently. Indicated before each dose as well as between doses to determine optimal dose and avoid toxicity. Nadirs occur 2 to 3 weeks after treatment, recovery should occur in 4 to 5 weeks. ▪ Monitor kidney function before and during therapy. ▪ Severe myelosuppression can occur with effective doses. Withhold further doses until blood cell counts have recovered if thrombocytopenia and/or leukopenia occur. ▪ Hypersensitivity reactions may occur with initial treatment but frequently are delayed and occur after multiple courses. Observe closely; anaphylaxis and death have occurred. ▪ Observe closely for all signs of infection or bleeding. Prophylactic antibiotics may be indicated pending results of C/S in a febrile neutropenic patient. ▪ Prophylactic antiemetics may reduce nausea and vomiting and increase patient comfort. ▪ Some facilities are using ice pops to help prevent stomatitis. ▪ Monitor for thrombocytopenia (platelet count less than 50,000/mm^3). Initiate precautions to prevent excessive bleeding (e.g., inspect IV sites, skin, and mucous membranes; use extreme care during invasive procedures; test urine, emesis, stool, and secretions for occult blood). ▪ See Drug/Lab Interactions.

Patient Education: Avoid pregnancy; nonhormonal birth control recommended. ▪ Report IV site burning or stinging promptly. ▪ See Appendix D, p. 1148.

Maternal/Child: Category D: avoid pregnancy. Can cause chromosomal damage and severe birth defects in the fetus and impairment of fertility in men and women. ■ Discontinue breast-feeding. ■ Safety and effectiveness for use in children not established; see Unlabeled Uses.

Elderly: No differences in response from younger patients. Consider age-related organ impairment and history of previous disease or drug therapy.

DRUG/LAB INTERACTIONS

Coadministration with cyclosporine (Sandimmune) may result in acute renal failure. May occur after the first dose of each drug. Renal toxicity. ■ Renal dysfunction and increased toxicity may occur with concurrent cisplatin. ■ Lung toxicity associated with carmustine (BiCNU) may be increased with concurrent use. ■ Interferon alfa may decrease serum concentrations of melphalan. ■ Use with nalidixic acid (NegGram) may cause severe hemorrhagic necrotic enterocolitis in pediatric patients.

SIDE EFFECTS

Reversible bone marrow suppression is dose-limiting. Irreversible bone marrow failure has been reported. Alopecia, diarrhea, hemolytic anemia, hepatic toxicity (including veno-occlusive disease), hypersensitivity reactions (2% [e.g., anaphylaxis, bronchospasm, dyspnea, edema, hypotension, pruritus, urticaria, tachycardia]), interstitial pneumonitis, nausea and vomiting, oral ulceration, pulmonary fibrosis, secondary malignancies (long-term use), skin ulceration at injection site, vasculitis.

Overdose: Severe bone marrow depression, cholinomimetic effects (e.g., bradycardia, increased peristalsis and salivation, incontinence), convulsions, decreased consciousness, hyponatremia (inappropriate secretion of ADH), muscular paralysis, severe nausea and vomiting.

ANTIDOTE

Keep physician informed of all side effects. Close monitoring of bone marrow may prevent most serious and potentially fatal side effects. WBC and platelet count nadirs occur 2 to 3 weeks after treatment with recovery in 4 to 5 weeks. Withhold further doses until blood cell counts have recovered if leukopenia or thrombocytopenia occur. There is no specific antidote, but adequate supportive care including administration of whole blood products (e.g., packed RBCs, platelets, leukocytes) and/or blood modifiers (e.g., darbepoetin alfa [Aranesp], epoetin alfa [Epogen, Procrit], filgrastim [Neupogen], pegfilgrastim [Neulasta], sargramostim [Leukine], oprelvekin [Neumega]) may be indicated to treat bone marrow toxicity. Appropriate antibiotics may be indicated. Monitor closely until recovery (6 weeks or more). Discontinue the infusion and treat allergic reactions with antihistamines, corticosteroids, pressor agents, or volume expanders; do not readminister melphalan (IV or oral). Hemodialysis probably not effective in overdose. For extravasation, elevate the extremity and apply intermittent ice packs over the area immediately and 4 times daily for ½ hour. Continue for several days.

MEPERIDINE HYDROCHLORIDE

(meh-per'ih-deen hye-droe-klor'id)

Narcotic analgesic (agonist)
Anesthesia adjunct

Demerol, Demerol HCl, Meperidine HCl PF

pH 3.5 to 6

USUAL DOSE

IV injection: 10 to 50 mg. Repeat every 2 to 4 hours as necessary. When seeking the required dose to achieve pain relief for an individual patient, increases in increments of at least 25% of the previous ineffective dose are suggested. Lower slightly if pain controlled but patient is too drowsy, or lower dose and increase frequency.

Infusion: Must be administered through a controlled infusion device. May be patient activated. ***Based on a 10 mg/ml dilution,*** an initial loading dose of 10 to 25 mg (1 to 2.5 ml) is average. The continuous background infusion to provide a level of pain relief and maintain patency of the vein may range from 10 to 35 mg/hr (1 to 3.5 ml/hr). Additional doses of 5 to 10 mg (0.5 to 1 ml) may be activated by the patient at selected intervals every 3 to 60 minutes (averaging 10 to 15 minutes). Additional boluses (averaging 5 to 10 mg [0.5 to 1 ml]) may be given by health care professionals (e.g., every 30 min prn). In selected patients all of these doses may be somewhat higher.

Supplement anesthesia: 1 mg/ml dilution. Titrate under the direct observation and control of the anesthesiologist. Dose dependent on premedication, type of anesthesia, and type and duration of procedure.

Treatment or prevention of shaking chills (unlabeled): 0.5 mg/kg 20 minutes before shaking chills are expected to begin or 50 mg after onset of chills. Up to 150 mg has been required within 30 minutes if administered after onset.

PEDIATRIC DOSE

1 to 1.5 mg/kg/dose. May repeat every 3 to 4 hours. Maximum dose 100 mg; see Maternal/Child.

DOSE ADJUSTMENTS

Reduced dose may be required in the elderly or debilitated, in hepatic or renal disease, or in numerous other disease entities; see Precautions. ■ Doses appropriate for the general population may cause serious respiratory depression in vulnerable patients. ■ See Drug/Lab Interactions.

DILUTION

IV injection: May be given undiluted; however, further dilution with 5 ml of SW, NS, or other IV solutions to facilitate titration is appropriate; see chart on inside back cover.

Infusion: Available as 10, 25, 50, 75, or 100 mg/ml for infusion. Each 10 mg must be diluted in at least 1 ml of NS, D5W, D5NS, or other compatible infusion solution. Usually diluted in NS for use in narcotic syringe infusor systems.

COMPATIBLE WITH

(Underline Indicates Conflicting Compatibility Information)

Consult pharmacist; specific conditions may apply; see Compatibilities, p. xvi.

Additive: Cefazolin (Kefzol), dobutamine (Dobutrex), metoclopramide (Reglan), ondansetron (Zofran), scopolamine, <u>sodium bicarbonate</u>, succinylcholine, triflupromazine, verapamil (Isoptin).

Syringe: Atropine, butorphanol (Stadol), chlorpromazine (Thorazine), cimetidine (Tagamet), dimenhydrinate (Dinate), diphenhydramine (Benadryl), droperidol (Inapsine), fentanyl (Sublimaze), glycopyrrolate, ketamine (Ketalar), metoclopramide (Reglan), midazolam (Versed), ondansetron (Zofran), pentazocine (Talwin), perphenazine (Trilafon), prochlorperazine (Compazine), promethazine (Phenergan), ranitidine (Zantac), scopolamine.

Y-site: Acyclovir (Zovirax), amifostine (Ethyol), amikacin (Amikin), ampicillin, ampicillin/sulbactam (Unasyn), atenolol (Tenormin), aztreonam (Azactam), bumetanide (Bumex), cefamandole (Mandol), cefazolin (Kefzol), cefotaxime (Claforan), cefotetan (Cefotan), cefoxitin (Mefoxin), ceftazidime (Fortaz), ceftizoxime (Cefizox), ceftriaxone (Rocephin), cefuroxime (Zinacef), chloramphenicol (Chloromycetin), cisatracurium (Nimbex), cladribine (Leustatin), clindamycin (Cleocin), dexamethasone (Decadron), diltiazem (Cardizem), diphenhydramine (Benadryl), dobutamine (Dobutrex), docetaxel (Taxotere), dopamine (Intropin), doxycycline (Vibramycin), droperidol (Inapsine), erythromycin lactobionate (Erythrocin), etoposide phosphate (Etopophos), famotidine (Pepcid IV), filgrastim (Neupogen), fluconazole (Diflucan), fludarabine (Fludara), furosemide (Lasix), gatifloxacin (Tequin), gemcitabine (Gemzar), gentamicin (Garamycin), granisetron (Kytril), heparin, hetastarch in electrolytes (Hextend), hydrocortisone sodium succinate (Solu-Cortef), insulin (regular), kanamycin (Kantrex), labetalol (Normodyne), lidocaine, linezolid (Zyvox), magnesium sulfate, melphalan (Alkeran), methyldopate (Aldomet), methylprednisolone (Solu-Medrol), metoclopramide (Reglan), metoprolol (Lopressor), metronidazole (Flagyl IV), nafcillin (Nafcil), ondansetron (Zofran), oxacillin (Bactocill), oxytocin (Pitocin), paclitaxel (Taxol), penicillin G potassium, piperacillin (Pipracil), piperacillin/tazobactam (Zosyn), potassium chloride (KCl), propofol (Diprivan), propranolol (Inderal), ranitidine (Zantac), remifentanil (Ultiva), sargramostim (Leukine), sulfamethoxazole-trimethoprim (Bactrim), teniposide (Vumon), thiotepa (Thioplex), ticarcillin (Ticar), ticarcillin/clavulanate (Timentin), tobramycin (Nebcin), vancomycin (Vancocin), verapamil (Isoptin), vinorelbine (Navelbine).

RATE OF ADMINISTRATION

IV injection: A single dose over 4 to 5 minutes. Frequently titrated according to symptom relief and respiratory rate.

Infusion: Must be administered through a controlled infusion device. May be patient activated. Initial loading dose, basal rate (continuous rate of infusion), patient self-administered dose and interval, additional boluses permitted, and total dose for 1 hour should be ordered by physician. Do not exceed direct IV rate. For continuous infusion note range of mg/hr under Usual Dose; distribute evenly via infusion device.

ACTIONS

A synthetic narcotic analgesic and descending CNS depressant, similar to but slightly less potent than morphine. Onset of action occurs in about 5 minutes and lasts for about 2 to 4 hours. Crosses the placental barrier. Readily absorbed and distributed throughout the body. Metabolized to an active, toxic metabolite (normeperidine) in the liver, its extended half-life (15 to 30 hours) may lead to cumulative effects. Excreted in the urine. Secreted in breast milk.

INDICATIONS AND USES

Short-term relief of most moderate to severe pain. ■ Preoperative medication. ■ Support of anesthesia. ■ Obstetric analgesia.

Unlabeled uses: Treatment or prevention of shaking chills (rigors) caused by some medications (e.g., amphotericin B [Fungizone], aldesleukin [Proleukin]).

CONTRAINDICATIONS

Acute bronchial asthma, hypersensitivity to meperidine, patients who have received MAO inhibitors (e.g., selegiline [Eldepryl]) in the previous 2 to 3 weeks, diarrhea resulting from poisoning until toxic material eliminated, pregnancy before labor, premature infants or labor and delivery of premature infants, pulmonary edema caused by chemical respiratory irritant, upper airway obstruction.

PRECAUTIONS

Use with caution in glaucoma, head injuries, increased intracranial pressure (elevates spinal fluid pressure), asthma, chronic obstructive pulmonary disease, decreased respiratory reserve or respiratory depression, supraventricular tachycardia, convulsions, acute abdominal conditions before diagnosis, the elderly and debilitated, and hepatic or renal insufficiency. ■ Use with caution in patients with renal dysfunction; normeperidine may accumulate resulting in increased CNS toxicity. ■ Cough reflex is suppressed. ■ Morphine is usually preferred for pain during cardiac arrhythmias. ■ IM route frequently used. Frequent IM injections may lead to severe fibrosis of muscle tissue. ■ Do not use in patients in sickle cell crisis or for any long-term pain relief (e.g., cancer).

Monitor: Oxygen, controlled respiratory equipment, and naloxone (Narcan) or nalmefene (Revex) must always be available. ■ Observe patient frequently to continuously based on amount of dose and monitor vital signs. ■ Keep patient supine; orthostatic hypotension and fainting may occur; less likely with continuous low doses, but observe closely during ambulation. ■ Uncontrolled pain causes sleep deprivation, decreases pain threshold, and increases pain. When pain is finally controlled, expect the patient to sleep more until recovery from sleep deprivation. ■ With use the active metabolite normeperidine accumulates to toxic levels; will lower seizure threshold. Monitor for twitching, jerking, shaky hands, tremors; may lead to grand mal seizure. ■ Stool softeners and/or laxatives may be required to avoid constipation and fecal impaction. Maintain adequate hydration.

Patient Education: Avoid alcohol or other CNS depressants (e.g., barbiturates, benzodiazepines [e.g., diazepam (Valium)]). ■ May cause blurred vision, dizziness, or drowsiness; use caution in tasks that require alertness. ■ Request assistance with ambulation. ■ May be habit forming.

Maternal/Child: Category C: see Contraindications. ■ Use caution during breast-feeding. Levels are low, but best to wait 4 to 6 hours before breast-feeding. ■ Not recommended for IV use in children but is used. May be more sensitive to effects (e.g., respiratory depression) and may cause paradoxical excitation.

Elderly: See Dose Adjustments, Precautions. ■ May be more sensitive to effects (e.g., respiratory depression, constipation, urinary retention). ■ Analgesia should be effective with lower doses. ■ Consider age-related organ impairment.

DRUG/LAB INTERACTIONS

Potentiated by antacids, anticholinergics, cimetidine (Tagamet), tricyclic antidepressants (e.g., amitriptyline [Elavil]), isoniazid (Nydrazid), neostigmine (Prostigmin), neuromuscular blocking agents, (e.g., tubocurarine), oral contraceptives, phenothiazines (e.g., promazine [Sparine]), general anesthetics, other narcotic analgesics, and CNS depressants including alcohol. Side effects (e.g., CNS depression, constipation, hypotension) may be additive. Reduced dosage of both drugs may be indicated. ■ Do not use with MAO inhibitors (e.g., selegiline [Eldepryl]); may cause cardiovascular collapse. ■ Concurrent use with protease inhibitors (e.g., saquinavir [Invirase], ritonavir [Norvir]) not recommended. May increase risk of side effects, including seizures and cardiac arrhythmias. ■ Inhibited by hydantoins (e.g., phenytoin [Dilantin]). ■ Metabolism increased and analgesic effects may be decreased or delayed in smokers. ■ May aggravate adverse effects of isoniazid with concomitant use.

SIDE EFFECTS

Dizziness, flushing, lightheadedness, nausea, postural hypotension, rash, restlessness, sedation, sweating, syncope, vomiting. Side effects associated with histamine release, convulsions, and constipation may be more common with meperidine than with most other narcotic analgesics.

Major: Allergic reactions, apnea, cardiac arrest, cardiovascular collapse, cold and clammy skin, convulsions, dilated pupils, normeperidine toxicity (jerking, tremor, twitching, shaky hands, grand mal seizure), respiratory depression, shock, tremor.

ANTIDOTE

With increasing severity of minor side effects or onset of any major side effect, discontinue the drug and notify the physician. Naloxone hydrochloride (Narcan) or nalmefene (Revex) will reverse serious reactions. A patent airway, artificial respiration, oxygen therapy, and other symptomatic treatment must be instituted promptly. Resuscitate as necessary.

MEROPENEM

(mer-oh-pen′em)

Merrem I.V.

Antibacterial (carbapenem)

pH 7.3 to 8.3

USUAL DOSE

Intraabdominal infections in adults and children weighing 50 kg or more: 1 Gm every 8 hours.

Febrile neutropenia in adults and children weighing 50 kg or more (unlabeled): 1 Gm every 8 hours.

PEDIATRIC DOSE

Intraabdominal infections in children over 3 months of age and less than 50 kg: 20 mg/kg every 8 hours.

Febrile neutropenia in children 3 months of age and older and less than 50 kg (unlabeled): 20 mg/kg every 8 hours.

Meningitis in children over 3 months of age and less than 50 kg: 40 mg/kg every 8 hours.

Meningitis in children weighing 50 kg or more: 2 Gm every 8 hours.

DOSE ADJUSTMENTS

Reduce dose required if CrCl is less than or equal to 51 ml/min based on the chart below:

Meropenem Recommended IV Dosage Schedule for Adults With Impaired Renal Function		
Creatinine Clearance (ml/min)	**Dose (dependent on type of infection)**	**Dosing Interval**
26-50	Recommended dose (1,000 mg)	Every 12 hours
10-25	One half recommended dose	Every 12 hours
<10	One half recommended dose	Every 24 hours

Consult package insert or front matter of this text for formula to convert SrCr to CrCl. ▪ No dose adjustment necessary in impaired hepatic function or in the elderly with a CrCl equal to or greater than 51 ml/min.

DILUTION

Available as vials for injection, vials for infusion, and ADD-Vantage vials for infusion.

Vials for injection: Reconstitute each 500 mg with 10 ml SW (1 Gm with 20 ml). Yields 50 mg/ml. Shake to dissolve and let stand until clear. May be given as an IV injection or further diluted with 50 to 250 ml of compatible infusion solutions (e.g., NS, D5W, D10W, D5NS, D5/¼NS, Ringer's, LR; see package insert for complete listing).

Vials for infusion: Reconstitute with 50 to 100 ml of compatible infusion solutions above.

ADD-Vantage vials for infusion: Must be reconstituted only with 50, 100, or 250 ml of D5W, ½NS, or NS. Instructions for preparation and use on packaging. Do not use flexible containers in series connections.

Storage: Store unopened vials at CRT. Use of freshly prepared solutions preferred. Vials for injection stable at room temperature for 2 hours after reconstitution and for 12 hours refrigerated. Stability of all other dilutions dependent on diluent and room temperature or refrigeration. Range is from 1 hour to 24 hours; see package insert or consult pharmacist. Do not freeze.

INCOMPATIBLE WITH

Manufacturer states, "Meropenem should not be mixed or physically added to solutions containing other drugs; compatibility not established."

COMPATIBLE WITH **(Underline Indicates Conflicting Compatibility Information)**

Consult pharmacist; specific conditions may apply; see Compatibilities, p. xvi.

Additive: ***See Incompatible With.*** <u>Acyclovir (Zovirax)</u>, aminophylline, atropine, cimetidine (Tagamet), dexamethasone (Decadron), dobutamine (Dobutrex), dopamine (Intropin), <u>doxycycline (Vibramycin)</u>, enalaprilat (Vasotec IV), fluconazole (Diflucan), furosemide (Lasix), gentamicin (Garamycin), heparin, insulin (regular), magnesium sulfate, metoclopramide (Reglan), morphine, norepinephrine (Levophed), <u>ondansetron (Zofran)</u>, phenobarbital (Luminal), ranitidine (Zantac), vancomycin (Vancocin), <u>zidovudine (AZT, Retrovir)</u>.

Y-site: <u>Acyclovir (Zovirax)</u>, aminophylline, atenolol (Tenormin), atropine, <u>calcium gluconate</u>, cimetidine (Tagamet), dexamethasone (Decadron), digoxin (Lanoxin), diphenhydramine (Benadryl), docetaxel (Taxotere), doxycycline (Vibramycin), enalaprilat (Vasotec IV), fluconazole (Diflucan), furosemide (Lasix), gentamicin (Garamycin), heparin, insulin (regular), linezolid (Zyvox), metoclopramide (Reglan), morphine, norepinephrine (Levophed), ondansetron (Zofran), phenobarbital (Luminal), vancomycin (Vancocin), zidovudine (AZT, Retrovir).

RATE OF ADMINISTRATION

Same rate is used for adults and children over 3 months of age.

IV injection: A single dose (up to 20 ml after dilution) over 3 to 5 minutes.

Intermittent infusion: A single dose over 15 to 30 minutes.

ACTIONS

A synthetic, broad-spectrum, carbapenem antibiotic. Bactericidal to selected gram-negative, gram-positive, and anaerobic organisms. Bactericidal activity results from the inhibition of cell wall synthesis. Readily penetrates the cell wall of susceptible organisms to reach penicillin-binding protein targets. Has significant stability to hydrolysis by penicillinases and cephalosporins produced by gram-positive and gram-negative bacteria. Peak plasma concentrations reached by the end of an infusion. Penetrates well into most body fluids and tissues, including cerebrospinal fluid. Peak fluid and tissue concentrations reached in 0.5 to 1.5 hours. Minimal protein binding. Elimination half-life averages 1 hour in adults, 1.5 hours in children age 3 months to 2 years. 70% recovered as unchanged drug in urine within 12 hours. Not yet known if it crosses the placental barrier or is secreted in breast milk.

INDICATIONS AND USES

Treatment of intraabdominal infections (e.g., complicated appendicitis, peritonitis) in adults and children caused by specific susceptible organisms (e.g., viridans group streptococci). ■ Treatment of bacterial meningitis in children 3 months of age and older caused by specific susceptible organisms. ■ Treatment of acute pulmonary exacerbations in cystic fibrosis patients with chronic lower respiratory tract infections with susceptible organisms (orphan drug status).

Unlabeled uses: Treatment of febrile neutropenia.

CONTRAINDICATIONS

History of hypersensitivity to meropenem, its components, any other carbapenem antibiotic (e.g., imipenem-cilastatin [Primaxin]), or patients with hypersensitivity to beta-lactams.

PRECAUTIONS

Specific sensitivity studies are indicated to determine susceptibility of the causative organism to meropenem. ■ Use extreme caution in patients with a history of allergic reactions to other beta-lactams (e.g., penicillins, cephalosporins, imipenem) and other allergens. ■ May cause seizures in patients with a history of CNS disorders (e.g., brain lesions, history of seizures) or with bacterial meningitis and/or compromised renal function. Use extreme caution; continue administration of anticonvulsants in patients with known seizure disorders. ■ Use with caution in patients with moderately severe impaired renal function (CrCl 10 to 26 ml/min); thrombocytopenia may occur and incidence of heart failure, kidney failure, and shock may be increased; see Dose Adjustments. ■ Staphylococci resistant to methicillin/oxacillin must be considered resistant to meropenem. ■ May have cross-resistance with strains resistant to other carbapenems (e.g., imipenem-cilastatin [Primaxin]). ■ Has been found to eliminate concurrent bacteremia associated with bacterial meningitis. ■ Avoid prolonged use of drug; superinfection caused by overgrowth of nonsusceptible organisms may result. ■ Pseudomembranous colitis has been reported; consider in patients that present with diarrhea during or after treatment with meropenem.

Monitor: Anaphylaxis has been reported. Emergency equipment must always be available. ■ Monitor infusion site for inflammation and/or extravasation. May cause thrombophlebitis. ■ Monitor for S/S of CNS reactions (e.g., focal tremors, myoclonus, seizures). ■ Monitor renal, hepatic, and hemopoietic systems in prolonged therapy. ■ Each 1 Gm contains 3.92 mEq of sodium; monitoring of electrolytes may be indicated. ■ See Side Effects.

Patient Education: Report any diarrhea, itching, rash, shortness of breath, or twitching sensation immediately. ■ Report any burning, pain, or stinging at injection site.

Maternal/Child: Category B: safety for use in pregnancy not established; use only if clearly needed. ■ Use caution during breast-feeding. Not known if meropenem is secreted in breast milk; safety not established. ■ Approved only for use in infants and children over 3 months of age.

Elderly: No differences in safety and effectiveness have been observed between patients over 65 years and younger patients. ■ Dose adjustments not indicated unless the CrCl is equal to or less than 51 ml/min; see Dose Adjustments.

DRUG/LAB INTERACTIONS

Probenecid inhibits renal excretion and increases serum levels of meropenem extending its half-life and increasing systemic exposure; coadministration is not recommended. ■ May be synergistic with aminoglycosides against some isolates of *Pseudomonas aeruginosa*. ■ May reduce serum concentrations of valproic acid to subtherapeutic levels.

SIDE EFFECTS

Toxicity rate is usually low. ***Children:*** Diarrhea, diaper area moniliasis, glossitis, oral moniliasis, rash, vomiting. ***Adults:*** Constipation, diarrhea, headache, nausea and vomiting, rash. Injection site reactions (e.g., edema, inflammation, pain, phlebitis, pruritus) are most common. Many other side effects including increases or decreases in hematologic, hepatic, and renal lab tests may occur in less than 1% of patients. ***Adults and children:*** Full scope of allergic reactions, including anaphylaxis, have occurred in a few patients. Agranulocytosis, angioedema, bleeding events (e.g., GI bleeding, epistaxis), erythema multiform, leukopenia, neutropenia, Stevens-Johnson syndrome, pseudomembranous colitis, seizures, shock, sepsis, thrombocytopenia, and toxic epidermal necrolysis can occur.

ANTIDOTE

Notify physician of all side effects. Most treated symptomatically. Discontinue immediately if an allergic reaction occurs; treat as indicated (e.g., oxygen, epinephrine, corticosteroids, diphenhydramine, vasopressors). If focal tremors, myoclonus, or seizures occur, evaluate neurologically, initiate anticonvulsant therapy, and decide whether to decrease or discontinue meropenem. Mild cases of colitis may respond to discontinuation of meropenem. Oral vancomycin (Vancocin) or metronidazole (Flagyl) is the treatment of choice for antibiotic-related pseudomembranous colitis. Adequate hydration and supplementation of electrolytes and proteins usually indicated. Hemodialysis may be helpful in overdose.

MESNA
(mez′nah)

Antidote
Antineoplastic adjunct
Prophylactic for hemorrhagic cystitis

Mesnex, ✤Uromitexan

pH 6.5 to 8.5

USUAL DOSE
Total daily dose is 60% of the ifosfamide dose equally divided into 3 doses. A single dose of mesna equal to 20% of the ifosfamide dose is given at the time of the ifosfamide injection and repeated 4 hours and 8 hours later (e.g., ifosfamide 1.2 Gm/M^2 would require mesna 240 mg/M^2 with the ifosfamide, 240 mg/M^2 in 4 hours, and again at 8 hours). The initial mesna dose each day may be mixed with the ifosfamide. Appears to be compatible. Available combined in solution with ifosfamide and as a single agent in tablet form.

DOSE ADJUSTMENTS
Dose of mesna must be repeated each day ifosfamide is administered and adjusted with each increase or decrease of the ifosfamide dose.

DILUTION
Each 100 mg (1 ml) must be diluted in a minimum of 4 ml D5W, D5NS, D5/½NS, NS, or LR. Desired concentration is 20 mg/ml.

Storage: Refrigerate diluted solutions and use within 6 hours. Discard any unused drug from the ampule. Mesna oxidizes to disulfide dimesna when exposed to oxygen.

COMPATIBLE WITH
Consult pharmacist; specific conditions may apply; see Compatibilities, p. xvi.

Additive: Bleomycin (Blenoxane), cyclophosphamide (Cytoxan), dexamethasone (Decadron), etoposide (VePesid), ifosfamide (Ifex), lorazepam (Ativan), potassium chloride.

Syringe: Ifosfamide (Ifex).

Y-site: Allopurinol (Aloprim, Zyloprim), amifostine (Ethyol), aztreonam (Azactam), cefepime (Maxipime), cladribine (Leustatin), docetaxel (Taxotere), doxorubicin liposome (Doxil), etoposide phosphate (Etopophos), filgrastim (Neupogen), fludarabine (Fludara), gatifloxacin (Tequin), gemcitabine (Gemzar), granisetron (Kytril), linezolid (Zyvox), melphalan (Alkeran), methotrexate (Folex), ondansetron (Zofran), paclitaxel (Taxol), piperacillin/tazobactam (Zosyn), sargramostim (Leukine), sodium bicarbonate, teniposide (Vumon), thiotepa (Thioplex), vinorelbine (Navelbine).

RATE OF ADMINISTRATION
A single dose over a minimum of 1 minute given as a single agent. Administer at rate for ifosfamide if given together.

ACTIONS
A detoxifying agent. Reacts chemically in the kidney with urotoxic ifosfamide metabolites to detoxify them and inhibit hemorrhagic cystitis. Remains in the intravascular compartment and much of a single dose is excreted within 4 hours in urine.

INDICATIONS AND USES
A prophylactic agent used to reduce the incidence of hemorrhagic cystitis caused by ifosfamide.

Unlabeled uses: May reduce the incidence of hemorrhagic cystitis caused by cyclophosphamide.

CONTRAINDICATIONS

Hypersensitivity to mesna or other thiol compounds.

PRECAUTIONS

Repeated doses are required to maintain adequate levels of mesna in the kidneys and bladder to detoxify urotoxic ifosfamide metabolites. ■ Hemorrhagic cystitis caused by ifosfamide is dose dependent. Mesna is most effective when ifosfamide dose is less than 1.2 $Gm/M^2/24$ hr. Somewhat less effective when ifosfamide dose is 2 to 4 $Gm/M^2/24$ hr. If hematuria develops with appropriate doses of mesna, ifosfamide dose may need to be reduced or discontinued. ■ Does not inhibit any other side effects or toxicities caused by ifosfamide therapy. ■ Not effective in preventing hematuria caused by other conditions (e.g., thrombocytopenia).

Maternal/Child: Category B: use during pregnancy only if benefits clearly outweigh risks. ■ Discontinue breast-feeding.

DRUG/LAB INTERACTIONS

May cause a false-positive reaction for urinary ketones. If a red-violet color develops, glacial acetic acid returns the coloring to violet.

SIDE EFFECTS

Average dose: Bad taste in the mouth, diarrhea, nausea, soft stool, vomiting.

Overdose: Allergic reactions, diarrhea, fatigue, headache, hematuria, hypotension, limb pain, nausea.

ANTIDOTE

No specific antidote. Keep physician informed of all side effects. Notify promptly if signs of overdose occur. Resuscitate as necessary.

METHOCARBAMOL

(meth-oh-kar′ba-mole)

Skeletal muscle relaxant (central acting)

Robaxin

pH 4 to 5

USUAL DOSE

1 Gm (10 ml) every 8 hours for no more than 3 days. May be repeated after an additional 2 days (days 6, 7, and 8) if indicated. In tetanus treatment, dose may be as high as 3 Gm every 6 hours. Initiate with 1 to 2 Gm by IV injection. Give balance of dose by infusion.

PEDIATRIC DOSE

Not recommended for children under 12 years of age except in tetanus. **Tetanus:** 15 mg/kg of body weight initially. Repeat every 6 hours as indicated.

DILUTION

May be given undiluted, or a single dose may be given as an IV infusion diluted in no more than 250 ml NS or D5W.

Storage: Store below 40° C. Do not refrigerate after dilution.

COMPATIBILITY

Specific information not available. Consult pharmacist. See Precautions.

RATE OF ADMINISTRATION

300 mg (3 ml) or fraction thereof over 1 minute or longer. Adjust infusion rate for patient comfort.

ACTIONS

A skeletal muscle relaxant. Action may be due to general CNS depression. Diminishes skeletal muscle hyperactivity without altering normal muscle tone. Widely distributed throughout the body. Metabolized in the liver and excreted in the urine.

INDICATIONS AND USES

Relief of discomfort from acute, painful musculoskeletal conditions. Adjunctive to other measures (e.g., rest, physical therapy). ■ Treatment of neuromuscular manifestations of tetanus. Adjunctive to other measures (e.g., tetanus antitoxin, fluid and electrolyte replacement). While FDA approved, this use is generally replaced by diazepam (Valium) or, in very severe cases, neuromuscular blocking agents (e.g., pancuronium [Pavulon]).

CONTRAINDICATIONS

Hypersensitivity to methocarbamol, known or suspected renal pathology.

PRECAUTIONS

Blood aspirated into syringe will not mix with medication; an expected phenomenon. ■ Use caution in known or suspected epileptic patients. ■ Maintenance doses should be oral even if the pills are crushed and given through a nasogastric tube.

Monitor: Observe site of injection continuously. A hypertonic solution; extravasation may cause thrombophlebitis or sloughing. ■ Keep patient in recumbent position for at least 15 minutes to avoid postural hypotension. ■ Monitor renal function if duration of treatment is 3 or more days. ■ See Drug/Lab Interactions.

Patient Education: Avoid alcohol or other CNS depressants (e.g., barbiturates, benzodiazepines [e.g., diazepam (Valium)]). ■ May cause dizziness, drowsiness, and visual disturbances. Request assistance for ambulation. ■ Use caution in any task that requires alertness. ■ Report fever, itching, nasal congestion, or rash promptly. ■ Urine may discolor to very dark green.

Maternal/Child: Use caution in pregnancy and breast-feeding. Safety for use not established. American Academy of Pediatrics considers it compatible with breast-feeding.

Elderly: Males may have sensitivity to anticholinergic effects (e.g., dry mouth, urinary retention). ■ Consider age-related renal impairment; may preclude use.

DRUG/LAB INTERACTIONS

Potentiated by alcohol, CNS depressants, MAO inhibitors (e.g., selegiline [Eldepryl]), and phenothiazines (e.g., chlorpromazine [Thorazine]). ■ May interfere with some laboratory tests (5-HIAA, VMA).

SIDE EFFECTS

Infrequent but more often associated with too-rapid injection.

Blurred vision, conjunctivitis, diplopia, dizziness, drowsiness, fainting, fever, flushing, headache, hypotension, GI upset, lightheadedness, metallic taste, muscular incoordination, nasal congestion, nystagmus, pruritus, rash, urticaria, vertigo.

Major: Anaphylactic reaction, bradycardia, convulsions, pain at injection site, sloughing at injection site, syncope, thrombophlebitis.

ANTIDOTE

Notify the physician of minor side effects. If these side effects progress or major side effects occur, discontinue the drug, notify the physician, and treat symptomatically. Epinephrine, steroids, and antihistamines should be readily available. Resuscitate as necessary.

METHOTREXATE SODIUM

(meth-oh-trex′ate so′de-um)

Antineoplastic (antimetabolite)
Antipsoriatic
Antirheumatic

Methotrexate PF, MTX

pH 8.5

USUAL DOSE

Many dose limitations based on patient condition, renal and hepatic function, and concomitant drugs or therapies; see Precautions/Monitor. Part of numerous protocols. Doses vary from 20 to 50 mg/M^2 every 1 to 2 weeks for treatment of solid tumors to 200 to 500 mg/M^2 every 2 to 4 weeks for treatment of leukemias or lymphomas. Any dose over 80 mg/week should be accompanied by leucovorin calcium rescue. Other examples outside of these dose ranges include:

Acute lymphoblastic leukemia: 3.3 mg/M^2 with prednisone 40 to 60 mg/M^2. Give daily if tolerated, and continue for up to 8 weeks or until satisfactory response (usually 4 to 6 weeks). Usually given PO. Maintenance dose individualized; 30 mg/M^2 IM or PO or 2.5 mg/kg IV every 14 days has been used. Any dose over 80 mg/week should be accompanied by leucovorin calcium rescue.

Gastric cancers (unlabeled): One regimen administers methotrexate 1.5 Gm/M^2 on day 1 followed by 1.5 Gm/M^2 of fluorouracil on day 1 (administer 1 hour after methotrexate infusion is complete), leucovorin calcium 15 mg/M^2 PO every 6 hours for 48 hours starting 24 hours after methotrexate, and doxorubicin 30 mg/M^2 IV on day 15. Repeated every 4 weeks.

Mycosis fungoides: 5 to 50 mg once weekly in the early stages of disease. Adjust dose or discontinue as indicated by patient response and hematologic monitoring. 15 to 37.5 mg twice weekly may be used in patients who respond poorly to weekly therapy. Usually given PO or IM, but combination chemotherapy regimens, including higher doses of IV methotrexate with leucovorin calcium rescue, have been used in advanced stages of the disease.

Breast cancer: 40 mg/M^2 on days 1 and 8 of each cycle. Given in combination with cyclophosphamide 100 mg/M^2 on days 1 through 14 of each cycle and fluorouracil 600 mg/M^2 on days 1 and 8 of each cycle. In patients over 60 years of age, reduce the initial methotrexate dose to 30 mg/M^2 and the initial fluorouracil dose to 400 mg/M^2. Repeat monthly (allows a 2-week rest period between cycles) for 6 to 12 cycles. Any dose over 80 mg/week should be accompanied by leucovorin calcium rescue. Doxorubicin (Adriamycin, Doxil) has been added to this regimen.

Psoriasis and rheumatoid arthritis: 10 to 25 mg once a week. Some references suggest an initial test dose of 10 mg followed by gradually increased doses until adequate response. Do not exceed 50 mg. Other sources suggest 20 to 30 mg/week as a maximum dose. Use smallest effective dose. Usually given PO or IM. May be used in combination with infliximab; see infliximab monograph.

Osteosarcoma: One regimen recommends 12 Gm/M^2 as a single dose given as an infusion over 4 hours. Begin the fourth week after surgery and repeat weekly at weeks 5, 6, 7, 11, 12, 15, 16, 29, 30, 44, and 45. A peak serum concentration of 1,000 micromolars/L at the end of the infusion is desired. Dose may be increased to 15 Gm/M^2 if required. Must be accompanied by leucovorin calcium rescue; begin 24 hours after start of methotrexate infusion and give 15 mg every 6 hours for 10 doses. Additional doses may be required; see leucovorin calcium monograph. Usually given PO. Osteosarcoma also requires combination chemotherapy. Protocols vary but may include methotrexate in combination with doxorubicin; methotrexate in combination with cisplatin and doxorubicin; methotrexate in combination with bleomycin, cyclophosphamide, and dactinomycin. These massive doses are highly individualized, require exacting calculations, and constant patient monitoring; see Precautions/Monitor.

PEDIATRIC DOSE

Safety for use in pediatric patients is limited to chemotherapy and in polyarticular-course juvenile rheumatoid arthritis. May contain benzyl alcohol; not recommended for use in neonates.

DOSE ADJUSTMENTS

Reduce dose by 25% if bilirubin is between 3 and 5 or aspartate aminotransferase (AST) above 180; if bilirubin above 5, omit dose. ■ Often used with other antineoplastic drugs to achieve tumor remission. ■ Reduced dose may be required with impaired renal function, in the very young or very elderly, the debilitated, and in other diseases; see Precautions. ■ See Drug/Lab Interactions.

DILUTION

Specific techniques required; see Precautions. 25 mg/ml is the maximum concentration that can be given IV. Reconstitution of each 5 mg with 2 ml of preservative-free D5W or NS is preferred. Each milliliter equals 2.5 mg of methotrexate. Available in preservative-free solution. Do not use formulations or diluents with preservatives (e.g., bacteriostatic) for experimental high-dose therapy or intrathecal injection. 1-Gm vial available for high-dose use with appropriate dilution. Not usually added to IV solutions when given in smaller doses (less than 100 mg). Discard solution if a precipitate forms. May be given through Y-tube or three-way stopcock of a free-flowing IV.

A single dose may be further diluted with D5W or NS immediately before use as an infusion with higher (100 mg or more) methotrexate doses.

Storage: If prepared without a preservative, use immediately. May be stable up to 14 days with a preservative.

COMPATIBLE WITH **(Underline Indicates Conflicting Compatibility Information)**

Consult pharmacist; specific conditions may apply; see Compatibilities, p. xvi.

Additive: Cyclophosphamide (Cytoxan), cytarabine (ARA-C), fluorouracil (5-FU), ondansetron (Zofran), sodium bicarbonate, vincristine (Oncovin). Other sources add dacarbazine (DTIC), furosemide (Lasix), hydrocortisone (Hydrocortone, Solu-Cortef), leucovorin calcium.

Syringe: Bleomycin (Blenoxane), cisplatin (Platinol), cyclophosphamide (Cytoxan), doxapram (Dopram), doxorubicin (Adriamycin), fluorouracil (5-FU), furosemide (Lasix), heparin, leucovorin calcium, <u>metoclopramide (Reglan)</u>, mitomycin (Mutamycin), vinblastine (Velban), vincristine (Oncovin).

Y-site: Allopurinol (Aloprim, Zyloprim), amifostine (Ethyol), amphotericin B cholesteryl (Amphotec), asparaginase (Elspar), aztreonam (Azactam), bleomycin (Blenoxane), cefepime (Maxipime), ceftriaxone (Rocephin), cimetidine (Tagamet), cisplatin (Platinol), cyclophosphamide (Cytoxan), cytarabine (ARA-C), daunorubicin (Cerubidine), dexamethasone (Decadron), diphenhydramine (Benadryl), doxorubicin (Adriamycin), doxorubicin liposome (Doxil), droperidol (Inapsine), etoposide (Etopophos, VePesid), famotidine (Pepcid IV), filgrastim (Neupogen), fludarabine (Fludara), fluorouracil (5-FU), furosemide (Lasix), ganciclovir (Cytovene), gatifloxacin (Tequin), granisetron (Kytril), heparin, hydromorphone (Dilaudid), imipenem-cilastatin (Primaxin), leucovorin calcium, linezolid (Zyvox), lorazepam (Ativan), melphalan (Alkeran), mesna (Mesnex), methylprednisolone (Solu-Medrol), metoclopramide (Reglan), mitomycin (Mutamycin), morphine, ondansetron (Zofran), oxacillin (Bactocill), paclitaxel (Taxol), piperacillin/tazobactam (Zosyn), prochlorperazine (Compazine), ranitidine (Zantac), sargramostim (Leukine), teniposide (Vumon), thiotepa (Thioplex), vancomycin (Vancocin), vinblastine (Velban), vincristine (Oncovin), vindesine (Eldisine), vinorelbine (Navelbine).

RATE OF ADMINISTRATION

IV injection: Each 10 mg or fraction thereof over 1 minute.

Infusion: A single dose equally distributed over 30 minutes to 4 hours or as prescribed by protocol.

ACTIONS

An antimetabolite and folic acid antagonist. Cell cycle–specific for the S phase, it interrupts the mitotic process during nucleic acid synthesis. Rapidly proliferating malignant cells are inhibited by a cytostatic effect. Widely distributed, average doses of methotrexate are excreted unchanged in the urine within 24 hours. Clearance rates decrease with higher doses. Does not cross blood-brain barrier. Secreted in breast milk.

INDICATIONS AND USES

Used for life-threatening neoplastic disease alone or in combination with other anti-cancer agents in the treatment of acute lymphocytic leukemia, breast cancer, epidermal tumors of the head and neck, small-cell and non–small-cell lung cancer, non-Hodgkin's lymphoma, advanced mycosis fungoides (cutaneous T-cell lymphoma). ■ Severe disabling psoriasis or rheumatoid arthritis unresponsive to other treatment. ■ High-dose regimen for treatment of osteosarcoma. ■ Given PO or IM for early-stage mycosis fungoides, trophoblastic disease, polyarticular-course juvenile rheumatoid arthritis, and other diagnoses and intrathecally for meningeal leukemia.

Unlabeled uses: Treatment of cancers of the cervix, ovaries, bladder, colon, rectum, esophagus, stomach, pancreas, and penis. Treatment of acute nonlymphocytic leukemia, Hodgkin's lymphomas, soft tissue sarcomas, and CNS lymphomas.

CONTRAINDICATIONS

Hypersensitivity to methotrexate; breast-feeding mothers. Not absolute, but methotrexate is not recommended during pregnancy or with hepatic, renal, or bone marrow damage.

PRECAUTIONS

Follow guidelines for handling cytotoxic agents. See Appendix A, p. 1142. ■ Administered by or under the direction of the physician specialist. ■ Evacuate excess fluid from ascites and pleural effusions before treatment. ■ Serious and sometimes fatal bone marrow suppression, aplastic anemia, and GI toxicity have been reported with concomitant use of methotrexate (usually high doses) and some NSAIDs; see Drug/Lab Interactions. ■

Methotrexate-induced lung disease or severe skin reactions can occur at any time and have been fatal. ■ Elevated liver enzymes may occur early during treatment, but hepatotoxicity (may be fatal) occurs more frequently with prolonged use. ■ Use with extreme caution in patients with ascites, bone marrow depression, folate deficiency, GI obstruction, infection, impaired renal or liver function, peptic ulcer, pleural effusion, or ulcerative colitis; in debilitated patients; and in the very young or very elderly. ■ Pseudomembranous colitis has been reported. May range from mild to life-threatening. Consider in patients that present with diarrhea during or after treatment with methotrexate. ■ Risk of soft tissue necrosis and osteonecrosis may be increased with concomitant use of methotrexate and radiotherapy. ■ Painful plaque erosions have been reported (rare) with use of methotrexate for treatment of psoriasis. ■ Nonreversible oliguric renal failure is likely to develop in patients who experience delayed early methotrexate elimination.

Monitor: Close patient observation is mandatory. Course of therapy is not repeated until all signs of toxicity from the previous course subside. ■ CBC with platelets, chest x-ray, and renal and liver function tests before, during, and after therapy are essential to comprehensive treatment. ■ Monitor closely for bone marrow, liver, lung, kidney, and skin toxicities. ■ Nadir of leukocyte and platelet count usually occurs after 7 to 10 days, with recovery 7 days later. Liver biopsy, pulmonary studies, and bone marrow studies may be indicated in high-dose or long-term therapy. ■ Monitor renal function closely; verify by CrCl levels; see Precautions. Maintain continuing adequate hydration and urine alkalinization. ■ May induce hyperuricemia, increased doses of antigout agents (e.g., allopurinol [Zyloprim], probenecid [Benemid]) may be necessary. Allopurinol preferred to reduce risk of uric acid nephropathy associated with uricosuric antigout agents. ■ Monitor serum methotrexate levels. ■ Use prophylactic antiemetics to reduce nausea and vomiting and increase patient comfort. ■ Observe closely for signs of infection. Prophylactic antibiotics may be indicated pending results of C/S in a febrile neutropenic patient. ■ Monitor for thrombocytopenia (platelet count less than 50,000/mm^3). Initiate precautions to prevent excessive bleeding (e.g., inspect IV sites, skin, and mucous membranes; use extreme care during invasive procedures; test urine, emesis, stool, and secretions for occult blood). ■ ***Administration of high-dose methotrexate*** requires a WBC count greater than 1,500 mm^3; neutrophil count greater than 200/mm^3; platelet count greater than 75,000 mm^3; serum bilirubin less than 1.2 mg/dl; alanine aminotransferase (ALT) level less than 450 units; any mucositis must be healing; ascites or pleural effusion must be drained dry; SrCr must be normal; CrCl greater than 60 ml/min; 1 L/M^2 of IV fluid over 6 hours before dosing and 3 L/M^2/day on day of infusion and for 2 days after; alkalinization of urine with sodium bicarbonate; and repeat serum methotrexate and SrCr levels at least daily until methotrexate level is below 0.05 micromolar. ■ See Drug/Lab Interactions.

Patient Education: Nonhormonal birth control recommended. Continue for at least 3 months after treatment completed. ■ Avoid alcohol and take only prescribed medications. Reactions can be lethal. ■ See Appendix D, p. 1148.

Maternal/Child: Category X: avoid pregnancy. Has caused fetal death and congenital anomalies. ■ Discontinue breast-feeding. ■ See Pediatric Dose.

Elderly: See Dose Adjustments. Diminished hepatic and renal function and increased folate stores may indicate much lower doses. Monitor for early signs of toxicity.

DRUG/LAB INTERACTIONS

The following drugs may enhance methotrexate toxicity when administered concomitantly: alcohol, amiodarone (Cordarone), antibacterials (e.g., tetracycline, chloramphenicol), cyclosporine (Sandimmune), any hepatotoxic drug (e.g., azathioprine [Imuran], retinoids [Vitamin A, sulfasalazine]), etretinate (Tegison), acetylated salicylates (e.g., aspirin), NSAIDs (e.g., ibuprofen [Advil, Motrin], ketoprofen, naproxen [Aleve, Naprosyn]), penicillins (e.g., amoxicillin, mezlocillin), probenecid, salicylates, sulfonamides, para-aminobenzoic acid (PABA), phenylbutazone, phenytoin (Dilantin), pyrimethamine, trimethoprim (component of sulfamethoxazole-trimethoprim [Bactrim, Septra]), and vancomycin (Vancocin [given up to 10 days prior to methotrexate]); interactions may be life threatening. Monitoring serum levels and/or reduced doses of methotrexate may be indicated or a longer duration of leucovorin calcium rescue may be required. One source suggests delaying administration of aspirin, NSAIDs, and probenecid for 48 hours after larger doses of methotrexate; see Precautions. ■ Omeprazole (Prilosec) increases serum levels of methotrexate. Discontinue several days before methotrexate administration. Consider an H_2 antagonist (e.g., ranitidine [Zantac]). ■ Asparaginase antagonizes methotrexate; separate administration by 24 hours. ■ Doxycycline may increase toxicity of methotrexate in high-dose regimens. ■ Vitamins with folic acid may inhibit the antifolate effects of methotrexate. ■ Methotrexate interacts with many drugs such as anticoagulants, antidiabetics, charcoal, corticosteroids, other antineoplastics (e.g., procarbazine), and others to produce potentially serious reactions. ■ Do not administer live vaccines to patients receiving antineoplastic drugs. ■ May decrease phenytoin (Dilantin) serum levels. ■ Procarbazine (Matulane) may increase nephrotoxicity of methotrexate. Allow 72 hours between last dose of procarbazine and first dose of methotrexate. ■ Monitor for signs of increased bone marrow suppression with sulfonamides (e.g., sulfisoxazole [Gantrisin], SMZ-TMP [Bactrim]), bone marrow–depressing agents (e.g., antineoplastics) and radiation therapy. May also cause SMZ-TMP (Bactrim)-induced megaloblastic anemia. ■ Urinary alkalinizers increase renal excretion and may reduce effectiveness.

SIDE EFFECTS

Toxicity usually dose related. Death can occur from average doses, high doses, drug interactions (e.g., NSAIDs), bone marrow toxicity, GI toxicity, hepatic toxicity, pulmonary toxicity, and/or severe skin reactions. Acne, alopecia (occasional), chills, cystitis, dehydration, depigmentation, diabetes, diarrhea, edema, enteritis, fever, GI ulceration, gingivitis, hematologic depression, hemorrhage from any site, hepatotoxicity, leukoencephalopathy, menstrual dysfunction, nausea, oliguric renal failure, oral ulceration, osteonecrosis, painful plaque erosions (psoriasis [rare]), pharyngitis, pruritus, pseudomembranous colitis, pulmonary disease (dry, nonproductive cough), rash, septicemia, soft-tissue necrosis, stomatitis, transient blindness, urticaria, vomiting.

ANTIDOTE

Discontinue methotrexate and notify the physician of any side effects. **Leucovorin calcium (citrovorum factor, folinic acid)** may be given PO, IM, or

IV promptly to counteract inadvertent overdose. Leucovorin calcium is also indicated as a planned rescue mechanism for large doses of methotrexate required to treat some malignancies. Doses equal to dose of methotrexate are frequently required. Should be given within 1 hour in overdose, 24 hours in rescue. See specific process for overdose and for rescue for high-dose MTX; in leucovorin calcium monograph. Doses up to 150 mg or 100 mg/M^2 every 3 hours may be required if SrCr is 50% or greater than baseline measurement before methotrexate administration. Serum methotrexate must come down to below 0.05 micromolar. Continuing hydration and urinary alkalinization are mandatory to prevent precipitation in renal tubules. Monitor fluid and electrolyte status until serum methotrexate has fallen to less than 0.05 micromolar and renal failure has resolved. Administration of whole blood products (e.g., packed RBCs, platelets, leukocytes) and/or blood modifiers (e.g., darbepoetin alfa [Aranesp], epoetin alfa [Epogen, Procrit], filgrastim [Neupogen], pegfilgrastim [Neulasta], sargramostim [Leukine], oprelvekin [Neumega]) may be indicated to treat bone marrow toxicity. Death may occur from the progression of most of these side effects. Symptomatic and supportive therapy is indicated. Charcoal hemoperfusion may be helpful, and/or acute intermittent hemodialysis with a high-flux dialyzer may be used to counteract toxicity or inadvertent overdose.

METHYLDOPATE HYDROCHLORIDE

Antihypertensive

(meth-ill-doe′pat hye-droe-klor′id)

Aldomet

pH 3 to 4.2

USUAL DOSE

250 to 500 mg every 6 hours. Up to 1 Gm every 6 hours is acceptable. Maximum dose is 4 Gm/24 hr. Maintain with oral medication in same dosage as soon as practical.

PEDIATRIC DOSE

2 to 4 mg/kg/dose up to 5 to 10 mg/kg of body weight/dose every 6 hours. Maximum dose is 65 mg/kg or 3 Gm/24 hr, whichever is less.

DOSE ADJUSTMENTS

Limit the initial dose of methyldopate to 500 mg/day in divided doses if given with antihypertensives other than thiazides; if added to a thiazide regimen, no dose adjustment of the thiazide is necessary. ▪ Reduced dose may be required in the elderly and with impaired liver and renal function. ▪ See Drug/Lab Interactions.

DILUTION

Single dose may be diluted in 100 ml of D5W or in sufficient D5W to achieve a final concentration of 10 mg/ml and given as an infusion. Also available in ADD-Vantage vials for use with ADD-Vantage infusion containers.

Storage: Store below 40° C.

COMPATIBLE WITH

Consult pharmacist; specific conditions may apply; see Compatibilities, p. xvi.

Additive: Aminophylline, ascorbic acid (Cenolate), chloramphenicol (Chloromycetin), diphenhydramine (Benadryl), heparin, magnesium sulfate, multivitamins (M.V.I.), potassium chloride (KCl), sodium bicarbonate, succinylcholine, verapamil (Isoptin).

Y-site: Esmolol (Brevibloc), heparin, meperidine (Demerol), morphine, theophylline.

RATE OF ADMINISTRATION

Each dose as an infusion is given over 30 to 60 minutes.

ACTIONS

A moderate antihypertensive drug. Exact mechanism of action is unknown, but is thought to be due to its metabolism to alpha-methylnorepinephrine, which lowers arterial BP through several processes. Reduces both supine and standing BP without affecting cardiac output, glomerular filtration rate, or renal blood flow. Onset of action is 4 to 6 hours and lasts 10 to 16 hours. Extensively metabolized and excreted in urine. Crosses placental barrier and is secreted in breast milk.

INDICATIONS AND USES

Hypertension when parenteral therapy is indicated. ■ Hypertensive crises, especially for patients with renal or coronary insufficiency. Because of delayed onset of action, other agents may be preferred.

CONTRAINDICATIONS

Hypersensitivity to any component, including sulfites; active liver disease (e.g., acute hepatitis or active cirrhosis); coadministration with MAO inhibitors (e.g., selegiline [Eldepryl]); history of previous methyldopa therapy being associated with liver disorders. One source lists pheochromocytoma.

PRECAUTIONS

More effective combined with diuretics. ■ Use caution in impaired liver and renal function.

Monitor: Check BP every 30 minutes until stabilized at desired level. Slow response lessens usefulness. ■ Liver function tests, CBC, and direct Coombs' test indicated. ■ Observe for adequate urine output. ■ See Drug/Lab Interactions.

Maternal/Child: Category B: use in pregnancy and breast-feeding with caution and only if clearly needed.

Elderly: Hypotensive and sedative effects and risk of syncope may be increased. ■ Consider age-related organ impairment.

DRUG/LAB INTERACTIONS

Antihypertensive effects may be reduced by barbiturates, and reduced or reversed by tricyclic antidepressants (e.g., amitriptyline [Elavil]). ■ Serious elevations in BP may occur with phenothiazines (e.g., promethazine [Phenergan]). ■ Potentiates oral antidiabetics (e.g., tolbutamide [Orinase]), levodopa, levarterenol (Levophed), and all antihypertensive drugs (e.g., hydralazine). ■ May produce adverse mental symptoms with haloperidol. ■ Capable of paradoxical reactions with cocaine, norepinephrine (Levophed), and phenylephrine (Neo-Synephrine). Severe hypertension can occur. ■ Concurrent use with MAO inhibitors (e.g., selegiline [Eldepryl]) is contraindicated, may produce hyperexcitability and hypertension. ■ Lithium toxicity has developed with concurrent use. ■ Causes false elevated urinary catecholamine response. ■ May potentiate anesthetics; reduced doses of anesthetics may be required. ■ Use with nonselective beta-blockers (e.g., propranolol [Inderal]) may cause paradoxical hypertension.

SIDE EFFECTS

Anaphylaxis, apprehension, depression, dizziness, dry mouth, edema, elevated alkaline phosphatase, elevated AST (SGOT), fever, hemolytic anemia, nasal congestion, nightmares, paradoxical hypertension, positive Coombs' test, postural hypotension (mild), sedation.

ANTIDOTE

Notify the physician of all side effects. Most can be decreased in severity by reducing dosage. Drug may be discontinued. Dopamine (Intropin) or levarterenol (Levophed) should reverse hypotension of overdose. Hemodialysis may be used in acute overdose.

METHYLERGONOVINE MALEATE

(meth-ill-er-gon′oh-veen ma′le-at)

Uterine stimulant (oxytocic)

Methergine

pH 2.7 to 3.5

USUAL DOSE

1 ml (0.2 mg); may be repeated every 2 to 4 hours as necessary. A maximum of 5 doses is usually not exceeded.

DILUTION

Check expiration date on vial; methylergonovine deteriorates with age. May be given undiluted. Some clinicians recommend dilution with 5 ml of NS. Do not add to IV solutions. May be given through Y-tube or three-way stopcock of infusion set.

Storage: Store at 15° to 30° C.

COMPATIBLE WITH

Consult pharmacist; specific conditions may apply; see Compatibilities, p. xvi.

Y-site: Heparin, hydrocortisone sodium succinate (Solu-Cortef), potassium chloride (KCl).

RATE OF ADMINISTRATION

0.2 mg or fraction thereof over 1 minute. Too-rapid injection may cause severe nausea and vomiting. See Precautions.

ACTIONS

A synthetic oxytocic. It exerts a direct stimulation on the smooth muscle of the uterus. Produces vasoconstriction, increases CVP, elevates BP, and may rarely produce peripheral ischemia. In therapeutic doses the prolonged initial contraction of the uterus is followed by periods of relaxation and contraction. Preferred because it is less likely to cause hypertension. Effective within 1 minute for up to 3 hours. It is probably metabolized in the liver and excreted in feces. Secreted in breast milk.

INDICATIONS AND USES

Routine management after delivery of the placenta. ■ Postpartum atony. ■ Hemorrhage. ■ Subinvolution.

CONTRAINDICATIONS

Hypersensitivity, hypertension, pregnancy before third stage of labor (delivery of the placenta), toxemia. Contraindicated with ritonavir.

PRECAUTIONS

Not recommended for use before the delivery of the placenta. Occasionally given after the anterior shoulder is delivered if the obstetrician directs and is present. ■ IV administration is for emergency use only. IM or oral routes are preferred and should be used after the initial IV dose. ■ IV use may induce hypotension and/or CVA. Give slowly and monitor BP. ■ Use caution in presence of sepsis, obliterative vascular disease, and cardiac, hepatic, or renal disease.

Monitor: Monitor BP. ■ Uterine response may be poor in calcium-deficient patients; calcium replacement may be required for effective response. Avoid or use extreme caution if calcium replacement is needed in patients taking digoxin. ■ See Drug/Lab Interactions.

Maternal/Child: Category C: see Contraindications and Precautions. Administration before delivery of the placenta may cause hypoxia and intracranial hemorrhage in the infant, captivation of the placenta, or missed diagnosis of a second infant. ■ May be given orally during breast-feeding for up to 1 week after delivery.

DRUG/LAB INTERACTIONS

Severe hypertension and cerebrovascular accidents can result with ephedrine, methoxamine (Vasoxyl), and other vasopressors. Chlorpromazine (Thorazine) or hydralazine IV will reduce this hypertension. ■ ***Contraindicated with ritonavir (Norvir);*** may cause acute ergot toxicity.

SIDE EFFECTS

Rare in therapeutic doses but may include the following:

Allergic phenomena, chest pain (temporary), diaphoresis, dilated pupils, dizziness, dyspnea, headache, hypertension (transient), hypotension, nausea, tinnitus, vomiting, weakness.

Overdose: Abortion, blindness, cerebrovascular accident, convulsions, excitement, gangrene, hypercoagulability, palpitations, severe nausea and vomiting, shock, tachycardia, thirst, tremor, uterine bleeding.

ANTIDOTE

Discontinue the drug immediately at the onset of any side effect and notify the physician. Most side effects are transient unless there is severe toxicity and will be treated symptomatically. Use antiemetics (e.g., prochlorperazine [Compazine], ondansetron [Zofran] for nausea and vomiting. Treat cardiac ischemia with nitroglycerin, seizures with diazepam (Valium) or phenytoin (Dilantin). Treat peripheral ischemia with nitroprusside sodium, tolazoline (Priscoline), or phentolamine (Regitine). Treat hypertension with nitroprusside sodium, chlorpromazine (Thorazine), or hydralazine. Severe poisoning is treated with vasodilator drugs, sedatives, calcium gluconate to relieve muscular pain, and other supportive treatment. Heparin is used to control hypercoagulability.

METHYLPREDNISOLONE SODIUM SUCCINATE

(meth-il-pred-niss'oh-lone so'de-um suk'suh-nat)

Hormone (adrenocorticoid/glucocorticoid) Antiinflammatory

Solu-Medrol **pH 7 to 8**

USUAL DOSE

Average dose range is 10 to 250 mg initially. May be repeated every 4 to 6 hours as necessary. IV methylprednisolone is usually given in an emergency situation or when oral dosing is not feasible. Larger doses may be justified by patient condition. Repeat until adequate response, then decrease dose as indicated. Total dose usually does not exceed 1.5 Gm/24 hr. Dose is individualized according to the severity of the disease and the response of the patient and is not necessarily reduced for children. High-dose treatment is utilized until patient condition stabilizes, usually no longer than 48 to 72 hours.

Antiinflammatory: 10 to 40 mg. May be repeated every 4 to 6 hours as necessary.

Life-threatening shock or septic shock (unlabeled and controversial): High-dose "pulse" therapy: Several regimens have been suggested:

30 mg/kg initially. Repeat every 4 to 6 hours *or*
100 to 250 mg initially. Repeat every 2 to 6 hours *or*
30 mg/kg as a loading dose, followed by a continuous infusion of 30 mg/kg every 12 hours for 24 to 48 hours.

Acute spinal cord injury high-dose therapy (unlabeled): Spinal cord injury must be less than 8 hours old and above L-2. The earlier methylprednisolone therapy begins, the better the results. ***Loading dose:*** 30 mg/kg of a specifically diluted solution (see Dilution) evenly distributed over 15 minutes. Maintain IV line with standard IV fluids for 45 minutes, then begin a ***maintenance dose*** of 5.4 mg/kg/hr for 23 hours. Discontinue 24 hours after loading dose initiated.

Status asthmaticus: 10 to 250 mg/dose every 4 to 6 hours.

Acute exacerbation of multiple sclerosis: 160 mg as a single dose each day for 7 days. Follow with 64 mg every other day for 1 month.

Pneumocystis carinii **pneumonia (unlabeled):** Initiate within 24 to 72 hours of initial antibiotic PCP therapy. 30 mg twice daily for 5 days. Follow with 30 mg once daily for 5 days (days 6-10). Then reduce to 15 mg once daily for 11 days (days 11-21) or until antibiotic regimen is complete.

Severe lupus nephritis (unlabeled): 1 Gm as an infusion over 1 hour for 3 days. Follow with long-term prednisolone oral therapy.

PEDIATRIC DOSE

Antiinflammatory/immunosuppressive: 0.16 to 0.8 mg/kg/24 hr in equally divided doses every 6 to 12 hours (0.08 to 0.4 mg/kg every 12 hours or 0.04 to 0.2 mg/kg every 6 hours). One source suggests that 0.5 mg/kg/day is the minimum dose.

Status asthmaticus: 1 to 2 mg/kg as a ***loading*** dose. ***Maintain*** with 0.5 to 1 mg/kg every 6 hours.

Severe lupus nephritis (unlabeled): 30 mg/kg every other day for 6 doses. Follow with long-term prednisolone oral therapy.

Continued

DOSE ADJUSTMENTS

Reduced dose may be required in the elderly, in patients with renal transplants, and with cyclophosphamide. See Precautions and Drug/Lab Interactions.

DILUTION

Available in Act-O-Vials containing 40 mg, 125 mg, 500 mg, 1,000 mg, and 2,000 mg. Each vial has an appropriate amount of diluent. Reconstitute by removing the protective cap, turning the rubber stopper a quarter turn, and pressing down, allowing the diluent into the lower chamber. Agitate gently. Using sterile technique, insert a needle through the center of the rubber stopper to withdraw diluted solution. To be diluted only with diluent supplied in Act-O-Vial. May be given direct IV, as an infusion, or further diluted in desired amounts of D5W, D5NS, D5/½NS, or NS. Best if minimally diluted to 0.25 mg/ml. With larger doses, this dilution could require large amounts of solution (up to 6 L/24 hr for 1.5 Gm); consult pharmacist. Discard unused solutions after 48 hours.

Acute spinal cord injury loading and maintenance doses: Each 1-Gm vial must be diluted to 16 ml with bacteriostatic water to maintain potency and avoid precipitation (62.5 mg/ml). Further dilute in D5W, D5NS, or NS with an amount to facilitate dose of 5.4 mg/kg/hr. (Example for a patient weighing 50 kg: [50 kg × 5.4 mg/hr = 270 mg/hr. 270 mg/hr × 23 hours = 6,210 mg total dose.] With a total dose of 6,210 mg at 62.5 mg/ml, you will have 99.36 [100] ml of reconstituted methylprednisolone. Add an additional 100 ml diluent to achieve 31.25 mg/ml. 270 mg/hr is the desired dose for this patient. 270 mg/hr divided by 31.25 mg/ml [strength of solution] equals 8.6. Administer at 8.6 ml/hr to achieve desired dose over 23 hours.)

COMPATIBLE WITH **(Underline Indicates Conflicting Compatibility Information)**

Consult pharmacist; specific conditions may apply; see Compatibilities, p. xvi.

Additive: Aminophylline, chloramphenicol (Chloromycetin), cimetidine (Tagamet), clindamycin (Cleocin), cytarabine (ARA-C), dopamine (Intropin), granisetron (Kytril), heparin, norepinephrine (Levophed), penicillin G potassium, ranitidine (Zantac), theophylline, verapamil (Isoptin).

Syringe: Granisetron (Kytril), metoclopramide (Reglan), selected contrast agents used in radiology.

Y-site: Acyclovir (Zovirax), amifostine (Ethyol), amphotericin B cholesteryl (Amphotec), aztreonam (Azactam), cefepime (Maxipime), cisatracurium (Nimbex), cisplatin (Platinol), cladribine (Leustatin), cyclophosphamide (Cytoxan), cytarabine (ARA-C), diltiazem (Cardizem), dopamine (Intropin), doxorubicin (Adriamycin), doxorubicin liposome (Doxil), enalaprilat (Vasotec IV), famotidine (Pepcid IV), fludarabine (Fludara), gatifloxacin (Tequin), granisetron (Kytril), heparin, hetastarch in electrolytes (Hextend), inamrinone (Inocor), linezolid (Zyvox), melphalan (Alkeran), meperidine (Demerol), methotrexate (Folex), metronidazole (Flagyl IV), midazolam (Versed), morphine, piperacillin/tazobactam (Zosyn), potassium chloride (KCl), remifentanil (Ultiva), sodium bicarbonate, tacrolimus (Prograf), teniposide (Vumon), theophylline, thiotepa (Thioplex), topotecan (Hycamtin).

RATE OF ADMINISTRATION

IV injection: Each 500 mg or fraction thereof over 2 to 3 minutes or longer. Direct IV administration is usually route of choice and eliminates possibility of overloading the patient with IV fluids. May be given as an ***infusion*** in its own diluent over 10 to 20 minutes. At the discretion of the physician, a continuous infusion may be given, properly diluted, over a specified time.

Shock: 30 mg over 15 to 30 min.

Acute spinal cord injury: See Usual Dose and Dilution.

ACTIONS

An adrenocortical steroid with potent metabolic, antiinflammatory actions and innumerable other effects. Has a greater antiinflammatory potency than prednisolone and less tendency to cause excessive potassium and calcium excretion and sodium and water retention. Has four times the potency of hydrocortisone sodium succinate. Has minimal mineralocorticoid activity. Primarily used for antiinflammatory and immunosuppressive effects. May be used in conjunction with other forms of therapy, such as epinephrine for acute allergic reactions or antibiotics in acute infections. Primarily metabolized in the liver and excreted in the urine and feces. 75% excretion occurs within 24 hours, allowing use of very large doses with reasonable safety. Crosses the placental barrier. Secreted in breast milk.

INDICATIONS AND USES

Supplementary therapy for severe allergic reaction (use epinephrine first). ■ Shock unresponsive to conventional therapy. ■ Acute exacerbation of multiple sclerosis. ■ Has numerous other uses when given IM or PO.

Unlabeled uses: High-dose therapy as an adjunct to traditional spinal cord injury management; to improve neurologic recovery in an acute (less than 8 hours old) spinal cord injury above L-2. ■ Treatment of *Pneumocystis carinii* pneumonia as an adjunct to antibiotics. ■ Treatment of severe lupus nephritis. ■ Treatment of septic shock (controversial).

CONTRAINDICATIONS

Absolute contraindications in long-term therapy, except in life-threatening situations: Hypersensitivity to any product component, including sulfites; newborns; systemic fungal infections.

Relative contraindications: Active or latent peptic ulcer, active or healed tuberculosis, acute psychoses, chickenpox, congestive heart failure, diabetes mellitus, diverticulitis, fresh intestinal anastomoses, hypertension, myasthenia gravis, ocular herpes simplex, osteoporosis, pregnancy, psychotic tendencies, renal insufficiency, septic shock, thromboembolic tendencies, vaccinia.

PRECAUTIONS

Not the drug of choice to treat acute adrenocortical insufficiency. ■ To avoid relative adrenocortical insufficiency, do not stop therapy abruptly; taper off. Patient is observed carefully, especially under stress, for up to 2 years; exception is very short-term therapy. ■ Prophylactic antacids may prevent peptic ulcer complications.

Monitor: Monitor electrolytes. May cause sodium retention and potassium and calcium excretion. May cause hypertension secondary to fluid and electrolyte disturbances. ■ May mask signs of infection. ■ May increase insulin needs in diabetics. ■ Administer single dose before 9 AM to reduce suppression of adrenocortical activity. ■ Periodic ophthalmic exams may be necessary with prolonged treatment. ■ See Drug/Lab Interactions.

Patient Education: Report edema, tarry stools, or weight gain promptly. Report anorexia, diarrhea, dizziness, fatigue, low blood sugar, nausea, weakness, weight loss, or vomiting; may indicate adrenal insufficiency after dose reduction or discontinuing therapy. ■ May mask signs of infection and/or decrease resistance. ■ Diabetics may have increased requirement for insulin or oral hypoglycemics. ■ Avoid immunizations with live vaccines. ■ Carry ID stating steroid dependent if receiving prolonged therapy.

Maternal/Child: Category C: see Contraindications. ■ Use caution in breast-feeding. Secretion into breast milk less than other glucocorticoids.■ Observe newborn for hypoadrenalism if mother received large doses. ■ Monitor growth and development of children receiving prolonged treatment. **Elderly:** Reduced muscle mass and plasma volume may require a reduced dose. Monitor BP, blood glucose, and electrolytes carefully. ■ Risk of hypertension and glucocorticoid-induced osteoporosis increased. ■ Avoid aluminum-based antacids (risk of Alzheimer's disease).

DRUG/LAB INTERACTIONS

Aminoglutethimide (Cytadren) and mitotane (Lysodren) suppress adrenal function of corticosteroids; monitor carefully if concurrent use is necessary. ■ Metabolism increased and effects reduced by hepatic enzyme–inducing agents (e.g., alcohol, barbiturates [e.g., phenobarbital], hydantoins [e.g., phenytoin (Dilantin)], rifampin [Rifadin]); dose adjustments may be required when adding or deleting from drug profile. ■ Risk of hypokalemia increased with amphotericin B, or potassium-depleting diuretics (e.g., thiazides, furosemide, ethacrynic acid). Monitor potassium levels and cardiac function. Increased risk of digitalis (e.g., digoxin) toxicity secondary to hypokalemia. ■ May decrease effectiveness of potassium supplements; monitor serum potassium. ■ Diuretics decrease sodium and fluid retention effects of corticosteroids; corticosteroids decrease sodium excretion and diuretic effects of diuretics. ■ Use with cyclosporine in organ transplants is therapeutic but may increase cyclosporine toxicity; use caution. ■ Clearance decreased and effects increased with estrogens, oral contraceptives, triazole antifungals (e.g., itraconazole [Sporanox]), macrolide antibiotics (e.g., azithromycin [Zithromax], erythromycin, troleandomycin [TAO]). ■ May interact with anticoagulants, nondepolarizing muscle relaxants (e.g., doxacurium [Nuromax]), or theophyllines; may inhibit or potentiate action, monitor carefully. ■ Monitor patients receiving insulin or thyroid hormones carefully; dose adjustments of either or both agents may be required. ■ Use with ritodrine (Yutopar) has caused pulmonary edema in the mother; discontinue both agents with onset of S/S of pulmonary edema. ■ May antagonize effects of anticholinesterases (e.g., neostigmine), isoniazid, salicylates, and somatrem; dose adjustments may be required. ■ Do not vaccinate with attenuated-virus vaccines (e.g., smallpox) during therapy. ■ Altered protein-binding capacity will impact effectiveness of this drug. ■ See Dose Adjustments.

SIDE EFFECTS

Do occur but are usually reversible: Cushing's syndrome; electrolyte and calcium imbalance; euphoria; glycosuria; hyperglycemia; hypersensitivity reactions, including anaphylaxis; hypertension; increased intracranial pressure; menstrual irregularities; peptic ulcer perforation and hemorrhage; protein catabolism; spontaneous fractures; transitory burning or tingling; sweating, headache, or weakness; thromboembolism and many others.

ANTIDOTE

Notify the physician of any side effect. Will probably treat the side effect if necessary. Resuscitate as necessary for anaphylaxis and notify physician. Keep epinephrine immediately available.

METOCLOPRAMIDE HYDROCHLORIDE

(met′oh-kloe-pra′mide hye-droe-klor′id)

GI stimulant
Antiemetic

✦Maxeran, Reglan

pH 4.5 to 6.5

USUAL DOSE

Small bowel intubation and/or radiologic examination of the small bowel: 10 mg (2 ml) as a single dose.

Antiemetic: High-dose regimen for highly emetogenic chemotherapy is rarely used, $5HT_3$ receptor antagonists (e.g., granisetron [Kytril], ondansetron [Zofran]) preferred. 2 mg/kg of body weight 30 minutes before giving emetogenic cancer chemotherapy (e.g., cisplatin, dacarbazine). Repeat every 2 hours for 2 doses, then every 3 hours for 3 doses; see Dose Adjustments. Another regimen calls for 3 mg/kg 30 minutes before and 90 minutes after emetogenic chemotherapy. Given in combination with dexamethasone and lorazepam or diphenhydramine.

Diabetic gastroparesis: 10 mg immediately before each meal and at bedtime. Use IV for up to 10 days if symptoms are severe. Continue treatment PO for 2 to 8 weeks.

Prevention of postoperative nausea and vomiting: 10 mg, usually given IM toward the end of surgery. Up to 20 mg may be used.

PEDIATRIC DOSE

Small bowel intubation and/or radiologic examination of the small bowel: ***6 to 14 years:*** 2.5 to 5 mg. ***Under 6 years:*** 0.1 mg/kg of body weight.

Gastroesophageal reflux or GI dysmotility (unlabeled): 0.2 to 0.4 mg/kg/24 hours in equally divided doses every 6 hours. Maximum dose 0.5 mg/kg/24 hr.

Antiemetic (unlabeled): Rarely used. $5HT_3$-receptor antagonists preferred. 0.22 to 0.46 mg/kg of body weight has been administered over 5 minutes. A high-dose regimen for highly emetogenic chemotherapy of 1 to 2 mg/kg/dose every 2 to 6 hours has also been administered but is rarely used. Premedicate with diphenhydramine (Benadryl) to reduce extrapyramidal symptoms.

DOSE ADJUSTMENTS

Dose may be reduced to 1 mg/kg if initial doses suppress vomiting. Initial doses may be reduced to 1 mg/kg for less emetogenic regimens. ■ Reduce initial dose by half in the elderly if indicated and in any patient with a CrCl less than 40 ml/min. Adjust subsequent doses as indicated. ■ See Drug/Lab Interactions.

DILUTION

May be given undiluted if dose does not exceed 10 mg. For doses exceeding 10 mg dilute in at least 50 ml of D5W, NS, D5/½NS, R, or LR, and give as an infusion.

Storage: Light sensitive; store in carton before use. Diluted solutions stable for 24 hours in normal light, 48 hours if protected from light. Do not freeze unless diluted in NS. Discard if color or particulate matter is observed.

INCOMPATIBLE WITH

Manufacturer lists chloramphenicol (Chloromycetin), sodium bicarbonate.

COMPATIBLE WITH (Underline Indicates Conflicting Compatibility Information)

Consult pharmacist; specific conditions may apply; see Compatibilities, p. xvi.

Additive: Manufacturer lists ampicillin, ascorbic acid (Cenolate), benztropine (Cogentin), cimetidine (Tagamet), cisplatin (Platinol), clindamycin (Cleocin), cyclophosphamide (Cytoxan), cytarabine (ARA-C), dexamethasone (Decadron), diphenhydramine (Benadryl), doxorubicin (Adriamycin), erythromycin lactobionate (Erythrocin), heparin, hydrocortisone sodium phosphate (Hydrocortone), insulin (regular), lidocaine, mannitol, methotrexate (Folex), multivitamins (M.V.I.), penicillin G potassium, potassium acetate, and potassium phosphate. Other sources add meperidine (Demerol), meropenem (Merrem IV), morphine, potassium chloride (KCl), verapamil (Isoptin).

Syringe: Aminophylline, ascorbic acid (Cenolate), atropine, benztropine (Cogentin), bleomycin (Blenoxane), butorphanol (Stadol), chlorpromazine (Thorazine), cisplatin (Platinol), cyclophosphamide (Cytoxan), cytarabine (ARA-C), dexamethasone (Decadron), dimenhydrinate (Dinate), diphenhydramine (Benadryl), doxorubicin (Adriamycin), droperidol (Inapsine), fentanyl (Sublimaze), fluorouracil (5-FU), heparin, hydrocortisone (Hydrocortone, Solu-Cortef), insulin (regular), leucovorin calcium, lidocaine, magnesium sulfate, meperidine (Demerol), methotrexate (Folex), methylprednisolone (Solu-Medrol), midazolam (Versed), mitomycin (Mutamycin), morphine, ondansetron (Zofran), pentazocine (Talwin), perphenazine (Trilafon), prochlorperazine (Compazine), promethazine (Phenergan), ranitidine (Zantac), scopolamine, sufentanil (Sufenta), vinblastine (Velban), vincristine (Oncovin).

Y-site: All drugs listed by the manufacturer as compatible under ***Additive.*** Other sources add acyclovir (Zovirax), aldesleukin (Proleukin, IL-2), amifostine (Ethyol), aztreonam (Azactam), bleomycin (Blenoxane), ciprofloxacin (Cipro IV), cisatracurium (Nimbex), cladribine (Leustatin), diltiazem (Cardizem), docetaxel (Taxotere), droperidol (Inapsine), etoposide phosphate (Etopophos), famotidine (Pepcid IV), fentanyl (Sublimaze), filgrastim (Neupogen), fluconazole (Diflucan), fludarabine (Fludara), fluorouracil (5-FU), foscarnet (Foscavir), gatifloxacin (Tequin), gemcitabine (Gemzar), granisetron (Kytril), hetastarch in electrolytes (Hextend), hydromorphone (Dilaudid), idarubicin (Idamycin), leucovorin calcium, levofloxacin (Levaquin), linezolid (Zyvox), melphalan (Alkeran), meperidine (Demerol), meropenem (Merrem IV), mitomycin (Mutamycin), morphine, ondansetron (Zofran), paclitaxel (Taxol), piperacillin/tazobactam (Zosyn), remifentanil (Ultiva), sargramostim (Leukine), sufentanil (Sufenta), tacrolimus (Prograf), teniposide (Vumon), thiotepa (Thioplex), topotecan (Hycamtin), vinblastine (Velban), vincristine (Oncovin), vinorelbine (Navelbine), zidovudine (AZT, Retrovir).

RATE OF ADMINISTRATION

Too-rapid IV injection will cause intense anxiety, restlessness, and then drowsiness.

IV injection: 10 mg or fraction thereof over 2 minutes. Reduce rate of injection in pediatric patients.

Infusion: Administer over a minimum of 15 minutes.

ACTIONS

A dopamine antagonist that blocks the stimulation of medullary chemoreceptor trigger zones by dopamine. Inhibits nausea and vomiting. Stimulates tone and amplitude of gastric contractions, relaxes the lower pyloric sphincter and duodenal bulb, and increases peristalsis of the duodenum and jejunum increasing gastric emptying. Does not stimulate gastric, biliary, or pancreatic secretions. Acts even if vagal innervation not present. Action negated by anticholinergic drugs. Onset of action occurs in 1 to 3 minutes and lasts 1 to 2 hours. Excreted in urine. Secreted in breast milk.

INDICATIONS AND USES

Facilitate small bowel intubation. ■ Stimulate gastric and intestinal emptying of barium to permit radiologic examination of the stomach and small intestine. ■ Prevention of nausea and vomiting associated with emetogenic cancer chemotherapy. ■ Prophylaxis of postoperative nausea and vomiting when nasogastric suction is not indicated. ■ Diabetic gastroparesis.

CONTRAINDICATIONS

Situations in which gastric motility is contraindicated, i.e., gastric hemorrhage, obstruction, or perforation; known hypersensitivity to metoclopramide; patients with epilepsy or patients taking drugs that may also cause extrapyramidal reactions; pheochromocytoma.

PRECAUTIONS

May produce sedation, extrapyramidal symptoms, or Parkinson-like symptoms, similar to those seen with phenothiazines. Use caution in patients with pre-existing disease. ■ Tardive dyskinesia (syndrome of potentially irreversible involuntary movements of the tongue, face, mouth, jaw, trunk, or extremities) is usually related to duration of treatment and total cumulative dose. ■ Produces a transient increase in plasma aldosterone, patients with cirrhosis or CHF may develop fluid retention and volume overload. If S/S occur, discontinue metoclopramide. ■ A prolactin-elevating compound; may be carcinogenic. Risk with a single dose almost nonexistent. ■ May cause serious depression and suicidal tendencies; use extreme caution in any patient with a history of depression. ■ See Maternal/Child.

Monitor: Monitor vital signs. ■ Pretreatment with diphenhydramine may reduce incidence of extrapyramidal symptoms with larger doses (e.g., antiemetic). ■ See Precautions and Drug/Lab Interactions.

Patient Education: Use caution performing any task that requires alertness, coordination, or physical dexterity; may produce dizziness and drowsiness. ■ If any involuntary movement of eyes, face, or limbs occurs, notify physician promptly. ■ Avoid alcohol or other CNS depressants (e.g., barbiturates, benzodiazepines [e.g., diazepam (Valium)]).

Maternal/Child: Category B: use caution in pregnancy and breast-feeding. ■ Depending on dose and frequency, may be within an acceptable range for breast-feeding infants. ■ May increase milk production (elevates prolactin). ■ Pharmacokinetics highly variable in children and neonates, similarity of safety profile to adults has not been established. ■ Extrapyramidal reactions are more common in pediatric patients. ■ Prolonged clearance in neonates may produce excessive serum concentrations. ■ May cause methemoglobinemia in premature and full-term neonates at doses exceeding 0.5 mg/kg/24 hr. ■ See Precautions and Side Effects.

Elderly: May be more sensitive to therapeutic or adverse effects. ■ Long-term use increases risk of extrapyramidal effects (e.g., parkinsonism, tardive dyskinesia). ■ See Dose Adjustments and Precautions.

DRUG/LAB INTERACTIONS

Antagonized by anticholinergic drugs (e.g., atropine) and narcotic analgesics (e.g., morphine). ■ Potentiates alcohol, cyclosporine, and succinylcholine. ■ Drugs ingested orally may be absorbed more slowly or more rapidly depending on the absorption site (e.g., inhibits cimetidine, digoxin). ■ Potentiates MAO inhibitors (e.g., selegiline [Eldepryl]); use extreme caution or do not use. ■ Insulin reactions may result from gastric stasis, making diabetic control difficult. Dose or timing of insulin may need adjustment. ■ Extrapyramidal effects may be potentiated with concomitant use of phenothiazines, butyrophenones, and thioxanthines (antipsychotic drugs). ■ Used concurrently, metoclopramide and levodopa have opposite effects on dopamine receptors; metoclopramide is inhibited and levodopa is potentiated.

SIDE EFFECTS

Usually mild, transient, and reversible after metoclopramide discontinued. Occur in 20% to 30% of patients. CNS and GI side effects occur in 81% and 43% respectively of patients treated for cisplatin-induced nausea. Allergic reactions can occur. Acute CHF, anxiety, arrhythmias, bowel disturbances, confusion, convulsions, depression (severe, may have suicidal tendencies), dizziness, drowsiness, extrapyramidal reactions, fatigue, fluid retention, hallucinations, headache, hypertension, hypotension, insomnia, methemoglobinemia in neonates, nausea, restlessness, sulfhemoglobinemia in adults, tardive dyskinesia. Numerous other side effects may occur.

Overdose: Disorientation, drowsiness, and extrapyramidal reactions.

ANTIDOTE

Notify physician of all side effects. Most will respond to a reduced dose or discontinuation of metoclopramide. Treat overdose or extrapyramidal reactions with diphenhydramine (Benadryl) or benztropine (Cogentin). Symptoms should disappear within 24 hours. Treat methemoglobinemia with IV methylene blue. Resuscitate as necessary.

METOPROLOL TARTRATE

(me-toe′pro-lole tahr′trat)

Beta-adrenergic blocking agent
Antiarrhythmic (post MI)

Lopressor

pH 7.5

USUAL DOSE

Treatment of myocardial infarction: 5 mg as an IV bolus dose. Initiate as soon as the patient's hemodynamic condition has stabilized. Repeat at 2-minute intervals for 2 more doses; a total dose of 15 mg (AHA recommends 5 mg at 5-minute intervals to a total dose of 15 mg). If IV doses are well tolerated, give 50 mg PO every 6 hours for 48 hours beginning 15 minutes after the last bolus. Follow with an oral maintenance dose of

100 mg twice daily. In patients who do not tolerate the full IV dose start 25 to 50 mg PO within 15 minutes of the last IV dose. Dosage based on degree of intolerance. May have to discontinue metoprolol. Best results achieved if administered within 2 to 4 hours of symptom onset or thrombolytic therapy.

Treatment of atrial fibrillation (unlabeled): 2.5 to 5 mg as an IV injection over 2 minutes. May repeat for 2 more doses if indicated.

Treatment of unstable angina (unlabeled): 5 mg as an IV injection over 5 minutes. May repeat for 2 more doses if indicated. Follow with 25 to 100 mg twice daily PO.

DOSE ADJUSTMENTS

See Drug/Lab Interactions. ■ Not required in impaired renal function.

DILUTION

May be given undiluted.

COMPATIBLE WITH

Consult pharmacist; specific conditions may apply; see Compatibilities, p. xvi.

Y-site: Alteplase (tPA), meperidine (Demerol), morphine.

RATE OF ADMINISTRATION

A single dose over 1 minute. Monitor ECG, HR, and BP and discontinue metoprolol if adverse symptoms occur (bradycardia less than 45 beats/min, heart block greater than first degree, systolic BP less than 100 mm Hg, or moderate to severe cardiac failure).

ACTIONS

Metoprolol is a cardioselective (B_1) adrenergic blocking agent. Its mechanism of action in patients with suspected or definite myocardial infarction is not known. It reduces the incidence of recurrent myocardial infarctions and reduces the size of the infarct and the incidence of fatal arrhythmias. Well distributed throughout the body, it acts within 1 to 2 minutes and lasts about 3 to 4 hours. Metabolized in the liver and throughout the body. Excreted as metabolites in the urine.

INDICATIONS AND USES

To reduce cardiac mortality in hemodynamically stable individuals with suspected or definite myocardial infarction. ■ Treatment of hypertension, angina pectoris, and CHF in oral dosage form.

Unlabeled uses: Treatment of atrial fibrillation and unstable angina.

CONTRAINDICATIONS

HR below 45 beats/min, second- or third-degree heart block, significant first-degree heart block (PR interval greater than 0.24 seconds), systolic BP below 100 mm Hg, or moderate to severe cardiac failure.

PRECAUTIONS

Use caution in presence of heart failure controlled by digitalis. Both drugs slow AV conduction. ■ May mask tachycardia occurring with hypoglycemia in diabetes and tachycardia of hyperthyroidism. ■ Use with extreme caution in any patient with asthma, bronchospasm, or lung disease. ■ Discontinuation of beta-blockers before OR is controversial (beta-blockade interferes with cardiac response to reflex stimuli); however, some authorities recommend administering throughout perioperative period. May cause arrhythmia, angina, MI, or death if stopped abruptly. ■ May cause severe bradycardia in patients with Wolff-Parkinson-White syndrome.

Monitor: Continuous ECG, HR, and BP monitoring is mandatory during administration of IV metoprolol. ■ See Drug/Lab Interactions.

Patient Education: Report any breathing difficulty promptly.
Maternal/Child: Category C: safety for use in pregnancy and breast-feeding and in children not established. Has caused some problems during delivery resulting in neonatal bradycardia and low APGAR scores. See literature for guidelines.
Elderly: Use with caution in age-related peripheral vascular disease; risk of hypothermia increased. ▪ May exacerbate mental impairment.

DRUG/LAB INTERACTIONS

Concurrent use with calcium channel blockers (e.g., diltiazem, verapamil) may potentiate both drugs and result in severe depression of myocardium and AV conduction and severe hypotension. ▪ Concurrent use with antihypertensive agents may result in excessive hypotension. Dose adjustment may be required. ▪ Effects decreased by cocaine; may result in hypertension, severe bradycardia, or heart block. ▪ Concurrent use within 14 days of MAO inhibitors (selegiline [Eldepryl]) may cause severe hypertension. ▪ Use with sympathomimetic agents (e.g., epinephrine, norepinephrine, phenylephrine) or xanthines (e.g., aminophylline) may negate therapeutic effects of both drugs. ▪ Effects of beta-adrenergic blocking agents may be decreased by ampicillin, antiinflammatory agents, barbiturates, calcium salts, rifampin, salicylates, and others. ▪ General anesthetics, cimetidine (Tagamet), furosemide, phenothiazines (e.g., promethazine [Phenergan]), phenytoin (Dilantin), and quinolone antibiotics (e.g., ciprofloxacin) may increase myocardial depressant effects and hypotension. ▪ Potentiates effects of oral antidiabetics, catecholamine-depleting drugs (e.g., reserpine), insulin, lidocaine, narcotics, and skeletal muscle relaxants; monitor carefully. Dose adjustment may be required. ▪ Concurrent use with clonidine may precipitate acute hypertension if one or both agents are stopped abruptly. Withdraw metoprolol first. ▪ Effects decreased when hypothyroid patient is converted to a euthyroid state; adjust dose as indicated. ▪ Used concurrently with digitalis or alpha-adrenergic blockers (e.g., phentolamine [Regitine]) as indicated. Use caution; both digitalis and metoprolol slow AV conduction. ▪ Concurrent use with diphenhydramine (Benadryl) may decrease metoprolol clearance and prolong effects.

SIDE EFFECTS

Bradyarrhythmias, bronchospasm, cardiac failure, confusion, dizziness, dyspnea, first-degree heart block, headache, hypotension, nightmares, pruritus, rash, respiratory distress, second- or third-degree heart block, syncopal attacks, tiredness, vertigo, visual disturbances.

ANTIDOTE

For any side effect, discontinue drug and notify physician immediately. Patients with myocardial infarction may be more hemodynamically unstable; treat with caution. Use atropine for bradycardia; use isoproterenol with caution if atropine not effective. Glucagon 5 to 10 mg IV may be effective if atropine and isoproterenol are not (investigational use). Transvenous cardiac pacing may be needed. Treat hypotension with IV fluids if indicated or vasopressors (dopamine [Intropin] or norepinephrine [Levarterenol]); treat cause of hypotension (e.g., bradycardia). Use all vasopressors with extreme caution; severe hypotension can result. Use digitalis and diuretics at first sign of cardiac failure; dobutamine, isoproterenol, or glucagon may be required. Use aminophylline or isoproterenol (with extreme care) for bronchospasm, glucagon or IV glucose for hypoglycemia. Treat other side effects symptomatically; resuscitate as necessary.

METRONIDAZOLE HYDROCHLORIDE

(meh-troh-nye′dah-zohl hye-droe-klor′id)

Antibacterial
Antiprotozoal

Flagyl IV, Flagyl IV RTU, Metronidazole RTU

pH 5 to 7

USUAL DOSE

Anaerobic infections: Begin with an initial loading dose of 15 mg/kg of body weight. Follow with 7.5 mg/kg (up to 1 Gm/dose) in 6 hours and every 6 hours thereafter for 7 to 10 days or longer if indicated. Do not exceed 4 Gm in 24 hours.

Complicated intraabdominal infections: 500 mg every 6 hours given in combination with ciprofloxacin 400 mg every 12 hours or cefepime 2 Gm every 12 hours.

Prevent postoperative infection in contaminated or potentially contaminated colorectal surgery: 15 mg/kg infused over 30 to 60 minutes and completed 1 hour before surgery. Follow with 7.5 mg/kg in 6 hours and in 12 hours. If *Bacteroides fragilis* is the suspected or confirmed organism, an alternate regimen is to give a 1,500-mg dose at the beginning of surgery to ensure adequate metronidazole levels.

Amebiasis (unlabeled): 500 to 750 mg every 8 hours for 5 to 10 days.

PEDIATRIC DOSE

Safety for use in infants and children not established, but is used for anaerobic infections.

Anaerobic infections: ***Children and infants more than 7 days of age:*** An initial loading dose of 15 mg/kg. Follow with 7.5 mg/kg every 6 hours. Another source suggests every 8 hours.

Preterm infants: An initial loading dose of 15 mg/kg. 48 hours after loading dose begin 7.5 mg/kg every 12 hours.

Term infants: Same as preterm except begin maintenance dose (7.5 mg/kg) 24 hours after loading dose.

DOSE ADJUSTMENTS

Reduce dose in hepatic disease and in the elderly. Increase intervals in neonates; see Pediatric Dose. ■ Dose adjustment not indicated in anuric patients; accumulated metabolites readily removed by dialysis.

DILUTION

All solutions are prediluted and ready to use (5 mg/ml) except Flagyl IV. Do not use plastic containers in series connections. Risk of air embolism is present. Avoid all contact with aluminum in needles and syringes in all situations. Color change will occur. Flagyl IV requires a specific dilution process; initially add 4.4 ml SW or NS for injection (100 mg/ml). Solution must be clear. Will be yellow to yellow-green in color with a pH of 0.5 to 2. Must be further diluted to at least 8 mg/ml with NS, D5W, or LR and be neutralized before infusion with 5 mEq of sodium bicarbonate per 500 mg metronidazole. Mix thoroughly. CO_2 gas will be generated and may require venting.

Storage: Store at room temperature before and after dilution. Discard diluted and neutralized solutions in 24 hours. Do not refrigerate; a precipitate will result. Protect from light when storing.

INCOMPATIBLE WITH

Manufacturer recommends, "Administer separately, discontinue the primary IV during administration, and do not introduce additives into the solution." Do not use equipment containing aluminum.

COMPATIBLE WITH **(Underline Indicates Conflicting Compatibility Information)**

Consult pharmacist; specific conditions may apply; see Incompatible With and Compatibilities, p. xvi.

METRONIDAZOLE READY TO USE (RTU)

Additive: ***Not recommended by manufacturer.*** Amikacin (Amikin), ampicillin, cefamandole (Mandol), cefazolin (Kefzol), cefepime (Maxipime), cefotaxime (Claforan), cefoxitin (Mefoxin), ceftazidime (Fortaz), ceftizoxime (Cefizox), ceftriaxone (Rocephin), cefuroxime (Zinacef), chloramphenicol (Chloromycetin), ciprofloxacin (Cipro IV), clindamycin (Cleocin), fluconazole (Diflucan), gentamicin (Garamycin), hydrocortisone sodium succinate (Solu-Cortef), penicillin G potassium, tobramycin (Nebcin).

Y-site: Acyclovir (Zovirax), allopurinol (Aloprim, Zyloprim), amifostine (Ethyol), cefepime (Maxipime), cisatracurium (Nimbex), cyclophosphamide (Cytoxan), diltiazem (Cardizem), docetaxel (Taxotere), dopamine (Intropin), doxorubicin liposome (Doxil), enalaprilat (Vasotec IV), esmolol (Brevibloc), etoposide phosphate (Etopophos), fluconazole (Diflucan), foscarnet (Foscavir), gatifloxacin (Tequin), gemcitabine (Gemzar), granisetron (Kytril), heparin, hetastarch in electrolytes (Hextend), hydromorphone (Dilaudid), labetalol (Normodyne), linezolid (Zyvox), lorazepam (Ativan), magnesium sulfate, melphalan (Alkeran), meperidine (Demerol), methylprednisolone (Solu-Medrol), midazolam (Versed), morphine, perphenazine (Trilafon), piperacillin/tazobactam (Zosyn), remifentanil (Ultiva), sargramostim (Leukine), tacrolimus (Prograf), teniposide (Vumon), theophylline, thiotepa (Thioplex), vinorelbine (Navelbine).

METRONIDAZOLE HYDROCHLORIDE, SINGLE-DOSE LYOPHILIZED VIALS

Additive: ***Not recommended by manufacturer.*** Amikacin (Amikin), aminophylline, cefamandole (Mandol), cefazolin (Kefzol), cefepime (Maxipime), cefotaxime (Claforan), cefoxitin (Mefoxin), ceftriaxone (Rocephin), chloramphenicol (Chloromycetin), clindamycin (Cleocin), gentamicin (Garamycin), heparin, hydrocortisone sodium succinate (Solu-Cortef), multivitamins (M.V.I.), penicillin G potassium, tobramycin (Nebcin).

Y-site: Amiodarone (Cordarone), diltiazem (Cardizem).

RATE OF ADMINISTRATION

Must be given as a slow intermittent or continuous IV infusion, each single dose evenly distributed over 1 hour. Discontinue primary IV during administration. Rate should be ordered by physician.

ACTIONS

A bactericidal agent with cytotoxic effects, active against specific anaerobic bacteria and protozoa. Widely distributed in therapeutic levels to all body fluids (including abscesses). Levels are directly proportional to dose given. Onset of action is prompt and lasts about 8 hours. Crosses placental and blood-brain barriers. Excreted in urine, some in feces. Secreted in breast milk.

INDICATIONS AND USES

Treatment of serious intraabdominal, skin and skin structure, gynecologic, bone and joint, CNS, and lower respiratory tract infections; bacterial septicemia; and endocarditis caused by susceptible anaerobic bacteria. ■ To provide anaerobic activity when used in combination with ciprofloxacin for the treatment of complicated intraabdominal infections. ■ Perioperative prophylaxis to reduce infection rates in contaminated or potentially contaminated colorectal surgery. ■ Given orally for antibiotic-related pseudomembranous colitis, amebiasis, and other indications.

Unlabeled uses: As a radiosensitizer to make resistant tumors more susceptible to radiation therapy. As an antiprotozoal in the treatment of amebiasis.

CONTRAINDICATIONS

Hypersensitivity to metronidazole or nitroimidazole derivatives; first trimester of pregnancy.

PRECAUTIONS

A mixed (anaerobic/aerobic) infection will require use of additional appropriate antibiotics. ■ Sensitivity studies indicated to determine susceptibility of the causative organism to metronidazole. ■ Avoid prolonged use of the drug; superinfection caused by overgrowth of nonsusceptible organisms may result. ■ Symptoms of candidiasis may be exacerbated and require treatment. ■ Use caution in patients predisposed to edema and/or taking corticosteroids, in patients with impaired cardiac function (contains 27 to 28 mEq sodium/Gm), CNS disease, or a history of blood dyscrasias. ■ Pseudomembranous colitis has been reported. May range from mild to life-threatening. Consider in patients that present with diarrhea during or after treatment with metronidazole. ■ Carcinogenic in rodents; use only when necessary.

Monitor: Rotate IV site frequently to avoid thrombophlebitis. Avoid extravasation. ■ Obtain total and differential leukocyte counts before and after therapy. ■ Monitor serum levels (suggested) and observe for toxicity in patients with hepatic disease receiving reduced doses and in the elderly. ■ Observe patients receiving high doses for extended periods; seizures and peripheral neuropathies may occur; neuropathy may not be reversible. ■ Transfer to oral dosing as soon as practical. ■ See Drug/Lab Interactions.

Patient Education: Avoid alcohol, alcohol-containing preparations, and disulfiram; toxic reactions will occur.

Maternal/Child: Safety for use in pregnancy, breast-feeding, children, and neonates not established. Half-life markedly extended in newborns; adjust intervals; see Pediatric Dose. ■ See Contraindications.

Elderly: Pharmacokinetics altered in the elderly; monitor serum levels if possible and adjust dose accordingly.

DRUG/LAB INTERACTIONS

Avoid alcohol, alcohol-containing preparations for at least 3 days after taking any dose of metronidazole; avoid for 2 weeks after disulfiram. Toxic reactions will occur. ■ Barbiturates (e.g., phenobarbital) may inhibit therapeutic action. ■ May be antagonized by bacteriostatic antibiotics (e.g., chloramphenicol, erythromycin, and tetracyclines); bactericidal action may be negated. ■ Cimetidine (Tagamet) may increase metronidazole serum levels. ■ Potentiates hydantoins (e.g., phenytoin [Dilantin]). ■ May decrease metabolism and increase anticoagulant effects of warfarin (Coumadin). Monitor PT/INR periodically. ■ May increase lithium levels and cause toxicity. ■ Neurotoxicity may be increased with concurrent use of other neurotoxic agents (e.g., ciprofloxacin [Cipro], cyclosporine [Sandimmune], imipenem-cilastatin [Primaxin]). ■ May cause decreased AST (SGOT) levels.

SIDE EFFECTS

Abdominal cramping, anorexia, constipation, cystitis, darkened deep red urine, decreased libido, diarrhea, dizziness, dryness of the mouth, vagina, or vulva; dysuria, epigastric distress, fever, fleeting joint pain, flushing, furry tongue, glossitis, headache, incontinence, metallic taste (expected), nasal congestion, nausea, neutropenia (reversible), painful coitus, pelvic pressure, peripheral neuropathy, polyuria, proctitis, pruritus, pseudomembranous colitis, rash, seizures, stomatitis, syncope, thrombocytopenia (reversible), thrombophlebitis, T-wave flattening, urticaria, vomiting.

ANTIDOTE

Notify physician of all side effects. Treatment will be symptomatic and supportive. Discontinue metronidazole with onset of seizures or signs of peripheral neuropathy (e.g., numbness or paresthesia of an extremity); benefit/risk of therapy must be reconsidered with onset of convulsions or peripheral neuropathy. Rapidly removed by hemodialysis. Treat anaphylaxis and resuscitate as necessary.

MIDAZOLAM HYDROCHLORIDE

(my-dayz'oh-lam hye-droe-klor'id)

Benzodiazepine
Sedative-hypnotic
Anesthetic adjunct
Amnestic

Versed

pH 3

USUAL DOSE

Dose requirements for each patient may vary and will depend on the type and amount of premedication used. Doses given below are general guidelines. Individualize dose and titrate slowly to effect. Allow 3 to 5 minutes between each small injection to evaluate the full effect before administering additional doses.

SEDATION, ANXIOLYSIS (ANTI-ANXIETY), AND/OR AMNESIA FOR SHORT DIAGNOSTIC, ENDOSCOPIC, AND THERAPEUTIC PROCEDURES

The desired endpoint for conscious sedation can usually be achieved in 3 to 6 minutes. Time will depend on total dose and type or dose of narcotic premedication used concomitantly.

Healthy adults less than 60 years of age: 1 to 2.5 mg immediately before the procedure.

Begin with 1 mg and titrate slowly up to slurred speech or 2.5 mg. Some patients respond adequately to 1 mg. If additional medication is needed wait a full 2 minutes, then titrate additional dosage slowly in small increments (usually no more than 1 mg). Wait a full 2 minutes between each increment. A total dose exceeding 5 mg is rarely necessary. Reduce dose by 30% in the presence of narcotic premedication or other CNS depressants. 25% of the sedating dose can be used for maintenance only when clearly indicated by clinical evaluation.

Patients over 60 years of age or debilitated or chronically ill patients: 1 to 1.5 mg. Begin with 1 mg and titrate slowly up to slurred speech or 1.5 mg. May respond adequately to 1 mg. If additional medication is needed wait a full 2 minutes, then titrate additional dosage in small increments (no more than 1 mg). Wait a full 2 minutes between each increment. A total dose exceeding 3.5 mg is rarely necessary. Reduce dose by 50% in the presence of narcotic premedication or other CNS depressants. 25% of the sedating dose can be used for maintenance only when clearly indicated by clinical evaluation.

Induction of Anesthesia Before Administration of Other Anesthetic Agents and/or Maintenance of Anesthesia as a Component of Balanced Anesthesia During Surgical Procedures

In all patients (unpremedicated and premedicated), allow 2 minutes from initial dose to reach peak effect. If necessary, complete induction with 25% of initial dose or use inhalational anesthesia (e.g., halothane). Doses of any agents used after induction of anesthesia with midazolam may need to be reduced to as little as 25% of the usual initial dose. 25% of the induction dose can be repeated when indicated by lightening of anesthesia.

Unpremedicated patients under 55 years of age: 0.3 to 0.35 mg/kg as an initial dose. A total dose of up to 0.6 mg/kg has been required; recovery may be prolonged.

Unpremedicated patients over 55 years of age (ASA I or II): 0.15 to 0.3 mg/kg as an initial dose.

Unpremedicated debilitated patients or those with severe systemic disease (ASA III or IV): 0.15 to 0.25 mg/kg as an initial dose. As little as 0.15 mg/kg may be adequate.

Patients premedicated with sedatives or narcotics under 55 years of age: 0.25 mg/kg as an initial dose may be adequate. Range is 0.15 to 0.35 mg/kg of body weight.

Patients premedicated with sedatives or narcotics over 55 years of age (Good risk [ASA I & II]): 0.2 mg/kg as an initial dose may be adequate.

Patients premedicated with sedatives or narcotics who are debilitated or those with severe systemic disease (ASA III or IV): 0.15 mg/kg as an initial dose may be adequate.

Premedication usually includes narcotics (e.g., fentanyl 1.5 to 2 mcg/kg IV 5 minutes before induction, or morphine [up to 0.15 mg/kg IM] or meperidine [up to 1 mg/kg IM]) 1 hour before induction with midazolam. Sedative premedication usually includes hydroxyzine (Vistaril) 100 mg PO or a barbiturate PO 1 hour before induction.

Sedation for Anesthesia or Treatment in a Critical Care Setting for Intubated and Mechanically Ventilated Patients

Continuous infusion (concentration 0.5 mg/ml): Begin with a ***loading dose*** of 0.01 to 0.05 mg/kg (0.5 to 4 mg for a typical adult) to rapidly initiate sedation. Infuse over several minutes. May be repeated at 10- to 15-minute intervals until adequate sedation achieved.

For maintenance of sedation: An initial infusion rate of 0.02 to 0.1 mg/kg/hr (1 to 7 mg/hr) may be used. Upper-end doses may be required, but use the lowest recommended doses in patients with residual effects from anesthetic drugs or in those concurrently receiving other sedatives or opioids. Initial infusion rate may be titrated up or down by 25% to 50% to maintain desired level of sedation. Decrease by 10% to 25% every few hours to find the minimum effective infusion rate. The lowest rate that produces the desired level of sedation is recommended. Agitation, hypertension, or tachycardia in response to stimulation in adequately sedated patients may

Continued

indicate need for an opioid analgesic. Reduced rate of midazolam infusion may be indicated with the addition of an opioid analgesic. Taper dose gradually if midazolam has been used for more than a few days. Abrupt discontinuation may result in withdrawal symptoms.

Adjunct to Local or Regional Anesthesia (Unlabeled)

0.03 to 0.06 mg/kg. Titrate dose slowly.

PEDIATRIC DOSE

In all situations dose is based on lean body weight in obese pediatric patients. See Precautions and Maternal/Child.

Sedation, Anxiolysis (Antianxiety), and/or Amnesia Before and During Procedures or Before Anesthesia

All increments of midazolam are on a mg/kg basis. Total dose will depend on patient response, type and duration of the procedure, and the type and dose of concomitant medications. Titrate dose of midazolam and other concomitant medications slowly to the desired clinical effect. With concomitant medications, dose of midazolam should be reduced (usually by 25% to 30%). Before beginning a procedure or repeating a dose, wait a full 2 to 3 minutes to fully evaluate the sedative effect. If further sedation is necessary, continue to titrate with small increments at 2- to 3-minute intervals until desired level of sedation achieved. Prolonged sedation and risk of hypoventilation may be associated with higher-end doses.

Nonintubated infants less than 6 months of age: Uncertain when patient transfers from neonatal physiology to pediatric physiology; manufacturer has no specific dosing recommendations. Titrate with very small increments to clinical effect and monitor very carefully for airway obstruction and hypoventilation.

Children 6 months to 5 years of age: Begin with an initial dose of 0.05 to 0.1 mg/kg. Up to 0.6 mg/kg may be required, but a total dose of 6 mg is usually not exceeded.

Children 6 to 12 years of age: Begin with an initial dose of 0.025 to 0.05 mg/kg. Up to 0.4 mg/kg may be required, but a total dose of 10 mg is usually not exceeded.

Children 12 to 16 years of age: See Usual Dose. May require higher-than-recommended adult doses, but total dose usually does not exceed 10 mg.

Sedation, Anxiolysis, Amnesia

Intubated children in critical care settings: Begin with a loading dose of 0.05 to 0.2 mg/kg. May be allowed to breathe on own through intubation tube but assisted ventilation recommended in children receiving other CNS depressants. In hemodynamically compromised children titrate the loading dose in small increments and monitor for hypotension, respiratory rate, and oxygen saturation. May be followed by a continuous IV infusion at 0.06 to 0.12 mg/kg/hr (1 to 2 mcg/kg/min). Increase or decrease infusion in 25% increments or use supplemental IV injection to maintain desired effect.

Sedation of Intubated Neonates in Critical Care Settings

Neonates less than 32 weeks: A continuous infusion at a rate of 0.03 mg/kg/hr (0.5 mcg/kg/min).

Neonates 32 weeks or older: A continuous infusion at a rate of 0.06 mg/kg/hr (1 mcg/kg/min).

Do not use loading doses in neonates. Infusion may be run more rapidly for the first several hours to establish therapeutic plasma levels. Reassess rate carefully and frequently to use the lowest possible effective dose and reduce the potential for drug accumulation. Midazolam contains benzyl alcohol and must be used with extreme caution in neonates.

DOSE ADJUSTMENTS

Reduce dose by 30% to 50%, depending on age, in the presence of narcotic premedication or other CNS depressants; see Usual Dose. ■ Reduce dose in congestive heart failure, chronic obstructive pulmonary disease, chronic renal failure, the debilitated, and patients over 55 years of age. Half-life is extended and depressant effects will be potentiated; see Usual Dose. ■ Dose based on lean body weight in obese pediatric patients. ■ See Drug/Lab Interactions.

DILUTION

Read Label Carefully and Confirm mg Dose. Available in Two Strengths, 1 mg/ml and 5 mg/ml.

IV injection: May be diluted with D5W or NS. Dilute in a sufficient amount to permit slow titration (i.e., 1 mg in 4 ml or 5 mg in 20 ml [0.25 mg/m]). Maximum concentration after dilution should not exceed 0.5 mg/ml.

Infusion: Dilute in either of the above solutions to a maximum concentration of 0.5 mg/ml. 5 ml of a 1 mg/ml (5 mg) in 5 ml of diluent yields 0.5 mg/ml. 5 ml of a 5 mg/ml (25 mg) in 45 ml diluent is usually a 24-hour supply and also yields 0.5 mg/ml. Use a controlled infusion device or at the very least a metriset (60 gtt/ml) to facilitate titration and control flow to prevent overdose.

COMPATIBLE WITH **(Underline Indicates Conflicting Compatibility Information)**

Consult pharmacist; specific conditions may apply; see Compatibilities, p. xvi.

Additive: Hydromorphone (Dilaudid).

Syringe: Alfentanil (Alfenta), atracurium (Tracrium), atropine, buprenorphine (Buprenex), butorphanol (Stadol), chlorpromazine (Thorazine), cimetidine (Tagamet), diphenhydramine (Benadryl), droperidol (Inapsine), fentanyl (Sublimaze), glycopyrrolate, hydromorphone (Dilaudid), meperidine (Demerol), metoclopramide (Reglan), morphine, nalbuphine (Nubain), ondansetron (Zofran), promethazine (Phenergan), scopolamine, sufentanil (Sufenta).

Y-site: Alatrofloxacin (Trovan IV), amikacin (Amikin), amiodarone (Cordarone), atracurium (Tracrium), calcium gluconate, cefazolin (Kefzol), cefotaxime (Claforan), cimetidine (Tagamet), ciprofloxacin (Cipro IV), cisatracurium (Nimbex), clindamycin (Cleocin), digoxin (Lanoxin), diltiazem (Cardizem), <u>dobutamine (Dobutrex)</u>, dopamine (Intropin), epinephrine (Adrenalin), erythromycin lactobionate (Erythrocin), esmolol (Brevibloc), etomidate (Amidate), famotidine (Pepcid IV), fentanyl (Sublimaze), fluconazole (Diflucan), gatifloxacin (Tequin), gentamicin (Garamycin), haloperidol (Haldol), heparin, hetastarch in electrolytes (Hextend), hydromorphone (Dilaudid), insulin (regular), labetalol (Normodyne), linezolid (Zyvox), lorazepam (Ativan), methylprednisolone (Solu-Medrol), metronidazole (Flagyl IV), milrinone (Primacor), morphine, nicardipine (Cardene IV), nitroglycerin (Nitro-Bid IV), nitroprusside sodium, norepinephrine (Levophed), pancuronium (Pavulon), piperacillin (Pipracil), potassium chloride (KCl), <u>propofol (Diprivan)</u>, ranitidine (Zantac), remifentanil (Ultiva), sufentanil (Sufenta), theophylline, tobramycin (Nebcin), vancomycin (Vancocin), vecuronium (Norcuron).

RATE OF ADMINISTRATION

IV injection: ***Sedation:*** Any single increment of a total dose titrated slowly over at least 2 minutes. Stop at any point that the speech becomes slurred.

Induction of anesthesia: Any single increment of a total dose over 20 to 30 seconds. Rapid injection in any situation may cause respiratory depression or apnea.

Infusion: See Usual Dose. The American Academy of Critical Care recommends limiting the use of midazolam in the critical care setting to 24 hours because its metabolites accumulate in peripheral tissue, especially with long-term infusion.

Pediatric rate: Any single increment of a total dose over a minimum of 2 to 3 minutes. Rapid injection or infusion may cause severe hypotension or seizures in infants and neonates; incidence increased with concomitant fentanyl. See comments under Infusion.

ACTIONS

A short-acting benzodiazepine CNS depressant 3 to 4 times as potent as diazepam. Has anxiolytic, hypnotic, anticonvulsant, muscle relaxant, and anterograde amnestic effects. Depressant effects are dependent on dose, route of administration, and the presence or absence of other premedications. Can depress the ventilatory response to CO_2 stimulation. Mechanics of respiration are not adversely affected with usual doses. Mean arterial pressure, cardiac output, stroke volume, and systemic vascular resistance may be slightly decreased. May cause HRs of less than 65/min to rise and more than 85/min to fall. Produces sleepiness and relief of apprehension, and diminishes patient recall very effectively. Widely distributed. Onset of action occurs within 1.5 to 5 minutes. Half-life is approximately 2.5 hours (range is 1 to 5 hours), shorter than that of diazepam (Valium). Time to recovery is usually within 2 hours but may take as long as 6 hours. Metabolized in the liver by cytochrome P_{450} mediation and excreted as metabolites in urine. Crosses the placental barrier. Secreted in breast milk.

INDICATIONS AND USES

To produce sedation, relieve anxiety, and impair memory of perioperative events. ■ May be used with or without narcotic sedation for conscious sedation before short diagnostic, endoscopic, or therapeutic procedures (e.g., bronchoscopy, gastroscopy, cystoscopy, coronary angiography, cardiac catheterization). ■ Induction of anesthesia before administration of other anesthetic agents. ■ As a component in the induction and maintenance of balanced anesthesia in short surgical procedures. ■ Continuous infusions may be used in intubated and mechanically ventilated patients for sedation as a component of anesthesia or during treatment in a critical care setting.

CONTRAINDICATIONS

Acute narrow-angle glaucoma, known hypersensitivity to midazolam, open-angle glaucoma unless receiving appropriate treatment. Not recommended in pregnancy, childbirth, breast-feeding, shock, coma, acute alcohol intoxication with depression of vital signs. Contraindicated with ritonavir (Norvir).

PRECAUTIONS

Should be used only in a hospital or ambulatory care setting with continuous monitoring of respiratory and cardiac function (e.g., pulse oximetry). Resuscitative drugs (including flumazenil [Romazicon]) and age- and size-appropriate equipment for bag/valve/mask ventilation and intubation must be immediately available. Personnel must be skilled in airway management. ■ A dedicated individual with no other responsibilities should monitor deeply sedated patients throughout any procedure. ■ A topical anesthetic agent should be used with midazolam during perioral endoscopy, and premedication with a narcotic is recommended in bronchoscopy since increased cough reflex and laryngospasm frequently occur. Premedication with a narcotic is also recommended with balanced anesthesia. ▪ For IV/IM use only. Contains benzyl alcohol. Do not use for intrathecal or epidural administration. ▪ Use caution in neonates. At recommended doses benzyl alcohol is not expected to be toxic, but excessive benzyl alcohol may result in hypotension, metabolic acidosis, and increased incidence of kernicterus, especially in small preterm infants. ▪ Use extreme caution in the elderly, in patients with chronic disease states, decreased pulmonary reserve, hepatic or renal impairment, neuromuscular disorders, and in those with uncompensated acute illness (e.g., severe fluid or electrolyte disturbances); may have increased risks of hypoventilation, airway obstruction, or apnea. Peak effect may take longer. ▪ Use with caution in obese patients and patients with CHF. Half-life is prolonged. ▪ See Pediatric Dose and Maternal/Child for additional precautions with infants and children. ▪ Does not protect against increased intracranial pressure or circulatory changes noted with succinylcholine or pancuronium or associated with intubation under light general anesthesia. ▪ Some clinicians prefer midazolam over diazepam because of effectiveness, minimum pain if any on injection, and miscibility with many drugs and solutions.

Monitor: Obtain a careful presedation history (e.g., medical conditions, concomitant meds), and complete a physical exam. Check for airway abnormalities. ▪ Monitor respiratory and cardiac function (e.g., BP, HR, pulse oximetry) continuously. ***Has caused apnea and cardiac arrest.*** Monitoring of ECG desirable. Maintain a patent airway and support adequate ventilation. Record assessments using standard assessment charts for scoring, especially in pediatric patients. ▪ Extravasation or arterial administration hazardous. ▪ Bed rest required for a minimum of 3 hours after IV injection. ▪ See Drug/Lab Interactions.

Patient Education: Do not drive or operate hazardous machinery until the day after surgery or longer. All effects must have subsided. Avoid use of alcohol or other CNS depressants (e.g., antihistamines, barbiturates) for 24 hours after last dose. ▪ May impair memory; request written postop instructions. ▪ Consider birth control options.

Maternal/Child: Category D: avoid pregnancy. ▪ Not recommended during pregnancy, labor and delivery, or breast-feeding. ▪ Elimination rate is faster in infants and children. ▪ Neonate has reduced or immature organ function. Clearance is decreased and half-life is increased in critically ill neonates. May be susceptible to profound and/or prolonged respiratory effects. ▪ See Precautions and Monitor.

Elderly: See Usual Dose and Dose Adjustments. Start with a small dose and increase gradually based on response. ▪ Clearance is reduced compared to younger adults, and time to recovery may be prolonged. ▪ All elderly are more sensitive to therapeutic and adverse effects (e.g., oversedation, ataxia, dizziness). Patients over 70 years of age may be particularly sensitive. IV injection may be more likely to cause apnea, bradycardia, hypotension, and cardiac arrest. ▪ See Precautions and Drug/Lab Interactions.

DRUG/LAB INTERACTIONS

Concurrent use with other CNS depressants (e.g., alcohol, antihistamines, barbiturates, inhalation anesthetics [e.g., halothane], MAO inhibitors [e.g., selegiline (Eldepryl)], narcotics [e.g., morphine, meperidine (Demerol), fentanyl], phenothiazines [e.g., prochlorperazine (Compazine)], thiopental, and tricyclic antidepressants [e.g., imipramine (Tofranil-PM)]) may result in additive effects for up to 48 hours. May produce apnea or prolonged effect, depress ventilatory response to CO_2, or cause hypotension. Reduce doses of midazolam. ■ Agents that inhibit cytochrome P_{450} activity (e.g., triazole antifungals [e.g., itraconazole (Sporanox), ketoconazole (Nizoral), miconazole (Monistat)], cimetidine [Tagamet], diltiazem [Cardizem], verapamil [Isoptin], macrolide antibiotics [e.g., erythromycin], omeprazole [Prilosec], and ranitidine [Zantac]) decrease clearance and increase effects of midazolam resulting in prolonged sedation. ■ Reduce doses of inhalation anesthetics (e.g., halothane) and/or thiopental when used with midazolam. ■ Protease inhibitors (e.g., indinavir [Crixivan], nelfinavir [Viracept], and saquinavir [Invirase]) may increase risk of prolonged sedation and respiratory depression. Concurrent use not recommended. Half-life may double with saquinavir. ***Contraindicated with ritonavir (Norvir);*** may cause life-threatening increased sedation and respiratory depression. Benzodiazepines metabolized by alternate routes may be safer (e.g., lorazepam [Ativan], oxazepam [Serax], temazepam [Restoril]). ■ May increase serum concentrations of digoxin; monitor digoxin serum levels. ■ Hypotensive effects of benzodiazepines may be increased by any agent that induces hypotension (e.g., antihypertensives, bretylium, CNS depressants, diuretics, lidocaine, paclitaxel). Monitor BP during and after use. ■ Use with rifampin (Rifadin) increases clearance and reduces effects of benzodiazepines. ■ Theophyllines (Aminophylline) antagonize sedative effects of benzodiazepines. ■ Smoking increases metabolism and clearance of midazolam, decreasing plasma levels and sedative effects.

SIDE EFFECTS

The incidence of cardiorespiratory events is higher in patients undergoing procedures involving the upper airway (e.g., upper endoscopy or dental procedures). Serious cardiorespiratory events may include airway obstruction, apnea, hypotension (especially with narcotic premedication), oxygen desaturation, respiratory arrest, and/or cardiac arrhythmias or arrest. Inadequate or excessive dosing may cause agitation, combativeness, involuntary movements (e.g., clonic, tonic, muscle tremor), and hyperactivity; may be caused by cerebral hypoxia or be true paradoxical reactions. Other common reactions are coughing, drowsiness, fluctuation in vital signs, headache, hiccups, nausea and vomiting, nystagmus (especially in children), induration, redness, or phlebitis at injection site. Capable of numerous other side effects. Has caused death and hypoxic encephalopathy. Withdrawal may be seen in patients receiving an infusion for extended periods of time.

Overdose: Sedation, somnolence, confusion, impaired coordination, diminished reflexes, coma, and untoward effect on vital signs.

ANTIDOTE

Notify the physician of all side effects. Reduction of dosage may be required or will be treated symptomatically. Discontinue the drug for major side effects or paradoxical reactions. Flumazenil (Romazicon) will reverse all sedative effects of benzodiazepines. A patent airway, artificial ventilation, oxygen therapy and other symptomatic treatment must be instituted promptly. Treat hypotension with IV fluids, Trendelenburg position, or vasopressors (e.g., dopamine [Intropin]) as indicated. May cause emesis; observe closely. Treat allergic reaction and resuscitate as necessary.

MILRONONE LACTATE

(mill′rih-nohn lak′tat)

Inotropic agent

Primacor

pH 3.2 to 4

USUAL DOSE

50 mcg/kg (0.05 mg/kg) of body weight as the initial loading dose (3.5 mg [3.5 ml of a 1 mg/ml solution] for a 70-kg person).

Milrinone Loading Dose (ml) Using 1 mg/ml Concentration										
Patient Body Weight (kg)										
kg	30	40	50	60	70	80	90	100	110	120
ml	1.5	2	2.5	3	3.5	4	4.5	5	5.5	6

Follow with a maintenance infusion of 0.5 mcg/kg/min (35 mcg/min for a 70-kg person). Titrate the infusion dose between 0.375 mcg/kg/min to 0.75 mcg/kg/min (26 mcg/min to 52 mcg/min for a 70-kg person) based on hemodynamic effect. Do not exceed a total dose of 1.13 mg/kg/24 hr, including boluses. Duration of infusion usually does not exceed 48 hours.

DOSE ADJUSTMENTS

Reduced dose required in impaired renal function based on CrCl; see literature.

DILUTION

Loading dose: May be given undiluted, or each 1 mg (1 ml) may be diluted in 1 ml NS or ½NS for injection.

Infusion: Dilute with NS, ½NS, or D5W. Available prediluted as 200 mcg/ml in D5W. Amount of diluent may be increased or decreased based on patient fluid requirements.

Guidelines for Dilution of Milrinone for Infusion			
Desired Infusion Concentration (mcg/ml)	Milrinone 1 mg/ml (ml)	Diluent (ml)	Total Volume (ml)
100	10	90	100
100	20	180	200
150	10	56.7	66.7
150	20	113	133
200	10	40	50
200	20	80	100

May be given through Y-tube or three-way stopcock of IV infusion set but should never come in contact with furosemide (Lasix) or bumetanide (Bumex). Use only freshly prepared solutions.

Storage: Store at room temperature before dilution; avoid freezing.

INCOMPATIBLE WITH

Manufacturer states, "Do not add supplementary medications." May form a precipitate with bumetanide (Bumex) or furosemide (Lasix).

COMPATIBLE WITH **(Underline Indicates Conflicting Compatibility Information)**

Consult pharmacist; specific conditions may apply; see Compatibilities, p. xvi.

Additive: ***Not recommended by manufacturer.*** Quinidine gluconate.

Syringe: ***Not recommended by manufacturer.*** Atropine, calcium chloride, digoxin (Lanoxin), epinephrine (Adrenalin), lidocaine, morphine, propranolol (Inderal), sodium bicarbonate, verapamil (Isoptin).

Y-site: Atracurium (Tracrium), bumetanide (Bumex), calcium gluconate, cimetidine (Tagamet), digoxin (Lanoxin), diltiazem (Cardizem), dobutamine (Dobutrex), dopamine (Intropin), epinephrine (Adrenalin), fentanyl (Sublimaze), heparin, hetastarch in electrolytes (Hextend), hydromorphone (Dilaudid), insulin (regular), isoproterenol (Isuprel), labetalol (Normodyne), lorazepam (Ativan), magnesium sulfate, midazolam (Versed), morphine, nicardipine (Cardene IV), nitroglycerin (Nitro-Bid IV), nitroprusside sodium, norepinephrine (Levophed), pancuronium (Pavulon), potassium chloride (KCl), propofol (Diprivan), propranolol (Inderal), quinidine gluconate, ranitidine (Zantac), rocuronium (Zemuron), sodium bicarbonate, theophylline, thiopental (Pentothal), torsemide (Demadex), vecuronium (Norcuron).

RATE OF ADMINISTRATION

Loading dose: A single dose over 10 minutes.

Infusion: Use a microdrip (60 gtt/ml) or an infusion pump to deliver milrinone in recommended doses. The following manufacturer's dose charts define selected dose in mcg/kg/min in infusion rate of ml/hr. Adjust as indicated by physician's orders and progress in patient's condition. Reduce rate or stop infusion for excessive drop in BP.

Milrinone Infusion Rate (ml/hr) Using 100 mcg/ml Concentration

Maintenance Dose (mcg/kg/min)	Patient Body Weight (kg) 30	40	50	60	70	80	90	100	110	120
0.375	6.8	9	11.3	13.5	15.8	18	20.3	22.5	24.8	27
0.4	7.2	9.6	12	14.4	16.8	19.2	21.6	24	26.4	28.8
0.5	9	12	15	18	21	24	27	30	33	36
0.6	10.8	14.4	18	21.6	25.2	28.8	32.4	36	39.6	43.2
0.7	12.6	16.8	21	25.2	29.4	33.6	37.8	42	46.2	50.4
0.75	13.5	18	22.5	27	31.5	36	40.5	45	49.5	54

Milrinone Infusion Rate (ml/hr) Using 150 mcg/ml Concentration										
Maintenance Dose	Patient Body Weight (kg)									
(mcg/kg/min)	30	40	50	60	70	80	90	100	110	120
0.375	4.5	6	7.5	9	10.5	12	13.5	15	16.5	18
0.4	4.8	6.4	8	9.6	11.2	12.8	14.4	16	17.6	19.2
0.5	6	8	10	12	14	16	18	20	22	24
0.6	7.2	9.6	12	14.4	16.8	19.2	21.6	24	26.4	28.8
0.7	8.4	11.2	14	16.8	19.6	22.4	25.2	28	30.8	33.6
0.75	9	12	15	18	21	24	27	30	33	36

Milrinone Infusion Rate (ml/hr) Using 200 mcg/ml Concentration										
Maintenance Dose	Patient Body Weight (kg)									
(mcg/kg/min)	30	40	50	60	70	80	90	100	110	120
0.375	3.4	4.5	5.6	6.8	7.9	9	10.1	11.3	12.4	13.5
0.4	3.6	4.8	6	7.2	8.4	9.6	10.8	12	13.2	14.4
0.5	4.5	6	7.5	9	10.5	12	13.5	15	16.5	18
0.6	5.4	7.2	9	10.8	12.6	14.4	16.2	18	19.8	21.6
0.7	6.3	8.4	10.5	12.6	14.7	16.8	18.9	21	23.1	25.2
0.75	6.8	9	11.3	13.5	15.8	18	20.3	22.5	24.8	27

ACTIONS

A new class of cardiac inotropic agent different in chemical structure and mode of action from digitalis glycosides and catecholamines. Similar to inamrinone (Inocor), with fewer side effects. With a loading dose, peak effect occurs within 10 minutes. Continuous administration is required to maintain serum levels. It has positive inotropic action with vasodilator activity. Reduces afterload and preload by direct relaxant effect on vascular smooth muscle. Produces slight enhancement of AV node conduction. Cardiac output is improved without significant increases in HR or myocardial oxygen consumption or changes in arteriovenous oxygen difference. Pulmonary capillary wedge pressure, total peripheral resistance, diastolic BP, and mean arterial pressure are decreased. HR generally remains the same. Primary route of excretion is in urine.

INDICATIONS AND USES

Short-term management of patients with acute decompensated heart failure.

CONTRAINDICATIONS

Severe aortic or pulmonary valvular disease in lieu of surgical relief of the obstruction. Hypersensitivity to milrinone or inamrinone (Inocor).

PRECAUTIONS

Not shown to be safe or effective for use longer than 48 hours. No improvement in symptoms and an increased risk of death have been reported. Use caution in impaired renal function; serum levels may increase considerably. ■ May be given to digitalized patients without causing signs of digitalis toxicity; correct hypokalemia with potassium supplements. ■ May increase ventricular response in atrial flutter/fibrillation. Consider pretreatment with digitalis. ■ Additional fluids and electrolytes may be required to facilitate appropriate response in patients who have been vigorously diuresed and may have insufficient cardiac filling pressure. Use caution. ■ Safety for use in the acute phase of myocardial infarction not established. ■ May aggravate outflow tract obstruction in hypertrophic subaortic stenosis or severe obstructive aortic or pulmonary valvular disease; see Contraindications.

Monitor: Observe patient continuously; monitoring of ECG, BP, urine output, renal function, fluid and electrolyte changes (especially potassium), and body weight are recommended. ■ Monitoring of cardiac index, pulmonary capillary wedge pressure, central venous pressure, and plasma concentration is very useful. ■ Observe for orthopnea, dyspnea, and fatigue. ■ Reduce rate or stop infusion for excessive drop in BP. ■ As cardiac output and diuresis improves, a reduction in diuretic dose may be indicated. ■ Possible risk of arrhythmias. Risk further increased with excessive diuresis and/or hypokalemia. Replace potassium as indicated.

Maternal/Child: Category C: safety for use during pregnancy, breastfeeding, and in children not established. Use during pregnancy only if potential benefit justifies potential risk.

Elderly: Consider impaired renal function; may require a reduced dose.

DRUG/LAB INTERACTIONS

Theoretical potential for interaction with calcium channel blockers (e.g., verapamil [Isoptin]); no clinical evidence to date. ■ May cause additive hypotensive effects with any drug that produces hypotension (e.g., alcohol, benzodiazepines [e.g., diazepam, Versed], lidocaine, paclitaxel). ■ See Monitor.

SIDE EFFECTS

Supraventricular and ventricular arrhythmias including nonsustained ventricular tachycardia do occur. Abnormal liver function tests, angina, chest pain, headaches, hypokalemia, hypotension, and tremor have been reported.

ANTIDOTE

Notify the physician of any side effect. Based on degree of severity and condition of the patient, may be treated symptomatically, and dose may remain the same, be decreased, or the milrinone may be discontinued. Reduce rate or discontinue the drug at the first sign of marked hypotension and notify the physician. May be resolved by these measures alone or vasopressors (e.g., dopamine [Intropin]) may be required. Treat dysrhythmias with the appropriate drug. Resuscitate as necessary.

MITOMYCIN
(mye-toe-mye'sin)

MTC, Mutamycin

Antineoplastic (antibiotic)

pH 6 to 8

USUAL DOSE

10 to 20 mg/M^2 as a single dose. May be repeated in 6 to 8 weeks after adequate bone marrow recovery; see Dose Adjustments. Discontinue drug if no response after two courses of treatment.

DOSE ADJUSTMENTS

Subsequent doses based on posttreatment leukocyte and platelet counts. Withhold dose for leukocytes below 4,000/mm^3 or platelet count below 100,000/mm^3. Adjust subsequent doses based on hematologic toxicity as follows; administer 70% of the previous dose with leukocytes between 2,000 to 2,999/mm^3 and platelet count between 25,000 to 74,999/mm^3 and 50% of the previous dose with leukocytes below 2,000/mm^3 and platelet count below 25,000/mm^3. ■ Lower usual dose range is indicated when used with other antineoplastic drugs and radiation.

DILUTION

Specific techniques required; see Precautions. Each 5 mg must be diluted with 10 ml SW for injection. Allow to stand at room temperature until completely in solution. May be given through the Y-tube or three-way stopcock of a free-flowing infusion of NS or D5W or further diluted in either of the same solutions or sodium lactate ⅙ M and given as an infusion.

Storage: Store unopened vial at CRT. Stable after initial reconstitution at room temperature for 7 days, up to 14 days if refrigerated. When further diluted to a concentration of 20 to 40 mcg/ml, it is stable at room temperature for 3 hours in D5W, 12 hours in NS, and 24 hours in sodium lactate ⅙ M.

COMPATIBLE WITH **(Underline Indicates Conflicting Compatibility Information)**

Consult pharmacist; specific conditions may apply; see Compatibilities, p. xvi.

Additive: Manufacturer states that mitomycin (5 to 15 mg) and heparin (1,000 to 10,000 units) in 30 ml NS is stable at CRT for 48 hours. Other sources list dexamethasone (Decadron), <u>heparin</u>, hydrocortisone sodium succinate (Solu-Cortef).

Syringe: Bleomycin (Blenoxane), cisplatin (Platinol), cyclophosphamide (Cytoxan), doxorubicin (Adriamycin), droperidol (Inapsine), fluorouracil (5-FU), furosemide (Lasix), heparin, leucovorin calcium, methotrexate (Folex), metoclopramide (Reglan), vinblastine (Velban), vincristine (Oncovin).

Y-site: Amifostine (Ethyol), bleomycin (Blenoxane), cisplatin (Platinol), cyclophosphamide (Cytoxan), doxorubicin (Adriamycin), droperidol (Inapsine), fluorouracil (5-FU), furosemide (Lasix), granisetron (Kytril), heparin, leucovorin calcium, melphalan (Alkeran), methotrexate (Folex), metoclopramide (Reglan), ondansetron (Zofran), teniposide (Vumon), thiotepa (Thioplex), vinblastine (Velban), vincristine (Oncovin).

RATE OF ADMINISTRATION

IV injection: A single dose over 5 to 10 minutes.

Infusion: Rate determined by amount and type of solution. Will maintain potency in D5W for 3 hours.

ACTIONS

A highly toxic antibiotic, antineoplastic agent. Cell cycle phase–nonspecific, it is most useful in G and S phases. Interferes with cell division by binding with DNA to slow production of RNA. Rapidly distributed to body tissues and ascitic fluid. Does not cross blood-brain barrier. Metabolized primarily in the liver, but some metabolism occurs in other tissues as well. Some excreted in urine.

INDICATIONS AND USES

Treatment of disseminated adenocarcinoma of the stomach or pancreas. Used in combination with other drugs. May be useful in bladder, cervical, breast, bronchogenic, gallbladder, lung, and head and neck carcinoma and malignant melanoma.

CONTRAINDICATIONS

Not recommended as single-agent primary therapy. Known hypersensitivity to mitomycin, thrombocytopenia, coagulation disorders, increased bleeding from other causes, potentially serious infections, SrCr greater than 1.7 mg/100 ml.

PRECAUTIONS

Follow guidelines for handling cytotoxic agents. See Appendix A, p. 1142. ■ Administered by or under the direction of the physician specialist. ■ Use extreme caution in impaired renal function; see Contraindications. ■ Acute shortness of breath and bronchospasm have occurred within minutes to hours following administration of vinca alkaloids (e.g., vincristine [Oncovin]) in patients who have received mitomycin previously or are receiving mitomycin simultaneously. Bronchodilators, steroids and/or oxygen may be used to treat respiratory distress. ■ Hemolytic Uremic Syndrome (hemolytic anemia, thrombocytopenia and irreversible renal failure) has occurred in patients receiving mitomycin as a single agent or in combination with other agents. It can occur at any time during treatment, but most cases have occurred with a cumulative dose greater than 60 mg. Administration of blood products may exacerbate the symptoms.

Monitor: Monitor WBC, RBC, platelet count, PT, bleeding time, differential, and hemoglobin before, during, and 7 to 10 weeks after therapy. ■ Monitor all patients, especially those nearing a cumulative dose of 60 mg, for unexplained anemia with fragmented cells on peripheral blood smear, thrombocytopenia, and decreased renal function; see Precautions. ■ Determine absolute patency of vein; use of an IV catheter is preferred because severe cellulitis and tissue necrosis will result from extravasation. If extravasation occurs, discontinue injection and use another vein. Elevate extremity and apply cold compresses to extravasated area. Delayed erythema with or without ulceration has occurred at or distant to the injection site. May occur weeks to months after mitomycin administration, even when no obvious evidence of extravasation was observed during administration. ■ May precipitate adult respiratory distress syndrome. Oxygen can be toxic to the lungs; monitor intake carefully and use only enough to provide adequate arterial saturation. ■ Monitor fluid balance; avoid overhydration. ■ Be alert for signs of bone marrow depression or infection. ■ Monitor for thrombocytopenia (platelet count less than 50,000/mm^3). Initiate precautions to prevent excessive bleeding (e.g., inspect IV sites, skin, and mucous membranes; use extreme care during invasive procedures; test urine, emesis, stool, and secretions for occult blood). ■ Prophylactic antibiotics may be indicated pending results of C/S in a febrile neutropenic patient. ■ Prophylactic antiemetics may reduce nausea and vomiting and increase patient comfort. ■ See Precautions and Drug/Lab Interactions.

Patient Education: Nonhormonal birth control recommended. ■ Report IV site burning and stinging promptly. ■ See Appendix D, p. 1148.

Maternal/Child: Avoid pregnancy; may produce teratogenic effects on the fetus. ■ Information on safety in breast-feeding or in children not available; discontinue breast-feeding.

Elderly: Consider diminished hepatic function; monitor for early signs of toxicity.

DRUG/LAB INTERACTIONS

Do not administer live vaccines to patients receiving antineoplastic drugs. ■ May cause shortness of breath, severe bronchospasm, and acute pneumonitis with vinca alkaloids (e.g., vinblastine [Velban]).

SIDE EFFECTS

Alopecia, anaphylaxis, anorexia, bleeding, blurring of vision, cellulitis at injection site, confusion, CHF (patient has usually received doxorubicin [Adriamycin, Doxil]); coughing, diarrhea, drowsiness, dyspnea with nonproductive cough, edema, elevated BUN or SrCr, fatigue, fever, headache, hematemesis, hemolytic uremic syndrome (microangiopathic hemolytic anemia [hematocrit less than 25%], irreversible renal failure [SrCr greater than 1.6 mg/dl], and thrombocytopenia [less than 100,000/mm^3]), hemoptysis, hypertension, leukopenia, mouth ulcers, nausea, paresthesias, pneumonia, pruritus, pulmonary edema, purple discoloration of vein, radiographic evidence of pulmonary infiltrates, rash, renal failure, respiratory distress syndrome (adult), skin toxicity, stomatitis, syncope, thrombocytopenia, thrombophlebitis, vomiting.

ANTIDOTE

Most side effects will be treated symptomatically. Keep the physician informed. All are potentially serious and many can be life threatening. Hematopoietic depression requires cessation of therapy until recovery occurs. Discontinue drug if dyspnea, nonproductive cough, or radiographic evidence of pulmonary infiltrates is present. Discontinue drug for any symptoms of hemolytic uremic syndrome. There is no specific antidote. Supportive therapy as indicated will help sustain the patient in toxicity. Administration of whole blood products (e.g., packed RBCs, platelets, leukocytes) and/or blood modifiers (e.g., darbepoetin alfa (Aranesp], epoetin alfa [Epogen, Procrit], filgrastim [Neupogen], pegfilgrastrim [Neulasta], sargramostim [Leukine], oprelvekin [Neumega]) may be indicated to treat bone marrow toxicity; see Precautions. If extravasation has occurred, L.A. dexamethasone injected into the indurated area with a fine hypodermic needle may be helpful; elevate extremity.

MITOXANTRONE HYDROCHLORIDE

(mye-toe-zan′trone hye-droe-klor′id)

Novantrone

Antineoplastic (antibiotic)

pH 3 to 4.5

USUAL DOSE

Acute nonlymphocytic leukemia: 10 to 12 mg/M²/day for 5 days.

Combination therapy in acute nonlymphocytic leukemia: ***Induction:*** 12 mg/M²/day of mitoxantrone on days 1 through 3 and cytarabine 100 mg/M²/day as a continuous 24-hour infusion on days 1 through 7. Should a complete remission not be achieved, repeat mitoxantrone, 12 mg/M²/day for only 2 days, and cytarabine 100 mg/M²/day for 5 days after all signs or symptoms of severe or life-threatening nonhematologic toxicity have cleared.

Consolidation: After full hematologic recovery, the second course doses may be repeated in approximately 6 weeks and again in 4 weeks. Severe myelosuppression occurred in these subsequent courses. See Monitor.

Other malignancies: 14 mg/M² once every 21 days. Reduce dose to 12 mg/M² in patients with inadequate bone marrow reserve.

Prostate cancer: 12 to 14 mg/M² as a short IV infusion once every 21 days. Used concurrently with steroids.

Multiple sclerosis (MS): 12 mg/M² as an infusion over 5 to 15 minutes. Repeat every 3 months. May be given for up to 2 years or until a cumulative dose of 140 mg/M² has been administered.

DOSE ADJUSTMENTS

Adjust dose based on clinical response and development and severity of toxicity. ■ Clearance is reduced by impaired hepatic function. Treat patients with impaired hepatic function with caution, dose adjustment may be indicated. Specific recommendations not available; see Precautions.

DILUTION

Specific techniques required; see Precautions. A single dose must be diluted with at least 50 ml of NS or D5W. May be further diluted in NS, D5W, or D5NS. Must be given through Y-tube or three-way stopcock of a free-flowing infusion of D5W or NS, or may be diluted in larger amounts of the same solutions and given as a continuous infusion.

Storage: Diluted solution should be used immediately. After penetration of the stopper on a multidose vial, the undiluted mitoxantrone may be stored at CRT for 7 days or refrigerated for up to 14 days. Do not freeze.

INCOMPATIBLE WITH

Manufacturer recommends not mixing in the same infusion with other drugs until compatibility data available, and states that it may form a precipitate if mixed in the same infusion with heparin.

COMPATIBLE WITH

(Underline Indicates Conflicting Compatibility Information)

Consult pharmacist; specific conditions may apply; see Compatibilities, p. xvi.

Additive: Cyclophosphamide (Cytoxan), cytarabine (ARA-C), etoposide (VePesid), fluorouracil (5-FU), hydrocortisone sodium phosphate (Hydrocortone), hydrocortisone sodium succinate (Solu-Cortef), potassium chloride (KCl).

Y-site: Allopurinol (Aloprim, Zyloprim), amifostine (Ethyol), cladribine Leustatin), etoposide (Etopophos, VePesid), filgrastim (Neupogen), fludarabine (Fludara), gatifloxacin (Tequin), gemcitabine (Gemzar), granisetron (Kytril), linezolid (Zyvox), melphalan (Alkeran), ondansetron (Zofran), sargramostim (Leukine), teniposide (Vumon), thiotepa (Thioplex), vinorelbine (Navelbine).

RATE OF ADMINISTRATION

IV injection: A single dose of properly diluted medication over at least 3 to 5 minutes.

Intermittent infusion: A single dose over 15 to 30 minutes.

Infusion: Sometimes a single dose is given as a continuous infusion over 24 hours. Is combined with cytarabine.

ACTIONS

An anthracenedione, a synthetic antibiotic antineoplastic agent. Has achieved complete remissions with a single course of combination therapy. Has a cytocidal effect on proliferating and nonproliferating cells. Probably not cell cycle specific. Inhibits DNA and RNA synthesis. Extensive distribution to tissue occurs rapidly. Partially metabolized. Thought to reduce the number of relapses and slow down progression of MS through its ability to suppress the activity of T-cells, B-cells, and macrophages. These cells attack the myelin sheath around nerve cells, causing the symptoms of MS. Improves the presentation of brain lesions on MRI studies. Half-life varies from 2.3 to 13 days. Slowly excreted in bile and urine.

INDICATIONS AND USES

Treatment of acute nonlymphocytic leukemia in adults. ▪ Treatment of bone pain in patients with advanced prostate cancer resistant to hormones. Used concurrently with steroids. ▪ To reduce neurologic disability and/or the frequency of clinical relapses in patients with secondary (chronic) progressive, progressive relapsing, or worsening relapsing-remitting multiple sclerosis (i.e., patients whose neurologic status is significantly abnormal between relapses). Not indicated in the treatment of patients with primary progressive MS.

Unlabeled uses: Treatment of solid tumors, including advanced breast cancers and hepatocellular carcinoma. Treatment of non-Hodgkin's lymphomas and acute lymphocytic leukemia.

CONTRAINDICATIONS

Hypersensitivity to mitoxantrone or other anthracyclines. Not indicated in the treatment of patients with primary progressive MS.

PRECAUTIONS

For IV use only. ▪ Follow guidelines for handling cytotoxic agents. See Appendix A, p. 1142. ▪ Use of goggles, gloves, and protective gown recommended. Flush skin copiously with warm water should any contact occur. Irrigate eyes immediately in case of contact. Clean spills with 5.5 parts calcium hypochlorite to 13 parts by weight of water for each 1 part of mitoxantrone. ▪ Usually administered by or under the direction of the physician specialist with facilities for monitoring the patient and responding to any medical emergency. ▪ Will cause severe myelosuppression; use extreme caution in pre-existing drug-induced bone marrow suppression. ▪ Except for treatment of acute nonlymphocytic leukemia, therapy generally should not be given to patients with baseline neutrophil counts of less than 1500 cells/mm^3. ▪ May cause acute congestive heart failure. May occur during therapy or months to years after completion. ▪ Use caution in impaired liver function. Clearance is decreased. Patients with MS who have hepatic impairment should ordinarily not be treated with mitoxantrone. See Dose Adjustments. ▪ Use caution if renal function impaired. ▪ Urine and sclera may turn bluish in color. ▪ Acute leukemia, myelodysplasia, and secondary leukemias have been reported in cancer patients treated with mitoxantrone in combination with other cytotoxic agents and/or radiotherapy. ▪ See Monitor.

Monitor: Monitoring of WBCs, RBCs, platelet count, liver function, and kidney function indicated before and during therapy. ▪ Use extreme caution and monitor ECG, chest x-ray, echocardiography, and systolic ejection fraction in patients with pre-existing heart disease, previous treatment with daunorubicin (Cerubidine), doxorubicin (Adriamycin), or radiation therapy encompassing the heart. ▪ Evaluation of left ventricular ejection fraction (LVEF) by echocardiogram or MUGA (Multiple Gated Acquisition) is recommended prior to initiating treatment in patients with MS. Patients with a baseline ejection fraction of less than 50% should not receive mitoxantrone. Repeat evaluations of LVEF are recommended if S/S of CHF develop and prior to all doses administered to patients that have received a cumulative dose of greater than 100 mg/M^2. Mitoxantrone should not ordinarily be administered to MS patients who have received a cumulative dose equal to or greater than 140 mg/M^2 or to those with either LVEF of less than 50% or a clinically significant reduction in LVEF. ▪ Because of rapid lysis of cancer cells, initiate hypouricemic therapy with allopurinol or similar agents before beginning treatment. Monitor uric acid levels, maintain hydration, and alkalinize urine if necessary. ▪ Observe closely and frequently for all signs of bleeding or infection. ▪ Prophylactic antibiotics may be indicated pending results of C/S in a febrile neutropenic patient. ▪ Has nonvesicant properties but extravasation has been reported; may result in tissue necrosis requiring debridement and skin grafting. Phlebitis at the infusion site has also been reported. Should extravasation or phlebitis occur, discontinue injection and use another vein. ▪ Prophylactic antiemetics may reduce nausea and vomiting and increase patient comfort. ▪ Monitor for thrombocytopenia (platelet count less than $50,000/mm^3$). Initiate precautions to prevent excessive bleeding (e.g., inspect IV sites, skin, and mucous membranes; use extreme care during invasive procedures; test urine, emesis, stool, and secretions for occult blood).

Patient Education: Nonhormonal birth control recommended; see Maternal/Child. ▪ Report IV site burning or stinging promptly. ▪ Urine may turn blue-green for 24 hours following administration. Bluish discoloration of sclera may also occur. ▪ See Appendix D, p. 1148.

Maternal/Child: Category D: avoid pregnancy. May produce teratogenic effects on the fetus. Women with MS who are biologically capable of becoming pregnant should have a pregnancy test before each dose of mitoxantrone regardless of other methods of birth control used including birth control pills. ▪ Excreted in breast milk. Discontinue breast-feeding. ▪ Safety for use in children not established.

Elderly: Specific age-related differences have not been identified; consider age-related organ impairment (e.g., bone marrow reserve, renal, hepatic).

DRUG/LAB INTERACTIONS

Additive bone marrow depression may occur with radiation therapy and/or other bone marrow–depressing agents (e.g., azathioprine [Imuran], chloramphenicol, melphalan [Alkeran]). Dose reduction may be required. ▪ Risk of cardiotoxicity increased in patients previously treated with maximum cumulative doses of other anthracyclines (e.g., doxorubicin [Adriamycin], epirubicin [Ellence], idarubicin [Idamycin]), and/or radiation encompassing the heart. ■ Leukopenic and/or thrombocytopenic effects may be increased with drugs that cause blood dyscrasias (e.g., anticonvulsants [e.g., carbamazepine (Tegretol), phenytoin (Dilantin)], NSAIDs [e.g., ibuprofen (Advil, Motrin), naproxen (Aleve, Naprosyn)]). ■ Do not administer live vaccines to patients receiving antineoplastic drugs.

SIDE EFFECTS

Abdominal pain, acute congestive heart failure, allergic reactions (e.g., dyspnea, hypotension, rash, urticaria), alopecia (reversible), altered liver function tests, arrhythmias, bleeding, bone marrow suppression (severe with standard doses), conjunctivitis, cough, decrease in systolic ejection fraction, diarrhea, dyspnea, erythema, fever, GI bleeding, headache, infections, injection site burning, jaundice, menstrual disorders, mucositis, nausea, phlebitis, renal failure, seizures, skin discoloration, stomatitis, swelling, vomiting. Interstitial pneumonitis has been reported. Anaphylaxis has been reported rarely.

ANTIDOTE

There is no specific antidote. Notify physician of all side effects. Most will be treated symptomatically. Blood and blood products, antibiotics and other adjunctive therapies must be available. Blood modifiers (e.g., darbepoetin alfa [Aranesp], epoetin alfa [Epogen, Procrit], filgrastim [Neupogen], pegfilgrastim [Neulasta], sargramostim [Leukine], oprelvekin [Neumega]) may be indicated to treat bone marrow toxicity. Nadir of leukocyte count occurs within 10 days. Recovery is within 21 days. Overdose has resulted in death. Peritoneal dialysis or hemodialysis not effective. Supportive therapy as indicated will help sustain the patient in toxicity.

MORPHINE SULFATE

(mor′feen sul′fat)

Narcotic analgesic (agonist)
Adjunct, pulmonary edema
Anesthesia adjunct

Astramorph PF, Duramorph **pH 2.5 to 7**

USUAL DOSE

IV injection: 2.5 to 15 mg/70 kg. Repeat every 2 to 4 hours as necessary. May be titrated to achieve pain relief with lowest dose (e.g., pain relief in myocardial infarction [1 to 3 mg every 5 min until desired response; AHA recommends 2 to 4 mg every 5 to 30 min]). 10 mg is adequate for most needs. Dose must be individualized based on response and tolerance. 8 to 15 mg is recommended for ***MI pain;*** repeat smaller doses every 3 to 4 hours.

When seeking the required dose to achieve pain relief for an individual patient, increases in increments of at least 25% of the previous ineffective dose are suggested. Lower slightly if pain controlled but patient is too drowsy, or lower dose and increase frequency. Cancer patients suffering with severe chronic pain often require higher doses because of increased tolerance (up to 150 mg/hr has been given). Very high doses (275 to 440 mg/hr) are occasionally used for short periods of time (hours to days) for extreme exacerbations of pain in these drug-tolerant individuals. 1 to 3 mg/kg over 15 to 20 minutes will induce unconsciousness.

Infusion: 1 mg/ml (range is 0.1 to 1 mg/ml) in NS or D5W per controlled infusion device (may be patient activated). ***Based on a 1 mg/ml dilution,*** an initial loading dose may be as high as 15 mg (15 ml). The continuous background infusion to provide a level of pain relief and maintain patency of the vein may range from 1 to 2.5 mg/hr (1 to 2.5 ml). Additional doses averaging 0.5 to 1.5 mg (0.5 to 1.5 ml) may be activated by the patient at selected intervals every 3 to 60 minutes (averaging 10 to 15 min). Additional boluses averaging 1 to 2 mg (1 to 2 ml) may be given by health care professionals (e.g., every 30 min prn). In selected cancer patients all of these doses may be considerably higher.

Open heart surgery: 0.5 to 3 mg/kg as the sole anesthetic or with an anesthetic agent. Cardiovascular function not depressed if oxygen is used and adequate ventilation maintained.

PEDIATRIC DOSE

Usual range is 0.05 to 0.1 mg/kg.

Selected children with severe chronic cancer pain: 0.025 to 2.6 mg/kg/hr (average 0.04 to 0.07 mg/kg/hr).

Selected children with severe pain during sickle cell crisis: 0.03 to 0.15 mg/kg/hr.

Selected children requiring postoperative analgesia: 0.01 to 0.04 mg/kg/hr. Reduce to 0.015 to 0.02 mg/kg/hr in neonates due to reduced elimination and susceptibility to CNS side effects.

DOSE ADJUSTMENTS

Reduced dose and/or extended intervals may be required in impaired renal or hepatic function and in the elderly. ■ Doses appropriate for the general population may cause serious respiratory depression in vulnerable patients. ■ See Drug/Lab Interactions.

DILUTION

IV injection: May be given undiluted; however, further dilution with 5 ml of SW or NS for injection or other IV solutions to facilitate titration is appropriate. May be given through Y-tube or three-way stopcock of infusion set.

Infusion: Each 0.1 to 1 mg is usually diluted in 1 ml NS or D5W and administered via a controlled infusion device that may be patient activated (e.g., a narcotic syringe infuser system). Available in 60-ml ampules containing 1 to 2 mg/ml for direct transfer to syringe infuser systems (Astramorph PF and Duramorph are preservative free and expensive; can be used IV, but are the only choice for epidural or intrathecal injection; see drug literature. Infumorph is **NOT** for IV use). Fluid restriction or high doses may require more concentrated solutions. Concentrations above 5 mg/ml are rarely exceeded. Available in vials containing 25 mg/ml, which must be further diluted before infusion. Also available in ADD-Vantage vials for use with ADD-Vantage infusion containers. Is sometimes added to larger amounts (500 ml to 1 L) of IV solution in selected situations and infused via a large volume controlled infusion pump (requires close titration).

Storage: Store at CRT. Protect from light and freezing.

COMPATIBLE WITH (Underline Indicates Conflicting Compatibility Information)

Consult pharmacist; specific conditions may apply; see Compatibilities, p. xvi.

Additive: Alteplase (tPA, Activase), atracurium (Tracrium), dobutamine (Intropin), fluconazole (Diflucan), furosemide (Lasix), ketamine (Ketalar), meropenem (Merrem IV), metoclopramide (Reglan), ondansetron (Zofran), succinylcholine, verapamil (Isoptin).

Syringe: Atropine, butorphanol (Stadol), chlorpromazine (Thorazine), cimetidine (Tagamet), dimenhydrinate (Dinate), diphenhydramine (Benadryl), droperidol (Inapsine), fentanyl (Sublimaze), glycopyrrolate, haloperidol (Haldol), heparin, ketamine (Ketalar), metoclopramide (Reglan), midazolam (Versed), milrinone (Primacor), ondansetron (Zofran), pentazocine (Talwin), pentobarbital (Nembutal), perphenazine (Trilafon), prochlorperazine (Compazine), promethazine (Phenergan), ranitidine (Zantac), scopolamine.

Y-site: Acyclovir (Zovirax), aldesleukin (Proleukin, IL-2), allopurinol (Aloprim, Zyloprim), amifostine (Ethyol), amikacin (Amikin), aminophylline, amiodarone (Cordarone), ampicillin, ampicillin/sulbactam (Unasyn), atenolol (Tenormin), atracurium (Tracrium), atropine, aztreonam (Azactam), bumetanide (Bumex), calcium chloride, cefamandole (Mandol), cefazolin (Kefzol), cefoperazone (Cefobid), cefotaxime (Claforan), cefotetan (Cefotan), cefoxitin (Mefoxin), ceftazidime (Fortaz), ceftizoxime (Cefizox), ceftriaxone (Rocephin), cefuroxime (Zinacef), chloramphenicol (Chloromycetin), cisatracurium (Nimbex), cisplatin (Platinol), cladribine (Leustatin), clindamycin (Cleocin), cyclophosphamide (Cytoxan), cytarabine (ARA-C), dexamethasone (Decadron), digoxin (Lanoxin), diltiazem (Cardizem), diphenhydramine (Benadryl), dobutamine (Dobutrex), docetaxel (Taxotere), dopamine (Intropin), doxorubicin (Adriamycin), doxycycline (Vibramycin), enalaprilat (Vasotec IV), epinephrine (Adrenalin), erythromycin lactobionate (Erythrocin), esmolol (Brevibloc), etomidate (Amidate), etoposide phosphate (Etopophos), famotidine (Pepcid IV), fentanyl (Sublimaze), filgrastim (Neupogen), fluconazole (Diflucan), fludarabine (Fludara), foscarnet (Foscavir), furosemide (Lasix), gatifloxacin (Tequin), gemcitabine (Gemzar), gentamicin (Garamycin), granisetron (Kytril), haloperidol (Haldol), heparin, hetastarch in electrolytes (Hextend), hydrocortisone sodium succinate (Solu-Cortef), hydromorphone (Dilaudid), insulin (regular), kanamycin (Kantrex), ketorolac (Toradol), labetalol (Normodyne), levofloxacin (Levaquin), lidocaine, linezolid (Zyvox), lorazepam (Ativan), magnesium sulfate, melphalan (Alkeran), meropenem (Merrem IV), methotrexate (Folex), methyldopate (Aldomet), methylprednisolone (Solu-Medrol), metoclopramide (Reglan), metoprolol (Lopressor), metronidazole (Flagyl IV), midazolam (Versed), milrinone (Primacor), nafcillin (Nafcil), nicardipine (Cardene IV), nitroglycerin (Nitro-Bid IV), nitroprusside sodium, norepinephrine (Levophed), ondansetron (Zofran), oxacillin (Bactocill), oxytocin (Pitocin), paclitaxel (Taxol), pancuronium (Pavulon), penicillin G potassium, phenobarbital (Luminal), piperacillin (Pipracil), piperacillin/tazobactam (Zosyn), potassium chloride (KCl), propofol (Diprivan), propranolol (Inderal), ranitidine (Zantac), remifentanil (Ultiva), scopolamine, sodium bicarbonate, sulfamethoxazole-trimethoprim (Bactrim), tacrolimus (Prograf), teniposide (Vumon), thiopental (Pentothal), thiotepa (Thioplex), ticarcillin (Ticar), ticarcillin/clavulanate (Timentin), tobramycin (Nebcin), vancomycin (Vancocin), vecuronium (Norcuron), vinorelbine (Navelbine), warfarin (Coumadin), zidovudine (AZT, Retrovir).

RATE OF ADMINISTRATION

Frequently titrated according to symptom relief and respiratory rate. Side effects markedly increased if rate of injection too rapid.

IV injection: 15 mg or fraction thereof over 4 to 5 minutes.

Infusion: Initial loading dose, basal rate (continuous rate of infusion), patient self-administered dose and interval, additional boluses permitted, and total dose for 1 hour should be ordered by physician. Administer initial dose and boluses at rate for IV injection. For continuous infusion and self-administered dose and interval, note range of ml/hr under Usual Dose.

ACTIONS

An opium-derivative, narcotic analgesic, which is a descending CNS depressant. It has definite respiratory depressant actions. Pain relief is effected almost immediately and lasts up to 4 to 5 hours (mean is 2 hours). Morphine induces sleep and inhibits perception of pain by binding to opiate receptors, decreasing sodium permeability, and inhibiting transmission of pain impulses. Depresses many other senses or reflexes. Relieves pulmonary congestion, lowers myocardial oxygen requirements, and reduces anxiety. Metabolized in the liver and primarily excreted in the urine. Crosses the placental barrier. Secreted in breast milk.

INDICATIONS AND USES

Relief of moderate to severe acute and chronic pain (e.g., postop or cancer pain). ■ Analgesic of choice in pain associated with myocardial infarction. ■ Treatment of acute pulmonary edema associated with left ventricular failure. ■ Preop to sedate, decrease anxiety and facilitate induction of anesthesia.

CONTRAINDICATIONS

Acute bronchial asthma, diarrhea caused by poisoning until toxic material eliminated, hypersensitivity to opiates, premature infants or labor and delivery of premature infants, pulmonary edema caused by a chemical respiratory irritant, respiratory depression, upper airway obstruction. Another source says use is not recommended in acute alcoholism, brain tumor, cardiac arrhythmias, convulsive states (e.g., status epilepticus, tetanus, strychnine poisoning), delirium tremens, heart failure secondary to chronic lung disease, idiosyncrasy to morphine, infection at pump site, paralytic ileus, and uncontrolled bleeding diathesis.

PRECAUTIONS

Use caution in the elderly, in patients with impaired hepatic or renal function, pulmonary disease, and patients on anticoagulation therapy. ■ Use extreme caution in craniotomy, head injury, and increased intracranial pressure; respiratory depression and intracranial pressure may be further increased. ■ May cause apnea in asthmatic patients. ■ Symptoms of acute abdominal conditions may be masked. ■ May increase ventricular response rate in presence of supraventricular tachycardias. ■ Cough reflex is suppressed. ■ Tolerance for the drug gradually increases, but abstinence for 1 to 2 weeks will restore effectiveness. ■ A marked increase in dose may precipitate seizures.

Monitor: Oxygen, controlled respiratory equipment, and naloxone (Narcan) or nalmefene (Revex) must always be available. ■ Observe patient frequently to continuously based on amount of dose and monitor vital signs. Keep patient supine; orthostatic hypotension and fainting may occur; less likely with continuous low doses, but observe closely during ambulation. ■ Uncontrolled pain causes sleep deprivation, decreases pain threshold, and increases pain. When pain is finally controlled, expect the patient to sleep more until recovery from sleep deprivation. ■ Stool softeners and/or laxatives will be required to avoid constipation and fecal impaction, especially with increased doses and extended use. Maintain adequate hydration. ■ See Drug/Lab Interactions.

Patient Education: Avoid alcohol or other CNS depressants (e.g., barbiturates, benzodiazepines [e.g., diazepam (Valium)]). ■ May cause blurred vision, dizziness, or drowsiness; use caution in tasks that require alertness. ■ Request assistance with ambulation. ■ May be habit forming.

Maternal/Child: Category C: safety for use in pregnancy or breast-feeding not established. Benefits must outweigh risks. ■ See Contraindications. ■ Pediatric patients may be more sensitive to effects, especially respiratory depressant effects. ■ May cause paradoxical excitation.

Elderly: See Dose Adjustments and Precautions. ■ May be more sensitive to effects (e.g., respiratory depression, constipation, urinary retention). ■ Analgesia should be effective with lower doses. ■ Consider age-related organ impairment.

DRUG/LAB INTERACTIONS

Alcohol, other CNS depressants (e.g., narcotic analgesics, general anesthetics, antidepressants [e.g., amitriptyline (Elavil), nortriptyline (Aventyl)], barbiturates, hypnotics, sedatives), H_2 antagonists (e.g., cimetidine [Tagamet]), and some phenothiazines (e.g., chlorpromazine [Thorazine]) may increase CNS depression, respiratory depression, and hypotension; reduced dose of one or both agents indicated. ■ Anticholinergics (e.g., atropine) and antidiarrheals may increase risk of constipation or paralytic ileus. ■ Hypotensive effects will be increased with diuretics (e.g., furosemide [Lasix]), antihypertensive agents (especially ganglionic blockers [e.g., guanethidine (Ismelin)]), or hypotension-producing agents (e.g., antidepressants, benzodiazepines [e.g., diazepam], adrenergic blocking agents [e.g., propranolol], calcium channel blocking agents [e.g., diltiazem], calcium, nitroprusside sodium, nitroglycerin). ■ Use with buprenorphine (Buprenex) may negate effects. ■ Concurrent use with rifampin (Rifadin) may decrease analgesic effects of morphine; an alternate analgesic may be required. ■ May antagonize effects of metoclopramide (Reglan). ■ Markedly reduced doses of MAO inhibitors (e.g., selegiline [Eldepryl]) required with opiates. ■ Administration of agonist/antagonist analgesics (e.g., butorphanol [Stadol] or buprenorphine [Buprenex]) to an opiate-dependent patient receiving a pure opiate may precipitate withdrawal symptoms. ■ May cause extended respiratory depression or prolonged blockade with neuromuscular blocking agents (e.g., mivacurium [Mivacron], succinylcholine, tubocurarine). ■ Avoid concurrent use with zidovudine (AZT); may increase toxicity of either or both. ■ After several weeks, hepatic metabolism increases and analgesic effect may decrease in smokers. ■ May potentiate anticoagulant effect of warfarin. ■ Plasma amylase and lipase determinations may be unreliable for 24 hours following narcotic administration.

SIDE EFFECTS

Average dose: Constipation, delayed absorption of oral medications, hypersensitivity reactions, hypothermia, increased intracranial pressure, nausea, neonatal apnea, orthostatic hypotension, respiratory depression (slight), urinary retention, vomiting. Side effects associated with histamine and constipation may be more common with morphine than with most other narcotic analgesics.

Overdose: Anaphylaxis, Cheyne-Stokes respiration, coma, excitation, hypotension (severe), inverted T-wave on ECG, myocardial depression (severe), pinpoint pupils, respiratory depression (severe), tachycardia, death.

ANTIDOTE

With increasing severity of any side effect or onset of symptoms of overdose, discontinue the drug and notify the physician. Naloxone (Narcan) or nalmefene (Revex) will reverse serious reactions. A patent airway, artificial ventilation, oxygen therapy, and other symptomatic treatment must be instituted promptly. Resuscitate as necessary.

MOXIFLOXACIN HYDROCHLORIDE

(moks-i-floks′a-sin hy-droe-klor′id)

Avelox

Antibacterial (fluoroquinolone)

pH 4.1 to 4.6

USUAL DOSE

400 mg once every 24 hours. Dose and duration of therapy are based on diagnosis as listed in the following chart. Serum levels similar by oral or IV route. Transfer to oral therapy as soon as practical; no dose adjustment necessary.

Moxifloxacin Dosing Guidelines		
Infection*	**Daily Dose**	**Duration**
Acute bacterial sinusitis	400 mg	10 days
Acute bacterial exacerbation of chronic bronchitis	400 mg	5 days
Community-acquired pneumonia	400 mg	7-14 days
Uncomplicated skin and skin structure infections	400 mg	7 days

*Due to the designated pathogens.

PEDIATRIC DOSE

Safety and effectiveness for use in children and adolescents under 18 years of age not established; see Maternal/Child.

DOSE ADJUSTMENTS

Dose adjustment is not indicated based on age, gender, or race; in impaired renal function; or in mild or moderate impaired hepatic function (Child Pugh Classes A and B). ■ Has not been studied in severe hepatic insufficiency (Child Pugh Class C) or in patients undergoing hemodialysis or peritoneal dialysis.

DILUTION

Available in ready-to-use latex-free plexibags containing 400 mg moxifloxacin in 0.8% saline. No further dilution is necessary.

Storage: Store at CRT. Do not refrigerate; a precipitate will form. Discard unused portions.

INCOMPATIBLE WITH

Limited compatibility data available. Manufacturer states, "Other IV substances, additives, or other medications should not be added to moxifloxacin or infused simultaneously through the same IV line." Flush line with a solution compatible to both drugs before and after administration of moxifloxacin and/or any other drug through the same IV line. May be administered through a Y-tube or three-way stopcock. Temporarily discontinue other solutions infusing at the same site.

COMPATIBLE WITH

Y-site: Manufacturer lists NS, D5W, D10W, SW, LR at ratios from 1:10 to 10:1.

RATE OF ADMINISTRATION

Single dose equally distributed over 60 minutes as an infusion. Avoid rapid or bolus IV infusion. Incidence and magnitude of QT prolongation may increase with increasing concentrations or increasing rates of infusion. Flush tubing before and after moxifloxacin with a compatible solution.

ACTIONS

A synthetic broad-spectrum methoxy fluoroquinolone antibacterial agent. Effective against a wide range of gram-negative and gram-positive organisms, including common respiratory pathogens such as *Streptococcus pneumoniae*, *Haemophilus influenzae*, and *Moraxella catarrhalis*, and atypicals such as *Chlamydia pneumoniae* and *Mycoplasma pneumoniae*. Bactericidal action results from inhibition of topoisomerase II and IV, which are required for bacterial DNA replication, transcription, repair, and recombination. Mode of action helps minimize selection of resistant mutants of gram-positive bacteria, which cause many respiratory tract infections. Mechanism of fluoroquinolones differs from that of aminoglycosides, cephalosporins, macrolides, penicillins, and tetracyclines, and fluoroquinolones may be active against pathogens resistant to these antibiotics. There is no cross-resistance between fluoroquinolones and these other antibiotics. Widely distributed throughout the body. Concentrations in most target tissues are higher than those found in serum. Half-life is 5 to 17 hours. Partially metabolized in the liver by glucuronide and sulfate conjugation. Excreted as unchanged drug and metabolites in feces and urine. May be secreted in breast milk.

INDICATIONS AND USES

Treatment of adults with infections caused by susceptible strains of microorganisms in conditions, including acute bacterial sinusitis, acute bacterial exacerbation of chronic bronchitis, community-acquired pneumonia (including pneumonia caused by penicillin-resistant *Streptococcus pneumoniae*), and uncomplicated skin and skin structure infections.

CONTRAINDICATIONS

History of hypersensitivity to moxifloxacin or other quinolone antibiotics (e.g., alatrofloxacin [Trovan IV], ciprofloxacin [Cipro], gatifloxacin [Tequin], levofloxacin [Levaquin], norfloxacin [Noroxin], ofloxacin [Floxin IV]).

PRECAUTIONS

For IV use only. ■ Culture and sensitivity studies indicated to determine susceptibility of the causative organism to moxifloxacin. ■ Prolonged use may cause superinfection because of overgrowth of nonsusceptible organisms. ■ Cross-resistance has been observed between moxifloxacin and other fluoroquinolones against gram-negative bacteria. However, gram-positive bacteria resistant to other fluoroquinolones may still be susceptible to moxifloxacin. ■ Prolongation of the QTc interval on ECG has been reported with moxifloxacin. Infrequent cases of arrhythmia (including torsades de pointes) have been reported with the use of other fluoroquinolones; not yet reported with moxifloxacin. The risk of arrhythmia may be reduced by avoiding quinolone use in patients with known prolongation of the QTc interval and in the presence of hypokalemia, significant bradycardia, acute myocardial ischemia, or concurrent treatment with class IA antiarrhythmic agents (e.g., quinidine [Quinidex], procainamide [Procanbid, Procan SR]) or class III antiarrhythmic agents (e.g., amiodarone [Cordarone], sotalol [Betapace]); see Rate of Administration. ■ Use with caution in patients receiving drugs that prolong the QTc interval (e.g., antipsychotics, cisapride [Propulsid], erythromycin, and tricyclic antidepressants). ■ Use with caution in patients with known or suspected CNS disorders, such as severe cerebral atherosclerosis, epilepsy, or other factors that may predispose to seizures. Convulsions, increased intracranial pressure, psychosis, and CNS stimulation have been reported; see Side Effects. ■ Rupture of the shoulder, hand, and Achilles tendons that required surgical repair or resulted in prolonged disability have been reported in patients receiving quinolones. May occur during or after completion of therapy. Risk may be increased in patients receiving concomitant steroids, especially in the elderly. ■ Pseudomembranous colitis has been reported and may range in severity from mild to life threatening. Consider this diagnosis in patients who present with diarrhea during or after treatment with moxifloxacin. ■ See Monitor.

Monitor: Serious and occasionally fatal hypersensitivity reactions have been reported in patients receiving quinolone therapy. May be seen with first or subsequent doses. Emergency equipment must be readily available; see Side Effects. Watch for early symptoms of allergic reaction. ▪ Obtain baseline and periodic CBC with differential. ▪ ECG monitoring for QT prolongation may be indicated in select patients. ▪ Maintain adequate hydration to prevent concentrated urine throughout treatment. Other quinolones have formed crystals. ▪ See Precautions, Drug/Lab Interactions, and Antidote.

Patient Education: Drink fluids liberally. ▪ Report skin rash or any other hypersensitivity reaction promptly. Report fainting spells or palpitations promptly. ▪ Photosensitivity has occurred in patients receiving other quinolones. It is best to avoid excessive sunlight or artificial ultraviolet light. May cause severe sunburn. Use sunscreen and wear dark glasses outdoors. ▪ Dizziness or lightheadedness may interfere with ambulation or motor coordination. Use caution in tasks that require alertness. ▪ Report tendon pain or inflammation promptly. ▪ May produce changes in ECG. ▪ Review medicines and disease states with physician or pharmacist before initiating therapy. ▪ See Precautions, Monitor, Drug/Lab Interactions, and Antidote.

Maternal/Child: Category C: safety for use in pregnancy not established. Benefit must outweigh risk to fetus. ▪ Has potential for harmful effects on breast-feeding infants; either discontinue breast-feeding or choose an alternate drug. ▪ Quinolones have caused erosion of cartilage in weight-bearing joints and other signs of arthropathy in juvenile animals.

Elderly: Overall response similar to that seen in younger patients; however, some ECG abnormalities were reported in elderly patients. ▪ See Precautions.

DRUG/LAB INTERACTIONS

May cause ventricular arrhythmias or torsades de pointes with drugs that prolong the QT interval; see Precautions. ▪ Risk of CNS stimulation and seizures may be increased with concurrent use of NSAIDs (e.g., ibuprofen [Advil, Motrin], naproxen [Aleve, Naprosyn]). ▪ Not metabolized by the cytochrome P_{450} isoenzyme system. Drug-drug interactions with digoxin, glyburide (DiaBeta), itraconazole (Sporanox), oral contraceptives, theophylline, and warfarin have not been observed. ▪ Does not inhibit the P_{450} isoenzyme system. Drugs metabolized by this system (e.g., cyclosporine [Sandimmune], midazolam [Versed], theophylline, or warfarin [Coumadin]) are not affected by co-administration of moxifloxacin. ▪ Digoxin, itraconazole, morphine, probenecid, ranitidine (Zantac), theophylline, and warfarin (Coumadin) have been shown not to alter the pharmacokinetics of moxifloxacin; dose adjustments are not indicated. ▪ Some quinolones may enhance the effects of warfarin (Coumadin); monitoring of PT or INR is recommended with concomitant use. ▪ See literature for additional drug/drug interactions on transfer to oral moxifloxacin. ▪ May cause a false-positive when testing for opiates.

SIDE EFFECTS

Diarrhea, dizziness, and nausea were most common and described as mild to moderate in severity. Capable of numerous other reactions in less than 1% of patients.

Major: Allergic reactions (e.g., anaphylaxis, cardiovascular collapse, death, dyspnea, edema [facial, laryngeal, or pharyngeal], hypotension, itching, rash, shock, urticaria), CNS stimulation (e.g., anxiety, confusion, depression, hallucinations, insomnia, nightmares, paranoia, restlessness, seizures, tremor), hyperglycemia, hypotension, increased intracranial pressure, increased prothrombin, and toxic psychoses have been reported; see Precautions. Pseudomembranous colitis and pain, inflammation, and ruptures of the shoulder, hand, and Achilles tendon have been reported in patients receiving quinolones.

ANTIDOTE

Keep physician informed of all side effects. Most minor side effects will be treated symptomatically or will resolve with continued dosing (e.g., dizziness, lightheadedness); monitor closely. Discontinue moxifloxacin at the first sign of hypersensitivity (e.g., skin rash). Treat allergic reactions as indicated with epinephrine, airway management, oxygen, IV fluids, antihistamines (e.g., diphenhydramine [Benadryl]), corticosteroids (e.g., Solu-Cortef), and pressor amines (e.g., dopamine [Intropin]). Treat CNS symptoms as indicated; may require anticonvulsants (e.g., phenytoin [Dilantin], diazepam [Valium]) for seizures and discontinuation of moxifloxacin. Mild cases of colitis may respond to discontinuation of drug. Treat antibiotic-related pseudomembranous colitis with fluid, electrolytes, protein supplements, and oral vancomycin (Vancocin) or metronidazole (Flagyl). Complete rest is indicated for an affected tendon until treatment is available. Discontinue if photosensitivity occurs. Monitoring of the ECG and adequate hydration are indicated in overdose. No specific antidote. Not known if moxifloxacin is removed by hemodialysis.

MULTIVITAMIN INFUSION

Nutritional supplement (vitamin)

(mul-ti vi′tah-min in-fu′zhun)

Cernevit, Cernevit-12, Infuvite, Infuvite Pediatric, M.V.I.-12, M.V.I. Pediatric

pH 5.9 (Cernevit)

USUAL DOSE

Multiples of the daily dose may be given for 2 or more days in patients (adults and children) with multiple vitamin deficiencies or markedly increased requirements. Individual components may be indicated in specific or long-standing deficiencies. Monitor blood vitamin concentrations to ensure maintenance of adequate levels.

One 5- to 10-ml dose every 24 hours.

PEDIATRIC DOSE

CERNEVIT

Age 1 to 11 years: 2.5 ml/day. Additional vitamin K and vitamin D required.

INFUVITE PEDIATRIC

Less than 1 kg: 30% of the contents of vial 1 and vial 2 (1.2 ml of vial 1 and 0.3 ml of vial 2).

1 to 3 kg: 65% of the contents of vial 1 and vial 2 (2.6 ml of vial 1 and 0.65 ml of vial 2).

Over 3 kg to 11 years of age: Entire contents of vial 1 (4 ml) and entire contents of vial 2 (1 ml).

MVI Pediatric

Less than 1 kg: 1.5 ml/24 hr.

1 to 3 kg: 3.25 ml/24 hr.

Over 3 kg to 11 years of age: 5 ml/24 hr.

DILUTION

Various preparations. Most may be reconstituted with 5 ml of SW or supplied diluent. ***Cernevit*** may be given through the Y-tube or 3-way stopcock of an infusion set after reconstitution. All other preparations must be further diluted in at least 500 ml but preferably 1,000 ml of IV fluids. Soluble in commonly used infusion fluids, including dextrose, saline, electrolyte replacement fluids, plasma, and selected protein amino acid products. Do not use if any crystals have formed.

Pediatric dilution: ***Intuvite Pediatric and MVI Pediatric:*** Each dose should be added to at least 100 ml of dextrose, saline, or other compatible infusion solution. When reconstituted as directed, M.V.I. Pediatric contains no more than 42 mcg/L of aluminum; see Precautions. See Maternal/Child.

Storage: Most preparations should be refrigerated. Protect from light. After reconstitution ***Cernevit*** may be refrigerated for up to 24 hours; immediate use preferred.

INCOMPATIBLE WITH

Incompatibilities may vary with preparation. Direct addition to IV fat emulsions is not recommended. Some manufacturers suggest that admixture or Y-site administration with vitamin solutions should be avoided. ***All formulations except Cernevit must be diluted in infusion solutions.*** Cernevit can be administered through the Y-site.

COMPATIBLE WITH

See Incompatible With. Consult pharmacist; specific conditions may apply; see Compatibilities, p. xvi.

Additive: Cefoxitin (Mefoxin), isoproterenol (Isuprel), methyldopate (Aldomet), metoclopramide (Reglan), norepinephrine (Levophed), sodium bicarbonate, verapamil (Isoptin).

Y-site: ***All formulations except Cernevit must be diluted in infusion solutions before administration at the Y-site.*** Acyclovir (Zovirax), ampicillin, cefazolin (Kefzol), diltiazem (Cardizem), erythromycin lactobionate (Erythrocin), fludarabine (Fludara), gentamicin (Garamycin), tacrolimus (Prograf).

RATE OF ADMINISTRATION

IV injection: ***Cernevit*** is the only multivitamin that may be given by IV injection. Give a single dose evenly distributed over 10 minutes or may be given as an infusion.

Other multivitamins: Give as an infusion at prescribed rate of infusion fluids.

ACTIONS

A multiple vitamin solution containing fat-soluble and water-soluble vitamins in an aqueous solution. Provides B complex and vitamins A, D, and E. Adult multivitamin preparations presently available do not contain vitamin K. ***Infuvite Pediatric and MVI Pediatric*** do contain vitamin K. Provides daily requirements or corrects an existing deficiency.

INDICATIONS AND USES

A daily multivitamin maintenance supplement for patients receiving parenteral nutrition. Provides the necessary vitamins required to maintain the body's normal resistance and repair processes. Used in situations such as surgery, trauma, burns, severe infectious disease, and comatose states which may provoke a stress response and alteration in the body's metabolic demands. Used when oral administration is contraindicated, not possible, or insufficient.

CONTRAINDICATIONS

Known hypersensitivity to thiamine hydrochloride or other product components; pre-existing hypervitaminosis. ■ Contraindicated prior to blood sampling for detection of megaloblastic anemia. Folic acid and cyanocobalamin in formulation may mask serum deficits.

PRECAUTIONS

Do not wait for the development of clinical signs of vitamin deficiency before initiating vitamin therapy. ■ Multivitamins contain vitamin B (thiamine); mild allergic reactions (e.g., sneezing, mild asthma) may intensify to anaphylaxis with further injections. ■ Use caution in patients receiving vitamin A from other sources. Use vitamin A in patients with renal failure with caution. ■ Elevated blood levels of vitamin E may result if doses larger than recommended or oral or parenteral vitamin E are administered. ■ Solutions containing multivitamins may contain aluminum. In impaired kidney function, aluminum may reach toxic levels. Premature neonates are particularly at risk because of their immature kidneys and requirement for calcium and phosphate, which also contain aluminum. Research indicates that patients with impaired renal function who receive more than 4 to 5 mcg/kg/day of parenteral aluminum are at risk for developing CNS or bone toxicity associated with aluminum accumulation. ■ See Drug/Lab Interactions.

Monitor: Monitor VS. ■ Monitor for any symptoms of allergic reaction. ■ Moderate increase in ALT (SGPT) may occur in patients with active inflammatory enterocolitis. Usually reversible following discontinuation of vitamin infusion. Monitoring of ALT levels suggested. ■ Monitor lipid-soluble vitamin levels in patients with impaired renal function. ■ Measure blood vitamin concentrations periodically in patients receiving parenteral nutrition to determine if vitamin deficiencies or excesses are developing. Blood levels of A, C, D, and folic acid may decline in patients receiving parenteral multivitamins as their sole source of vitamins for 4 to 6 months. ■ See Precautions and Maternal/Child.

Maternal/Child: Category C: safety for use in pregnancy not established. ■ Not recommended for use in breast-feeding. ■ Vitamin A may adhere to plastic resulting in inadequate vitamin A administration in the doses recommended in MVI Pediatric. Additional vitamin A supplementation may be necessary, especially in low-birth-weight infants. ■ Polysorbates (a component of some multivitamins) have been associated with E-Ferol syndrome (ascites, cholestasis, hepatomegaly, hypotension, metabolic acidosis, renal dysfunction, and thrombocytopenia) in low-birth-weight infants; however, this has not been reported with the use of pediatric multivitamins. ■ See Precautions.

Elderly: Consider age-related decreased organ function and/or medical problems.

DRUG/LAB INTERACTIONS

Folic acid may lower serum concentration of phenytoin, resulting in increased seizure frequency; monitor serum levels of both drugs. ■ Phenytoin may decrease serum folic acid concentrations; avoid during pregnancy. ■ Folic acid may obscure pernicious anemia and may decrease the patient's response to methotrexate therapy. ■ Pyridoxine may reduce effectiveness of levodopa. ■ Concomitant administration of hydralazine or isoniazid (INH) may increase pyridoxine requirements. ■ Vitamin K may antagonize oral anticoagulants (e.g., warfarin [Coumadin]) reducing their effectiveness; monitor INR/PT. ■ The hematologic response to vitamin B_{12} therapy in patients with pernicious anemia may be inhibited by concomitant administration of chloramphenicol. ■ Thiamine, riboflavin, pyridoxine, niacinamide, and ascorbic acid may decrease the antibiotic activity of erythromycin, kanamycin, streptomycin, doxycycline, and lincomycin. ■ Bleomycin is inactivated in vitro by ascorbic acid and riboflavin. ■ Ascorbic acid in the urine may cause false-negative urine glucose determinations.

SIDE EFFECTS

Rare when administered as recommended: Agitation; allergic reactions including anaphylaxis, angioedema, shortness of breath, urticaria, and wheezing; anxiety; diplopia; dizziness; erythema; fainting; headache; pruritus; rash. Vitamin A and vitamin D hypervitaminosis (symptomatology related to hypercalcemia) may occur with prolonged use of significant doses.

ANTIDOTE

With onset of any side effect, discontinue administration immediately and notify physician. Treat anaphylaxis or resuscitate as necessary.

MUROMONAB-CD3

(mur-oo-mon′ab)

Orthoclone OKT3

Monoclonal antibody
Immunosuppressant

pH 6.5 to 7.5

USUAL DOSE

Do not give initial or subsequent doses unless patient temperature is less than 37.8° C (100° F). Administration of IV methylprednisolone sodium succinate 8 mg/kg of body weight 1 to 4 hours before muromonab-CD3 is recommended to reduce side effects of cytokine release syndrome (CRS) associated with the first two to three doses. Acetaminophen and antihistamines may also be used concomitantly. See Monitor.

Renal allograph rejection: 5 mg/24 hr for 10 to 14 days. Initiate on diagnosis of acute renal rejection.

Cardiac/hepatic allograph rejections: 5 mg/24 hr for 10 to 14 days if rejection has not been reversed by corticosteroid therapy.

PEDIATRIC DOSE

Manufacturer states that it has been used in infants and children at doses less than 5 mg/day. Dose based on immunologic monitoring. Another source recommends 0.1 mg/kg/24 hr for 10 to 14 days.

DOSE ADJUSTMENTS

Doses of concomitant immunosuppressive therapy must be reduced to the lowest level compatible with a therapeutic response during muromonab-CD3 therapy. Resume maintenance doses 3 days before completion of muromonab-CD3 therapy.

DILUTION

May be given undiluted. Must be withdrawn from vial through a low protein-binding 0.2- or 0.22-micron filter. Discard filter and attach needle for direct IV administration. Do not shake.

Storage: Keep unopened vials under refrigeration. May have some fine translucent particles. Will not affect potency, and use of filter will clear.

COMPATIBILITY

Until specific data are available, the manufacturer states, "Other IV medications/substances should not be added or infused simultaneously through the same IV line," and recommends flushing line with NS before and after administration of muromonab-CD3 and/or any other drug through the same IV line. Also states, "Do not give by IV infusion or in conjunction with other drug solutions."

RATE OF ADMINISTRATION

A single dose as an IV bolus in less than 1 minute.

ACTIONS

A murine monoclonal antibody to the T3 (CD3) antigen of human T cells. An immunosuppressive agent that reverses graft rejection by blocking all known T-cell functions. Onset of action is within minutes. CD3-positive cells reappear within several days and reach pretreatment levels in 1 week after daily injections are stopped.

INDICATIONS AND USES

Treatment of acute allograft rejection in renal transplant patients. ■ Treatment of acute rejection in heart and liver transplant patients resistant to standard steroid therapy.

CONTRAINDICATIONS

Hypersensitivity to muromonab-CD3 or any product of murine origin; anti-mouse antibody titer equal to or greater than 1:1,000; patients in fluid overload as evidenced by chest x-ray or greater than 3% weight gain within the week before treatment; history of seizures or patients who may be predisposed to seizures; pregnancy and breast-feeding.

PRECAUTIONS

Usually administered in the hospital by or under the direction of a physician experienced in immunosuppressive therapy and management of organ transplant patients. Adequate laboratory and supportive medical resources including airway management, emergency drugs, and equipment must be available. ■ A protein substance that induces antibodies; use extreme caution if a second course of therapy is needed. ■ May cause lymphomas, skin cancers, or lymphoproliferative disorders. ■ Neuropsychiatric events including seizures, encephalopathy, cerebral edema, aseptic meningitis, and headache have been reported.

Monitor: To reduce incidence of serious side effects, evaluate patients for fluid overload. Must have a clear chest x-ray within 24 hours and have gained no more than 3% above minimal weight present 7 days before injection. ■ Monitor WBC count and differential, circulating T cells as CD3 antigen, and 24-hour trough values of muromonab-CD3 (rise rapidly for the first 3 days of treatment and then average 0.9 mcg/ml thereafter during treatment). ■ Monitor renal and hepatic function. ■ Testing for human-mouse antibody titers is strongly recommended; see Contraindications. ■ Observe for fever, chills, dyspnea, and malaise, which frequently occur 30 minutes to 6 hours after a dose. Symptoms of cytokine release syndrome (CRS) may range from flu-like to a life-threatening shock-like reaction. ■ Anaphylaxis may occur immediately. ■ May be difficult to distinguish between CRS and anaphylaxis. If hypersensitivity is suspected, do not reexpose patient to muromonab-CD3. ■ Increased susceptibility to infection; observe closely. Prophylactic antibiotics may be indicated pending results of C/S in a febrile neutropenic patient. ■ Treat any fever over 37.8° C (100° F) with antipyretics to lower before giving any single dose. ■ See Dose Adjustments.

Patient Education: Side effects from first few doses are expected. Incidence lessens with subsequent doses. ■ Avoid pregnancy; consider birth control options. ■ See Appendix D, p. 1148. ■ Review potentially serious symptoms of CRS. ■ Report difficulty in breathing, swallowing, rapid heartbeat, rash, or itching immediately. ■ Use caution performing tasks that require mental alertness.

Maternal/Child: Category C: safety for use in pregnancy and men and women capable of conception not established. Use only when absolutely necessary. ■ Discontinue breast-feeding. ■ Has been used in children over 2 years of age, but safety not established; monitor closely.

DRUG/LAB INTERACTIONS

Do not administer live vaccines to patients receiving immunosuppressive drugs. ■ Immunosuppressive agents (e.g., azathioprine, cyclophosphamide, corticosteroids, cyclosporine) increase risk of infection and development of lymphoproliferative disorders. Use reduced doses with caution.

SIDE EFFECTS

Cytokine release syndrome (chills, dyspnea, fever, and malaise) is very common with early doses and can progress to shock; incidence lessens with subsequent doses. Anaphylaxis, chest pain, diarrhea, infections (e.g., cytomegalovirus, Epstein Barr, herpes simplex, *Staphylococcus epidermidis, Pneumocystis carinii, Legionella, Cryptococcus, Serratia*), lymphomas, nausea, serum sickness, severe pulmonary edema, tremors, vomiting, and wheezing have occurred.

ANTIDOTE

Notify the physician of all side effects. Most can be treated symptomatically. Pretreat as indicated in Usual Dose to reduce side effects with early doses. Use antipyretics and antihistamines as indicated. Proper patient screening should reduce incidence of pulmonary edema. Shock from CRS may require O_2, IV fluids, corticosteroids, pressor amines (e.g., dopamime [Intropin]), antihistamines (e.g., diphenhydramine [Benadryl]), and intubation. Drug may be decreased or discontinued or other immunosuppressive agents utilized. Resuscitate as necessary.

MYCOPHENOLATE MOFETIL HYDROCHLORIDE

Immunosuppressant

(my-co-fen′o-late mah′fuh-teel hye-droe-klor′id)

CellCept Intravenous

pH 2.4 to 4.1

USUAL DOSE

Used in combination with cyclosporine (Sandimmune) and corticosteroids. IV and oral doses are therapeutically equivalent. Oral form should be used as soon as tolerated by the patient. Initial dose should be given within 24 hours of transplantation. The IV preparation may be used for up to 14 days.

Kidney or liver transplant: 1 Gm as an infusion twice daily (total daily dose of 2 Gm).

Heart transplant: 1.5 Gm as an infusion twice daily (total daily dose of 3 Gm).

PEDIATRIC DOSE

Limited data available; see Indications and product insert. Safety and efficacy not established.

DOSE ADJUSTMENTS

No dose adjustments are indicated in renal transplant patients who experience delayed graft function postoperatively. ■ Avoid doses greater than 1 Gm twice a day in renal transplant patients with severe chronic renal impairments (GFR less than 25 ml/min/1.73 M^2) outside the immediate posttransplant period. ■ Data not available for cardiac transplant patients with severe chronic renal impairment; potential benefits must outweigh risks. ■ Reduce dose or interrupt the dosing cycle if neutropenia (ANC less than 1.3×10^3 [1,300 cells/mm^3]) occurs. ■ Dose adjustment not indicated in impaired liver function. ■ See Precautions/Monitor.

DILUTION

Specific techniques required; see Precautions. Use caution in handling and preparation. Avoid skin contact with the solution. If skin contact occurs, wash thoroughly with soap and water; rinse eyes with plain water.

Reconstitute each 500-mg vial with 14 ml of D5W (500 mg/15 ml). Shake gently to dissolve. Discard if particulate matter or discoloration is observed. To achieve a final concentration of 6 mg/ml, each 500 mg must be further diluted with 70 ml of D5W (1 Gm with 140 ml; 1.5 Gm with 210 ml).

Storage: Store powder and reconstituted or diluted solutions at 15° to 30° C (59° to 86° F). Most desired storage temperature is 25° C (77° F). Reconstituted or diluted solutions are best used immediately after preparation, but the infusion must begin within 4 hours of reconstitution/dilution.

COMPATIBILITY

Manufacturer states, "Mycophenolate is incompatible with other IV solutions and should not be mixed or administered concurrently via the same infusion catheter with other intravenous drugs or infusion admixtures."

RATE OF ADMINISTRATION

A single dose must be given as an infusion over a minimum of 2 hours.

ACTIONS

A hydrochloride salt of mycophenolate mofetil. A potent immunosuppressive agent, inhibiting proliferation of both B- and T-lymphocytes. Has been shown to prolong the survival of allogenic transplants (kidney, heart, liver, intestine, limb, small bowel, pancreatic islets, and bone marrow) and to reverse ongoing acute rejection episodes in animal models. Rapidly and completely metabolized to MPA, its active metabolite. MPA is then metabolized predominantly to its inactive metabolite, MPAG. Secondary peak in plasma MPA concentration is usually noted 6 to 12 hours postdose. Enterohepatic recirculation is thought to contribute to MPA concentrations. Both MPA and MPAG are highly bound to albumin. In patients with renal impairment or delayed graft function, levels of MPAG may be elevated. Binding of MPA may then be reduced as a result of competition between MPAG and MPA. Plasma concentrations of metabolites are increased in patients with renal impairment. Half-life is 11.4 to 24.8 hours. Excreted primarily as MPAG in urine. Small amount excreted in feces. May cross the placental barrier. May be secreted in breast milk.

INDICATIONS AND USES

Used as part of an immunosuppressive regimen that includes cyclosporine and corticosteroids. ■ Prophylaxis of acute organ rejection in patients receiving allogenic kidney, heart or liver transplants. ■ Capsules, tablets, and oral solution approved for prevention of acute rejection in pediatric renal transplant patients.

CONTRAINDICATIONS

Hypersensitivity to mycophenolate mofetil, mycophenolic acid, any component of the drug product, or polysorbate 80 (TWEEN).

PRECAUTIONS

For IV use only. ■ Use caution in handling and preparation. Avoid skin contact of the solution. If contact occurs, wash thoroughly with soap and water; rinse eyes with plain water. Follow guidelines for handling cytotoxic agents. See Appendix A, p. 1142. ■ Usually administered by or under the direction of a physician experienced in immunosuppressive therapy and management of organ transplant patients. Adequate laboratory and supportive medical resources must be available. ■ Use caution; allergic reactions have been observed; emergency equipment and drugs for treatment of severe hypersensitivity reactions must be immediately available. ■ Risk of developing lymphomas and other malignancies, particularly of the skin, is increased. Appears to be related to the intensity and duration of immunosuppression rather than to any specific agent. ■ Oversuppression of the immune system can also increase susceptibility to infection, including opportunistic infections, sepsis, and fatal infections. ■ Has been associated with an increased incidence of GI adverse effects. Use caution in patients with active serious digestive system disease. ■ Use with caution in patients with hepatic insufficiency. Metabolism of MPA may be affected by certain types of hepatic disease. ■ See Monitor, Patient Education, and Maternal/Child.

Monitor: Obtain baseline CBC with differential before treatment. Repeat weekly during the first month, twice monthly for the second and third months, then monthly thereafter. ■ Monitor for neutropenia. Has been observed most frequently in the period from 31 to 180 days posttransplant. May be due to mycophenolate, concomitant medications, viral infections, or some combination of these causes. If neutropenia develops (ANC less than 1,300 cells/mm^3), mycophenolate should be interrupted or the dose reduced. Appropriate diagnostic tests and treatment should be instituted. ■ Monitor patients with severe chronic renal impairment and patients with delayed graft function closely. See Dose Adjustments and Actions.

Patient Education: In women of childbearing age, effective contraception must be used before beginning mycophenolate, during therapy, and for 6 weeks following cessation of therapy. Either total abstinence is required or two reliable forms of contraception must be used simultaneously even in patients with a history of infertility unless due to hysterectomy. Birth control pills may be ineffective. ■ Report any S/S of infection or bone marrow depression (e.g., unexpected bruising, bleeding) promptly. ■ May increase risk of lymphoproliferative disease and some other malignancies. ■ Although most vaccinations may be less effective, the manufacturer suggests that flu vaccinations may be of value. ■ Risk of skin cancer may be increased. Reduce exposure to sunlight and UV light. Wear protective clothing and use a sunscreen with a high protection factor. ■ Cooperation with repeated laboratory tests imperative. ■ See Appendix D, p. 1148.

Maternal/Child: Category C: may cause fetal harm. Avoid pregnancy. A negative serum or urine pregnancy test with a sensitivity of at least 50 mIU/ml within 1 week of beginning therapy is indicated in all women of childbearing age. Contraception required before, during, and after use. See Patient Education. Use during pregnancy only if benefit justifies risk; should pregnancy occur during treatment, discuss the desirability of continuing the pregnancy. ■ Discontinue breast-feeding. ■ Safety and effectiveness for use in children not established; see Indications.

Elderly: No specific recommendations. Consider age-related decreased organ function and/or additional medical problems and medications. May be at increased risk of adverse reactions. Observe carefully.

DRUG/LAB INTERACTIONS

Salicylates (e.g., aspirin) increase the free fraction of MPA. Cyclosporine, digoxin, naproxen (Naprosyn), prednisone, propranolol (Inderal), tacrolimus (Prograf), theophylline (aminophylline), tolbutamide (Orinase), and warfarin (Coumadin) did not increase the free fraction of MPA. ■ Cyclosporine (Sandimmune) may decrease serum levels of mycophenolate. Monitor levels closely when cyclosporine is added or removed from a drug regimen containing mycophenolate. ■ Tacrolimus may increase serum levels of mycophenolate. Monitor serum levels and adjust dose as indicated. ■ MPA has little effect on the binding of digoxin, propranolol, or warfarin but may slightly decrease protein binding of phenytoin (Dilantin) and theophylline, increasing the free fraction of these drugs. ■ Has been administered in combination with antithymocyte globulin (ATGAM), cyclosporine, corticosteroids, muromonab CD3 (Orthoclone). Safety for use with other agents has not been determined. ■ Manufacturer recommends not administering concomitantly with azathioprine. Both agents may cause bone marrow suppression and concomitant administration has not been studied. ■ Use caution with drugs that interfere with enterohepatic recirculation or alter the intestinal flora (e.g., cholestyramine [Questran]). ■ In impaired renal function, acyclovir (Zovirax) and/or ganciclovir (Cytovene) and mycophenolate may compete for tubular secretion, further increasing the serum levels of both drugs, monitor patients closely. ■ Coadministration with probenicid (Benemid) results in an increase in the AUC of MPAG and MPA. Other agents that undergo renal tubular secretion (e.g., acyclovir, ganciclovir) may also result in increased serum levels of mycophenolate. ■ Oral contraceptives may be ineffective, use additional birth control measures. ■ Do not use live vaccines in patients receiving mycophenolate; other types of vaccinations may be less effective. See Patient Education.

SIDE EFFECTS

Principle side effects include diarrhea, infection, leukopenia, phlebitis, thrombosis, and vomiting occur most frequently. Abdominal pain, acne, asthenia, back pain, bone marrow depression (e.g., anemia, hypochromic anemia, leukocytosis, leukopenia, neutropenia, thrombocytopenia), chest pain, colitis, constipation, cough, dizziness, dyspepsia, dyspnea, edema, fever, GI hemorrhage (3%), headache, hematuria, hypercholesterolemia, hyperglycemia, hyperkalemia, hypertension, hypokalemia, hypophosphatemia, infection (a higher frequency of opportunistic infections including TB and atypical mycobacterial infections [fatal infections occurred in less than 2% of patients]), insomnia, kidney tubular necrosis, nausea, oral moniliasis, pain, pancreatitis, peripheral edema, pharyngitis, rash, severe neutropenia (2% to 3% of patients), tremor, and UTI may occur. In renal transplant patients, those receiving 2 Gm/day demonstrated an overall better safety profile than those receiving 3 Gm/day. In addition, arrhythmias, abnormal kidney function, accidental injury, bradycardia, ecchymosis, heart failure, hypotension, increased kidney and liver function tests, oliguria, pericardial effusion, tachycardia, and other side effects occurred in cardiac transplant patients.

ANTIDOTE

Notify the physician of all side effects. Most can be treated symptomatically. Drug may be decreased or discontinued or other immunosuppressive agents utilized. Some side effects (e.g., neutropenia) may require temporary reduction of dosage or withholding of treatment. At clinically encountered concentrations, MPA and MPAG are not usually removed by hemodialysis. However, at high concentrations (greater than 100 mcg/ml) small amounts of MPAG are removed. MPA may be removed by bile and acid sequestrants such as cholestyramine (Questran).

NAFCILLIN SODIUM

(naf'sill-in so'de-um)

Antibacterial
(penicillinase-resistant penicillin)

Nafcil, Nallpen

pH 6 to 8.5

USUAL DOSE

500 mg to 1 Gm every 4 hours. Up to 18 Gm in 24 hours has been used in severe infections.

Endocarditis or osteomyelitis: 1 to 2 Gm every 4 hours.

Meningitis: 100 to 200 mg/kg/24 hr in equally divided doses every 4 to 6 hours (16.6 to 33.3 mg/kg every 4 hours or 25 to 50 mg/kg every 6 hours).

PEDIATRIC DOSE

Children less than 40 kg and over 1 month of age: 50 to 100 mg/kg/24 hr in equally divided doses every 6 hours (12.5 to 25 mg/kg every 6 hours) in moderate infections. 100 to 200 mg/kg of body weight/24 hr in equally divided doses every 4 to 6 hours (16.6 to 33.3 mg/kg every 4 hours or 25 to 50 mg/kg every 6 hours) has been used in serious infections (e.g., osteomyelitis, pericarditis, endocarditis). IM route preferred; rarely used IV in children.

NEONATAL DOSE

10 to 20 mg/kg every 8 to 12 hours or dosing specific to age and weight.

Over 2,000 Gm; age up to 7 days: 25 mg/kg every 8 hours. 50 mg/kg every 8 hours for meningitis.

Over 2,000 Gm; over 7 days of age: 25 mg/kg every 6 hours. 50 mg/kg every 6 hours for meningitis.

Under 2,000 Gm; age up to 7 days: 25 mg/kg every 12 hours. 50 mg/kg every 12 hours for meningitis.

Under 2,000 Gm; over 7 days of age: 25 mg/kg every 8 hours. 50 mg/kg every 8 hours for meningitis.

DOSE ADJUSTMENTS

May need to decrease dose in patients with severe renal and hepatic impairment.

DILUTION

Each 500-mg vial is diluted with 1.7 ml of SW for injection (1-Gm vial with 3.4 ml, 2-Gm vial with 6.8 ml). Each 1 ml equals 250 mg. Further dilute each dose with a minimum of 15 to 30 ml of SW, NS, or ½NS, or other compatible IV solutions (see chart on inside back cover or literature). Concentration should be 2 to 40 mg/ml. Available prediluted and in ADD-Vantage vials for use with ADD-Vantage infusion containers. May be given through Y-tube, three-way stopcock, or with additive tubing, or may be added to larger volume of compatible solutions.

Storage: Refrigerate unused medication after initial dilution and discard after 7 days. Stable in specific solutions at concentrations of 2 to 40 mg/ml for 24 hours at room temperature and 96 hours if refrigerated.

INCOMPATIBLE WITH

Inactivated in solution with aminoglycosides (e.g., amikacin [Amikin], gentamicin [Garamycin]). Do not mix in the same solution. Appropriate spacing and/or separate sites required. See Drug/Lab Interactions.

COMPATIBLE WITH (Underline Indicates Conflicting Compatibility Information)

Consult pharmacist; specific conditions may apply; see Compatibilities, p. xvi.

Additive: ***See Incompatible With.*** Aminophylline, chloramphenicol (Chloromycetin), chlorothiazide (Diuril), dexamethasone (Decadron), diphenhydramine (Benadryl), ephedrine sulfate, heparin, lidocaine, potassium chloride (KCl), prochlorperazine (Compazine), sodium bicarbonate, sodium lactate, verapamil (Isoptin).

Syringe: Cimetidine (Tagamet), heparin.

Y-site: Acyclovir (Zovirax), atropine, cyclophosphamide (Cytoxan), diazepam (Valium), diltiazem (Cardizem), enalaprilat (Vasotec IV), esmolol (Brevibloc), famotidine (Pepcid IV), fentanyl (Sublimaze), fluconazole (Diflucan), foscarnet (Foscavir), heparin, hydromorphone (Dilaudid), magnesium sulfate, meperidine (Demerol), morphine, perphenazine (Trilafon), propofol (Diprivan), theophylline, vancomycin (Vancocin), zidovudine (AZT, Retrovir).

RATE OF ADMINISTRATION

IV injection: Each 500 mg or fraction thereof properly diluted over 5 to 10 minutes.

Intermittent IV: Administration over 30 to 60 minutes may decrease incidence of thrombophlebitis.

Infusion: When diluted in large volumes of infusion fluids, give at rate prescribed.

ACTIONS

A semisynthetic penicillin, used for its bactericidal action against gram-positive organisms, primarily penicillinase-producing staphylococci. Readily distributed into most body fluids and tissues except spinal fluid. Crosses the placental barrier. Primarily excreted through bile; a small amount is excreted in the urine. Secreted in breast milk.

INDICATIONS AND USES

Treatment of infections caused by penicillinase-producing staphylococci.

CONTRAINDICATIONS

Known hypersensitivity to any penicillin or cephalosporin (not absolute).

PRECAUTIONS

Sensitivity studies necessary to determine susceptibility of the causative organism to nafcillin; sometimes difficult to determine accurately. ■ Avoid prolonged use of the drug; superinfection caused by overgrowth of nonsusceptible organisms may result. ■ Pseudomembranous colitis has been reported. May range from mild to life-threatening. Consider in patients that present with diarrhea during or after treatment with nafcillin.

Monitor: Watch for early symptoms of allergic reaction, especially in individuals with a history of allergic problems. ■ Renal, hepatic, and hematopoietic function should be checked during long-term therapy. ■ Test patients with syphilis for HIV. ■ May cause thrombophlebitis, especially in the elderly or with too-rapid injection. Limit IV treatment to 24 to 48 hours when possible. Change to oral therapy as soon as practical. ■ Electrolyte imbalance and cardiac irregularities from sodium content are possible. Contains up to 3.3 mEq sodium/Gm. May aggravate CHF. Observe for hypokalemia. ■ See Drug/Lab Interactions.

Patient Education: May require alternate birth control.

Maternal/Child: Category B: use only if clearly needed. ■ May cause diarrhea, candidiasis, or allergic response in nursing infants. ■ Elimination rate markedly reduced in neonates.

Elderly: Response similar to that seen in younger patients. Consider age-related organ impairment and concomitant disease or drug therapy. See Precautions/Monitor and Dose Adjustments.

DRUG/LAB INTERACTIONS

May be antagonized by bacteriostatic antibiotics (e.g., chloramphenicol, erythromycin, tetracyclines), may interfere with bactericidal action. ■ Potentiated by probenecid (Benemid); toxicity may result. ■ Synergistic when used in combination with aminoglycosides (e.g., amikacin [Amikin], gentamicin [Garamycin]). Synergism may be inconsistent; see Incompatible With. ■ Concomitant use with beta-adrenergic blockers (e.g., propranolol [Inderal]) may increase risk of anaphylaxis and inhibit treatment. ■ Risk of bleeding with anticoagulants (e.g., heparin) is increased. ■ May decrease serum levels and effectiveness of cyclosporine (Sandimmune). ■ Inhibits effectiveness of oral contraceptives; breakthrough bleeding or pregnancy could result. ■ High doses (9 to 12 Gm daily) may decrease serum half-life of warfarin; monitor PT up to 30 days after nafcillin completed. ■ May decrease clearance and increase toxicity of methotrexate. ■ May cause false values in common lab tests; see literature.

SIDE EFFECTS

Relatively infrequent except for sensitivity reactions such as anaphylaxis, skin rashes, and urticaria. Bleeding abnormalities, diarrhea, nausea, pruritus, and vomiting have been reported. Hypersensitivity myocarditis (fever, eosinophilia, rash, sinus tachycardia, ST-T changes, and cardiomegaly) or pseudomembranous colitis can occur. Higher-than-normal doses may cause neurologic adverse reactions, including convulsions, especially with impaired renal function.

ANTIDOTE

Notify physician immediately of any adverse symptoms. For severe symptoms discontinue the drug, treat allergic reaction (antihistamines, epinephrine, corticosteroids), and resuscitate as necessary. Hemodialysis or peritoneal dialysis is minimally effective in overdose. Hyaluronidase (Wydase) has been used to treat extravasation.

NALBUPHINE HYDROCHLORIDE

(nal′byoo-feen hye-droe-klor′id)

Narcotic analgesic (agonist-antagonist) Anesthesia adjunct

Nubain

pH 3.5

USUAL DOSE

Pain control: 10 mg/70 kg. May repeat every 3 to 6 hours. Up to 20 mg can be given in a single dose if required. Maximum total daily dose is 160 mg.

Adjunct to balanced anesthesia: A loading dose of 300 mcg (0.3 mg) to 3 mg/kg over 10 to 15 minutes. Maintain desired level of balanced anesthesia with 250 to 500 mcg (0.25 to 0.5 mg)/kg as required. Administered only under the direction of the anesthesiologist.

DOSE ADJUSTMENTS

Reduce dose to one fourth if previous medication a narcotic. Observe for symptoms of withdrawal. Increase to effective dose gradually. ■ Reduced dose may be required in the elderly or debilitated; in impaired liver or renal function; in patients with limited pulmonary reserve; and in the presence of other CNS depressants. ■ See Drug/Lab Interactions.

DILUTION

May be given undiluted.

Storage: Store at CRT. Avoid freezing and/or prolonged exposure to light.

INCOMPATIBLE WITH

Manufacturer lists nafcillin (Nafcil) and ketorolac (Toradol).

COMPATIBLE WITH

(Underline Indicates Conflicting Compatibility Information)

Consult pharmacist; specific conditions may apply; see Compatibilities, p. xvi.

Syringe: Atropine, cimetidine (Tagamet), diphenhydramine (Benadryl), droperidol (Inapsine), glycopyrrolate, lidocaine, midazolam (Versed), prochlorperazine (Compazine), <u>promethazine (Phenergan)</u>, ranitidine (Zantac), scopolamine.

Y-site: Amifostine (Ethyol), aztreonam (Azactam), cisatracurium (Nimbex), cladribine (Leustatin), D5NS, D10W, etoposide phosphate (Etopophos), filgrastim (Neupogen), fludarabine (Fludara), gatifloxacin (Tequin), gemcitabine (Gemzar), granisetron (Kytril), hetastarch in electrolytes (Hextend), LR, linezolid (Zyvox), melphalan (Alkeran), NS, paclitaxel (Taxol), propofol (Diprivan), remifentanil (Ultiva), teniposide (Vumon), thiotepa (Thioplex), vinorelbine (Navelbine).

RATE OF ADMINISTRATION

Pain control: Each 10 mg or fraction thereof over 3 to 5 minutes. Frequently titrated according to symptom relief and respiratory rate.

Anesthesia adjunct: See Usual Dose.

ACTIONS

A synthetic narcotic agonist-antagonist analgesic. It equals morphine in analgesic effect and has one fourth the antagonist effect of naloxone. Does produce respiratory depression, but this does not increase markedly with increased doses. Pain relief is effected in 2 to 3 minutes and lasts about 3 to 6 hours. Metabolized in the liver. Some excretion in urine. Crosses the placental barrier. Secreted in breast milk.

INDICATIONS AND USES

Relief of moderate to severe pain. ■ Preoperative analgesia. ■ Surgical anesthesia supplement. ■ Obstetric analgesia during labor.

Unlabeled uses: 10 mg SC to reduce pruritus from epidural morphine.

CONTRAINDICATIONS

Hypersensitivity to nalbuphine or its components (may contain sulfites).

PRECAUTIONS

May precipitate withdrawal symptoms if stopped too quickly after prolonged use or if patient has been on opiates. ■ Use caution in respiratory depression or difficulty from any source: head injury, increased intracranial pressure, biliary surgery, history of drug abuse, the elderly or debilitated, and in impaired liver or kidney function. Reduced doses may be indicated. ■ Use caution in patients with myocardial infarction or compromised cardiac function; effect on heart not fully evaluated.

Monitor: Naloxone (Narcan), oxygen, and controlled respiratory equipment must be available. ■ Observe frequently; monitor vital signs. ■ Keep patient supine to minimize side effects; orthostatic hypotension and fainting may occur. Observe closely during ambulation. ■ Pain control usually more effective with routinely administered doses. Determine appropriate interval through clinical assessment ■ See Drug/Lab Interactions.

Patient Education: Avoid use of alcohol or other CNS depressants (e.g., antihistamines, diazepam [Valium]). ■ Request assistance for ambulation. ■ Use caution performing any task that requires alertness; may cause dizziness, euphoria, and sedation. ■ May be habit forming.

Maternal/Child: Category C: safety for use in pregnancy or breast-feeding not established. ■ Has been used safely during labor and delivery of term infants, but use caution during labor and delivery of premature infants. ■ Not recommended for children under 18 years of age.

Elderly: May be more sensitive to effects (e.g., respiratory depression, constipation, dizziness, urinary retention). ■ Analgesia should be effective with lower doses. ■ Consider age-related organ impairment.

DRUG/LAB INTERACTIONS

Potentiated by cimetidine (Tagamet), phenothiazines (e.g., chlorpromazine [Thorazine]), by other CNS depressants such as narcotic analgesics, general anesthetics, alcohol, anticholinergics, antihistamines, barbiturates, hypnotics, neuromuscular blocking agents (e.g., mivacurium [Mivacron]), psychotropic agents, and sedatives. Reduced doses of both drugs may be indicated. ■ May decrease analgesic effects of other narcotics; avoid concurrent use. ■ Plasma amylase and lipase determinations may be unreliable for 24 hours following narcotic administration.

SIDE EFFECTS

Anaphylaxis, blurred vision, bradycardia, clammy skin, dizziness, dry mouth, headache, hypertension, hypotension, nausea, psychotomimetic effect (symptoms resembling a psychosis), respiratory depression, sedation, symptoms associated with histamine release, tachycardia, urinary urgency, vertigo, vomiting.

ANTIDOTE

With increasing severity of any side effect or onset of symptoms of overdose, discontinue the drug and notify the physician. Naloxone hydrochloride (Narcan) will reverse severe reactions. A patent airway, artificial ventilation, oxygen therapy, and other symptomatic treatment must be instituted promptly.

NALMEFENE HYDROCHLORIDE

(nal′me-feen hye-droe-klor′id)

Antidote
Narcotic antagonist

Revex

pH 3.9

USUAL DOSE

Manage known or suspected narcotic overdose: nonopioid dependent: (fully reversing dose) 0.5 mg/70 kg. May be followed by 1 mg/70 kg in 2 to 5 minutes if indicated. If no clinical response, additional nalmefene is not indicated.

Suspicion of opioid dependency: Begin with a challenge dose of 0.1 mg/70 kg. If no evidence of withdrawal (e.g., abdominal cramps, anxiety, chills, diaphoresis, gooseflesh, joint pain, myalgia, restlessness, rhinorrhea, vomiting, yawning) in 2 minutes, follow dose recommendations for nonopioid dependent.

Reverse postoperative narcotic depression: (partially reversing dose) 0.25 mcg/kg. Repeat at 2- to 5-minute intervals until ventilation is adequate and the patient is alert without significant pain or discomfort. A total dose above 1 mcg/kg does not provide additional therapeutic effect.

Nalmefene Guidelines for Reversal of Postoperative Opioid Depression

Body Weight	ml of Nalmefene 100 mcg/ml Solution
50 kg	0.125
60 kg	0.15
70 kg	0.175
80 kg	0.2
90 kg	0.225
100 kg	0.25

PEDIATRIC DOSE

Safety for use in children and neonates not established.

DOSE ADJUSTMENTS

Reduce dose to 0.1 mcg/kg if reversing postoperative narcotic depression in a patient known to be at increased cardiovascular risk. Increments should also be reduced to 0.1 mcg/kg. ■ Reduced doses not indicated for single episodes of reversal in impaired hepatic or renal function or in the elderly.

DILUTION

Available in two concentrations. Blue label contains 100 mcg/ml and is primarily used postoperatively. Green label contains 1 mg/ml and is primarily used to manage or reverse known or suspected narcotic overdose. May be given undiluted except in the postoperative patient at increased cardiac risk (1:1 dilution with NS or SW is recommended).

Storage: Store at CRT.

COMPATIBILITY

Specific information not available; consult pharmacist. May be compatible in solution or at Y-site with D5W, D5LR, D5/½NS, LR, 5% sodium bicarbonate, ½NS, NS.

RATE OF ADMINISTRATION

Give the initial dose over 15 to 30 seconds. Extend to 60 seconds to prevent dizziness and hypertension in patients with renal failure. Titrate subsequent doses required to desired effect.

ACTIONS

A potent narcotic antagonist similar to naloxone and naltrexone. Prevents or reverses the effects of opioids (e.g., respiratory depression, sedation, hypotension) by competing for opioid receptors. Has no narcotic agonist activity. Onset of action occurs within 2 minutes. Partially reversing doses (1 mcg/kg) have a duration of 30 to 60 minutes. Fully reversing doses (1 mg/70 kg) have an elimination half-life of 10.8 hours (naloxone's is 1.1 hours) so the duration of action is as long as that of most narcotics. It provides protection against renarcotization, sustains reversal of respiratory depression, and reduces the need for repeat doses. Actions are dose proportional. Rapidly distributed. Metabolized in the liver and excreted in urine. Probably crosses the placental barrier. Secreted in breast milk.

INDICATIONS AND USES

Management of known or suspected narcotic overdose. ▪ Complete or partial reversal of narcotic drug effects, including respiratory depression, induced by both natural and synthetic narcotics (including propoxyphene, nalbuphine, pentazocine, and butorphanol).

Unlabeled uses: Reverse the systemic effects of intrathecal opioids.

CONTRAINDICATIONS

Known hypersensitivity to nalmefene.

PRECAUTIONS

Use with caution in patients with opioid dependence; may cause acute withdrawal symptoms. ▪ Use caution in patients at high cardiovascular risk or patients receiving potentially cardiotoxic drugs; arrhythmias (including bradycardia, tachycardia, VT, and VF), hypertension, hypotension, and pulmonary edema have occurred with opioid reversal. ▪ With recommended low doses (incremental doses of 0.25 mcg/kg titrated to desired effect) maintenance of opioid analgesia is maintained. Larger doses or fully reversing doses may produce long-lasting antianalgesic effects; use caution in postop patients or surgical outpatients. ▪ Withdrawal symptoms may occur in nonopioid dependent patients if high doses of opioids are used during surgery. ▪ Serious adverse cardiovascular or respiratory effects may occur if opioids are used to overcome full blockade in treatment of withdrawal reactions.

Monitor: Before administration, establish a patent airway. Controlled artificial ventilation with oxygen may be indicated. Establish an IV line. ▪ Monitor vital signs and pupil dilation closely; ECG monitoring may be indicated. ▪ Continue to monitor until no reasonable risk of recurrent respiratory depression. ▪ See Precautions and Drug/Lab Interactions.

Patient Education: Notify physician if pain control medication not adequately effective.

Maternal/Child: Category B: use only if clearly needed. ■ Human studies not available, but was secreted into rat's milk; probably best to postpone breast-feeding for 12 to 24 hours. ■ Safety for use in children and neonates not yet established.

Elderly: No specific recommendations for single episodes of reversal. ■ See Precautions.

DRUG/LAB INTERACTIONS

Propoxyphene, methadone, and levo-alpha-acetylmethadol (LAMM) have longer half-lives than nalmefene; observe patient closely. ■ Reversal of buprenorphine (Buprenex)-induced respiratory depression may be incomplete and require mechanically assisted ventilation. ■ No adverse interactions to this date with benzodiazepines (e.g., diazepam [Valium], midazolam [Versed]), inhalation anesthetics (e.g., halothane), muscle relaxants (e.g., doxacurium [Nuromax]), and muscle relaxant antagonists (e.g., edrophonium [Enlon], neostigmine [Prostigmin]). ■ May be an increased risk of seizures with flumazenil (Romazicon).

SIDE EFFECTS

Incidence of side effects is dose related. Many side effects may be caused by abrupt reversal of the effects of the opioid. Hypertension, nausea and vomiting, and tachycardia occur most frequently. Blurred vision, chills, diarrhea, dizziness, drowsiness, fatigue, fever, headache, hypotension, irritability, pain, paranoia, tremor, and vasodilation may occur. Arrhythmias (including bradycardia, tachycardia, VT, and VF) and pulmonary edema have occurred.

ANTIDOTE

Notify the physician of any side effect. Treatment will probably be symptomatic. Resuscitate as necessary.

NALOXONE HYDROCHLORIDE

(nal-oks′one hye-droe-klor′id)

Narcan

Antidote
Narcotic antagonist
pH 3 to 4

USUAL DOSE

Narcotic overdose: 0.4 to 2 mg. Repeat in 2 to 3 minutes if indicated. The diagnosis of narcotic overdose should be questioned if no response is observed after 10 mg of naloxone. If effective, dosage may be repeated as necessary for recurrence of symptoms.

Postoperative narcotic depression: 0.1 to 0.2 mg at 2- to 3-minute intervals to desired response. Titrate to avoid excessive reduction of narcotic analgesic action.

Challenge test for suspected opioid dependence: 0.2 mg. Observe for 30 seconds for S/S of withdrawal (e.g., abdominal cramps, diaphoresis, dysphoria, nausea and vomiting, rhinorrhea). If no evidence of withdrawal, inject 0.6 mg of naloxone and observe for an additional 20 minutes. Monitor VS and observe patient again for S/S of opiate withdrawal.

PEDIATRIC DOSE

Ampules containing 0.02 mg/ml are available, but larger doses are frequently required. Adult strength is often used to reduce amount of injection and to effect desired response, which may require increased or repeat doses. One source states "up to 10 times a dose has been required."

Narcotic overdose: ***Less than 20 kg:*** 0.01 to 0.1 mg/kg of body weight initially. Based on estimated degree of overdose and respiratory depression. May repeat every 2 to 3 minutes. May dilute with SW. American Academy of Pediatrics recommends 0.1 mg/kg. Manufacturer recommends 0.01 mg/kg.

Over 20 kg or over 5 years of age: 2 mg. Repeat every 2 to 3 minutes as necessary. A continuous infusion may be used after the initial effective dose. Add 75% to 100% of effective dose to a specific amount of IV fluid and infuse evenly distributed over 1 hour. For some overdoses (e.g., methadone) weaning in 50% increments may take up to 48 hours. In other situations 6 to 12 hours is adequate. If symptoms recur, rebolus and go back to 100%.

Postoperative narcotic depression: 0.005 to 0.01 mg IV at 2- to 3-minute intervals to desired response.

NEONATAL DOSE

Neonatal opiate depression: Administration into umbilical vein is preferred. 0.01 to 0.1 mg/kg of body weight initially. Based on estimated degree of overdose and respiratory depression. May repeat every 2 to 3 minutes to achieve a satisfactory response. May dilute with SW. American Academy of Pediatrics recommends 0.1 mg/kg repeated every 2 to 3 minutes. Manufacturer recommends 0.01 mg/kg repeated every 2 to 3 minutes. Another source suggests an initial dose of 0.01 mg/kg. If response is not satisfactory, increase subsequent doses to 0.1 mg/kg.

DILUTION

May be given undiluted, diluted with SW for injection, or further diluted in NS or D5W and given as an infusion (2 mg in 500 ml equals a concentration of 0.004 mg/ml). Discard infusions after 24 hours.

Storage: Store below 40° C. Protect from light.

INCOMPATIBLE WITH

Bisulfites, sulfites, long-chain or high-molecular-weight anions, solutions with an alkaline pH.

COMPATIBLE WITH

Consult pharmacist; specific conditions may apply; see Compatibilities, p. xvi.

Additive: Verapamil (Isoptin).

Syringe: Heparin, ondansetron (Zofran).

Y-site: Gatifloxacin (Tequin), linezolid (Zyvox), propofol (Diprivan).

RATE OF ADMINISTRATION

Each 0.4 mg or fraction thereof over 15 seconds. Titrate infusion to patient response.

ACTIONS

A potent narcotic antagonist. Overcomes effects of narcotic overdose including respiratory depression, sedation, and hypotension. Unlike other narcotic antagonists, it does not have any narcotic effect itself. Onset of action is within 2 minutes. Duration of action is dependent on dose and route of naloxone administration. Requirement for repeat doses is dependent on amount, type, and route of narcotic administration. Metabolized in the liver and excreted in urine.

INDICATIONS AND USES

Reversal of narcotic depression. ■ Antidote for natural and synthetic narcotics (e.g., butorphanol, methadone, nalbuphine, pentazocine, and propoxyphene). ■ Diagnosis of suspected opioid tolerance or acute opiate overdose.

Unlabeled uses: Reversal of alcoholic coma and improvement of circulation in refractory shock.

CONTRAINDICATIONS

Known hypersensitivity to naloxone. ■ The naloxone challenge test should not be performed in patients showing S/S of withdrawal or whose urine contains opioids.

PRECAUTIONS

Does not produce respiratory depression with nonnarcotic drug overdose, a beneficial action. ■ It is ineffective against respiratory depression caused by barbiturates, anesthetics, other nonnarcotic agents, or pathologic conditions. ■ Will precipitate acute withdrawal symptoms in narcotic addicts; use caution, especially with newborns of narcotic-dependent mothers. ■ Use caution in patients with cardiac disease or those receiving cardiotoxic drugs.

Monitor: Symptomatic treatment with oxygen and artificial ventilation as necessary should be continued until naloxone is effective. Observe patient continuously. Duration of narcotic action may exceed that of naloxone.

Maternal/Child: Category B: use in pregnancy and breast-feeding only when clearly needed. Safety for use not established. ■ See Precautions.

SIDE EFFECTS

Elevated PTT (occasional), hypertension, irritability and increased crying in the newborn, nausea and vomiting, sweating, tachycardia, tremulousness. Overdose postoperatively may result in excitement, hypertension, hypotension, reversal of analgesia, pulmonary edema, ventricular tachycardia and fibrillation.

ANTIDOTE

Notify the physician of any side effect. Treatment will probably be symptomatic. Resuscitate as necessary.

NEOSTIGMINE METHYLSULFATE

(neo-stig′meen meth′il-sul′fat)

Cholinergic
Cholinesterase inhibitor
Antidote
Antimyasthenic

Prostigmin **pH 5.9**

USUAL DOSE

Muscle relaxant antagonist: 0.5 to 2 mg. Repeat as required to restore voluntary respiration. 5 mg is the normal maximum total dose. Administer atropine sulfate, 0.6 to 1.2 mg for each 0.5 to 2 mg of neostigmine. Administer in a separate syringe a few minutes before neostigmine. Use caution and monitor pulse rate. Pulse rate must be at least 80 beats/min. Alternately, glycopyrrolate 0.2 mg for each 1 mg of neostigmine can be used and can be mixed in the same syringe as neostigmine.

Treatment of myasthenia gravis: 0.5 mg; titrate carefully; usually given IM.

PEDIATRIC DOSE

Muscle relaxant antagonist: 40 mcg (0.04 mg)/kg of body weight with 20 mcg (0.02 mg)/kg of atropine. An alternate dose regimen is:

Infants: 0.025 to 0.1 mg/kg with atropine 0.0125 to 0.05 mg/kg.

Children: 0.025 to 0.08 mg/kg with atropine 0.0125 to 0.04 mg/kg. Maximum dose is 2.5 mg. Glycopyrrolate 0.2 mg for each 1 mg of neostigmine can be used instead of atropine. See all comments under Usual Dose.

Treatment of myasthenia gravis: 0.01 to 0.04 mg/kg. May repeat every 2 to 3 hours. Usually given IM.

DOSE ADJUSTMENTS

Use extreme caution and minimum effective dose in small children, cardiac disease, asthma, epilepsy, hypothyroidism, vagotonia, peptic ulcer, and severely ill patients. Titrate exact dose; evaluate response with a peripheral nerve stimulator device.

DILUTION

Confirm ampule or vial is for IV use. May be given undiluted. Do not add to IV solutions. May be given through Y-tube or three-way stopcock of infusion set.

Storage: Store below 40° C. Protect from light.

COMPATIBLE WITH

Consult pharmacist; specific conditions may apply; see Compatibilities, p. xvi. Consider specific use and potential toxicity.

Syringe: Glycopyrrolate, heparin, ondansetron (Zofran), pentobarbital (Nembutal), thiopental (Pentothal).

Y-site: Heparin, hydrocortisone sodium succinate (Solu-Cortef), potassium chloride (KCl).

RATE OF ADMINISTRATION

0.5 mg or fraction thereof over 1 minute.

ACTIONS

An anticholinesterase and antagonist of nondepolarizing neuromuscular blocking agents. Inhibits the enzyme cholinesterase, allowing acetylcholine to accumulate at the myoneural junction. Restores normal transmission of nerve impulses and makes muscle contraction stronger and more prolonged. Onset of action is 4 to 8 minutes. Duration of action is 2 to 4 hours. Hydrolyzed by cholinesterases and metabolized by microsomal enzymes in the liver. Excreted primarily in urine.

INDICATIONS AND USES

Antidote for nondepolarizing muscle relaxants (e.g., doxacurium [Nuromax], mivacurium [Mivacron], tubocurarine [Curare]), atropine, hyoscine. ■ Treatment of myasthenia gravis.

CONTRAINDICATIONS

High concentrations of inhalant anesthesia (e.g., halothane, cyclopropane); known sensitivity to bromides and neostigmine, mechanical intestinal or urinary obstruction, peritonitis.

PRECAUTIONS

A physician should be present when this drug is used IV. ■ Has many additional uses given IM or orally. ■ Edrophonium (Tensilon) can differentiate between myasthenic and cholinergic crisis. ■ See Dose Adjustments.

Monitor: A peripheral nerve stimulator device should be used to monitor effectiveness. ■ ***Caution:*** Atropine may mask symptoms of neostigmine overdose. ■ Epinephrine should always be available. ■ Hyperventilate the patient. ■ See Dose Adjustments and Drug/Lab Interactions.

Maternal/Child: Category C: may induce premature labor in pregnancy near term. ■ Transient muscular weakness in swallowing, sucking, and breathing has been observed in neonates of myasthenic mothers. Confirm distinction between cholinergic or myasthenic crisis in neonate with edrophonium test. Treat neonate with IM pyridostigmine 0.05 to 0.15 mg/kg of body weight if indicated. ■ Discontinue breast-feeding.

Elderly: Duration of antagonism of neuromuscular blockade prolonged.

DRUG/LAB INTERACTIONS

Potentiates narcotic analgesics (e.g., morphine, codeine, meperidine) and succinylcholine. ■ Antagonized by ganglionic blocking agents (e.g., trimethaphan [Arfonad], guanethidine [Ismelin], mecamylamine [Inversine]) and aminoglycoside antibiotics (e.g., gentamicin [Garamycin]). ■ May be inhibited by corticosteroids and magnesium.

SIDE EFFECTS

Usually caused by overdose: abdominal cramps, anorexia, anxiety, bradycardia, cardiac arrhythmias and arrest, cholinergic crises, cold moist skin, convulsion, diaphoresis, diarrhea, hypotension, increased bronchial secretions, increased lacrimation, increased salivation, miosis, muscle cramps, muscle weakness, nausea, pulmonary edema, vomiting.

ANTIDOTE

Atropine sulfate. If side effects occur, discontinue drug and notify the physician. Atropine sulfate in doses of 0.6 mg IV will counteract most side effects and may be repeated every 3 to 10 minutes. Endotracheal intubation or tracheostomy is considered prophylactic in anesthesia or crises. Artificial ventilation, oxygen therapy, cardiac monitoring, adequate suctioning, and treatment of shock or convulsions must be instituted and maintained as necessary. Treat allergic reactions with epinephrine. Pralidoxime chloride (PAM) 2 Gm IV followed by 250 mg every 5 minutes may be required to reactivate cholinesterase and reverse paralysis.

NESIRITIDE

(neh-sir'i-tide)

Natrecor

Cardiotonic
Vasodilator

USUAL DOSE

Prime the IV tubing with the diluted nesiritide solution before connecting to the patient and before giving the bolus dose and infusion.

An initial dose of 2 mcg/kg of diluted solution is given as an IV bolus over 60 seconds. Follow immediately with the diluted solution as an infusion of 0.01 mcg/kg/min (0.1 ml/kg/hr); see Dilution and Rate of Administration. Experience is limited in the use of the infusion for more than 48 hours. Use only the recommended dose; see Dose Adjustments and Precautions.

PEDIATRIC DOSE

Safety and effectiveness for use in pediatric patients not established.

DOSE ADJUSTMENTS

Reduced doses are not required in impaired renal function or based on age, gender, race, baseline endogenous human B-type natriuretic peptide (hBNP) concentration, severity of CHF, or concomitant administration of an ACE inhibitor (e.g., enalapril [Vasotec, Lexxel]). ■ During clinical studies, if indicated and after 3 hours had passed, a bolus of 1 mcg/kg was given and the infusion was increased by 0.005 mcg/kg/min in select patients (with central hemodynamic monitoring, a pulmonary capillary wedge pressure [PCWP] equal to or greater than 20 mm Hg, and a systolic blood pressure [SBP] equal to or greater than 100 mm Hg). Bolus and infusion increase of 0.005 mcg/kg/min may be repeated only once every 3 hours to a maximum dose of 0.03 mcg/kg/min; see Precautions. ■ See Antidote.

DILUTION

Each 1.5-mg vial must be reconstituted with 5 ml of diluent withdrawn from a pre-filled, preservative-free, 250 ml plastic IV bag of D5W, NS, D5/½NS, or D5/¼NS. Do not shake. Ensure complete dilution by rotating the vial gently so all surfaces, including the stopper, are in contact with the diluent. Withdraw the entire contents of the vial and add to the 250-ml plastic IV bag used for the initial reconstitution. Invert several times to ensure complete mixing. Yields a concentration of 6 mcg/ml. Withdraw the bolus dose from this final dilution. Use the remaining solution for the infusion.

Storage: Vials should be stored in the carton at CRT or refrigerated (2° to 8° C [36° to 46° F]). Reconstituted vials may be stored at CRT or refrigerated for up to 24 hours.

INCOMPATIBLE WITH

Manufacturer lists bumetanide (Bumex), enalaprilat (Vasotec IV), ethacrynate sodium (Edecrin), furosemide (Lasix), heparin, hydralazine, insulin (regular), and any injectable drug that contains the preservative sodium metabisulfite. Manufacturer states, "Do not co-administer as infusions with nesiritide through the same IV catheter." If an incompatible drug has been administered, the IV catheter must be flushed with a compatible solution (see Dilution) before and after the administration of nesiritide. Do not administer through a heparin-coated catheter (central or peripheral). Binds to heparin and could bind to the lining of a heparin-coated catheter and decrease the amount of nesiritide delivered to the patient.

COMPATIBLE WITH

Specific information not available. Consider specific use; consult pharmacist.

RATE OF ADMINISTRATION

If the IV line has been used to administer other drugs, flush it with a solution compatible to nesiritide before administration and then prime it with nesiritide solution.

IV bolus: A single dose over 60 seconds through an IV port in the tubing.

IV infusion: Use a volume-controlled infusion pump and administer at a flow rate of 0.1 ml/kg/hr to deliver the desired dose of 0.01 mcg/kg/min.

Adjust bolus volumes and rates of infusion by weight according to the following chart.

Nesiritide Weight-Adjusted Bolus Volume and Infusion Flow Rate (2 mcg/kg Bolus Followed by a 0.01 mcg/kg/min Infusion)		
Patient Weight (kg)	Volume of Bolus (ml)	Rate of Infusion (ml/hr)
60	20	6
70	23.3	7
80	26.7	8
90	30	9
100	33.3	10
110	36.7	11

Alternately, the following formulas can be used to calculate the correct bolus volume and infusion rate:

$$\text{Bolus volume (ml)} = 0.33 \times \text{Patient weight (kg)}$$

$$\text{Infusion flow rate (ml/hr)} = 0.1 \times \text{Patient weight (kg)}$$

ACTIONS

A recombinant form of human B-type natriuretic peptide (hBNP). Has the same 32–amino acid sequence as the endogenous peptide produced by the ventricular myocardium. Binds to specific receptors of vascular smooth muscle and endothelial cells, resulting in increased intracellular concentrations of cGMP and smooth muscle cell relaxation. Dilates veins and arteries. Produces dose-dependent reductions in PCWP and systemic arterial pressure in patients with heart failure. Has no effect on cardiac contractility or measures of cardiac electrophysiology (e.g., atrial and ventricular refractory times or atrioventricular node conduction) in animals. 60% of the 3-hour effect on PCWP reduction and 70% of the 3-hour effect on SBP reduction is achieved within 15 minutes. Half-life is approximately 18 minutes. Duration of action may be longer than predicted based on half-life and may be dose dependent. At steady state, plasma hBNP levels increase from baseline levels by 3-fold to 6-fold, with infusion doses ranging from 0.01 to 0.03 mcg/kg/min. Cleared from circulation through three independent mechanisms: binding to cell surface receptors, proteolytic cleavage by endopeptidases, and renal filtration.

INDICATIONS AND USES

Treatment of acutely decompensated CHF in patients who have dyspnea at rest or with minimal activity. Has been shown to reduce PCWP and improve dyspnea.

CONTRAINDICATIONS

Hypersensitivity to nesiritide or its components (a recombinant protein manufactured using *Escherichia coli*). ■ Not recommended as primary therapy for patients with cardiogenic shock or patients with a systolic BP less than 90 mm Hg. ■ Not recommended in patients for whom vasodilating agents are not appropriate (e.g., restrictive or obstructive cardiomyopathy, constrictive pericarditis, pericardial tamponade, significant valvular stenosis), for other conditions in which cardiac output is dependent on venous return, or for patients who may have or are known to have low cardiac filling pressures.

PRECAUTIONS

Safety and effectiveness for use longer than 48 hours not established. ■ Administered by or under the supervision of a physician experienced in its use and in a facility equipped to monitor the patient and respond to any medical emergency. ■ Use caution in patients with allergies; anaphylaxis has not been reported but is possible (a protein substance). ■ May cause azotemia in patients with severe CHF whose renal function may depend on the activity of the renin-angiotensin-aldosterone system. Some patients have required first-time dialysis. ■ Use with caution in patients with a baseline SBP of less than 100 mm Hg; risk of hypotension may be increased. ■ Increased risk of hypotensive episodes of greater intensity and duration with bolus doses larger than 2 mcg/kg and infusion doses ranging from 0.015 to 0.03 mcg/kg/min.

Monitor: Incidence of hypotension is similar to nitroglycerin, but duration of hypotension is longer. Monitor BP closely. Reduce rate or stop infusion for excessive drop in BP; see Antidote. ■ Observe patient continuously; monitor ECG, urine output, renal function, fluid and electrolyte changes, and body weight. Monitoring of cardiac index and PCWP useful. ■ Observe for orthopnea, dyspnea, and fatigue. ■ As cardiac output and diuresis improves, a reduction in diuretic dose may be indicated. ■ Possible risk of arrhythmias. Risk increased with excessive diuresis and/or hypokalemia. Replace potassium as indicated. ■ See Precautions and Drug/Lab Interactions.

Patient Education: Report dizziness or faintness; request assistance for ambulation.

Maternal/Child: Pregnancy Category C: use only if potential benefit justifies possible risk to the fetus. ■ Not known if nesiritide is secreted in breast milk; use caution in women who are breast-feeding.

Elderly: Response similar to that found in younger patients; however, use with caution in the elderly; may have a greater sensitivity to its effects.

DRUG/LAB INTERACTIONS

May cause additive hypotension with oral ACE inhibitors (e.g., enalapril [Vasotec, Lexxel]) and other drugs that may cause hypotension (e.g., antidepressants [e.g., amitriptyline (Elavil)], antihypertensives, benzodiazepines [e.g., diazepam (Valium), lorazepam (Ativan)], magnesium sulfate). ■ Has been administered with angiotensin II receptor antagonists, anticoagulants, beta-blockers (e.g., atenolol [Tenormin]), calcium channel blockers (e.g., diltiazem [Cardizem], verapamil [Isoptin]), class III antiarrhythmic agents (e.g., amiodarone [Cordarone], sotalol [Betapace]), digoxin, diuretics, dobutamine (Dobutrex), dopamine (Intropin), oral ACE inhibitors, oral nitrates, and statins (e.g., simvastatin [Zocor]). No specific effect on the action of nesiritide was noted, but hypotensive effects are additive. ■ Effects of concurrent use with other IV vasodilators (e.g., IV ACE inhibitors, milrinone, nitroglycerin, or nitroprusside sodium) have not been studied, but hypotensive effects would be additive.

SIDE EFFECTS

Hypotension is the primary side effect; may be symptomatic and can be dose limiting; see Antidote. Other reported side effects include abdominal pain, amblyopia (vision impairment), anemia, angina, anxiety, apnea, arrythmias (e.g., atrial fibrillation, AV node conduction abnormalities, bradycardia, PVCs, tachycardia, VT), back pain, catheter pain, confusion, dizziness, fever, headache, hemoptysis, increased cough, increased serum creatinine, injection site reaction, insomnia, leg cramps, nausea, paresthesia, pruritus, rash, somnolence, sweating, tremor, and vomiting. Allergic reactions and anaphylaxis may occur.

ANTIDOTE

Notify the physician of any side effects. Based on degree of severity and condition of the patient; may be treated symptomatically; dose may remain the same, be decreased, or be discontinued. Reduce rate or discontinue nesiritide at the first sign of marked hypotension and notify the physician. Hypotension may respond to a Trendelenburg position and IV fluids (avoid fluid overload). Hypotension may last for hours; observation for a prolonged period may be indicated before restarting nesiritide. After hypotension is stabilized, nesiritide may be restarted; do not administer a bolus dose and reduce the rate of infusion by 30%. Treat allergic reactions as indicated. Treat arrhythmias with the appropriate drug.

NICARDIPINE HYDROCHLORIDE

(nye-card′i-peen hye-droe-klor′id)

Calcium channel blocker
Antihypertensive

Cardene IV

pH 3.5

USUAL DOSE

Must be individualized based on the severity of hypertension and the response of each patient. Blood pressure decrease is dependent on the rate of infusion and frequency of dose adjustments. Gradual reduction based on clinical situation is best. Avoid too-rapid or excessive drop in BP.

To substitute for oral nicardipine therapy: 5 ml diluted solution/hr (0.5 mg/hr) will achieve similar plasma concentration to an oral dose of 20 mg every 8 hours; 12 ml/hr (1.2 mg/hr) to an oral dose of 30 mg every 8 hours; 22 ml/hr (2.2 mg/hr) to an oral dose of 40 mg every 8 hours.

Gradual reduction of BP in a drug-free patient: Initiate therapy with diluted solution at 50 ml/hr (5 mg/hr). May be increased by 25 ml/hr (2.5 mg/hr) every 15 minutes until desired BP reduction is achieved. Do not exceed 150 ml/hr (15 mg/hr).

Rapid reduction of BP in a drug-free patient: Initiate at 50 ml/hr as above, but increases of 25 ml/hr may be given every 5 minutes until desired BP reduction is achieved. Do not exceed 150 ml/hr of diluted solution.

Maintenance: When desired BP is achieved, reduce rate to 30 ml/hr (3 mg/hr). This is the average maintenance rate. Adjust as needed to maintain desired response.

Transfer to an oral antihypertensive agent: The first dose of oral Cardene should be given 1 hour before discontinuing infusion. Initiate any other oral antihypertensive agent on discontinuation of infusion.

DOSE ADJUSTMENTS

Lower doses and slower titration suggested in congestive heart failure and impaired hepatic or renal function.

DILUTION

Each ampule (25 mg in 10 ml) must be diluted with 240 ml of compatible infusion solution to equal a concentration of 0.1 mg/ml. Compatible in ½NS, NS, D5W, D5/½NS, D5NS. Also compatible in D5W with 40 mEq of potassium added.

Storage: Store ampules in carton, protected from light at CRT. Has a light yellow color. Diluted solution is stable at room temperature for 24 hours.

COMPATIBLE WITH

Consult pharmacist; specific conditions may apply; see Compatibilities, p. xvi.

Y-site: Diltiazem (Cardizem), dobutamine (Dobutrex), dopamine (Intropin), epinephrine (Adrenalin), fentanyl (Sublimaze), gatifloxacin (Tequin), hydromorphone (Dilaudid), labetalol (Normodyne), linezolid (Zyvox), lorazepam (Ativan), midazolam (Versed), milrinone (Primacor), morphine, nitroglycerin (Nitro-Bid IV), norepinephrine (Levophed), ranitidine (Zantac), vecuronium (Norcuron).

RATE OF ADMINISTRATION

Must be administered as a slow continuous infusion in a concentration of 0.1 mg/ml (25 mg in 250 ml). Adjust as indicated in Usual Dose and Dose Adjustments.

ACTIONS

The first dihydropyridine calcium channel blocker for IV use. Lowers BP by blocking the entry of calcium ions into the blood vessels. Does not alter serum calcium. Causes coronary and peripheral blood vessels to dilate and relax, reducing systemic vascular resistance. Increases cardiac output, coronary blood flow, and myocardial oxygen supply without increasing cardiac oxygen demand. Reduces BP without significantly affecting cardiac conduction and usually does not depress cardiac function. Begins to reduce BP in minutes; achieves 50% of ultimate decrease in 45 minutes but may not reach final steady state for 24 to 48 hours. When discontinued, can lose 50% of effect within 30 minutes, but gradually decreasing effects persist for up to 50 hours. Effects more prominent in hypertensive than in normotensive volunteers. Extensively metabolized in the liver. Excreted in urine and feces. Crosses placental barrier. Secreted in breast milk.

INDICATIONS AND USES

Short-term treatment of hypertension when oral therapy is not feasible or not desirable. ■ Continuation of hypertensive therapy in chronic hypertensive patients in critical care, surgery, or emergency room.

CONTRAINDICATIONS

Advanced aortic stenosis (reduced diastolic pressure may worsen rather than improve myocardial oxygen balance), hypersensitivity.

PRECAUTIONS

Use caution in patients with coronary artery disease. May cause increase in frequency, duration, or severity of angina. ■ Has improved left ventricle function after beta-blockade. ■ Can lead to worsened failure in congestive heart failure, especially with severe left ventricle dysfunction or use of beta-blockers. ■ Use caution in hypertension of pheochromocytoma; limited experience. ■ May increase hepatic venous pressure; use caution in patients with portal hypertension. ■ Use caution in impaired hepatic or renal function; lower doses indicated. ■ Continue regular dosing on day of surgery and thereafter unless otherwise specified by physician. May cause severe angina or MI if discontinued.

Monitor: Avoid too-rapid or excessive reduction in either systolic or diastolic BP. Monitor BP during and after infusion. ■ If administered via a peripheral vein, change infusion site every 12 hours. ■ Transfer to oral therapy as soon as clinical condition permits. ■ See Precautions and Drug/Lab Interactions.

Patient Education: Request assistance to change position or ambulate.

Maternal/Child: Category C: use during pregnancy only if benefit justifies risk. ■ Discontinue breast-feeding. ■ Safety for use in children under 18 years of age not established.

Elderly: Half-life may be prolonged. ■ May cause drug-induced tinnitus.

DRUG/LAB INTERACTIONS

Not a beta-blocker; when used in conjunction with beta-blockers (e.g., atenolol [Tenormin], metoprolol [Lopressor]), beta-blocker withdrawal must be gradual. ■ Cimetidine (Tagamet) increases nicardipine plasma concentrations; monitor carefully. ■ May alter digoxin plasma levels; monitor serum digoxin. ■ May cause hypotension during fentanyl anesthesia if used concomitantly with a beta-blocker; an increased volume of circulating fluids may be required. ■ Will increase plasma levels of cyclosporine (Sandimmune); monitor and decrease cyclosporine dose if indicated. ■ Plasma protein binding of nicardipine not altered with therapeutic concentrations of furosemide (Lasix), propranolol (Inderal), dipyridamole (Persantine), warfarin (Coumadin), quinidine, or naproxen (Naprosyn).

SIDE EFFECTS

Average dose: Generally not serious and are expected consequences of vasodilation; dizziness (1.4%), ECG abnormality including PVCs (1.4%), headache (14.6%), hypotension (5.6%), nausea and vomiting (4.8%), polyuria (1.4%), postural hypotension (1.4%), sweating (1.4%), tachycardia (3.5%). Many other side effects occurred in less than 1% of patients.

Overdose: Bradycardia, confusion, drowsiness, flushing, hypotension (marked), palpitations, slurred speech. Progressive AV block may occur with lethal overdose.

ANTIDOTE

Keep physician informed of all side effects. Headache, hypotension, and tachycardia have required a reduction in dose or discontinuation of nicardipine. When symptoms subside, nicardipine may be restarted at low doses (e.g., 30 to 50 ml/hr) and adjusted to maintain desired BP. In overdose monitor BP, cardiac and respiratory functions; put patients in Trendelenburg position; use vasopressors (e.g., dopamine [Intropin]) for excessive hypotension. IV calcium gluconate may reverse effects of calcium entry blockade.

NITROGLYCERIN IV

(nye-troe-gli′ser-in)

Antianginal
Antihypertensive
Vasodilator

Nitro-Bid IV, Tridil

pH 3 to 6.5

USUAL DOSE

5 mcg/min initially. Increase by 5 mcg/min increments every 3 to 5 minutes until some BP response is noted. Reduce increments and/or increase time to fine-tune to desired hemodynamic response. If no response at 20 mcg/min, 10 mcg/min increases may be used. Increases of up to 20 mcg/min have been used to achieve desired effect. No fixed optimum dose. Tolerance may develop if administered over 12 to 24 hours.

Unstable angina and congestive heart failure associated with MI: 10 to 20 mcg/min; increase by 5 to 10 mcg/min every 5 to 10 minutes until desired hemodynamic response. AHA recommends an IV bolus of 12.5 to 25 mcg followed by an infusion at 10 to 20 mcg/min.

PEDIATRIC DOSE

0.25 to 0.5 mcg/kg/min initially. May increase by 0.5 to 1 mcg/kg/min increments every 3 to 5 minutes until desired response. See Maternal/Child.

DOSE ADJUSTMENTS

Reduced dose may be required with persistent headache unrelieved by analgesics. Reduce dose gradually when weaning to prevent rebound symptoms. ■ Lower-end initial doses may be appropriate in the elderly based on potential for decreased organ function, concomitant disease, or other drug therapy.

DILUTION

Available premixed in D5W with various concentrations of nitroglycerin. All other preparations must be diluted and administered as an infusion. Use only non-PVC plastic or glass infusion bottles and specific (nonpolyvinyl chloride) infusion tubing (provided by manufacturer). Do not use filters. Dilute in a given amount of D5W or NS for infusion. Concentration dependent on initial preparation (0.5 mg/ml or 5 mg/ml) and patient fluid tolerances. 10 ml of 0.5 mg/ml in 250 ml diluent equals 20 mcg/ml (in 1,000 ml, 5 mcg/ml). 10 ml of 5 mg/ml in 250 ml diluent equals 200 mcg/ml (in 1,000 ml, 50 mcg/ml). See dilution chart below.

Guidelines for Dilution of Nitroglycerin IV for Infusion

Diluent Volume (ml)	Quantity of Nitroglycerin (5 mg/ml)	Approximate Final Concentration (mcg/ml)
100	10 mg (2 ml)	100
100	20 mg (4 ml)	200
100	40 mg (8 ml)	400
250	25 mg (5 ml)	100
250	50 mg (10 ml)	200
250	100 mg (20 ml)	400
500	50 mg (10 ml)	100
500	100 mg (20 ml)	200
500	200 mg (40 ml)	400

May be used in dilutions from 25 to 400 mcg/ml.

Pediatric dilution: 6 mg/kg nitroglycerin in 100 ml D5W at an infusion rate of 1 ml/hr equals 1 mcg/kg/min.

Storage: Protect vials from light. Solution stable for up to 24 hours.

INCOMPATIBLE WITH

Manufacturer states, "Do not admix with any other drug." See Dilution. Non-PVC plastic or glass infusion bottles and nonpolyvinyl chloride infusion tubing is required to deliver accurate dosing with minimal adsorption. Calculated dose will not be correct if other infusion containers or tubing are used because of excess adsorption.

COMPATIBLE WITH

(Underline Indicates Conflicting Compatibility Information)

Consult pharmacist; specific conditions may apply; see Compatibilities, p. xvi.

Additive: ***Not recommended by manufacturer; see Incompatible With.*** Alteplase (tPA, Activase), aminophylline, <u>bretylium (Bretylate)</u>, dobutamine (Dobutrex), dopamine (Intropin), enalaprilat (Vasotec IV), furosemide (Lasix), lidocaine, verapamil (Isoptin).

Y-site: Alatrofloxacin (Trovan IV), amiodarone (Cordarone), amphotericin B cholesteryl (Amphotec), atracurium (Tracrium), cisatracurium (Nimbex), diltiazem (Cardizem), dobutamine (Dobutrex), dopamine (Intropin), epinephrine (Adrenalin), esmolol (Brevibloc), famotidine (Pepcid IV), fentanyl (Sublimaze), fluconazole (Diflucan), furosemide (Lasix), gatifloxacin (Tequin), haloperidol (Haldol), heparin, hetastarch in electrolytes

(Hextend), hydralazine, hydromorphone (Dilaudid), inamrinone (Inocor), insulin (regular), labetalol (Normodyne), lidocaine, linezolid (Zyvox), lorazepam (Ativan), midazolam (Versed), milrinone (Primacor), morphine, nicardipine (Cardene IV), nitroprusside sodium, norepinephrine (Levophed), pancuronium (Pavulon), propofol (Diprivan), ranitidine (Zantac), remifentanil (Ultiva), streptokinase, tacrolimus (Prograf), theophylline, thiopental (Pentothal), vecuronium (Norcuron), warfarin (Coumadin).

RATE OF ADMINISTRATION

Dependent on patient response and effective dose. Specific adjustments required; see Usual Dose. Use extreme caution in patients responsive to initial 5 mcg/min dose. Decrease adjustments and increase time between doses as patient begins to respond. Use of an infusion pump or microdrip (60 gtt/ml) required. Exact and constant delivery mandatory. See chart below.

Nitroglycerin IV Guidelines for Infusion

Concentration (mcg/ml)	50	100	200	400
Desired Dose (mcg/min)	60 Microdrops = 1 ml Flow Rate (microdrops/min = ml/hr)			
5	6	3	—	—
10	12	6	3	—
15	18	9	—	—
20	24	12	6	3
30	36	18	9	—
40	48	24	12	6
60	72	36	18	9
80	96	48	24	12
120	—	72	36	18
160	—	96	48	24
240	—	—	72	36
320	—	—	96	48
480	—	—	—	72
640	—	—	—	96

ACTIONS

A vascular smooth-muscle relaxant and vasodilator. Affects arterial and venous beds. Reduces myocardial oxygen consumption, preload, and afterload by reducing systolic, diastolic, and mean arterial blood pressure; central venous and pulmonary capillary wedge pressures; and pulmonary and systemic vascular resistance. Effective coronary perfusion is usually maintained. Low doses (30 to 40 mcg/min) produce venodilation; high doses (150 to 500 mcg/min) produce arteriolar dilation. Widely distributed throughout the body. Onset of action occurs in 1 to 2 minutes and lasts 3 to 5 minutes. Metabolized in the liver and excreted in urine.

INDICATIONS AND USES

Control of BP in perioperative hypertension (especially cardiovascular procedures). ■ Drug of choice in unstable angina or congestive heart failure associated with acute myocardial infarction. May be used in combination with dobutamine (Dobutrex) 2 to 20 mcg/kg/min to produce hemodynamic improvement while reducing risk of ischemic damage. ■ Treatment of angina pectoris if patient unresponsive to therapeutic doses of organic nitrates and/or a beta-blocker. ■ Controlled hypotension during surgical procedures.

CONTRAINDICATIONS

Anemia (severe), hypersensitivity to nitrates, hypotension or uncorrected hypovolemia, cerebral hemorrhage, closed-angle glaucoma, head trauma, increased intracranial pressure, patients taking sildenafil (Viagra), pericardial tamponade, constrictive pericarditis.

PRECAUTIONS

Special tubing causes problems with infusion pump control. Patient may still be receiving nitroglycerin even though pump is off or tubing clamped. Low flow rates may actually be higher and not deliver accurate dosage. ■ Plastic (polyvinyl chloride) tubing or containers will absorb up to 80% of diluted nitroglycerin. Use extreme caution and adjust dose if changing tubing, using extension tubings, etc. Absorption greatest with slowest rate. ■ If changing preparations from 0.8 mg/ml to 5 mg/ml, use new tubing or clear tubing with a minimum of 15 ml, adjust dose carefully, and observe effects. ■ Use caution in patients with low left ventricular filling pressure or low pulmonary capillary wedge pressure. May have exaggerated response to low dosage. ■ Use caution in hepatic or renal disease, pericarditis, or postural hypotension.

Monitor: Maintain adequate systemic BP and coronary perfusion pressure. HR and BP measurements mandatory; pulmonary wedge pressure recommended. ■ Observe for tachycardia, which can decrease diastolic filling time. ■ Observe for fall in pulmonary wedge pressure. Precedes arterial hypotension and impending shock. Reduce or discontinue drug temporarily. ■ Headache may improve with analgesics or slightly lower dose; usually improves with time. ■ See Drug/Lab Interactions.

Maternal/Child: Category C: safety for use in pregnancy, breast-feeding, and in children not established.

Elderly: Hypotensive effects may be increased. ■ Differences in response compared to younger patients not identified. ■ Lower-end initial doses may be indicated; see Dose Adjustments.

DRUG/LAB INTERACTIONS

May cause irreversible hypotension if given within 24 hours of sildenafil citrate (Viagra). Potentiated by alcohol (may cause hypotension and cardiovascular collapse), antihypertensives, aspirin, beta-adrenergic blockers (e.g., propranolol [Inderal]), other vasodilators, phenothiazines (e.g., prochlorperazine [Compazine]), and tricyclic antidepressants. ■ Inhibited by dihydroergotamine and sympathomimetics (e.g., vasopressors [phenylephrine], bronchodilators, decongestants, glaucoma agents, mydriatics). ■ Inhibits acetylcholine, histamine, norepinephrine. ■ Potentiates nondepolarizing muscle relaxants (e.g., tubocurarine [Curare]); may cause apnea. ■ May cause marked orthostatic hypotension with calcium channel blockers (e.g., verapamil [Isoptin]). ■ May antagonize anticoagulant effects of heparin; monitor. ■ Concurrent use with alteplase (tPA); reduces the thrombolytic effects of alteplase.

SIDE EFFECTS

Abdominal pain, allergic reactions (e.g., itching, tracheobronchitis, wheezing), angina, apprehension, dizziness, headache, hypotension, methemoglobinemia, muscle twitching, nausea, palpitations, postural hypotension, restlessness, retrosternal discomfort, tachycardia, vomiting.

Overdose: Bloody diarrhea, colic, confusion, diaphoresis, dyspnea, flushing, heart block, paralysis, tachycardia, visual disturbances. Severe hypotension may result in shock, reflex paradoxical bradycardia, inadequate cerebral circulation, constrictive pericarditis, pericardial tamponade, decreased organ perfusion, and death.

ANTIDOTE

Notify physician of all side effects. Discontinue if blurred vision or dry mouth occur. For accidental overdose with severe hypotension and reflex tachycardia and/or fall in pulmonary wedge pressure, reduce rate or temporarily discontinue until condition stabilizes. Lower head of bed (Trendelenburg position). Administer IV fluids. Use O_2 and assisted ventilation if indicated. An alpha-adrenergic agonist (methoxamine [Vasoxyl] or phenylephrine [Neo-Synephrine]) is rarely required. Epinephrine and related compounds (dopamine) are contraindicated. Monitor levels and treat methemoglobinemia if indicated with methylene blue 0.2 ml/kg of body weight (1 to 2 mg/kg) IV and high-flow oxygen. Treat anaphylaxis and resuscitate as necessary.

NITROPRUSSIDE SODIUM

(nye-troh-prus′eyed so′de-um)

Antihypertensive
Vasodilator

pH 3.5 to 6

USUAL DOSE

Begin with 0.3 mcg/kg of body weight/min. Under continuous BP monitoring, titrate upward very gradually (small increments every 2 to 3 minutes). 3 mcg/kg/min is the average effective dose; range is 0.1 to 5 mcg/kg/min. AHA guidelines recommend beginning with 0.1 mcg/kg/min. Titrate upward every 3 to 5 minutes to desired effect (up to 5 mcg/kg/min). Small adjustments can lead to major fluctuations in BP. Never exceed 10 mcg/kg/min. If 10 mcg/kg/min does not promote adequate BP reduction in 10 minutes, discontinue administration and use another antihypertensive agent. Cyanide toxicity can occur with as little as 2 mcg/kg/min and could begin to occur after 10 minutes at the maximum dose.

Acute CHF: Titrate as above until one of the following occurs: cardiac output is no longer increasing, perfusion of vital organs would be compromised by further reduction of BP, or maximum infusion rate (10 mcg/kg/min) is reached.

PEDIATRIC DOSE

Begin with 0.3 mcg/kg/min. Adjust slowly to individual response as in Usual Dose. AHA guidelines recommend 1 mcg/kg/min initially. Titrate as needed up to 8 mcg/kg/min.

DOSE ADJUSTMENTS

Average effective dose may be as little as 0.5 mcg/kg/min in patients who are receiving other antihypertensive agents by any route. ■ Reduced dose may be required in the elderly.

DILUTION

Available in a liquid formulation (25 mg/ml), or each 50 mg must be reconstituted with 2 to 3 ml of D5W or SW for injection without a preservative. Further dilute in a minimum of 250 ml of D5W (manufacturer's recommendation). JAMA suggests NS may be used. Must be administered as an infusion. Larger amounts of solution may be used. 50 mg in 250 ml equals 200 mcg/ml. 50 mg in 500 ml equals 100 mcg/ml. Immediately after mixing, wrap infusion bottle in opaque material (e.g., aluminum foil) to protect from light. Use only freshly prepared solutions; usually discard infusion within 4 hours of mixing. (Literature now states, "Stable for 24 hours if properly protected.") ■ Solution has a faint brownish tint; discard immediately if highly colored, blue, green, or dark red. **Pediatric dilution:** Add 0.6 mg/kg to 100 ml diluent. 1 ml/hr equals 0.1 mcg/kg/min.

COMPATIBLE WITH **(Underline Indicates Conflicting Compatibility Information)**

Consult pharmacist; specific conditions may apply; see Compatibilities, p. xvi.

Additive: Cimetidine (Tagamet), enalaprilat (Vasotec IV), esmolol (Brevibloc), ranitidine (Zantac), verapamil (Isoptin).

Syringe: Heparin.

Y-site: Atracurium (Tracrium), cisatracurium (Nimbex), diltiazem (Cardizem), dobutamine (Dobutrex), dopamine (Intropin), enalaprilat (Vasotec IV), esmolol (Brevibloc), famotidine (Pepcid IV), haloperidol (Haldol), heparin, hetastarch in electrolytes (Hextend), inamrinone (Inocor), indomethacin (Indocin), insulin (regular), labetalol (Normodyne), lidocaine, midazolam (Versed), milrinone (Primacor), morphine, nitroglycerin (Nitro-Bid IV), pancuronium (Pavulon), propofol (Diprivan), tacrolimus (Prograf), theophylline, vecuronium (Norcuron).

RATE OF ADMINISTRATION

Use of an infusion pump (volumetric preferred) required to regulate dose accurately. Increase mcg/kg/min rate as outlined in Usual Dose to reduce BP gradually to preset or desired levels. Do not exceed maximum dose. Response should be noted almost immediately. Manufacturer provides an infusion rate chart in ml/hr to achieve initial (0.3 mcg/kg/min) and maximal (10 mcg/kg/min) for 50-, 100-, and 200-mcg/ml dilutions.

Nitroprusside Sodium Guidelines for Infusion							
Volume		250 ml		500 ml		1,000 ml	
Nitroprusside Sodium		50 mg		50 mg		50 mg	
Injection Concentration		200 mcg/ml		100 mcg/ml		50 mcg/ml	
Patient Weight		Infusion Rate (ml/hr)					
kg	lbs	Initial	Maximal	Initial	Maximal	Initial	Maximal
10	22	1	30	2	60	4	120
20	44	2	60	4	120	7	240
30	66	3	90	5	180	11	360
40	88	4	120	7	240	14	480
50	110	5	150	9	300	18	600
60	132	5	180	11	360	22	720
70	154	6	210	13	420	25	840
80	176	7	240	14	480	29	960
90	198	8	270	16	540	32	1,080
100	220	9	300	18	600	36	1,200

ACTIONS

A potent, rapid-acting antihypertensive agent. Produces peripheral vasodilation through direct action on smooth muscle of the blood vessels. Effective almost immediately. Will lower diastolic BP 30% to 40% or more below pretreatment levels. May increase HR and/or cardiac output slightly. Effectiveness ends when IV infusion is stopped. BP will return to pretreatment levels in 1 to 10 minutes. Rapidly converted to thiocyanate and eventually excreted in the urine.

INDICATIONS AND USES

Drug of choice for hypertensive emergencies. ■ Cardiogenic shock. ■ Controlled hypotension during surgery. ■ Acute congestive heart failure. **Unlabeled uses:** In combination with dopamine to reduce afterload in hypertensive patient with myocardial infarction. ■ Treatment of left ventricular failure in combination with oxygen, morphine, and a loop diuretic.

CONTRAINDICATIONS

Compensatory hypertension, e.g., arteriovenous shunt or coarctation of the aorta; known inadequate cerebral circulation; emergency surgery on moribund patients.

PRECAUTIONS

Use only when adequate personnel and appropriate equipment are available for continuous monitoring. ■ Precipitous decreases in BP can occur quickly. Can lead to irreversible ischemic injuries or death. ■ Cyanide toxicity can occur with doses less than the average effective dose and will begin to occur as the maximum dose of 10 mcg/kg/min is approached. May be rapid, serious, and lethal. ■ Methemoglobinemia may begin to occur within 16 hours if larger doses are required. ■ Use caution in hypothyroidism, increased intracranial pressure, liver or renal impairment, and the elderly. ■ May increase ischemia in myocardial infarction.

Monitor: Determine patency of vein; avoid extravasation. ■ Continuous automatic BP monitoring is mandatory (intraarterial pressure sensor preferred). Never allow systolic BP to fall below 60 mm Hg. ■ Monitor pulmonary wedge pressure in patients with myocardial infarction or severe congestive heart failure. ■ Oral antihypertensive agents may be given concomitantly to maintain ongoing BP regulation. Reduced nitroprusside sodium dose may be indicated; see Dose Adjustments. ■ Measure blood thiocyanate levels daily if dose is 3 mcg/kg/min (1 mcg/kg/min in the anuric patient). Desired level of steady-state thiocyanate is less than 1 mmol/L. Coadministration of sodium thiosulfate in doses 5 to 10 times that of nitroprusside sodium has been used to avoid toxicity with larger doses or necessary long-term therapy. May potentiate hypotensive action; use with extreme caution. ■ In controlled hypotension, monitor blood loss and correct hypovolemia before and during surgery. ■ Persistent hypotension (lasting more than 1 to 10 minutes) after nitroprusside sodium is discontinued is due to another source. Monitor for sodium retention.

Patient Education: Report IV site burning or stinging promptly. ■ Request assistance to ambulate.

Maternal/Child: Category C: safety for use in pregnancy and in children not yet established. Has caused cyanide toxicity in fetuses of ewes, but not in humans. ■ Discontinue breast-feeding.

Elderly: See Dose Adjustments and Precautions. ■ Hypotensive effects may be increased. ■ Consider age-related renal impairment.

DRUG/LAB INTERACTIONS

Potentiated by ganglionic blocking agents (e.g., trimethaphan [Arfonad]), volatile liquid anesthesia (e.g., halothane), and circulatory depressants. ■ Will cause profound hypotension with diazoxide (Hyperstat IV).

SIDE EFFECTS

Usually occur with too-rapid rate of infusion and are reversible: abdominal pain, apprehension, bradycardia, coma, decreased platelet aggregation, diaphoresis, dizziness, ECG changes, flushing, headache, hypotension (profound), ileus, increased intracranial pressure, muscle twitching, nausea, palpitations, rash, restlessness, retching, retrosternal discomfort, venous streaking. With prolonged therapy or overdose, cyanide intoxication (air hunger, bright red venous blood, confusion, elevated cyanide levels, marked clinical deterioration, metabolic acidosis, and death), hypothyroidism, or methemoglobinemia (chocolate brown blood, impaired oxygen delivery even though cardiac output and arterial pO_2 are adequate) can occur.

ANTIDOTE

At first sign of side effects, decrease rate of administration. Never allow systolic BP to fall below 60 mm Hg. If BP begins to rise or side effects persist, notify the physician. Hemodialysis or peritoneal dialysis may be indicated for thiocyanate levels over 10 mg/dl. For massive overdose with signs of cyanide toxicity or tachyphylaxis, discontinue nitroprusside sodium. Cyanide antidote kits contain all needed medications (see sodium nitrite/sodium thiosulfate monograph for complete information). Administer amyl nitrite inhalations for 15 to 30 seconds each minute until 3% sodium nitrite solution can be initiated as an IV infusion or immediately start the infusion (4 to 6 mg/kg) over 2 to 4 minutes. Monitor BP carefully; may cause hypotension that will also require treatment. Next, inject sodium thiosulfate 150 to 200 mg/kg (usually about 12.5 Gm or 50 ml of the 25% solution) in 50 ml of 5% dextrose in water IV over 10 minutes. Observe patient. If signs of overdose reappear, may repeat the above process after 2 hours; but use one half the original dosage. Sodium nitrite provides a buffer for cyanide by converting HgB into methemoglobin; sodium thiosulfate converts cyanide into thiocyanate, which is then excreted in urine. For hypotension, slow or discontinue the IV and put the patient in Trendelenburg position. Should improve in 1 to 10 minutes. Correct hypotension with vasopressors (e.g., dopamine [Intropin]). Treat methemoglobinemia with methylene blue 1 to 2 mg/kg. Use with caution if considerable amounts of cyanide are bound to methemoglobin.

NOREPINEPHRINE

(nor-ep-i-nef′rin)

Vasopressor

Levarterenol Bitartrate, Levophed

pH 3 to 4.5

USUAL DOSE

8 to 12 mcg/min initially (AHA recommendation is 0.5 to 1 mcg/min up to 30 mcg/min), then adjust to maintain desired BP range, usually 2 to 4 mcg/min. Another source suggests 0.5 to 1 mcg/min. Adjust gradually to achieve desired BP. Follow with a maintenance infusion of 2 to 12 mcg/min. Larger doses may be given safely as long as the patient remains hypotensive and blood volume depletion is corrected. Up to 30 mcg/min may be required in patients with refractory shock. 2 mg bitartrate equals 1 mg of norepinephrine. All doses are expressed in terms of norepinephrine.

PEDIATRIC DOSE

Begin with an initial dose of 0.05 to 0.1 mcg/kg/min. Titrate up to a maximum dose of 2 mcg/kg/min to maintain desired BP. AHA recommends 0.1 to 2 mcg/kg/min in advanced life support. Another source suggests 1 to 2 mcg/min adjusted to maintain desired BP.

DOSE ADJUSTMENTS

Lower-end initial doses may be indicated in the elderly based on potential for decreased organ function and concomitant disease or drug therapy.

DILUTION

Must be diluted in 250 to 1,000 ml of D5W or D5NS and given as an infusion. 4 mg (4 ml) in 1 L of diluent equals 4 mcg/ml. Final concentration based on fluid volume requirements of the patient. Administration in a dextrose solution reduces loss of potency resulting from oxidation. NS without dextrose is not recommended. Phentolamine (Regitine) 5 to 10 mg and/or heparin sodium to provide 100 to 200 units/hr may be added to the diluent to prevent any sloughing, necrosis, and/or thrombosis from slight leakage along the vein pathway.

Storage: Before dilution, store at CRT; protect from light.

INCOMPATIBLE WITH

Consult pharmacist; may be inactivated by solutions with a pH above 6. Incompatible with whole blood; administer through Y-tube or a separate IV line.

COMPATIBLE WITH (Underline Indicates Conflicting Compatibility Information)

Consult pharmacist; specific conditions may apply; see Compatibilities, p. xvi.

Additive: Amikacin (Amikin), calcium chloride, calcium gluconate, cimetidine (Tagamet), dimenhydrinate (Dinate), dobutamine (Dobutrex), heparin, hydrocortisone sodium succinate (Solu-Cortef), magnesium sulfate, meropenem (Merrem IV), methylprednisolone (Solu-Medrol), multivitamins (M.V.I.), nafcillin (Nafcil), potassium chloride (KCl), ranitidine (Zantac), succinylcholine, verapamil (Isoptin).

Syringe: Heparin.

Y-site: Amiodarone (Cordarone), cisatracurium (Nimbex), diltiazem (Cardizem), dobutamine (Dobutrex), dopamine (Intropin), epinephrine (Adrenalin), esmolol (Brevibloc), famotidine (Pepcid IV), fentanyl (Sublimaze), furosemide (Lasix), haloperidol (Haldol), heparin, hetastarch in electrolytes (Hextend), hydrocortisone sodium succinate (Solu-Cortef), hydromorphone (Dilaudid), inamrinone (Inocor), labetalol (Normodyne), lorazepam (Ativan), meropenem (Merrem IV), midazolam (Versed), milrinone (Primacor), morphine, nicardipine (Cardene IV), nitroglycerin (Nitro-Bid IV), potassium chloride (KCl), propofol (Diprivan), ranitidine (Zantac), remifentanil (Ultiva), vecuronium (Norcuron).

RATE OF ADMINISTRATION

See Usual Dose. Use the slowest possible flow rate to correct hypotension gradually and maintain adequate or preset BP. Some response should be noted within 1 to 2 minutes of IV administration. Use of an infusion pump or microdrip (60 gtt/ml) is an aid to correct evaluation of dose. Reduce infusion rate gradually. Avoid sudden discontinuation.

Norepinephrine (Levophed) Infusion Rate						
Desired Dose	4 mg in 1,000 ml D5W or D5NS 2 mg in 500 ml D5W or D5NS 4 mcg/ml			8 mg in 1,000 ml D5W or D5NS 4 mg in 500 ml D5W or D5NS 8 mcg/ml		
mcg/min	mcg/hr	ml/min	ml/hr	mcg/hr	ml/min	ml/hr
2	120	0.5	30	120	0.25	15
3	180	0.75	45	180	0.375	22.5
4	240	1	60	240	0.5	30
6	360	1.5	90	360	0.75	45
8	480	2	120	480	1	60
9	540	2.25	135	540	1.125	67.5
10	600	2.5	150	600	1.25	75
11	660	2.75	165	660	1.375	82.5
12	720	3	180	720	1.5	90

ACTIONS

Levarterenol is the levo-isomer of norepinephrine. It is a sympathomimetic drug that functions as a peripheral vasoconstrictor (alpha-adrenergic action) and inotropic stimulator of the heart and dilator of coronary arteries (beta-adrenergic action). Dilates the coronary arteries more than twice as much as epinephrine can. It is rapidly inactivated in the body by various enzymes and excreted in changed form in the urine.

INDICATIONS AND USES

All hypotensive states, including those associated with spinal anesthesia, blood reactions, drug reactions, hemorrhage, myocardial infarction, pheochromocytomectomy, septicemia, surgery, sympathectomy, and trauma. ■ Adjunct in treatment of cardiac arrest and profound hypotension.

CONTRAINDICATIONS

Do not use in hypotension from blood loss unless an emergency, in mesenteric or peripheral vascular thrombosis, or with cyclopropane or halothane (inhalant) anesthesia.

PRECAUTIONS

Whole blood or plasma should be given in a separate IV site. May be given through Y-tube connection. ■ Use caution in the elderly and in those with peripheral vascular disease or ischemic heart disease. ■ Use caution in previously hypertensive patients. Raise BP no more than 40 mm Hg below pre-existing systolic pressure. ■ Use caution in patients with allergies; some formulations contain sulfites. ■ Therapy may be continued until the patient can maintain own BP. Decrease dosage gradually.

Monitor: Check BP every 2 minutes until stabilized at the desired level. Check every 5 minutes thereafter during therapy. Avoid hypertension. One source suggests limiting rise in BP in previously hypertensive patients to no more than 40 mm Hg below previously systolic normal. ■ Observe for hypovolemia and replace fluids immediately. In an emergency, norepinephrine can be effective in a hypovolemic state before fluid replacement has been accomplished. ■ Check flow rate and injection site constantly. ■ Infusion should be through a large vein, preferably the antecubital vein, to prevent complications of prolonged peripheral vasoconstriction. Avoid veins in the hands, ankles, and legs. Use of the femoral vein may be considered. ■ Causes severe tissue necrosis, sloughing, and gangrene. Insert a plastic IV catheter or similar intravascular device at least 6 inches long well into the large vein chosen to prevent extravasation into any surrounding tissue; see Dilution. ■ Blanching along the vein pathway is a preliminary sign of extravasation. Change the injection site. ■ See Drug/Lab Interactions.

Patient Education: Report IV site burning or stinging promptly. ■ Request assistance to ambulate.

Maternal/Child: Category C: use only if clearly needed; benefits must outweigh risks. ■ Use caution in breast-feeding.

Elderly: See Precautions. ■ Lower-end initial doses may be indicated; see Dose Adjustments. ■ Differences in response versus younger patients not documented.

DRUG/LAB INTERACTIONS

Pressor effects may be potentiated by amphetamines, anesthetics, antihistamines, tricyclic antidepressants (e.g., desipramine [Norpramin]), rauwolfia alkaloids (e.g., reserpine), thyroid preparations, and methylphenidate (Ritalin). ■ May cause severe hypertension with ergot alkaloids and guanethidine (Ismelin), and severe prolonged hypertension with MAO inhibitors (e.g., selegiline [Eldepryl]). ■ May cause hypotension and bradycardia with hydantoins (e.g., phenytoin [Dilantin]). ■ Bretylium and halogenated hydrocarbon anesthetics (e.g., halothane) may cause serious arrhythmias. ■ Interacts in numerous and sometimes contradictory ways with many drugs.

SIDE EFFECTS

Rare when used as directed; anxiety, arrhythmias (e.g., bradycardia and VT), chest pain, decreased cardiac output, dyspnea, headache, ischemia, necrosis caused by extravasation, pallor, photophobia, seizures, vomiting. Persistent headache may indicate overdose and severe hypertension. Gangrene has been reported.

ANTIDOTE

To prevent sloughing and necrosis in areas where extravasation has occurred, with a fine hypodermic needle inject 5 to 10 mg of phentolamine (Regitine) diluted in 10 to 15 ml of NS liberally throughout the tissue in the extravasated area. Treatment should be started as soon as extravasation is recognized. Atropine may be used to counteract the bradycardia. Notify physician of any side effect. Should a sudden or uncontrolled hypertensive state occur, discontinue levarterenol, notify the physician, and if necessary, treat with an adrenergic blocking agent (e.g., phentolamine [Regitine] or phenoxybenzamine [Dibenzyline]).

OCTREOTIDE ACETATE
(ok-tree′oh-tide as′ah-tat)

Sandostatin

Antidiarrheal
Growth hormone suppressant

pH 3.9 to 4.5

USUAL DOSE

Usually given SC. Check label, confirm for IV use; Sandostatin LAR Depot is for IM use only; see Precautions. In most situations begin with a lower dose to allow gradual tolerance to GI side effects. Increase gradually based on patient response and tolerance. Begin SC or IM (LAR Depot) dosing as soon as practical.

Antidiarrheal (GI tumor): 50 mcg once or twice daily. Increase gradually if indicated.

Antidiarrheal (unlabeled for AIDS): 100 mcg as an IV bolus over 10 minutes. Follow with a continuous infusion, intermittent infusion, or bolus dose of 10 mcg/hr. Increase gradually to 100 mcg/hr. When adequate control is achieved, decrease to 75 mcg/hr. SC dose range is from 100 mcg up to 3,000 mcg/24 hr.

Carcinoid tumors: 100 to 600 mcg/24 hr in equally divided doses 2 to 4 times daily during first 2 weeks of therapy. Average total daily dose ranges from 300 to 450 mcg, but therapeutic response is obtained with ranges from 50 to 750 mcg. Up to 1,500 mcg/day has been used in selected patients.

Carcinoid crisis (unlabeled): 100 mcg as an IV bolus. May be given to treat carcinoid crisis during anesthesia or given before induction of anesthesia as a prophylactic measure.

Vasoactive intestinal peptide tumors: Average dose range is 200 to 300 mcg/24 hr in equally divided doses 2 to 4 times daily during first 2 weeks of therapy. Average total daily dose ranges from 150 to 750 mcg but therapeutic response usually achieved with doses under 450 mcg/24 hr. IV doses of 25 to 50 mcg/hr for 2 to 4 days have been used.

Treatment of GI bleeding (unlabeled): Begin with a loading dose of 50 to 100 mcg. Follow with a continuous infusion of 25 to 50 mcg/hr for 1 to 5 days. Intermittent infusion or bolus doses may be substituted for the continuous infusion.

Growth hormone suppression: 50 mcg every 8 hours is the initial dose. Increase dose gradually as indicated by IGF-1 levels; see Monitor. Another study suggests an initial dose of 100 mcg equally distributed over 24 hours as a continuous infusion. Increase by 100 mcg each 24-hour period. Acromegaly has been suppressed at doses of 300 to 500 mcg/24 hr. May be maintained at home with infusions through an implantable IV or SC pump or SC dosing of 50 to 100 mcg every 8 hours.

Antihypoglycemic: Life-threatening hypoglycemia secondary to insulinoma (unlabeled): 100 mcg as an IV bolus.

Reduce output from GI or pancreatic fistulas (unlabeled): 50 to 200 mcg every 8 hours. In one study, 250 mcg/hr was given as a continuous infusion for 48 hours, followed with SC dosing. Fistula became dry within 72 hours and eventually closed.

PEDIATRIC DOSE

Experience is limited, but seems to be well tolerated in infants and young children.

1 to 10 mcg/kg of body weight/24 hours has been effective in various conditions (e.g., as an antidiarrheal).

Nesidioblastosis (pancreatic tumors [unlabeled]): 1 mcg/kg/hr as an IV infusion until vasoactive intestinal peptide (VIP) levels fall and fluid absorption is normal. Follow with SC dosing.

DOSE ADJUSTMENTS

In all situations dose adjustment may be required on a daily basis to maintain symptomatic control. After initial 2 weeks of therapy, gradually decrease dose to achieve therapeutically effective maintenance dose. ■ Reduce dose in the elderly; half-life extended and clearance decreased. ■ Half-life markedly extended in severe renal failure requiring dialysis. Reduction of maintenance dose indicated. ■ See Drug/Lab Interactions.

DILUTION

May be given undiluted or may be diluted with 50 to 200 ml of NS or D5W and given as an intermittent infusion or further diluted and given as a continuous infusion.

Storage: Before use store in refrigerator (2° to 8° C [36° to 46° F]) or at CRT for 14 days; protect from light. May store at room temperature on day of use. Diluted solution stable for 24 hours. Multi-dose vial must be dated on opening and discarded after 14 days.

INCOMPATIBLE WITH

Manufacturer lists TPN (forms a conjugate that decreases effectiveness). If used as an additive with insulin, octreotide markedly increases adsorption of insulin and reduces insulin availability.

COMPATIBLE WITH

Consult pharmacist; specific conditions may apply; see Compatibilities, p. xvi.

Additive: Heparin.

RATE OF ADMINISTRATION

IV injection: A single dose over 3 minutes.

Intermittent infusion: A single dose over 15 to 30 minutes.

Continuous infusion: Give at a rate consistent with the required hourly dose in an amount of fluid appropriate for the specific patient.

ACTIONS

A long-acting octapeptide. Mimics the actions of the natural hormone somatostatin, suppressing secretion of serotonin, gastroenteropancreatic peptides (e.g., gastrin, vasoactive intestinal peptide, insulin, glucagon, secretin, motilin, pancreatic polypeptide), and growth hormone. Decreases splanchnic blood flow. Stimulates fluid and electrolyte absorption from GI tract and prolongs GI transit time. Readily absorbed from subcutaneous injection site, and about 65% bound to plasma protein. Half-life longer than the natural hormone (1.5 hours compared to 1 to 3 minutes). Action may extend to 12 hours. Some excreted unchanged in urine.

INDICATIONS AND USES

To suppress or inhibit the severe diarrhea and flushing episodes associated with carcinoid syndrome. ■ Treatment of profuse watery diarrhea associated with vasoactive intestinal peptide tumors (VIPomas). ■ Treatment of acromegaly to suppress growth hormone and achieve normalization of growth hormone and IGF-1 levels.

Unlabeled uses: Treatment of severe diarrhea in patients with AIDS. Carcinoid crisis during anesthesia, adjunct to treatment of life-threatening hypoglycemia, treatment of GI bleeding. Adjunct to pancreatectomy and treatment of GI or pancreatic fistulas.

CONTRAINDICATIONS

Sensitivity to octreotide acetate or any of its components.

PRECAUTIONS

IV use is limited to emergency situations. SC injection with rotation of injection sites is preferred route of administration. ■ Sandostatin LAR Depot must be administered intragluteally but has the advantage of extending the interval between injections to every 4 weeks. ■ May decrease size of tumors and slow rate of growth and metastases. Data not definitive. ■ Use caution in patients with diabetes; requirements for insulin, sulfonylureas, and diazoxide may be altered.

Monitor: Observe for transient hyperglycemia or hypoglycemia during induction and dose changes because of changes in balance of hormones (e.g., insulin, glucagon, and growth hormone). ■ Monitor fluids and electrolytes carefully. ■ 5-HIAA, plasma serotonin, and plasma substance P may be useful lab studies to evaluate patient response with carcinoid tumor. Measurement of plasma vasoactive intestinal peptide will be helpful in VIPoma. ■ In acromegaly, initial response may be monitored with growth hormone levels at 1- to 4-hour intervals for 8 to 12 hours after a dose. IGF-1 levels every 2 weeks and/or multiple growth hormone levels taken 0 to 8 hours after administration may be used to make dose adjustments. ■ Can alter fat absorption and decrease gallbladder motility; observe for gallbladder disease. Baseline and periodic ultrasound of gallbladder and bile ducts indicated in long-term SC therapy. Periodic fecal fat and carotene studies also indicated. ■ Monitor baseline and periodic thyroid function tests, especially in long-term SC therapy. ■ See Dose Adjustments and Drug/Lab Interactions.

Patient Education: Instruct patient and/or family in appropriate skills if self-administration indicated. To avoid or lessen incidence of GI side effects, schedule injections between meals and at bedtime.

Maternal/Child: Category B: although studies do not indicate harm to the fetus, use in pregnancy and breast-feeding only if clearly needed. ■ Has been used at doses of 3 to 40 mcg/kg/day in infants over 1 month and children, but safety and efficacy are not established; see Literature.

Elderly: See Dose Adjustments. ■ May be more sensitive to side effects; observe carefully.

DRUG/LAB INTERACTIONS

Use caution in patients receiving concomitant beta-blockers (e.g., atenolol [Tenormin], propranolol [Inderal]) calcium channel blockers (e.g., diltiazem [Cardizem], verapamil [Isoptin]), or any agents used for fluid and electrolyte balance. Will require adjustment in these therapies as symptoms are controlled by octreotide. ■ May inhibit effectiveness of cyclosporine and may result in transplant rejection. ■ Markedly increases adsorption of insulin and reduces availability. ■ Concurrent use with oral antidiabetic agents, glucagon, growth hormone, or insulin may cause hypoglycemia or hyperglycemia. Monitor patient carefully and give adjunct dose of these agents as indicated.

SIDE EFFECTS

Most side effects are of mild to moderate severity and of short duration. Abdominal pain/discomfort, abnormal stools, anorexia, anxiety, biliary sludge, cholelithiasis, constipation, convulsions, depression, diarrhea, dizziness, drowsiness, fatigue, fat malabsorption, flatulence, fluttering sensation, GI bleeding, headache, heartburn, hepatitis, hyperesthesia, hyperglycemia, hypoglycemia, increase in liver enzymes, insomnia, irritability, jaundice, nausea, pounding in the head, rectal spasm, swollen stomach, vomiting. Many other side effects occur in less than 1% of patients.

ANTIDOTE

Keep physician informed of all side effects. A dose adjustment of either octreotide or other concomitant therapies may be required. Symptomatic and supportive treatment may be indicated. Overdose will cause hyperglycemia or hypoglycemia depending on tumor involved and endocrine status of patient. Discontinue octreotide temporarily, notify the physician, and monitor the patient carefully. Symptomatic treatment should be sufficient.

OFLOXACIN

(o-flox′a-sin)

Floxin I.V.

Antibacterial (fluoroquinolone)

pH 3.5 to 5.8

USUAL DOSE

200 to 400 mg every 12 hours. Dose and duration of treatment are based on mild to moderate infection and specific diagnosis. Normal renal function required. Dose and serum levels similar by oral or IV route. Transfer to oral dose as soon as practical. IV administration should not be used for more than 10 days (no studies available on longer use).

Exacerbation of chronic bronchitis, community-acquired pneumonia, and uncomplicated skin and skin structure infections: 400 mg every 12 hours for 10 days.

Acute uncomplicated gonorrhea: A single dose of 400 mg.

Cervical and urethral infections due to *C Trachomatis* and/or *W gonorrhoeae:* 300 mg every 12 hours for 7 days.

Pelvic inflammatory disease: 400 mg every 12 hours for 10 to 14 days.

Cystitis: 200 mg every 12 hours for 3 to 7 days depending on causative organism (see literature).

Complicated urinary tract infections: 200 mg every 12 hours for 10 days.

Prostatitis due to E. coli: 300 mg every 12 hours for up to 6 weeks.

DOSE ADJUSTMENTS

After a normal initial dose increase interval between doses to 24 hours if CrCl is between 20 and 50 ml/min. Reduce subsequent dose by one half and increase interval to 24 hours if CrCl less than 20 ml/min. ■ Do not exceed a maximum dose of 400 mg/day in patients with severe liver function disorders (e.g., cirrhosis with or without ascites). See Drug/Lab Interactions.

DILUTION

Available premixed and ready for use in infusion bottles and in plastic infusion containers. All contain 4 mg/ml. Do not hang plastic containers in a series; may cause air embolism; see packaging for specific preparation and administration directions. Also available in 10-ml vials (40 mg/ml). Vials must be diluted to a final maximum concentration of 4 mg/ml. May be further diluted to concentrations as low as 0.4 mg/ml. To yield 4 mg/ml, dilute 200-mg dose (5 ml of 40 mg/ml) with 50 ml diluent; 300-mg dose (7.5 ml of 40 mg/ml) with 75 ml diluent; and 400-mg dose (10 ml of 40 mg/ml) with 100 ml diluent. Compatible diluents are NS, D5W, D5/½NS, D5NS, D5LR, or D5 in Plasma-Lyte 56; D5/½NS with 0.15% potassium chloride; 5% sodium bicarbonate; sodium lactate (⅙ M lactate); and SW for injection.

Storage: A clear, colorless to slightly yellow solution. Vials stable to expiration date at room temperature before opening. Contains no preservative; all preparations are intended for single use only. If using a vial that will yield more than one dose, dilute all at one time. Diluted solutions stable at CRT for 3 days, up to 14 days if refrigerated. May be frozen for up to 6 months. Do not force thaw (e.g., microwave or water bath) and do not refreeze. Discard any unused portion of premixed solutions and/or opened vials.

INCOMPATIBLE WITH

Manufacturer recommends ofloxacin be administered separately. Always flush line before and after administration of any other drug through the same IV line. Never administer in the same IV or through the same tubing with any solution containing metal ions (e.g., calcium, copper, iron, magnesium, zinc); may chelate with these ions.

COMPATIBLE WITH

Consult pharmacist; specific conditions may apply; see Compatibilities, p. xvi.

Additive: Ceftazidime (Fortaz), clindamycin (Cleocin), gentamicin (Garamycin), piperacillin (Pipracil), tobramycin (Nebcin), vancomycin (Vancocin).

Syringe: Cefotaxime (Claforan).

Y-site: Ampicillin, cisatracurium (Nimbex), docetaxel (Taxotere), etoposide phosphate (Etopophos), gemcitabine (Gemzar), granisetron (Kytril), linezolid (Zyvox), propofol (Diprivan), remifentanil (Ultiva), thiotepa (Thioplex).

RATE OF ADMINISTRATION

A single dose must be equally distributed over 60 minutes as an infusion. Too-rapid administration may cause hypotension, increase incidence of anaphylaxis, local site inflammation, or other side effects. May be given through a Y-tube or three-way stopcock of infusion set. Temporarily discontinue other solutions infusing at the same site and flush tubing before and after ofloxacin.

ACTIONS

A synthetic broad-spectrum antimicrobial agent, a fluoroquinolone. Bactericidal to a wide range of aerobic and anaerobic gram-negative and gram-positive organisms through interference with an enzyme needed for synthesis of bacterial DNA. Onset of action is prompt, and serum levels are dose related. Steady state is achieved after 4 doses. Half-life averages 4 to 6 hours. Readily distributed to body fluids and tissue. Therapeutic levels found in blister fluid, cervix, lung tissue, ovary, prostatic fluid and tissue, skin, and sputum. Well absorbed in patients with cystic fibrosis. Activity not affected by beta-lactamase production. Resistant chlamydia strains may emerge. Minimal metabolism occurs in the liver (less than other quinolones). Excreted as unchanged drug in the urine. Small amounts found in bile and feces. Crosses placental barrier. Secreted in breast milk.

INDICATIONS AND USES

Treatment of mild to moderate lower respiratory, skin and skin structure, urinary tract and prostate infections, pelvic inflammatory disease, and sexually transmitted diseases. Effective against specific organism (see literature). ■ Used in multi-drug–resistant organism infections when other antiinfectives are ineffective or cannot be used. ■ Additional appropriate therapy required if anaerobic organisms are suspected of contributing to the infection. ■ Not effective in the treatment of syphilis.

CONTRAINDICATIONS

Known hypersensitivity to ofloxacin or any other quinolone antimicrobial agent (e.g., norfloxacin [Noroxin], ciprofloxacin [Cipro]).

PRECAUTIONS

For IV use only. ■ Safety and effectiveness in severe infections not established. ■ Culture and sensitivity studies indicated to determine susceptibility of the causative organism to ofloxacin. ■ *Pseudomonas aeruginosa* may develop resistance during treatment. Ongoing culture and sensitivity studies indicated. ■ Prolonged use may cause superinfection because of overgrowth of nonsusceptible organisms. ■ Pseudomembranous colitis has been reported. May range from mild to life-threatening. Consider in patients that present with diarrhea during or after treatment with ofloxacin. ■ Use with caution in patients with known CNS disorders that predispose to seizures (e.g., epilepsy, severe cerebral arteriosclerosis, concomitant drug therapy). ■ May cause ophthalmologic abnormalities (e.g., cataracts). Incidence increases with length of treatment. ■ Prolongation of the QT interval on ECG and infrequent cases of arrhythmia (including torsades de pointes) have been reported with the use of fluoroquinolones. The risk of arrhythmia may be reduced by avoiding their use in the presence of hypokalemia, significant bradycardia, cardiomyopathy, or concurrent treatment with class 1A antiarrhythmic agents (e.g., quinidine, procainamide [Pronestyl]) or with class III antiarrhythmic agents (e.g., amiodarone [Cordarone], sotalol [Betapace]). ■ Ruptures of shoulder, hand, and/or Achilles tendons that required surgical repair or resulted in prolonged disability have been reported in patients receiving quinolones.

Monitor: May cause anaphylaxis with the first or succeeding doses, even in patients without known hypersensitivity. Emergency equipment and drugs must always be available. ■ Maintain adequate hydration to prevent concentrated urine throughout treatment. May form crystals in alkaline urine. ■ Test all patients with gonorrhea for syphilis at time of diagnosis and in 3 months. Requires additional treatment. ■ Monitor hematopoietic, hepatic, and renal systems during prolonged treatment. ■ Use of larger veins will help to reduce incidence of allergic reactions with incidence of local irritation. Symptoms of local irritation do not preclude further administration of ofloxacin unless they recur or worsen. Generally resolve when infusion complete. ■ See Drug/Lab Interaction.

Patient Education: Consider birth control options. ■ Report skin rash or any other hypersensitivity reaction promptly. ■ Avoid excessive sunlight or artificial ultraviolet light. Potential for photosensitivity may cause severe sunburn. Wear dark glasses outdoors. ■ Dizziness or light-headedness may interfere with ambulation and motor coordination. Use caution in tasks that require alertness. ■ Effects of caffeine or theophylline preparations may be increased. Limit or eliminate concurrent use. Monitor if use necessary. ■ Report tendon pain or inflammation promptly. ■ See Precautions/Monitor and Drug/Lab Interactions.

Maternal/Child: Category C: not recommended. Benefits must outweigh risks. High doses have caused maternal and fetal toxicity. ■ Discontinue breast-feeding. ■ Safety for use in children under 18 years of age not established. Has caused arthropathy and osteochondrosis in juvenile animals.

Elderly: Percent of side effects similar to younger adults. Half-life extended to 6 or 7 hours with normal renal function.

DRUG/LAB INTERACTIONS

Other quinolones have caused serious or fatal reactions with theophylline (e.g., cardiac arrhythmia or arrest, respiratory failure, seizures, status epilepticus). If must be used concomitantly, monitor serum levels of theophylline and decrease dose as appropriate. No problems have occurred, but observe closely with caffeine. ■ Serum levels may be increased with cimetidine (Tagamet). ■ Serum levels may be decreased with antineoplastics agents (e.g., cisplatin, doxorubicin [Adriamycin]). ■ Cyclosporine serum levels and nephrotoxic effects may be increased with concomitant use. ■ Risk of CNS stimulation and seizures may be increased with concurrent use of NSAIDs (e.g., ibuprofen [Advil, Motrin], naproxen [Aleve, Naprosyn]). ■ May potentiate oral anticoagulants (e.g., warfarin [Coumadin]); monitor PT/INR. ■ Probably potentiated by probenicid; may require dose adjustment based on ofloxacin serum levels. ■ Concurrent administration with procainamide may decrease procainamide levels. ■ See Side Effects. ■ May cause a false-positive when testing for opiates.

SIDE EFFECTS

Abdominal pain and cramps, altered sense of taste, chest pain, decreased appetite, diarrhea, dizziness, dry mouth, external genital pruritus in women, fatigue, flatulence, GI distress, headache, insomnia, local site reactions (e.g., erythema, phlebitis, swelling), nausea, nervousness, pharyngitis, phototoxicity, pruritus, pseudomembranous colitis, pyrexia, rash, somnolence, taste disturbances, trunk pain, vaginal discharge, vaginitis, visual disturbances, and vomiting. Capable of numerous other reactions in less than 1% of patients. Allergic reactions (anaphylaxis, cardiovascular collapse, death, dyspnea, edema [facial, laryngeal, or pharyngeal], eosinophilia, fever, hepatic necrosis, itching, jaundice, loss of consciousness, rash, urticaria); cardiac arrest; CNS stimulation (confusion, hallucinations, light-headedness, restlessness, seizures, tingling, toxic psychosis, tremors) can occur.

Overdose: Disorientation, dizziness, drowsiness, facial swelling and numbness, hot and cold flushes, nausea, slurring of speech.

ANTIDOTE

Keep physician informed of all side effects. Many will require symptomatic treatment; monitor closely. Discontinue ofloxacin at the first appearance of a skin rash or any other sign of hypersensitivity or at the onset of any CNS symptom, pseudomembranous colitis, or phototoxicity. Treat allergic reactions with epinephrine (Adrenalin), airway management, oxygen, IV fluids, antihistamines (e.g., diphenhydramine [Benadryl]), corticosteroids (e.g., Solu-Cortef), and pressor amines (e.g., dopamine [Intropin]) as indicated. Treat CNS symptoms as indicated. May require diazepam (Valium) for seizures. Mild cases of colitis may respond to discontinuation of ofloxacin. Oral vancomycin (Vancocin) or metronidazole (Flagyl) is the treatment of choice for antibiotic-related pseudomembranous colitis. Adequate hydration and supplementation of electrolytes and proteins usually indicated. Maintain hydration in overdose. No specific antidote; not removed by hemodialysis or peritoneal dialysis. Maintain patient until drug is excreted.

ONDANSETRON HYDROCHLORIDE

(on-dan-seh′tron hye-droe-klor′id)

Antiemetic
$5HT_3$ receptor antagonist

Zofran

pH 3.3 to 4

USUAL DOSE

Nausea associated with emetogenic agents: A single 32-mg dose or 0.15 mg/kg of body weight (first in a sequence of three doses) 30 minutes before giving emetogenic cancer chemotherapy (e.g., cisplatin, methotrexate). Given as an intermittent infusion. Repeat 0.15 mg/kg dose at 4 and 8 hours after the first dose. Concurrent use with dexamethasone may improve the effectiveness of ondansetron in controlling cisplatin-induced nausea and vomiting.

Alternate ***unlabeled regimens*** are 10 to 15 mg every 3 hours as an intermittent infusion; *or*

An infusion containing 8 mg of ondansetron in combination with 20 mg of dexamethasone diluted in 50 ml of D5W; *or*

A continuous infusion of 1 mg/hr for 24 hours.

In selected situations doses are used every 3 hours to supplement the continuous infusion, based on symptoms, response, and tolerance of individual patient. These doses exceed present FDA approvals. For non-cisplatin chemotherapeutic regimens, another source suggests an initial dose of 8 mg (may be half IV and half PO) followed by PO doses for 1 to 5 days.

Postoperative nausea in adults and children weighing 40 kg or more: 4 mg before anesthesia induction or immediately after surgery. Although repeat doses are not recommended by the manufacturer, they have been given.

PEDIATRIC DOSE

Nausea associated with emetogenic agents in children 4 to 18 years of age: 0.15 mg/kg of body weight 30 minutes before giving emetogenic cancer chemotherapy. Given as an intermittent infusion. Repeat 0.15 mg/kg/dose at 4 and 8 hours after the first dose. Another source suggests 3 to 5 mg/M^2 as an intermittent infusion immediately before emetogenic chemotherapy followed by 4 mg PO every 8 hours for up to 5 days. For highly emetogenic cancer chemotherapy, one source suggests 0.45 mg/kg 30 minutes before administration. Maximum dose is 32 mg. This source suggests following all of the above doses with 0.15 mg/kg/dose every 4 hours as needed.

Postoperative nausea in children 2 to 12 years of age: Given before anesthesia induction or immediately after surgery. See comments under Usual Dose.

Weight 40 kg or less: 0.1 mg/kg.

Weight more than 40 kg: See Adult dose.

DOSE ADJUSTMENTS

No dose adjustment required for the elderly or in renal disease. ■ A single maximum daily dose of 8 mg is suggested for patients with severe hepatic disease.

DILUTION

IV injection: 4 mg dose may be given undiluted.

Intermittent IV: A single dose should be diluted in 50 ml of NS, D5W, D5/½NS, D5NS. Also available as 32 mg in 50 ml D5W.

Infusion: Available prediluted and ready to use or may be further diluted in larger amounts of the above solutions. Also compatible in 10% mannitol and Ringer's injection. A precipitate will form in alkaline solutions.
Storage: Store unopened vials at CRT or refrigerate. Protect from light. Stable at CRT for 48 hours after dilution.

COMPATIBLE WITH **(Underline Indicates Conflicting Compatibility Information)**

Consult pharmacist; specific conditions may apply; see Compatibilities, p. xvi.

Additive: Cisplatin (Platinol), cyclophosphamide (Cytoxan), cytarabine (ARA-C), dacarbazine (DTIC), dexamethasone (Decadron), doxorubicin (Adriamycin), etoposide (VePesid), hydromorphone (Dilaudid), meperidine (Demerol), meropenem (Merrem IV), methotrexate (Folex), morphine.

Syringe: Alfentanil (Alfenta), atropine, dexamethasone (Decadron), fentanyl (Sublimaze), glycopyrrolate, meperidine (Demerol), metoclopramide (Reglan), midazolam (Versed), morphine, naloxone (Narcan), neostigmine (Prostigmin), propofol (Diprivan).

Y-site: Alatrofloxacin (Trovan IV), aldesleukin (Proleukin, IL-2), amifostine (Ethyol), amikacin (Amikin), aztreonam (Azactam), bleomycin (Blenoxane), carboplatin (Paraplatin), carmustine (BiCNU), cefazolin (Kefzol), cefotaxime (Claforan), cefoxitin (Mefoxin), ceftazidime (Fortaz), ceftizoxime (Cefizox), cefuroxime (Zinacef), chlorpromazine (Thorazine), cimetidine (Tagamet), cisatracurium (Nimbex), cisplatin (Platinol), cladribine (Leustatin), clindamycin (Cleocin), cyclophosphamide (Cytoxan), cytarabine (ARA-C), dacarbazine (DTIC), dactinomycin (Cosmegen), daunorubicin (Cerubidine), dexamethasone (Decadron), diphenhydramine (Benadryl), docetaxel (Taxotere), dopamine (Intropin), doxorubicin (Adriamycin), doxorubicin liposome (Doxil), doxycycline (Vibramycin), droperidol (Inapsine), etoposide (Etopophos, VePesid), famotidine (Pepcid IV), filgrastim (Neupogen), fluconazole (Diflucan), fludarabine (Fludara), fluorouracil (5-FU), gatifloxacin (Tequin), gemcitabine (Gemzar), gentamicin (Garamycin), haloperidol (Haldol), heparin, hetastarch in electrolytes (Hextend), hydrocortisone (Hydrocortone, Solu-Cortef), hydromorphone (Dilaudid), ifosfamide (Ifex), imipenem-cilastatin (Primaxin), linezolid (Zyvox), magnesium sulfate, mannitol, mechlorethamine (nitrogen mustard), melphalan (Alkeran), meperidine (Demerol), meropenem (Merrem IV), mesna (Mesnex), methotrexate (Folex), metoclopramide (Reglan), mitomycin (Mutamycin), mitoxantrone (Novantrone), morphine, paclitaxel (Taxol), pentostatin (Nipent), piperacillin/tazobactam (Zosyn), potassium chloride (KCl), prochlorperazine (Compazine), promethazine (Phenergan), ranitidine (Zantac), remifentanil (Ultiva), sodium acetate, streptozocin (Zanosar), teniposide (Vumon), thiotepa (Thioplex), ticarcillin (Ticar), ticarcillin/clavulanate (Timentin), topotecan (Hycamtin), vancomycin (Vancocin), vinblastine (Velban), vincristine (Oncovin), vinorelbine (Navelbine), zidovudine (AZT, Retrovir).

RATE OF ADMINISTRATION

IV injection: (Postop N/V): A single 4-mg dose over at least 30 seconds; 2 to 5 minutes preferred.
Intermittent IV adults and children: A single dose equally distributed over 15 minutes.
Infusion: Evenly distributed over 12 to 24 hours.

ACTIONS

A selective antagonist of serotonin ($5HT_3$) receptors. Chemotherapeutic agents such as cisplatin increase the release of serotonin from specific cells in the GI tract, causing emesis. By antagonizing these receptors, chemotherapy-induced nausea and vomiting are prevented. Lacks the activity at dopamine receptors of metoclopramide (Reglan), so it does not cause sedation. No correlation between plasma levels and antiemetic activity. Metabolized by specific hepatic enzymes; onset of action is prompt and lasts about 4 hours. May last only 2 to 3 hours in children under 15 years of age. Excreted in feces and urine. May be secreted in breast milk.

INDICATIONS AND USES

Prevention of nausea and vomiting associated with initial and repeat courses of emetogenic cancer chemotherapy, including high-dose cisplatin, nonplatinum agents, and radiation therapy. Has been shown to be effective with cyclophosphamide (Cytoxan), doxorubicin (Adriamycin), etoposide (VePesid), fluorouracil (Adrucil), ifosfamide (Ifex), methotrexate (Folex), mitoxantrone (Novantrone), and vincristine (Oncovin). Concurrent use with dexamethasone has been shown to improve the effectiveness of ondansetron in controlling cisplatin-induced nausea and vomiting. ■ Prevention or treatment of postoperative nausea. ■ Used orally (available as liquid, tablets, and orally disintegrating tablets) for prevention of nausea and vomiting, including postoperative N/V, and N/V associated with chemotherapy and radiotherapy. Recently approved for IM injection as an alternative to IV in the prevention of postoperative nausea and vomiting.

Unlabeled uses: Treatment of panic disorder.

CONTRAINDICATIONS

Hypersensitivity to ondansetron.

PRECAUTIONS

Sterile technique imperative in withdrawing a single dose from the multidose vial. Available as a single-dose vial and in 4- and 8-mg tablets. ■ Cross-sensitivity has been reported between ondansetron and other $5HT_3$ receptor agonists (e.g., dolasetron [Anzemet] or granisetron [Kytril]). ■ Use with caution in patients with hepatic impairment. Clearance is decreased; see Dose Adjustments. ■ Not indicated instead of gastric suction or intestinal peristalsis. Use in abdominal surgery or in patients with chemotherapy induced nausea and vomiting may mask a progressive ileus or gastric distension.

Monitor: Observe closely. Ambulate slowly to avoid orthostatic hypotension. ■ Stool softeners or laxatives may be required to prevent constipation.

Patient Education: May cause dizziness or fainting; request assistance to ambulate. ■ Report promptly difficulty breathing, tightness in the chest, or wheezing.

Maternal/Child: Category B: no evidence of impaired fertility or harm to fetus. Use in pregnancy only if potential benefit justifies potential risk. ■ Use caution if required during breast-feeding. ■ Safety for use in children under 2 to 3 years of age not established.

Elderly: See Dose Adjustments.

DRUG/LAB INTERACTIONS

Even though metabolized in the liver and changes in clearance rates do occur, no specific drug interactions requiring dose adjustments have been identified.

SIDE EFFECTS

Abdominal pain or discomfort, arrhythmias (including ventricular and superventricular tachycardia, PVCs, atrial fibrillation, and bradycardia), chest pain, constipation, cramps, diarrhea, dizziness, ECG alterations (including second-degree heart block and ST segment depression), faintness, flushing, headache, hypersensitivity reactions (e.g., anaphylaxis, angioedema, bronchospasm, cardiopulmonary arrest, hypotension, laryngospasm, shock, shortness of breath, stridor, urticaria), hiccups, hypokalemia, light-headedness, pain at injection site, palpitations, transient blurred vision, transient elevation of AST (SGOT) or ALT (SGPT). Other side effects have occurred (e.g., extrapyramidal reaction, rash) in fewer than 1% of patients. Overdose caused sudden blindness in one patient.

ANTIDOTE

Most side effects will be treated symptomatically. Keep physician informed as indicated. Overdose of 10 times the usual dose has not caused significant problems. Treat anaphylaxis and resuscitate as necessary.

ORPHENADRINE CITRATE

(or-fen′a-dreen sit′rat)

Skeletal muscle relaxant (central acting)

Norflex

pH 5 to 6

USUAL DOSE

60 mg (2 ml) every 12 hours.

DILUTION

May be given undiluted, or a single dose may be diluted in 5 to 10 ml of SW for injection.

Storage: Store at CRT.

COMPATIBILITY

Specific information not available. Consult pharmacist.

RATE OF ADMINISTRATION

60 mg or fraction thereof over 5 minutes.

ACTIONS

A diphenhydramine derivative with anticholinergic effects. Exact mechanism of action is unknown, but may be related to its analgesic properties. Does not directly relax tense skeletal muscles. Onset of action is immediate. Half-life of parent compound is 14 hours. Metabolized in the liver. Excreted in feces and urine.

INDICATIONS AND USES

Acute spasm of voluntary muscle, especially posttraumatic, discogenic, and tension spasms. ■ Treatment of nicotine-induced convulsions.

CONTRAINDICATIONS

Achalasia, bladder neck obstruction, cardiospasm, glaucoma, hypersensitivity to orphenadrine citrate or its components (contains bisulfites), myasthenia gravis, prostatic hypertrophy, pyloric or duodenal obstruction, stenosing peptic ulcer.

PRECAUTIONS

Equal effectiveness produced by IM or oral route. Use IV only when necessary for rapid onset of action. ▪ Use caution in tachycardia, cardiac arrhythmias, cardiac decompensation, coronary insufficiency, pregnancy, and breast-feeding. ▪ Norflex contains sulfites; use caution to prevent allergic response.

Monitor: Keep patient in recumbent position for at least 15 minutes to avoid postural hypotension.

Patient Education: Avoid alcohol and other CNS depressants. ▪ May cause dizziness, drowsiness, and visual disturbances. ▪ Request assistance for ambulation. ▪ Use caution in any task requiring alertness.

Maternal/Child: Safety for use in pregnancy and breast-feeding not established; benefits must outweigh risks. ▪ Not recommended for children.

Elderly: May cause confusion. ▪ Sensitivity to anticholinergic effects (dry mouth, urinary retention). ▪ Consider age-related renal impairment; may preclude use.

DRUG/LAB INTERACTIONS

Absorption of many oral drugs inhibited or potentiated due to decreased GI motility. ▪ Not recommended for concomitant use with propoxyphene (Darvon) or perphenazine (Trilafon). ▪ Potentiates anticholinergic drugs and thiazide diuretics. ▪ Inhibits haloperidol and phenothiazines (e.g., prochlorperazine [Compazine]).

SIDE EFFECTS

Usually associated with higher doses or too-rapid administration: blurred vision, dizziness, drowsiness, dry mouth, excitation, headache, lightheadedness, nausea, palpitations, pupil dilation, tachycardia, urinary retention, urticaria, vomiting, weakness. Anaphylactic reactions can occur (rare).

Overdose: Deep coma, cardiac arrhythmias, tonic and clonic seizures, shock, respiratory arrest, death.

ANTIDOTE

Notify the physician of any side effects. Reduction of dosage will probably relieve them. For symptoms of hypersensitivity, discontinue the drug, notify physician, and treat symptomatically. Treat overdose promptly. Resuscitate as necessary.

OXACILLIN SODIUM

(ox-a-sill'in so'de-um)

Antibacterial (penicillinase-resistant penicillin)

Bactocill, Prostaphlin

pH 6 to 8.5

USUAL DOSE

Over 40 kg (88 lb): 250 mg to 1 Gm or more every 4 to 6 hours. Maximum dose is 20 Gm/24 hr.

PEDIATRIC DOSE

Under 40 kg: 50 to 100 mg/kg of body weight/24 hr in equally divided doses every 6 hours (12.5 to 25 mg/kg of body weight every 6 hours). Maximum dose is 100 to 300 mg/kg/24 hr.

INFANT DOSE

Under 2,000 Gm; less than 7 days of age: 25 mg/kg every 12 hr.
Under 2,000 Gm; over 7 days of age: 25 mg/kg every 8 hr.
Over 2,000 Gm; less than 7 days of age: 25 mg/kg every 12 hr.
Over 2,000 Gm; over 7 days of age: 25 mg/kg every 6 hr.

Increase dose to 50 mg/kg every 6, 8, or 12 hours in meningitis.

DOSE ADJUSTMENTS

Decreased dose may be required in severe renal impairment.

DILUTION

Each 500 mg or fraction thereof should be diluted in 5 ml of SW or NS for injection. May be further diluted for intermittent or continuous infusion in 50 to 1,000 ml of D5W, D5NS, NS, LR, or other compatible IV solutions to a final concentration of 0.5 to 40 mg/ml (see literature or chart on inside back cover). Available prediluted and in ADD-Vantage vials for use with ADD-Vantage infusion containers.

Storage: Diluted solution stable for at least 6 hours. See literature.

INCOMPATIBLE WITH

Manufacturer states, "Do not physically mix with other agents." May degrade in infusion solutions containing acidic agents. Inactivated in solution with aminoglycosides (e.g., amikacin [Amikin], gentamicin [Garamycin]). Do not mix in the same solution. Appropriate spacing and/or separate sites required. See Drug/Lab Interactions.

COMPATIBLE WITH

(Underline Indicates Conflicting Compatibility Information)

Consult pharmacist; specific conditions may apply; see Compatibilities, p. xvi.

Additive: ***See Incompatible With.*** <u>Amikacin (Amikin)</u>, chloramphenicol (Chloromycetin), dopamine (Intropin), potassium chloride (KCl), sodium bicarbonate, <u>verapamil (Isoptin)</u>.

Y-site: Acyclovir (Zovirax), cyclophosphamide (Cytoxan), diltiazem (Cardizem), famotidine (Pepcid IV), fluconazole (Diflucan), foscarnet (Foscavir), heparin, hydrocortisone sodium succinate (Solu-Cortef), hydromorphone (Dilaudid), labetalol (Normodyne), levofloxacin (Levaquin), magnesium sulfate, meperidine (Demerol), methotrexate (Folex), morphine, perphenazine (Trilafon), potassium chloride (KCl), tacrolimus (Prograf), zidovudine (AZT, Retrovir).

RATE OF ADMINISTRATION

Too-rapid rate may cause seizures.

IV injection: 1 Gm (10 ml) or fraction thereof slowly over 10 minutes.

Intermittent IV: A single dose over 10 to 30 minutes.

Infusion: May be administered in specific IV solutions (check literature) over up to a 6-hour period.

ACTIONS

A semisynthetic penicillin with bactericidal effect against penicillinase-producing organisms. Easily distributed into most body fluids, including trace amounts in spinal fluid. Crosses the placental barrier. Excreted primarily in the urine. Secreted in breast milk.

INDICATIONS AND USES

Infection caused by penicillinase-producing staphylococci.

CONTRAINDICATIONS

Known sensitivity to any penicillin or cephalosporin (not absolute).

PRECAUTIONS

Sensitivity studies necessary to determine susceptibility of the causative organism to oxacillin. ■ Superinfection caused by overgrowth of nonsusceptible organisms is a possibility. ■ Pseudomembranous colitis has been reported. May range from mild to life-threatening. Consider in patients that present with diarrhea during or after treatment with oxacillin. ■ Change to oral therapy as soon as practical.

Monitor: Periodic liver, kidney, and hematopoietic studies are advised. ■ Test patients with syphilis for HIV. ■ Electrolyte imbalance and cardiac irregularities from sodium content are possible. Contains up to 4.02 mEq sodium/Gm. May aggravate CHF. Observe for hypokalemia. ■ May cause thrombophlebitis; observe carefully and rotate infusion sites. ■ See Drug/Lab Interactions.

Patient Education: May require alternate birth control.

Maternal/Child: Category B: use only if clearly needed. ■ May cause diarrhea, candidiasis, or allergic response in nursing infants. ■ Limited experience in use on premature infants and neonates. Use with caution. Elimination rate markedly reduced in neonates.

Elderly: Response similar to that seen in younger patients. Consider age-related organ impairment and concomitant disease or drug therapy. ■ See Precautions/Monitor and Dose Adjustments.

DRUG/LAB INTERACTIONS

Synergistic when used in combination with aminoglycosides (e.g., amikacin [Amikin], gentamicin [Garamycin]). Synergism may be inconsistent; see Incompatible With. ■ May be antagonized by bacteriostatic antibiotics (e.g., chloramphenicol, erythromycin, tetracyclines); may interfere with bactericidal action. ■ Potentiated by probenecid (Benemid); toxicity may result. ■ May potentiate heparin. ■ Concomitant use with beta-adrenergic blockers (e.g., propranolol [Inderal]) may increase risk of anaphylaxis and inhibit treatment. ■ May decrease clearance and increase toxicity of methotrexate. ■ May inhibit effectiveness of oral contraceptives; breakthrough bleeding or pregnancy could result. ■ May cause false values in common lab tests; see literature.

SIDE EFFECTS

Relatively infrequent: diarrhea, elevated AST (SGOT), hepatic dysfunction, hypersensitivity with anaphylaxis, nausea, pruritus, skin rash, thrombophlebitis, transient hematuria in newborns, urticaria, vomiting. Hypersensitivity myocarditis (fever, eosinophilia, rash, sinus tachycardia, ST-T changes, and cardiomegaly) and pseudomembranous colitis can occur. Higher-than-normal doses may cause neurologic adverse reactions including convulsions, especially with impaired renal function.

ANTIDOTE

Notify the physician of any adverse symptoms. For severe symptoms, discontinue the drug, treat allergic reaction (antihistamines, epinephrine, corticosteroids), and resuscitate as necessary. Hemodialysis or peritoneal dialysis are minimally effective in overdose.

OXALIPLATIN

Antineoplastic

(oks-al'i-pla-tin)

Eloxatin

USUAL DOSE

Given in combination with 5-FU and leucovorin calcium in a dose schedule that repeats every 2 weeks. For information on 5-FU and leucovorin calcium, see respective monographs. Prehydration is not required. Premedication with antiemetics recommended; see Monitor.

Day 1: Oxaliplatin 85 mg/m^2 and leucovorin calcium 200 mg/m^2, both given as an IV infusion over 120 minutes at the same time in separate bags using a Y-line. Follow with 5-FU 400 mg/m^2 IV bolus given over 2 to 4 minutes, followed by 5-FU 600 mg/m^2 in 500 ml D5W (recommended) as a 22-hour continuous infusion.

Day 2: Leucovorin calcium 200 mg/m^2 IV infusion over 120 minutes. Follow with 5-FU 400 mg/m^2 IV bolus given over 2 to 4 minutes, followed by 5-FU 600 mg/m^2 in 500 ml D5W (recommended) as a 22-hour continuous infusion.

PEDIATRIC DOSE

Safety and effectiveness in pediatric patients not studied; not indicated for pediatric patients.

DOSE ADJUSTMENTS

Dose adjustments are based on clinical toxicities. Reduce dose of oxaliplatin to 65 mg/m^2 in patients who experience persistent Grade 2 neurosensory events that do not resolve. (See Monitor for study-specific neurotoxicity scale.) Consider discontinuing therapy in patients with persistent Grade 3 neurosensory events. The infusional 5-FU/leucovorin calcium regimen need not be altered. ■ Reduce dose of oxaliplatin to 65 mg/m^2 and 5-FU by 20% (300 mg/m^2 bolus and 500 mg/m^2 as a 22-hour infusion) in patients who develop grade 3 or 4 gastrointestinal toxicity (despite prophylactic treatment) or grade 3 or 4 hematologic toxicity (neutrophils less than 1.5×10^9/L [1,500 cells/mm^3], platelets less than 100×10^9/L [100,000 cells/mm^3]). Allow recovery from given toxicity before continuing therapy.

DILUTION

Specific techniques required; see Precautions.

Do not reconstitute or dilute with a sodium chloride solution (e.g., NS, ½NS, ¼NS) or other chloride-containing solutions. To reconstitute, add 10 ml (for the 50-mg vial) or 20 ml (for the 100-mg vial) of SW or D5W. The reconstituted solution must be further diluted with 250 to 500 ml of D5W. Do not use needles or administration sets with aluminum parts; a precipitate may form, and potency may decrease.

Storage: Store unopened vials under normal lighting conditions at CRT; excursions permitted to 15° to 30° C (59° to 86° F). The reconstituted solution may be stored up to 24 hours under refrigeration. After final dilution with 250 to 500 ml of D5W, the solution may be stored for up to 6 hours at CRT or up to 24 hours under refrigeration.

INCOMPATIBLE WITH

Manufacturer states oxaliplatin "is incompatible in solution with alkaline medications or media (such as basic solutions of 5-FU) and must not be mixed with these or administered simultaneously through the same infusion line. *The infusion line should be flushed with D5W prior to administration of any concomitant medication."* Reconstitution or final dilution must not be performed with a sodium chloride solution or other chloride-containing solutions. Do not use needles or administration sets with aluminum parts; a precipitate may form, and potency may decrease.

COMPATIBLE WITH

Y-site: Manufacturer lists leucovorin calcium.

RATE OF ADMINISTRATION

The infusion line should be flushed with D5W prior to administration of any concomitant medication.

Day 1: Oxaliplatin and leucovorin calcium are given as infusions and equally distributed over 120 minutes. Given at the same time in separate bags using a Y-line. When complete, flush the IV line with D5W. Follow with a **5-FU bolus** administered over 2 to 4 minutes, followed by a **5-FU continuous infusion** equally distributed over 22 hours. ■ Increasing the infusion time of oxaliplatin from 2 to 6 hours may mitigate acute toxicities. The infusion times for 5-FU and leucovorin calcium need not be altered.

Day 2: Leucovorin calcium is given as an infusion equally distributed over 120 minutes. Follow with a **5-FU bolus** administered over 2 to 4 minutes, followed by a **5-FU continuous infusion** equally distributed over 22 hours.

ACTIONS

A platinum-based antineoplastic agent. Undergoes nonenzymatic conversion to active derivatives that inhibit DNA replication and transcription. Cytotoxicity is cell-cycle nonspecific. Rapidly distributed into tissues or eliminated in the urine. Highly protein bound. Undergoes rapid and extensive nonenzymatic biotransformation. No evidence of cytochrome P_{450}-mediated metabolism. Major route of elimination is renal excretion.

INDICATIONS AND USES

Used in combination with infusional 5-FU and leucovorin calcium for the treatment of patients with metastatic carcinoma of the colon or rectum whose disease has recurred or progressed during or within 6 months of completion of first-line therapy with the combination of bolus 5-FU/leucovorin calcium and irinotecan.

CONTRAINDICATIONS

Hypersensitivity to oxaliplatin or other platinum-containing compounds (e.g., carboplatin [Paraplatin], cisplatin [Platinol]).

PRECAUTIONS

Follow guidelines for handling cytotoxic agents. See Appendix A, p. 1142. Administered by or under the direction of the physician specialist. ■ Adequate diagnostic and treatment facilities and emergency resuscitation equipment and supplies must always be available. ■ Hypersensitivity and anaphylactic-like reactions have been reported and may occur within minutes of administration. See Side Effects and Antidote. ■ Use with caution in patients with renal impairment. Safety and effectiveness have not been evaluated. ■ Associated with two types of neuropathy. *The first type is an acute, reversible, primarily peripheral sensory neuropathy that is of early onset, occurs within hours or 1 to 2 days of dosing, resolves within 14 days, and frequently recurs with further dosing.* Symptoms may be precipitated or exacerbated by exposure to cold temperature or cold objects. Usually presents as transient paresthesia (abnormal sensation [e.g., burning, prickling]), dysesthesia (decreased sensitivity to stimulation), and hypoesthesia (impairment of any sense, especially touch) in the hands, feet, perioral area, or throat. *The second type is a persistent (lasting more than 14 days), primarily peripheral, sensory neuropathy that is usually characterized by paresthesias, dysesthesias, and hypoesthesias but may also include deficits in proprioception (stimulus of the sensory end organs [e.g., muscles, tendons]), which can interfere with daily activities (e.g., writing, buttoning, swallowing, and walking).* May occur without any prior acute neuropathy event. Symptoms may or may not improve with discontinuation of oxaliplatin. ■ Has been associated with pulmonary fibrosis, which may be fatal; see Monitor. ■ See Drug/Lab Interactions.

Monitor: CBC with differential, platelet count and blood chemistries (including ALT, AST, bilirubin and creatinine) are recommended before each cycle. See Dose Adjustments and Precautions. ■ Monitor for unexplained respiratory symptoms such as nonproductive cough, dyspnea, crackles, or radiologic pulmonary infiltrates. Discontinue oxaliplatin until pulmonary investigation rules out interstitial lung disease or pulmonary fibrosis. ■ Monitor for S/S of neuropathy (e.g., transient paresthesia [abnormal sensation (e.g., burning, prickling)], dysesthesia [decreased sensitivity to stimulation], and hypoesthesia [impairment of any sense, especially touch] in the hands, feet, perioral area, or throat). Neurotoxicity scale used during studies differed from the National Cancer Institute toxicity grading. The grading scale for paresthesias/dysesthesias was as follows: Grade 1, resolved and did not interfere with functioning; Grade 2, interfered with function but not daily activities; Grade 3, pain or functional impairment that interfered with daily activities; Grade 4, persistent impairment that is disabling or life-threatening. ■ Nausea and vomiting may be severe. Prophylactic administration of antiemetics, including $5HT_3$ blockers (e.g., ondansetron [Zofran]), is recommended. ■ Observe closely for signs of infection. Prophylactic antibiotics may be indicated pending results of C/S in a febrile neutropenic patient.

Patient Education: Avoid pregnancy. Nonhormonal birth control recommended. ■ Report any neurologic toxicities. Acute neurosensory toxicity may be precipitated or exacerbated by exposure to cold. Avoid cold drinks and use of ice. Cover exposed skin prior to exposure to cold temperature. ■ Promptly report persistent vomiting, diarrhea, breathing difficulty, cough, or any sign or infection, allergic reaction, or dehydration. ■ Manufacturer supplies a patient information leaflet. ■ See Appendix D, p. 1148.

Maternal/Child: Category D: avoid pregnancy; may cause fetal harm. ■ Discontinue breast-feeding.

Elderly: The overall rates of adverse events, including grade 3 and 4 events, were similar for all age groups. However, the incidence of dehydration, diarrhea, fatigue, and hypokalemia were higher in patients 65 years of age or older.

DRUG/LAB INTERACTIONS

Formal studies have not been performed. ■ Do not administer live-virus vaccines to patients receiving antineoplastic agents. ■ Platinum-containing species are eliminated primarily through the kidney; clearance of these products may be decreased by co-administration of potentially nephrotoxic compounds (e.g., aminoglycosides [e.g., gentamicin (Garamycin)], amphotericin B [all formulations (e.g., Amphotec, Fungizone)], NSAIDs [e.g., ibuprofen (Advil, Motrin), naproxen (Aleve, Naprosyn), phenylbutazone (Butazolidin)], pamidronate [Aredia], tacrolimus [Prograf]). ■ Oxaliplatin is not metabolized by, nor does it inhibit, cytochrome P_{450} isoenzymes. P_{450}-mediated interactions are not anticipated.

SIDE EFFECTS

Are frequent and numerous. Most common adverse reactions are diarrhea, nausea, neutropenia, and peripheral sensory neuropathies; see Precautions. Other reported reactions include abdominal pain, alopecia, angioedema, anorexia, arthralgia, back pain, chest pain, constipation, coughing, deafness, dehydration, dizziness, dyspepsia, dyspnea, dysuria, edema, elevated serum creatinine, epistaxis, fatigue, fever, flushing, gastroesophageal reflux, headache, hand-foot syndrome, hematuria, hemolytic uremic syndrome, hematologic toxicities (e.g., anemia, leukopenia, neutropenia, thrombocytopenia), hepatic toxicity (e.g., elevated ALT, AST, total bilirubin), hypersensitivity reactions (e.g., anaphylaxis, bronchospasm, erythema, hypotension, pruritis, rash, urticaria), hypokalemia, injection site reaction, insomnia, pain, persistent vomiting, pharyngitis, pulmonary fibrosis, rhinitis, rigors, stomatitis, thromboembolism, visual disorders (e.g., decrease of visual acuity, visual field disturbance, optic neuritis). Many other side effects have been reported and may occur.

ANTIDOTE

Notify physician of all side effects. Oxaliplatin may need to be discontinued permanently or until recovery. Slowing of infusion rate may help mitigate acute toxicities. Symptomatic and supportive treatment is indicated. Administration of whole blood products (e.g., packed RBCs, platelets, leukocytes) and/or blood modifiers (e.g., darbepoetin alfa [Aranesp], epoetin alfa [Epogen, Procrit], filgrastim [Neupogen], oprelvekin [Neumega], pegfilgrastim [Neulasta], sargramostim [Leukine]) may be indicated to treat bone marrow toxicity. Treat anaphylaxis with epinephrine, corticosteroids, oxygen, and antihistamines (diphenhydramine). There is no specific antidote. Resuscitate as indicated.

OXYMORPHONE HYDROCHLORIDE

(ox-ee-mor′fone hye-droe-klor′id)

Narcotic analgesic (agonist)

Numorphan

pH 2.7 to 4.5

USUAL DOSE

0.5 mg initially. May repeat every 2 to 4 hours. Up to 1.5 mg may be required.

When seeking the required dose to achieve pain relief for an individual patient, increases in increments of at least 25% of the previous dose are suggested. Lower slightly if pain controlled but patient is too drowsy, or lower dose and increase frequency.

DOSE ADJUSTMENTS

Reduced dose or extended intervals may be required in the elderly, in hepatic or renal disease, and in emphysema. ■ Doses appropriate for the general population may cause serious respiratory depression in vulnerable patients. ■ See Drug/Lab Interactions.

DILUTION

May be given undiluted; however, further dilution with 5 ml of SW or NS to facilitate titration is appropriate. May give through Y-tube or three-way stopcock of infusion set.

Storage: Store below 40° C. Protect from light.

COMPATIBLE WITH

Consult pharmacist; specific conditions may apply; see Compatibilities, p. xvi.

Syringe: Glycopyrrolate, ranitidine (Zantac).

RATE OF ADMINISTRATION

A single dose over 2 to 5 minutes. Usually titrated according to symptom relief and respiratory rate.

ACTIONS

An opium derivative and CNS depressant closely related to morphine. Ten times more potent than morphine milligram for milligram. Onset of action is prompt and lasts 3 to 4 hours. Detoxified in the liver and excreted in the urine. Crosses placental barrier. Secreted in breast milk.

INDICATIONS AND USES

Relief of moderate to severe pain. ■ Support of anesthesia. ■ Obstetric analgesia. ■ Relief of anxiety in dyspnea of acute left ventricular failure and pulmonary edema (rarely used; morphine is the preferred agent).

CONTRAINDICATIONS

Acute bronchial asthma, children under 12 years of age, diarrhea caused by poisoning until toxic material eliminated, known hypersensitivity to opiates, paralytic ileus, premature infants and labor and delivery of premature infants, pulmonary edema caused by chemical respiratory irritant, upper airway obstruction.

PRECAUTIONS

Use caution in the elderly and in patients with impaired hepatic or renal function and pulmonary disease. ■ Use extreme caution in craniotomy, head injury, and increased intracranial pressure; respiratory depression and intracranial pressure may be further increased. ■ May cause apnea in the asthmatic. ■ Symptoms of acute abdominal conditions may be masked. ■ May increase ventricular response rate in presence of supraventricular tachycardias. ■ Cough reflex is suppressed. ■ Tolerance to oxymorphone gradually increases. A marked increase in dose may precipitate seizures.

Monitor: Oxygen, controlled respiratory equipment, and naloxone (Narcan) or nalmefene (Revex) must be available. ■ Observe patient frequently and monitor vital signs. Keep patient supine; orthostatic hypotension and fainting may occur. Uncontrolled pain causes sleep deprivation, decreases pain threshold, and increases pain; when pain is finally controlled, expect the patient to sleep more until recovery from sleep deprivation.

Patient Education: Avoid alcohol or other CNS depressants (e.g., barbiturates, benzodiazepines [e.g., diazepam (Valium)]). ■ May cause blurred vision, dizziness, or drowsiness; use caution in tasks that require alertness. ■ Request assistance with ambulation. ■ May be habit forming.

Maternal/Child: Category C: safety for use in pregnancy or breast-feeding not established; see Contraindications. ■ Safety for use in adolescents under 18 years of age not established.

Elderly: See Dose Adjustments and Precautions. ■ May be more sensitive to effects (e.g., respiratory depression, constipation, urinary retention). ■ Analgesia should be effective with lower doses. ■ Consider age-related organ impairment.

DRUG/LAB INTERACTIONS

Potentiated by phenothiazines and other CNS depressants such as narcotic analgesics, alcohol, antihistamines, barbiturates, cimetidine (Tagamet), hypnotics, sedatives, MAO inhibitors (e.g., selegiline [Eldepryl]), neuromuscular blocking agents (e.g., tubocurarine), and psychotropic agents. Reduced dosages of both drugs may be indicated. ■ Plasma amylase and lipase determinations may be unreliable for 24 hours following narcotic administration.

SIDE EFFECTS

At equianalgesic doses, may cause more nausea, vomiting, and euphoria than morphine.

Anorexia, constipation, dizziness, skin rash, urinary retention, urticaria.

Major: Anaphylaxis, hypotension, respiratory depression, somnolence.

ANTIDOTE

Notify the physician of any side effect. If minor side effects progress or any major side effect occurs, discontinue the drug and notify the physician. Treat anaphylaxis as indicated or resuscitate as necessary. Naloxone hydrochloride (Narcan) or nalmefene (Revex) will reverse serious reactions.

OXYTOCIN INJECTION

(ox-ee-toe'sin in-jek'shun)

Oxytocic
Antihemorrhagic

Pitocin, Syntocinon

pH 2.5 to 4.5

USUAL DOSE

Determined by uterine response and intended use, dilution, and rate of administration. Oxytocins must be administered by only one route at a time. For instance, do not combine oral and IV routes. Piggyback oxytocin into a NS IV without oxytocins; see Precautions.

Induction of labor: Begin with 0.5 to 2 milliunits/min (mU/min). See Dilution and Rate of Administration.

Control of postpartum bleeding: 10 units at 10 to 40 mU/min, following delivery of the infant(s) and preferably the placenta(s). See Dilution and Rate of Administration.

Incomplete or inevitable abortion: 10 units at 10 to 20 mU/min; a second source says 10 to 40 mU/min. See Dilution and Rate of Administration.

Postabortion hemorrhage (unlabeled): 10 units at 20 to 100 mU/min. See Dilution and Rate of Administration.

Oxytocin challenge test (unlabeled): Infuse properly diluted oxytocin (10 mU/ml) at an initial rate of 0.5 mU/min. Gradually increase rate until contractions are every 3 to 4 minutes. Monitor fetal HR concurrently. Observe signs of fetal distress with contractions. Distress indicates inadequate placental reserve. Stop infusion.

DILUTION

In all situations rotate gently to distribute medication through solution.

Induction of labor: Dilute 1 ml (10 units) in 1 liter of NS, D5W, LR, or D5NS for infusion (10 mU/ml). This dilution is also used for the ***oxytocin challenge test.***

Control of postpartum bleeding: Dilute 1 to 4 ml (10 to 40 units) in 1 liter of above infusion fluids (10 to 40 mU/ml).

Incomplete or inevitable abortion/postabortion hemorrhage: Dilute 1 ml (10 units) in 500 ml of above infusion fluids (20 mU/ml).

Storage: Check package insert; if refrigeration is required, some preparations may be stored at CRT for up to 30 days.

INCOMPATIBLE WITH

Rapidly decomposes in the presence of sodium bisulfate.

COMPATIBLE WITH

Consult pharmacist; specific conditions may apply; see Compatibilities, p. xvi.

Additive: Chloramphenicol (Chloromycetin), sodium bicarbonate, thiopental (Pentothal), verapamil (Isoptin).

Y-site: Heparin, hydrocortisone sodium succinate (Solu-Cortef), insulin (regular), meperidine (Demerol), morphine, potassium chloride (KCl), warfarin (Coumadin).

RATE OF ADMINISTRATION

Given only as an IV infusion. Use of an infusion pump or other accurate control device is required. In all situations, use the minimum effective rate and monitor strength, frequency, and duration of contractions; resting uterine tone, fetal HR (in induction of labor), and maternal BP at least every 15 minutes or more often if indicated.

Induction of labor: Begin with 0.5 to 2 mU/min (0.05 to 0.2 ml), increase in increments of 1 to 2 mU/min at 30- to 60-minute intervals until contractions simulate normal labor. Maximum dose rarely exceeds 9 to 10 mU/min at term, average is 2 to 5 mU/min. Reduce by similar increments when desired frequency of contractions is reached and labor has progressed to 5 to 6 cm. 6 mU/min provides oxytocin levels similar to spontaneous labor. Preterm inductions may require somewhat higher doses (one source suggests a maximum of 20 mU/min); use caution.

Control of postpartum bleeding: Rate of infusion must control uterine atony. Begin with 10 to 40 mU/min. Increase or decrease rate as indicated. Proceed quickly but with caution because of strength of solution.

Incomplete or inevitable abortion: 10 to 40 mU/min.

Postabortion hemorrhage: 20 to 100 mU/min.

ACTIONS

A synthetic posterior pituitary hormone that will produce rhythmic contraction of uterine smooth muscle. Its effectiveness depends on the level of uterine excitability, which usually increases as a pregnancy progresses. Very rapid acting, it has a shorter duration of action than ergot derivatives (half-life of 1 to 6 minutes). Duration of action is approximately 1 hour. Is the drug of choice for induction of delivery. Probably detoxified in the liver and through enzymatic processes and excreted in the urine. Has a weak antidiuretic effect.

INDICATIONS AND USES

After selective patient evaluation by the physician, it is used to induce or stimulate labor at term or before. ■ To control postpartum bleeding. ■ To treat incomplete or inevitable abortion. ■ Treatment of postabortion hemorrhage.

Unlabeled uses: Oxytocin challenge test.

CONTRAINDICATIONS

Cephalopelvic disproportion, fetal malpresentation, hypersensitivity, hypertonic uterine contractions, lack of satisfactory progress with adequate uterine activity, obstetrical emergencies (e.g., abruptio placentae), prolonged use in uterine inertia, serious medical or obstetric conditions (past or present), toxemia (severe), vaginal delivery contraindicated (e.g., active herpes genitalis, cord presentation or prolapse, invasive cervical carcinoma, total placenta previa and vasa previa). See Precautions.

PRECAUTIONS

A NS IV without oxytocins must be hung, connected by Y-tube or three-way stopcock, and ready for use in adverse reactions. ■ Should be administered only in the hospital; the physician must be immediately available. ■ Use in fetal distress, hydramnios, partial placenta previa, prematurity, borderline cephalopelvic disproportion, and any condition that may cause uterine rupture (e.g., cesarean section [previous], uterine surgery, uterine overdistention, past history of uterine sepsis) is not recommended except in unusual circumstances. ■ Oxytocin challenge test is an antepartum test of uteroplacental insufficiency in high-risk pregnancy. Test done only by a qualified physician.

Monitor: Monitor BP, fetal heart tones, strength and timing of contractions, and resting uterine tone at least every 15 minutes or more often if indicated. Continuous observation of patient required. ■ Monitor oral fluid intake and observe for signs of fluid retention. Water intoxication has caused maternal death. ■ See Precautions and Drug/Lab Interactions.

Maternal/Child: Has no use before induction of labor; see Contraindications. ▪ May be found in breast milk; consider postponing breast-feeding for 24 hours after discontinued.

DRUG/LAB INTERACTIONS

Severe hypertension can result in the presence of local anesthesia, regional anesthesia (caudal or spinal), and with dopamine (Intropin), ephedrine, epinephrine, methoxamine (Vasoxyl), and other vasopressors. Chlorpromazine (Thorazine) IV will reduce this hypertension.

SIDE EFFECTS

Maternal: Anaphylaxis, cardiac arrhythmias, fatal afibrinogenemia, fluid retention leading to water intoxication and coma, convulsion, and death; hypertension, increased blood loss, nausea, pelvic hematoma, PVCs, postpartum hemorrhage, severe uterine hypertonicity, spasm or contraction; subarachnoid hemorrhage, uterine rupture, vomiting.

Fetal: Bradycardia, brain damage, CNS damage, death, low Apgar scores, neonatal jaundice, retinal hemorrhage.

ANTIDOTE

Nausea and vomiting are tolerable and can be treated symptomatically. Immediately call the physician's attention to any side effect noted or suspected; many can be fatal. Discontinue the drug immediately for any signs of fetal distress, uterine hyperactivity, tetanic contractions, uterine resting tone exceeding 15 to 20 mm H_2O, or water intoxication. Use of a Y-connection or three-way stopcock, allowing the oxytocin drip to be discontinued while the vein is kept open, is required. Turn mother on side (to prevent fetal anoxia) and administer oxygen. Restriction of fluids, diuresis, hypertonic saline solutions IV, correction of electrolyte imbalance, control of convulsions with cautious use of barbiturates, or the use of magnesium sulfate may be required. These side effects can occur during labor and delivery and into the postpartum period. Careful evaluation and selection of patients eliminate many hazards, but be prepared for an emergency.

PACLITAXEL

(pa-kli-tax'el)

Onxol, Taxol

Antineoplastic (miscellaneous)

pH 4.4 to 5.6

USUAL DOSE

Several regimens of paclitaxel, alone or in combination with other antineoplastics, are in use. Doses vary, depending on the regimen used. Consult literature. ■ For all uses, premedication, specific parameters, and specific equipment are required before or during administration; see Premedication, Dose Adjustments, and Precautions/Monitor.

Premedication: Must be premedicated before each dose to prevent severe hypersensitivity reactions. Usual regimen includes IV or oral dexamethasone (Decadron) 20 mg 12 and 6 hours before; IV diphenhydramine (Benadryl) 50 mg 30 to 60 minutes before; and an H_2 antagonist (e.g., IV cimetidine [Tagamet] 300 mg, ranitidine [Zantac] 50 mg, or famotidine [Pepcid IV] 20 mg) 30 to 60 minutes before dosing with paclitaxel. When premedicating patients with AIDS-related Kaposi's sarcoma, reduce the dose of dexamethasone to 10 mg at 12 and 6 hours before paclitaxel. The doses of IV diphenhydramine and IV H_2 antagonists remain as above.

Ovarian cancer in previously untreated patients: 135 mg/M^2 as an infusion over 24 hours. Follow with cisplatin 75 mg/M^2 as an infusion over 6 to 8 hours. Repeat every 3 weeks. An alternative regimen is paclitaxel 175 mg/M^2 as an infusion over 3 hours. Follow with cisplatin 75 mg/M^2 (one source suggests an infusion over 24 hours, another suggests 6 to 8 hours which would allow for outpatient therapy). Repeat every 3 weeks. See comments under Usual Dose.

Ovarian cancer in patients previously treated with chemotherapy: 135 or 175 mg/M^2 as an infusion over 3 hours. An alternate regimen suggests the same dose(s) given as a 24-hour infusion. Repeat every 3 weeks. Larger doses, with or without filgrastim (G-CSF, Neupogen), have produced similar responses. See comments under Usual Dose.

Adjuvant treatment of node-positive breast cancer: 175 mg/M^2 as an infusion over 3 hours. Repeat every 3 weeks for four courses. Administered sequentially to doxorubicin-containing combination therapy. Clinical trials used four courses of doxorubicin and cyclophosphamide. Administer filgrastim (G-CSF) 5 mcg/kg/dose on days 3 through 10. See comments under Usual Dose.

Breast cancer in patients previously treated with chemotherapy: 175 mg/M^2 as an infusion over 3 hours. Alternate regimen suggests same dose(s) given as a 24-hour infusion. Repeat every 3 weeks. See comments under Usual Dose.

First-line treatment of non–small-cell lung cancer: 135 mg/M^2 as an infusion over 24 hours. Follow with cisplatin 75 mg/M^2 over 6 to 8 hours. Repeat every 3 weeks. See comments under Usual Dose. A Canadian source recommends 175 mg/M^2 as an infusion over 3 hours followed with cisplatin 75 mg/M^2 over 6 to 8 hours and repeated every 3 weeks.

AIDS-related Kaposi's sarcoma: 135 mg/M^2 as an infusion over 3 hours. An alternate regimen suggests the same dose(s) given as a 24-hour infusion. Repeat every 3 weeks. Another regimen is 100 mg/M^2 as an infusion over 3 hours repeated every 2 weeks. Toxicity somewhat increased with 135 mg/M^2 dose in clinical studies. See comments under Usual Dose.

Fallopian tube and peritoneal cancers of ovarian origin (unlabeled): 135 to 175 mg/M^2 as a 3-hour infusion in combination with carboplatin AUC 5 to 6, every 3 weeks. Repeat for 5 to 9 cycles. Extend infusion time of paclitaxel if appropriate (e.g., patient comfort, level of toxicity).

DOSE ADJUSTMENTS

Reduce dose by 20% for subsequent courses in patients who experience severe peripheral neuropathy or severe neutropenia (neutrophils less than 500 cells/mm^3) for 1 week or longer. ▪ Withhold therapy if neutrophils below 1,500/mm^3 or platelets below 100,000/mm^3. ▪ Dose reduction not required in impaired renal function. Consider dose adjustment in patients with moderate to severe hepatic impairment. ▪ In AIDS-related Kaposi's sarcoma the parameters are slightly different. Initiate or repeat paclitaxel only if neutrophil count is equal to or greater than 1,000/mm^3; reduce dose of dexamethasone to 10 mg/dose; reduce dose of paclitaxel by 20% in patients who experience severe neutropenia (neutrophils less than 500/mm^3 for a week or longer); use concomitant filgrastim (G-CSF) as clinically indicated.

DILUTION

Specific techniques required; see Precautions. Must be diluted and given as an infusion. May leach the toxic plasticizer DEHP from PVC infusion bags or sets; prepare and store in bottles (glass, polypropylene) or plastic bags (polypropylene, polyolefin) and administer through polyethylene-lined administration sets. Compatible with NS, D5W, D5NS, or D5R. Final concentration of 0.3 to 1.2 mg/ml required. For a 135 mg/M^2 dose, a large adult (body surface about 2 M^2) will receive 270 mg (45 ml of paclitaxel at 6 mg/ml). Will require dilution in an additional 180 ml to make a 1.2 mg/ml concentration or 855 ml to make a 0.3 mg/ml concentration. Solution may appear hazy. Do not use a chemo-dispensing pin, can cause the stopper to collapse and result in loss of sterility.

Storage: May be stored at CRT or refrigerated before dilution (may appear precipitated under refrigeration, will redissolve at room temperature). Diluted for infusion, it is stable at room temperature for up to 27 hours.

INCOMPATIBLE WITH

Leaches out plasticizers; see Dilution.

COMPATIBLE WITH (Underline Indicates Conflicting Compatibility Information)

Consult pharmacist; specific conditions may apply; see Compatibilities, p. xvi.

Additive: Carboplatin (Paraplatin), <u>cisplatin (Platinol)</u>, doxorubicin (Adriamycin); see Drug/Lab Interactions.

Y-site: Acyclovir (Zovirax), amikacin (Amikin), aminophylline, ampicillin/sulbactam (Unasyn), bleomycin (Blenoxane), butorphanol (Stadol), calcium chloride, carboplatin (Paraplatin), cefepime (Maxipime), cefotetan (Cefotan), ceftazidime (Fortaz), ceftriaxone (Rocephin), cimetidine (Tagamet), cisplatin (Platinol), cladribine (Leustatin), cyclophosphamide (Cytoxan), cytarabine (ARA-C), dacarbazine (DTIC), dexamethasone (Decadron), diphenhydramine (Benadryl), doxorubicin (Adriamycin), droperidol (Inapsine), etoposide (Etopophos, VePesid), famotidine (Pepcid

IV), fluconazole (Diflucan), fluorouracil (5-FU), furosemide (Lasix), ganciclovir (Cytovene), gatifloxacin (Tequin), gemcitabine (Gemzar), gentamicin (Garamycin), granisetron (Kytril), haloperidol (Haldol), heparin, hydrocortisone (Hydrocortone, Solu-Cortef), hydromorphone (Dilaudid), ifosfamide (Ifex), linezolid (Zyvox), lorazepam (Ativan), magnesium sulfate, mannitol, meperidine (Demerol), mesna (Mesnex), methotrexate (Folex), metoclopramide (Reglan), morphine, nalbuphine (Nubain), ondansetron (Zofran), pentostatin (Nipent), potassium chloride (KCl), prochlorperazine (Compazine), propofol (Diprivan), ranitidine (Zantac), sodium bicarbonate, thiotepa (Thioplex), topotecan (Hycamtin), vancomycin (Vancocin), vinblastine (Velban), vincristine (Oncovin), zidovudine (AZT, Retrovir).

RATE OF ADMINISTRATION

A single dose properly diluted must be equally distributed over 3 hours or as indicated in Usual Dose. Use of an in-line filter not greater than 0.22 microns required. Use of a metriset (60 gtt/ml) or an infusion pump appropriate to control flow. Rate extended to 24 hours in some regimens.

ACTIONS

An antineoplastic. A novel antimicrotubule agent. Paclitaxel derived from the bark of pacific yew has now been replaced by paclitaxel produced semisynthetically from a renewable source (needles and twigs of the Himalayan yew). Both are chemically identical. Through specific processes it stabilizes microtubules, thus preventing depolymerization. This action inhibits the normal dynamic reorganization of the microtubule network essential for vital interphase and mitotic cellular functions. Also induces abnormal bundles of microtubules throughout the cell cycle and multiple asters of microtubules during mitosis. More active in patients who have not received previous chemotherapy. Distribution and/or tissue (protein) binding is extensive. Evidence suggests metabolism in the liver via the P_{450} system. Half-life ranges from 4.6 to 17.4 hours. High concentrations occur and are probably excreted through bile. Minimal excretion of unchanged drug occurs in urine.

INDICATIONS AND USES

Treatment of metastatic carcinoma of the ovary after failure of first-line or subsequent chemotherapy. ■ First-line treatment for ovarian cancer in combination with cisplatin. ■ Adjuvant treatment of node-positive breast cancer administered sequentially to standard doxorubicin-containing combination chemotherapy. Most effective in estrogen- and progesterone-receptor–negative tumors. ■ Metastatic breast cancer refractory to initial chemotherapy or for a relapse within 6 months. ■ First-line treatment, in combination with cisplatin, for non–small-cell lung cancer in patients who are not candidates for potentially curative surgery or radiation therapy. ■ Second-line treatment of AIDS-related Kaposi's sarcoma.

Unlabeled uses: Advanced head and neck cancer. ■ Cancers of the bladder, cervix, endometrium, esophagus, and upper GI tract. ■ Hormone-refractory prostate cancer. ■ Previously untreated extensive-stage small-cell lung cancer. ■ Non-Hodgkin's lymphomas. ■ Treatment of fallopian tube and peritoneal cancer of ovarian origin. ■ First-line therapy alone and in combination with other agents for treatment of metastatic breast cancer. ■ Treatment of testicular germ cell tumors in patients refractory to cisplatin-based therapy.

CONTRAINDICATIONS

Baseline neutropenia less than 1,500 cells/mm^3 in patients with solid tumors or baseline neutropenia less than 1,000 cells/mm^3 in patients with AIDS-related Kaposi's sarcoma. History of prior severe hypersensitivity reactions to paclitaxel or other drugs formulated in polyoxyethylated castor oil (Cremophor EL [e.g., cyclosporine, teniposide]).

PRECAUTIONS

Follow guidelines for handling cytotoxic agents. See Appendix A, p. 1142. ■ Usually administered by or under the direction of the physician specialist. ■ Adequate diagnostic and treatment facilities must be readily available. ■ Use caution in patients with cardiac conduction abnormalities, CHF, and MI within previous 6 months. ■ Myelosuppression may be more frequent and more severe in patients who have received prior radiation therapy. ■ Pre-existing neuropathies resulting from prior therapies are not a contraindication for paclitaxel therapy. ■ Various studies show that incidence and severity of neurotoxicity and hematologic toxicity increase with dose, especially above 190 mg/M^2. ■ Use with caution in patients with moderate to severe hepatic impairment; see Dose Adjustments.

Monitor: ■ Use caution to prevent bone marrow depression, primarily neutropenia. Dose dependent and is the dose-limiting toxicity. Obtain baseline CBC with differential and platelet count. Monitor frequently during therapy and before each dose. Neutrophil nadir occurs around day 11; see Dose Adjustments. ■ Obtain baseline ECG; arrhythmias occur frequently. Continuous cardiac monitoring required for all patients with an abnormal baseline ECG or those who experienced conduction arrhythmias during administration of a previous dose. ■ Anaphylaxis and severe hypersensitivity reactions have been reported. Fatal reactions have occurred despite premedication. ■ Most severe hypersensitivity reactions occur in the first hour; monitor all vital signs, including BP continuously for the first 30 minutes of the infusion and at frequent intervals after that. Incidence seems to decrease with subsequent doses. ■ Treatment can often be continued in patients with mild hypersensitivity reactions if proper premedication is given. ■ Observe closely for signs of infection. Prophylactic antibiotics may be indicated pending results of C/S in a febrile neutropenic patient. ■ Use prophylactic antiemetics to reduce nausea and vomiting and increase patient comfort. ■ Monitor injection site carefully; avoid extravasation. Incidence of inflammation increased with 24-hour infusions. Injection site reactions may occur during administration or be delayed by 7 to 10 days. ■ Monitor for thrombocytopenia (platelet count less than 50,000/mm^3). Initiate precautions to prevent excessive bleeding (e.g., inspect IV sites, skin, and mucous membranes; use extreme care during invasive procedures; test urine, emesis, stool, and secretions for occult blood).

Patient Education: Avoid pregnancy; nonhormonal birth control recommended. ■ Review of monitoring requirements and adverse events before therapy imperative. ■ Report any unusual or unexpected symptoms, side effects, pain or burning at injection site, signs of infection (e.g., chills, fever, night sweats), or signs of bleeding (e.g., bruising, tarry stools, blood in urine, pinpoint red spots on skin) as soon as possible. ■ See Appendix D, p. 1148. ■ Obtain name and telephone number of a contact person for

emergencies, questions, or problems. ■ Seek resources for counseling or supportive therapy. ■ Manufacturer provides a patient information booklet.
Maternal/Child: Category D: avoid pregnancy. May cause fetal harm. ■ Discontinue breast-feeding. ■ Safety for use in children not established. ■ CNS toxicity (rarely associated with death) was reported in one pediatric trial using high-dose paclitaxel. Use of antihistamines and the ethanol contained in the paclitaxel may have contributed to toxicity noted.
Elderly: Studies suggest response is similar to that seen in younger patients. However, incidence of side effects, including myelosuppression, neuropathy, and cardiovascular events, may be increased in the elderly.

DRUG/LAB INTERACTIONS

Dexamethasone, diphenhydramine, cimetidine, and ranitidine do not affect protein binding of paclitaxel. ■ To reduce potential for profound myelosuppression when using paclitaxel and cisplatin concurrently, give paclitaxel first, then cisplatin. ■ Ketoconazole (Nizoral) concomitantly may inhibit metabolism and increase toxicity. ■ Other inhibitors of cytochrome P_{450} isoenzyme CYP2C8 (e.g., cyclosporine [Sandimmune], dexamethasone [Decadron], diazepam [Valium], etoposide, quinidine, teniposide [Vumon], testosterone, verapamil [Isoptin]) may also inhibit metabolism of paclitaxel and increase toxicity. ■ Neurotoxicity and symptomatic motor dysfunction occurring with higher doses (greater than 250 mg/M^2) may be potentiated by cisplatin and filgrastim (G-CSF). ■ May cause additive effects with bone marrow–depressing agents, radiation therapy or agents that cause blood dyscrasias (e.g., amphotericin B, antithyroid agents [Methimazole (Tapazole)], azathioprine [Imuran], chloramphenicol, ganciclovir [Cytovene], interferon, plicamycin [Mithracin], zidovudine [AZT]). Reduced doses may be required. ■ May increase levels of doxorubicin and its active metabolite when drugs are used in combination. ■ Do not administer chloroquine or live virus vaccines to patients receiving antineoplastic agents.

SIDE EFFECTS

Dose dependent and generally reversible, but may be fatal. All patients were premedicated to prevent hypersensitivity reactions. Abnormal ECG, alopecia, arthralgia/myalgia, bleeding, bone marrow depression (anemia, leukopenia, neutropenia, thrombocytopenia), bleeding, bradycardia, diarrhea, elevated bilirubin, elevated alkaline phosphatase, elevated AST (SGOT), fever, hypersensitivity reactions (moderate, [e.g., dyspnea, flushing, hypotension, rash, tachycardia]; severe [e.g., chest pain, dyspnea requiring bronchodilators, hypotension requiring treatment, generalized urticaria]), hypertension, hypotension, infections (chills, fever, nightsweats), injection site reactions (cellulitis, fibrosis, induration, necrosis, phlebitis, skin exfoliation), mucositis, nausea and vomiting, numbness, peripheral neuropathy, respiratory reactions (interstitial pneumonia, lung fibrosis, pulmonary embolism), Stevens-Johnson syndrome, and toxic epidermal necrolysis. A grand mal seizure occurred in one patient.

ANTIDOTE

Keep physician informed of all side effects. Most will be treated symptomatically as indicated. Most hypersensitivity reactions will subside with temporary discontinuation of paclitaxel, and incidence seems to decrease with subsequent doses. Moderate reactions such as dyspnea, flushing, hypotension, skin reactions, or tachycardia do not usually require interruption of treatment. Severe reactions may require epinephrine (Adrenalin), antihistamines (e.g., diphenhydramine [Benadryl]), corticosteroids (e.g., dexamethasone [Decadron]), or bronchodilators (e.g., albuterol [Ventolin], theophylline [aminophylline]). Most severe reactions should not be rechallenged, but some patients tolerated subsequent doses. Neutropenia can be profound, and the nadir usually occurs about day 11. Recovery is generally rapid and spontaneous but may be treated with filgrastim (G-CSF, Neupogen, pegfilgrastim [Neulasta]). Severe thrombocytopenia (nadir day 8 or 9) may require platelet transfusions; has been treated with oprelvekin (Neumega). Severe anemia (less than 8 Gm/dl) may require packed cell transfusions, moderate anemia (less than 11 Gm/dl) may be treated with darbepoetin alfa [Aranesp] or epoetin alfa (Epogen). Hypotension and bradycardia do not usually occur at the same time except in hypersensitivity. Treat only if symptomatic. Some arrhythmias (e.g., nonspecific repolarization abnormalities, sinus tachycardia, and PVCs) are common and may not require intervention. Treat any serious or symptomatic arrhythmia (e.g., conduction abnormalities, ventricular tachycardia) promptly and monitor continuously during subsequent doses. Neurologic symptoms tend to worsen with each course; see Dose Adjustments. Usually improve within several months. Severe peripheral neuropathies or seizure may necessitate discontinuation of paclitaxel. There is no specific antidote for overdose. Supportive therapy will help sustain the patient in toxicity. Resuscitate if indicated.

PAMIDRONATE DISODIUM

(pam-id′drow-nate dye-so′de-um)

APD, Aredia

Antihypercalcemic (bisphosphonate)

pH 6 to 7.4

USUAL DOSE

Prehydration required. Do not exceed a single dose of 90 mg. See Precautions and Monitor.

Moderate hypercalcemia (corrected serum calcium of 12 to 13.5 mg/dl): One dose of 60 to 90 mg as an infusion.

Severe hypercalcemia (corrected serum calcium greater than 13.5 mg/dl): One dose of 90 mg as an infusion. Serum calcium levels should fall into the normal range (8.5 to 10.5 mg/100 ml [1 dl], corrected for serum albumin).

Experience is limited, but retreatment with the same dose may be considered if hypercalcemia recurs; wait at least 7 days from completion of first infusion to allow full response. Always used in conjunction with adequate hydration and appropriate testing. See Precautions/Monitor.

Paget's disease: 30 mg/day as an infusion for 3 consecutive days. Selected patients have been retreated with the same dose when indicated. Experience limited; see note above.

Osteolytic bone lesions of multiple myeloma: 90 mg as an infusion once every 30 days. Optimal duration of therapy not known. Withhold dose if renal function has deteriorated; see Dose Adjustments, Precautions, and Monitor.

Osteolytic bone metastases of breast cancer: 90 mg as an infusion every 3 to 4 weeks. Withhold dose if renal function has deteriorated; see Dose Adjustments, Precautions, and Monitor.

DOSE ADJUSTMENTS

Lower-dose regimen may be appropriate in impaired renal or hepatic function. No experience with creatinine above 5 mg/100 ml (1 dl). ■ See Precautions.

Osteolytic bone lesions of multiple myeloma and osteolytic bone metastases of breast cancer: Withhold dose if renal function has deteriorated. Renal deterioration is defined as an increase of 0.5 mg/dl in patients with a *normal* baseline creatinine or an increase of 1 mg/dl in patients with *abnormal* baseline creatinine. One study suggests that treatment should not be resumed until SrCr has returned to within 10% of baseline value.

DILUTION

Reconstitute each 30-, 60-, or 90-mg vial with 10 ml SW for injection. Dissolve completely (3, 6, or 9 mg/ml).

Hypercalcemia of malignancy: Further dilute a single daily dose in 1,000 ml NS (preferred), ½NS, or D5W. A minimum of 500 ml diluent may be used if absolutely necessary in patients with compromised cardiovascular status.

Paget's disease: Further dilute a single daily dose in 500 ml of the above solutions.

Osteolytic bone lesions of multiple myeloma: Further dilute each 90 mg dose in 500 ml of above solutions.

Osteolytic bone metastases of breast cancer: Further dilute each 90-mg dose in 250 ml of above solutions.

Storage: Before reconstitution, store at CRT. After reconstitution, may be refrigerated for up to 24 hours. Stable after dilution for 24 hours at room temperature.

COMPATIBILITY

Manufacturer states, "Should be given in a single intravenous solution and line separate from all other drugs, and do not mix with calcium-containing solutions (e.g., Ringer's solutions)."

RATE OF ADMINISTRATION

Use of a microdrip (60 gtt/ml) or an infusion pump recommended for even distribution. Do not exceed recommended rate of infusion. Duration should be no less than 2 hours. Too-rapid infusion rate may lead to overdose, elevated BUN and creatinine levels, and renal tubular necrosis. Rate recommendations vary considerably. They are based on specific clinical trials for each diagnosis. In some trials a rate of up to 1 mg/min has been used with caution.

Hypercalcemia of malignancy: A 60-mg dose or 90-mg dose equally distributed over 2 to 24 hours. Longer infusion times (i.e., greater than 2 hours) may reduce the risk of renal toxicity, particularly in patients with pre-existing renal insufficiency.

Paget's disease: A single dose over 4 hours.

Osteolytic bone lesions of multiple myeloma: A single dose over 4 hours.

Osteolytic bone metastases of breast cancer: A single dose over 2 hours.

ACTIONS

A bisphosphonate hypocalcemic agent. Reduces serum calcium concentrations by inhibiting accelerated bone resorption. Binds to preformed bone surfaces and may block bone mineral dissolution. Effectively inhibits accelerated bone resorption resulting from osteoclast hyperactivity induced by various tumors. Does not inhibit bone formation and mineralization. Plasma levels achieve some reduction in calcium levels in 24 to 48 hours, and maximal response in 4 to 7 days. In two studies a single dose normalized serum calcium by day 7 in 61% to 70% of patients treated with 60 mg and 100% of those treated with 90 mg. Maintains duration of normocalcemia/hypocalcemia longer than etidronate (Didronel). Rapidly adsorbed by bone with some transit through the liver. Slowly excreted in urine.

INDICATIONS AND USES

Treatment of moderate to severe hypercalcemia of malignancy in patients with or without bone metastasis, in conjunction with adequate hydration. Symptoms of hypercalcemia may include anorexia, bone pain, confusion, constipation, dehydration, depression, fatigue, lethargy, muscle weakness, nausea and vomiting, and polyuria. Severe dehydration may lead to renal insufficiency. With high levels of serum calcium, cardiac manifestations (e.g., bradycardia, cardiac arrest, ventricular arrhythmias), and neurologic symptoms (e.g., coma, seizures, and death) may occur. ■ Treatment of Paget's disease. ■ Adjunct in treatment of osteolytic lesions of multiple myeloma and osteolytic bone metastases of breast cancer.

Unlabeled uses: Prevent or decrease bone loss in women undergoing chemotherapy.

CONTRAINDICATIONS

Hypersensitivity to pamidronate or other bisphosphonates (e.g., etidronate [Didronel], alendronate [Fosamax]).

PRECAUTIONS

Calcium is bound to serum protein; concentration fluctuates with changes in blood volume. Changes in serum calcium (especially during rehydration) may not reflect true plasma levels. Measurement with ionized calcium levels is preferred. If unavailable, all calcium measurement should be corrected for albumin to establish a basis for treatment and evaluation of treatment. ■ Mild or asymptomatic hypercalcemia will be treated with conservative measures (e.g., saline hydration, with or without diuretics [after correcting hypovolemia]). Consider patient's cardiovascular status. Corticosteroids may be indicated if the underlying cancer is sensitive (e.g., hematologic cancers). ■ Use in the treatment of hypercalcemia associated with hyperparathyroidism or with other non–tumor-related conditions has not been adequately studied. ■ May be used adjunctively with chemotherapy, radiation, or surgery. ■ May cause renal toxicity. Deterioration in renal function progressing to renal failure has been reported. Patients with pre-existing renal impairment may be at increased risk for developing toxicity. Do not exceed dose of 90 mg. ■ ***Osteolytic bone lesions of multiple myeloma and osteolytic bone metastases of breast cancer:*** Patients being treated for multiple myeloma and bone metastases should have the dose withheld if renal function has deteriorated. Renal deterioration is defined as an increase of 0.5 mg/dl in patients with a *normal* baseline creatinine or an increase of 1 mg/dl in patients with *abnormal* baseline creatinine. One study suggests that treatment should not be resumed until SrCr has returned to within 10% of baseline value. Use is not recommended in patients with severe renal impairment being treated for bone metastases. See Monitor and Dose Adjustments. Limited information available on use in multiple myeloma patients with a SrCr above 3 mg/dl.

Monitor: Obtain baseline measurements of serum calcium (corrected for serum albumin), electrolytes, phosphate, magnesium, and creatinine and CBC with differential and hematocrit/hemoglobin. Monitor all closely as indicated by baseline results (may be daily). Serum phosphate levels will decrease and usually require treatment. ■ Monitor renal function prior to each treatment; nephropathy has been reported; see Precautions. ■ Monitor serum alkaline phosphatase during therapy for Paget's disease. ■ Patients with cancer-related hypercalcemia are frequently dehydrated. Must be adequately hydrated orally and/or IV before treatment is initiated. Hydration with saline is preferred to facilitate renal excretion of calcium and correct dehydration. A pretreatment urine output of 2 L/day is recommended. Maintain adequate hydration and urine output throughout treatment. ■ Avoid overhydration in patients with compromised cardiovascular status. Observe frequently for signs of fluid overload. Correct hypovolemia before using diuretics. ■ Monitor patients with pre-existing anemia, leukopenia, or thrombocytopenia very carefully during treatment and the first 2 weeks following treatment. ***Osteolytic bone lesions of multiple myeloma:*** Adequately hydrate patients with marked Bence-Jones proteinuria and dehydration before pamidronate infusion.

Patient Education: Regular visits and assessment of lab tests imperative. ■ Dietary restriction of calcium and vitamin D may be required. ■ Take only prescribed meds. ■ Report abdominal cramps, chills, confusion, fever, muscle spasms, sore throat and/or any new medical problems promptly. ■ Avoid pregnancy; use of nonhormonal birth control suggested.

Maternal/Child: Category D: should not be used during pregnancy. May cause fetal harm. Avoid pregnancy; use of birth control necessary. ■ Safety for use during breast-feeding not established. ■ Safety for use in children not established.

Elderly: Monitor fluid and electrolyte status carefully to avoid overhydration. Use of lower fluid volume may be required; see Dilution.

DRUG/LAB INTERACTIONS

Use caution when administered with other potentially nephrotoxic drugs (e.g., aminoglycosides [tobramycin (Nebcin), gentamicin (Garamycin)], cisplatin [Platinol]). ■ Use with furosemide (Lasix) does not affect calcium-lowering action. ■ Does not interfere with any known primary cancer therapy. ■ Effects may be antagonized by calcium-containing preparations or vitamin D; avoid use.

SIDE EFFECTS

Average dose: Abdominal pain, anemia, anorexia, bone pain, constipation, fever (mild and transient), generalized pain, hypertension, hypocalcemia (abdominal cramps, confusion, muscle spasms), infusion site reaction (e.g., induration and pain on palpation, redness, swelling), renal toxicity, seizures, urinary tract infections, vomiting. Fluid overload, hypokalemia, hypomagnesemia, and hypophosphatemia occur frequently with use of concurrent fluid and diuretics. Rare instances of allergic reactions, including anaphylaxis, angioedema, dyspnea, and hypotension, have occurred.

Overdose: Occurs less frequently with lower dose range (30 to 60 mg). Fever (high), hypocalcemia, hypotension, leukopenia or lymphopenia (fever, chills, sore throat), transient taste perversion. Elevated BUN and CrCl levels and renal tubular necrosis may occur with excessive dose or rate of administration.

ANTIDOTE

Keep physician informed of side effects. Some may respond to symptomatic treatment. Magnesium, phosphorus, and potassium may require replacement if depletion too severe. If mild, all will probably return toward normal in 7 to 10 days. For asymptomatic or mild to moderate hypocalcemia (6.5 to 8 mg/100 ml [1 dl] corrected for serum albumin), short-term calcium therapy (e.g., calcium gluconate) may be indicated. Discontinue drug for any symptoms of overdose. Monitor serum calcium and use vigorous IV hydration, with or without diuretics, for 2 to 3 days. Monitor intake and output to ensure adequacy and balance. Use short-term IV calcium therapy if indicated. High fever may respond to steroids. RBC transfusions may be required in anemia. Treat anaphylaxis and resuscitate as indicated.

PANCURONIUM BROMIDE
(pan-kyoo-roe′nee-um bro′mid)

Pavulon

Neuromuscular blocking agent (nondepolarizing)
Anesthesia adjunct

pH 4

USUAL DOSE

Adjunct to general anesthesia for adults and children: Must be individualized, depending on previous drugs administered and degree and length of muscle relaxation required. Must be used with adequate anesthesia and/or sedation and after unconsciousness induced. Succinylcholine must show signs of wearing off before pancuronium is given. 0.04 to 0.1 mg/kg of body weight initially. 0.01 mg/kg in increments as required to maintain muscle relaxation; usually 25- to 60-minute intervals.

Endotracheal intubation: 0.06 to 0.1 mg/kg.

Support of intubated mechanically ventilated or respiratory-controlled adult ICU patients (unlabeled): ***IV bolus injection:*** 0.1 to 0.2 mg/kg every 1 to 3 hours. ***Continuous infusion:*** begin with a ***loading dose*** of 0.03 to 0.1 mg/kg followed by a ***maintenance dose*** of 0.06 to 0.1 mg/kg/hr. A lower-end or reduced dose may be indicated if administered more than 5 minutes after the start of an inhalation agent, when steady-state has been achieved, or in patients with organ dysfunction (e.g., impaired renal function). Adjust dose according to clinical assessment of the patient's response. Use of a peripheral nerve stimulator is recommended.

NEONATAL DOSE

Adjunct to general anesthesia: Extreme sensitivity to pancuronium exists during the first month of life. Begin with a test dose of 0.02 mg/kg and assess responsiveness.

DOSE ADJUSTMENTS

See Drug/Lab Interactions; marked reduction of pancuronium dose may be required. ■ A higher total dose may be required in biliary or hepatic disease, but onset is slower and neuromuscular block is prolonged.

DILUTION

May be given undiluted or diluted in D5W, D5/½NS, D5NS, NS, or LR for use as an infusion.

Storage: Best if stored in refrigerator. Will maintain potency at room temperature for up to 6 months.

COMPATIBLE WITH

(Underline Indicates Conflicting Compatibility Information)

Consult pharmacist; specific conditions may apply; see Compatibilities, p. xvi.

Additive: Verapamil (Isoptin).

Syringe: Heparin.

Y-site: Aminophylline, cefazolin (Kefzol), cefuroxime (Zinacef), cimetidine (Tagamet), dobutamine (Dobutrex), dopamine (Intropin), epinephrine (Adrenalin), esmolol (Brevibloc), etomidate (Amidate), fentanyl (Sublimaze), fluconazole (Diflucan), gentamicin (Garamycin), heparin, hetastarch in electrolytes (Hextend), hydrocortisone sodium succinate (Solu-Cortef), isoproterenol (Isuprel), levofloxacin (Levaquin), lorazepam (Ativan), midazolam (Versed), milrinone (Primacor), morphine, nitroglycerin (Nitro-Bid IV), nitroprusside sodium, propofol (Diprivan), ranitidine (Zantac), sulfamethoxazole-trimethoprim (Bactrim), vancomycin (Vancocin).

RATE OF ADMINISTRATION

Adjunct to general anesthesia: A single dose over 60 to 90 seconds.

Mechanical ventilation support in ICU: See Usual Dose for specific rates and criteria.

ACTIONS

A skeletal muscle relaxant five times as potent as tubocurarine chloride (curare). Causes paralysis by interfering with neural transmission at the myoneural junction. Onset of action is dose dependent. Peak effect occurs in 3 to 4 minutes and lasts 30 to 45 minutes. It may take another 30 minutes or up to several hours before complete recovery occurs. Excreted in the urine.

INDICATIONS AND USES

Adjunctive to general anesthesia to facilitate endotracheal intubation and to relax skeletal muscles during surgery or mechanical ventilation.

Unlabeled uses: Support of intubated, mechanically ventilated, or respiratory-controlled patients in ICU.

CONTRAINDICATIONS

Known hypersensitivity to pancuronium or bromides; first trimester of pregnancy.

PRECAUTIONS

Usually administered by or under the direct observation of the anesthesiologist. ■ Repeated doses may produce a cumulative effect. ■ Impaired pulmonary function or respiratory deficiencies can cause critical reactions. ■ Use caution in impaired liver or kidney function, in patients with tachycardia, and in any patient who might develop adverse effects from an increase in HR. ■ Myasthenia gravis increases sensitivity to drug. ■ Long-term use (i.e., intensive care) may result in prolonged paralysis or skeletal muscle weakness. ■ Acid base and/or electrolyte imbalance, debilitation, hypoxic episodes, and/or the use of other drugs (e.g., broad-spectrum antibiotics, narcotics, steroids) may prolong the effects of pancuronium.

Monitor: ***All uses:*** This drug produces apnea. Controlled artificial ventilation with oxygen must be continuous and under direct observation at all times. Maintain a patent airway. ■ Use a peripheral nerve stimulator to monitor response to pancuronium and avoid overdose. ■ Patient may be conscious and completely unable to communicate by any means. Pancuronium has no analgesic or sedative properties. ■ Action is altered by dehydration, electrolyte imbalance, body temperatures, and acid-base imbalance. ■ Hyperkalemia may cause cardiac arrhythmias and increased paralysis. ■ See Precautions and Drug/Lab Interactions.

Mechanical ventilation support in ICU: Physical therapy is recommended to prevent muscular weakness, atrophy, and joint contracture. Muscular weakness may first be noticed during attempts to wean patients from the ventilator.

Maternal/Child: Category C: unknown potential hazards to fetus. Benefits must outweigh risks. Not recommended in first trimester. ■ Has caused rare severe skeletal muscle weakness in neonates undergoing mechanical ventilation.

Elderly: Delay in onset time may be caused by slower circulation time in cardiovascular disease, old age, or edematous states; allow more time for drug to achieve maximum effect.

DRUG/LAB INTERACTIONS

May cause severe arrhythmias with inhalant anesthetics (e.g., enflurane, halothane), and in patients on chronic tricyclic antidepressant therapy (e.g., amitriptyline [Elavil]). ■ Potentiated by hypokalemia, some carcinomas, many antibiotics (e.g., aminoglycosides [kanamycin (Kantrex), gentamicin (Garamycin)], bacitracin, colistin [Coly-Mycin S], colistimethate [Coly-Mycin M], polymixin-B [Aerosporin], tetracyclines, piperacillin), calcium salts, CO_2, diuretics, diazepam (Valium) and other muscle relaxants, digitalis, magnesium sulfate, quinidine, morphine, lidocaine, meperidine, propranalol (Inderal), succinylcholine, and others. May need to reduce dose of pancuronium; use with caution. ■ Recurrent paralysis may occur with quinidine. ■ Effects may be decreased by acetylcholine, anticholinesterases, aminophylline, azathioprine, carbamazepine, and potassium. ■ Succinylcholine must show signs of wearing off before pancuronium is given. Use caution.

SIDE EFFECTS

Increased HR, decrease in mean arterial pressure, prolonged action resulting in respiratory insufficiency or apnea and tachycardia. Airway closure caused by relaxation of epiglottis, pharynx, and tongue muscles. Hypersensitivity reactions are possible. Anaphylaxis, histamine release (e.g., bronchospasm, vasodilation, hypotension, cutaneous flushing), and shock may occur. Muscular weakness and atrophy may occur with long-term use (1 to 3 weeks).

ANTIDOTE

All side effects are medical emergencies. Treat symptomatically. Controlled artificial ventilation must be continuous. Pyridostigmine (Mestinon) or neostigmine (Prostigmin) given with atropine will probably reverse the muscle relaxation. Not effective in all situations; may aggravate severe overdose. Resuscitate as necessary.

PANTOPRAZOLE SODIUM

(pan-toe-pra′zole so′de-um)

Protonix IV

Proton pump inhibitor (Gastric acid inhibitor)

pH 9 to 10

USUAL DOSE

Given as an alternative to continued oral therapy. Resume oral therapy as soon as practical.

Treatment of gastroesophageal reflux disease (GERD): 40 mg as an infusion once daily for 7 to 10 days.

Treatment of Zollinger-Ellison syndrome (ZES): 80 mg as an infusion every 12 hours. Adjust to patient needs based on acid output measurements. If an increased dose is required, 80 mg every 8 hours is expected to maintain gastric acid output at less than 10 mEq/hr. Daily doses in excess of 240 mg or for more than 6 days have not been studied.

DOSE ADJUSTMENTS

No dose adjustments are necessary based on race or gender, in the elderly, or in patients with mild, moderate, or severe renal insufficiency, on hemodialysis; or with mild to moderate impaired hepatic function.

DILUTION

Reconstitute each single dose with 10 ml NS. Must be further diluted with 100 ml D5W, NS, or LR to achieve a final concentration of approximately 0.4 mg/ml for infusion. Must be administered through a 1.2 micron filter (supplied by manufacturer).

Storage: Refrigerate vials in carton to protect from light. Do not freeze. Store supplied filters at CRT. Reconstituted solution stable for 2 hours at CRT. Fully diluted solution is stable at CRT for up to 12 hours prior to actual infusion. Protection from light is not required for reconstituted or fully diluted solutions.

COMPATIBILITY

Manufacturer states, "Administer through a dedicated line, should not be simultaneously administered through the same line with other intravenous solutions." See Rate of Administration.

RATE OF ADMINISTRATION

Use of an in line 1.2 micron filter required. Filter is supplied by the manufacturer and must be used to remove precipitates that may form when the reconstituted drug is further diluted with IV solution. A dedicated line is preferred but if a Y-site is used, the filter must be positioned below the Y-site that is closest to the patient. In all situations the IV line must be flushed before and after administration of pantoprazole with compatible infusion solutions (D5W, NS, or LR).

Each single dose should be evenly distributed as an infusion over 15 minutes but the rate per minute should not exceed 3 mg/min (7 ml/min).

ACTIONS

A proton pump inhibitor (PPI) that suppresses the final step in gastric acid production. Acts at the secretory surface of the gastric parietal cell. Its effect is dose-related up to a daily dose of 80 mg and leads to inhibition of both basal and stimulated gastric acid secretion irrespective of the stimulus. Does not accumulate and pharmacokinetics are not altered with multiple daily dosing. Half-life is approximately one hour. Duration of antisecretory effect persists longer than 24 hours. Distributed mainly in extracellular fluid. Highly bound by serum protein (primarily albumin). Extensively metabolized in the liver through the cytochrome P_{450} (CYP) system. Metabolism is independent of the route of administration (intravenous or oral). Primarily excreted in urine with some excretion in feces.

INDICATIONS AND USES

Short-term treatment (7 to 10 days) of gastroesophageal reflux disease (GERD), as an alternative to oral therapy in patients who are unable to continue taking pantoprazole delayed-release tablets. Safety and effectiveness for use in the initial treatment of GERD has not been demonstrated. ■ Treatment of pathological hypersecretion associated with Zollinger-Ellison syndrome.

CONTRAINDICATIONS

Known hypersensitivity to pantoprazole or its components.

PRECAUTIONS

For IV use only; do not give IM or SC. ■ Gastric malignancy may be present even though patient's symptoms improve with pantoprazole therapy. ■ Use caution in patients with severe hepatic impairment. Half-life is prolonged (range is 3.5 to 10 hours). Some accumulation (equal to or less than 23% with once-daily dosing) occurs but no dose adjustment is indicated. ■ A prolonged half-life with similar accumulation may also occur in Asian (17% to 23%), African American (3%), and Caucasian (3%) populations, dose adjustment is not indicated. ■ May have carcinogenic potential. ■ Should be discontinued as soon as the patient is able to resume treatment with pantoprazole delayed-release tablets. ■ Data on safe and effective dosing for other conditions (including life-threatening upper GI bleeds) is not available. 40 mg IV of pantoprazole daily does not raise gastric pH levels sufficiently to treat such life-threatening conditions.

Monitor: Observe for S/S of allergic reaction, anaphylaxis has been reported in post-marketing reports. ■ Monitor vital signs and pain levels. ■ Concomitant use of antacids may be indicated. ■ In hypersecretory states, acid output measurements may be indicated to guide dose adjustment. ■ Change to oral dosing when appropriate.

Patient Education: Review prescription and non-prescription drugs with your physician. ■ Oral route preferred.

Maternal/Child: Category B: use during pregnancy only when clearly needed. ■ Has potential for serious harm to nursing infants, discontinue breast-feeding. ■ Safety and effectiveness for pediatric patients under 18 years of age is not established.

Elderly: Safety and effectiveness similar to that of younger patients.

DRUG/LAB INTERACTIONS

Because of profound and long lasting inhibition of gastric acid secretion, pantoprazole may interfere with absorption of drugs where gastric pH is an important determinant of their bioavailability (e.g., ampicillin [Omnipen], esters, iron salts [ferrous sulfate], ketoconazole [Nizoral]). Studies suggest that with concurrent use the metabolism and serum concentrations of pantoprazole are not significantly altered by other drugs metabolized by the Cytochrome P_{450} system (e.g., diazepam [Valium], diclofenac [Apo-Diclo], metoprolol [Lopressor], nifedipine [ProCardia XL], phenytoin [Dilantin], theophylline). ■ Studies also suggest that concurrent use with pantoprazole has not been found to significantly alter the metabolism and serum concentrations of the above agents as well as other drugs metabolized by a similar process (e.g., carbamazepine [Tegretol], cisapride [Propulsid], oral contraceptives). Concurrent administration should not require dose adjustment of either drug. ■ Antipyrine (Allergen), caffeine, digoxin (Lanoxin), and glyburide (DiaBeta) had no clinically relevant interactions during clinical studies. ■ May cause false-positive for tetrahydrocannabinol (THC) with urine screening tests.

SIDE EFFECTS

Abscess, abdominal pain, blurred vision, chest pain, confusion, diarrhea, dyspnea, gastroenteritis, headache, hemorrhage, hyperglycemia, hypokinesia, increased salivation, injection site reactions including thrombophlebitis, nausea, pruritus, rash, speech disorder, tinnitus, urinary tract infection, and vertigo have been reported. Numerous other side effects have been associated with oral pantoprazole. Post-marketing reports include allergic reactions (e.g., anaphylaxis, angioedema), anterior ischemic optic neuropathy, hepatocellular damage leading to jaundice and hepatic failure, pancreatitis, severe dermatologic reactions (e.g., erythema multiforme, Stevens-Johnson syndrome, toxic epidermal necrolysis [some fatal]).

ANTIDOTE

Keep physician informed of all side effects. May be treated symptomatically. Discontinue and initiate appropriate treatment if S/S associated with post-marketing reports occur; see Side Effects. Adverse effects from overdose (up to 240 mg/day in healthy subjects) did not occur during clinical trials. Not removed by hemodialysis.

PAPAVERINE HYDROCHLORIDE

(pa-pav′er-een hye-droe-klor′id)

Vasodilator (peripheral)

pH 3 to 4.5

USUAL DOSE

1 to 4 ml (30 to 120 mg) every 3 hours as indicated. Second dose may be given in 10 minutes only when treating extrasystoles.

PEDIATRIC DOSE

1.5 mg/kg of body weight every 6 hours.

DOSE ADJUSTMENTS

See Drug/Lab Interactions.

DILUTION

May be given undiluted or may be diluted in an equal amount of SW for injection. Usually not added to IV solutions. May be given through Y-tube or three-way stopcock of infusion set.

INCOMPATIBLE WITH

Will form a precipitate with LR.

COMPATIBLE WITH

Consult pharmacist; specific conditions may apply; see Compatibilities, p. xvi.

Additive: Theophylline.

Syringe: Phentolamine (Regitine).

RATE OF ADMINISTRATION

1 ml (30 mg) or fraction thereof over 2 minutes. Rapid IV injection may cause death.

ACTIONS

A nonnarcotic opium alkaloid, it is a direct smooth muscle relaxant and antispasmodic. Relaxation is noted in vascular system and bronchial musculature and in GI, biliary, and urinary tracts. More effective on muscle in spasm, it has an affinity for the smooth muscle of blood vessels. Affects cardiac muscle to depress conduction and increase refractory period. Improved circulation and muscle relaxation decrease pain. Metabolized in the liver and excreted in the urine.

INDICATIONS AND USES

Vascular spasm associated with an acute myocardial infarction. ■ Peripheral or pulmonary embolism. ■ Peripheral vascular disease and cerebral angiospastic states. ■ Visceral spasm of ureteral, biliary, or GI colic. ■ Angina pectoris.

CONTRAINDICATIONS

Complete AV heart block.

PRECAUTIONS

Rarely used; active therapeutic value is questioned. ■ Rapid IV injection may cause death. ■ IM injection is preferred. ■ Use with caution in glaucoma and impaired liver function. ■ Large doses can depress AV and intraventricular conduction, resulting in arrhythmias.

Monitor: Observe patient continuously; monitor vital signs. ■ See Drug/Lab Interactions.

Patient Education: Avoid alcohol and other CNS depressants. ■ May cause dizziness and drowsiness; request assistance for ambulation. ■ Use caution in any task requiring alertness.

Maternal/Child: Category C: safety for use in pregnancy and breast-feeding and in children not established.

Elderly: Risk of hypothermia may be increased.

DRUG/LAB INTERACTIONS

May be used with narcotics if the relaxant effect is not adequate to relieve discomfort. Narcotic dosage should be reduced. ■ Antagonizes effects of levodopa.

SIDE EFFECTS

Blurred or double vision, diaphoresis, discomfort (generalized), flushing, hypertension (slight), hypotension, respiratory depth increase, scleral jaundice, sedation, tachycardia.

Major: Respiratory depression, seizures, ventricular ectopic rhythms, sudden death.

ANTIDOTE

Notify the physician of any minor side effects. If minor symptoms progress or any major side effect appears, discontinue the drug immediately and notify the physician. Treatment of toxicity will be symptomatic and supportive. Consider diazepam (Valium) or phenytoin (Dilantin) for convulsions. Anesthesia with thiopental and paralysis with a neuromuscular blocking agent (e.g., tubocurarine [curare]) may be required. Use dopamine (Intropin) for hypotension. Calcium gluconate may reduce toxic cardiovascular effects. Monitor ECG. Resuscitate as necessary.

PARICALCITOL

(pare-i-cal′sih-tal)

Vitamin D analog

Zemplar

USUAL DOSE

The currently accepted target range for intact parathyroid hormone (iPTH) in chronic renal failure (CRF) patients is no more than 1.5 to 3 times the non-uremic upper limit of normal.

Recommended initial dose is 0.04 to 0.1 mcg/kg administered no more frequently than every other day at any time during dialysis. Doses as high as 0.24 mcg/kg have been safely administered.

Information supplied by the manufacturer suggests that the relative dosing of paricalcitol to calcitriol is 4:1. When converting a patient from calcitriol to paricalcitol, the initial dose of paricalcitol should be four times greater than the patient's dose of calcitriol.

DOSE ADJUSTMENTS

Adjust dosing based on patient response. If a satisfactory response is not observed, dose may be increased by 2 to 4 mcg at 2- to 4-week intervals. Monitor serum calcium, phosphorus, and calcium × phosphorus product (Ca × P) frequently during any dose adjustment period. See Monitor. ■ Reduce dose or interrupt therapy if elevated calcium level or a Ca × P product of greater than 75 is noted. Reinitiate therapy at a lower dose when parameters have normalized. ■ Paricalcitol dose may need to be reduced as parathyroid hormone (PTH) levels decrease in response to therapy. The following chart is a suggested approach to dose titration:

Paricalcitol Suggested Dosing Guidelines	
PTH Level	**Paricalcitol Dose**
The same or increasing	Increase
Decreasing by <30%	Increase
Decreasing by >30%, <60%	Maintain
Decreasing by >60%	Decrease
One and one-half to three times upper limit of normal	Maintain

DILUTION

May be given undiluted. Available as 5 mcg/ml solution in 1- and 2-ml vials.

Storage: Store unopened vials at 25° C (77° F); range: 15° to 30° C (59° to 86° F).

COMPATIBILITY

Specific information not available. Consider specific use; consult pharmacist.

RATE OF ADMINISTRATION

Administer as a bolus dose at any time during dialysis.

ACTIONS

A synthetic vitamin D analog. Suppresses PTH levels with no significant difference in the incidence of hypercalcemia or hyperphosphatemia when compared to placebo. However, serum phosphorus, calcium, and the Ca × P product may increase when paricalcitol is administered. Studies suggest that paricalcitol may cause less hypercalcemia and hyperphosphatemia than calcitriol. Serum paricalcitol levels decrease rapidly after a bolus injection. Mean half-life is approximately 15 hours. Eliminated primarily by hepatobiliary excretion in feces and, to a much smaller extent, by the kidneys. Protein binding is extensive.

INDICATIONS AND USES

Prevention and treatment of secondary hyperparathyroidism associated with chronic renal failure.

CONTRAINDICATIONS

Patients with evidence of vitamin D toxicity, hypercalcemia, or hypersensitivity to any ingredient in this product; see Precautions.

PRECAUTIONS

Acute overdose may cause hypercalcemia and require emergency attention. If clinically significant hypercalcemia develops, dose should be reduced or held. Chronic administration may place patient at risk of hypercalcemia, elevated Ca × P product, and metastatic calcification. See Side Effects and Antidote. ▪ Phosphate or vitamin D–related compounds should not be taken concomitantly with paricalcitol. ▪ Adynamic bone lesions may develop if PTH levels are suppressed to abnormal levels.

Monitor: During initiation of therapy, obtain baseline serum calcium and phosphorus levels and determine levels at least twice a week. Once dosage has been established, serum calcium and phosphorus should be monitored at least monthly. See Dose Adjustments. ▪ Calculate Ca × P (should be less than 75). ▪ Measurement of serum or plasma PTH (iPTH assay recommended) is suggested every 3 months. ▪ Monitor for signs and symptoms of hypercalcemia. See Side Effects.

Patient Education: Report symptoms of hypercalcemia promptly. Dose adjustment or treatment may be required. Strict adherence to dietary supplementation of calcium and restriction of phosphorus is required to ensure optimal effectiveness of therapy. Phosphate-binding compounds (e.g., calcium acetate [Phos-lo]) may be needed to control serum phosphorus levels in patients with CRF, but excessive use of aluminum-containing products (e.g., aluminum hydroxide gel [Alternagel]) should be avoided.

Maternal/Child: Category C: safety for use in pregnancy and breast-feeding not established. Benefits must outweigh risks. ▪ Safety and effectiveness have not been established for children.

Elderly: No overall differences in effectiveness or safety have been observed in the elderly.

DRUG/LAB INTERACTIONS

Specific interaction studies have not been performed. ▪ Digitalis toxicity is potentiated by hypercalcemia. Use caution when paricalcitol is prescribed concomitantly with digitalis compounds. ▪ Phosphate or vitamin D–related compounds should not be taken concomitantly with paricalcitol. ▪ May reduce serum total alkaline phosphatase levels.

SIDE EFFECTS

Overdose or chronic administration may lead to hypercalcemia. Signs and symptoms of vitamin D intoxication associated with hypercalcemia include: **Early:** bone pain, constipation, dry mouth, headache, metallic taste, muscle pain, nausea, somnolence, vomiting, and weakness. **Late:** Anorexia, cardiac arrhythmias, conjunctivitis (calcific), death, decreased libido, ectopic calcification, elevated AST and ALT, elevated BUN, hypercholesterolemia, hypertension, hyperthermia, overt psychosis (rare), pancreatitis, photophobia, pruritus, rhinorrhea, somnolence, and weight loss. The following adverse events were documented in clinical studies and represent adverse events occurring with greater frequency in the paricalcitol group at a frequency of 2% or greater (causality not necessarily established): chills, dry mouth, edema, fever, flu, gastrointestinal bleed, lightheadedness, nausea, palpitations, pneumonia, sepsis, and vomiting.

ANTIDOTE

Notify physician of any side effects. Treatment of patients with clinically significant hypercalcemia consists of immediate dose reduction or interruption of the therapy and includes a low-calcium diet, withdrawal of calcium supplements, patient mobilization, attention to fluid and electrolyte imbalances, assessment of electrocardiographic abnormalities (critical in patients receiving digitalis), and hemodialysis or peritoneal dialysis against a calcium-free dialysate, as warranted. Monitor serum calcium levels frequently until calcium levels return to within normal limits.

PEGASPARGASE

(peg-as′per-gase)

Antineoplastic (miscellaneous)

Oncaspar, PEG-L-Asparaginase

pH 7.3

USUAL DOSE

2,500 international units (IU)/M^2 every 14 days as an infusion. Most frequently used as a component of a multiple agent protocol. Infrequently used in the same dose as a single agent. See Precautions.

PEDIATRIC DOSE

Over 1 year of age with body surface area less than 0.6 M^2: 82.5 IU/kg of body weight every 14 days.

Body surface area greater than 0.6 M^2: Same as adult dose.

DOSE ADJUSTMENTS

Adjust dose based on patient response and toxicity.

DILUTION

Specific techniques required; see Precautions. Available preservative free in 5-ml vials containing 750 IU/ml. Must be further diluted with 100 ml of NS or D5W and administered through the Y-tube or three-way stopcock of a free-flowing infusion of similar solutions. Do not shake; mix gently. Use only clear solutions.

Storage: Appearance the same but activity is destroyed if accidentally frozen. ***Do not administer!*** Refrigerate before dilution. For single-dose use only. Do not reenter vial; discard unused portions. Discard any time solution is cloudy or after 48 hours at room temperature.

COMPATIBILITY

Specific information not available. Consider specific use and toxicity; consult pharmacist.

RATE OF ADMINISTRATION

A single dose evenly distributed over 1 to 2 hours. Slow rate of infusion as indicated by side effects.

ACTIONS

An oncolytic agent. A modified version of L-asparaginase (native asparaginase derived from *Escherichia coli*) that rapidly depletes asparagine from cells. Some malignant cells have a metabolic defect that makes them unable to synthesize asparagine as normal cells do. They are dependent on exogenous asparagine for survival. Plasma half-life does not appear to be influenced by dose levels, nor does it correlate with age, sex, surface area, renal or hepatic function, diagnosis, or extent of disease. Measurable for up to 15 days. Cannot be detected in urine.

INDICATIONS AND USES

Treatment of acute lymphoblastic leukemia in patients who require L-asparaginase but have developed hypersensitivity to its native form. Primarily used as part of a multiple agent protocol with other chemotherapeutic agents (e.g., cytarabine, daunorubicin, doxorubicin, methotrexate, vincristine). Should be used as a single agent only when multiagent chemotherapy is considered inappropriate. Safety and effectiveness have been established in patients between 1 and 21 years of age with known previous hypersensitivity to native L-asparaginase.

Unlabeled uses: Treatment of acute lymphocytic leukemia.

CONTRAINDICATIONS

Pancreatitis, past history of pancreatitis, significant hemorrhagic events associated with prior L-asparaginase therapy, and patients who have had previous serious allergic reactions (e.g., bronchospasm, generalized urticaria, hypotension, laryngeal edema, hypotension) or other unacceptable adverse reactions to pegaspargase (Oncaspar).

PRECAUTIONS

Follow guidelines for handling cytotoxic agents. See Appendix A, p. 1142. ■ Must be administered by or under the direction of the physician specialist (e.g., medical oncologist). ■ Freezing destroys activity; see Storage. ■ Intramuscular is the preferred route of administration; incidence of allergic reactions, hepatotoxicity, coagulopathy, and gastrointestinal and renal disorders are lower. ■ May cause severe hepatic and central nervous system toxicity; use caution. ■ May be at increased risk for bleeding or thrombosis. ■ See Drug/Lab Interactions.

Monitor: Observe patient carefully during and for at least 1 hour after infusion. ■ Appropriate treatment for resuscitation and/or anaphylaxis must always be available. Risk may be increased if patient has had reactions to native asparaginase or is over 21 years of age. ■ Frequent monitoring of blood cell counts, bone marrow evaluation, serum amylase, blood sugar, uric acid, and liver and kidney function are necessary. ■ Monitoring of fibrinogen, PT, and PTT may be indicated to determine effects on plasma proteins. ■ Allopurinol, increased fluid intake, and alkalinization of the urine may be required to reduce uric acid levels. ■ Nausea and vomiting can be severe. Prophylactic administration of antiemetics recommended to increase patient comfort. ■ Predisposition to infection probable. ■ Prophylactic antibiotics may be indicated pending results of C/S in febrile neutropenic patient. ■ Monitor for thrombocytopenia (platelet count less than 50,000/mm^3). Initiate precautions to prevent excessive bleeding (e.g., inspect IV sites, skin, and mucous membranes; use extreme care during invasive procedures; test urine, emesis, stool, and secretions for occult blood).

Patient Education: Report all symptoms promptly; incidence of allergic reaction is significant and risk of bleeding is increased. ■ All meds including nonprescription drugs must be evaluated. Contact physician before changing any meds. ■ Verbalize all questions. ■ Assess birth control requirements. ■ See Appendix D, p. 1148.

Maternal/Child: Category C: effect on fetus unknown. Evaluation of benefit versus risk is necessary for anyone who is pregnant or may become pregnant. ■ Discontinue breast-feeding.

Elderly: Consider age-related organ toxicity.

DRUG/LAB INTERACTIONS

Potential for increased risk of bleeding or thrombosis; may be exacerbated with concurrent administration of drugs with anticoagulant effects (e.g., heparin, coumadin, dipyridamole [Persantine], aspirin, or NSAIDs [e.g., ibuprofen (Advil, Motrin), naproxen (Aleve, Naprosyn)]). ■ Use extreme caution with hepatotoxic agents (e.g., other chemotherapeutic agents, alcohol, NSAIDs, phenytoin [Dilantin]), especially in the presence of liver dysfunction. May cause severe hepatic and CNS toxicity. ■ May inhibit action of drugs dependent on protein synthesis or cell replication (e.g., methotrexate). ■ May interfere with the enzymatic detoxification of other drugs, particularly in the liver. ■ Depletes serum protein; may increase the toxicity of protein-bound drugs.

SIDE EFFECTS

May be more toxic in adults than in children. Allergic reactions occur more frequently in patients hypersensitive to native asparaginase (60% versus 12% in nonsensitized patients) and may be dose limiting. Allergic reactions (e.g., bronchospasm, chills, dyspnea, edema, erythema, fever, pain, rash, urticaria), coagulopathy, fever, hepatotoxicity, increased ALT (SGPT), malaise, nausea and vomiting (over 5%), hyperglycemia requiring insulin therapy (3%), pancreatitis (clinical) (1%), thrombosis (4%). Has caused fatal fulminating pancreatitis. Capable of causing numerous other side effects in 1% to 5% of all patients.

ANTIDOTE

Notify physician of all side effects. Reduced rate of administration may be helpful. Pegaspargase may have to be discontinued until recovery or permanently discontinued. Symptomatic and supportive treatment is indicated. Treat allergic reactions promptly with epinephrine, corticosteroids, oxygen, and antihistamines. There is no specific antidote.

PENICILLIN G AQUEOUS

(pen-i-sill′in a′kwe-us)

Antibacterial (penicillin)

Penicillin G Potassium, Penicillin G Sodium, Pfizerpen

pH 6 to 8.5

USUAL DOSE

1 to 20 million units/24 hr equally distributed over 24 hours as a continuous infusion or equally divided in 4 to 6 intermittent infusions. Doses up to 80 million units/24 hr have been given in life-threatening infections. (400,000 units equals approximately 250 mg.) See package insert for specific indications.

PEDIATRIC DOSE

100,000 to 400,000 units/kg of body weight/24 hr in equally divided doses every 4 to 6 hours as an intermittent infusion. Dosage can vary greatly and must be adjusted according to the severity of the infection. Treat congenital syphilis for 10 to 14 days. Maximum dose is 24,000,000 units/24 hr.

NEONATAL DOSE

Administration by intermittent infusion over 15 to 30 minutes is preferred.

Under 1,200 Gm: 25,000 units/kg of body weight every 12 hours (meningitis 50,000 units).

Under 2,000 Gm; *age 0 to 7 days:* 25,000 units/kg every 12 hours (meningitis, 50,000 units). ***Over 7 days:*** 25,000 units/kg every 8 hours (meningitis, 75,000 units).

Over 2,000 Gm; *age 0 to 7 days:* 25,000 units/kg every 8 hours (meningitis, 50,000 units). ***Over 7 days:*** 25,000 units/kg every 6 hours (meningitis, 56,250 units).

Congenital syphilis: Treat for 10 to 14 days.

Age 0 to 7 days: 50,000 units/kg every 12 hours.

Age 7 to 28 days: 50,000 units/kg every 8 hours.

Over 28 days of age: 50,000 units/kg every 6 hours.

DOSE ADJUSTMENTS

Reduce dose in severe impaired renal function; additional reductions may be indicated if liver function is also impaired. ■ If CrCl is greater than 10 ml/min in uremic patients, give a full loading dose followed by one-half loading dose every 4 to 5 hours. ■ See Drug/Lab Interactions.

DILUTION

Available premixed, or reconstitute each vial with SW for injection or NS. Direct flow of diluent against sides of the vial while gently rotating vial. Shake vigorously. Directions on vial should be followed to provide desired number of units per milliliter. Available with 1, 5, 10, and 20 million units per vial. May be added to NS or dextrose solutions for infusion. See chart on inside back cover.

Storage: Dry powder stored at CRT. Reconstituted solutions stable for 1 week if refrigerated. Infusion solutions stable at CRT for 24 hours.

INCOMPATIBLE WITH

Penicillins are rapidly inactivated in alkaline carbohydrate solutions, reducing agents, alcohols, and glycols; optimum pH range is 6 to 7. To preserve bactericidal action, consult pharmacist before mixing other agents with penicillin in the infusion solution. May form a precipitate with vancomycin (Vancocin). Inactivated in solution with aminoglycosides (e.g., amikacin [Amikin], gentamicin [Garamycin]). Do not mix in the same solution. Appropriate spacing and/or separate sites required. See Drug/Lab Interactions.

COMPATIBLE WITH (Underline Indicates Conflicting Compatibility Information)

Consult pharmacist; specific conditions may apply; see Compatibilities, p. xvi.

PENICILLIN G POTASSIUM

Additive: ***See Incompatible With.*** Amikacin (Amikin), ascorbic acid (Cenolate), calcium chloride, calcium gluconate, chloramphenicol (Chloromycetin), cimetidine (Tagamet), clindamycin (Cleocin), dimenhydrinate (Dinate), diphenhydramine (Benadryl), ephedrine, erythromycin lactobionate (Erythrocin), furosemide (Lasix), heparin, hydrocortisone sodium succinate (Solu-Cortef), kanamycin (Kantrex), lidocaine, lincomycin (Lincocin), magnesium sulfate, methylprednisolone (Solu-Medrol), metronidazole (Flagyl IV), potassium chloride (KCl), prochlorperazine (Compazine), promethazine (Phenergan), ranitidine (Zantac), sodium bicarbonate, verapamil (Isoptin).

Syringe: Heparin.

Y-site: Acyclovir (Zovirax), amiodarone (Cordarone), cyclophosphamide (Cytoxan), diltiazem (Cardizem), enalaprilat (Vasotec IV), esmolol (Brevibloc), fluconazole (Diflucan), foscarnet (Foscavir), heparin, hydromorphone (Dilaudid), labetalol (Normodyne), magnesium sulfate, meperidine (Demerol), morphine, perphenazine (Trilafon), potassium chloride (KCl), tacrolimus (Prograf), theophylline, verapamil (Isoptin).

PENICILLIN G SODIUM

Additive: ***See Incompatible With.*** Calcium chloride, calcium gluconate, chloramphenicol (Chloromycetin), clindamycin (Cleocin), diphenhydramine (Benadryl), erythromycin lactobionate (Erythrocin), furosemide (Lasix), gentamicin (Garamycin), heparin, hydrocortisone sodium succinate (Solu-Cortef), kanamycin (Kantrex), lincomycin (Lincocin), potassium chloride (KCl), ranitidine (Zantac), verapamil (Isoptin).

Syringe: Chloramphenicol (Chloromycetin), cimetidine (Tagamet), gentamicin (Garamycin), heparin, kanamycin (Kantrex), lincomycin (Lincocin), streptomycin.

Y-site: Levofloxacin (Levaquin).

RATE OF ADMINISTRATION

Penicillin is not given by IV injection. Administer as ordered as continuous IV drip; for example, 5 million units in 1,000 ml of D5W over 12 hours. Is sometimes given by intermittent infusion ($\frac{1}{6}$ or $\frac{1}{4}$ of a daily dose in 100 ml over 1 to 2 hours every 4 to 6 hours). Dosage level must be maintained to provide therapeutic serum levels. Too-rapid administration or excessive doses may cause electrolyte imbalance and/or seizures. Stable at room temperature for at least 24 hours.

Pediatric rate: Administration by intermittent infusion over 15 to 30 minutes is preferred for infants and children.

ACTIONS

Bactericidal against penicillin-sensitive microorganisms during the stage of active multiplication. Distributed into most body fluids. Distribution into spinal fluid is minimal unless inflammation is present. Crosses the placental barrier. Excreted in the urine. Secreted in breast milk.

Available in a potassium salt containing 1.7 mEq of potassium and 0.3 mEq sodium in 1 million units or a sodium salt containing 2 mEq sodium in 1 million units.

INDICATIONS AND USES

Severe infections caused by penicillin G–sensitive gram-positive, gram-negative, and anaerobic microorganisms (e.g., streptococcal, pneumococcal, Vincent's gingivitis, spirochetal infections, meningitis, endocarditis).

Unlabeled uses: Arthritis, carditis.

CONTRAINDICATIONS

Known sensitivity to any penicillin or cephalosporin (not absolute).

PRECAUTIONS

Sensitivity studies necessary to determine susceptibility of the causative organism to penicillin. ■ Avoid prolonged use of drug; superinfection caused by overgrowth of nonsusceptible organisms may result. ■ Allergic reactions are most likely to occur in patients with a history of sensitivity to multiple allergens. ■ Pseudomembranous colitis has been reported. May range from mild to life-threatening. Consider in patients that present with diarrhea during or after treatment with penicillin. ■ Potassium penicillin most frequently used. Doses over 10,000,000 units may cause fatal hyperkalemia, especially in patients with renal insufficiency.

Monitor: Periodic evaluation of renal and hematopoietic systems is recommended in prolonged therapy. ■ Test patients with syphilis for HIV. ■ Electrolyte imbalance from potassium or sodium content is very possible. Monitor closely. Penicillin G potassium contains 1.02 mEq sodium/million units. May aggravate CHF. ■ May cause thrombophlebitis; observe carefully and rotate infusion sites. ■ See Drug/Lab Interactions.

Patient Education: May require alternate birth control.

Maternal/Child: Category B: use only if clearly needed. ■ May cause diarrhea, candidiasis, or allergic response in nursing infants. ■ Elimination rate markedly reduced in neonates.

Elderly: Response similar to that seen in younger adults. ■ Consider age-related organ impairment and concomitant disease or drug therapy. Monitor renal function. ■ See Dose Adjustments.

DRUG/LAB INTERACTIONS

Synergistic when used in combination with aminoglycosides (e.g., amikacin [Amikin], gentamicin [Garamycin]). Synergism may be inconsistent; see Incompatible With. ■ May be antagonized by bacteriostatic antibiotics (e.g., chloramphenicol, erythromycin, tetracyclines); may interfere with bactericidal action. ■ Risk of bleeding with anticoagulants (e.g., heparin) is increased. ■ Probenecid decreases elimination of penicillin resulting in prolonged half-life and increased serum levels. May be desirable or may cause toxicity. ■ May decrease effectiveness of oral contraceptives; breakthrough bleeding or pregnancy could result. ■ Concomitant use with potassium supplements, potassium-sparing diuretics (e.g., spironolactone [Aldactone]), or ACE inhibitors (e.g., enalaprilat [Vasotec IV]) may increase risk of hyperkalemia. ■ May decrease clearance and increase toxicity of methotrexate. ■ May cause false values in common lab tests; see literature.

SIDE EFFECTS

Arthralgia, chills, edema, fever, prostration, skin rash, urticaria.

Major: Acute interstitial nephritis, anaphylaxis, convulsions, hemolytic anemia, hyperreflexia, neurotoxicity, potassium poisoning with coma, sodium-induced congestive heart failure. Hypersensitivity myocarditis (fever, eosinophilia, rash, sinus tachycardia, ST-T changes and cardiomegaly) and pseudomembranous colitis can occur. Higher-than-normal doses may cause neurologic adverse effects including convulsions, especially with impaired renal function.

ANTIDOTE

For all side effects, discontinue the drug, treat the allergic reaction or resuscitate as necessary, and notify the physician. Treat minor side effects symptomatically according to physician's order. Removed by hemodialysis.

PENTAMIDINE ISETHIONATE

Antiprotozoal

(pen-tam′i-deen is-ah-thi′o-nat)

♣Pentacarinat **pH 4.09 to 5.4**

USUAL DOSE

Treatment of pneumocystis carinii: 4 mg/kg of body weight once daily for 14 days. See Precautions/Monitor. Has been used up to 21 days; benefits not defined.

Pneumocystis prophylaxis: 4 mg/kg once each month. May be given every 2 weeks if indicated.

Leishmania, visceral (unlabeled): 2 to 4 mg/kg once daily for up to 15 days.

Leishmania, cutaneous (unlabeled): 2 to 4 mg/kg once or twice a week until lesions heal.

Trypanosoma gambiense (unlabeled): 4 mg/kg once daily for 10 days.

PEDIATRIC DOSE

Pneumocystis carinii: 4 mg/kg once daily for 12 to 14 days.

Pneumocystis prophylaxis: See Usual Dose.

Leishmania donovani: 2 to 4 mg/kg once daily for 15 days. Up to 21 days have been suggested, but risks with therapy over 14 days may be increased.

Trypanosoma gambiense: See Usual Dose.

DOSE ADJUSTMENTS

Reduced dose in renal failure may be indicated.

DILUTION

Initially dilute each 300 mg or fraction thereof in 3 to 5 ml SW or D5W. Dilute 200 mg vial of ♣Pentacarinat with 2 ml. A single dose must be further diluted in 50 to 250 ml of D5W (♣Pentacarinat 200 or 300 mg in 500 ml) and given as an infusion.

Storage: Stable at room temperature for 24 hours. Discard unused portion. Protect dry product and reconstituted solution from light.

INCOMPATIBLE WITH

Will form a precipitate with NS; do not use for dilution or infusion. Manufacturer states, "Do not mix pentamidine solutions with any other drugs."

COMPATIBLE WITH

Consult pharmacist; specific conditions may apply; see Compatibilities, p. xvi.

Y-site: Diltiazem (Cardizem), gatifloxacin (Tequin), zidovudine (AZT, Retrovir).

RATE OF ADMINISTRATION

A single dose should be evenly distributed over 60 minutes.

Leishmania, visceral and cutaneous: A single dose evenly distributed over 1 to 2 hours.

ACTIONS

An antiprotozoal agent. Specifically active against *Pneumocystis carinii.* It is thought to interfere with nuclear metabolism and inhibit the synthesis of DNA, RNA, phospholipids, and proteins. Route of metabolism is unknown. Excreted partially in urine. May accumulate in renal failure.

INDICATIONS AND USES

Treatment and prophylaxis of *Pneumocystis carinii* pneumonia (PCP).

Unlabeled uses: Treatment of trypanosomiasis and visceral and cutaneous leishmaniasis. Aerosol used prophylactically to prevent PCP in high-risk patients.

CONTRAINDICATIONS

None if the diagnosis of *Pneumocystis carinii* pneumonia is confirmed.

PRECAUTIONS

Specific use only; establish correct diagnosis. ■ Sulfamethoxazole-trimethoprim is the drug of choice for treatment of *Pneumocystis* pneumonia. Pentamidine causes numerous and serious side effects and is indicated only if the patient does not respond to or tolerate SMX-TMP. ■ Use extreme caution in patients with hypertension, hypotension, hypoglycemia, hyperglycemia, hypocalcemia, leukopenia, thrombocytopenia, anemia, hepatic or renal dysfunction, ventricular tachycardia, pancreatitis, and Stevens-Johnson syndrome.

Monitor: Before, during, and after therapy obtain a BUN and SrCr (daily), CBC, platelet count, alkaline phosphatase, bilirubin, AST (SGOT), ALT (SGPT), serum calcium, and ECG. ■ Has caused fatalities resulting from severe hypotension, hypoglycemia, and cardiac arrhythmias even with the administration of the first dose. Keep patient supine, observe continuously for any sign of adverse reaction, and monitor BP continuously during infusion and afterward until stable. ■ Emergency equipment for resuscitation must be immediately available. ■ Monitor blood glucose levels daily during therapy and several times after therapy is complete. Pancreatic necrosis and very high plasma insulin levels have occurred. May also cause hyperglycemia and diabetes mellitus.

Patient Education: May cause severe hypotension; remain lying down until BP is stable. ■ Report any unusual bleeding or bruising.

Maternal/Child: Category C: use only when clearly needed during pregnancy and breast-feeding. Hazards to fetus or infant are unknown. ■ Discontinue breast-feeding.

SIDE EFFECTS

Occur in over 50% of patients and may be life threatening. Some occur after course of treatment is completed. Acute renal failure, anemia, anorexia, bad taste in mouth, cardiac arrhythmias including ventricular tachycardia, confusion, dizziness, elevated SrCr and liver function tests, fever, hallucinations, hyperglycemia, hyperkalemia, hypocalcemia, hypoglycemia, hypotension, leukopenia, nausea, neuralgia, phlebitis, rash, thrombocytopenia.

ANTIDOTE

Discontinue drug for any life-threatening side effects. Notify physician of all side effects. Symptomatic treatment indicated. Resuscitate as necessary.

PENTAZOCINE (LACTATE)

(pen-taz'oh-seen lak'tat)

Narcotic analgesic (agonist-antagonist) Anesthesia adjunct

Talwin

pH 4 to 5

USUAL DOSE

30 mg. May repeat every 3 to 4 hours or decrease to 5 to 15 mg and repeat every 2 hours. 360 mg equals maximum dose in 24 hours. Use oral form of pentazocine when appropriate.

Patients in labor: 20 mg when contractions become regular. May repeat every 2 to 3 hours as needed for two or three additional doses.

PEDIATRIC DOSE

Safety and effectiveness for IV use in children under 12 years of age not established. See Maternal/Child.

DOSE ADJUSTMENTS

Reduced dose may be required in the elderly or debilitated, in impaired hepatic or renal function, in patients with limited pulmonary reserve, and in the presence of other CNS depressants; use caution. ■ Increased dose may be required in smokers. ■ See Precautions, Drug/Lab Interactions, and Elderly.

DILUTION

May be given undiluted. It is preferable to dilute each 5 mg with at least 1 ml of SW for injection.

Storage: Store at CRT. Avoid freezing.

INCOMPATIBLE WITH

Manufacturer states, "Do not mix in the same syringe with soluble barbiturates (e.g., phenobarbital [Luminal]); precipitation will occur."

COMPATIBLE WITH

Consult pharmacist; specific conditions may apply; see Compatibilities, p. xvi.

Syringe: Atropine, butorphanol (Stadol), chlorpromazine (Thorazine), cimetidine (Tagamet), dimenhydrinate (Dinate), diphenhydramine (Benadryl), droperidol (Inapsine), fentanyl (Sublimaze), hydromorphone (Dilaudid), meperidine (Demerol), metoclopramide (Reglan), morphine, perphenazine (Trilafon), prochlorperazine (Compazine), promethazine (Phenergan), propiomazine, ranitidine (Zantac), scopolamine.

Y-site: Heparin, hydrocortisone sodium succinate (Solu-Cortef), potassium chloride (KCl).

RATE OF ADMINISTRATION

Each 5 mg or fraction thereof over 1 minute.

ACTIONS

A synthetic narcotic agonist-antagonist with a potent analgesic action, pentazocine is somewhat less effective than morphine and meperidine in equivalent doses. May produce respiratory depression, but does not increase markedly with increased doses. Onset of action is prompt, 2 to 3 minutes, and lasts about 2 to 3 hours. Metabolized in the liver. Excreted in urine. Crosses the placental barrier. Secreted in breast milk.

INDICATIONS AND USES

Relief of moderate to severe pain. ■ Preoperative medication. ■ Support of anesthesia. ■ Obstetric analgesia.

CONTRAINDICATIONS

Hypersensitivity to pentazocine or its components (contains sulfites); pathologic brain conditions.

PRECAUTIONS

Use with caution in bronchial asthma, relief of biliary pain, history of drug abuse, decreased renal or hepatic function, respiratory depression from any cause, a history of seizures, and in patients with head injury or increased intracranial pressure. ■ Some formulations contain sulfites, use caution in patients with allergies; see Contraindications. ■ Use with caution in patients with acute MI accompanied by hypertension or left ventricular failure. May increase systemic and pulmonary arterial pressure and systemic vascular resistance. ■ Mild narcotic antagonist. May precipitate withdrawal symptoms in patients accustomed to narcotics. ■ May provide less effective analgesia in heavy smokers.

Monitor: Naloxone (Narcan), oxygen, and controlled respiratory equipment must always be available. ■ Observe patient continuously during injection and frequently thereafter. Monitor vital signs. Keep patient supine to minimize side effects; orthostatic hypotension and fainting may occur. Observe closely during ambulation. ■ Pain control usually more effective with routinely administered doses. Determine appropriate interval through clinical assessment. ■ See Drug/Lab Interactions.

Patient Education: Avoid use of alcohol or other CNS depressants (e.g., antihistamines, diazepam [Valium]). ■ Request assistance for ambulation. ■ May be habit forming.

Maternal/Child: Category C: safety for use in pregnancy, (other than labor) and breast-feeding not established. ■ Respiratory depression, dyspnea, and transient apnea have been reported in a small number of newborn infants whose mothers received pentazocine during labor. ■ Use extreme caution if necessary during delivery of premature infants.

Elderly: May be more sensitive to effects (e.g., respiratory depression, confusion, constipation, dizziness, oversedation, urinary retention). ■ Analgesia should be effective with lower doses. ■ Consider age-related organ impairment, monitoring of renal function may be indicated. ■ Half-life longer and clearance lower compared to younger patients. ■ See Dose Adjustments.

DRUG/LAB INTERACTIONS

Potentiated by cimetidine (Tagamet), and other CNS depressants such as narcotic analgesics, general anesthetics, alcohol, anticholinergics, antihistamines, barbiturates, hypnotics, sedatives, psychotropic agents, MAO inhibitors, and neuromuscular blocking agents (e.g., mivacurium [Mivacron]). Reduced doses of both drugs may be indicated. ■ May decrease analgesic effects of other narcotics; avoid concurrent use. ■ Metabolism and clearance increased in smokers; analgesic effects may be decreased.

SIDE EFFECTS

Allergic reactions, apprehension, blurred vision, circulatory depression, confusion, constipation, cramps, depression, diarrhea, disorientation, dizziness, double vision, dreams, drug dependence, dry mouth, dyspnea, euphoria, facial edema, floating feeling, flushing, hallucinations, headache, hypertension, injection site reactions, insomnia, muscle tremor, nausea, neonatal apnea, nervousness, nystagmus, paresthesias, perspiration, pruritus, respiratory depression, sedation, seizures, shock, tachycardia, taste alteration, urinary retention, uterine contraction depression.

ANTIDOTE

For any side effect, discontinue the drug and notify the physician. Treat side effects symptomatically. For overdose or respiratory depression, naloxone hydrochloride (Narcan) is the antidote of choice. If naloxone is not available, methylphenidate (Ritalin) may be of value in respiratory depression (only available in oral form).

PENTOBARBITAL SODIUM

(pen-toe-bar′bi-tal so′de-um)

Barbiturate
Sedative-hypnotic
Anticonvulsant

Nembutal Sodium

pH 9 to 10.5

USUAL DOSE

100 mg initially. Wait 1 full minute between each dose to determine drug effect. Additional doses in increments of 25 to 50 mg may be given as indicated. Maximum dosage ranges from 200 to 500 mg.

Barbiturate coma: ***Loading dose:*** 3 to 10 mg/kg over 30 minutes to 3 hours. ***Maintenance dose:*** 1.5 to 2 mg/kg every 1 to 2 hours or an infusion of 0.5 to 3 mg/kg/hr. Adjust to maintain pentobarbital blood level between 110 and 177 mm/l (25 to 40 mg/dl) or ICP below 25 Torr.

PEDIATRIC DOSE

1 to 3 mg/kg slowly until asleep. Maximum dose 100 mg/24 hr.

Barbiturate coma: See Usual Dose. An alternate source suggests ***Loading dose:*** 10 to 15 mg/kg over 1 to 2 hours. ***Maintenance dose:*** Begin with 1 mg/kg/hr; increase to 2 to 3 mg/kg/hr to maintain EEG burst suppression.

DOSE ADJUSTMENTS

Reduce dose in impaired renal or hepatic function; usually required in the debilitated or elderly. ■ See Drug/Lab Interactions.

DILUTION

May be given undiluted or, preferably, may be further diluted in SW, NS, or Ringer's injection. Any desired amount of diluent may be used. 9 ml of diluent with 1 ml of pentobarbital (50 mg) equals 5 mg/ml. Use only absolutely clear solutions.

INCOMPATIBLE WITH

Manufacturer states, "Should not be admixed with any other medication or solution." Do not mix in a syringe with pentazocine (Talwin); precipitation will occur.

COMPATIBLE WITH **(Underline Indicates Conflicting Compatibility Information)**

Consult pharmacist; specific conditions may apply; see Compatibilities, p. xvi.

Additive: ***Not recommended by manufacturer.*** Amikacin (Amikin), aminophylline, calcium chloride, chloramphenicol (Chloromycetin), dimenhydrinate (Dinate), erythromycin lactobionate (Erythrocin), lidocaine, <u>sodium bicarbonate</u>, <u>succinylcholine</u>, thiopental (Pentothal), verapamil (Isoptin).

Syringe: Aminophylline, atropine, ephedrine, hydromorphone (Dilaudid), morphine, neostigmine (Prostigmin), scopolamine, sodium bicarbonate, thiopental (Pentothal).

Y-site: Acyclovir (Zovirax), gatifloxacin (Tequin), insulin (regular), linezolid (Zyvox), propofol (Diprivan).

RATE OF ADMINISTRATION

50 mg or fraction thereof over 1 minute. Titrate slowly to desired effect. Rapid injection rate may cause symptoms of overdose (e.g., serious respiratory depression).

Barbiturate coma: See specific dose recommendations.

ACTIONS

A sedative, hypnotic barbiturate of short duration with anticonvulsant effects. Pentobarbital is a CNS depressant. Onset of action is prompt by the IV route and lasts about 3 to 4 hours. Will effectively depress the motor cortex if adequate doses are administered. Pain perception is unimpaired. Reportedly reduces cerebral blood flow and thus reduces cerebral edema and intracranial pressure. Detoxified in the liver and excreted fairly quickly in the urine in changed form. Crosses the placental barrier. Secreted in breast milk.

INDICATIONS AND USES

Preanesthetic sedation. ■ Dental and minor surgical sedation. ■ Control of convulsions caused by disease and drug poisoning. ■ Short-term hypnotic. ■ Sedation in psychotic states.

Unlabeled uses: High doses have been used to induce coma in the management of cerebral ischemia and increased intracranial pressure. Has been most effective in patients under 35 years of age or in closed head injuries.

CONTRAINDICATIONS

Acute or chronic pain, delivery (when maximum drug effect would be at the time of delivery), history of porphyria, known hypersensitivity to barbiturates, severely impaired liver function especially with any signs of hepatic coma, severe respiratory disease or depression.

PRECAUTIONS

IV route usually reserved for critical situations. ■ Use caution in status asthmaticus, shock, severe renal or liver disease, depressive states after convulsions, shock, and in the elderly. ■ Use caution in acute or chronic pain. ■ Status epilepticus can occur from too-rapid withdrawal. ■ May be habit forming. Use caution in the presence of fever, diabetes, hyperthyroidism, or severe anemia; may increase side effects. ■ Benzodiazepines (diazepam [Valium], midazolam [Versed]) generally preferred for sedation.

Monitor: Record BP, pulse, and respirations every 3 to 5 minutes. Keep patient under constant observation. ■ Maintain a patent airway. ■ Treat the cause of a convulsion. ■ Highly alkaline; determine absolute patency of vein; use of large veins preferred to prevent thrombosis. Avoid extravasation. Intraarterial injection will cause gangrene. ■ Monitor phenytoin and barbiturate levels when both drugs are used concurrently. ■ Monitor hematopoietic, renal, and hepatic systems in extended therapy. ■ See Drug/Lab Interactions.

Patient Education: Avoid alcohol and other CNS depressants (e.g., antihistamines, diazepam [Valium]). ■ May be habit forming. ■ May require alternate birth control.

Maternal/Child: Category D: avoid pregnancy; will cause birth defects. ■ May cause drowsiness in the nursing infant. ■ See Contraindications. ■ May cause paradoxical excitement in children.

Elderly: Often have increased sensitivity to barbiturates; may cause marked excitement, depression, confusion, and increased risk of barbiturate-induced hypothermia. ■ See Dose Adjustments and Precautions. ■ Consider age-related hepatic or renal impairment and concomitant disease or drug therapy.

DRUG/LAB INTERACTIONS

Use extreme caution if any other CNS depressants have been given, such as alcohol, narcotic analgesics, anesthetics, antidepressants, antihistamines, hypnotics, MAO inhibitors, phenothiazines, sedatives, aminoglycoside antibiotics, or tranquilizers; potentiation with respiratory depression may occur. ■ Inhibits effectiveness of propranolol (Inderal), corticosteroids, doxycycline (Vibramycin), oral anticoagulants, oral contraceptives, quinidine, and theophylline. Capable of innumerable interactions with many drugs. ■ May increase orthostatic hypotension with furosemide (Lasix). ■ Monitor phenytoin and barbiturate levels when both drugs are used concurrently. ■ May inhibit vitamin D metabolism with extended use.

SIDE EFFECTS

Average dose: Depression, dermatitis, facial edema, fever, hypotension, neonatal apnea, pain at or below injection site, respiratory depression (hypoventilation), thrombocytopenic purpura.

Overdose: Apnea, coma, cough reflex depression, flat EEG (reversible unless hypoxic damage has occurred), hypotension, laryngospasm, lowered body temperature, pulmonary edema, renal shutdown, respiratory depression, sluggish or absent reflexes.

ANTIDOTE

Discontinue drug immediately for pain at or below injection site. Notify the physician of any side effects. Symptomatic and supportive treatment are most important in overdose. Maintain an adequate airway with artificial ventilation if indicated. Keep the patient warm. IV volume expanders (dextran) and IV fluids will help maintain adequate circulation. Diuretics or hemodialysis will promote the elimination of the drug. Vasopressors (dopamine [Intropin]) will maintain BP.

PENTOSTATIN

(pen-toh-stah′tin)

Antineoplastic (antibiotic)

2-Deoxycoformycin, Nipent

pH 7 to 8.5

USUAL DOSE

4 mg/M^2 every other week. Evaluation and prehydration is required before administration; see Monitor. If there is no major toxicity and improvement is continuous, treat until a complete response is achieved, then administer two additional doses. Do not treat beyond 12 months.

DOSE ADJUSTMENTS

Reduced dose and benefit-versus-risk assessment may be required with impaired renal function (CrCl below 60 ml/min); insufficient data available. ■ Withhold dose if SrCr elevated; obtain CrCl. ■ Withhold dose if the absolute neutrophil count falls from a baseline of greater than 500 cells/mm^3 before therapy to less than 200 cells/mm^3 during treatment. Resume treatment when count returns to predose levels.

DILUTION

Specific techniques required; see Precautions. Diluent (5 ml SW) provided; dissolve completely; will yield 2 mg/ml. May be given by IV injection or further diluted in 25 to 50 ml NS or D5W; 25 ml yields 0.33 mg/ml, 50 ml yields 0.18 mg/ml. Treat spills or waste with a 5% sodium hypochlorite solution before disposal.

Storage: Refrigerate before initial reconstitution. Store at room temperature and use within 8 hours after initial reconstitution or dilution for infusion.

COMPATIBLE WITH

Consult pharmacist; specific conditions may apply; see Compatibilities, p. xvi. Does not interact with PVC infusion containers or administration sets at concentrations specified for dilution.

Y-site: Fludarabine (Fludara), melphalan (Alkeran), ondansetron (Zofran), paclitaxel (Taxol), sargramostim (Leukine).

RATE OF ADMINISTRATION

Follow each dose with an additional 500 ml of prehydration infusion fluids.

IV injection: A single dose over 1 minute.

Infusion: A single dose over 20 to 30 minutes.

ACTIONS

Mechanism of action is not known, but it is cytotoxic as a result of its potent inhibition of the enzyme adenosine deaminase (ADA). Blocks DNA and RNA synthesis and causes DNA damage. Average terminal half-life of 6 hours is extended to 18 hours in patients with impaired renal function (CrCl less than 50 ml/min). Inhibits ADA for up to 1 week; actual response may not occur for months. Crosses blood-brain barrier. Primarily excreted in urine.

INDICATIONS AND USES

Treatment of hairy cell leukemia (HCL).

Unlabeled uses: May be used in combination or sequentially with SC interferon-alpha-2b (Intron A). Treatment of non-Hodgkin's lymphoma, mycosis fungoides, adult T-cell lymphoma, chronic lymphocytic leukemia, rheumatoid arthritis.

CONTRAINDICATIONS

Hypersensitivity to pentostatin.

PRECAUTIONS

Follow guidelines for handling cytotoxic agents. See Appendix A, p. 1142. ■ Assess drug profile before administration. ■ Myelosuppression, especially neutropenia, is most severe during the first few courses of treatment. ■ Must consider risk/benefit in patients with some bone marrow depression, the possibility of chickenpox or herpes zoster, a history of gout or urate renal stones, renal function impairment, or previous cytotoxic drug or radiation therapy. Use extreme caution. ■ After 6 months of treatment, assess for response; if partial or complete response is not evident, discontinue treatment. If partial response is evident, reevaluate as indicated but do not treat beyond 12 months.

Monitor: Monitor CBC (including differential and platelet count) and SrCr before each dose and as indicated. Blood chemistries including serum uric acid, and a CrCl assay is required before and during treatment. ■ Prehydration with 500 to 1,000 ml 5% dextrose in half-NS or an equivalent is required. An additional 500 ml is required postadministration. ■ Treatment of patients with infection may exacerbate symptoms and cause death. Control infection before treatment initiated. Withhold treatment if an active infection occurs; resume when infection is controlled. ■ Prophylactic antiemetics recommended (e.g., prochlorperazine [Compazine], ondansetron [Zofran]); continue for 48 to 72 hours. ■ Observe closely for severe rashes, nervous system toxicity, and myelosuppression (especially after initial cycles); pentostatin may have to be withheld or discontinued. ■ For severe neutropenia beyond the initial cycles, evaluate for disease status, including a bone marrow examination. ■ Assess response to treatment with periodic monitoring of peripheral blood for hairy cells. Bone marrow aspirates and biopsies may be required at 2- to 3-month intervals. ■ Monitor for thrombocytopenia (platelet count less than 50,000/mm^3). Initiate precautions to prevent excessive bleeding (e.g., inspect IV sites, skin, and mucous membranes; use extreme care during invasive procedures; test urine, emesis, stool, and secretions for occult blood).

Patient Education: Consider birth control options; nonhormonal birth control recommended. ■ Report rashes, symptoms of infection, or bruising and bleeding immediately. ■ See Appendix D, p. 1148.

Maternal/Child: Category D: avoid pregnancy; can cause fetal harm. ■ Discontinue breast-feeding. ■ Safety for use in children and adolescents under 18 years of age not established.

Elderly: Consider decreased renal function.

DRUG/LAB INTERACTIONS

Assess drug profile before administration. ■ Do not use with fludarabine (Fludara); may increase risk of fatal pulmonary toxicity. ■ May cause skin rash with allopurinol. ■ Elevates liver function tests; usually reversible. ■ Do not administer live vaccines to patients receiving antineoplastic drugs. ■ Uric acid levels may increase, increased dose of gout agents (e.g., colchicine, probenicid, sulfinpyrazone [Anturane]) may be indicated. ■ Leukopenia and thrombocytopenia increased by agents causing blood dyscrasias (e.g., anticonvulsants [phenytoin (Dilantin)], penicillins, phenothiazines, and many others).

SIDE EFFECTS

Allergic reactions, anemia, anorexia, chills, cough, diarrhea, fatigue, fever, GU disorders, headache, hepatic disorders/elevated liver function tests, infection, leukopenia, lung disorders, myalgia, nausea, neurologic disorders/CNS, pain, rashes, skin disorders, thrombocytopenia, upper respiratory infections, and vomiting occur in 10% of patients and may require discontinuation of treatment. Abdominal pain, abnormal thinking, abnormal vision, abnormal ECG, anxiety, arthralgia, asthenia, back pain, bronchitis, cardiac arrhythmias, chest pain, confusion, conjunctivitis, constipation, depression, dizziness, dry skin, dyspnea, dysuria, ear pain, ecchymosis, eczema; elevated BUN, creatinine, and LDH; epistaxis, eye pain, flatulence, flu syndrome, hematuria, hemorrhage, herpes simplex, herpes zoster, insomnia, lung edema, lymphadenopathy, maculopapular rash, malaise, neoplasm, nervousness, paresthesia, peripheral edema, petechia, pharyngitis, pneumonia, pruritus, rhinitis, seborrhea, sinusitis, skin discoloration, somnolence, stomatitis, sweating, thrombophlebitis, vesiculobullous rash, weight loss, and death have occurred in 3% to 10% of patients.

ANTIDOTE

Keep physician informed of all side effects; most will be treated symptomatically if indicated. Withhold dose and notify physician for elevated SrCr, absolute neutrophil count below 200 cells/mm^3, myelosuppression, infection, CNS toxicity, or severe rash. Administration of whole blood products (e.g., packed RBCs, platelets, leukocytes) and/or blood modifiers (e.g., darbepoetin alfa [Aranesp], epoetin alfa [Epogen, Procrit], filgrastim [Neupogen], pegfilgrastim [Neulasta], sargramostim [Leukine], oprelvekin [Neumega]) may be indicated to treat bone marrow toxicity. Overdose may cause death due to severe renal, hepatic, pulmonary, or CNS toxicity. There is no specific antidote. Supportive therapy as indicated will help sustain the patient.

PERPHENAZINE

(per-fen′a-zeen)

Phenothiazine
Antipsychotic
Antiemetic

Trilafon

pH 4.2 to 5.6

USUAL DOSE

1 mg, repeat as necessary, allowing 1 to 2 minutes between doses, only until symptoms are controlled. Do not exceed 5 mg.

DOSE ADJUSTMENTS

Dose selection should be cautious in the elderly and in emaciated or debilitated patients. Reduced dose (one third to one half) may be indicated based on the potential for increased sensitivity to side effects, decreased organ function, and concomitant disease or drug therapy; see Elderly. ■ See Drug/Lab Interactions.

DILUTION

Check label on ampule. Only single-dose, 5-mg ampules may be given IV. Handle carefully; may cause contact dermatitis. Each 5 mg (1 ml) must be diluted with 9 ml of NS. Shake well. 1 ml will equal 0.5 mg. May be further diluted and given as an infusion under observation of anesthesiologist (use an infusion pump or a microdrip, 60 gtt/ml).

Storage: Store at CRT. Slightly yellow color does not affect potency. Discard if markedly discolored. Protect from light and freezing.

COMPATIBLE WITH

Consult pharmacist; specific conditions may apply; see Compatibilities, p. xvi.

Syringe: Atropine, benztropine (Cogentin), butorphanol (Stadol), chlorpromazine (Thorazine), cimetidine (Tagamet), dimenhydrinate (Dinate), diphenhydramine (Benadryl), droperidol (Inapsine), fentanyl (Sublimaze), meperidine (Demerol), metoclopramide (Reglan), morphine, pentazocine (Talwin), prochlorperazine (Compazine), promethazine (Phenergan), ranitidine (Zantac), scopolamine.

Y-site: Acyclovir (Zovirax), amikacin (Amikin), ampicillin, cefamandole (Mandol), cefazolin (Kefzol), cefotaxime (Claforan), cefoxitin (Mefoxin), cefuroxime (Zinacef), chloramphenicol (Chloromycetin), clindamycin (Cleocin), doxycycline (Vibramycin), erythromycin lactobionate (Erythocin), famotidine (Pepcid IV), gentamicin (Garamycin), kanamycin (Kantrex), metronidazole (Flagyl IV), minocycline (Minocin), nafcillin (Nafcil), oxacillin (Bactocill), penicillin G potassium, piperacillin (Pipracil), sulfamethoxazole-trimethoprim (Bactrim), tacrolimus (Prograf), ticarcillin (Ticar), ticarcillin/clavulanate (Timentin), tobramycin (Nebcin), vancomycin (Vancocin).

RATE OF ADMINISTRATION

0.5 mg or fraction thereof over 1 minute.

ACTIONS

A phenothiazine derivative said to be approximately 10 times more potent than chlorpromazine (Thorazine) with effects on the central, autonomic, and peripheral nervous systems. Has weak to moderate sedative and anticholinergic effects; and strong antiemetic and extrapyramidal effects. Onset of action is prompt and lasting. Metabolized by the liver and excreted in urine and feces. Crosses the placental barrier. Secreted in breast milk.

INDICATIONS AND USES

Control of severe nausea and vomiting, intractable hiccups, or acute symptoms such as violent retching during surgery.

CONTRAINDICATIONS

Comatose or severely depressed states; hypersensitivity to phenothiazines or its components (contains bisulfites), in the presence of existing blood dyscrasias, bone marrow depression or liver disease, or in patients receiving large doses of other CNS depressants (e.g., antihistamines, barbiturates, or narcotics).

PRECAUTIONS

Use IV only when absolutely necessary. ■ May mask diagnosis of brain tumor, drug intoxication, and intestinal obstruction. ■ Use caution in coronary disease, respiratory disease, severe hypertension or hypotension, and glaucoma. ■ Use caution in patients with epilepsy; may lower seizure threshold. ■ Use caution in patients with bone marrow depression, liver or renal dysfunction. ■ May produce ECG changes (e.g., prolonged QT interval, changes in T waves). ■ Anticholinergic and cardiac effects may be troublesome during anesthesia. For patients receiving phenothiazines, discontinue preoperatively if they will not be continued after surgery.

■ Reexposure of patients who have experienced jaundice, skin reactions, or blood dyscrasias with a phenothiazine is not recommended. Cross-sensitivity may occur. ■ Extrapyramidal symptoms caused by phenothiazines may be confused with CNS signs of an undiagnosed disease (e.g., Reye's syndrome or encephalopathy). ■ Tardive dyskinesia (potentially irreversible involuntary dyskinetic movements) may develop. Use smallest doses and shortest duration of therapy to minimize risk. ■ Neuroleptic malignant syndrome (NMS) characterized by hyperpyrexia, muscle rigidity, altered mental status, and autonomic instability has been reported; see Antidote. ■ May contain sulfites; use with caution in patients with asthma. ■ Metabolized through the P_{450} 2D6 isoenzyme. 10% of Caucasians have reduced activity of this enzyme and will have higher plasma concentrations of perphenazine at usual doses. Correlation with the incidence of side effects has been documented.

Monitor: Keep patient in supine position and monitor BP and pulse between doses. ■ Observe elderly patients closely post-operatively; may be at greater risk for falling. ■ Cough reflex is often depressed; monitor closely if nauseated or vomiting to prevent aspiration. ■ Fever without etiology indicates drug intolerance.

Patient Education: Request assistance for ambulation; may cause dizziness or fainting. ■ Possible skin and eye sensitivity; avoid unprotected exposure to sun. ■ Avoid use of alcohol or other CNS depressants (e.g., antihistamines, barbiturates). ■ Use caution performing tasks requiring alertness.

Maternal/Child: Safety for use in pregnancy and breast-feeding not established. ■ May cause paradoxical excitement in children. ■ Not recommended for use in children under 12 years.

Elderly: Response similar to that seen in younger adults; however, dose selection should be cautious; see Dose Adjustments. ■ May have increased sensitivity to side effects (e.g., postural hypotension, anticholinergic and sedative effects). ■ May be at increased risk for falls and consequent hip fractures. ■ May have an increased risk of extrapyramidal side effects (e.g., tardive dyskinesia, parkinsonism). ■ May cause paradoxical excitement. ■ See Precautions and Monitor.

DRUG/LAB INTERACTIONS

Increased CNS, respiratory depression and hypotensive effects with CNS depressants (e.g., narcotics, barbiturates, alcohol, anesthetics). Reduced dose of these agents usually indicated; may have less potentiating effect than other phenothiazines. ■ Additive effects with MAO inhibitors (e.g., selegiline [Eldepryl]), anticholinergics, antihistamines, antihypertensives, hypnotics, muscle relaxants, rauwolfia alkaloids, and thiazide diuretics; dose adjustment may be necessary. ■ Risk of cardiotoxicity increased with pimozide (Orap) and sparfloxacin (Zagam); concurrent use not recommended. ■ Risk of additive QT interval prolongation, cardiac depressant effects, and cardiac arrhythmias increased with amiodarone (Cordarone), cisapride (Propulsid), disopyramide (Norpace), erythromycin, probucol (Lorelco), procainamide (Pronestyl) and quinidine. ■ Concurrent use with antidepressants (e.g., fluoxetine [Prozac], paroxetine [Paxil]), tricyclic antidepressants (e.g., amitriptyline [Elavil]) or MAO inhibitors may increase effects of both drugs; risk of neuroleptic malignant syndrome may be increased. Monitor closely. Dose reduction of one or both agents may be indicated. ■ Encephalopathic syndrome has been reported with concurrent use of lithium, monitor for S/S of neurologic toxicity. ■ Use of epinephrine not recommended; may cause precipitous hypotension. ■ Use caution during anesthesia with barbiturates (e.g., methohexital, thiopental); may increase frequency and severity of hypotension and neuromuscular excitation. ■ Capable of innumerable other interactions.

SIDE EFFECTS

Usually transient if drug is discontinued, but may require treatment if severe: anaphylaxis, blurring of vision, cardiac arrest, dermatitis, dizziness, dryness of mouth, dysphagia, extrapyramidal symptoms (e.g., abnormal positioning, extreme restlessness, pseudoparkinsonism, weakness of extremities), elevated BP, excitement, hypersensitivity reactions, hypotension, slurred speech, spastic movements (especially about the face), tachycardia, temperature without etiology, tightness of the throat, tongue discoloration, tongue protrusion, and many others. Overdose can cause convulsions, hallucinations, and death.

ANTIDOTE

Discontinue the drug at onset of any side effect and notify the physician. Counteract hypotension with IV fluids, or norepinephrine (Levophed) or phenylephrine (Neo-Synephrine), and extrapyramidal symptoms with benztropine mesylate (Cogentin) or diphenhydramine (Benadryl). Epinephrine is contraindicated for hypotension; further hypotension will occur. Use diazepam (Valium) followed by phenytoin for convulsions or hyperactivity. Phenytoin may be helpful in ventricular arrhythmias; extended monitoring of cardiac function may be required. In treating respiratory depression and unconsciousness, avoid analeptics such as doxapram (Dopram); they may cause convulsions. Signs of arousal from coma may not occur for 48 hours. Not removed by hemodialysis. Resuscitate as necessary.

PHENOBARBITAL SODIUM

(fee-noe-bar′bi-tal so′de-um)

Barbiturate
Sedative-hypnotic
Anticonvulsant

Luminal Sodium

pH 8.5 to 10.5

USUAL DOSE

Use only enough medication to achieve the desired effect. May take up to 15 minutes to reach peak levels in the brain; guard against overdose and excessive respiratory depression.

Hypnotic: 100 to 325 mg.

Sedative: 30 to 120 mg/day in 2 or 3 divided doses.

Anticonvulsant: 200 to 320 mg. May be repeated if necessary. Maximum dose usually does not exceed 600 mg.

Status epilepticus: ***Loading dose:*** 10 to 20 mg/kg in single or divided doses. May give an additional 5 mg/kg every 15 to 30 minutes up to a maximum dose of 30 mg/kg.

Maintenance dose: 1 to 3 mg/kg/24 hr or 0.5 to 1.5 mg/kg every 12 hours.

PEDIATRIC DOSE

See comments under Usual Dose.

Preoperative sedation: 1 to 3 mg/kg of body weight 60 to 90 minutes before procedure.

Status epilepticus: ***Loading dose:*** 15 to 18 mg/kg as a single dose or in divided doses. May give an additional 5 mg/kg every 15 to 30 minutes up to a maximum dose of 30 mg/kg.

Maintenance dose: Infants: 2.5 to 3 mg/kg every 12 hours.

Ages 1 to 5: 3 to 4 mg/kg every 12 hours.

Ages 6 to 12: 2 to 3 mg/kg every 12 hours.

Over 12 years of age: 0.5 to 1.5 mg/kg every 12 hours. Up to 12 mg/kg/24 hours has been used in maintenance doses.

NEONATAL DOSE

See comments under Usual Dose.

Status epilepticus: ***Loading dose:*** 15 to 20 mg/kg as a single dose or in divided doses.

Maintenance dose: 1.5 to 2 mg/kg every 12 hours; may be increased to 2.5 mg/kg every 12 hours if needed.

DOSE ADJUSTMENTS

Reduce dose in impaired renal or hepatic function; usually required in the debilitated or elderly. ■ See Drug/Lab Interactions.

DILUTION

Sterile powder must be slowly diluted with SW for injection. Use a minimum of 3 ml of diluent. Also available in sterile vials and tubexes. Best if further diluted up to 10 ml with SW for injection. Solutions from powder form must be freshly prepared. Use only absolutely clear solutions. Discard powder or solution exposed to air for 30 minutes.

COMPATIBLE WITH

Consult pharmacist; specific conditions may apply; see Compatibilities, p. xvi.

Additive: Amikacin (Amikin), aminophylline, calcium chloride, calcium gluconate, dimenhydrinate (Dinate), meropenem (Merrem IV), sodium bicarbonate, thiopental (Pentothal), verapamil (Isoptin).

Syringe: Heparin.

Y-site: Enalaprilat (Vasotec IV), fentanyl (Sublimaze), fosphenytoin (Cerebyx), gatifloxacin (Tequin), hydromorphone (Dilaudid), levofloxacin (Levaquin), linezolid (Zyvox), meropenem (Merrem IV), morphine, propofol (Diprivan), sufentanil (Sufenta).

RATE OF ADMINISTRATION

60 mg (gr 1) or fraction thereof over 1 minute. Titrate slowly to desired effect. Rapid injection rate may cause symptoms of overdose (e.g., serious respiratory depression).

Status epilepticus: A single loading dose over 10 to 15 minutes.

ACTIONS

A sedative, hypnotic barbiturate of long duration with potent anticonvulsant effects. Phenobarbital is a CNS depressant. Onset of action is prompt by the IV route and becomes rapidly more intense. Effects last from 6 to 10 hours. Will effectively depress the motor cortex with small doses. Pain perception is unimpaired. Rapidly absorbed by all body tissues and excreted in changed form in the urine. Excreted more readily in alkaline urine. Crosses the placental barrier. Secreted in breast milk.

INDICATIONS AND USES

Prolonged sedation (medical and psychiatric). ■ Anticonvulsant.

CONTRAINDICATIONS

History of porphyria, impaired renal function, impaired hepatic function especially with any signs of hepatic coma, known hypersensitivity to barbiturates, previous addiction, severe respiratory depression including dyspnea, obstruction, or cor pulmonale.

PRECAUTIONS

IV route usually reserved for critical situations. ■ Use caution in elderly and debilitated patients and those with asthma, pulmonary disease, shock, and impaired renal or hepatic function. ■ Status epilepticus can occur from too-rapid withdrawal. ■ May be habit forming. Use caution in acute or chronic pain. ■ Benzodiazepines (diazepam [Valium], midazolam [Versed]) generally preferred for sedation.

Monitor: Keep patient under constant observation. Record vital signs every hour, or more often if indicated. ■ Maintain a patent airway. ■ Monitor hematopoietic, renal and hepatic systems in any extended therapy. ■ Treat the cause of a convulsion. ■ Keep equipment for artificial ventilation available. ■ Highly alkaline. Determine absolute patency of vein; use of large veins preferred to prevent thrombosis. Avoid extravasation. Intra-arterial injection will cause gangrene. ■ Monitor phenytoin and barbiturate levels when both drugs are used concurrently. ■ See Drug/Lab Interactions.

Patient Education: Avoid alcohol or other CNS depressants (e.g., antihistamines, diazepam [Valium]). May be habit forming. ■ May require alternate birth control.

Maternal/Child: Category D: avoid pregnancy; will cause birth defects. ■ May cause drowsiness in the nursing infant. ■ See Precautions.

Elderly: See Dose Adjustments and Precautions. ■ Often have increased sensitivity to barbiturates; may cause marked excitement, depression, confusion, and increased risk of barbiturate-induced hypothermia. ■ Consider age-related hepatic or renal impairment and concomitant disease or drug therapy.

DRUG/LAB INTERACTIONS

Use extreme caution if any other CNS depressants have been given, such as alcohol, narcotic analgesics, anesthetics, antidepressants, antihistamines, hypnotics, MAO inhibitors, phenothiazines, sedatives, aminoglycoside antibiotics, tranquilizers. Potentiation with respiratory depression may occur. ■ Inhibits effectiveness of propranolol (Inderal), corticosteroids, doxycycline (Vibramycin), oral anticoagulants, oral contraceptives, quinidine, and theophylline. Capable of innumerable interactions with many drugs. ■ May increase orthostatic hypotension with furosemide (Lasix). ■ Monitor phenytoin (Dilantin), felbamate (Felbatol), carbamazepine (Tegretol), and barbiturate levels when any combination of these drugs is used concurrently. ■ May inhibit vitamin D metabolism with extended use. ■ May decrease plasma concentrations and effectiveness of triazole antifungals (e.g., itraconazole [Sporanox]).

SIDE EFFECTS

Rarely occur with slow injection of average doses.

Average dose: Depression, dermatitis, facial edema, fever, headache, hypotension, nausea, neonatal apnea, respiratory depression (hypoventilation), thrombocytopenic purpura, vertigo.

Overdose: Apnea, coma, cough reflex depression, delirium, flat EEG (reversible unless hypoxic damage has occurred), hypotension, laryngospasm, lowered body temperature, pulmonary edema, renal shutdown, respiratory depression, sluggish or absent reflexes, stupor.

ANTIDOTE

Notify the physician of any side effects. Symptomatic and supportive treatment is most important in overdose. Maintain an adequate airway with artificial ventilation if indicated. Keep the patient warm. IV volume expanders (dextran) and other IV fluids will help maintain adequate circulation. Diuretics may promote the elimination of the drug. Vasopressors (e.g., dopamine [Intropin]) will maintain BP.

PHENTOLAMINE MESYLATE

(fen-tole′a-meen mes′uh-lat)

Alpha-adrenergic blocking agent
Antihypertensive
Vasodilator

Regitine

pH 4.5 to 6.5

USUAL DOSE

Phentolamine is available on an allocation basis from the manufacturer (Novartis). Hospitals are allowed to keep two boxes on hand; otherwise request must be faxed to manufacturer at (973) 781-5508 (24 hours). Include a copy of the prescription (doctor's order), a written request for the required supply, and the name and address of a wholesaler for billing purposes. Telephone (888) 669-6682.

Preoperative: 5 mg 1 to 2 hours before surgery. May be repeated. During surgery the same doses are used as indicated to control epinephrine intoxication.

Prevent necrosis caused by norepinephrine (Levophed): Add 10 mg to each 1,000 ml of IV solution containing norepinephrine or dopamine.

Test dose for diagnosis of pheochromocytoma: 2.5 to 5 mg.

Treatment of congestive heart failure (unlabeled): 5 to 10 mg in 500 ml of D5W given at a rate of 0.17 to 0.4 mg/min.

PEDIATRIC DOSE

Preoperative: 1 mg, 0.1 mg/kg of body weight, or 3 mg/M^2 1 to 2 hours before surgery. Repeat as indicated; see Usual Dose.

Prevent necrosis caused by norepinephrine (Levophed): Add 0.1 to 0.2 mg/kg up to a maximum of 10 mg to each 1,000 ml of IV solution containing norepinephrine.

Test dose for diagnosis of pheochromocytoma: 1 mg.

DILUTION

Each 5 mg should be reconstituted with 1 ml of SW for injection. May be further diluted with 5 to 10 ml of SW or NS. Use only freshly prepared solutions.

Storage: Store below 40° C.

COMPATIBLE WITH

Consult pharmacist; specific conditions may apply; see Compatibilities, p. xvi.

Additive: Dobutamine (Dobutrex), verapamil (Isoptin).

Syringe: Papaverine hydrochloride.

Y-site: Amiodarone (Cordarone).

RATE OF ADMINISTRATION

Each 5 mg or fraction thereof over 1 minute.

Test dose: Inject rapidly after pressor response to venipuncture has subsided.

ACTIONS

An alpha-blocking agent that competitively antagonizes endogenous and exogenous alpha agents (e.g., epinephrine and norepinephrine). Has positive chronotropic and inotropic effects on cardiac muscle, as well as vasodilator effects on vascular smooth muscle. Onset of action is prompt. Half-life is approximately 19 minutes. Metabolic fate is undetermined.

INDICATIONS AND USES

Prevention and treatment of hypertensive episodes of pheochromocytoma preoperatively and during surgery. ■ Prevention and treatment of necrosis and sloughing occurring with dopamine (Intropin) and norepinephrine (Levophed). ■ Definitive diagnosis of pheochromocytoma.

Unlabeled uses: Treatment of congestive heart failure, hypertensive crisis due to MAO inhibitor/sympathomimetic amine interactions, and rebound hypertension after discontinuation of clonidine, propranolol, or other hypertensive agents.

CONTRAINDICATIONS

Coronary artery disease, coronary insufficiency, hypersensitivity to phentolamine, myocardial infarction (previous or present).

PRECAUTIONS

Use caution in gastritis or peptic ulcer disease. ■ Use care in the presence of any arrhythmia. It is preferable to have a normal sinus rhythm. ■ MI, cerebrovascular spasm and cerebrovascular occlusion have occurred following administration, usually in association with marked hypotensive episodes. ■ For diagnosis of pheochromocytoma, urinary tests such as vanillylmandelic acid (VMA) are safer and more accurate. Phentolamine is used only when absolutely necessary. Specific procedure must be followed. Consult with physician and pharmacist.

Monitor: Monitor vital signs every 2 minutes.

Maternal/Child: Category C: safety for use during pregnancy and breast-feeding not established. Use with extreme caution and only when clearly indicated.

Elderly: Risk of phentolamine-induced hypothermia may be increased.

DRUG/LAB INTERACTIONS

Antagonizes effects of epinephrine and ephedrine.

SIDE EFFECTS

Abdominal pain, diarrhea, dizziness, hypotension, nasal stuffiness, nausea, tachycardia, tingling of skin, weakness, vomiting.

Major: Cardiac arrhythmias, cerebrovascular occlusion, cerebrovascular spasm, hypotension (severe), myocardial infarction, shock, tachycardia, vomiting under anesthesia.

ANTIDOTE

For minor side effects, notify the physician. If symptoms progress or any major side effect occurs, discontinue drug and notify the physician immediately. Elevation of legs, volume expanders (e.g., albumin, hetastarch), and administration of norepinephrine are recommended for treatment of hypotension. Do not use epinephrine. Maintain the patient as indicated. If tachycardia or cardiac arrhythmias occur, defer use of digitalis derivatives if possible until rhythm returns to normal.

PHENYLEPHRINE HYDROCHLORIDE

Vasopressor

(fen-ill-ef′rin hye-droe-klor′id)

Neo-Synephrine

pH 3 to 6.5

USUAL DOSE

Mild to moderate hypotension or hypotensive emergencies during spinal anesthesia: 0.2 mg. From 0.1 to 0.5 mg may be used initially. May be repeated every 10 to 15 minutes. Never exceed 0.5 mg in a single dose. Highly individualized. Start with a small dose, giving only as much of the drug as required to alleviate undesirable symptoms.

Severe hypotension and shock- or drug-related hypotension: Begin infusion at 100 to 180 mcg/min (0.1 to 0.18 mg/min) until BP stabilized at a low normal for specific individual. Maintain with 40 to 60 mcg/min (0.04 to 0.06 mg/min). Titrate to desired effect.

Paroxysmal supraventricular tachycardia: 0.25 to 0.5 mg has been given as a rapid IV bolus. If additional doses are required to achieve adequate response, increase in increments of 0.1 to 0.2 mg and never exceed a total single dose of 1 mg. Adenosine may be the drug of choice.

PEDIATRIC DOSE

Mild to moderate hypotension: 5 to 20 mcg/kg of body weight per dose. May be repeated every 10 to 15 minutes. Do not exceed adult dose.

Severe hypotension and shock- or drug-related hypotension: Begin an infusion at 0.1 to 0.5 mcg/kg/min. Titrate to desired effect. Do not exceed a maximum total dose of 5 mg.

Paroxysmal supraventricular tachycardia: 5 to 10 mcg/kg/dose as a rapid IV bolus. May repeat dose or double a dose and repeat every 5 minutes until desired systolic BP reached.

DOSE ADJUSTMENTS

Hypotension of powerful peripheral adrenergic blocking agents, chlorpromazine, or pheochromocytomectomy may require carefully calculated increased dose therapy.

DILUTION

IV injection: Dilute 1 ml of a 10 mg/ml solution with 9 ml of SW for injection to prepare a final concentration of 1 mg/ml.

Infusion: Dilute 10 mg in 500 ml of NS or D5W to provide a 1:50,000 solution (20 mcg/ml). May increase to 20 or 30 mg in 500 ml if necessary (40 to 60 mcg/ml).

Pediatric infusion: Add 0.6 mg/kg to 100 ml diluent. 1 ml/hr equals 0.1 mcg/kg/min.

Storage: Protect from light.

COMPATIBLE WITH (Underline Indicates Conflicting Compatibility Information)

Consult pharmacist; specific conditions may apply; see Compatibilities, p. xvi.

Additive: Chloramphenicol (Chloromycetin), dobutamine (Dobutrex), lidocaine, potassium chloride (KCl), sodium bicarbonate.

Y-site: Amiodarone (Cordarone), cisatracurium (Nimbex), etomidate (Amidate), famotidine (Pepcid IV), haloperidol (Haldol), hetastarch in electrolytes (Hextend), inamrinone (Inocor), levofloxacin (Levaquin), propofol (Diprivan), remifentanil (Ultiva), zidovudine (AZT, Retrovir).

RATE OF ADMINISTRATION

IV injection: Single dose over 20 to 30 seconds to treat paroxysmal supraventricular tachycardia; over 1 minute in other situations.

Infusion: Regulate drip rate to provide and maintain individual's low normal BP. Use an infusion pump or microdrip (60 gtt/ml) to administer.

ACTIONS

A sympathomimetic, similar to epinephrine. Acts primarily on alpha-adrenergic receptors. A potent, long-lasting vasoconstrictor. Unique in that it slows HR, increases stroke volume, and does not induce any change in rhythm of the pulse. Renal vessel constriction will occur. Repeated injections produce comparable results. Effective within seconds and lasts about 15 minutes. Metabolic fate and route of excretion have not been determined. Uptake of drug into tissue and some metabolism by the liver have been documented.

INDICATIONS AND USES

Maintain adequate BP in inhalation and spinal anesthesia, shocklike states, drug-induced hypotension, and hypersensitivity reactions. ■ Treat paroxysmal supraventricular tachycardia. ■ Prolong anesthesia.

Unlabeled use: Specific antidote for hypotension produced by chlorpromazine hydrochloride (Thorazine).

CONTRAINDICATIONS

Hypertension, ventricular tachycardia and hypersensitivity to phenylephrine.

PRECAUTIONS

Blood volume depletion should be corrected. May be administered concurrently with blood volume replacement. ■ Use extreme caution in the elderly, hyperthyroidism, bradycardia, partial heart block, myocardial disease, or severe arteriosclerosis. ■ Contains bisulfites; use caution in allergic individuals.

Monitor: Check BP every 2 minutes until stabilized at the desired level. ■ Discontinue IV administration if vein infiltrates or is thrombosed; can cause tissue necrosis and sloughing. ■ See Precautions, Drug/Lab Interactions.

Maternal/Child: Category C: safety for use in pregnancy or breast-feeding not established.

Elderly: See Precautions; may have increased sensitivity to effects.

DRUG/LAB INTERACTIONS

Potentiated by tricyclic antidepressants (e.g., desipramine [Norpramin]), guanethidine, MAO inhibitors (e.g., selegiline [Eldepryl]), other vasopressors (epinephrine [Adrenalin]); ergot alkaloids or oxytocic agents (e.g., ergonovine, oxytocin); hypertensive crisis and death can result. ■ Use caution with digitalis, bretylium, or halogenated hydrocarbon anesthetics (e.g., halothane, isoflurane); arrhythmias may occur.

SIDE EFFECTS

Bradycardia, fullness of head, headache, hypertension, tingling of extremities, tremulousness, ventricular extrasystoles, ventricular tachycardia (short paroxysms), vertigo.

ANTIDOTE

To prevent sloughing and necrosis in areas where extravasation has occurred, with a fine hypodermic needle inject 5 to 10 mg of phentolamine (Regitine) diluted in 10 to 15 ml of NS liberally throughout the tissue in the extravasated area. Treatment should be started as soon as extravasation is recognized. Notify the physician of all side effects. IM injection may be preferable. Treat hypertension with phentolamine (Regitine). Treat cardiac arrhythmias as indicated. Treat bradycardia with atropine. Resuscitate as necessary.

PHENYTOIN SODIUM

(fen′ih-toyn so′de-um)

Hydantoin
Anticonvulsant
Antiarrhythmic

Dilantin, Dilantin Sodium

pH 12

USUAL DOSE

In all situations, transfer to oral therapy 12 to 24 hours after a loading dose or as soon as practical. See Precautions.

Status epilepticus, anticonvulsant: A ***loading dose*** of 10 to 20 mg/kg. Follow with ***maintenance doses*** of 100 mg every 6 to 8 hours. Do not exceed a total dose of 1.5 Gm. Lethal dose estimated at 2 to 5 Gm. If seizure not terminated, consider other anticonvulsants, barbiturates, or anesthesia. IV diazepam may be the drug of choice for initial treatment. Concurrent administration of phenytoin in the lesser doses is suggested by clinicians to maintain control.

Antiarrhythmic: 50 to 100 mg at 5- to 15-minute intervals until the arrhythmia is abolished or side effects occur. Do not exceed a total dose of 15 mg/kg or 1 Gm.

PEDIATRIC DOSE

Status epilepticus, anticonvulsant: 250 mg/M^2 as a ***loading dose,*** followed by ***maintenance doses*** of 4 to 8 mg/kg/24 hr in divided doses every 8 to 12 hours (2 to 4 mg/kg every 12 hours or 1.33 to 2.66 mg/kg every 8 hours). An alternate regimen for children of all ages is a ***loading dose*** of 15 to 20 mg/kg. Follow with a ***maintenance dose for age*** (listed below):

Neonates: Begin with 5 mg/kg/24 hr in equally divided doses every 8 to 12 hours (2.5 to 4 mg/kg every 12 hours or 1.6 to 2.67 mg/kg every 8 hours). Range is 5 to 8 mg/kg/24 hr.

Infants and children: Begin with 5 mg/kg/24 hr in equally divided doses every 8 to 12 hours (2.5 mg/kg every 12 hours or 1.67 mg/kg every 8 hours). Range varies according to age:

6 months to 3 years: 8 to 10 mg/kg/24 hr (4 to 5 mg/kg every 12 hours or 2.67 to 3.33 mg/kg every 8 hours).

4 to 6 years: 7.5 to 9 mg/kg/24 hr (3.75 to 4.5 mg/kg every 12 hours or 2.5 to 3 mg/kg every 8 hours).

7 to 9 years: 7 to 8 mg/kg/24 hr (3.5 to 4 mg/kg every 12 hours or 2.3 to 2.6 mg/kg every 8 hours).

10 to 16 years: 6 to 7 mg/kg/24 hr (3 to 3.5 mg/kg every 12 hours or 2 to 2.3 mg/kg every 8 hours).

Maintenance dose should not exceed 20 mg/kg/24 hr. Loading dose not included in this total. See comments in Usual Dose.

Antiarrhythmic: 1.25 mg/kg every 5 minutes until arrhythmia abolished or side effects occur. Do not exceed a total dose of 15 mg/kg. Maintenance dose is 2.5 to 5 mg/kg every 12 hours.

DOSE ADJUSTMENTS

Use caution, lower dose, and slower rate of administration in the seriously ill, elderly, cachetic patients, and in impaired liver or renal function. ■ In obesity calculate dose on ideal body weight plus 1.33 of excess over ideal; phenytoin preferentially distributes into fat. ■ Dose adjustment may be required based on serum albumin levels. ■ See Drug/Lab Interactions.

DILUTION

Available as 100- or 250-mg ampules, syringes, or vials. Usually not added to IV solutions. May be injected through Y-tube or three-way stopcock of infusion set of a compatible solution. Use solution only when completely dissolved and clear; discard if hazy or if a precipitate forms. May be light yellow in color. Recent studies have utilized NS for infusion solutions that should be prepared immediately before use in suitable concentrations (less than 6.7 mg/ml) to facilitate required rate and fluid limitations or requirements. Method not recommended by manufacturer but is in common use; see Incompatible With. According to most studies, a 0.22-micron in-line filter is required, and use within 1 to 2 hours is recommended.

Storage: Store between 15° and 30° C.

INCOMPATIBLE WITH

Manufacturer recommends not adding to IV solutions or mixing with other medications. May precipitate if pH is altered. Always flush line with NS before and after administration of any other drug through the same IV line. See Dilution.

COMPATIBLE WITH

See Incompatible With. Consult pharmacist; specific conditions may apply; see Compatibilities, p. xvi.

Additive: Bleomycin (Blenoxane), sodium bicarbonate, verapamil (Isoptin).

Y-site: Esmolol (Brevibloc), famotidine (Pepcid IV), fluconazole (Diflucan), foscarnet (Foscavir), tacrolimus (Prograf).

RATE OF ADMINISTRATION

Very alkaline; follow each injection with sterile NS to reduce local venous irritation. Best to flush before and after with NS.

Anticonvulsant: ***Adults:*** 25 to 50 mg or fraction thereof over 1 minute. ***Neonates and pediatric patients:*** A rate of 0.5 to 3 mg/kg/min (not to exceed 25 mg/min) has been suggested. Another source suggests 1 mg/min. ***Elderly:*** Limit rate to 25 mg/min.

Antiarrhythmic: 25 mg or fraction thereof over 2 to 3 minutes.

Infusion: Should be completed within 1 hour. Do not exceed 25 to 50 mg/min rate. Best if piggybacked to a compatible primary IV so phenytoin can be discontinued if side effects occur, but IV can be kept open.

ACTIONS

A synthetic anticonvulsant, chemically related to barbiturates. Selectively stabilizes seizure threshold and depresses seizure activity in the motor cortex. Effective control in emergency treatment of seizures may take 15 to 20 minutes because of rate of injection required. Also exerts a depressant effect on the myocardium by selectively elevating the excitability threshold of the cell, reducing the cell's response to stimuli. Readily absorbed, phenytoin is metabolized in the liver and excreted in changed form in the urine. Crosses placental barrier. Secreted in breast milk.

INDICATIONS AND USES

Control of grand mal and psychomotor seizures. ■ Treatment of status epilepticus (grand mal seizures).

Unlabeled use: Treatment of supraventricular and ventricular arrhythmias, including those caused by digitalis intoxication. Especially useful for patients who are unable to tolerate quinidine or procainamide.

CONTRAINDICATIONS

Bradycardia, sinoatrial, second- or third-degree heart block, Stokes-Adams syndrome; known sensitivity to hydantoin derivatives.

PRECAUTIONS

Because of benefits provided by fosphenytoin (Cerebyx)—e.g., solubility in IV solutions, improved infusion site tolerance, more rapid rate of administration, and well-tolerated IM option—Parke-Davis wants to discontinue injectable phenytoin (Dilantin). Generic products will still be available. ■ Status epilepticus can occur from abrupt withdrawal of hydantoins. ■ Not effective for petit mal seizures; combined therapy required if both conditions present. ■ Use caution in hypotension and severe myocardial insufficiency. ■ Use caution with low serum albumin level, and adjust dose as indicated. Phenytoin is 90% bound to serum protein, and a reduced albumin causes an increase in free drug availability. ■ Lymphadenopathy has been reported. Monitoring and change in anticonvulsant therapy may be indicated. ■ Discontinue phenytoin if skin rash appears. ■ Hyperglycemia and blood dyscrasias have been reported.

Monitor: Narrow margin of error between therapeutic and toxic dose. Plasma levels above 10 mcg/ml usually control seizure activity. The acceptable range is 5 to 20 mcg/ml. Toxicity begins with nystagmus and may be seen at levels less than 20 mcg/ml. ■ Periodic monitoring of CBC, platelets, albumin, urinalysis, hepatic and renal function is recommended. ■ Monitor ECG and BP continuously. ■ Observation of patient symptoms and effectiveness of all medications is imperative. ■ Determine absolute patency of vein. Avoid extravasation. Very alkaline; follow each injection with sterile NS to reduce local venous irritation. ■ Patients maintained with phenytoin should be given a dose the morning of surgery to maintain adequate serum levels. ■ See Drug/Lab Interactions.

Maternal/Child: Capable of numerous interactions in pregnant women. May cause birth defects (see literature). ■ Alterations in phenytoin kinetics in pregnant women may necessitate periodic monitoring of serum levels. ■ Discontinue nursing. ■ May decrease folic acid serum concentrations; avoid during pregnancy.

Elderly: See Dose Adjustments and Rate of Administration. ■ May have elevated serum concentrations because of slow metabolism. ■ Low serum albumin causing a decrease in protein binding may result in increased sensitivity to phenytoin.

DRUG/LAB INTERACTIONS

Interactions are numerous and potentially life threatening. Review of drug profile by pharmacist imperative. ■ Serum levels may be increased by alcohol (acute ingestion), anticoagulants, antidepressants, antifungal agents (e.g., fluconazole, miconazole, ketoconazole), antihistamines, benzodiazepines (e.g., diazepam [Valium]), chloramphenicol, cimetidine (Tagamet), disulfiram (Antabuse), estrogens, fluorouracil, fluoxetine (Prozac), metronidazole, myocardial depressants, paroxetine (Paxil), phenothiazines, sulfonamides, tacrolimus (Prograf), valproic acid, and others. Toxicity and fatality may result. ■ Serum levels may be decreased by chronic alcohol ingestion, antineoplastics, antituberculosis drugs, barbiturates, folic acid, leucovorin calcium, rifampin, theophylline, and others resulting in reduced phenytoin effect. ■ Phenytoin serum levels may be increased or decreased by carbamazepine (Tegretol). ■ May increase serum levels of CNS depressants, folic acid antagonists, and muscle relaxants. ■ May decrease effectiveness of corticosteroids, digitalis, diuretics, itraconazole (Sporanox), levodopa, quetiapine (Seroquel), quinidine, ranitidine (Zantac), and others. ■ Severe hypotension and bradycardia result with concomitant administration with dopamine (Intropin) and all other sympathomimetic antihypertensive drugs. ■ In one case report, a patient stabilized on phenytoin and valproic acid experienced seizures and a reduction in antiepileptic drug serum concentration when acyclovir was added to the regimen. ■ Alters some clinical laboratory tests.

SIDE EFFECTS

Ataxia, confusion, dizziness, drowsiness, fever, hyperplasia of gums, nervousness, nystagmus, skin eruptions, tremors, visual disturbances.

Major: Bradycardia, cardiac arrest, heart block, hypotension, respiratory arrest, tonic seizures, ventricular fibrillation.

ANTIDOTE

Notify the physician of any side effects. If minor symptoms progress or any major side effect occurs, discontinue the drug and notify the physician. Maintain a patent airway and resuscitate as necessary. Symptoms of heart block or bradycardia may be reversed with IV atropine. Epinephrine may also be useful. Hemodialysis may be required in overdose.

PHOSPHATE
(fos′fat)

Electrolyte replenisher
Antihypophosphatemic

Potassium Phosphate, Sodium Phosphate **pH 5 to 7.8**

USUAL DOSE

Dependent on individual needs of the patient. In total parenteral nutrition (TPN), 10 to 15 mM (310 to 465 mg) of phosphorus/liter of TPN solution should maintain normal serum phosphate. Larger amounts may be required. 1 mM equals 31 mg.

Acute hypophosphatemia: Adults and children: 0.16 to 0.32 mM/kg (5 to 10 mg/kg) of body weight as a ***loading dose*** equally distributed over 6 hours. ***Maintain children*** with 0.5 to 1.5 mM/kg/24 hr (15 to 45 mg/kg/24 hr). ***Maintain adults*** with 48.4 to 64.5 mM/24 hr (1.5 to 2 Gm/24 hr).

INFANT DOSE

Infants receiving TPN: 1.5 to 2 mM/kg (46.5 to 62 mg) of body weight/day.

DOSE ADJUSTMENTS

Lower-end initial doses may be indicated in the elderly based on the potential for decreased organ function and concomitant disease or drug therapy.

DILUTION

Must be diluted in a larger volume of suitable IV solution and given as an infusion. Soluble in most commonly used IV solutions (see chart on inside back cover) except protein hydrolysate. Mix thoroughly. See Incompatible With.

INCOMPATIBLE WITH

ALL FORMULATIONS

Mix thoroughly after each addition of supposedly compatible drugs or solutions. TPN solutions requiring the addition of phosphates and calcium salts must be mixed by the pharmacist to avoid a precipitate of calcium phosphate. Specific amounts, calculations, order and temperature (precipitate forms more readily at room temperature) are required. Deaths have been reported.

COMPATIBLE WITH

See Incompatible With. Consult pharmacist; specific conditions may apply; see Compatibilities, p. xvi.

POTASSIUM PHOSPHATE

Additive: Mix thoroughly. Magnesium sulfate, metoclopramide (Reglan), verapamil (Isoptin).

Y-site: Diltiazem (Cardizem), enalaprilat (Vasotec IV), esmolol (Brevibloc), famotidine (Pepcid IV), labetalol (Normodyne).

SODIUM PHOSPHATE

Y-site: Gatifloxacin (Tequin).

RATE OF ADMINISTRATION

0.2 mM of phosphate/kg/hr is the maximum infusion rate. Potassium phosphate will be further limited by the maximum rate for potassium. Consider sodium/potassium content. Infuse slowly. Rapid infusion may cause phosphate or potassium intoxication. Serum calcium may be reduced rapidly, causing hypocalcemic tetany.

ACTIONS

Involved in bone deposition. Helps to maintain calcium levels, has a buffering effect on acid-base equilibrium, and influences renal excretion of the hydrogen ion. Normal levels in adults, 3 to 4.5 mg/dl of serum; in children, 4 to 7 mg/dl. Excreted in urine.

INDICATIONS AND USES

To prevent or correct hypophosphatemia in patients with restricted or no oral intake.

CONTRAINDICATIONS

Any disease with high phosphate or low calcium levels, hyperkalemia (potassium phosphate), hypernatremia (sodium phosphate).

PRECAUTIONS

Rapid infusion may cause phosphate, sodium, or potassium intoxication. Serum calcium may be reduced, rapidly causing hypocalcemic tetany. ■ Use sodium phosphate with caution in renal impairment, cirrhosis, cardiac failure, or any edematous, sodium-retaining state. ■ Use potassium phosphate with caution in cardiac disease, renal disease, and digitalized patients. ■ See Incompatible With.

Monitor: Monitor serum calcium, potassium, phosphate, chlorides, and sodium. Discontinue when serum phosphate exceeds 2 mg/dl. ■ See Drug/Lab Interactions.

Maternal/Child: Category C: safety for use in pregnancy not established.

Elderly: Differences in response between elderly and younger patients have not been identified. Lower end initial doses may be appropriate in the elderly; see Dose Adjustments.

DRUG/LAB INTERACTIONS

May cause hyperkalemia with potassium-sparing diuretics (e.g., amiloride) or angiotensin-converting enzyme inhibitors (e.g., enalapril [Vasotec]).

SIDE EFFECTS

Elevated phosphates; reduced calcium levels and hypocalcemic tetany; elevated potassium levels causing cardiac arrhythmias; flaccid paralysis; heaviness of the legs; hypotension; listlessness; mental confusion; paresthesia of the extremities.

ANTIDOTE

For any side effect, discontinue the drug and notify the physician. Restore serum calcium with calcium gluconate or chloride. Shift potassium from serum to cells with 150 ml of ⅙ M sodium lactate or 10% to 20% dextrose with 10 units regular insulin for each 20 Gm dextrose at 300 to 500 ml/hr. Correct acidosis with sodium bicarbonate. Reduce sodium by restriction, diuretics, or hemodialysis. Resuscitate as necessary.

PHYSOSTIGMINE SALICYLATE

(fye-zoh-stig′meen sah-lis′a-lat)

Cholinergic
Cholinesterase inhibitor
Antidote

Antilirium

pH 5.8

USUAL DOSE

Anticholinergic toxicity: 0.5 to 2 mg initially. 1 to 4 mg may be repeated as necessary as life-threatening signs recur (arrhythmias, convulsions, deep coma). Maximum dose is 4 mg in 30 minutes.

Postanesthesia: 0.5 to 1 mg initially. Repeat at 10- to 30-minute intervals until desired results obtained.

PEDIATRIC DOSE

To be used in life-threatening situations only. 0.02 mg/kg/dose. May be repeated at 5- to 10-minute intervals only if toxic effects persist and there is no sign of cholinergic effects. Maximum total dose is 2 mg.

DILUTION

May be given undiluted. Do not add to IV solutions. May be given through Y-tube or three-way stopcock of infusion set.

COMPATIBILITY

Specific information not available. Consider specific use; consult pharmacist.

RATE OF ADMINISTRATION

Rapid IV administration may cause bradycardia, hypersalivation, respiratory distress, and convulsions.

1 mg or fraction thereof over 1 to 3 minutes.

Pediatric rate: 0.5 mg or fraction thereof over at least 1 minute.

ACTIONS

An extract of *Physostigma venenosum* seeds. It inhibits the destructive action of acetylcholinesterase and prolongs and exaggerates the effects of acetylcholine. Stimulates parasympathetic nerve stimulation (pupil contraction, increased intestinal musculature tonus, bronchial constriction, salivary and sweat gland stimulation). Does enter the CNS. Onset of action occurs in 5 minutes and lasts about 1 hour. Rapidly hydrolyzed by cholinesterases.

INDICATIONS AND USES

To reverse CNS toxic effects caused by drugs capable of producing anticholinergic poisoning (e.g., atropine, scopolamine), other anticholinergic/antispasmodic agents (e.g., phenothiazines, antihistamines) and anticholinergic antiparkinson agents (e.g., benztropine [Cogentin], trihexyphenidyl [Artane]).

Unlabeled uses: Treatment of delirium tremens and Alzheimer's disease.

CONTRAINDICATIONS

Asthma, cardiovascular disease, diabetes, gangrene, mechanical obstruction of the intestines or urogenital tract, vagotonic states, patients receiving choline esters, depolarizing neuromuscular blocking agents (succinylcholine), or tricyclic antidepressants (e.g., amitriptyline [Elavil]).

PRECAUTIONS

Rapid IV administration may cause bradycardia, hypersalivation, respiratory distress, and convulsions. ■ Contains bisulfites; use caution in allergic individuals.

Monitor: Atropine must always be available. ■ Monitor vital signs. ■ See Drug/Lab Interactions.

Maternal/Child: Safety for use in pregnancy and breast-feeding not established. ■ Has caused muscular weakness in neonates of mothers treated with other cholinesterase inhibitors for myasthenia gravis. ■ May contain benzyl alcohol; do not use in neonates.

DRUG/LAB INTERACTIONS

Potentiates succinylcholine and other choline esters (e.g., bethanecol). ■ May antagonize CNS depressant effects of diazepam (Valium). May cause serious complications, including death, with tricyclic antidepressants (e.g., amitriptyline [Elavil]).

SIDE EFFECTS

Anxiety, bradycardia, cholinergic crisis (overdose), coma, convulsions, defecation, delirium, disorientation, emesis, hallucinations, hyperactivity, hypersalivation, hypersensitivity, nausea, respiratory distress, salivation, seizures, sweating, urination.

ANTIDOTE

Keep physician informed of side effects. For excessive nausea or sweating, reduce dose. Discontinue drug for bradycardia, convulsions, excessive defecation, emesis, salivation, or urination, or respiratory distress. Treat cholinergic side effects (e.g., arrhythmias, bronchoconstriction) or hypersensitivity with the specific antagonist atropine sulfate in doses of 0.6 mg IV. May be repeated every 3 to 10 minutes. Endotracheal intubation or tracheostomy are considered prophylactic in anesthesia or crisis. Artificial ventilation, oxygen therapy, cardiac monitoring, adequate suctioning, and treatment of shock or convulsions must be instituted and maintained as necessary.

PHYTONADIONE

(fye-toe-na-dye'one)

Vitamin (prothrombinogenic)
Antidote
Antihemorrhagic

Aquamephyton, Vitamin K_1 **pH 5 to 7**

USUAL DOSE

Should be given by the SC route whenever possible; IV and IM routes have caused death; see Precautions. A single dose is preferred, but it may be repeated if clinically indicated. Use the smallest dose that achieves effective results to prevent clotting hazards.

Vitamin K deficiency: Up to 10 mg may be added to TPN solutions as indicated.

Anticoagulant-induced (warfarin or dicumarol) hypoprothrombinemia: 2.5 to 10 mg. Doses up to 25 mg and, rarely, 50 mg may be needed. May repeat in 6 to 8 hours if initial response is not adequate.

Hypoprothrombinemia from other causes: 2 to 25 mg (rarely 50 mg), depending on the severity of the deficiency and the response obtained.

PEDIATRIC DOSE

See Usual Dose, Precautions, and Maternal/Child.

Vitamin K deficiency: 1 to 2 mg may be added to TPN solutions as indicated.

Anticoagulant-induced (warfarin or dicumarol) hypoprothrombinemia in infants and children: 1 to 2 mg/dose.

Hypoprothrombinemia from other causes in infants and children: A single dose of 1 to 2 mg.

NEWBORN DOSE

See Usual Dose, Precautions, and Maternal/Child. Rarely given IV in the newborn; use extreme caution if administered IM. SC injection preferred.

Prophylaxis of hemorrhagic disease of the newborn: 0.5 to 1 mg IM or SC within 1 hour of birth.

Treatment of hemorrhagic disease of the newborn: 1 to 2 mg/24 hr. Higher doses may be necessary if the mother has been receiving oral anticoagulants. Whole blood or blood components may be indicated for excessive bleeding. Give phytonadione concurrently to correct the underlying disorder.

DOSE ADJUSTMENTS

See Drug/Lab Interactions.

DILUTION

Use only preservative-free solutions. May be diluted only with NS, D5NS, or D5W. Dilution with at least 10 ml of diluent is recommended to facilitate prescribed rate of administration. Photosensitive; protect from light in all dilutions. Discard after single use.

COMPATIBLE WITH

Consult pharmacist; specific conditions may apply; see Compatibilities, p. xvi.

Additive: Amikacin (Amikin), chloramphenicol (Chloromycetin), cimetidine (Tagamet), sodium bicarbonate.

Syringe: Doxapram (Dopram).

Y-site: Ampicillin, epinephrine (Adrenalin), famotidine (Pepcid IV), heparin, hydrocortisone sodium succinate (Solu-Cortef), potassium chloride (KCl).

RATE OF ADMINISTRATION

Each 1 mg or fraction thereof over 1 minute or longer.

ACTIONS

Vitamin K, a fat-soluble vitamin, is essential for hepatic production of four blood coagulation factors including prothrombin. These are required for normal blood clotting. Results should be detectable in 1 to 2 hours. Usually controls hemorrhage in 3 to 6 hours; normal prothrombin levels should be obtained in 12 to 14 hours. Metabolized completely by the body.

INDICATIONS AND USES

Coagulation disorders due to faulty formation of factors II, VII, IX, and X when caused by vitamin K deficiency or interference with vitamin K activity. Indicated in anticoagulant-induced prothrombin deficiency (warfarin or dicumarol). ■ Prophylaxis and treatment of hemorrhagic disease of the newborn. ■ Hypoprothrombinemia resulting from antibacterial therapy. ■ Hypoprothrombinemia secondary to factors limiting the absorption or synthesis of vitamin K (e.g., obstructive jaundice, biliary fistula, sprue, ulcerative colitis, celiac disease, intestinal resection, cystic fibrosis of the pancreas, and regional enteritis). ■ Other drug-induced hypoprothrombinemia where it is definitely shown that the result is due to interference with vitamin K metabolism (e.g., salicylates).

CONTRAINDICATIONS

Hypersensitivity to components.

PRECAUTIONS

IV and IM are not routes of choice; used only when SC route cannot be used. Use extreme caution; has caused severe reactions, including death, with the first injection. ■ As an alternative to administering phytonadione, discontinuation or reduction of the doses of drugs interfering with coagulation mechanisms (e.g., antibiotics, salicylates) should be considered. The severity of the coagulation disorder should determine if phytonadione is required in addition to discontinuing or reducing the doses of interfering drugs. ■ Supplement with whole blood transfusion or blood components if indicated. ■ Now the only vitamin K product for IV use. ■ Do not use to counteract anticoagulant effects of heparin, not effective; protamine sulfate is indicated. ■ When phytonadione is used in a patient for whom anticoagulant therapy is indicated, the same clotting hazards that existed before beginning anticoagulant therapy will recur. Use the smallest dose of phytonadione possible and monitor PT.

Monitor: See Neonatal Dose, Precautions, and Drug/Lab Interactions. ■ Dose and effect determined by PT. Keep the physician informed. ■ Pain and swelling at injection site can occur.

Maternal/Child: Category C: safety for use not established. ■ Use caution during breast-feeding. ■ Use extreme caution in premature infants and neonates. Hemolysis, jaundice, and hyperbilirubinemia in newborns may be related to the dose of phytonadione. The recommended dose should not be exceeded. Severe hemolytic anemia, hemoglobinuria, kernicterus, brain damage, and death may occur.

DRUG/LAB INTERACTIONS

Discontinue drugs adversely affecting the coagulation mechanism if possible (e.g., salicylates, antibiotics). ■ May cause temporary resistance to prothrombin-depressing oral anticoagulants by increasing amount of phytonadione in the liver and blood. Anticoagulation will require larger doses of same or use of heparin sodium.

SIDE EFFECTS

Cyanosis, diaphoresis, dizziness, dyspnea, hyperbilirubinemia, hypotension, injection site reactions, peculiar taste sensations, rapid and weak pulse, tachycardia, transient flushing sensation. Anaphylaxis, shock, and death have occurred with IV and IM injection.

ANTIDOTE

Should not be necessary if dosage is accurately calculated before administration. Action can be reversed by warfarin or heparin if indicated. Discontinue the drug and notify the physician of any side effects. For most side effects the physician will probably choose to continue the drug at a decreased rate of administration. Treat allergic reactions as necessary.

PIPERACILLIN SODIUM

(pi-per′a-sill-in so′de-um)

Antibacterial (extended-spectrum penicillin)

Pipracil

pH 5.5 to 7.5

USUAL DOSE

3 to 4 Gm every 4, 6, 8, or 12 hours depending on severity of infection. Maximum dose usually 24 Gm/24 hr. Usual duration of therapy is 7 to 10 days. Continue at least 2 days after symptoms of infection disappear.

Empirical therapy in febrile neutropenic patients: 50 mg/kg every 4 hours, not to exceed 24 Gm/day or 300 mg/kg/day. Given in combination with ciprofloxacin 400 mg every 8 hours.

Perioperative prophylaxis: 2 to 4 Gm 30 minutes to 1 hour before incision. Repeat every 4 to 6 hours for up to 24 hours if indicated. Specific doses for specific procedures (see literature).

PEDIATRIC DOSE

200 to 300 mg/kg/24 hr in equally divided doses every 4 to 6 hours (33.3 to 50 mg/kg every 4 hours or 50 to 75 mg/kg every 6 hours).

Cystic fibrosis in children under 12 years of age: 300 to 600 mg/kg/24 hr in equally divided doses every 4 to 6 hours (50 to 100 mg/kg every 4 hours or 75 to 150 mg/kg every 6 hours).

NEONATAL DOSE

Premature infants (less than 36 weeks' gestation) less than 7 days of age: 75 mg/kg every 12 hours. **7 days of age or older:** 75 mg/kg every 8 hours.

Full-term infants less than 7 days of age: 75 mg/kg every 8 hours. **7 days of age or older:** 75 mg/kg every 6 hours.

Another source suggests:

7 days of age or younger and 2 kg or less: 50 mg every 12 hours; **over 2 kg:** 50 mg every 8 hours.

Over 7 days of age and 2 kg or less: 50 mg every 8 hours; **over 2 kg:** 50 mg every 6 hours.

DOSE ADJUSTMENTS

Reduce dose only in severe renal impairment with CrCl temporarily below 40 ml/min. May be given to patients undergoing hemodialysis and peritoneal dialysis (see literature for dose).

DILUTION

Each 1 Gm or fraction thereof should be reconstituted with at least 5 ml of SW or NS. Shake vigorously to dissolve. May be further diluted to desired volume (50 to 100 ml) with D5W, NS, D5NS, or LR, and given as an intermittent infusion. Also available in ADD-Vantage vials for use with ADD-Vantage infusion containers.

Storage: Stable at room temperature for 24 hours. Use solutions diluted with LR within 2 hours.

INCOMPATIBLE WITH

Inactivated in solution with aminoglycosides (e.g., amikacin [Amikin], gentamicin [Garamycin]). Do not mix in the same solution. Appropriate spacing and/or separate sites required. See Drug/Lab Interactions.

COMPATIBLE WITH (Underline Indicates Conflicting Compatibility Information)

Consult pharmacist; specific conditions may apply; see Compatibilities, p. xvi.

Additive: ***See Incompatible With.*** <u>Ciprofloxacin (Cipro IV)</u>, clindamycin (Cleocin), fluconazole (Diflucan), hydrocortisone sodium succinate (Solu-Cortef), linezolid (Zyvox), ofloxacin (Floxin IV), potassium chloride (KCl), verapamil (Isoptin).

Syringe: Heparin.

Y-site: Acyclovir (Zovirax), aldesleukin (Proleukin, IL-2), allopurinol (Aloprim, Zyloprim), amifostine (Ethyol), aztreonam (Azactam), ciprofloxacin (Cipro IV), <u>cisatracurium (Nimbex)</u>, cyclophosphamide (Cytoxan), diltiazem (Cardizem), docetaxel (Taxotere), doxorubicin liposome (Doxil), enalaprilat (Vasotec IV), esmolol (Brevibloc), etoposide phosphate (Etopophos), famotidine (Pepcid IV), fludarabine (Fludara), foscarnet (Foscavir), granisetron (Kytril), heparin, hetastarch in electrolytes (Hextend), hydromorphone (Dilaudid), labetalol Normodyne), linezolid (Zyvox), lorazepam (Ativan), magnesium sulfate, melphalan (Alkeran), meperidine (Demerol), midazolam (Versed), morphine, perphenazine (Trilafon), propofol (Diprivan), ranitidine (Zantac), remifentanil (Ultiva), tacrolimus (Prograf), teniposide (Vumon), theophylline, thiotepa (Thioplex), <u>vancomycin (Vancocin)</u>, verapamil (Isoptin), zidovudine (AZT, Retrovir).

RATE OF ADMINISTRATION

Too-rapid injection may cause seizures.

IV injection: A single dose over 3 to 5 minutes.

Intermittent infusion: A single dose properly diluted over 30 minutes. Discontinue primary IV infusion during administration. Slow infusion rate for pain along venipuncture site.

ACTIONS

An extended-spectrum penicillin. Bactericidal against a variety of gram-negative and gram-positive bacteria, including aerobic and anaerobic strains. Especially effective against *Klebsiella* and *Pseudomonas*. Well distributed in all body fluids, tissue, and bone and through inflamed meninges. Onset of action is prompt. Excreted in bile and urine. Crosses the placental barrier. Secreted in breast milk.

INDICATIONS AND USES

Treatment of serious lower respiratory tract, intraabdominal, urinary tract, gynecologic, hepatobiliary, skin and skin structure, bone and joint, and gonococcal infections and septicemia caused by susceptible organisms. May be used in either liver or renal impairment since excretion occurs in bile and urine. Frequently used to initiate therapy in serious infections because of broad spectrum. ■ Perioperative prophylaxis.

CONTRAINDICATIONS

History of allergic reaction to any penicillin or cephalosporin (not absolute).

PRECAUTIONS

Sensitivity studies indicated to determine susceptibility of the causative organism to piperacillin. ■ Avoid prolonged use of drug; superinfection caused by overgrowth of nonsusceptible organisms may result. ■ Incidence of side effects increased in patients with cystic fibrosis. ■ Pseudomembranous colitis has been reported. May range from mild to life-threatening. Consider in patients that present with diarrhea during or after treatment with piperacillin.

Monitor: Watch for early symptoms of allergic reaction. ■ Periodic evaluation of renal, hepatic, and hematopoietic systems and serum potassium is recommended in prolonged therapy. Observe for hypokalemia and increased bleeding tendencies. Test patients with syphilis for HIV. ■ Observe for electrolyte imbalance and cardiac irregularities. Contains 1.85 mEq sodium/Gm. May aggravate CHF. ■ May cause thrombophlebitis; observe carefully and rotate infusion sites. ■ See Drug/Lab Interactions.

Patient Education: May require alternate birth control.

Maternal/Child: Category B: use only if absolutely necessary in pregnancy and breast-feeding. ■ May cause diarrhea, candidiasis, or allergic response in nursing infants. ■ Safety for use in children under 12 years not established but is used.

Elderly: No problems documented. Age-related decrease in renal function may require decreased dose.

DRUG/LAB INTERACTIONS

Synergistic when used in combination with aminoglycosides (e.g., amikacin [Amikin], gentamicin [Garamycin]). Synergism may be inconsistent; see Incompatible With. ■ Concomitant use with beta-adrenergic blockers (e.g., propranolol [Inderal]) may increase risk of anaphylaxis and inhibit treatment. ■ Risk of bleeding may be increased with anticoagulants (e.g., heparin); monitoring of coagulation tests may be indicated. Use caution. ■ May be antagonized by bacteriostatic antibiotics (e.g., chloramphenicol, erythromycin, tetracyclines); may interfere with bactericidal action. ■ May inhibit effectiveness of oral contraceptives; could result in breakthrough bleeding or pregnancy. ■ Probenecid decreases rate of piperacillin elimination resulting in higher and more prolonged blood levels. May be desirable or may cause toxicity. ■ May prolong neuromuscular blockade with vecuronium (Norcuron). ■ May decrease clearance and increase toxicity of methotrexate. ■ May cause false urine protein reactions with various tests; see Side Effects and/or literature.

SIDE EFFECTS

Anaphylaxis, convulsions, diarrhea, dizziness, elevated SrCr, BUN, alkaline phosphatase, LDH, serum bilirubin, AST (SGOT), and ALT (SGPT); fatigue, headache, hypokalemia, increased creatinine or BUN, leukopenia, muscle relaxation (prolonged), nausea, neutropenia, pruritus, pseudomembranous colitis, thrombocytopenia, thrombophlebitis, skin rash, vomiting. Hypersensitivity myocarditis can occur (fever, eosinophilia, rash, sinus tachycardia, ST-T changes and cardiomegaly). Higher than normal doses may cause neurologic adverse reactions, including convulsions, especially with impaired renal function.

ANTIDOTE

Notify the physician immediately of any adverse symptoms. For severe symptoms, discontinue the drug, treat allergic reaction (antihistamines, epinephrine, corticosteroids), and resuscitate as necessary. Hemodialysis is effective in overdose.

PIPERACILLIN SODIUM AND TAZOBACTAM SODIUM

(pi-per′a-sill-in so′de-um, taz′o-bac-tam so′de-um)

Antibacterial (extended-spectrum penicillin and beta-lactamase inhibitor)

Zosyn

USUAL DOSE

Measurement of both drugs is included in the total dose; for every 1 Gm of piperacillin there is 0.125 Gm of tazobactam (8:1 ratio). 12 Gm piperacillin/1.5 Gm tazobactam/24 hours given as 3.375 (3 Gm piperacillin/0.375 Gm tazobactam) every 6 hours. Doses up to 4.5 Gm every 4 to 8 hours have been used. Usual duration of therapy is 7 to 10 days, based on severity of infection and patient progress.

Nosocomial pneumonia: 3.375 Gm every 4 hours. Use an aminoglycoside also. Continue aminoglycoside if *P. aeruginosa* is isolated; discontinue if it is not isolated. Usual duration of therapy is 7 to 14 days.

PEDIATRIC DOSE

Safety for use in pediatric patients under 12 years of age not established.

DOSE ADJUSTMENTS

Reduce dose in renal impairment with a CrCl between 20 and 40 ml/min to 2.25 Gm every 6 hours; below 20 ml/min to 2.25 Gm every 8 hours. May be given to patients undergoing hemodialysis and peritoneal dialysis. Dose in hemodialysis is 2.25 Gm every 8 hours, with a single dose of 0.75 Gm following each dialysis period. Supplemental doses not required in peritoneal dialysis. Measure serum levels further to adjust dose as needed. ■ No dose adjustment needed in impaired liver function. ■ Dose reduction may be required in the elderly.

DILUTION

Each 1 Gm of piperacillin content should be reconstituted with at least 5 ml of suitable diluent (e.g., SW or NS with or without preservatives, D5W). May be further diluted to desired volume (50 to 100 ml) with the compatible infusion solutions above or 6% dextran in saline and given as an intermittent infusion. Also available premixed and in ADD-Vantage vials for use with ADD-Vantage infusion containers.

Storage: Use single-dose vials immediately after reconstitution; discard any unused portion after 24 hours at room temperature or 48 hours if refrigerated. Stable for up to 7 days after dilution if refrigerated, 3 months if frozen. Do not refrigerate or freeze ADD-Vantage vials after reconstitution.

INCOMPATIBLE WITH

One source recommends temporarily discontinuing other solutions infusing at the same site to avoid compatibility problems. May be inactivated in solution with aminoglycosides (e.g., amikacin [Amikin], gentamicin [Garamycin]). Do not mix in the same solution. Appropriate spacing and/or separate sites required. See Drug/Lab Interactions.

COMPATIBLE WITH **(Underline Indicates Conflicting Compatibility Information)**

Consult pharmacist; specific conditions may apply; see Compatibilities, p. xvi.

Y-site: Aminophylline, aztreonam (Azactam), bleomycin (Blenoxane), bumetanide (Bumex), buprenorphine (Buprenex), butorphanol (Stadol), calcium gluconate, carboplatin (Paraplatin), carmustine (BiCNU), cefepime (Maxipime), cimetidine (Tagamet), <u>cisatracurium (Nimbex)</u>, clindamycin (Cleocin), cyclophosphamide (Cytoxan), cytarabine (ARA-C), dexamethasone (Decadron), diphenhydramine (Benadryl), docetaxel (Taxotere), dopamine (Intropin), enalaprilat (Vasotec IV), etoposide (Etopophos, VePesid), fluconazole (Diflucan), fludarabine (Fludara), fluorouracil (5-FU), furosemide (Lasix), granisetron (Kytril), heparin, hetastarch in electrolytes (Hextend), hydrocortisone (Hydrocortone, Solu-Cortef), hydromorphone (Dilaudid), ifosfamide (Ifex), leucovorin calcium, linezolid (Zyvox), lorazepam (Ativan), magnesium sulfate, mannitol, meperidine (Demerol), mesna (Mesnex), methotrexate (Folex), methylprednisolone (Solu-Medrol), metoclopramide (Reglan), metronidazole (Flagyl IV), morphine, ondansetron (Zofran), plicamycin (Mithracin), potassium chloride (KCl), ranitidine (Zantac), remifentanil (Ultiva), sargramostim (Leukine), sodium bicarbonate, sulfamethoxazole-trimethoprim (Bactrim), thiotepa (Thioplex), <u>vancomycin (Vancocin)</u>, vinblastine (Velban), vincristine (Oncovin), zidovudine (AZT, Retrovir).

RATE OF ADMINISTRATION

A single dose over 30 minutes as an intermittent infusion. Slow infusion rate for pain along venipuncture site. See Incompatible With.

ACTIONS

An antimicrobial agent that combines the extended-spectrum penicillin piperacillin with the potent beta-lactamase inhibitor tazobactam. May be used in suspected polymicrobial infections due to its broad spectrum of activity; spectrum is superior to many other agents. Bactericidal against all three classes of bacterial pathogens; gram-positive and gram-negative aerobes, anaerobes, and enterococci that may be resistant to other antibiotics. Well distributed in all body fluids and tissues. Mean tissue concentrations are 50% to 100% of plasma concentrations. Peak levels are achieved immediately at the completion of an infusion. Plasma half-life ranges from 0.7 to 1.2 hours. Extended two-fold (piperacillin) to four-fold (tazobactam) if CrCl less than 40 mcg/ml. Primarily excreted rapidly in urine. Crosses the placental barrier. Secreted in breast milk.

INDICATIONS AND USES

Treatment of infections caused by piperacillin-resistant beta-lactamase–producing strains of specific microorganisms in the following conditions: intraabdominal (e.g., appendicitis complicated by rupture or abscess and peritonitis), gynecologic (e.g., postpartum endometritis and pelvic inflammatory disease), skin and skin structure (complicated and uncomplicated, e.g., cellulitis, cutaneous abscesses, and ischemic/diabetic foot infection), and pneumonia. ■ Used in combination with aminoglycosides for infections in neutropenic patients or nosocomial pneumonia.

Unlabeled uses: Treatment of septicemia.

CONTRAINDICATIONS

History of allergic reaction to any penicillin, cephalosporin, or beta-lactamase inhibitors (not absolute).

PRECAUTIONS

Sensitivity studies indicated determine susceptibility of the causative organism to piperacillin. ■ Avoid prolonged use of drug; superinfection caused by overgrowth of nonsusceptible organisms may result. ■ Use caution in patients with CHF or those with a history of bleeding disorders or GI disease (e.g., colitis). ■ Pseudomembranous colitis has been reported. May range from mild to life threatening. Consider in patients who present with diarrhea during or after treatment with piperacillin/tazobactam. ■ Incidence of side effects may be increased in patients with cystic fibrosis. ■ Continue at least 2 days after symptoms of infection disappear.

Monitor: Watch for early symptoms of allergic reaction. ■ Periodic evaluation of renal, hepatic, and hematopoietic systems and serum potassium recommended in prolonged therapy. May cause hypokalemia; observe closely. ■ Test patients with syphilis for HIV. ■ Contains 2.35 mEq of sodium/Gm. Observe for electrolyte imbalance and cardiac irregularities. May aggravate CHF. ■ May cause thrombophlebitis; observe carefully, rotate infusion sites. ■ Observe for increased bleeding tendencies in all patients, especially those with impaired renal function. ■ See Drug/Lab Interactions.

Patient Education: Report promptly: fever, rash, sore throat, unusual bleeding or bruising, severe stomach cramps, and/or diarrhea, seizures. ■ May require alternate birth control.

Maternal/Child: Category B: use during pregnancy only if clearly needed. ■ May cause diarrhea, candidiasis, or allergic response in nursing infants.

Elderly: No problems documented. Consider age-related impaired renal function.

DRUG/LAB INTERACTIONS

Synergistic when used in combination with aminoglycosides (e.g., amikacin [Amikin], gentamicin [Garamycin]). Synergism may be inconsistent; see Incompatible With. ■ Does not affect pharmacokinetics of vancomycin; may be given without dose adjustment. ■ Concomitant administration with probenecid decreases rate of elimination resulting in higher and more prolonged blood levels. May be desirable or may cause toxicity. ■ Use caution with anticoagulants (e.g., heparin), thrombolytic agents (e.g., alteplase [tPA], anistreplase [Eminase]), platelet aggregation inhibitors (e.g., aspirin, NSAIDs [such as ibuprofen (Advil, Motrin), naproxen (Aleve, Naprosyn)], dextran, dipyridamole, plicamycin). Risk of bleeding is increased. Monitoring of coagulation tests may be indicated. Concurrent use with thrombolytic agents is not recommended; may increase risk of severe hemorrhage. ■ May be antagonized by bacteriostatic antibiotics (e.g., chloramphenicol, erythromycin, and tetracyclines); may interfere with bactericidal action. ■ May decrease clearance and increase toxicity of methotrexate. ■ May inhibit effectiveness of oral contraceptives; could result in breakthrough bleeding or pregnancy. ■ May prolong neuromuscular blockade with vecuronium (Norcuron). ■ May cause false urine protein reactions with various tests and false-positive glucose with Clinitest. ■ See Side Effects.

SIDE EFFECTS

Hypokalemia, increased PTT, and prolonged PT. Most other side effects are usually mild moderate and transient. Abdominal pain, agitation, anxiety, chest pain, cholestatic jaundice, constipation, diarrhea, dizziness, dyspnea, dyspepsia, edema, elevated liver function tests, fever, headache, hemolytic anemia, hepatitis, hypertension, insomnia, moniliasis, nausea, pain, positive Coombs' test, pruritus, pseudomembranous colitis, rash (e.g., bullous, eczematoid, erythema multiforme, maculopapular, Stevens-Johnson syndrome, urticarial), rhinitis, vomiting. Anaphylaxis can occur. Transient leukopenia and eosinophilia can occur with prolonged therapy. Higher-than-normal doses may cause neurologic adverse reactions, including convulsions.

ANTIDOTE

Notify the physician immediately of any adverse symptoms. For severe symptoms, discontinue the drug, treat allergic reaction (antihistamines, epinephrine, corticosteroids, airway management, oxygen), and resuscitate as necessary. Use anticonvulsants (e.g., diazepam [Valium]) or barbiturates (e.g., phenobarbital) for seizures. Hemodialysis is effective in overdose.

PLASMA PROTEIN FRACTION

Plasma volume expander

(plaz′ma pro′teen frak′shun)

Plasmanate, Plasmatein, Protenate

pH 6.7 to 7.3

USUAL DOSE

Variable, depending on indication for use, condition of patient, and response to therapy. Range is from 250 to 1,500 ml/24 hr. Each 500-ml bottle yields 25 Gm of plasma protein. Suggested initial doses are as follows:

Shock: 250 to 500 ml.

Burns: 500 to 1,000 ml.

Hypoproteinemia: 1,000 to 1,500 ml/24 hr.

PEDIATRIC DOSE

Treatment of acute shock: 6.6 to 30 ml/kg of body weight.

DILUTION

Available as a 5% solution buffered with saline in 250- and 500-ml bottles with injection sets. Plasmanate also available in a 50-ml size. No further dilution is required. Do not use if solution is turbid or a sediment is visible. Use immediately after opening and discard any unused portion. Contains no preservatives.

Storage: Store at CRT.

INCOMPATIBLE WITH

Solutions containing alcohol, protein hydrolysates, or amino acid products.

COMPATIBLE WITH

Solution: Manufacturer states, "Compatible with the usual carbohydrate and electrolyte solutions."

RATE OF ADMINISTRATION

Variable, depending on indication, present blood volume, and patient response. Adjust or slow rate according to clinical response and rising BP. Averages are:

Normal blood volume: 1 ml/min.

Treatment of shock and burns in adult: 5 to 8 ml/min. Higher rates may be tolerated if necessary. Rapid infusion (over 10 ml/min) may cause hypotension. Decrease flow rate as patient improves.

Treatment of shock in infants and children: 5 to 10 ml/min. Do not exceed 10 ml/min in children.

Treatment of hypoproteinemia: Single 500-ml dose over 1 hour. For larger amounts the maximum rate is 100 ml/hr.

ACTIONS

A sterile, natural, plasma protein substance containing at least 83% albumin, no more than 17% alpha and beta globulins, and no more than 1% gamma globulin. Contains 130 to 160 mEq sodium/liter. It expands intravascular volume, prevents marked hemoconcentration, and maintains appropriate electrolyte balance in burns.

INDICATIONS AND USES

Emergency treatment of hypovolemic shock caused by burns, infections, surgery, or trauma (may also be due to dehydration in infants and children). ■ Temporary treatment of hemorrhage when whole blood unavailable. ■ Hypoproteinemia until cause determined and corrected. ■ Prevention of hemoconcentration and maintenance of electrolyte balance in burn patients.

CONTRAINDICATIONS

Cardiac failure, cardiopulmonary bypass, history of allergic reactions to albumin, normal or increased intravascular volume, severe anemia.

PRECAUTIONS

May be given without regard to blood group or type. ■ Not effective for coagulation mechanism defects. ■ Added protein, fluid, and sodium load requires caution in hepatic or renal impairment. ■ If continuous protein loss occurs or edema is present, normal serum albumin (25%) may be the preferred product.

Monitor: Monitor vital signs (including central venous pressure if possible) and urine output every 5 to 15 minutes for 1 hour and hourly thereafter depending on condition. ■ For treatment of shock, observe carefully for bleeding points that may not have been evident at lower pressures. ■ Whole blood may be indicated for considerable RBC loss or anemia caused by administration of large amounts of plasma protein fraction. ■ Additional fluids are required for dehydrated patients. Tissue dehydration caused by osmotic action of plasma proteins can be acute. ■ May cause vascular overload; monitor for signs of pulmonary edema or heart failure (e.g., dyspnea, fluid in the lungs, abnormal increases in BP or CVP). ■ Hemoglobin, hematocrit, electrolyte, and serum protein evaluations are necessary during therapy.

Maternal/Child: Category C: safety for use in pregnancy not established.

DRUG/LAB INTERACTIONS

May cause an elevated alkaline phosphatase level.

SIDE EFFECTS

Allergic and/or pyrogenic reactions can occur. Incidence of toxicity is low when administered with appropriate caution. Slight nausea can occur. Hypotension can be sudden if administered too rapidly.

ANTIDOTE

Notify the physician of all symptoms and side effects. Discontinue infusion for sudden hypotension. Decrease flow rate if indicated and treat symptomatically. Resuscitate as necessary.

PLICAMYCIN

(ply-ka-my′sin)

Antineoplastic (antibiotic)
Antihypercalcemic

Mithracin

pH 7

USUAL DOSE

Testicular tumors: 25 to 30 mcg/kg of body weight/24 hr. Repeat daily for 8 to 10 days unless significant side effects or toxicity occur. Repeat at monthly intervals if indicated.

Hypercalcemia and hypercalciuria: 25 mcg/kg of body weight/24 hr for 3 or 4 days. Repeat weekly as required to maintain normal calcium levels.

PEDIATRIC DOSE

Hypercalcemia with malignancies: 25 mcg/kg/dose as an infusion daily for 1 to 4 days. Repeat at weekly intervals as needed or maintain with 1 to 3 doses weekly.

DOSE ADJUSTMENTS

Dose based on average weight in presence of edema or ascites.

DILUTION

Specific techniques required; see Precautions. Each 2.5-mg vial must be initially diluted with 4.9 ml of SW for injection (1 ml equals 500 mcg). A single daily dose must be further diluted in 1,000 ml of D5W or NS and given as an infusion. Do not use a filter smaller than 5 microns. Loss of potency will occur. Prepare fresh daily and discard any unused portion.

Pediatric dilution: Same as for adults.

Storage: Store in refrigerator before dilution.

COMPATIBLE WITH

Consult pharmacist; specific conditions may apply; see Compatibilities, p. xvi.

Y-site: Allopurinol (Aloprim, Zyloprim), amifostine (Ethyol), aztreonam (Azactam), etoposide phosphate (Etopophos), filgrastim (Neupogen), gemcitabine (Gemzar), granisetron (Kytril), melphalan (Alkeran), piperacillin/tazobactam (Zosyn), teniposide (Vumon), thiotepa (Thioplex), vinorelbine (Navelbine).

RATE OF ADMINISTRATION

A single dose every 24 hours over 4 to 6 hours. Extend to 4 to 8 hours in children.

ACTIONS

A potent antibiotic, antineoplastic agent. Interferes with cell division by binding with DNA to inhibit and slow production of RNA. Exact mechanism unknown. Well distributed to kidney, liver, bone, and cerebrospinal fluid. Cytotoxic to HeLa cell tissue culture and some animal tumors. Also acts to lower serum calcium in patients with cancer. Metabolized in the liver. Some excretion in urine.

INDICATIONS AND USES

Testicular tumors not treatable with surgery and/or radiation. ■ Hypercalcemia and hypercalciuria associated with many advanced neoplasms.

CONTRAINDICATIONS

Thrombocytopenia, thrombocytopathy, coagulation disorders or any susceptibility to bleeding, impairment of bone marrow function, lack of hospital and laboratory facilities.

PRECAUTIONS

Follow guidelines for handling cytotoxic agents. See Appendix A, p. 1142. ■ Administered by or under the direction of the physician specialist. ■ Use extreme caution in impaired renal or hepatic function.

Monitor: Determine absolute patency of vein; cellulitis and tissue necrosis may result from extravasation. Discontinue injection; use another vein. Elevate extremity and apply warm, moist heat to the extravasated area. ■ Severe sudden onset of hemorrhage and even death can result from use. ■ Maintain hydration and correct any electrolyte imbalance before treatment. ■ Monitor renal and hepatic function and electrolytes (especially calcium, potassium, and phosphorus). ■ Monitor platelet count, PT, and bleeding time during and after therapy. ■ Monitor for thrombocytopenia (platelet count less than $50,000/mm^3$). Initiate precautions to prevent excessive bleeding (e.g., inspect IV sites, skin, and mucous membranes; use extreme care during invasive procedures; test urine, emesis, stool, and secretions for occult blood). ■ Observe closely for all signs of infection. ■ Prophylactic antibiotics may be indicated pending results of C/S in a febrile neutropenic patient. ■ Prophylactic antiemetics may reduce nausea and vomiting and increase patient comfort.

Patient Education: Consider birth control options; nonhormonal birth control recommended. ■ Report IV site burning or stinging promptly. ■ Calcium and vitamin D supplementation or restriction may be necessary depending on indication. ■ Report unusual bleeding or bruising, bloody nose, chills, dark urine, fever, rashes, sore throat, tarry stools, or yellowing of eyes or skin. ■ Do not lie down after eating. ■ See Appendix D, p. 1148.

Maternal/Child: Category X: avoid pregnancy. ■ Discontinue breastfeeding.

Elderly: Monitor fluid and electrolyte status carefully to avoid overhydration. ■ Monitor for early signs of toxicity. ■ Consider age-related organ impairment.

DRUG/LAB INTERACTIONS

Risk of bleeding increased with anticoagulants (e.g., heparin, warfarin [Coumadin]), thrombolytic agents (e.g., alteplase [tPA]), NSAIDs (e.g., indomethacin [Indocin], ibuprofen [Advil, Motrin], naproxen [Aleve, Naproxyn]), aspirin, dextran, dipyridamole (Persantine), sulfinpyrazone (Anturane), or valproic acid. Concurrent use not recommended. ■ Potential for toxicity increased with bone marrow depressants (e.g., antineoplastics [e.g., cisplatin], colchicine, eflornithine [Orindyl]), hepatotoxic agents (e.g., alcohol, estrogens), or nephrotoxic agents (e.g., acyclovir, aminoglycosides [e.g., tobramycin], amphotericin B). May be antagonized by calcium or vitamin D preparations. ■ Do not administer live-virus vaccines to patients receiving antineoplastic drugs.

SIDE EFFECTS

Anorexia, depression, diarrhea, drowsiness, fever, flushing, headache, nausea, skin rash, stomatitis, vomiting.

Major: Abnormal clot retraction, abnormal liver function tests, abnormal renal function tests, bone marrow depression (e.g., anemia, neutropenia, thrombocytopenia), elevation of bleeding and clotting time, epistaxis (severe), hematemesis, hemoglobin depression, leukopenia (unusual), platelet count depression, prothrombin content depression, serum calcium, phosphorus, and potassium depression.

ANTIDOTE

Minor side effects will be treated symptomatically. Discontinue the drug and notify the physician immediately of any major side effects. Administration of whole blood products (e.g., packed RBCs, platelets, leukocytes) and/or blood modifiers (e.g., darbepoetin alfa [Aranesp], epoetin alfa [Epogen, Procrit], filgrastim [Neupogen], pegfilgrastim [Neulasta], sargramostim [Leukine], oprelvekin [Neumega]) may be indicated to treat bone marrow toxicity. Provide immediate treatment or supportive therapy as indicated; bleeding episodes can be fatal. If extravasation has occurred, long-acting dexamethasone injected into the indurated area with a fine hypodermic needle may be helpful. Apply moderate heat.

PORFIMER SODIUM

(pour′fi-mur so′de-um)

Photofrin

Photosensitizing agent
Antineoplastic

pH 7 to 8

USUAL DOSE

A course is a two-stage process requiring administration of both drug and light.

A single IV injection of 2 mg/kg of porfimer sodium is the ***first stage.*** No further injection of porfimer sodium should be given in any one course of therapy.

Illumination with nonthermal laser light at 40 to 50 hours postinjection is the ***second stage.*** Standard endoscopic techniques are used for light administration and débridement. The laser system must be approved for delivery of a stable power output at a wavelength of 630± nm. Light is delivered to the tumor by cylindrical Optiguide fiber-optic diffusers passed through the operating channel of an endoscope/bronchoscope. The choice of diffuser tip length depends on the length of the tumor. Diffuser length should be sized to avoid exposure of nonmalignant tissue to light and to prevent overlapping of previously treated malignant tissue. A second laser light application may be given 96 to 120 hours after injection. Before providing a second laser light treatment, the residual tumor should be gently débrided. Vigorous débridement may cause esophageal tumor bleeding.

Up to three courses may be given, but each must be separated by at least 30 days. Evaluate patients with esophageal cancer for the presence of a tracheoesophageal or bronchoesophageal fistula before each course. Evaluate all patients for possible erosion of the tumor into a major blood vessel.

Esophageal cancer: 2 mg/kg of porfimer sodium as an IV injection. A light dose of 300 joules/cm of tumor length should be delivered by the specific process outlined above. Light exposure time is set to 12 minutes and 30 seconds. Débridement of tumor should be performed 2 days later; see Precautions.

Endobronchial non–small-cell lung cancer: 2 mg/kg of porfimer sodium as an IV injection. A light dose of 200 joules/cm of tumor length should be delivered by the specific process outlined above. Light exposure time is set to 8 minutes and 20 seconds. Débridement of tumor should be performed 2 to 3 days later; see Precautions.

PEDIATRIC DOSE

Safety and effectiveness for use in children not established.

DOSE ADJUSTMENTS

No adjustments required.

DILUTION

Specific techniques required; see Precautions. Prepare immediately before use. Each vial of porfimer sodium must be reconstituted with 31.8 ml of D5W or NS. Concentration will be 2.5 mg/ml. Shake well until dissolved. An opaque solution; detection of particulate matter by visual inspection is difficult. Withdraw desired dose. Must be protected from bright light and used immediately.

Storage: Store unopened vials at CRT in carton to protect from light.

COMPATIBILITY

Manufacturer states, "Do not mix porfimer sodium with other drugs in the same solution."

RATE OF ADMINISTRATION

A single dose equally distributed over 3 to 5 minutes.

ACTIONS

The first light-activated drug (photosensitizing agent) for use in photodynamic therapy (PDT) to be approved in the United States. After IV infusion it is allowed to circulate. It accumulates and is retained in tumors, skin, and organs of the reticuloendothelial system (e.g., liver, spleen) while largely clearing from other tissues. Has no apparent effect on tumors until it is activated by selective delivery of light (usually 40 to 50 hours postinfusion). Light activation induces a photochemical, not a thermal, effect that produces an active form of oxygen and releases thromboxane A_2. This process causes vasoconstriction, activation and aggregation of platelets, and increased clotting that contribute to ischemic necrosis leading to tissue and tumor death. In patients with esophageal cancer, ability to swallow is improved, as is quality of life. Elimination half-life is very prolonged, up to several weeks. Highly protein bound.

INDICATIONS AND USES

Palliative treatment of patients with completely obstructing esophageal cancer or partially obstructing esophageal cancers that are unsuitable for treatment with thermal laser therapy. ■ Treatment of microinvasive endobronchial non–small-cell lung cancer (NSCLC) in patients for whom surgery and radiotherapy are not indicated. ■ Reduction of obstruction and palliation of symptoms in patients with completely or partially obstructing non–small-cell lung cancer.

Unlabeled uses: Treatment of bladder cancer (approved for use in Canada). Studies are in progress on other tumors accessible by scope and fiberoptics to deliver light (e.g., Barrett's esophagus, various cutaneous carcinomas, head and neck carcinomas).

CONTRAINDICATIONS

Known allergies to porphyrins, an existing tracheoesophageal or bronchoesophageal fistula, porphyria, or tumors eroding into a major blood vessel.

PRECAUTIONS

Use rubber gloves and eye protection during preparation and administration. Avoid any skin or eye contact since that area will become photosensitive. Wipe up spills with a damp cloth. Dispose of all contaminated materials in a polyethylene bag to avoid accidental contact by others. Protection from light will be necessary if accidental exposure or overexposure occurs. See process in Patient Education. ■ Administered by or under the direction of the physician specialist with appropriate knowledge of the selected laser system. Facilities for monitoring the patient and responding to any medical emergency must be available. ■ Requires laser systems and a fiber-optic diffuser to activate. The FDA has approved several photodynamic lasers and the Optiguide fiber-optic diffuser for use with porfimer sodium. ■ Avoid exposure of skin and eyes to direct sunlight or bright indoor light; see Patient Education. ■ In the original studies for esophageal tumors, some experienced investigators indicated that natural sloughing action in the esophagus might be sufficient and débridement could needlessly traumatize the area. However, débridement is now recommended after each light activation to minimize the potential for obstruction caused by necrotic debris. ■ A minimum of 4 weeks after radiation therapy is complete is recommended before treatment with PDT (photodynamic therapy). This allows the acute inflammation produced by radiotherapy to subside. ■ 2 to 4 weeks should be allowed after PDT is complete before beginning any radiotherapy.

Esophageal tumors: Not recommended if the esophageal tumor is eroding into the trachea or bronchial tree; tracheoesophageal or bronchoesophageal fistula may result from treatment. ■ Use extreme caution in patients with esophageal varices. Light should not be given directly to the variceal area because of the high risk of bleeding.

Endobronchial cancer: Interstitial fiber placement is preferred to intraluminal activation in noncircumferential endobronchial tumors that are soft enough to penetrate. Results in less exposure of the normal bronchial mucosa to light. ■ Patients with obstructing lung cancer who have received prior radiation therapy have a higher incidence of fatal hemoptysis. ■ An endobronchial tumor that invades deeply into the bronchial wall may create a fistula as the tumor resolves. ■ Use with extreme caution in endobronchial tumors located where treatment-induced inflammation could obstruct the airway (e.g., long or circumferential tumors of the trachea, tumors of the carina that involve both mainstem bronchi circumferentially, or circumferential tumors in the mainstem bronchus in patients with prior pneumonectomy).

Monitor: Obtain baseline CBC and monitor for anemia due to tumor bleeding. ■ Prevent extravasation at the injection site. Should extravasation occur, area must be protected from light. ■ Opiates may be required to control pain. ■ Observe patients carefully; most are critically ill, and many complications could occur. Monitor patients with ***endobronchial tumors*** closely between the laser light therapy and the mandatory débridement bronchoscopy for any evidence of respiratory distress, inflammation, mucositis, or necrotic debris that may cause obstruction of the airway. Immediate bronchoscopy may be required to remove secretions and debris to open the airway. ■ Monitor for hemoptysis; may be a sign of progressive disease, or may result from resolution of a tumor that has eroded into a pulmonary artery. ▪ Photosensitivity not transferable through skin to caregivers. ▪ See Precautions, Patient Education, and Drug/Lab Interactions.

Patient Education: Must observe precautions to avoid exposure of skin and eyes to direct sunlight or bright indoor light for at least 30 days. Some patients may remain photosensitive for up to 90 or more days. Photosensitivity is due to residual drug, which is present in all parts of the skin. Ambient indoor light is beneficial as it gradually inactivates the remaining drug through a photobleaching reaction. Do not remain in a darkened room. Do expose skin to ambient indoor light. Avoid bright indoor light from examination lamps, dental lamps, operating room lamps, and unshaded light bulbs. Limit time outdoors to necessary excursions and completely cover body with clothing and shade face before going out. Conventional ultraviolet sunscreens are of no value because photoactivation is caused by visible light, not UV rays. Eyes will be sensitive to sun, bright lights, and car headlights; wear dark sunglasses with an average white light transmittance of less than 4%. After several weeks and before exposing any area of skin to direct sunlight or bright indoor light, test a small area of skin (not the face) for residual photosensitivity. Expose the small area of skin for 10 minutes. If no photosensitivity reaction (redness, swelling, or blistering) occurs within 24 hours, gradually resume normal outdoor activities. Exercise caution and increase skin exposure gradually. If some photosensitivity reaction occurs, continue precautions for 2 more weeks and then retest. Retest level of photosensitivity if traveling to a different geographic area with greater sunshine. ▪ Report chest pain (caused by inflammatory response within the area of treatment); may require prescription pain medication. ▪ Effective contraception necessary for women of childbearing age.

Maternal/Child: Category C: use during pregnancy only if benefits justify potential risk to fetus. Effective contraception necessary for women of childbearing age. Has caused maternal and fetal toxicity in rats and rabbits (increased resorptions, decreased litter size, and reduced fetal body weight). ▪ Discontinue breast-feeding; not known if it is secreted in breast milk, but serious reactions could occur in the infant. ▪ Safety and effectiveness in children not established.

Elderly: Dose modification based on age is not required.

DRUG/LAB INTERACTIONS

No specific studies have been completed, but the following interactions are likely to occur. ▪ Use with other photosensitizing agents (e.g., griseofulvin, phenothiazines [e.g., prochlorperazine (Compazine)], sulfonamides [sulfisoxazole (Gantrisin), ophthalmic solutions (AK-Sulf)], sulfonylurea hypoglycemic agents [tolbutamide (Orinase)], tetracyclines [doxycycline (Vibramycin)], thiazide diuretics [chlorothiazide (Diuril)]) could increase the photosensitivity reaction. ▪ Antitumor activity may be decreased by dimethyl sulfoxide, beta-carotene, ethanol, formate, mannitol. ▪ Antitumor activity may also be decreased by allopurinol (Zyloprim), calcium channel blockers (e.g., diltiazem [Cardizem]), prostaglandin synthesis inhibitors (NSAIDs [e.g., ibuprofen (Advil, Motrin), naproxen (Aleve, Naprosyn)]), and tissue ischemia. ▪ Effectiveness may be reduced by drugs that decrease clotting (e.g., heparin, alteplase [tPA]), vasoconstriction (e.g., nicardipine [Cardene]), or platelet aggregation (e.g., dipyridamole [Persantine], ticlopidine [Ticlid]). ■ Glucocorticoid hormones (e.g., dexamethasone [Decadron]) given before or with PDT may reduce the effectiveness of porfimer by inhibiting the production of thromboxane A_2.

SIDE EFFECTS

May cause constipation. Most toxicities are local effects in the region of illumination and occasionally in surrounding tissues. Usually an inflammatory response induced by the photodynamic effects. Photosensitivity reactions occurred in 20% of patients in clinical studies. Reactions were usually mild to moderate erythema, but also included blisters, burning sensation, itching, and swelling. Less common skin manifestations included increased hair growth, skin discoloration, skin nodules, increased wrinkles, and skin fragility.

Esophageal tumors: Bronchoesophageal or tracheoesophageal fistula can occur as a result of the disease or treatment, including débridement. Abdominal pain, anemia (more prevalent if tumor is located in the lower third of the esophagus), anorexia, arrhythmias (atrial fibrillation [more prevalent if tumor is located in the middle third of the esophagus], tachycardia), candidiasis, chest pain, coughing, dyspepsia, dysphagia, dyspnea, edema, eructation, esophageal edema (more prevalent if tumor is located in the upper third of the esophagus), esophageal tumor bleeding, esophageal stricture, esophagitis, fever, hematemesis, hypertension, hypotension, insomnia, nausea, pleural effusion, and vomiting may occur, as well as numerous others.

Endobronchial tumors: Coughing, dysphagia, dyspnea (may be life threatening), mucositis reaction (e.g., edema, exudate, and mucous plug obstruction), stricture, ulceration. Fatal hemoptysis has occurred (higher incidence in patients who have received radiation therapy).

ANTIDOTE

If an overdose of porfimer sodium is given, do not give the laser light treatment. Porfimer sodium is not dialyzable. Increased side effects and damage to normal tissue can be expected if an overdose of light is given. Keep physician informed of all side effects; most will be treated symptomatically. Some may be life threatening. Respiratory obstruction may require immediate bronchoscopy and removal of the obstruction with suction or forceps. Stent placement may be required in endobronchial stricture. Chest pain may require the use of opiates.

POTASSIUM ACETATE AND POTASSIUM CHLORIDE

(po-taah'see-um as'ah-tat, po-taah'see-um klor'id)

Electrolyte replenisher
Antihypokalemic

pH 4 to 8

USUAL DOSE

Starting dose based on losses, desired replacement, or maintenance. 20 to 60 mEq/24 hr. 200 mEq/24 hr is usually not exceeded. Up to 400 mEq/24 hr has been given in selected situations (e.g., serum potassium less that 2 mEq/L) with extreme caution. Potassium acetate may contain up to 200 mcg/L of aluminum; see Precautions.

PEDIATRIC DOSE

1 to 4 mEq/kg of body weight/24 hr. Do not exceed 40 mEq/day. Potassium acetate may contain up to 200 mcg/L of aluminum; see Precautions.

DOSE ADJUSTMENTS

Reduce dose in impaired renal function. ■ Lower-end initial doses may be appropriate in the elderly based on potential for decreased organ function and concomitant disease or drug therapy.

DILUTION

Each individual dose must be diluted in a larger volume of suitable IV solution and given as an infusion. Check labels for aluminum content; see Precautions. Soluble in commonly used IV solutions; see chart on inside back cover. 40 mEq/L is the preferred dilution. 80 mEq/L is the usual maximum concentration and must be administered with caution. In replacement therapy more concentrated doses may be used and must be administered with extreme caution. 40 mEq/100 ml is commonly used and must be controlled by an infusion pump. *Up to 100 mEq/100 ml has been administered through a central line (to avoid phlebitis); must be controlled by an infusion pump.* ***Direct injection of any concentrated solution can be instantly fatal.*** Avoid layering of potassium by thoroughly agitating the prepared IV solution. Do not add potassium to an IV bottle in the hanging position; remove from hanger to guarantee dispersion throughout solution. In severe hypokalemia, solutions without dextrose are preferred (dextrose might decrease serum potassium level). Use only clear solutions.

COMPATIBLE WITH

(Underline Indicates Conflicting Compatibility Information)

Consult pharmacist; specific conditions may apply; see Compatibilities, p. xvi.

POTASSIUM ACETATE

Additive: Metoclopramide (Reglan).

Y-site: Ciprofloxacin (Cipro IV).

POTASSIUM CHLORIDE

Additive: <u>Amikacin (Amikin)</u>, aminophylline, amiodarone (Cordarone), atracurium (Tracrium), bretylium (Bretylate), calcium gluconate, cefepime (Maxipime), chloramphenicol (Chloromycetin), cimetidine (Tagamet), ciprofloxacin (Cipro IV), clindamycin (Cleocin), cytarabine (ARA-C), dimenhydrinate (Dinate), <u>dobutamine (Dobutrex)</u>, dopamine (Intropin), enalaprilat (Vasotec IV), erythromycin lactobionate (Erythrocin), fluconazole (Diflucan), foscarnet (Foscavir), fosphenytoin (Cerebyx), furosemide (Lasix), heparin, hydrocortisone sodium succinate (Solu-Cortef), isoproterenol (Isuprel), lidocaine, methyldopate (Aldomet), metoclopramide (Reglan), mitoxantrone (Novantrone), nafcillin (Nafcil), norepinephrine (Levophed), oxacillin (Bactocill), penicillin G potassium, penicillin G sodium, phenylephrine (Neo-Synephrine), piperacillin (Pipracil), ranitidine (Zantac), sodium bicarbonate, thiopental (Pentothal), vancomycin (Vancocin), verapamil (Isoptin).

Y-site: Acyclovir (Zovirax), alatrofloxacin (Trovan IV), aldesleukin (Proleukin, IL-2), allopurinol (Aloprim, Zyloprim), amifostine (Ethyol), aminophylline, amiodarone (Cordarone), ampicillin, atropine, aztreonam (Azactam), calcium gluconate, chlordiazepoxide (Librium), chlorpromazine (Thorazine), ciprofloxacin (Cipro IV), cisatracurium (Nimbex), cladribine (Leustatin), dexamethasone (Decadron), digoxin (Lanoxin), diltiazem (Cardizem), diphenhydramine (Benadryl), dobutamine (Dobutrex), docetaxel (Taxotere), dopamine (Intropin), doxorubicin liposome (Doxil), droperidol (Inapsine), edrophonium (Enlon), enalaprilat (Vasotec IV), epinephrine (Adrenalin), esmolol (Brevibloc), estrogens, conjugated (Premarin), ethacrynate sodium (Edecrin), etoposide phosphate (Etopophos), famotidine (Pepcid IV), fentanyl (Sublimaze), filgrastim (Neupogen), fludarabine (Fludara), fluorouracil (5-FU), furosemide (Lasix), gatifloxacin (Tequin), gemcitabine (Gemzar), granisetron (Kytril), heparin, hetastarch in electrolytes (Hextend), hydralazine, idarubicin (Idamycin), inamrinone (Inocor), indomethacin (Indocin), insulin (regular), isoproterenol (Isuprel), kanamycin (Kantrex), labetalol (Normodyne), lidocaine, linezolid (Zyvox), lorazepam (Ativan), magnesium sulfate, melphalan (Alkeran), meperidine (Demerol), methylergonovine (Methergine), methylprednisolone (Solu-Medrol), midazolam (Versed), milrinone (Primacor), minocycline (Minocin), morphine, neostigmine (Prostigmin), norepinephrine (Levophed), ondansetron (Zofran), oxacillin (Bactocill), oxytocin (Pitocin), paclitaxel (Taxol), penicillin G potassium, pentazocine (Talwin), phytonadione (Aquamephyton), piperacillin/tazobactam (Zosyn), procainamide (Pronestyl), prochlorperazine (Compazine), promethazine (Phenergan), propofol (Diprivan), propranolol (Inderal), pyridostigmine (Mestinon), remifentanil (Ultiva), sargramostim (Leukine), scopolamine, sodium bicarbonate, succinylcholine, tacrolimus (Prograf), teniposide (Vumon), theophylline, thiotepa (Thioplex), tirofiban (Aggrastat), vinorelbine (Navelbine), warfarin (Coumadin), zidovudine (AZT, Retrovir).

RATE OF ADMINISTRATION

A maximum of 10 mEq/hr of potassium chloride in any given amount of infusion fluid should not be exceeded. With serious potassium depletion (under 2 mEq/L serum), 20 to 40 mEq/hr has been given with extreme caution. Use of an infusion pump is recommended in all situations and required with any dose exceeding 60 mEq/24 hr.

Pediatric rate: 0.5 to 1 mEq/kg/hr. Do not exceed 10 mEq/hr.

ACTIONS

Helps to maintain osmotic pressure and ion balance. Flow of potassium into the cell (serum deficiency) increases membrane resting potential and decreases membrane permeability. Flow of potassium out of the cell (serum excess) decreases resting membrane potential and increases membrane permeability. Essential for intracellular tonicity; nerve impulse transmission; cardiac, skeletal, and smooth muscle contraction; normal renal function; metabolism of carbohydrates and proteins; and enzyme reactions. Excreted in urine.

INDICATIONS AND USES

Prophylaxis or treatment of potassium deficiency (e.g., hypokalemia due to diuretic therapy, digitalis intoxication, low dietary potassium intake, vomiting and diarrhea, diabetic acidosis, metabolic alkalosis, corticosteroid therapy, increased renal excretion resulting from acidosis, hemodialysis).

CONTRAINDICATIONS

Any disease or condition in which high potassium levels may occur through potassium retention or other processes (e.g., acute dehydration, adrenocortical insufficiency [untreated Addison's disease]), adynamica episodica hereditaria [periodic loss of strength or weakness], anuria, azotemia, crush syndrome, heat cramps, hyperkalemia from any cause, oliguria, patients on digitalis with severe or complete heart block, postoperative oliguria (early [except during GI drainage]), renal failure, severe hemolytic reactions.

PRECAUTIONS

Impaired renal function or adrenal insufficiency can cause potassium intoxication, which can develop rapidly and without symptoms. ■ Loss of chloride usually accompanies potassium depletion and may cause hypochloremic alkalosis. Treat cause of potassium depletion in addition to giving potassium. ■ Potassium phosphate is preferred for specific intracellular deficiency not caused by alkalosis, since phosphate is the usual ion attached to potassium in the body. Not used in the presence of kidney failure. ■ Alkalyzing potassiums (e.g., acetate, citrate) are preferred for potassium-deficient patients with renal tubular acidosis. Metabolic acidosis and hyperchloremia are most likely present. ■ Use potassium acetate with caution in patients with metabolic or respiratory alkalosis. ■ Some solutions of potassium acetate contain aluminum. In impaired kidney function, aluminum may reach toxic levels. Premature neonates are particularly at risk because of their immature kidneys and requirement for calcium and phosphate, which also contain aluminum. Research indicates that patients with impaired renal function who receive more than 4 to 5 mcg/kg/day of parenteral aluminum are at risk for developing CNS or bone toxicity associated with aluminum accumulation.

Monitor: Routine serum potassium, calcium, and sodium levels; pH; ECGs; adequate hydration; and evaluation of adequate urine output are mandatory. Only extracellular potassium can be measured; intracellular potassium equals 98% of total body potassium. Entire clinical picture must be considered. ■ Normal daily requirements; ***newborn,*** 2 to 6 mEq/kg/24 hr; ***children,*** 2 to 3 mEq/kg/24 hr; ***adults,*** 40 to 80 mEq/24 hr. ■ Continuous cardiac monitoring is preferable for infusion of over 10 mEq of potassium in 1 hour. ■ Confirm absolute patency of vein. Extravasation will cause necrosis. Local pain and phlebitis may occur with concentrations greater than 40 mEq/L. ■ See Drug/Lab Interactions.

Patient Education: Report burning or stinging at IV site promptly.

Maternal/Child: Category C: effect unknown; use caution and only if clearly needed in pregnancy and breast-feeding.

Elderly: See Dose Adjustments. Monitoring of renal function suggested. ■ Increased risk of hyperkalemia.

DRUG/LAB INTERACTIONS

Potentiated by angiotensin-converting enzyme inhibitors (e.g., captopril [Capoten], enalaprilat [Vasotec], lisinopril [Prinivil, Zestril]). ■ Digitalis intoxication may occur with hypokalemia. Use caution if discontinuing potassium after stabilization in patients taking digitalis. ▪ Potassium-sparing diuretics (e.g., spironolactone [Aldactone], triamterene [Dyrenium, and a component of Dyazide and Maxzide]) may cause hyperkalemia.

SIDE EFFECTS

Abdominal pain, bradycardia, cardiac arrest, confusion, diarrhea, dysphagia, ECG changes (including increased amplitude of T wave, decreased amplitude of R wave, below-baseline depression of S wave, disappearing P wave, PR prolongation), hyperkalemia, nausea, respiratory distress, weakness, ventricular fibrillation, voluntary muscle paralysis, vomiting. Progression of side effects may cause death.

ANTIDOTE

For any side effect, discontinue the drug and notify the physician. Death may result from potassium levels of 8 mEq/L. For severe hyperkalemia (over 6.5 mEq/L plasma), use IV sodium bicarbonate 40 to 160 mEq over 5 minutes to correct acidosis. Repeat in 10 to 15 minutes if ECG still abnormal. Initially, one ampule of 50% dextrose may be given into a large vein. Follow with IV dextrose, 10% to 20%, with 1 unit of regular insulin for every 3 Gm of dextrose (or 5 to 10 units insulin for each 20 Gm of dextrose) and infuse at 300 to 500 ml over 1 hour. 150 ml of ⅙ M sodium lactate is rarely used as a substitute. Eliminate potassium-containing foods and medicines. Monitor ECG continuously. If P waves are absent, give calcium gluconate or chloride 0.5 to 1 Gm over 2 minutes (exceeds usual rate of administration). Do not use if patient receiving digitalis. All of these measures cause a shift of potassium into the cells and may be used simultaneously. Sodium polystyrene sulfonate (Kayexalate) orally or as retention enemas is used to actually remove potassium from the body. Hemodialysis or peritoneal dialysis may be useful. Use caution in the digitalized patient; too-rapid removal of potassium may cause digitalis toxicity. Resuscitate as necessary. For extravasation, apply warm, moist compresses.

PRALIDOXIME CHLORIDE

(pra-li-dox'eem klor'id)

Antidote (anticholinesterase antagonist)

Protopam Chloride

pH 3.5 to 4.5

USUAL DOSE

In poisonings, correct any existing hypoxemia, then administer atropine as directed in the following paragraphs. After the effects of atropine have become apparent, pralidoxime may be administered. See Contraindications. If IV administration is not possible, may be given IM or SC.

ORGANOPHOSPHATE PESTICIDE POISONING

Atropine: Must be given before pralidoxime and as soon as possible after adequate ventilation has been established (hypoxemia corrected). Ventricular fibrillation can occur if oxygenation is inadequate. Give atropine, 2 to 4 mg IV, after cyanosis disappears, then give initial dose of pralidoxime. Repeat atropine every 10 minutes until atropine toxicity (delirium, dilated pupils, dry mouth, muscle twitching, pulse 140 beats/min). Maintain atropinization for at least 48 hours.

Pralidoxime: 1 to 2 Gm initially after hypoxemia has been corrected, initial dose of atropine has been given, and effects of atropine are apparent (secretions are inhibited). Repeat in 1 hour if indicated. If muscle weakness continues, additional doses can be given with extreme caution, usually every 8 to 12 hours (has been given more frequently).

ORGANOPHOSPHATE CHEMICAL POISONING

Usually administered IM by an autoinjector system (survival technology). Atropine must be given first. After the effects of atropine are apparent (e.g., dry mouth), give pralidoxime 600 mg. Repeat both drugs at 15-minute intervals times 2 if indicated. If muscle weakness persists, seek medical help; IV doses may be required.

ANTICHOLINESTERASE OVERDOSE (E.G., NEOSTIGMINE, PYRIDOSTIGMINE)

1 to 2 Gm followed by 250 mg every 5 minutes.

PEDIATRIC DOSE

Organophosphate pesticide or chemical poisoning: Give atropine 0.05 to 0.1 mg/kg. See Usual Dose for order of administration and specific criteria. Dose of pralidoxime is 20 to 50 mg/kg initially. Repeat in 1 hour and at 8- to 12-hour intervals (or more frequently) if muscle weakness persists.

DOSE ADJUSTMENTS

Reduce dose in renal impairment. ■ Lower-end initial doses may be indicated in the elderly. Dose selection should be cautious in the elderly. Consider age-related organ impairment and concomitant disease or drug therapy.

DILUTION

Each 1 Gm of sterile powder is diluted with 20 ml of SW for injection. Should be further diluted in 100 ml of NS and given as an IV infusion. If reduced fluids are indicated (e.g., pulmonary edema is present), a 5% solution (1 Gm in 20 ml SW) given over no less than 5 minutes may be used.

Storage: Store at CRT. Use promptly after reconstitution; discard remaining solution.

COMPATIBILITY

Specific information not available. Consider specific use; consult pharmacist.

RATE OF ADMINISTRATION

Too-rapid injection may cause laryngospasm, muscle rigidity, or tachycardia. Do not exceed a rate of 200 mg/min.

IV injection diluted in 20 ml SW: Each 1 Gm or fraction thereof over no less than 5 minutes. Used only if pulmonary edema present or infusion not practical.

Infusion (diluted in 100 ml NS, preferred): A single dose over 15 to 30 minutes.

ACTIONS

An anticholinesterase antagonist that reactivates cholinesterase inhibited by phosphate esters. Slows the conversion of phosphorylated cholinesterase to a nonreactivatable form and detoxifies certain organophosphates by direct chemical reaction. It reverses nicotinic effects (e.g., muscle weakness, respiratory depression, and CNS effects caused by organophosphate poisoning) while atropine reverses muscarinic effects (e.g., bradycardia, bronchoconstriction, excessive secretions). Relieves paralysis of the respiratory muscles. Rapidly dispersed throughout body fluids. Onset of action is within 10 to 40 minutes; half-life is short (about 1.2 hours), requiring repeated doses as more poison is absorbed into the GI tract. Partially metabolized by the liver. Most of a single dose is excreted within 6 hours in the urine.

INDICATIONS AND USES

Principal indications for the use of pralidoxime are muscle weakness and respiratory depression. In severe poisoning, respiratory depression may be due to muscle weakness. ■ An antidote (treatment adjunct) in organophosphate pesticide or chemical poisoning. Primarily useful for many phosphate ester insecticide poisons with anticholinesterase activity (e.g., diazinon, malathion) or chemicals with anticholinesterase activity (e.g., nerve gas). ■ Control of overdose of anticholinesterase drugs used to treat myasthenia gravis. Confirm diagnosis with edrophonium (Tensilon).

CONTRAINDICATIONS

Hypersensitivity to any component of the product. Not recommended in carbamate poisoning (increases toxicity of Sevin [carbamate insecticide]). ■ Not effective for treatment of poisoning due to phosphorus, inorganic phosphates, or organophosphates not having anticholinesterase activity.

PRECAUTIONS

In poisoning: Most effective if administered immediately after poisoning. May be ineffective if more than 24 to 48 hours has passed since exposure; some response may be obtained in severe poisoning; see Contraindications. ■ Caregivers must protect themselves from contamination. Wear gowns and gloves. ■ Remove contaminated clothing and cleanse contaminated skin surfaces, hair, and fingernails with water, sodium bicarbonate solution, or alcohol. ■ Gently flush eyes with water for at least 15 minutes. ■ Diazepam (Valium) may be required to stop convulsions. ■ Use caution in myasthenia gravis; may cause a myasthenic crisis.

Monitor: Before any medication is given, establish and maintain an adequate airway and controlled respiration as indicated. Suctioning of secretions and oxygen usually required. Correction of acidosis may be required. Draw blood samples for baseline RBC acetylcholinesterase and pseudocholinesterase concentrations. ■ In suspected poisoning, initiate treatment without waiting for lab confirmation of diagnosis. Combined with a history of possible poisoning, a RBC cholinesterase concentration less than 50% of normal is indicative of organophosphate ester poisoning. ■ Gastric lavage and activated charcoal are indicated if organophosphates are ingested; most effective if started within 30 minutes of ingestion. Avoid emesis as patient may lose consciousness and aspirate. ■ Monitor vital signs and ECG continuously. ■ Maintain adequate urine output. ■ In cases of ingested poison, toxicity may recur as poison is absorbed from bowel; monitor for 48 to 72 hours. ■ In all cases of organophosphate poisoning, patient should be observed for at least 24 hours. ■ See Drug/Lab Interactions.

Maternal/Child: Category C: effects not known; use only if clearly needed. ■ Safety for breast-feeding and children not established.

Elderly: Response similar to younger adults. ■ Dose selection should be cautious; see Dose Adjustments.

DRUG/LAB INTERACTIONS

Used in combination with atropine. Signs of atropinization (e.g., dryness of mouth and nose, flushing, mydriasis, tachycardia) may occur earlier than when atropine is used alone. ■ Potentiates barbiturates, increasing

CNS depression. ■ CNS depressants (e.g., anticonvulsants, antihistamines, muscle relaxants, narcotics, reserpine compounds, phenothiazines) and xanthines (e.g., aminophylline, caffeine) will intensify the effects of organophosphate poisoning and defeat effectiveness of treatment. ■ Succinylcholine may cause prolonged respiratory paralysis. ■ Thiamine delays excretion of pralidoxime.

SIDE EFFECTS

Blurred vision, diplopia, dizziness, drowsiness, headache, hyperventilation, impaired accommodation, increased diastolic and systolic BP, laryngospasm, muscle rigidity, muscular weakness, nausea, pharyngeal pain, tachycardia, transient elevated AST, ALT, and CPK. Excitement and manic behavior may occur (atropinization) if pralidoxime is delayed after atropine has been given.

ANTIDOTE

Has not been needed. Patient should be observed for atropine intoxication. Artificial ventilation and other supportive therapy should be administered as needed.

PROCAINAMIDE HYDROCHLORIDE

Antiarrhythmic

(proe-kane′a-mide hye-droe-klor′id)

Pronestyl

pH 4 to 6

USUAL DOSE

Loading dose: 0.2 to 1 Gm (100 mg/ml). 100 mg every 5 minutes or 20 mg every 1 minute may be given as an infusion until arrhythmia suppressed or 500 mg is administered. Wait 10 minutes to allow adequate distribution, then resume dosing until arrhythmia suppressed or maximum initial dose (1 Gm or 17 mg/kg) is reached, or side effects appear (e.g., hypotension, QRS complex widening by 50%). ***Maintenance dose:*** After arrhythmia suppressed or maximum dose reached, follow initial dose with an infusion of 1 to 4 mg/min (may require up to 6 mg/min). Titrate to control arrhythmias. Maintain with oral procainamide as soon as possible but at least 4 hours after last IV dose.

Cardiac arrest: AHA recommends 20 mg/min as an infusion to a maximum total dose of 17 mg/kg for intermittent or recurrent VF/VT.

PEDIATRIC DOSE

2 to 5 mg/kg of body weight. Do not exceed 100 mg/dose. Repeat as indicated every 10 to 30 minutes. Maximum dose in 24 hours is 30 mg/kg or 2 Gm. An alternate dose regimen is 2 to 6 mg/kg as a ***loading dose*** given over 5 minutes; follow with a ***maintenance infusion*** of 20 to 80 mcg/kg/min to control arrhythmias.

DOSE ADJUSTMENTS

Maintenance dose may be reduced in impaired or reduced renal function and in individuals over age 50. ■ See Drug/Lab Interactions.

DILUTION

IV injection: Dilute each 100 mg with 5 to 10 ml of D5W.

Infusion: Add 1 Gm of procainamide to 50, 250, or 500 ml of D5W. Yields

20 mg/ml, 4 mg/ml, or 2 mg/ml respectively. 20 mg/ml should only be used as a loading dose. 2 and 4 mg/ml dilutions may be used for loading or maintenance based on fluid restrictions. Solution should be clear; may be light yellow. Discard if darker than light amber.

Pediatric infusion: ***Loading dose:*** Add a calculated loading dose (2 to 5 mg/kg) to a minimum of 10 ml D5W for each 100 mg or fraction thereof. More diluent may be used based on size of child and fluid restriction.

Maintenance infusion: See chart under Rate of Administration (Pediatric).

Storage: Photosensitive; protect from light. Store at CRT.

COMPATIBLE WITH **(Underline Indicates Conflicting Compatibility Information)**

Consult pharmacist; specific conditions may apply; see Compatibilities, p. xvi.

Additive: *Consider individualized rate adjustments necessary to achieve desired effects.* Amiodarone (Cordarone), atracurium (Tracrium), bretylium (Bretylate), dobutamine (Dobutrex), flumazenil (Romazicon), lidocaine, verapamil (Isoptin).

Y-site: Amiodarone (Cordarone), cisatracurium (Nimbex), diltiazem (Cardizem), famotidine (Pepcid IV), heparin, hetastarch in electrolytes (Hextend), hydrocortisone sodium succinate (Solu-Cortef), inamrinone (Inocor), potassium chloride (KCl), ranitidine (Zantac), remifentanil (Ultiva).

RATE OF ADMINISTRATION

20 mg or fraction thereof over 1 minute. Use an infusion pump or a microdrip (60 gtt/ml) for infusion to deliver a constant rate. Up to 50 mg may be given by IV injection over 1 minute with extreme caution. After stabilized with loading dose, follow with a maintenance infusion at 1 to 6 mg/min.

Procainamide Infusion Rate (Adults)

Desired Dose	1 Gm in 500 ml D5W 2 mg/ml			1 Gm in 250 ml D5W 4 mg/ml		
mg/min	mg/hr	ml/min	ml/hr	mg/hr	ml/min	ml/hr
1	60	0.5	30	60	0.25	15
2	120	1	60	120	0.5	30
3	180	1.5	90	180	0.75	45
4	240	2	120	240	1	60
5	300	2.5	150	300	1.25	75
6	360	3	180	360	1.5	90

Procainamide Infusion Rate (Pediatric)

Desired Dose	200 mg in 500 ml D5W 400 mcg/ml	200 mg in 125 ml D5W 1,600 mcg/ml
mcg/kg/min	ml/kg/min × kg = ml/min	ml/kg/min × kg = ml/min
20	0.05 × wt in kg	0.0125 × wt in kg
30	0.075 × wt in kg	0.01875 × wt in kg
40	0.1 × wt in kg	0.025 × wt in kg

Continued

Procainamide Infusion Rate (Pediatric)—cont'd		
Desired Dose	200 mg in 500 ml D5W 400 mcg/ml	200 mg in 125 ml D5W 1,600 mcg/ml
mcg/kg/min	ml/kg/min × kg = ml/min	ml/kg/min × kg = ml/min
50	0.125 × wt in kg	0.03125 × wt in kg
60	0.15 × wt in kg	0.0375 × wt in kg
70	0.175 × wt in kg	0.04375 × wt in kg
80	0.2 × wt in kg	0.05 × wt in kg
Example: To deliver 30 mcg/kg/min of a 400 mg/ml solution to a child weighing 20 kg, multiply 0.075 (ml/kg/min) × 20 (wt in kg) = an infusion rate of 1.5 ml/min.		

ACTIONS

A procaine derivative. Exerts a depressing antiarrhythmic action on the heart, slowing the rate, slowing conduction, reducing myocardial irritability, and prolonging the refractory period. Decreases membrane permeability of the cell and prevents loss of sodium and potassium ions. Onset of action should occur in 2 to 3 minutes. Half-life is 3 to 4 hours. Crosses the placental barrier. Plasma levels decrease slowly; partially metabolized to the active metabolite NAPA; remaining drug excreted in the urine.

INDICATIONS AND USES

Suppress PVCs and recurrent ventricular tachycardia when lidocaine is contraindicated or has not suppressed ventricular arrhythmias. ■ Treat wide-complex tachycardias difficult to distinguish from VT (lidocaine preferred). ■ Rarely used in atrial fibrillation, paroxysmal atrial tachycardia, or arrhythmias caused by anesthesia. Safer drugs (e.g., verapamil, diltiazem) are readily available.

CONTRAINDICATIONS

Complete atrioventricular heart block, second- and third-degree AV block unless an electrical pacemaker is operative, pre-existing QT prolongation, torsades de pointes, known sensitivity to procainamide or any other local anesthetic of the ester type, myasthenia gravis, systemic lupus erythematosus.

PRECAUTIONS

Oral or IM administration is the route of choice; IV route for emergencies only. ■ Use extreme caution in first- or second-degree blocks, ventricular tachycardia after a myocardial infarction, digitalis intoxication, CHF, any structural heart disease, and impaired liver or reduced kidney function. ■ Predigitalize or cardiovert patients with atrial flutter or fibrillation to reduce incidence of sudden increase in ventricular rate as atrial rate is slowed. Use caution if used concurrently with other drugs that prolong QT interval (e.g., amiodarone [Cordarone]). ■ Some clinicians recommend giving a dose the night before surgery and then discontinuing until after surgery. If an arrhythmia occurs, use lidocaine for ventricular arrhythmias and calcium channel blockers (e.g., diltiazem, verapamil) or beta-blockers (e.g., atenolol, propranolol) for supraventricular arrhythmias. Resume dosing postop and utilize oral dosing as soon as possible. **Monitor:** Monitor the patient's ECG and BP continuously. Keep patient in a supine position. Avoid a hypotensive response. ■ Discontinue IV use when the cardiac arrhythmia is interrupted or when the ventricular rate slows without regular atrioventricular conduction. ▪ Small emboli may be dislodged when atrial fibrillation is corrected. ▪ Monitor blood levels of procainamide and NAPA (active metabolite) in patients with renal impairment and in any patient receiving a constant infusion over 3 mg/min for more than 24 hours. ▪ Monitor CBC, including WBC, differential, and platelets with continued use; fatal blood dyscrasis have occurred with usual doses. ▪ See Drug/Lab Interactions.

Maternal/Child: Category C: safety for use in pregnancy and breast-feeding and in children not established. Consider quinidine as an alternate for use during pregnancy.

Elderly: Half-life prolonged; renal excretion reduced about 25% at age 50 and 50% at age 75. ▪ Increased risk of hypotension.

DRUG/LAB INTERACTIONS

Potentiates or is potentiated by neuromuscular blocking antibiotics (e.g., kanamycin [Kantrex]), anticholinergics (e.g., atropine), thiazide diuretics, antihypertensive agents, muscle relaxants, succinylcholine, cimetidine (Tagamet), and others. ▪ May cause serious arrhythmias (e.g., prolongation of QT interval or other additive effects) with other antiarrhythmic agents (e.g., amiodarone [Cordarone], digitalis, disopyramide [Norpace], lidocaine [Xylocaine], quinidine). Lower doses of both drugs may be required. ▪ Antagonizes anticholinesterases (e.g., neostigmine). ▪ Alcohol may increase hepatic metabolism. ▪ Concurrent use with ofloxacin (Floxin IV) may decrease procainamide serum levels. ▪ May elevate AST (SGOT) levels.

SIDE EFFECTS

Anorexia, bleeding, bruising, chills, dizziness, fever, flushing, giddiness, hallucinations, joint swelling or pain, mental confusion, nausea, skin rash, tremor, vomiting, weakness. May indicate onset of more serious side effects.

Major: Blood dyscrasias (e.g., agranulocytosis, bone marrow depression, hypoplastic anemia, neutropenia, thrombocytopenia); hypotension with a BP drop over 15 mm Hg, lupus erythematosus-like symptoms, PR interval prolongation, QRS complex widening, QT interval prolongation, ventricular asystole, ventricular fibrillation, ventricular tachycardia.

ANTIDOTE

Notify the physician of any side effect. If minor symptoms progress or any major side effect appears, discontinue the drug immediately and notify the physician. Use dopamine (Intropin) or phenylephrine hydrochloride (Neo-Synephrine) to correct hypotension. Treatment of toxicity is symptomatic and supportive. Infusion of ⅙ M sodium lactate injection may reduce cardiotoxic effects. Hemodialysis may be indicated or urinary acidifiers may increase renal clearance. Resuscitate as necessary. Depending on arrhythmia, quinidine or lidocaine is an effective alternate. Consider insertion of a ventricular pacing electrode as a precautionary measure in case serious AV block develops.

PROCHLORPERAZINE EDISYLATE

(proe-klor-per′a-zeen ah-dis′ah-lat)

Phenothiazine
Antiemetic
Antipsychotic

Compazine, ✤Stemetil

pH 4.2 to 6.2

USUAL DOSE

A single IV dose should not exceed 10 mg. The maximum daily IV dose should not exceed 40 mg.

Control of severe nausea and vomiting: 2.5 to 10 mg; may be repeated one time in 1 to 2 hours if indicated.

Control of severe nausea and vomiting in adult surgical patients: 5 to 10 mg 15 to 30 minutes before induction of anesthesia or to control symptoms during or after surgery. Repeat once if necessary. Another source suggests 20 mg diluted in 1 L solution (see Dilution) during and/or after surgery.

Management of nausea and vomiting in emetic-inducing chemotherapy (unlabeled): One source suggests 10 to 20 mg 30 minutes before and 3 hours after treatment. Another source suggests 30 to 40 mg 30 minutes before and 3 hours after treatment. A third source suggests 0.8 mg/kg 30 minutes before and 3 hours after treatment and cites precipitous hypotension with larger doses; but another source suggests 2 mg/kg for highly emetogenic agents (e.g., cisplatin, dacarbazine) and 1 mg/kg for less emetogenic agents. Begin 30 minutes before chemotherapy, repeat every 2 hours for 2 doses, then every 3 hours for 3 doses. Treat extrapyramidal symptoms with diphenhydramine (Benadryl) IM. These doses have not been recommended by the manufacturer and exceed the recommended maximum daily IV dose of 40 mg/24 hr. In addition, recommended doses of newer agents (e.g., ondansetron [Zofran]) may be more effective.

Control of severe vascular and tension headaches (unlabeled): 10 mg given as an injection over 2 minutes. Sometimes given concurrently with dihydroergotamine 1 mg as an infusion over 30 minutes. Another regimen administers 3.5 mg of prochlorperazine over 5 minutes followed by dexamethasone 20 mg over 10 minutes.

PEDIATRIC DOSE

IV route not recommended for children; safety has not been established; see Contraindications, Precautions/Maternal/Child.

DOSE ADJUSTMENTS

Lower-end initial doses and more gradual adjustments may be indicated in the elderly and in debilitated or emaciated patients. ■ See Drug/Lab Interactions.

DILUTION

May be given undiluted or each 5 mg (1 ml) may be diluted with 9 ml of NS to facilitate titration. 1 ml will equal 0.5 mg. Larger amounts of NS may be used. May add doses over 10 mg to 50 ml to 1 liter of commonly used IV solution (e.g., D5W, NS, D5/½NS, Ringer's or LR), and give as an intermittent or prolonged infusion. Handle carefully; may cause contact dermatitis. Slightly yellow color does not affect potency. Discard if markedly discolored.

Storage: Store below 40° C and protect from light and freezing.

INCOMPATIBLE WITH

Manufacturer recommends not mixing with other agents in a syringe.

COMPATIBLE WITH **(Underline Indicates Conflicting Compatibility Information)**

Consult pharmacist; specific conditions may apply; see Compatibilities, p. xvi.

Additive: Amikacin (Amikin), ascorbic acid (Cenolate), calcium gluconate, dexamethasone (Decadron), dimenhydrinate (Dinate), erthyromycin lactobionate (Erythrocin), ethacrynate sodium (Edecrin), lidocaine, nafcillin (Nafcil), penicillin G potassium, sodium bicarbonate.

Syringe: ***Not recommended by manufacturer.*** Atropine, butorphanol (Stadol), chlorpromazine (Thorazine), cimetidine (Tagamet), diphenhydramine (Benadryl), droperidol (Inapsine), fentanyl (Sublimaze), glycopyrrolate, hydromorphone (Dilaudid), meperidine (Demerol), metoclopramide (Reglan), morphine, nalbuphine (Nubain), pentazocine (Talwin), perphenazine (Trilafon), promethazine (Phenergan), ranitidine (Zantac), scopolamine, sufentanil (Sufenta).

Y-site: Calcium gluconate, cisatracurium (Nimbex), cisplatin (Platinol), cladribine (Leustatin), cyclophosphamide (Cytoxan), cytarabine (ARA-C), docetaxel (Taxotere), doxorubicin (Adriamycin), doxorubicin liposome (Doxil), fluconazole (Diflucan), gatifloxacin (Tequin), granisetron (Kytril), heparin, hetastarch in electrolytes (Hextend), hydrocortisone sodium succinate (Solu-Cortef), linezolid (Zyvox), melphalan (Alkeran), methotrexate (Folex), ondansetron (Zofran), paclitaxel (Taxol), potassium chloride (KCl), propofol (Diprivan), remifentanil (Ultiva), sargramostim (Leukine), sufentanil (Sufenta), teniposide (Vumon), thiotepa (Thioplex), topotecan (Hycamtin), vinorelbine (Navelbine).

RATE OF ADMINISTRATION

IV injection: Each 5 mg or fraction thereof over 1 minute.

Infusion: May be given at ordered rate, or rate may be increased or decreased as symptoms indicate. Use an infusion pump or a microdrip (60 gtt/ml) for infusion.

Management of nausea and vomiting associated with emetic-inducing chemotherapy: A single dose over 15 to 20 minutes as an ***intermittent IV.***

ACTIONS

A phenothiazine derivative approximately six times more potent than chlorpromazine (Thorazine), with effects on the central, autonomic, and peripheral nervous systems. Has weak anticholinergic effects, moderate sedative effects, and strong extrapyramidal effects. A potent antiemetic, acting both centrally at the chemoreceptor trigger zone and peripherally by blocking the vagus nerve in the GI tract. Onset of action is prompt and lasting. Metabolized in the liver and excreted in urine and feces. Crosses placental barrier. Secreted in breast milk.

INDICATIONS AND USES

Control of severe nausea and vomiting. ■ Used IM or PO in the treatment of schizophrenia and nonpsychotic anxiety.

Unlabeled uses: Use of higher doses to control nausea and vomiting associated with emetic-inducing chemotherapy. ■ Treatment of severe vascular and tension headaches.

CONTRAINDICATIONS

Children under 2 years or 10 kg (22 lb); children with conditions that do not have an established dose; comatose or severely depressed states or in the presence of large amounts of CNS depressants (e.g., alcohol, barbiturates, narcotics); hypersensitivity to phenothiazines; breast-feeding and pregnancy, except labor and delivery; do not use in pediatric surgery.

PRECAUTIONS

Use IV only when absolutely necessary. IV not recommended for children. ■ Extrapyramidal symptoms caused by prochlorperazine may be confused with undiagnosed disease (e.g., Reye's syndrome, encephalopathy). ■ May mask diagnosis of other conditions including Reye's syndrome, brain tumor, drug intoxication, and intestinal obstruction. ■ May produce ECG changes (e.g., prolonged QT interval, changes in T waves). ■ Use caution in coronary disease, glaucoma, severe hypertension or hypotension, and in patients with bone marrow depression. ■ Use caution in patients with epilepsy. May lower the seizure threshold. ■ Neuroleptic malignant syndrome, characterized by hyperpyrexia, muscle rigidity, autonomic instability, and altered mental status has been reported with phenothiazine use. ■ Tardive dyskinesia (potentially irreversible involuntary dyskinetic movements) may develop. Use the smallest doses and shortest duration of therapy to minimize risk. ■ Anticholinergic and cardiac effects may be troublesome during anesthesia. For patients receiving phenothiazines, taper and discontinue preoperatively if they will not be continued after surgery. ■ May discolor urine pink to reddish brown. ■ Photosensitivity of skin is possible. ■ May cause paradoxical excitation in children and the elderly. ■ Do not re-expose patients who have experienced jaundice, skin reactions, or blood dyscrasias in reaction to a phenothiazine. Cross-sensitivity may occur. ■ May contain sulfites; use caution in patients with allergies.

Monitor: Keep patient in supine position and monitor BP and pulse before administration and between doses. ■ Cough reflex may be suppressed. Monitor closely if nauseated or vomiting to prevent aspiration. ■ See Drug/Lab Interactions.

Patient Education: Avoid use of alcohol or other CNS depressants (e.g., antihistamines, barbiturates). ■ Request assistance for ambulation; may cause dizziness or fainting. ■ Use caution performing tasks that require alertness. ■ May cause skin and eye photosensitivity. Avoid unprotected exposure to sun.

Maternal/Child: Safety for use in pregnancy, breast-feeding, and children not established; see Contraindications. ■ Has been used during pregnancy, for intractable nausea and vomiting; physician must decide if benefit outweighs risk. ■ Use near term may cause maternal hypotension and adverse neonatal effects (e.g., extrapyramidal syndrome, hyperreflexia, hyporeflexia, jaundice). ■ Fetuses and infants have a reduced capacity to metabolize and eliminate. ■ Children may metabolize antipsychotic agents more rapidly than adults. ■ Incidence of extrapyramidal reactions is relatively high in children, especially in the presence of acute illness (e.g., measles, chickenpox, gastroenteritis).

Elderly: See Dose Adjustments and Precautions. ■ Have a reduced capacity to metabolize and eliminate and may have increased sensitivity to postural hypotension, anticholinergic and sedative effects. ■ Increased risk of extrapyramidal side effects (e.g., tardive dyskinesia, parkinsonism).

DRUG/LAB INTERACTIONS

Use with epinephrine not recommended; may cause precipitous hypotension. ■ Increased CNS respiratory depression and hypotensive effects with narcotics, alcohol, anesthetics, barbiturates; reduced doses of these agents usually indicated. ■ Additive effects with MAO inhibitors (e.g., selegiline [Eldepryl]), anticholinergics, antihistamines, antihypertensives, hypnotics, muscle relaxants, phenytoin (Dilantin), propranolol (Inderal), rauwolfia alkaloids, and thiazide diuretics; dose adjustment may be necessary. ■ Risk of cardiotoxicity increased with pimozide (Orap) and sparfloxacin (Zagam); concurrent use not recommended. ■ Risk of additive QT interval prolongation, cardiac depressant effects, and cardiac arrhythmias increased with amiodarone (Cordarone), cisapride (Propulsid), disopyramide (Norpace), erythromycin, probucol (Lorelco), procainamide (Pronestyl), and quinidine. ■ Concurrent use with antidepressants (e.g., fluoxetine [Prozac], paroxetine [Paxil]), tricyclic antidepressants (e.g., amitriptyline [Elavil]), or MAO inhibitors may increase effects of both drugs; risk of neuroleptic malignant syndrome may be increased. ■ Encephalopathic syndrome has been reported with concurrent use of lithium, monitor for S/S of neurologic toxicity. ■ May diminish effects of oral anticoagulants. ■ May lower seizure threshold. Dose adjustment of anticonvulsants may be necessary. ■ Use with metrizamide (Amipaque) may lower seizure threshold; discontinue prochlorperazine 48 hours before myelography, and do not resume for 24 hours after test is completed. ■ Use caution during anesthesia with barbiturates (e.g., methohexital, thiopental); may increase frequency and severity of hypotension and neuromuscular excitation. ■ Capable of innumerable other interactions.

SIDE EFFECTS

Usually transient if drug discontinued but may require treatment if severe: anaphylaxis, blurring of vision, cardiac arrest, dermatitis, dizziness, drowsiness, dryness of mouth, dysphagia, elevated BP, extrapyramidal symptoms (e.g., abnormal positioning, extreme restlessness, pseudoparkinsonism, weakness of extremities), excitement, fever without etiology, hematologic toxicities (e.g., agranulocytosis, aplastic anemia, leukopenia, thrombocytopenia), hypersensitivity reactions, hypotension, photosensitivity, slurred speech, spastic movements (especially about the face), tachycardia, tardive dyskinesia, tightness of the throat, tongue discoloration, tongue protrusion, and many others. Overdose can cause convulsions, hallucinations, and death.

ANTIDOTE

Discontinue the drug at onset of any side effect and notify the physician. Discontinue prochlorperazine and all drugs not essential to concurrent therapy immediately if NMS occurs. Will require intensive symptomatic treatment, medical monitoring, and management of concomitant medical problems. Counteract hypotension with IV fluids and norepinephrine (Levophed) or phenylephrine (Neo-Synephrine) and extrapyramidal symptoms with benztropine mesylate (Cogentin), or diphenhydramine (Benadryl). Maintain a clear airway and adequate hydration. ***Epinephrine is contraindicated for hypotension.*** Further hypotension will occur. Use diazepam (Valium) for convulsions or hyperactivity. Follow with phenytoin. Phenytoin may be helpful in ventricular arrhythmias. In treating respiratory depression and unconsciousness, avoid analeptics such as doxapram (Dopram); they may cause convulsions. Not removed by dialysis. Resuscitate as necessary.

PROMETHAZINE HYDROCHLORIDE

(proe-meth′a-zeen hye-droe-klor′id)

Phenothiazine
Antiemetic
Sedative-hypnotic

Phenergan

pH 4 to 5.5

USUAL DOSE

Nausea and vomiting: 12.5 to 25 mg every 4 to 6 hours as needed.

Allergic conditions: 25 mg. May repeat in 2 hours if necessary. Change to oral therapy as soon as possible.

Sedation, nighttime: 25 to 50 mg.

Sedation, perioperative: 25 to 50 mg. May combine with a reduced dose of narcotic analgesic and an anticholinergic drug (e.g., atropine).

Sedation, labor and delivery: 50 mg during early stage of labor. When labor fully established, may administer 25 to 75 mg with a reduced dose of a narcotic analgesic. May repeat every 4 hours to a maximum dose of 100 mg.

PEDIATRIC DOSE

IV rarely used; see Maternal/Child.

Nausea and vomiting: 0.25 to 0.5 mg/kg of body weight every 4 to 6 hours. Do not exceed one half of adult dose.

Preoperative sedation: 0.5 to 1.1 mg/kg. May be combined with a reduced dose of narcotic analgesic and an anticholinergic drug (e.g., atropine).

Postoperative sedation: 10 to 25 mg. May be combined with a reduced dose of narcotic.

DOSE ADJUSTMENTS

Reduced dose may be indicated in the elderly. See Drug/Lab Interactions.

DILUTION

May be given undiluted or may dilute with NS. Concentration should not exceed 25 mg/ml. 1 ml (25 to 50 mg) diluted with 9 ml of NS equals 2.5 to 5 mg/ml. Slightly yellow color does not alter potency. Discard if greatly discolored. Administer through Y-tube or three-way stopcock of a free-flowing IV.

Storage: Store at CRT. Protect from light.

INCOMPATIBLE WITH

May form a precipitate with heparin; flush heparinized infusion sets with SW or NS before and after administration.

COMPATIBLE WITH

(Underline Indicates Conflicting Compatibility Information)

Consult pharmacist; specific conditions may apply; see Compatibilities, p. xvi.

Additive: Amikacin (Amikin), ascorbic acid (Cenolate), hydromorphone (Dilaudid), <u>penicillin G potassium</u>.

Syringe: Atropine, butorphanol (Stadol), chlorpromazine (Thorazine), cimetidine (Tagamet), dihydroergotamine (D.H.E. 45), diphenhydramine (Benadryl), droperidol (Inapsine), fentanyl (Sublimaze), glycopyrrolate, hydromorphone (Dilaudid), meperidine (Demerol), metoclopramide (Reglan), midazolam (Versed), <u>morphine</u>, <u>nalbuphine (Nubain)</u>, pentazocine (Talwin), perphenazine (Trilafon), prochlorperazine (Compazine), ranitidine (Zantac), scopolamine, selected contrast agents used in radiology.

Y-site: Amifostine (Ethyol), aztreonam (Azactam), ciprofloxacin (Cipro IV), cisatracurium (Nimbex), cisplatin (Platinol), cladribine (Leustatin), cyclophosphamide (Cytoxan), cytarabine (ARA-C), docetaxel (Taxotere), doxorubicin (Adriamycin), etoposide phosphate (Etopophos), filgrastim (Neupogen), fluconazole (Diflucan), fludarabine (Fludara), gatifloxacin (Tequin), gemcitabine (Gemzar), granisetron (Kytril), heparin, hetastarch in electrolytes (Hextend), hydrocortisone sodium succinate (Solu-Cortef), linezolid (Zyvox), melphalan (Alkeran), ondansetron (Zofran), potassium chloride (KCl), remifentanil (Ultiva), sargramostim (Leukine), teniposide (Vumon), thiotepa (Thioplex), vinorelbine (Navelbine).

RATE OF ADMINISTRATION

Each 25 mg or fraction thereof over 1 minute.

ACTIONS

A phenothiazine derivative with effects on the central, autonomic, and peripheral nervous systems. It has antihistaminic, antiemetic, anticholinergic and sedative effects. As an antihistamine, it competitively blocks the H_1 histamine receptor, antagonizing most of the effects of histamine to at least some degree. Potentiates respiratory depression, sedative, and hypotensive effects of narcotics and other CNS depressants. Has no analgesic effects and does not potentiate analgesic effects of narcotics. Onset of action is prompt. Duration of action is 4 to 6 hours. Primarily metabolized in the liver and excreted in the urine.

INDICATIONS AND USES

Prophylaxis or treatment of minor transfusion reactions. ■ Treatment of hypersensitivity reactions. ■ Treatment of acute nausea, vomiting, and motion sickness. ■ Sedation to meet surgical and obstetric needs. ■ Adjunct to analgesics for control of postoperative pain.

CONTRAINDICATIONS

Bone marrow depression, comatose or severely depressed states, hypersensitivity to phenothiazines, jaundice, breast-feeding, pregnancy. Never inject into an artery or SC.

PRECAUTIONS

Ampule must state "for IV use." Use with extreme caution in children and the elderly; see Maternal/Child and Elderly. ■ May cause paradoxical excitation in children and the elderly. ■ Use phenothiazines with extreme caution in children with a history of sleep apnea, a family history of sudden infant death syndrome, or in the presence of Reye's syndrome. ■ Use with caution in patients with asthma, bladder neck obstruction, bone marrow depression, cardiovascular disease, glaucoma, liver dysfunction, prostatic hypertrophy, or stenosing peptic ulcer disease. ■ May produce ECG changes (e.g., prolonged QT interval, changes in T waves). ■ May mask diagnosis of other conditions, including Reye's syndrome, brain tumor, drug intoxication, and intestinal obstruction. ■ May lower seizure threshold; use extreme caution in patients with known seizure disorders and with narcotics or local anesthetics that also lower seizure threshold. ■ Do not re-expose patients who have experienced jaundice to a phenothiazine. ■ May contain sulfites; use caution in patients with allergies. ■ Anticholinergic and cardiac effects may be troublesome during anesthesia. For patients receiving phenothiazines, taper and discontinue preoperatively if they will not be continued after surgery.

Monitor: Determine absolute patency of vein; extravasation will cause necrosis. ■ Keep patient in supine position. Monitor BP and pulse before administration and between doses. ■ Sedative effect may require ambulation to be monitored. ■ See Drug/Lab Interactions.

Patient Education: Avoid use of alcohol or other CNS depressants (e.g., antihistamines, barbiturates). ■ Request assistance for ambulation; may cause dizziness or fainting. ■ Use caution performing tasks that require alertness. ■ May cause skin and eye photosensitivity. Avoid unprotected exposure to sun. ■ Report stinging or burning at IV site promptly.

Maternal/Child: Category C: safety for use in pregnancy, breast-feeding, and children not established. Use only when clearly needed. ■ Use near term may cause maternal hypotension and adverse neonatal effects (e.g., extrapyramidal syndrome, hyperreflexia, hyporeflexia, jaundice). ■ Do not use in premature infants or neonates; they have a reduced capacity to metabolize and eliminate. ■ Do not use for vomiting of unknown etiology in children. ■ Excessively large doses of antihistamines in children have caused hallucination, convulsions, and death. ■ Children metabolize antipsychotic agents more rapidly than adults. ■ Incidence of extrapyramidal reactions is relatively high in children, especially in the presence of acute illness (e.g., measles, chickenpox, gastroenteritis). ■ See Precautions and Contraindications.

Elderly: See Dose Adjustments and Precautions. ■ Have a reduced capacity to metabolize and eliminate. ■ May cause confusion, dizziness, hyperexcitability, hypotension, and/or sedation. ■ Increased sensitivity to anticholinergic effects (e.g., dry mouth, urinary retention). ■ Increased risk of extrapyramidal side effects (e.g., tardive dyskinesia, parkinsonism).

DRUG/LAB INTERACTIONS

Increased CNS respiratory depression and hypotensive effects with narcotics, alcohol, anesthetics, and barbiturates; reduced doses of these agents usually indicated. ■ Additive effects with MAO inhibitors (e.g., selegiline [Eldepryl]), anticholinergics, antihistamines, antihypertensives, hypnotics, muscle relaxants, phenytoin (Dilantin), propranolol (Inderal), rauwolfia alkaloids, and thiazide diuretics; dose adjustment may be necessary. ■ Use with epinephrine not recommended; may cause precipitous hypotension. ■ Risk of cardiotoxicity increased with pimozide (Orap) and sparfloxacin (Zagam); concurrent use not recommended. ■ Risk of additive QT interval prolongation, cardiac depressant effects, and cardiac arrhythmias increased with amiodarone (Cordarone), cisapride (Propulsid), disopyramide (Norpace), erythromycin, probucol (Lorelco), procainamide (Pronestyl), and quinidine. ■ Concurrent use with antidepressants (e.g., fluoxetine [Prozac], paroxetine [Paxil]), tricyclic antidepressants (e.g., amitriptyline [Elavil]), or MAO inhibitors may increase effects of both drugs; risk of neuroleptic malignant syndrome may be increased. ■ Encephalopathic syndrome has been reported with concurrent use of lithium, monitor for S/S of neurologic toxicity. ■ May lower seizure threshold. Dose adjustment of anticonvulsants may be necessary. ■ Does not potentiate analgesic effects of narcotics. ■ May produce apnea with neuromuscular blocking antibiotics (e.g., gentamicin). ■ Contraindicated with quinidine, epinephrine, and thiazide diuretics. ■ Use caution during anesthesia with barbiturates (e.g., methohexital, thiopental); may increase frequency and severity of hypotension and neuromuscular excitation. ■ Capable of innumerable other interactions.

SIDE EFFECTS

Average dose: Blurring of vision, dizziness, dryness of mouth, hyperexcitability, hypersensitivity reactions, hypertension (rare), hypotension (mild), nightmares, photosensitivity, spastic movements of upper extremities.

Overdose: Anaphylaxis, cardiac arrest, coma, convulsions, deep sedation, respiratory depression. All side effects of phenothiazines are possible, but rarely occur. See prochlorperazine (Compazine).

ANTIDOTE

Discontinue the drug at onset of any side effect and notify the physician. Counteract hypotension with norepinephrine (Levophed) or phenylephrine (Neo-Synephrine) and IV fluids; extrapyramidal symptoms with benztropine mesylate (Cogentin) or diphenhydramine (Benadryl). Epinephrine is contraindicated for hypotension; further hypotension will occur. Use diazepam (Valium) or phenobarbital for convulsions or hyperactivity. Phenytoin may be helpful in ventricular arrhythmias. In treating respiratory depression and unconsciousness, avoid analeptics such as doxapram (Dopram); they may cause convulsions. Resuscitate as necessary.

PROPOFOL INJECTION

(pro′poh-fole in-jek′shun)

Diprivan

General anesthetic
Anesthesia adjunct
Sedative-hypnotic

pH 7 to 8.5

USUAL DOSE

Induction of Anesthesia

Must be individualized and titrated to desired response.

Healthy adults less than 55 years of age: 40 mg every 10 seconds until induction onset (approximately 2 to 2.5 mg/kg).

Adults over 55 years of age, debilitated, or ASA III or IV risk patients: 20 mg every 10 seconds until induction onset (approximately 1 to 1.5 mg/kg).

Cardiac anesthesia: 20 mg every 10 seconds until induction onset (0.5 to 1.5 mg/kg).

Neurosurgical patients: 20 mg every 10 seconds until induction onset (approximately 1 to 2 mg/kg). Infusion or slow injection (20 mg over 10 seconds) is used to avoid significant hypotension and decrease in cerebral perfusion pressure.

Maintenance of Anesthesia

Must be titrated to desired clinical effect.

Adults less than 55 years of age: Immediately follow induction with an infusion of 100 to 200 mcg/kg/min (6 to 12 mg/kg/hr) or an intermittent bolus in increments of 25 to 50 mg as needed.

Adults over 55 years of age, debilitated, or ASA III or IV risk patients: Immediately follow induction with an infusion of 50 to 100 mcg/kg/min (3 to 6 mg/kg/hr). Do NOT use a rapid intermittent bolus in these patients.

Cardiac anesthesia: Most patients require 100 to 150 mcg/kg/min in combination with an opioid (primary propofol with an opioid secondary). An alternate regimen is an opioid primary with low-dose propofol 50 to 100 mcg/kg/min.

Neurosurgical patients: Immediately follow induction with an infusion of 100 to 200 mcg/kg/min (6 to 12 mg/kg/hr). Do NOT use a rapid intermittent bolus in these patients.

INITIATION OF MAC SEDATION

MAC sedation rates are approximately 25% of those used for anesthesia. Must be individualized.

Healthy adults less than 55 years of age: An infusion of 100 to 150 mcg/kg/min (6 to 9 mg/kg/hr) or a slow injection of 0.5 mg/kg over 3 to 5 minutes. Slow infusion or slow injection techniques are preferable to rapid bolus administration.

Adults over 55 years of age, debilitated, or ASA III or IV risk patients: Most patients require doses similar to healthy adults. Must be given as a slow infusion (preferred) or as a slow injection over 3 to 5 minutes. Do NOT give as a rapid bolus.

MAINTENANCE OF MAC SEDATION

Healthy adults less than 55 years of age: Maintain with an infusion (preferred) of 25 to 75 mcg/kg/min (1.5 to 4.5 mg/kg/hr) or incremental bolus doses of 10 to 20 mg.

Adults over 55 years of age, debilitated, or ASA III or IV risk patients: Most patients require 20% reduction of the adult dose; an infusion of 20 to 60 mcg/kg/min (1.2 to 3.6 mg/kg/hr). Do NOT use bolus doses.

SEDATION OF INTUBATED MECHANICALLY VENTILATED OR RESPIRATORY CONTROLLED ICU PATIENTS

Given as a continuous infusion. Begin with an initial dose of 5 mcg/kg/min (0.3 mg/kg/hr) over 5 minutes. Allow at least 5 minutes between adjustments to reach peak drug effect and to avoid hypotension. Increase slowly over 5 to 10 minutes by 5 to 10 mcg/kg/min (0.3 to 0.6 mg/kg/hr) to desired level of sedation. Individualize to patient condition, response, blood lipid profile, and vital signs. Some clinicians recommend reducing dose by approximately one half for elderly (over 55 years) and debilitated.

MAINTENANCE OF SEDATION IN MECHANICALLY VENTILATED OR RESPIRATORY-CONTROLLED ICU PATIENTS

5 to 50 mcg/kg/min as a continuous infusion slowly titrated to desired level of sedation. Temporarily reduce dose once each day to assess neurologic and respiratory function. Average maintenance dose ***under 55 years*** is 38 mcg/kg/min; ***over 55 years,*** 20 mcg/kg/min. Average maintenance dose for ***post–coronary artery bypass graft (CABG) patients*** is usually low (median of 11 mcg/kg/min) because of high intraoperative opiates.

RELIEF OF CHOLESTATIC PRURITUS (UNLABELED)

1 to 1.5 mg/kg/hr as a continuous infusion for 3 days.

PEDIATRIC DOSE

To minimize pain on injection of propofol in pediatric patients, administer through anticubital or larger veins or pretreat smaller veins with lidocaine.

INDUCTION OF ANESTHESIA IN HEALTHY CHILDREN 3 TO 16 YEARS OF AGE

Must be individualized and titrated to desired response. 2.5 to 3.5 mg/kg administered over 20 to 30 seconds. ***Induction with propofol is indicated only in children 3 years of age or older. In children from 2 months to 3 years of age, induction must be achieved by supplementing with another agent (literature suggests nitrous oxide 60% to 70%).*** See Dose Adjustments.

Continued

MAINTENANCE OF ANESTHESIA IN HEALTHY CHILDREN FROM 2 MONTHS TO 16 YEARS OF AGE

Must be titrated to desired clinical effect. (See statement under induction in healthy children in the previous paragraph.)

Children 3 years and older: Immediately follow induction dose with an infusion of 125 to 300 mcg/kg/min (7.5 to 18 mg/kg/hr). Initially, a rate of 200 to 300 mcg/kg/min may be indicated and can be reduced to 125 to 150 mcg/kg/min after the first half-hour.

Children 2 months to 3 years: Similar doses in a variable rate infusion supplemented by nitrous oxide 60% to 70% usually provides satisfactory general anesthesia.

All children: Decrease infusion rate if clinical signs of light anesthesia are not present after 30 minutes of maintenance; see Rate of Administration. Younger pediatric patients may require higher maintenance infusion rates than older pediatric patients. See Dose Adjustments.

DOSE ADJUSTMENTS

All situations: Reduce induction and maintenance doses for pediatric patients classified as ASA III or IV. ▪ See Usual Dose for specific reduced doses required for adults over 55 years of age, debilitated, or ASA III or IV risk patients. ▪ Reduced dose required in presence of other CNS depressants. See Drug/Lab Interactions. ▪ No dose adjustment required for gender, chronic hepatic cirrhosis, or chronic renal failure.

ICU sedation: Adjust infusion to maintain a light level of sedation through the wake-up assessment or weaning process.

DILUTION

Supplied in ready-to-use vented vials containing 10 mg/ml. Shake well before use. May be further diluted only with D5W. Do not dilute to a concentration less than 2 mg/ml (4 ml diluent to 1 ml propofol yields 2 mg/ml). More stable in glass than in plastic. Strict aseptic technique imperative; emulsion supports rapid growth of microorganisms. Do not use with evidence of emulsion separation. Prepare immediately before each use. Flush IV line at end of every 6 hours in extended procedures to remove residual propofol.

Storage: Protect from light and store below 22° C (72° F) but do not refrigerate. Discard infusion and tubing every 12 hours.

INCOMPATIBLE WITH

Manufacturer states, "Should not be mixed with other therapeutic agents prior to administration. Compatibility with blood/serum/plasma has not been established."

COMPATIBLE WITH **(Underline Indicates Conflicting Compatibility Information)**

Consult pharmacist; specific conditions may apply; see Compatibilities, p. xvi.

Syringe: ***Not recommended by manufacturer; see Incompatible With.*** Ondansetron (Zofran), thiopental (Pentothal).

Y-site: Acyclovir (Zovirax), alatrofloxacin (Trovan IV), alfentanil (Alfenta), aminophylline, ampicillin, <u>atracurium (Tracrium)</u>, <u>atropine</u>, aztreonam (Azactam), bumetanide (Bumex), buprenorphine (Buprenex), butorphanol (Stadol), calcium gluconate, carboplatin (Paraplatin), cefazolin (Kefzol), cefepime (Maxipime), cefoperazone (Cefobid), cefotaxime (Claforan), cefotetan (Cefotan), cefoxitin (Mefoxin), ceftazidime (Fortaz), ceftizoxime (Cefizox), ceftriaxone (Rocephin), cefuroxime (Zinacef), chlorpromazine (Thorazine), cimetidine (Tagamet), <u>cisatracurium (Nimbex)</u>, cisplatin (Platinol), clindamycin (Cleocin), cyclophosphamide (Cytoxan), cyclosporine (Sandimmune), cytarabine (ARA-C), D5LR, D5W, dexamethasone (Decadron), diphenhydramine (Benadryl), dobutamine (Dobutrex), dopamine (Intropin), doxycycline (Vibramycin), droperidol (Inapsine), enalaprilat (Vasotec IV), ephedrine, epinephrine (Adrenalin), esmolol (Brevibloc), famotidine (Pepcid IV), fentanyl (Sublimaze), fluconazole (Diflucan), fluorouracil (5-FU), furosemide (Lasix), ganciclovir (Cytovene), glycopyrrolate, granisetron (Kytril), haloperidol (Haldol), heparin, hydrocortisone sodium succinate (Solu-Cortef), hydromorphone (Dilaudid), ifosfamide (Ifex), imipenem-cilastatin (Primaxin), inamrinone (Inocor), insulin (regular), isoproterenol (Isuprel), ketamine (Ketalar), labetalol (Normodyne), levorphanol (Levo-Dromoran), lidocaine, lorazepam (Ativan), LR, magnesium sulfate, mannitol, meperidine (Demerol), midazolam (Versed), milrinone (Primacor), morphine, nafcillin (Nafcil), nalbuphine (Nubain), naloxone (Narcan), nitroglycerin (Nitro-Bid IV), nitroprusside sodium, norepinephrine (Levophed), ¼NS, ½NS, NS, ofloxacin (Floxin IV), paclitaxel (Taxol), pancuronium (Pavulon), pentobarbital (Nembutal), phenobarbital (Luminal), phenylephrine (Neo-Synephrine), piperacillin (Pipracil), potassium chloride (KCl), prochlorperazine (Compazine), propranolol (Inderal), ranitidine (Zantac), scopolamine, sodium bicarbonate, succinylcholine, sufentanil (Sufenta), thiopental (Pentothal), ticarcillin (Ticar), ticarcillin/clavulanate (Timentin), vancomycin (Vancocin), vecuronium (Norcuron).

RATE OF ADMINISTRATION

Use of a syringe pump or volumetric pump recommended to provide controlled infusion rates. See Usual Dose for specific rates for specific age and/or indication. Extend rate based on age, debilitation, or calculated risk. Must be individualized and titrated to desired level of sedation and changes in vital signs. Monitor respiratory function continuously. Continuous administration preferable to intermittent to avoid periods of undersedation or oversedation. Too-rapid administration (bolus dosing, too-rapid increase in infusion rate, overdose) can cause severe cardiorespiratory complications, especially in children, adults over 55 years, debilitated or ASA III or IV risk patients. In all anesthesia, higher rates are generally required for the first 15 minutes, then appropriate responses can usually be maintained with a decrease of 30% to 50%. Always titrate rates downward until there is a mild response to surgical stimulation. This avoids administration at rates higher than clinically necessary. Control increased response to surgical stimulation or lightening of anesthesia (increased pulse rate, BP, sweating and/or tearing) with bolus injections of 25 to 50 mg ***(adults under 55 years of age only);*** slow injection of reduced doses, or by increasing the infusion rate ***(adults under or over 55 years of age)*** or by increasing the infusion rate ***(pediatric patients).*** If control not effective within 5 minutes, consider use of an opioid, barbiturate, vasodilator, or inhalation agent.

ACTIONS

A potent emulsified IV sedative hypnotic agent. Action is dose and rate dependent. Can provide conscious (verbal contact maintained) or unconscious sedation, depending on dose. Produces hypnosis rapidly and smoothly with minimal excitation, usually within 40 seconds. Depth of sedation easily and rapidly controlled by adjusting rate of infusion. Rapid onset of action facilitates accurate titration and minimizes oversedation. Due to extensive redistribution from the central nervous system to other tissues and high metabolic clearance, recovery from anesthesia or sedation is rapid. Most patients are awake and responsive to verbal commands and oriented in 8 minutes. Metabolized in the liver and excreted as metabolites in urine. Has minimal impact on cardiac output, but changes may occur because of assisted or controlled ventilation, additional opioids or other CNS depressants, intubation, or surgical stimulation. Crosses placental barrier. Secreted in breast milk.

INDICATIONS AND USES

Adults: Induce and/or maintain anesthesia as part of a balanced anesthetic technique for inpatient and outpatient surgery. ■ Initiate and maintain monitored anesthesia care (MAC) during diagnostic procedures (e.g., colonoscopy, dental procedures) and in conjunction with local/regional anesthesia during surgical procedures. ■ Continuous sedation and control of stress responses in intubated or respiratory controlled ICU patients (e.g., post-CABG, postsurgical, neuro/head trauma, ARDS, COPD, asthma, status epilepticus, tetanus). Continuous infusions of low doses allows controlled recovery of consciousness when required and for assessment.
Children: Induction of anesthesia as a part of a balanced anesthetic technique for inpatient and outpatient surgery in pediatric patients over 3 years of age. ■ Maintenance of anesthesia as part of a balanced anesthetic technique for inpatient and outpatient surgery in pediatric patients over 2 months of age. Not recommended for induction of anesthesia below the age of 3 years or for maintenance of anesthesia below the age of 2 months. Not indicated for use in pediatric patients for ICU sedation or for MAC sedation for surgical, nonsurgical, or diagnostic procedures.

Unlabeled uses: Subhypnotic doses used to treat morphine-induced (cholestatic) pruritus. ■ Treatment of status epilepticus refractory to standard anticonvulsant therapy.

CONTRAINDICATIONS

Known hypersensitivity to propofol or its components (e.g., soybean oil, glycerol, egg lecithin, sodium hydroxide) or any time general anesthesia or sedation is contraindicated.

PRECAUTIONS

All situations: For IV use only. ■ Administered by or under the direct observation of the anesthesiologist. Must have responsibility only for anesthesia during surgery and/or procedures. ■ Staff must be skilled in medical management of critically ill patients, cardiovascular resuscitation, and airway management. ■ Use caution in patients with compromised myocardial function, intravascular volume depletion, or abnormally low vascular tone (e.g., sepsis); may be more susceptible to hypotension. ■ An emulsion; use caution in patients with lipid metabolism disorders (e.g., diabetic hyperlipidemia, pancreatitis, and primary hyperlipoproteinemia). ■ May cause convulsions during recovery phase in patients with epilepsy. ■ Use caution in patients with increased intracranial pressure or impaired cerebral circulation. Decrease in mean arterial pressure may cause decreases in cerebral perfusion. ■ Has no analgesic properties; provide pain relief or local anesthetic as indicated. Has been used successfully with midazolam (Versed), 1 to 3 mg, for initial induction. Midazolam provides better amnesia and causes less pain on injection, whereas propofol sustains sedation and allows more rapid recovery. ■ May contain sulfites; use caution in patients with allergies.

ICU sedation: Monitor triglycerides with long-term use (ICU sedation). Adjust if fat inadequately cleared from body and reduce other lipid administration.

Monitor: ***All situations:*** Correct fluid volume deficiencies before administration. ■ Will cause transient local pain during IV injection; minimize by using larger veins and lidocaine previous to injection. Use with midazolam reduces awareness of this pain. ■ Apnea may occur during induction and last for more than 60 seconds. Intubation equipment, controlled ventilation equipment, oxygen, and facilities for resuscitation and life support must be available. Maintain a patent airway and ascertain adequate ventilation at all times. ■ All vital signs must be monitored continuously. Use of a respiratory monitor required. ■ Hypotension common during first 60 minutes; monitor closely. Significant hypotension or cardiovascular depression can be profound. ■ To prevent profound bradycardia, anticholinergic agents (e.g., atropine, glycopyrrolate) may be required to modify increases in vagal tone due to concomitant agents (e.g., succinylcholine) or surgical stimulation. ■ Bed rest required for a minimum of 3 hours after IV injection, or satisfy specific hospital rules for discharge. ■ See Drug/Lab Interactions.

ICU sedation: Observe for signs and symptoms of pain; may indicate need for opioids or analgesia, not an increase in propofol dose. ■ Benzodiazepines (e.g., diazepam [Valium]) and/or neuromuscular blocking agents (e.g., mivacurium [Mivacron], succinylcholine) may also be used. ■ Dose may be reduced carefully to allow patient to awaken to a lighter level of sedation allowing neurologic and respiratory assessment daily. Avoid rapid awakening; will cause anxiety, agitation, and resistance to mechanical ventilation. ■ Discontinue opioids and paralytic agents and optimize respiratory function before weaning from mechanical ventilation. ■ Maintain light sedation until 15 minutes before extubation.

Patient Education: Avoid alcohol or other CNS depressants (e.g., antihistamines, benzodiazepines) for 24 hours following anesthesia. ■ Do not perform tasks requiring mental alertness (e.g., driving, operating hazardous machinery, or signing legal documents) until the day after surgery or longer. All effects must have subsided.

Maternal/Child: Category B: use during pregnancy only if clearly needed. ■ Not recommended for use in obstetric procedures, including cesarean section; no assurance of safety for fetus. ■ Not recommended for use during breast-feeding. ■ Has been approved for induction of anesthesia in children 3 years to 16 years of age. Has been approved for maintenance of anesthesia in children 2 months to 16 years of age. ■ Distribution and clearance in children 3 years to 12 years of age is similar to that seen in adults. ■ Serious bradycardia may result with concomitant administration of fentanyl. ■ Serious adverse effects, including fatalities occurred during ICU sedation in children with respiratory infections and/or with doses in excess of recommendations for adults. ■ A recent study identified an increase in deaths with propofol versus standard sedative agents. Manufacturer has issued a warning letter stating that propofol should not be used for sedation of pediatric patients in ICU. ■ See Side Effects.

Elderly: Dose requirements decrease after age 55 due to reduced clearance and higher blood levels. Minimize undesirable cardiorespiratory depression (hypotension, apnea, airway obstruction, and/or oxygen desaturation) by using reduced doses and rates of administration. See Usual Dose and Dose Adjustments.

DRUG/LAB INTERACTIONS

Potentiated by inhalational anesthetics (e.g., enflurane, halothane, isoflurane, nitrous oxide), narcotics (e.g., morphine, meperidine [Demerol], fentanyl [Sublimaze]), sedatives (e.g., barbiturates, benzodiazepines [e.g., diazepam (Valium), midazolam (Versed)], chloral hydrate, droperidol [Inapsine]). Anesthetic and sedative effects increased; systolic, diastolic, mean arterial pressure, and cardiac output are decreased. Reduce dose of propofol to maintain desired level of anesthesia or sedation. ■ No significant adverse interactions noted to date with neuromuscular blocking agents (e.g., succinylcholine, pipecuronium [Arduran], tubocurarine [Curare]). ■ Neuroexcitatory effects of propofol may cause seizures in patients receiving chlordiazepoxide (Librium) or antidepressants (e.g., fluoxetine [Prozac], maprotilene [Ludiomil]). ■ In pediatric patients serious bradycardia may result with concomitant administration of fentanyl.

SIDE EFFECTS

Adults and children: More likely to occur during loading boluses, with supplemental boluses or higher rate of administration. Apnea; bradycardia (profound); cough; dyspnea; headache; hypotension; hypoventilation; injection site burning, pain, stinging; nausea, and upper airway obstruction are most common. Urine may be green. Abdominal cramping, anaphylaxis (including bronchospasm, erythema, and hypotension), bucking/jerking/thrashing, clonic/myclonic movement (rarely including convulsions and opisthotonus), dizziness, fever, flushing, hiccough, hypertension, tingling/numbness/coldness at injection site, twitching, and vomiting may occur. **Children:** Increased incidences of agitation, bradycardia, and jitteriness have occurred; apnea has been observed frequently. Abrupt discontinuation following prolonged infusion may result in agitation, flushing of the hands and feet, hyperirritability, and tremulousness.

Overdose: Cardiorespiratory depression (hypotension, apnea, airway obstruction, and/or oxygen desaturation).

ANTIDOTE

Keep physician informed of all side effects. Reduction of dose may be required or will be treated symptomatically. Discontinue the drug for major side effects, paradoxical reactions, or accidental overdose. A short-acting drug, a patent airway, and continuous controlled ventilation with oxygen until normal function assured should be adequate. Treat bradycardia and/or hypotension with increased rate of IV fluids, Trendelenburg position, vasopressors (e.g., dopamine [Intropin]). Anticholinergic agents (e.g., atropine or glycopyrrolate) may be required. Treat allergic reaction and resuscitate as necessary.

PROPRANOLOL HYDROCHLORIDE

(proe-pran′oh-lole hye-droe-klor′id)

Beta-adrenergic blocking agent
Antiarrhythmic

Inderal

pH 2.8 to 3.5

USUAL DOSE

0.5 to 3 mg given 1 mg at a time. If there is no change in rhythm for at least 2 minutes after the initial dose, cycle may be repeated one time. (AHA recommends 0.1 mg/kg divided into 3 equal doses and given at 2- to 3-minute intervals.) ***No further propranolol may be given by any route for at least 4 hours.*** Best results achieved if administered within 2 to 4 hours of symptom onset or thrombolytic therapy.

PEDIATRIC DOSE (UNLABELED)

0.01 to 0.1 mg/kg. Maximum dose is 1 mg. Repeat at 6- to 8-hour intervals if needed.

Tetralogy spells: 0.15 to 0.25 mg/kg/dose may be given slowly. May repeat once in 15 minutes.

DOSE ADJUSTMENTS

Lower-end initial doses may be indicated in the elderly based on potential for decreased organ function and concomitant disease or drug therapy. ▪ See Drug/Lab Interactions. ▪ Reduce dose gradually to avoid rebound angina, myocardial infarction, or ventricular arrhythmias.

DILUTION

Each 1 mg can be diluted in 10 ml of D5W or may be given undiluted. May be diluted in 50 ml of NS for infusion.

COMPATIBLE WITH

Consult pharmacist; specific conditions may apply; see Compatibilities, p. xvi.

Additive: Dobutamine (Dobutrex), verapamil (Isoptin).

Syringe: Inamrinone (Inocor), milrinone (Primacor).

Y-site: Alteplase (tPA, Activase), gatifloxacin (Tequin), heparin, hydrocortisone sodium succinate (Solu-Cortef), inamrinone (Inocor), linezolid (Zyvox), meperidine (Demerol), milrinone (Primacor), morphine, potassium chloride (KCl), propofol (Diprivan), tacrolimus (Prograf).

RATE OF ADMINISTRATION

Each 1 mg or fraction thereof must be given over 1 minute to avoid excessive hypotension and/or cardiac standstill. A single dose may be given as an infusion over 10 to 15 minutes. Allow adequate time for distribution. Observe monitor and discontinue propranolol as soon as rhythm change occurs.

Pediatric rate: Extend rate of administration of a single dose by injection to a minimum of 5 minutes in pediatric patients.

ACTIONS

Propranolol is a beta-adrenergic blocker with antiarrhythmic effects. Cardiac response to sympathetic nerve stimulation is inhibited, slowing the HR (especially ventricular rate) by inhibiting atrioventricular conduction, decreasing the force of cardiac contractility, and decreasing arterial pressure and cardiac output. Well distributed throughout the body, the onset of action occurs within 1 to 2 minutes and lasts about 4 hours. Metabolized in the liver. Some excreted in the urine.

INDICATIONS AND USES

Management of cardiac arrhythmias such as paroxysmal atrial tachycardia, sinus tachycardia, atrial or ventricular extrasystoles, atrial flutter and fibrillation, and/or arrhythmias associated with Wolff-Parkinson-White syndrome. ■ Management of tachyarrhythmia caused by digitalis intoxication, anesthesia (other than chloroform and ether, etc.), thyrotoxicosis, and catecholamines (epinephrine, norepinephrine). Reserve IV use for life-threatening situations. ■ Treatment of ventricular tachycardia and arrhythmias caused by tumor manipulation during excision of pheochromocytoma after treatment with an alpha-adrenergic blocking agent. ■ Reduce cardiac mortality, recurrent MI, and incidence of ventricular fibrillation in hemodynamically stable individuals with suspected or definite myocardial infarction. ■ Reduce BP in systolic hypertension caused by hyperdynamic beta-adrenergic circulatory state that occurs in younger persons. ■ Not the drug of choice to treat VT with the exception of those induced by catecholamines (e.g., epinephrine) or digitalis, but may be used in critical situations when cardioversion and/or other drugs are not effective or are not indicated. ■ Used orally to treat migraine and essential tremor.

CONTRAINDICATIONS

Allergic rhinitis, bronchial asthma, bronchospasm, cardiogenic shock, complete heart block, congestive heart failure (unless caused by tachycardia), chronic obstructive pulmonary disease, hypersensitivity to beta-adrenergic blocking agents, right ventricular failure caused by pulmonary hypertension, second-degree heart block, sinus bradycardia.

PRECAUTIONS

Oral administration is preferred. Use IV administration only when necessary. ■ Not considered the drug of choice for arrhythmias in myocardial infarction. ■ Used concurrently with digitalis or alpha-adrenergic blockers as indicated. ■ Use with extreme caution in asthmatics, patients with lung disease or bronchospasm, diabetics, or patients with a history of hypoglycemia. May cause hypoglycemia and mask the symptoms. ■ Discontinuation of beta-blockers before OR is controversial (beta blockade interferes with cardiac response to reflex stimuli); however, some authorities recommend administering throughout the perioperative period. May cause arrhythmia, angina, MI, or death if stopped abruptly. ■ IV dose used during surgery to replace an oral dose should be 1/10 of the oral dose. ■ May cause severe bradycardia in patients with Wolff-Parkinson-White syndrome.

Monitor: Continuous ECG and BP monitoring is mandatory during administration of IV propranolol. Monitoring of pulmonary wedge pressure or central venous pressure is recommended. Discontinue the drug when a rhythm change is noted and wait to note full effect before giving additional medication if indicated. ■ See Precautions and Drug/Lab Interactions.

Patient Education: Report any breathing difficulty promptly.

Maternal/Child: Category C: safety for use in pregnancy and breast-feeding and in children not established. Use only when clearly indicated.

Elderly: Lower-end initial doses may be indicated; see Dose Adjustments. ■ Response of elderly vs. younger patients not documented. ■ Use with caution in age-related peripheral vascular disease; risk of hypothermia increased. ■ May exacerbate mental impairment.

DRUG/LAB INTERACTIONS

Effects of both drugs may be reduced with xanthines (e.g., aminophylline) or theophylline levels may increase; monitor carefully. ▪ Cimetidine (Tagamet), haloperidol (Haldol), propafenone (Rythmol), and quinolone antibiotics (e.g., ciprofloxacin [Cipro IV]) inhibit propranolol metabolism; reduced dose may be required. Hypotension and bradycardia may be life-threatening with haloperidol. ▪ Potentiates benzodiazepines (e.g., diazepam [Valium]) by inhibiting their metabolism; consider use of atenolol (Tenormin). ▪ Potentiates ergot alkaloids (e.g., dihydroergotamine [D.H.E. 45]); monitor for peripheral ischemia; reduce ergot dose or discontinue beta-blocker. ▪ May be synergistic, additive, or toxic with other cardiac agents (e.g., calcium channel blockers [e.g., verapamil (Isoptin), diltiazem (Cardizem)], digitalis, lidocaine, phenytoin [Dilantin], procainamide [Pronestyl], quinidine). Arrhythmias, severe hypotension, and/or severe depression of the myocardium and AV conduction can result. Monitor cardiac function; decrease dose of both drugs as indicated. ▪ Added hypotensive effect with disopyramide (Norpace), diuretics (e.g., furosemide), other antihypertensive agents (e.g., enalaprilat, nitroglycerin), some phenothiazines (e.g., chlorpromazine [Thorazine]), and reserpine. Reduced dose of one or both drugs may be indicated or consider use of atenolol. ▪ Will cause severe bradycardia with MAO inhibitors (e.g., selegiline [Eldepryl]). ▪ Use with clonidine may precipitate acute hypertension or aggravate rebound hypertension if clonidine stopped abruptly; discontinue propranolol several days before gradual withdrawal of clonidine. Monitor BP with concurrent use. ▪ Antihypertensive effects inhibited by NSAIDs (e.g., ibuprofen [Advil, Motrin], indomethacin [Indocin], naproxen [Aleve, Naprosyn]); avoid combination. ▪ Effects antagonized by atropine (counteract bradycardia) and somewhat by tricyclic antidepressants (e.g., amitryptyline [Elavil]) or nefazodone (Serzone). ▪ Large doses of isoproterenol (Isuprel) may be required to overcome effects of propranolol; use extreme caution. Glucagon is safer. ▪ Use extreme caution with sympathomimetics (e.g., epinephrine); alpha receptor stimulation may be unopposed. Severe hypertension, bradycardia, and heart block can result from concurrent use (will require use of chlorpromazine, hydralazine, aminophylline, and/or atropine to treat). May be indicated in overdose of propranolol. ▪ May increase postural hypotension with prazosin (Minipress). ▪ May prolong or counteract effects of nondepolarizing muscle relaxants (e.g., pancuronium (Pavulon). ▪ May increase anticoagulant effects of warfarin. ▪ May mask symptoms of hypoglycemia with insulin and sulfonylureas and result in prolonged hypoglycemia. ▪ Reduce dose of propranolol when patients on thioamines (e.g., propylthiouracil [PTU], methimazole [Tapazole]) become euthyroid. ▪ Some authorities recommend that beta-adrenergic blockers be discontinued 48 hours before major surgery (beta blockade interferes with cardiac response to reflex stimuli). If continued, use caution administering general anesthetics that depress the myocardium (e.g., cyclopropane, trichlorethylene). ▪ BUN may be elevated in patients with impaired renal function. ▪ May increase triglycerides. ▪ Can interfere with numerous diagnostic and physiologic tests. Consult literature. ▪ Metabolism and release of catecholamines increased in smokers; increased doses may be required. May also interfere with therapeutic effects in treatment of angina.

SIDE EFFECTS

AV conduction delays, bradyarrhythmias, bronchospasm, cardiac failure, cardiac standstill, erythematous rash, hallucination, hypotension, laryngospasm, paresthesia of the hands, respiratory distress, syncopal attacks, vertigo, visual disturbances.

ANTIDOTE

For any side effect or excessive dosage, discontinue the drug and notify the physician immediately. Treat bradycardia with atropine 0.25 to 1 mg. Isoproterenol (Isuprel) may be used with caution if no response to vagal blockade. Treat cardiac failure with digitalization and diuretics. Treat hypotension with vasopressors (e.g., epinephrine [evidence suggests as the drug of choice], norepinephrine [Levophed]). Dose cautiously and monitor closely; protracted severe hypotension may result. Unresponsive hypotension and bradycardia may be reversed by glucagon 5 to 10 mg over 30 seconds, followed by a continuous infusion of 5 mg/hr (see glucagon monograph). Treat bronchospasm with isoproterenol and aminophylline. Treat other side effects symptomatically. Not significantly removed by hemodialysis or peritoneal dialysis. Resuscitate as necessary.

PROTAMINE SULFATE

(proe′ta-meen sul′fat)

Antidote (heparin antagonist)

pH 6 to 7

USUAL DOSE

1 mg for approximately every 100 USP units of heparin. May be repeated if needed in 10 to 15 minutes. Never exceed 50 mg in any 10-minute period or 100 mg in 2 hours. Dose adjusted as indicated by coagulation studies. Any dose over 100 mg in 2 hours should be justified by coagulation studies (has its own anticoagulant effect). The dose of protamine required decreases rapidly with the time elapsed after heparin injection. (30 minutes after IV heparin, 0.5 mg of protamine will neutralize 100 USP units of heparin.)

DOSE ADJUSTMENTS

Because heparin disappears rapidly from the system, reduce dose of protamine based on length of time elapsed since heparin dose (up to one half if 30 minutes has elapsed). ■ Prompt administration of protamine sulfate may also decrease dose requirements.

DILUTION

Most preparations are prediluted and ready for use. Each 50 mg of powder is diluted with 5 ml SW or bacteriostatic SW for injection. Shake vigorously. May be further diluted with at least an equal volume of NS or D5W. May be given as an infusion by diluting in a given amount of the same infusion solutions.

Storage: Refrigerate before dilution. Use immediately after dilution. Discard remaining medication. Some literature states, "Stable for 72 hr diluted with bacteriostatic water if refrigerated."

INCOMPATIBLE WITH

Manufacturer recommends not mixing with other drugs unless compatibility is known, and lists as incompatible with some antibiotics, including several cephalosporins and penicillins. Consider individualized rate adjustment necessary to produce desired effects.

COMPATIBLE WITH

Consult pharmacist; specific conditions may apply; see Compatibilities, p. xvi.

Additive: Cimetidine (Tagamet), ranitidine (Zantac), verapamil (Isoptin).

RATE OF ADMINISTRATION

50 mg (5 ml) or fraction thereof over 10 minutes. Do not exceed 50 mg in 10 minutes. As an infusion, may be given over 2 to 3 hours with dosage titrated according to coagulation studies. Use infusion pump or microdrip (60 gtt/ml) to administer. Too-rapid administration can cause anaphylaxis, bradycardia, dyspnea, flushing, sensation of warmth, or severe hypotension. Hypertension has also occurred.

ACTIONS

An anticoagulant if administered alone. In the presence of heparin, protamine forms a stable salt, neutralizing the anticoagulant effect of both drugs. Each 1 mg of protamine can neutralize approximately 100 USP units of heparin. Onset of action is within 0.5 to 1 minute. Duration of action is about 2 hours.

INDICATIONS AND USES

To neutralize the anticoagulant activity of heparin in severe heparin overdosage. ■ Neutralization of heparin administered during extracorporeal circulation in arterial and cardiac surgery or dialysis procedures.

CONTRAINDICATIONS

None when used as indicated.

PRECAUTIONS

Potential for hypersensitivity increased in patients with allergies to fish, previous exposure to protamine (e.g., protamine insulin), and in infertile or vasectomized men (may have antiprotamine antibodies). ■ Pulmonary edema and/or circulatory collapse may occur in patients undergoing cardiac bypass surgery; etiology unknown.

Monitor: Facilities to treat shock must be available. ■ After cardiac surgery, even with adequate neutralization, further bleeding may occur any time within 24 hours (heparin "rebound"). Observe the patient continuously. Additional protamine sulfate may be indicated.

Maternal/Child: Category C: safety for use in pregnancy, breast-feeding, or children not established.

SIDE EFFECTS

Occur more frequently with too-rapid injection; anaphylaxis, back pain, bradycardia, dyspnea, feeling of warmth, flushing, lethargy, nausea, severe hypertension or hypotension, vomiting. Acute pulmonary hypertension, capillary leak and noncardiogenic pulmonary edema, circulatory collapse, or pulmonary edema may occur.

ANTIDOTE

Discontinue the drug and notify the physician, who may recommend a decrease in rate of administration or, if side effects are severe, symptomatic treatment such as administration of whole blood, vasopressors (e.g., dopamine [Intropin]) for hypotension, atropine for bradycardia, and oxygen for dyspnea. Resuscitate as necessary.

PROTEIN (AMINO ACID) PRODUCTS

Nutritional therapy

(pro′ten [ah-me′no as′id] prod′ukts)

Aminess 5.2% with histadine ▪ Aminosyn 3.5%, 3.5% M, 5%, 7%, 8.5% ▪ Aminosyn 7%, 8.5%, and 10% with electrolytes ▪ Aminosyn (pH 6) 7%, 8.5%, and 10% ▪ Aminosyn HBC 7% ▪ Aminosyn HF 8% ▪ Aminosyn II 7%, 8.5%, 10%, and 15% ▪ Aminosyn II 8.5% and 10% with electrolytes ▪ Aminosyn II 3.5% in D5 or D25 ▪ Aminosyn II 5% in D25 ▪ Aminosyn II 4.25% in D10, D20, and D25 ▪ Aminosyn II 3.5% in D25 with electrolytes and calcium ▪ Aminosyn II 4.25% in D20, D25 with electrolytes and calcium ▪ Aminosyn PF 7% and 10% ▪ Aminosyn RF 5.2% ▪ 4% Branch Amin ▪ Clinimix 2.75% (sulfite free [SF]) in D5, D10, and D25 ▪ Clinimix 4.25% (SF) in D5, D10, D20, and D25 ▪ Clinimix 5% (SF) in D10, D15, D20, D25, and D35 ▪ Clinimix E 2.75% (SF) in D5, D10, D25 with electrolytes and calcium ▪ Clinimix E 4.25% (SF) in D5, D10, D20, and D25 with electrolytes and calcium ▪ Clinimix E 5% (SF) in D10, D15, D20, D25, and D35 with electrolytes and calcium ▪ Clinisol 15% (SF) ▪ Crystalline amino acid infusions ▪ FreAmine HBC 6.9% ▪ FreAmine III 8.5%, 10%, and 3% and 8.5% with electrolytes ▪ HepaAmine 8% ▪ Hepatosol 8% ▪ Hyperalimentation ▪ NephrAmine 5.4% ▪ Novamine 11.4% and 15% ▪ ProcalAmine ▪ ProSol 20% (sulfite free) ▪ Protein hydrolysates ▪ RenAmin without electrolytes ▪ Total parenteral nutrition ▪ Travasol 2.75% and 4.25% in D5, D10, D15, D20, and D25 ▪ Travasol 2.75% and 4.25% (SF) in D5, D10, D15, D20, and D25 with electrolytes ▪ Travasol 5.5%, 8.5%, and 10% without electrolytes ▪ Travasol 5.5% and 8.5% with electrolytes ▪ Travasol (SF) 3.5%, 5.5%, and 10% with electrolytes ▪ TrophaAmine 6% and 10%

pH 5 to 7

USUAL DOSE

0.5 to 2 Gm/kg of body weight/24 hr. Actual dose will depend on several factors including protein requirements, disease state, physical condition, and weight. Protein amino acid products are available in general, renal failure, hepatic failure/encephalopathy, and metabolic stress formulations. See Precautions/Monitor.

PEDIATRIC INFANT DOSE

Consult pharmacist; not all products approved for use in pediatric patients. Amino acid formulations developed specifically for nutritional support of infants and children are available (e.g., Aminosyn P/F sulfite free).

1.5 to 3 Gm/kg of body weight/24 hr. Actual dose will depend on several factors including age, protein requirements, disease state, physical condition, and weight. Infants and children require different percentages of all components. Another source suggests an average TPN maintenance dose of 2.5 Gm amino acids/kg/day. Dextrose kcal (nutritional calories) must be added (range is from 100 to 300 kcal/kg/day). Another source recommends specific total nonprotein calories by weight; ***less than 10 kg,*** 100 cal/kg; ***10 to 20 kg,*** 1,000 calories plus 50 cal/kg for each kg over 10; ***greater than 20 kg,*** 1,500 calories plus 20 cal/kg for each kg over 20. Total may include IV fat calories.

DILUTION

Dilute under strict aseptic techniques according to manufacturer's specific instructions. Some solutions are very concentrated; are for compounding only, not for direct infusion. Check label for aluminum content; see Precautions. Most commonly mixed with dextrose (nonprotein calorie source), electrolytes, vitamins, and trace elements to provide total parenteral nutrition (TPN) or peripheral parenteral nutrition (PPN). Intravenous lipids, providing a second nonprotein calorie source and a source of essential fatty acids, may be mixed with the dextrose/amino acid solution or run simultaneously. Use promptly after mixing; laminar flow hood preferred; refrigerate briefly if necessary, and discard any unused portion. Use only clear solutions; observe against adequate light for particulate matter or evidence of container damage.

Storage: Manufacturer recommends refrigeration after any additives (e.g., IV lipids, electrolytes, minerals) are added. Some preparations can be refrigerated for only short periods, preferably no more than 24 hours. When prepared for home use, some preparations have been refrigerated for up to 14 days (dextrose and amino acids) or up to 7 days with lipids added. Leave vitamins (e.g., M.V.I.) out until time of administration. Consult pharmacist.

INCOMPATIBLE WITH

Most incompatibilities relate to the preparation (chloride as opposed to phosphate), amount of medication added, other additives present, and thoroughness of mixing. Consult with the pharmacist before mixing any drugs in protein (amino acid) products. Many TPN solutions contain some phosphate. The addition of calcium salts may cause a precipitate. These additives must be mixed by the pharmacist. Specific amounts, calculations, temperature (precipitate forms more readily at room temperature), and order of dilution are required.

COMPATIBLE WITH **(Underline Indicates Conflicting Compatibility Information)**

Consult pharmacist; specific conditions may apply; see Compatibilities, p. xvi. Manufacturers suggest that only required nutritional products should be added, but H_2 receptors (e.g., cimetidine [Tagamet], ranitidine [Zantac]), insulin, and heparin are frequently added to selected products. Other drugs may be compatible for specific lengths of time.

Solution: <u>Fat emulsion 10% IV.</u>

Additive: Amikacin (Amikin), aminophylline, <u>ampicillin</u>, aztreonam (Azactam), calcium gluconate, cefamandole (Mandol), cefazolin (Kefzol), cefepime (Maxipime), cefotaxime (Claforan), cefoxitin (Mefoxin), ceftazidime (Fortaz), ceftriaxone (Rocephin), cefuroxime (Zinacef), cimetidine (Tagamet), clindamycin (Cleocin), cyclophosphamide (Cytoxan), cyclosporine (Sandimmune), cytarabine (ARA-C), dopamine (Intropin), epoetin alfa (Epogen, Procrit), famotidine (Pepcid IV), fluorouracil (5-FU), folic acid (Folvite), fosphenytoin (Cerebyx), furosemide (Lasix), gentamicin (Garamycin), heparin, hydrochloric acid, insulin (regular), iron dextran, isoproterenol (Isuprel), kanamycin (Kantrex), lidocaine, meperidine (Demerol), methotrexate (Folex), methyldopate (Aldomet), methylprednisolone (Solu-Medrol), metoclopramide (Reglan), midazolam (Versed), morphine, multivitamins (M.V.I.), nafcillin (Nafcil), norepinephrine (Levophed), octreotide (Sandostatin), ondansetron (Zofran), oxacillin (Bactocill), penicillin G potassium and sodium, phytonadione (Aquamephyton), potassium phosphate, ranitidine (Zantac), sodium bicarbonate, tacrolimus (Prograf), ticarcillin (Ticar), tobramycin (Nebcin), vancomycin (Vancocin).

Y-site: Aldesleukin (Proleukin, IL-2), amikacin (Amikin), aminophylline, ampicillin, ampicillin/sulbactam (Unasyn), ascorbic acid (Cenolate), atracurium (Tracrium), aztreonam (Azactam), bumetanide (Bumex), buprenorphine (Buprenex), butorphanol (Stadol), calcium gluconate, carboplatin (Paraplatin), cefamandole (Mandol), cefazolin (Kefzol), cefoperazone (Cefobid), cefotaxime (Claforan), cefotetan (Cefotan), cefoxitin (Mefoxin), ceftazidime (Fortaz), ceftizoxime (Cefizox), ceftriaxone (Rocephin), cefuroxime (Zinacef), chloramphenicol (Chloromycetin), chlorpromazine (Thorazine), cimetidine (Tagamet), ciprofloxacin (Cipro IV), cisplatin (Platinol), clindamycin (Cleocin), cyclophosphamide (Cytoxan), cyclosporine (Sandimmune), cytarabine (ARA-C), dexamethasone (Decadron), diazepam (Valium), digoxin (Lanoxin), diphenhydramine (Benadryl), dobutamine (Dobutrex), dopamine (Intropin), doxycycline (Vibramycin), droperidol (Inapsine), enalaprilat (Vasotec IV), epinephrine (Adrenalin), erythromycin lactobionate (Erythrocin), famotidine (Pepcid IV), fentanyl (Sublimaze), fluconazole (Diflucan), fluorouracil (5-FU), folic acid (Folvite), foscarnet (Foscavir), furosemide (Lasix), ganciclovir (Cytovene), gentamicin (Garamycin), granisetron (Kytril), haloperidol (Haldol), heparin, hydrocortisone (Hydrocortone, Solu-Cortef), hydromorphone (Dilaudid), idarubicin (Idamycin), ifosfamide (Ifex), imipenem/cilastatin (Primaxin), insulin (regular), isoproterenol (Isuprel), kanamycin (Kantrex), leucovorin calcium, levorphanol (Levo-Dromoran), lidocaine, linezolid (Zyvox), lorazepam (Ativan), magnesium sulfate, mannitol, meperidine (Demerol), meropenem (Merrem IV), mesna (Mesnex), methotrexate (Folex), methyldopate (Aldomet), methylprednisolone (Solu-Medrol), metoclopramide (Reglan), metronidazole (Flagyl IV), milrinone (Primacor), mitoxantrone (Novantrone), morphine, multivitamins (M.V.I.), nafcillin (Nafcil), nalbuphine (Nubain), nitroglycerin (Nitro-Bid IV), nitroprusside sodium, norepinephrine (Levophed), octreotide (Sandostatin), ofloxacin (Floxin IV), ondansetron (Zofran), oxacillin (Bactocill), paclitaxel (Taxol), penicillin G potassium, pentobarbital (Nembutal), phenobarbital (Luminal), piperacillin (Pipracil), piperacillin/tazobactam (Zosyn), potassium chloride (KCl), prochlorperazine (Compazine), promethazine (Phenergan), propofol (Diprivan), ranitidine (Zantac), sargramostim (Leukine), sodium bicarbonate, sulfamethoxazole-trimethoprim (Bactrim), tacrolimus (Prograf), thiotepa (Thioplex), ticarcillin (Ticar), ticarcillin/clavulanate (Timentin), tobramycin (Nebcin), vancomycin (Vancocin), vecuronium (Norcuron), zidovudine (AZT, Retrovir).

RATE OF ADMINISTRATION

Begin parenteral nutrition at 1 to 2 ml/min and increase gradually as tolerated until the target rate is reached. With the correct parenteral nutrition formulation, fluid, protein, and calorie requirements should be met at the target rate. ***Total daily dose should be evenly distributed over the 24-hour period. Maintain a constant drip rate.*** Use of infusion pump and microfilter (0.22 micron for dextrose and amino acids, 1.2 micron for solutions with lipids [3 in 1]) recommended. Precipitate very difficult to detect in solutions that contain lipids. There are specific situations (e.g., cyclic TPN primarily used in home care patients) where a daily dose is given over less than 24 hours. Range is from 10 to 14 hours. Usually administered overnight, allowing individuals requiring prolonged TPN to maintain their daytime activities.

Pediatric rate: Usually begin with a one-half strength nutritional solution at 60 to 70 ml/kg/day. May be gradually increased over 48 hours until full strength and increased to 125 to 150 ml/kg/day. See all comments under Rate of Administration/Adult.

ACTIONS

Supplies essential and nonessential amino acids and calories with the intent of promoting protein production (anabolism) and preventing protein breakdown (catabolism), promotes wound healing, and acts as a buffer in intracellular and extracellular body fluids. Various brands supply additional calories with alcohol, fructose, or glucose. These additional calories permit available protein to be used for repair of tissue in addition to meeting basic caloric needs.

INDICATIONS AND USES

To prevent nitrogen loss or to reverse negative nitrogen balance in severe illness when oral alimentation is not practical for prolonged periods or normal GI absorption is impaired.

CONTRAINDICATIONS

Hypersensitivity to any component, acidosis, anuria, azotemia, decreased circulating blood volume, severe liver disease, metabolic disorders with impaired amino acid metabolization.

PRECAUTIONS

Catheter insertion for administration of central parenteral nutrition is a sterile surgical procedure (must be a large vein [subclavian or superior vena cava preferred]; 50% glucose is a sclerosing solution). ■ Peripheral veins are suitable for specific products (peripheral parenteral nutrition) when amino acid products are diluted with 2.5%, 5%, or 10% dextrose. ■ Amino acids given without carbohydrates may cause ketone accumulation. ■ Use caution in impaired hepatic function; may cause serum amino acid imbalances, metabolic alkalosis, prerenal azotemia, hyperammonemia, stupor, and coma. ■ Use caution in impaired renal function; may further increase BUN. ■ Fatty infiltration of the liver, acute respiratory failure, and difficulty in weaning hypermetabolic patients from the respirator may be caused by excessive carbohydrate calories. ■ Some solutions may contain aluminum. In impaired kidney function, aluminum may reach toxic levels. Premature neonates are particularly at risk because of their immature kidneys and requirement for calcium and phosphate, which also contain aluminum. Research indicates that patients with impaired renal function who receive greater than 4 to 5 mcg/kg/day of parenteral aluminum are at risk for developing CNS or bone toxicity associated with aluminum accumulation. ■ Essential fatty acid deficiency has been observed in patients on long-term TPN (more than 5 days). The use of fat emulsion to provide 4% to 10% of total caloric intake as linoleic acid may help to prevent this deficiency.

Monitor: Specific baseline studies required before administration: CBC, platelet count, PT, BUN, SrCr, electrolytes, glucose, triglycerides, cholesterol, albumin, bilirubin, liver function tests (e.g., AST, ALT, LDH), weight, body length and head circumference (in infants), and immunocompetence. Repeat lab tests as indicated during therapy. ■ Monitor intake and output, weight, and during stabilization (3 to 5 days), measure urine glucose, and ketones every shift. After stabilization, measurement of urine glucose and ketones every 8 hours is suggested. ■ Follow a strict, regular aseptic routine to care for insertion site. ■ Single-port central venous catheters to be used only for the nutritional regimen. Do not draw blood samples, transfuse blood, or administer other medications. Pseudoagglutination and thrombosis can occur, risk of contamination is great, and validity of results is compromised. Multiple-port central venous catheters may be used for these additional procedures. Observe specific protocols. ■ Monitor BUN frequently. Discontinue infusion if BUN exceeds normal postprandial limits and continues to rise. ■ Blood ammonia levels important, especially in infants. ■ Check frequently for any signs of extravasation. ■ Observe for any signs of infection. ■ Additional insulin coverage may be required, especially when dosage is increased too rapidly or with maximum doses. ■ To prevent rebound hypoglycemia, decrease rate gradually over at least 24 hours to discontinue administration. Follow with use of fluids containing 5% to 10% dextrose for several days. ■ Discard any single bottle after 24 hours. Replace administration set every 24 to 48 hours.

Maternal/Child: Use hypertonic dextrose (component of parenteral nutrition) with extreme caution in low-birth-weight or septic infants. May cause hyperglycemia, hypoglycemia, or increased serum osmolality with possible intracerebral hemorrhage. Monitor serum glucose frequently. Solutions administered by peripheral vein should not exceed 718 mOsm/L. ■ Hyperammonemia is of particular significance in infants. Can cause mental retardation; measure blood ammonia frequently.

Elderly: Differences in responses between elderly and younger patients have not been identified. ■ Lower end initial doses may be appropriate in the elderly based on the potential for decreased organ function and concomitant disease or drug therapy.

DRUG/LAB INTERACTIONS

Tetracycline may reduce protein-sparing effects.

SIDE EFFECTS

Abdominal pains, anaphylaxis, bone demineralization, changes in levels of consciousness, convulsions, dehydration, edema at the site of injection, electrolyte imbalances, glycosuria, hyperammonemia, hyperglycemia, hyperpyrexia, hypertension, metabolic acidosis and/or alkalosis, osmotic dehydration, phlebitis and thrombosis, pulmonary edema, rebound hypoglycemia, septicemia, vasodilation, vomiting, weakness.

ANTIDOTE

Notify the physician of all side effects. An alternate brand may cause fewer problems, or amounts of glucose or additives may be adjusted to correct the problem. Many of the side effects listed will respond to a reduced rate. Some will require catheter insertion at a new site. Treat symptomatically and resuscitate as necessary. Stop infusion immediately for any signs of acute respiratory distress. May represent pulmonary embolus or interstitial pneumonitis, which may be caused by a precipitate of electrolytes (e.g., calcium and phosphates) in the solution.

PYRIDOXINE HYDROCHLORIDE

(peer-i-dox′een hye-droe-klor′id)

Nutritional supplement (vitamin)
Antidote

Vitamin B_6

pH 2 to 3.8

USUAL DOSE

Pyridoxine dependency syndrome: 30 to 600 mg/day.

Drug-induced pyridoxine deficiency: 50 to 200 mg/day for 3 weeks. Follow with 25 to 100 mg/day as needed.

Prophylaxis or treatment of pyridoxine deficiency in patients receiving parenteral nutrition: May be added to parenteral nutrition; dose will depend on patient condition.

INH poisoning (greater than 10 Gm) (unlabeled): 4 Gm IV followed by 1 Gm IM every 30 minutes. Total pyridoxine dose should equal ingested INH dose.

Cycloserine poisoning (unlabeled): 300 mg/day. Higher doses may be required.

Hydrazine poisoning (unlabeled): 25 mg/kg. Give one third of dose IM and remainder as a 3-hour infusion.

Gyrometra mushroom poisoning (unlabeled): 25 mg/kg over 15 to 30 minutes. Repeat as needed.

PEDIATRIC DOSE

Pyridoxine-dependent seizures: 10 to 100 mg.

DOSE ADJUSTMENTS

Removed by hemodialysis. Dialysis patients may require higher doses.

DILUTION

May be given by IV injection undiluted or added to most IV solutions and given as an infusion. See chart on inside back cover.

Storage: Store below 40° C unless otherwise stated by manufacturer. Deteriorates in excessive heat; protect from heat and light.

INCOMPATIBLE WITH

Manufacturer lists alkaline solutions, iron salts, oxidizing solutions.

COMPATIBLE WITH

Consult pharmacist; specific conditions may apply; see Compatibilities, p. xvi.

Solution: Fat emulsion 10% IV.

Syringe: Doxapram (Dopram).

RATE OF ADMINISTRATION

50 mg or fraction thereof over 1 minute if given undiluted.

ACTIONS

Vitamin B_6 is water soluble. It is a coenzyme necessary for the metabolism of proteins, carbohydrates, and lipids. Involved in many reactions including the conversion of tryptophan to nicotinamide and serotonin, breakdown to glucose-1-phosphate, synthesis of gamma aminobutyric acid (GABA) in the CNS (energy transformation in brain and nerve cells), and synthesis of heme. Metabolized by the liver, and excreted in the urine.

INDICATIONS AND USES

Prophylaxis and treatment of pyridoxine deficiency. Deficiency may be due to inadequate diet, inborn error of metabolism or concomitant drug use.

Unlabeled uses: Treatment of INH, hydrazine, and cycloserine poisoning. Treatment of neurologic effects of Gyrometra mushroom poisoning. Nausea and vomiting associated with pregnancy.

CONTRAINDICATIONS

Known sensitivity to pyridoxine.

PRECAUTIONS

Used IV only when oral dosage not acceptable. ■ Deficiency can cause abnormal EEG. ■ Need for pyridoxine increases with amount of protein in diet. Chronic administration of large doses may cause adverse neurologic effects.

Maternal/Child: Category A: requirements are increased in pregnancy and breast-feeding. Do not exceed RDA. ■ Large doses in utero can cause pyridoxine-dependency syndrome in newborn. ■ May inhibit breast-feeding. ■ Safety for use in children not established.

DRUG/LAB INTERACTIONS

An antagonist to levodopa. Does not antagonize carbidopa/levodopa combination (Sinemet). ■ Isoniazid is a vitamin B_6 antagonist and will cause deficiency disease. ■ Cycloserine, penicillamine, hydralazine, oral contraceptives may increase pyridoxine requirements. ■ May decrease phenobarbital and phenytoin (Dilantin) levels. ■ Excessive doses may elevate AST.

SIDE EFFECTS

Almost nonexistent; some slight flushing or feeling of warmth may occur. With larger doses, ataxia, low folic acid levels, paresthesias, somnolence, and withdrawal seizures in infants with high maternal doses may occur.

ANTIDOTE

No antidote is known or has been needed. Symptomatic treatment of side effects may be indicated.

QUINIDINE GLUCONATE INJECTION

Antiarrhythmic

(kwin′i-deen glu-ko′nat in-jek′shun)

pH 5.5 to 7

USUAL DOSE

Antiarrhythmic: A test dose of 200 mg IM for idiosyncrasy is desired if time permits. 200 mg. Repeat as indicated to control arrhythmia. 330 mg or less effective in most patients. Up to 1 Gm has been required. Maintain with an oral quinidine preparation. Do not exceed 5 Gm total dose in 24 hours. ***Plasmodium falciparum* malaria:** A loading dose of 15 mg/kg in 250 ml NS as an infusion over 4 hours. 24 hours from initial dose begin 7.5 mg/kg in 125 to 250 ml NS over 4 hours. Repeat every 8 hours for 7 days or transfer to oral therapy. An alternate regimen is a loading dose of 10 mg/kg in 250 ml NS as an infusion over 1 to 2 hours. Follow immediately with 0.02 mg/kg/min for up to 72 hours, until parasitemia less than 1% or transferred to oral therapy.

PEDIATRIC DOSE

2 to 10 mg/kg every 3 to 6 hours. Use IV only when other routes not possible.

DOSE ADJUSTMENTS

Reduced dose may be indicated in the elderly based on potential for decreased organ function and concomitant disease or drug therapy. ■ See Drug/Lab Interactions.

DILUTION

800 mg (10 ml) must be diluted in at least 40 ml of D5W. 1 ml of properly diluted solution equals 16 mg quinidine. Use only clear, colorless solutions. May be adsorbed to PVC tubing; minimize tubing length.

Storage: Store at CRT. Protect from light.

COMPATIBLE WITH

(Underline Indicates Conflicting Compatibility Information)

Consult pharmacist; specific conditions may apply; see Compatibilities, p. xvi.

Additive: Bretylium (Bretylate), cimetidine (Tagamet), milrinone (Primacor), ranitidine (Zantac), verapamil (Isoptin).

Y-site: <u>Diazepam (Valium)</u>, <u>heparin</u>, milrinone (Primacor).

RATE OF ADMINISTRATION

1 ml (16 mg) or fraction thereof of properly diluted solution over 1 minute. Do not exceed a rate of 0.25 mg/kg/min. Use an infusion pump or microdrip (60 gtt/ml). Too-rapid administration may cause a marked decrease in arterial pressure.

ACTIONS

A dextro-isomer of quinine. Exerts a depressing antiarrhythmic action on the heart, slowing the rate, slowing conduction, reducing myocardial contractility, and prolonging the refractory period. Increases potassium levels within the cells while it decreases sodium levels. Can have a vasodilating effect. Onset of action occurs when an effective blood concentration has been reached (15 to 30 minutes usually) and lasts 4 to 6 hours. Metabolized in the liver; most of the drug is excreted in the urine. Crosses placental barrier. Secreted in breast milk.

INDICATIONS AND USES

Cardiac arrhythmias, including atrial fibrillation, atrial flutter, premature asystoles, supraventricular tachycardia, ventricular tachycardia, and paroxysmal rhythms. ■ Treatment of life-threatening *Plasmodium falciparum* malaria.

CONTRAINDICATIONS

Partial AV or complete heart block, any severe intraventricular conduction defects (including digitalis toxicity), aberrant impulses and abnormal rhythms due to escape mechanism, history of drug-induced torsades de pointes, history of long QT syndrome, known hypersensitivity to quinidine or cinchona (e.g., febrile reactions, skin eruption, thrombocytopenia), myasthenia gravis, history of thrombocytopenic purpura with quinidine administration. ***Contraindicated with ritonavir (Norvir).***

PRECAUTIONS

Oral or IM administration is route of choice. ■ Use extreme caution in first- or second-degree blocks, extensive myocardial damage, digitalis intoxication, and impaired liver or kidney function. ■ Use caution in atrial flutter or fibrillation; may require pretreatment with digitalis to prevent progressive reduction of AV block and an extremely rapid ventricular rate. ■ Any other antiarrhythmic agent may cause new, increased, or more severe arrhythmias (e.g., more frequent PVCs, ventricular tachycardia or fibrillation, torsades de pointes). ■ Lidocaine or procainamide is generally used in preference to quinidine. ■ Doses used for *P. falciparum* malaria may cause hypotension, increased QRS and QT intervals, and cinchonism (e.g., dizziness, ringing in ears). ■ Some clinicians recommend giving a dose the night before surgery and then discontinuing until after surgery. If arrhythmia occurs, use lidocaine for ventricular arrhythmias and calcium channel blockers (e.g., verapamil) or beta-blockers (e.g., atenolol, propranolol) for supraventricular arrhythmias. Resume dosing postop and utilize oral dosing as soon as possible. ■ See Drug/Lab Interactions.

Monitor: Monitor patient's ECG and BP continuously (plus parasitemia in malaria). Too-rapid administration may cause a marked decrease in arterial pressure. ■ Keep patient in supine position. ■ Discontinue IV use when the normal sinus rhythm returns, HR falls to 120 beats/min, or any signs of cardiac toxicity occur (increased PR and QT intervals, over a 50% prolongation of QRS complex, or P waves disappear). ■ Monitor serum levels if quinidine is used over 48 hours. ■ See Drug/Lab Interactions.

Patient Education: Report breathing difficulty, dizziness, headache, nausea, ringing in the ears, skin rash, or visual disturbances promptly.

Maternal/Child: Category C: safety for use in pregnancy not established, but no congenital defects have been reported in years of use. ■ Safety for use in breast-feeding and in children not established.

Elderly: Reduced dose may be indicated; see Dose Adjustments. ■ Half-life prolonged; frequency and severity of side effects may be increased. ■ Response of elderly vs. younger patients not documented.

DRUG/LAB INTERACTIONS

Potentiates or is potentiated by other antiarrhythmics (e.g., amiodarone [Cordarone]), anticholinergics (e.g., atropine), anticoagulants, antihypertensive agents, cimetidine (Tagamet), nondepolarizing neuromuscular blockers (e.g., tubocurarine, mivacurium), neuromuscular blocking antibiotics (e.g., kanamycin [Kantrex]), phenothiazines (e.g., prochlorperazine [Compazine]), reserpine, succinylcholine, thiazide diuretics, tricyclic antidepressants (e.g., amitriptyline [Elavil]), urinary alkalinizers, and others. May produce fatal cardiac arrhythmias, prolonged neuromuscular block, and other serious side effects. ■ Contraindicated with ritonavir (Norvir); may cause life-threatening arrhythmias. ■ Use caution with digoxin, procainamide, metoprolol, and propranolol. Lower doses of both drugs may be required. ■ Inhibited by barbiturates (e.g., phenobarbital), cholinergic agents (e.g., edrophonium, neostigmine), nifedipine, phenytoin (Dilantin), and rifampin; adjust dose. ■ May cause severe hypotension with verapamil, especially in patients with hypertrophic cardiomyopathy. ■ Increased levels of disopyramide (Norpace) and decreased levels of quinidine occur when used together. ■ May decrease analgesic activity of codeine. ■ Metabolism may be decreased and serum levels increased with concurrent use of itraconazole (Sporanox); monitoring of quinidine levels suggested. ■ A case report suggests concurrent use with erythromycin may increase serum levels of quinidine. ■ May cause increased serum skeletal muscle creatine phosphokinase. ■ Triamterene (Dyrenium) interferes with fluorescent measurement of serum levels. ■ Grapefruit juice may affect certain enzymes of the P_{450} enzyme system and should be avoided.

SIDE EFFECTS

Apprehension, cramps, deafness (transitory), diaphoresis, fever, headache, nausea, rash, tinnitus, urge to defecate, urge to void, vertigo, visual disturbances, vomiting.

Major: Potentially fatal arrhythmias including atrioventricular heart block, cardiac standstill, prolonged PR or QT intervals, or 50% widening of QRS complex, tachycardia, ventricular fibrillation, acidosis, arthralgia, coma, confusion, hypokalemia, hypotension (acute), lethargy, myalgia, paresthesia, respiratory depression or arrest, thrombocytopenia purpura, seizures, urticaria.

ANTIDOTE

Notify the physician of any side effects. If minor symptoms progress or any major side effect appears, discontinue the drug immediately and notify the physician. Use fluid replacement and dopamine (Intropin) or norepinephrine (Levophed) to correct hypotension and ⅙ M sodium lactate to block effects of quinidine on the myocardium. Use phenytoin (Dilantin) or lidocaine for tachyarrhythmias. In overdose, monitoring of blood gases, electrolytes, and acidification of urine (avoid alkalinization) are indicated; cardiac pacing may be required. Treatment of toxicity is symptomatic and supportive. Hemodialysis may be indicated. Do not administer CNS depressants in overdose. Resuscitate as necessary. Depending on original arrhythmia, procainamide or lidocaine is effective alternate.

QUINUPRISTIN/DALFOPRISTIN

(kwin′oo-pris′tin/dal′foh-pris-tin)

Synercid

Antibacterial (Streptogramin)

pH 4.5 to 4.75

USUAL DOSE

Vancomycin-resistant *Enterococcus faecium:* 7.5 mg/kg every 8 hours. Duration of therapy based on site and severity of infection.

Complicated skin and skin structure infection: 7.5 mg/kg every 12 hours. Minimum recommended duration of therapy is 7 days.

PEDIATRIC DOSE

Safety and effectiveness for use in patients under 16 years of age have not been established. Doses of 7.5 mg/kg every 8 or 12 hours have been used under emergency-use conditions in a limited number of pediatric patients; see Maternal/Child.

DOSE ADJUSTMENTS

No dose adjustments required in the elderly, pediatric patients, patients with renal insufficiency, or patients undergoing hemodialysis or peritoneal dialysis. See Maternal/Child. ■ Dose reduction may be required in patients with hepatic cirrhosis (Child Pugh A or B). Exact recommendations are not currently available, but one source recommends decreasing dose to 5 mg/kg in patients who cannot tolerate the usual dose. ■ Patients experiencing arthralgias and myalgias may respond to a reduction in dose frequency to every 12 hours; see Precautions. ■ See Drug/Lab Interactions.

DILUTION

Available in 500-mg vials (150 mg quinupristin and 350 mg dalfopristin). Reconstitute single-dose vial by slowly adding 5 ml of D5W or SW. Swirl gently to limit foam formation. Do not shake. Allow solution to sit until foam has disappeared. Final concentration of reconstituted solution is 100 mg/ml. Must be further diluted, withdraw calculated dose and add to 250 ml of D5W. Desired concentration is approximately 2 mg/ml. If moderate to severe venous irritation occurs following peripheral administration, consideration should be given to increasing infusion volume to 500 to 750 ml of D5W; see Precautions. An infusion volume of 100 ml may be used for central line infusions.

Storage: Store unopened vials in refrigerator at 2° to 8° C (36° to 46° F). Reconstituted solution should be used within 30 minutes. Diluted solution is stable for 5 hours at CRT and for 54 hours if refrigerated.

INCOMPATIBLE WITH

Manufacturer lists saline solutions and heparin and recommends administering separately. Always flush line with D5W before and after administration of any other drug through the same IV line.

COMPATIBLE WITH

Consult pharmacist; specific conditions may apply; see Compatibilities, p. xvi.

Y-site: Manufacturer lists specific concentrations of aztreonam (Azactam [20 mg/ml]), ciprofloxacin (Cipro IV [1 mg/ml]), fluconazole (Diflucan [2 mg/ml]), haloperidol (Haldol [0.2 mg/ml]), metoclopramide (Reglan [5 mg/ml]), and potassium chloride (KCl [40 mEq/L]).

RATE OF ADMINISTRATION

Flush IV line with D5W before and after administration. A single dose properly diluted over 60 minutes. Use of an infusion pump or device to control rate of infusion is recommended. In animal studies toxicity was higher when administered as a bolus. Studies in humans have not been performed.

ACTIONS

A streptogramin antimicrobial agent composed of two semisynthetic pristinamycin derivatives, quinupristin and dalfopristin, in a ratio of 30:70 (w:w). Streptogramins are functionally related to the macrolide (e.g., erythromycin) and lincosamide (e.g., clindamycin) classes of antibiotics through their proposed mechanism of action. Quinupristin and dalfopristin are thought to enter bacterial cells and irreversibly bind to different sites on the 50 S ribosomal subunit. Binding leads to inhibition of protein synthesis and often results in cell death. Each component alone is bacteriostatic. When combined, the two components work synergistically and are bactericidal against specific gram-positive organisms including vancomycin-resistant and multi-drug resistant strains of *Enterococcus faecium, Staphylococcus aureus* (methicillin-susceptible strains only), and *Streptococcus pyogenes.* Recent studies show that it may be active against additional organisms; consult manufacturer. Cross resistance between quinupristin/dalfopristin and other antibacterial agents such as beta-lactams, aminoglycosides, glycopeptides, quinolones, macrolides, lincosamides and tetracyclines has not been reported. The bactericidal activity seen with quinupristin/dalfopristin is not seen with the macrolide and lincosamide antibiotics. Quinupristin/dalfopristin has improved activity against pathogens resistant to macrolides and lincosamides as well as some pathogens resistant to beta-lactams and glycopeptide antibiotics. Metabolized in the liver via non-enzymatic processes to several active metabolites. Elimination half-life of quinupristin and dalfopristin is approximately 0.85 and 0.7 hours, respectively. Although the elimination half-life for each component is short, the combination exhibits a prolonged post-antibiotic effect of 10 hours with *Staphylococcus aureus* and 9.1 hours with *Streptococcus pneumoniae.* Fecal excretion is the primary elimination route for both components and their metabolites. Urinary excretion accounts for about 15% of the quinupristin and 19% of the dalfopristin dose.

INDICATIONS AND USES

Treatment of adult patients with serious or life-threatening infections associated with vancomycin-resistant *Enterococcus faecium* (VREF) bacteremia. ■ Treatment of complicated skin and skin structure infections caused by *Staphylococcus aureus* (methicillin susceptible) or *Streptococcus pyogenes.*

CONTRAINDICATIONS

Known hypersensitivity to quinupristin/dalfopristin or to other streptogramins (e.g., pristinamycin or virginiamycin).

PRECAUTIONS

Not active against *Enterococcus faecalis.* Differentiation of enterococcal species is important to avoid misidentification of *Enterococcus faecalis* as *Enterococcus faecium.* ■ C/S indicated to determine susceptibility of causative organism to quinupristin/dalfopristin. ■ Quinupristin/dalfopristin's approval for the treatment of patients with serious or life-threatening infections associated with VREF bacteremia was approved for marketing under the FDA accelerated approval regulations that allow marketing of products for use in life-threatening conditions when other therapies are not available. Approval of drugs under these regulations is based on a demonstrated effect on a surrogate endpoint that is likely to predict clinical benefit. Quinupristin/dalfopristin's ability to clear VREF from the bloodstream is the surrogate endpoint. There are currently no well-controlled studies that confirm the validity of this surrogate endpoint. However, a study to verify the clinical benefit of therapy using traditional clinical endpoints (such as cure of underlying infection) is currently under way. ■ Flush line with D5W after completion of peripheral infusion to minimize vein irritation. If moderate to severe venous irritation occurs with 250-ml infusion, consider increasing volume to 500 or 750 ml of D5W, changing the infusion site, or infusing by a peripherally inserted central catheter (PICC) or a central venous catheter; see Dilution. Concomitant administration of hydrocortisone or diphenhydramine does ***not*** appear to alleviate venous irritation. ■ Episodes of arthralgia and myalgia have been reported. In some patients, improvement was noted with a reduction in dose frequency to every 12 hours; see Dose Adjustments. ■ Superinfection caused by the overgrowth of nonsusceptible organisms may occur with antibiotic use. Treat as indicated. ■ Pseudomembranous colitis has been reported and may range from mild to life threatening. Consider in patients that present with diarrhea during or after treatment with quinupristin/dalfopristin. ■ Emerging resistance to quinupristin/dalfopristin during treatment of VREF infections has occurred and was associated with resistance to both components.

Monitor: Monitor total bilirubin. Levels greater than 5 times the upper limit of normal were reported in approximately 25% of patients. ■ Monitor infusion site for any sign of irritation or inflammation; see Precautions.

Patient Education: Report pain at injection site or any other side effect promptly.

Maternal/Child: Category B: safety for use in pregnancy and breast-feeding not established. Use caution. ■ Safety and effectiveness in patients under 16 years of age not established. Has been used in a limited number of pediatric patients under emergency-use conditions. Dose adjustment does not appear to be required; see Pediatric Dose.

Elderly: No apparent differences in frequency, type, or severity of side effects. Dose adjustment not required.

DRUG/LAB INTERACTIONS

Quinupristin/dalfopristin significantly inhibits cytochrome P_{450} 3A4 metabolism of cyclosporin A (Sandimmune), midazolam (Versed), nifedipine (Procardia), and tacrolimus (Prograf) and increases their plasma concentrations, dose adjustments may be indicated. Monitoring of cyclosporine and/or tacrolimus serum levels to determine therapeutic dose should be performed when cyclosporine or tacrolimus must be used concomitantly with quinupristin/dalfopristin. ■ It is reasonable to expect that quinupristin/dalfopristin would inhibit other drugs that are metabolized by the P_{450} 3A4 enzyme system. Use caution if being co-administered with drugs that have a narrow therapeutic index (e.g., cyclosporine) and are metabolized via this pathway. Effects may be prolonged, side effects may be increased, dose adjustments may be indicated. Some drugs that are predicted to have elevated plasma concentrations when co-administered with quinupristin/dalfopristin are carbamazepine (Tegretol), cisapride (Propulsid), delavirdine (Rescriptor), diazepam (Valium), dihydropyridines (e.g., nifedipine [Procardia]), diltiazem (Cardizem), disopyramide (Norpace), docetaxel (Taxotere), HMA-CoA reductase inhibitors (e.g., lovastatin [Mevacor], simvastatin [Zocor]), lidocaine, quinidine, indinavir (Crixivan), methylprednisolone (Solu-Medrol), nevirapine (Viramune), paclitaxel (Taxol), ritonavir (Norvir), tacrolimus (Prograf), verapamil (Isoptin), vinca alkaloids (e.g., vinblastine). ■ Concomitant medications metabolized by the P_{450} 3A4 enzyme system that may prolong the QTc interval should be avoided. ■ May increase digoxin levels. If S/S of digoxin toxicity occur, monitor digoxin levels. ■ In vitro combination testing of quinupristin/dalfopristin with aztreonam, cefotaxime (Claforan), ciprofloxacin, and gentamicin (Garamycin) against *Enterobacteriaceae* and *Pseudomonas aeruginosa* did not show antagonism. ■ In vitro combination testing of quinupristin/dalfopristin prototype drugs of the following classes: aminoglycosides (gentamicin), beta-lactams (cefepime, ampicillin, and amoxicillin), glycopeptides (vancomycin), quinolones (ciprofloxacin), tetracyclines (doxycycline), and also chloramphenicol against enterococci and staphylococci did not show antagonism. See Actions.

SIDE EFFECTS

Allergic reaction; arthralgia; diarrhea; edema, inflammation, and/or pain at infusion site; edema, elevated total and conjugated bilirubin; headache; myalgia; nausea; pain; pruritus; rash; thrombophlebitis; thrombus; and vomiting are reported most frequently. Numerous other side effects have been reported in less than 1% of patients. Pseudomembranous colitis has been reported. ■ Numerous laboratory abnormalities were noted during studies but were not significantly different than those seen in the comparator group. See literature.

ANTIDOTE

Notify physician of any side effects. Discontinue drug if indicated. Treat antibiotic-related pseudomembranous colitis with fluids, electrolytes, protein supplements, and oral vancomycin (Vancocin) or metronidazole (Flagyl) as indicated. Treat allergic reaction as indicated. Observation and supportive therapy are indicated in an overdose situation. Is not removed by hemodialysis or peritoneal dialysis. Resuscitate as necessary.

RANITIDINE

(ra-ni′ti-deen)

Zantac

H_2 antagonist
Antiulcer agent
Gastric acid inhibitor

pH 6.7 to 7.3

USUAL DOSE

IV injection or intermittent infusion: 50 mg (2 ml) every 6 to 8 hours. Increase frequency of dose, not amount, if necessary for pain relief. 50 mg every 8 to 12 hours may be used short term to replace an oral dose of 150 mg every 12 hours in patients unable to take oral meds. Do not exceed 400 mg/day.
Continuous infusion: 150 mg may be given as a continuous infusion equally distributed over 24 hours. To maintain intergastric acid secretion rates at 10 mEq/hr or less, dose range may be higher in patients with pathologic hypersecretory syndrome (Zollinger-Ellison). Literature suggests an initial dose of 1 mg/kg/hr. Measure gastric acid output in 4 hours. If above 10 mEq/hr or symptoms recur, adjust dose upward in 0.5 mg/kg/hr increments. Up to 2.5 mg/kg/hr has been used.
Additive for total parental nutrition (TPN): 70% to 100% of an average 24-hour dose has been used equally distributed over 24 hours as a continuous infusion. May be supplemented with intermittent doses as needed.
Prevention of pulmonary aspiration during anesthesia: 50 mg 60 to 90 minutes before anesthesia.
Control of acute upper GI bleeding: 150 mg over 24 hours.
Prevention of stress ulcers: 0.125 to 0.25 mg/kg/hr.

PEDIATRIC DOSE

Safety for selective use in children from 1 month to 16 years of age established; see Indications.
One source suggests:
Infants and children: 2 to 4 mg/kg/24 hr in equally divided doses every 6 to 8 hours (0.5 to 1 mg/kg every 6 hours or 0.67 to 1.3 mg/kg every 8 hours). Do not exceed 50 mg/dose.

NEONATAL DOSE

Safety for use of IV ranitidine in neonates less than 1 month of age not established; see Maternal/Child.
1 to 2 mg/kg/24 hr in equally divided doses every 6 to 8 hours (0.25 to 0.5 mg/kg every 6 hours or 0.33 to 0.67 mg/kg every 8 hours). Another source suggests 2 mg/kg every 12 to 24 hours or as a continuous infusion.

DOSE ADJUSTMENTS

Dose selection should be cautious in the elderly. ▪ If the CrCl is less than 50 ml/min, reduce dose to 50 mg every 18 to 24 hours. Gradually increase to 50 mg every 12 hours, or 6 hours with caution if indicated. Adjust schedule to be given after dialysis.

DILUTION

IV injection: Each vial containing 50 mg (2 ml) must be diluted with 20 ml of NS or other compatible infusion solution for injection (D5W, D10W, LR, 5% sodium bicarbonate). Concentration of solution must be no greater than 2.5 mg/ml. Additional diluent may be used.
Intermittent infusion: Available premixed as a 1 mg/ml solution in 50 ml. May be given without further dilution. Or each 50 mg may be diluted in

100 ml (0.5 mg/ml) of D5W or other compatible infusion solution and given piggyback. Concentration of solution should be no greater than 0.5 mg/ml. Manufacturer recommends discontinuing primary IV during intermittent infusion to avoid incompatibilities. Do not use premixed plastic containers in series connections; may cause air embolism.

Continuous infusion: Total daily dose may be diluted in 250 ml of D5W or other compatible infusion solution. For Zollinger-Ellison patients, concentration of solution must be no greater than 2.5 mg/ml.

In all situations, avoid any contact with aluminum during administration (e.g., needles). Inspect for color and clarity. Slight darkening of solution does not affect potency. Compatible in selected TPN solutions for 24 hours (consult pharmacist).

Storage: Stable at room temperature for 48 hours after dilution.

INCOMPATIBLE WITH

Manufacturer states, "Additives should not be introduced into the premixed solution, and the primary IV should be discontinued during ranitidine infusion."

COMPATIBLE WITH **(Underline Indicates Conflicting Compatibility Information)**

See Incompatible With. Consult pharmacist; specific conditions may apply; see Compatibilities, p. xvi.

Solution: Selected TNA and TPN solutions; see Dilution.

Additive: Acetazolamide (Diamox), amikacin (Amikin), aminophylline, <u>ampicillin</u>, chloramphenicol (Chloromycetin), chlorothiazide (Diuril), ciprofloxacin (Cipro IV), <u>clindamycin (Cleocin)</u>, dexamethasone (Decadron), digoxin (Lanoxin), dobutamine (Dobutrex), dopamine (Intropin), doxycycline (Vibramycin), epinephrine (Adrenalin), erythromycin lactobionate (Erythrocin), flumazenil (Romazicon), furosemide (Lasix), gentamicin (Garamycin), heparin, <u>insulin (regular)</u>, isoproterenol (Isuprel), lidocaine, lincomycin (Lincocin), meropenem (Merrem IV), methylprednisolone (Solu-Medrol), nitroprusside sodium, <u>norepinephrine (Levophed)</u>, penicillin G potassium and sodium, potassium chloride (KCl), protamine sulfate, quinidine gluconate, ticarcillin (Ticar), tobramycin (Nebcin), vancomycin (Vancocin).

Syringe: Atropine, <u>chlorpromazine (Thorazine)</u>, dexamethasone (Decadron), dimenhydrinate (Dinate), diphenhydramine (Benadryl), dobutamine (Dobutrex), dopamine (Intropin), fentanyl (Sublimaze), glycopyrrolate, heparin, hydromorphone (Dilaudid), isoproterenol (Isuprel), meperidine (Demerol), metoclopramide (Reglan), morphine, nalbuphine (Nubain), oxymorphone (Numorphan), pentazocine (Talwin), perphenazine (Trilafon), prochlorperazine (Compazine), promethazine (Phenergan), scopolamine.

Y-site: Acyclovir (Zovirax), aldesleukin (Proleukin, IL-2), allopurinol (Aloprim, Zyloprim), amifostine (Ethyol), aminophylline, atracurium (Tracrium), aztreonam (Azactam), bretylium (Bretylate), cefazolin (Kefzol), cefepime (Maxipime), cefoperazone (Cefobid), cefoxitin (Mefoxin), ceftazidime (Fortaz), ceftizoxime (Cefizox), ciprofloxacin (Cipro IV), cisatracurium (Nimbex), cisplatin (Platinol), cladribine (Leustatin), cyclophosphamide (Cytoxan), cytarabine (ARA-C), diltiazem (Cardizem), dobutamine (Dobutrex), docetaxel (Taxotere), dopamine (Intropin), doxorubicin (Adriamycin), doxorubicin liposome (Doxil), enalaprilat (Vasotec IV), epinephrine (Adrenalin), esmolol (Brevibloc), etoposide phosphate (Etopophos), fentanyl (Sublimaze), filgrastim (Neupogen), fluconazole

(Diflucan), fludarabine (Fludara), foscarnet (Foscavir), furosemide (Lasix), gatifloxacin (Tequin), gemcitabine (Gemzar), granisetron (Kytril), heparin, hetastarch in electrolytes (Hextend), hydromorphone (Dilaudid), idarubicin (Idamycin), labetalol (Normodyne), linezolid (Zyvox), lorazepam (Ativan), melphalan (Alkeran), meperidine (Demerol), methotrexate (Folex), midazolam (Versed), milrinone (Primacor), morphine, nicardipine (Cardene IV), nitroglycerin (Nitro-Bid IV), norepinephrine (Levophed), ondansetron (Zofran), paclitaxel (Taxol), pancuronium (Pavulon), piperacillin (Pipracil), piperacillin/tazobactam (Zosyn), procainamide (Pronestyl), propofol (Diprivan), remifentanil (Ultiva), sargramostim (Leukine), tacrolimus (Prograf), teniposide (Vumon), theophylline, thiopental (Pentothal), thiotepa (Thioplex), vecuronium (Norcuron), vinorelbine (Navelbine), warfarin (Coumadin), zidovudine (AZT, Retrovir).

RATE OF ADMINISTRATION

Too-rapid administration has precipitated rare instances of bradycardia, tachycardia, and PVCs.

IV injection: Each 50 mg or fraction thereof at a rate not to exceed 4 ml/min diluted solution (20 ml over 5 min).

Intermittent infusion: Each 50-mg dose over 15 to 20 minutes. Should not exceed a rate of 5 to 7 ml/min.

Continuous infusion: Total daily dose equally distributed over 24 hours. Should not exceed a rate of 6.25 mg/hr (10.7 ml/hr if 150 mg [6 ml ranitidine] is diluted in 250 ml). Use of infusion pump preferred to avoid complications of overdose or too-rapid administration.

ACTIONS

A histamine H_2 antagonist, it inhibits both daytime and nocturnal basal gastric acid secretion. It also inhibits gastric acid secretion stimulated by food, histamine, bentazole, and pentagastrin. Not an anticholinergic agent. Does not lower calcium levels in hypercalcemia. Onset of action is prompt and effective for 6 to 8 hours. 5 to 12 times more potent than cimetidine. Half-life is 2 to 2.5 hours. Metabolized in the liver. Excreted in the urine. 70% of a dose is recovered in urine as unchanged drug. Crosses placental barrier. Secreted in breast milk.

INDICATIONS AND USES

Short-term treatment of intractable duodenal ulcers and pathologic hypersecretory conditions in the hospitalized patient. ■ Treatment of active benign gastric ulcers in those patients unable to take oral medication. ■ Treatment of erosive gastroesophageal reflux disease (GERD) and erosive esophagitis diagnosed by endoscopy. ■ Additive to TPN to simplify fluid and electrolyte management (decreases the volume and chloride content of gastric secretions). ■ Treatment of duodenal ulcers in pediatric patients from 1 month to 16 years of age. Safety for use in pathologic hypersecretory conditions not established. ■ Oral dosing for treatment of duodenal and gastric ulcers, maintenance of healing of duodenal and gastric ulcers, and treatment of GERD and erosive esophagitis has been approved for pediatric patients from 1 month to 16 years of age; see package insert.

Unlabeled uses: Preoperatively to prevent pulmonary aspiration of acid during anesthesia. ■ Control of acute upper GI bleeding. ■ Prevention of stress ulcers.

CONTRAINDICATIONS

Known hypersensitivity to ranitidine or its components or other H_2 receptor antagonists (e.g., cimetidine [Tagamet], famotidine [Pepcid IV]).

PRECAUTIONS

Use antacids concomitantly to relieve pain. ■ Gastric malignancy may be present even though patient's symptoms improve on ranitidine therapy. ■ Use caution in patients with impaired hepatic or renal function. ■ Gastric pain and ulceration may recur after medication stopped. ■ Effects maintained with oral dosage. Total treatment usually discontinued after 6 weeks.

Monitor: Observe frequently; monitor vital signs and pain levels. ■ Obtain baseline SrCr. Monitor periodically during extended course of treatment. ■ Monitor ALT (SGPT) if therapy exceeds 400 mg for over 5 days. ■ Change to oral dose when appropriate. ■ See Drug/Lab Interactions.

Patient Education: Stop smoking or at least avoid smoking after the last dose of the day. ■ May increase blood alcohol levels.

Maternal/Child: Category B: use during pregnancy or breast-feeding only when clearly needed. ■ Safety for use of IV ranitidine in neonates less than 1 month of age not established; however, limited data suggest that ranitidine may be useful and safe in increasing gastric pH for infants at risk of GI hemorrhage. ■ Half-life in neonates averages 6.6 hours.

Elderly: Use caution in dose selection; monitoring of renal function suggested; see Dose Adjustments. ■ Half-life is prolonged (3.1 hours) and total clearance is decreased due to reduced renal function. ■ Differences in response between elderly and younger patients not identified; greater sensitivity of some elderly cannot be ruled out. ■ Agitation, confusion (reversible), depression, and hallucination have been reported.

DRUG/LAB INTERACTIONS

Concurrent use with warfarin may result in increased or decreased PT and/or INR. ■ Potentiates effects of alcohol, procainamide (Pronestyl), sulfonylureas (Glipizide). ■ May potentiate theophyllines (e.g., aminophylline). ■ May inhibit gastric absorption of ketoconazole (Nizoral). ■ Clinical effect (inhibition of nocturnal gastric secretions) may be reversed by cigarette smoking. ■ Elevated ALT (SGOT), slight elevation in SrCr, and a false-positive for urine protein with Multistix may occur.

SIDE EFFECTS

Abdominal discomfort, burning and itching at IV site, constipation, diarrhea, headache (severe), and nausea and vomiting are the most common side effects. Allergic reactions (bronchospasm, fever, rash, eosinophilia) can occur. Agitation, alopecia, arthralgias, bradycardia, confusion, depression, dizziness, elevated SGPT, erythema multiforme, hallucinations, hepatitis (reversible), impotence, insomnia, malaise, muscular pain, PVCs, somnolence, tachycardia, vasculitis, and vertigo occur rarely. See Drug/Lab Interactions.

ANTIDOTE

Notify physician of all side effects. May be treated symptomatically or may respond to decrease in frequency of dosage. Discontinue ranitidine if S/S of hepatitis with or without jaundice occur. Resuscitate as necessary for overdose. Hemodialysis or peritoneal dialysis may be indicated in overdose.

RASBURICASE

(ras-ber′i-case)

Antihyperuricemic

Elitek

USUAL DOSE

Prehydration required; see Monitor.

0.15 or 0.2 mg/kg as a single daily dose each day for 5 days. Chemotherapy should be initiated 4 to 24 hours after the first dose. Safety and effectiveness of other schedules have not been evaluated. Dosing beyond 5 days and/or administration of more than one course of rasburicase is not recommended.

PEDIATRIC DOSE

See Usual Dose.

DOSE ADJUSTMENTS

No dose adjustments recommended.

DILUTION

Each vial contains 1.5 mg of rasburicase. Determine the number of vials needed to provide the calculated dose. Reconstitute each vial with 1 ml of the diluent provided (SW and Poloxamer 188). Mix by swirling gently. ***Do not shake.*** Withdraw the calculated dose of reconstituted solution and inject into an infusion bag containing the appropriate volume of NS to achieve a final total volume of 50 ml. (For example a 20-kg child would receive a dose of 4 mg [20 kg × 0.2 mg/kg = 4 mg]. Reconstitute 3 vials, each with 1 ml of the diluent provided. Withdraw 2.7 ml of reconstituted solution and add to an infusion bag containing 47.3 ml of NS.)

No filters should be used for the infusion.

Storage: Refrigerate unopened lyophilized drug product and diluent. Do not freeze; protect from light. Both the reconstituted and diluted product may be stored for 24 hours if refrigerated. Discard any unused product.

COMPATIBILITY

Manufacturer states, "Should be infused through a different line than that used for the infusion of other concomitant medications. If use of a separate line is not possible, the line should be flushed with at least 15 ml of NS prior to and after infusion with rasburicase."

RATE OF ADMINISTRATION

A single dose as an infusion equally distributed over 30 minutes.

Do not administer as a bolus infusion. Do not filter infusion.

ACTIONS

A recombinant urate-oxidase enzyme produced by genetic engineering. Catalyzes enzymatic oxidation of uric acid into an inactive and soluble metabolite (allantoin). Half-life is 18 hours.

INDICATIONS AND USES

Initial management of plasma uric acid levels in pediatric patients with leukemia, lymphoma, and solid tumor malignancies who are receiving anti-cancer therapy expected to result in tumor lysis and subsequent elevation of plasma uric acid.

CONTRAINDICATIONS

Glucose-6-phosphatase dehydrogenase (G6PD) deficiency or a history of hypersensitivity, hemolytic reactions, or methemoglobinemia reactions to rasburicase or any of its components.

PRECAUTIONS

May cause severe hypersensitivity reactions, including anaphylaxis. ■ Is immunogenic in healthy volunteers. May elicit antibodies that inhibit the activity of rasburicase. ■ Has caused severe hemolytic reactions in patients with G6PD deficiency. It is recommended that patients at higher risk for G6PD deficiency (e.g., patients of African or Mediterranean descent) be screened prior to starting rasburicase therapy. See Contraindication and Antidote. ■ Methemoglobinemia has been reported. Patients developed serious hypoxemia, requiring intervention and medical support. See Antidote.

Monitor: Monitor serum uric acid levels, electrolytes, and renal function before and during therapy. ■ Patients should be hydrated intravenously according to standard medical practice for the management of plasma uric acid in patients at risk for tumor lysis syndrome (TLS). ■ Maintain urine at neutral or slightly alkaline pH. To increase solubility of uric acid, alkalinity of urine may be increased with sodium bicarbonate. ■ Observe for symptoms of TLS (e.g., hyperuricemia, hyperkalemia, hyperphosphatemia, and hypocalcemia). If untreated, may develop acute uric acid nephropathy, leading to renal failure. ■ Monitor for S/S of an allergic reaction (e.g., anaphylaxis, chest pain, dyspnea, hypotension, urticaria). ■ Will cause enzymatic degradation of uric acid within blood samples left at room temperature, resulting in falsely low uric acid levels. To ensure accurate measurement, blood must be collected into pre-chilled tubes containing heparin anticoagulant and immediately *immersed and maintained* in an ice water bath. Plasma samples must be prepared by centrifugation in a pre-cooled centrifuge (4° C). Plasma samples must be analyzed within 4 hours of sample collection.

Patient Education: Report blood in urine, painful urination, or signs of allergic reactions promptly.

Maternal/Child: Category C: studies have not been performed. Potential benefits must justify potential risks to fetus. ■ Discontinue breast-feeding. ■ Studied in children from 1 month to 17 years of age. Children less than 2 years of age had a higher mean uric acid AUC and a lower rate of success at achieving maintenance uric acid concentrations by 48 hours than older pediatric patients. They also experienced more toxicity (e.g., diarrhea, fever, rash, and vomiting).

Elderly: There are insufficient data to determine whether geriatric subjects, or adults in general, respond differently than pediatric patients.

DRUG/LAB INTERACTIONS

Studies have not been conducted. ■ Does not metabolize allopurinol (Aloprim, Zyloprim), cytarabine (ARA-C), methylprednisolone (Solu-Medrol), methotrexate, 6-mercaptopurine (Purinethol), thioguanine, etoposide (Etopophos, VePesid), daunorubicin (Cerubidine), cyclophosphamide, or vincristine (Oncovin) *in vitro*. Metabolic-based drug interactions are not anticipated with these agents. ■ Did not affect the activity of P_{450} isoenzymes in preclinical *in vivo* studies. Clinically relevant P_{450}-mediated drug-drug interactions are not anticipated. ■ Will cause enzymatic degradation of uric acid within blood samples left at room temperature, resulting in falsely low uric acid levels; see Monitor.

SIDE EFFECTS

The most serious adverse reactions observed are allergic reactions (e.g., anaphylaxis, chest pain, dyspnea, hypotension, urticaria), hemolysis, methemoglobinemia, and severe rash. Other, more commonly observed reactions include abdominal pain, acute renal failure, constipation, diarrhea, fever, headache, mucositis, nausea, neutropenia with or without fever, rash, respiratory distress, sepsis, and vomiting. Several other reactions have been observed in a small number of patients. Causality is uncertain. See product literature.

ANTIDOTE

Notify physician of all side effects. Should be immediately and permanently discontinued in patients who experience severe hypersensitivity reactions, hemolysis, or methemoglobinemia. Do not rechallenge. Treat anaphylaxis with epinephrine, corticosteroids (e.g., dexamethasone [Decadron]), oxygen, and antihistamines (diphenhydramine [Benadryl]). Hemolysis or methemoglobinemia may require transfusion support. Methylene blue may be required for treatment of methemoglobinemia. There is no specific antidote. Resuscitate as indicated.

REMIFENTANIL HYDROCHLORIDE

(rem-ih-fin′ta-nill hye-droe-klor′id)

Ultiva

Narcotic analgesic (agonist)
Anesthesia adjunct

pH 2.5 to 3.5

USUAL DOSE

General anesthesia and continuing as an analgesic into the immediate postoperative period: Not recommended as the sole anesthetic agent because it may not cause loss of consciousness and it has a high incidence of apnea, muscle rigidity, and tachycardia. Given concomitantly with reduced doses of other anesthetics (e.g., isoflurane, midazolam [Versed], propofol [Diprivan], and/or thiopental [Pentothal]); see Dose Adjustments and Drug/Lab Interactions. Individualize based on patient response. May be premedicated with benzodiazepines (e.g., diazepam [Valium], midazolam [Versed]). See the following charts:

Remifentanil Dosing Guidelines in Adults for General Anesthesia

Phase	Continuous IV Infusion (mcg/kg/min)	Infusion Dose Range (mcg/kg/min)	Supplemental IV Bolus Dose (mcg/kg)
Induction of anesthesia (through intubation)	0.5-1*		

*If intubation is to occur less than 8 minutes after the start of a remifentanil infusion, an initial dose of 1 mcg/kg may be administered over 30 to 60 seconds.

Continued

Remifentanil Dosing Guidelines in Adults for General Anesthesia—cont'd			
Phase	Continuous IV Infusion (mcg/kg/min)	Infusion Dose Range (mcg/kg/min)	Supplemental IV Bolus Dose (mcg/kg)
Maintenance of anesthesia with:			
Nitrous oxide (66%)	0.4	0.1-2	1
Isoflurane (0.4 to 1.5 MAC)	0.25	0.05-2	1
Propofol (100 to 200 mcg/kg/min)	0.25	0.05-2	1
Continuation as an analgesic into the immediate post-operative period	0.1	0.025-0.2	not recommended

Remifentanil Dosing Guidelines for Monitored Anesthesia Care (MAC)			
Method	Timing	Remifentanil Alone	Remifentanil + 2 mg Midazolam
Single IV dose	Given 90 seconds before local anesthetic	1 mcg/kg over 30 to 60 seconds	0.5 mcg/kg over 30 to 60 seconds
Continuous IV infusion	Beginning 5 minutes before local anesthetic	0.1 mcg/kg/min	0.05 mcg/kg/min
	After local anesthetic	0.05 mcg/kg/min (Range: 0.025-0.2 mcg/kg/min)	0.025 mcg/kg/min (Range: 0.025-0.2 mcg/kg/min)

PEDIATRIC DOSE

Children 1 to 12 years of age: Note all comments under Usual Dose. Effectiveness and safety established only for use in maintenance of general anesthesia. 20 or 25 mcg/ml dilution recommended. See the chart below.

Remifentanil Dosing Guidelines in Pediatric Patients for General Anesthesia			
Phase	Continuous IV Infusion (mcg/kg/min)	Infusion Dose Range (mcg/kg/min)	Supplemental IV Bolus Dose (mcg/kg)
Maintenance of anesthesia with:			
Halothane (0.3 to 1.5 MAC)	0.25	0.05-1.3	1
Sevoflurane (0.3 to 1.5 MAC)	0.25	0.05-1.3	1
Isoflurane (0.4 to 1.5 MAC)	0.25	0.05-1.3	1

Continued

DOSE ADJUSTMENTS

Reduce starting dose by 50% in the elderly (over 65 years of age), then cautiously titrate to effect. ■ Base starting dose on ideal body weight in obese patients (more than 30% over their IBW). ■ No dose adjustment required in patients with atypical cholinesterase or in chronic or severe renal or hepatic dysfunction. ■ Dose may be reduced up to 75% with other anesthetic agents; see Drug/Lab Interactions. ■ See Precautions.

DILUTION

To reconstitute add 1 ml of diluent for each mg of remifentanil (1 mg/ml). Compatible with SW, D5W, D5NS, NS, ½NS, and D5LR. Shake well. Must be further diluted to a final concentration of 20, 25, 50, or 250 mcg/ml with additional amounts of the above solutions (see chart below). When used for MAC anesthesia the 25 mcg/ml dilution is recommended. When used for ***pediatric dilution:*** 20 or 25 mcg/ml dilution recommended.

Remifentanil Reconstitution and Dilution

Amount of Reconstituted Remifentanil in Each Vial	Amount of Diluent	Final Volume After Reconstitution and Dilution	Final Concentration
1 mg	49 ml	50 ml	
2 mg	98 ml	100 ml	20 mcg/ml
5 mg	245 ml	250 ml	
1 mg	39 ml	40 ml	
2 mg	78 ml	80 ml	25 mcg/ml
5 mg	195 ml	200 ml	
1 mg	19 ml	20 ml	
2 mg	38 ml	40 ml	50 mcg/ml
5 mg	95 ml	100 ml	
5 mg	15 ml	20 ml	250 mcg/ml

Storage: Store between 2° to 25° C (34° to 80° F). Stable for 24 hours at CRT after reconstituted and diluted with above solutions. Stability reduced to 4 hours with LR injection.

INCOMPATIBLE WITH

Do not administer into the same IV tubing as blood or blood products.

COMPATIBLE WITH (Underline Indicates Conflicting Compatibility Information)

Consult pharmacist; specific conditions may apply; see Compatibilities, p. xvi.

Y-site: Acyclovir (Zovirax), alfentanil (Alfenta), amikacin (Amikin), aminophylline, amphotericin B (Fungizone), ampicillin, ampicillin/sulbactam (Unasyn), aztreonam (Azactam), bretylium (Bretylate), bumetanide (Bumex), buprenorphine (Buprenex), butorphanol (Stadol), calcium gluconate, cefazolin (Kefzol), cefoperazone (Cefobid), cefotaxime (Claforan), cefotetan (Cefotan), cefoxitin (Mefoxin), ceftazidime (Fortaz), ceftizoxime (Cefizox), ceftriaxone (Rocephin), cefuroxime (Zinacef), chlorpromazine (Thorazine), cimetidine (Tagamet), ciprofloxacin (Cipro IV), cisatracurium (Nimbex), clindamycin (Cleocin), dexamethasone (Decadron), diazepam (Valium), digoxin (Lanoxin), diphenhydramine (Benadryl), dobutamine (Dobutrex), dopamine (Intropin), doxycycline (Vibramycin), droperidol (Inapsine), enalaprilat (Vasotec IV), epinephrine (Adrenalin), esmolol (Brevibloc), famotidine (Pepcid IV), fentanyl (Sublimaze), fluconazole (Diflucan), furosemide (Lasix), ganciclovir (Cytovene), gatifloxacin (Tequin), gentamicin (Garamycin), haloperidol (Haldol), heparin, hydrocortisone sodium succinate (Solu-Cortef), hydromorphone (Dilaudid), imipenem-cilastatin (Primaxin), inamrinone (Inocor), isoproterenol (Isuprel), ketorolac (Toradol), lidocaine, linezolid (Zyvox), lorazepam (Ativan), magnesium sulfate, mannitol, meperidine (Demerol), methylprednisolone (Solu-Medrol), metoclopramide (Reglan), metronidazole (Flagyl IV), mezlocillin (Mezlin), midazolam (Versed), minocycline (Minocin), morphine, nalbuphine (Nubain), nitroglycerin (Nitro-Bid IV), norepinephrine (Levophed), oflaxacin (Floxin IV), ondansetron (Zofran), phenylephrine (Neo-Synephrine), piperacillin (Pipracil), piperacillin/tazobactam (Zosyn), potassium chloride (KCl), procainamide (Pronestyl), prochlorperazine (Compazine), promethazine (Phenergan), propofol (Diprivan), ranitidine (Zantac), sodium bicarbonate, sufentanil (Sufenta), sulfamethoxazole-trimethoprim (Bactrim), theophylline, thiopental (Pentothal), ticarcillin (Ticar), ticarcillin/clavulanate (Timentin), tobramycin (Nebcin), vancomycin (Vancocin), zidovudine (AZT, Retrovir).

RATE OF ADMINISTRATION

Use of an infusion device required. Injection site should be close to the venous cannula, and all IV tubing should be flushed when the infusion is discontinued to prevent delayed effects. Rapid elimination and lack of accumulation permits titration of infusion rate without concern for prolonged duration. Every 0.1 mcg/kg/min change in the infusion rate will lead to a 2.5 ng/ml change in blood concentration within 5 to 10 minutes; see Precautions. Skeletal muscle rigidity is related to the dose and speed of administration. In any situation infusion rates greater than 0.2 mcg/kg/min may cause respiratory depression.

Anesthesia induction: If intubation is to occur less than 8 minutes after the start of a remifentanil infusion, an initial dose of 1 mcg/kg over 30 to 60 seconds may be given.

Anesthesia maintenance: Titrate upward in 25% to 100% increments or downward in 25% to 50% increments every 2 to 5 minutes to attain desired level of opioid effect. Supplemental bolus doses of 1 mcg/kg may be given every 2 to 5 minutes in response to light anesthesia or episodes of intense surgical stress. If infusion rates greater than 1 mcg/kg/min are required, consider increasing concomitant anesthetic agents to increase the depth of anesthesia.

Continuation as an analgesic during the immediate postoperative period: Adjust rate in 0.025 mcg/kg/min increments every 5 minutes to balance level of analgesia and respiratory rate. Administer alternate analgesics to control postoperative pain before discontinuing remifentanil.

Monitored anesthesia care (MAC): See table in Usual Dose. 25 mcg/ml dilution recommended. Titrate to patient comfort, analgesia, and adequate respiration; do not use sedation as a criteria for titration. May cause muscle rigidity and respiratory depression. See Contraindications and Precautions.

After placement of a local or regional block with MAC: To reduce risk of hypoventilation, decrease infusion rate to 0.05 mcg/kg/min; thereafter titrate in increments of 0.025 mcg/kg/min at 5-minute intervals to balance level of analgesia and respiratory rate.

Remifentanil IV Infusion Rates (ml/hr) for a 20-mcg/ml Solution

Desired Infusion Rate (mcg/kg/min)	Patient Weight (kg)						
	5	10	20	30	40	50	60
0.0125	0.188	0.375	0.75	1.125	1.5	1.875	2.25
0.025	0.375	0.75	1.5	2.25	3	3.75	4.5
0.05	0.75	1.5	3	4.5	6	7.5	9
0.075	1.125	2.25	4.5	6.75	9	11.25	13.5
0.1	1.5	3	6	9	12	15	18
0.15	2.25	4.5	9	13.5	18	22.5	27
0.2	3	6	12	18	24	30	36
0.25	3.75	7.5	15	22.5	30	37.5	45
0.3	4.5	9	18	27	36	45	54
0.35	5.25	10.5	21	31.5	42	52.5	63
0.4	6	12	24	36	48	60	72

Remifentanil IV Infusion Rates (ml/hr) for a 25-mcg/ml Solution

Desired Infusion Rate (mcg/kg/min)	Patient Weight (kg)									
	10	20	30	40	50	60	70	80	90	100
0.0125	0.3	0.6	0.9	1.2	1.5	1.8	2.1	2.4	2.7	3
0.025	0.6	1.2	1.8	2.4	3	3.6	4.2	4.8	5.4	6
0.05	1.2	2.4	3.6	4.8	6	7.2	8.4	9.6	10.8	12
0.075	1.8	3.6	5.4	7.2	9	10.8	12.6	14.4	16.2	18
0.1	2.4	4.8	7.2	9.6	12	14.4	16.8	19.2	21.6	24
0.15	3.6	7.2	10.8	14.4	18	21.6	25.2	28.8	32.4	36
0.2	4.8	9.6	14.4	19.2	24	28.8	33.6	38.4	43.2	48

Remifentanil IV Infusion Rates (ml/hr) for a 50-mcg/ml Solution

Desired Infusion Rate (mcg/kg/min)	Patient Weight (kg)							
	30	40	50	60	70	80	90	100
0.025					2.1	2.4	2.7	3
0.05		2.4	3	3.6	4.2	4.8	5.4	6
0.075	2.7	3.6	4.5	5.4	6.3	7.2	8.1	9
0.1	3.6	4.8	6	7.2	8.4	9.6	10.8	12

Continued

Remifentanil IV Infusion Rates (ml/hr) for a 50-mcg/ml Solution—cont'd								
Desired Infusion Rate (mcg/kg/min)	Patient Weight (kg)							
	30	40	50	60	70	80	90	100
0.15	5.4	7.2	9	10.8	12.6	14.4	16.2	18
0.2	7.2	9.6	12	14.4	16.8	19.2	21.6	24
0.25	9	12	15	18	21	24	27	30
0.5	18	24	30	36	42	48	54	60
0.75	27	36	45	54	63	72	81	90
1	36	48	60	72	84	96	108	120
1.25	45	60	75	90	105	120	135	150
1.5	54	72	90	108	126	144	162	180
1.75	63	84	105	126	147	168	189	210
2	72	96	120	144	168	192	216	240

Remifentanil IV Infusion Rates (ml/hr) for a 250-mcg/ml Solution								
Desired Infusion Rate (mcg/kg/min)	Patient Weight (kg)							
	30	40	50	60	70	80	90	100
0.1	0.72	0.96	1.2	1.44	1.68	1.92	2.16	2.4
0.15	1.08	1.44	1.8	2.16	2.52	2.88	3.24	3.6
0.2	1.44	1.92	2.4	2.88	3.36	3.84	4.32	4.8
0.25	1.8	2.4	3	3.6	4.2	4.8	5.4	6
0.5	3.6	4.8	6	7.2	8.4	9.6	10.8	12
0.75	5.4	7.2	9	10.8	12.6	14.4	16.2	18
1	7.2	9.6	12	14.4	16.8	19.2	21.6	24
1.25	9	12	15	18	21	24	27	30
1.5	10.8	14.4	18	21.6	25.2	28.8	32.4	36
1.75	12.6	16.8	21	25.2	29.4	33.6	37.8	42
2	14.4	19.2	24	28.8	33.6	38.4	43.2	48

ACTIONS

An opioid agonist analgesic with rapid onset (1 minute) and peak effect (3 to 5 minutes) and short duration of action (5 to 10 minutes). Effects and side effects are dose dependent. There is direct correlation between dose, blood levels, and response. Blood concentration decreases 50% in 3 to 6 minutes after a 1-minute infusion or after prolonged continuous infusion due to rapid distribution and elimination and is independent of duration of drug administration. Recovery from effects occurs within 5 to 10 minutes. New steady-state concentrations occur within 5 to 10 minutes after changes in infusion rates. Serum concentrations, volume of distribution, clearance, and half-life in children 2 to 12 years were similar to adults. Rapidly metabolized by specific blood and tissue esterases.

INDICATIONS AND USES

An analgesic agent for use during induction and maintenance of general anesthesia for inpatient and outpatient procedures and for continuation as an analgesic in a postoperative anesthesia care unit or intensive care setting. ■ Analgesic component of monitored anesthesia care. ■ Not studied in pediatric patients for use in the immediate postoperative period or for use as a component of monitored anesthesia care.

CONTRAINDICATIONS

Known hypersensitivity to remifentanil or other fentanyl analogs (e.g., alfentanil, fentanyl, sufentanil). ■ Contains glycine; do not use for epidural or intrathecal administration. ■ ***IV bolus doses should be used only during the maintenance of general anesthesia. Administration of bolus doses simultaneously with a continuous infusion to spontaneously breathing patients is not recommended.***

PRECAUTIONS

For IV use only. ■ Intended for use by or under the direct supervision of the anesthesiologist. Must have responsibility only for anesthesia during surgery and/or procedures. Staff must be skilled in medical management of critically ill patients, cardiovascular resuscitation, and airway management. ■ Analgesia usually achieved with minimal decrease in respiratory rate with infusions of 0.05 to 0.1 mcg/kg/min producing blood concentrations of 1 to 3 ng/ml. Supplemental doses of 0.5 to 1 mcg/kg, incremental increases in infusion rate greater than 0.05 mcg/kg/min, and blood concentrations exceeding 5 ng/ml (typically produced by infusions of 0.2 mcg/kg/min) have caused transient and reversible respiratory depression, apnea, and muscle rigidity. ■ May cause chest wall rigidity (inability to ventilate) after single doses of more than 1 mcg/kg administered over 30 to 60 seconds or infusion rates greater than 0.1 mcg/kg/min; peripheral muscle rigidity may occur at lower doses. May also cause chest wall rigidity with doses lower than 1 mcg/kg when given concurrently with a continuous infusion of remifentanil. May be prevented or lessened by prior or concurrent administration of a hypnotic (propofol or thiopental) or a neuromuscular blocking agent (e.g., atracurium). ■ With a 1-minute infusion of less than 2 mcg/kg, remifentanil will cause dose-dependent hypotension and bradycardia in premedicated patients undergoing anesthesia. Additional doses greater than 2 mcg/kg do not produce further decreases, but may increase duration of hemodynamic effect. ■ Respiratory depression is dose related, but due to a lack of drug accumulation recovery of respiratory drive is more rapid and less variable than other similar agents. Rate of respiratory recovery will vary depending on concurrent anesthetics (e.g., N_2O, propofol, isoflurane). ■ Use caution in very obese patients; may have increased potential for cardiovascular or respiratory problems. ■ Increased risk of respiratory depression in patients with impaired respiratory function; use caution. ■ Use caution in patients with bradycardia; HR may decrease further. ■ Intraoperative awareness has been reported. ■ Has not been used for longer than 16 hours in ICU patients.

Monitor: Oxygen, intubation equipment, controlled ventilation equipment, nalmefene (Revex), naloxone (Narcan), neuromuscular blocking agents (e.g., mivacurium [Mivacron]), and facilities for resuscitation and life support must always be available. Maintain a patent airway and ascertain adequate ventilation at all times. A conscious patient will appear to be asleep and may forget to breathe unless commanded to do so. ■ Can cause rigidity of respiratory muscles; may require a muscle relaxant (benzodiazepine) or neuromuscular blocking agent to relax muscles and permit artificial ventilation. ■ All vital signs must be monitored continuously. Use of a respiratory monitor and monitoring of oxygen saturation required. Supplemental oxygen always required for general anesthesia; strongly recommended for MAC. ■ Keep patient supine; orthostatic hypotension and fainting may occur. ■ Flush IV line before discontinuing an infusion of remifentanil. ■ Establish adequate postoperative analgesia before discontinuing an infusion of remifentanil. ■ See Precautions. ■ Monitor for 30 to 60 minutes after anesthesia complete. Effect of remifentanil will be offset within 5 to 10 minutes, but respiratory depression may still occur from concomitant anesthetics.

Patient Education: Avoid alcohol or other CNS depressants (e.g., antihistamines, diazepam [Valium]). ■ Blurred vision, dizziness, drowsiness, or lightheadedness may occur; request assistance with ambulation. ■ Do not perform tasks requiring mental alertness (e.g., driving, operating hazardous machinery, or signing legal documents) until the day after surgery or longer.

Maternal/Child: Category C: use during pregnancy only when clearly needed; benefit must justify risk to fetus. ■ May cause respiratory depression and other opioid effects in the newborn if used before or during labor and delivery; safety not demonstrated. ■ Other fentanyl analogs are secreted in breast milk; remifentanil not yet studied. Use caution during breast-feeding. ■ Safety for use in infants and children under 1 year of age not established. ■ Not studied in pediatric patients for use in the immediate postoperative period or for use as a component of monitored anesthesia care.

Elderly: See Dose Adjustments. Increased sensitivity to effects and clearance reduced by 25%, but blood concentrations fall as rapidly after remifentanil is discontinued. Incidence of hypotension may be increased; nausea and vomiting may be decreased.

DRUG/LAB INTERACTIONS

Respiratory depression increased and prolonged with other concurrent anesthetics (e.g., N_2O, propofol, isoflurane). ■ Nonspecific esterases in blood products may inactivate remifentanil. ■ Clearance is not altered by concomitant use of thiopental, isoflurane, propofol, or temazepam (Restoril) during anesthesia; is synergistic with hypnotics (e.g., propofol, thiopental), inhaled anesthetics (e.g., isoflurane), and benzodiazepines (e.g., midazolam). Risk of hypotension and respiratory depression increased. Doses of these agents have been reduced by up to 75%. ■ No drug interactions to date with atracurium (Tracium), mivacurium (Mivacron), esmolol (Brevibloc), antiglaucoma agents (echothiophate), neostigmine (Prostigmin), or physostigmine (Antilirium). ■ During monitored anesthesia care concurrent administration with midazolam greater than 2 mg (4 to 8 mg) increased the rate of respiratory depression even when the dose of remifentanil was reduced by 50%. ■ Does not prolong the duration of muscle paralysis from succinylcholine in animals. ■ Hypothermic cardiopulmonary bypass may reduce clearance by 20%, increasing effects.

SIDE EFFECTS

Chills, dizziness, fever, flushing, headache, nausea, pain at IV site, postoperative pain, pruritus, shivering, sweating, vomiting, warm sensation.

Major: Apnea, bradycardia, hypertension, hypotension, respiratory depression, skeletal muscle rigidity, tachycardia. Many other serious side effects can occur, including other arrhythmias.

Overdose: Apnea, bradycardia, chest wall rigidity, hypoxemia, hypotension, seizures.

ANTIDOTE

Keep physician informed of all side effects. Minor side effects will be tolerated or treated symptomatically. Major side effects or overdose may be life threatening and must be treated immediately. Antagonized by opioid antagonists; short-acting opioid antagonists should be adequate (e.g., nalmefene [Revex], naloxone [Narcan]). Reversal of opioid effects may lead to acute pain and sympathetic hyperactivity. Maintain a patent airway, with oxygen and artificial ventilation as needed. Respiratory depression in spontaneously breathing patients is usually managed by decreasing the rate of infusion by 50% or temporarily discontinuing remifentanil. Bradycardia and hypotension can be reversed by reducing the rate of infusion or the dose of concurrent anesthetics. Bradycardia may require atropine or glycopyrrolate. Hypotension may require IV fluids or catecholamines (e.g., ephedrine, epinephrine, norepinephrine). Treat excessive muscle rigidity during induction of anesthesia by administering a neuromuscular blocking agent (e.g., succinylcholine) and concurrent induction medications (e.g., thiopental). Treat excessive muscle rigidity in spontaneously breathing patients by decreasing the rate, discontinuing remifentanil, or administering a neuromuscular blocking agent or naloxone. Hypertension may require antihypertensives (e.g., nitroglycerin). Treatment of seizures may require benzodiazepines (e.g., diazepam [Valium]).

RESPIRATORY SYNCYTIAL VIRUS IMMUNE GLOBULIN INTRAVENOUS

Immunizing agent (passive)

(res′pir-ah-tor-e sin-sish′ti-al vi′rus im-myoun′ gloh′byou-lin in′trah-ve-nes)

RespiGam, RSV-IGIV

PEDIATRIC DOSE

750 mg/kg as a single-dose IV infusion. Administer the first dose prior to the respiratory syncytial virus (RSV) season (early November through April in the northern hemisphere). Repeat monthly throughout the season. Another source suggests starting in September or October and continuing for a total of 5 doses. Palivizumab (Synagis) is an agent for the same indication that can be given IM.

DILUTION

No dilution required; ready to infuse in a 50 mg/ml solution. Should be clear and colorless. Do not shake vial; avoid foaming. Remove the tab portion of the vial cap and clean with 70% alcohol before puncturing with infusion set. See Compatibility.

Storage: Refrigerate unopened vials. Begin infusion within 6 hours and complete within 12 hours after single-use vial is entered.

COMPATIBILITY

Manufacturer states, "Should be administered through a separate IV line. If piggybacking is necessary, the pre-existing line must contain only 2½%, 5%, 10%, or 20% dextrose in water or NS. Dilution must not exceed 1 part RSV-IGIV to 2 parts dextrose solution at the Y-connection.

RATE OF ADMINISTRATION

An infusion pump is required to deliver a constant rate; an in-line filter larger than 15 microns may be used. Slow rate of infusion at onset of patient discomfort or for any adverse reactions (e.g., anxiety, dizziness, hypotension, pruritus). Begin with 1.5 ml/kg/hr for the first 15 minutes. If no discomfort or adverse effects, may be increased 3 ml/kg/hr from 15 to 30 minutes and 6 ml/kg/hr from 30 minutes to the end of the infusion. Monitor closely during and after each rate change. Slower rates of infusion may be indicated in ill children. Never exceed 6 ml/kg/hr.

ACTIONS

A specialty immunoglobulin (IgG) containing neutralizing and protecting antibodies to RSV. Provides passive immunity to RSV. Capable of neutralizing each of 62 different RSV clinical isolates of subgroups A and B. Pooled from adult human plasma selected for high titers of neutralizing antibody against RSV. RSV antibody content is 5 to 10 times that of standard Intravenous Immune Globulin. Purified and standardized by several specific methods (e.g., solvent-detergent viral inactivation process decreases the possibility of transmission of blood-borne pathogens [e.g., HIV, hepatitis]). Mean half-life of a single dose is 22 to 28 days.

INDICATIONS AND USES

Prevention of serious lower respiratory tract infection caused by RSV in children under 24 months of age with bronchopulmonary dysplasia (BPD) or a history of premature birth (35 weeks' gestation or less). Has reduced the incidence and duration of RSV hospitalization and severity of RSV illness in these high-risk infants. ■ Has not been shown to be effective for the treatment of RSV infection.

CONTRAINDICATIONS

History of a prior severe hypersensitivity reaction to RSV-IGIV or other immunoglobulin preparations, patients with isolated IgA deficiency or pre-existing antibodies to IgA.

PRECAUTIONS

Use caution; infants with underlying pulmonary disease may be more susceptible to fluid overload; may respond to rate reduction or require loop diuretics (e.g., bumetanide [Bumex] or furosemide [Lasix]). ■ Not recommended for use in children with clinically apparent fluid overload. ■ Aseptic meningitis syndrome (AMS) has been reported in a few patients. Symptoms (e.g., drowsiness, fever, headache, [severe], muscle rigidity, nausea and vomiting, painful eye movements) may occur within a few hours or up to 2 days following infusion. Other causes of meningitis must be ruled out. Seems to occur with higher doses (2 Gm/kg) and subsides with discontinuation of IGIV.

Monitor: Assess vital signs and cardiopulmonary status. At a minimum, must be done before infusion, before each rate increase, and thereafter at 30-minute intervals until 30 minutes after the infusion is complete. Observe for symptoms of fluid overload (e.g., increases in HR, respiratory rate, retractions, and rales). ■ Loop diuretics, epinephrine, and diphenhydramine must be readily available. See Antidote.

Patient Education: Inform parent of possible side effects. ■ Review possible alteration of immunization schedule.

Maternal/Child: Category C: use only if clearly indicated. ■ Safety for use in infants with congenital heart disease (CHD) has not been established. A somewhat larger number of life-threatening adverse events occurred during trial in infants with CHD with right-to-left shunts who underwent surgery.

DRUG/LAB INTERACTIONS

May interfere with immune response to live-virus vaccines (e.g., measles, mumps, rubella). Reimmunization is recommended at least 10 months after RSV-IGIV is discontinued, if appropriate. The American Association of Pediatrics (AAP) recommends deferring primary immunization with these agents until 9 months after the last dose of RSV-IGIV. ■ Effect on antibody responses to DPT, haemophilus influenza type b (Hib), and oral polio virus is unknown; booster doses may be indicated 3 to 4 months after RSV-IGIV is discontinued. The AAP states, "Current data do not support the need for supplemental doses of these vaccines in infants receiving RSV-IGIV."

SIDE EFFECTS

Most side effects (except hypersensitivity reactions) are related to rate of administration. Abdominal cramps, anxiety, arthralgia, chest tightness, dizziness, dyspnea, flushing, hypotension, myalgia, palpitations, pruritus may occur and may be related to the rate of infusion. Mild fluid overload and/or mild decreases in oxygen saturation may occur. Full range of allergic symptoms, including anaphylaxis, may occur. Is made from human plasma; process attempts to eliminate risk of hepatitis or HIV infection.

Overdose: Fluid overload.

ANTIDOTE

Reduce rate or temporarily stop infusion immediately for patient discomfort, mild hypotension, S/S of fluid overload, or other signs of adverse reaction. Keep physician informed. Treat fluid overload with loop diuretics (e.g., bumetanide, furosemide) if indicated. Treat mild hypersensitivity reactions with diphenhydramine (Benadryl) and if necessary, corticosteroids. Discontinue immediately for precipitous hypotension, anaphylaxis, or severe allergic reaction, and treat acute allergic symptoms with epinephrine, diphenhydramine, and corticosteroids as needed. Hypotension should resolve quickly; may require dopamine (Intropin).

RETEPLASE RECOMBINANT

(ree'teh-place re-kom'buh-nant)

Thrombolytic agent (recombinant)

Retavase, r-PA

pH 7 to 7.4

USUAL DOSE

Administered concomitantly with heparin. Give a 5,000-unit IV bolus of heparin before the initial injection of reteplase, then give 10 units (10 ml) of reteplase as an IV injection. Follow with a 1,000 unit/hr continuous IV infusion of heparin for at least 24 hours. Give a second 10-unit bolus of reteplase 30 minutes after the first. See Dilution, Incompatible With, and Rate of Administration. Aspirin is also used either during or following heparin treatment; an initial dose of 160 to 350 mg is followed by doses of 75 to 350 mg.

DOSE ADJUSTMENTS

The second bolus should not be given if serious bleeding in a critical location (e.g., intracranial, gastrointestinal, retroperitoneal, pericardial) occurs before it is due to be given.

DILUTION

Supplied in a kit with all components for reconstitution. Each kit contains a package insert and two of each of the following: single-use reteplase vials (10.8 units each), single-use diluent vials of SW (10 ml each), sterile 10-ml syringes with 20-gauge needles attached, sterile dispensing pins, sterile 20-gauge needles for administration, and alcohol swabs. Withdraw diluent with 20-gauge needle. Discard needle and put dispensing pin on syringe of diluent. Transfer diluent to vial of reteplase. Pin and syringe should remain in place while vial is swirled to dissolve reteplase. ***Do not shake.*** When completely dissolved, withdraw 10 ml reconstituted solution into the syringe (vials are 0.7 ml overfilled). Remove dispensing pin and replace with a 20-gauge needle for administration.

Storage: Kit should remain sealed to protect contents from light. Store at 2° to 25° C (36° to 77° F). Do not use beyond expiration date. Contains no preservatives; should be reconstituted immediately before use, but may be stored at room temperature if used within 4 hours. Discard all unused solution and supplies.

COMPATIBILITY

Manufacturer states, "Should be given via an IV line in which no other medication is being simultaneously injected or infused. No other medication should be added to the injection solution containing reteplase. Incompatible with heparin; do not administer heparin in the same IV line unless the line is flushed through with NS or D5W before and after reteplase."

RATE OF ADMINISTRATION

Heparin: First 1,000 units over 1 minute. After this test dose, the balance of 4,000 units may be given over 1 minute. Follow with an infusion of 1,000 units/hr.

Reteplase: A single dose evenly distributed over 2 minutes. To avoid incompatibilities and ensure delivery of both doses, be sure to flush line with a minimum of 30 to 50 ml NS or D5W before and after each injection.

ACTIONS

A recombinant plasminogen activator. Exerts its thrombolytic action by generating plasmin from plasminogen through a specific process. Plasmin then degrades the fibrin matrix of the thrombus. Potency is expressed in units that are specific to reteplase. With therapeutic doses, a decrease in circulating fibrinogen makes the patient susceptible to bleeding. Onset of action is prompt, effecting patency of the vessel within 90 minutes in most patients. The FDA has allowed the manufacturer to claim superiority over alteplase at achieving patency within 90 minutes. Prompt opening of arteries increases probability of improved cardiac function. Half-life is 13 to 16 minutes. Cleared from the plasma by the liver and kidneys. Mean fibrinogen level should return to baseline value within 48 hours.

INDICATIONS AND USES

Management of acute myocardial infarction (AMI) in adults for the improvement of ventricular function following AMI, the reduction of the incidence of congestive failure, and the reduction of mortality associated with AMI. Treatment should begin as soon as possible after the onset of symptoms of AMI. ■ Current AHA and JAMA recommendations identify thrombolytic agents as Class 1 therapy in patients younger than 70 years with recent onset of chest pain (within 6 hours) consistent with AMI and at least 0.1 mV of ST segment elevation in at least two ECG leads. Use in all other patients based on age, accurate diagnosis, and time from onset of chest pain.

CONTRAINDICATIONS

Active internal bleeding, arteriovenous malformation or aneurysm, bleeding diathesis, history of cerebral vascular accident, intracranial or intraspinal surgery or trauma within 2 months, intracranial neoplasm, severe uncontrolled hypertension.

PRECAUTIONS

Administered under the direction of a physician knowledgeable in its use and with appropriate emergency drugs, diagnostic and laboratory facilities available. ■ Reperfusion arrhythmias occur frequently (e.g., sinus bradycardia, accelerated idioventricular rhythm, PVCs, ventricular tachycardia); have antiarrhythmic meds available at bedside. ■ A greater alteration of hemostatic status than with heparin. Strict bed rest indicated to reduce risk of bleeding. Use extreme care with the patient; avoid any excessive or rough handling or pressure (including too-frequent BPs); avoid invasive procedures (e.g., arterial puncture, venipuncture, IM injection). If these procedures are absolutely necessary, use extreme precautionary methods (use radial artery instead of femoral; small-gauge catheters and needles, and sites that are easily observed and compressible where bleeding can be controlled; avoid handling of catheter sites, and use extended pressure application of up to 30 minutes). Minor bleeding occurs often at catheter insertion sites. Avoid use of razors and toothbrushes. ■ Use extreme caution and weigh risks against anticipated benefits in the following situation: recent major surgery (e.g., coronary artery bypass graft, obstetric delivery, organ biopsy), previous puncture of noncompressible vessels (e.g., jugular, subclavian), cerebrovascular disease, recent GI or GU bleeding, recent trauma, hypertension (e.g., systolic BP equal to or greater than 180 mm Hg and/or diastolic BP equal to or greater than 110 mm Hg), high likelihood of left heart thrombus (e.g., mitral stenosis with atrial fibrillation), acute pericarditis, subacute bacterial endocarditis, hemostatic defects including those secondary to severe hepatic or renal disease, severe hepatic or renal dysfunction, pregnancy, diabetic hemorrhagic retinopathy or other hemorrhagic ophthalmic conditions, septic thrombophlebitis or occluded AV cannula at a seriously infected site, advanced age, patients currently receiving oral anticoagulants (e.g., warfarin [Coumadin]), any other condition in which bleeding constitutes a significant hazard or would be particularly difficult to manage because of its location. ■ Simultaneous therapy with continuous infusion of heparin is used to reduce the risk of rethrombosis. Markedly increases risk of bleeding. ■ Standard treatment for myocardial infarction continues simultaneously with reteplase therapy except if temporarily contraindicated (e.g., arterial blood gases) unless absolutely necessary. ■ No experience with patients receiving repeat courses of reteplase. ■ Cholesterol embolization has been reported and may be fatal.

Monitor: Best to establish separate IV lines for reteplase and heparin. If not appropriate, be sure to flush the IV line before and after each injection of reteplase. ■ Baseline ECG, CPK, and clotting studies (TT, PTT, CBC, fibrinogen level, platelets) and baseline assessment (patient condition, pain, hematomas, petechiae, or recent wounds) should be completed before administration. Type and cross-match may also be ordered. ■ Monitor ECG continuously, and record strips with greatest ST segment elevation initially and every 15 minutes for at least 4 hours. A 12-lead ECG is indicated when therapy is complete. ■ Maintain strict bed rest; monitor the patient carefully and frequently for anginal pain and signs of bleeding; observe catheter sites at least every 15 minutes and apply pressure dressings to any recently invaded site; watch for hematuria, hematemesis, bloody stool, petechiae, hematoma, flank pain, muscle weakness; do neuro checks every hour. Continue until normal clotting function returns. ■ Watch for extravasation. ■ See Precautions and Drug/Lab Interactions.

Patient Education: Compliance with all measures to minimize bleeding (e.g., strict bed rest) is very important. ■ Avoid use of razors, toothbrushes, and other sharp items. ■ Use caution while moving to avoid excessive bumping. ■ Report all episodes of bleeding and apply local pressure if indicated. Expect oozing from IV sites.

Maternal/Child: Category C: has resulted in hemorrhage leading to spontaneous abortions in rabbits. Safety for use in pregnancy, breast-feeding, and children not established.

Elderly: See Indications and Precautions. ■ May have poorer prognosis following AMI and pre-existing conditions that may increase risk of intracranial bleeding. Select patients carefully to maximize benefits.

DRUG/LAB INTERACTIONS

Interaction of reteplase with other cardioactive drugs has not been studied. Risk of bleeding may be increased by any medicine that affects blood clotting including anticoagulants (e.g., heparin, lepirudin [Refludan], warfarin [Coumadin]); Glycoprotein GPIIb/IIIa receptor antagonists (e.g., abciximab [ReoPro], eptifibatide [Integrilin], tirofiban [Aggrastat]; any medication that may cause hypoprothrombinemia, thrombocytopenia, or GI ulceration or bleeding (e.g., selected antibiotics such as cefamandole [Mandol], cefoperazone [Cefobid], cefotetan [Cefotan], ticarcillin [Ticar], aspirin, NSAIDs [e.g., ibuprofen (Advil, Motrin), naproxen (Aleve, Naprosyn), phenylbutazone [Butazolidin]); and/or any other medication that inhibits platelet aggregation (e.g., clopidogrel [Plavix], dipyridamole [Persantine], plicamycin [Mithracin], sulfinpyrazone [Anturane], ticlopidine [Ticlid], valproic acid [Depacon]). Concurrent use not recommended with the exception of heparin and aspirin (in AMI) to reduce the risk of rethrombosis. If concurrent or subsequent use indicated (e.g., management of acute coronary syndrome, percutaneous coronary intervention) monitor PT and aPTT closely. ■ Coagulation tests will be unreliable; specific procedures can be used; notify the lab of reteplase use.

SIDE EFFECTS

Bleeding is most common: internal (GI tract, GU tract, intracranial, respiratory, or retroperitoneal sites), epistaxis, gingival, and superficial or surface bleeding (venous cutdowns, arterial punctures, sites of recent surgical intervention). Reperfusion arrhythmias are common; other serious arrhythmias may occur. A few allergic reactions, as well as fever, hypotension, nausea, and vomiting, have occurred. Cholesterol embolism has been reported and may be fatal. Clinical S/S may include acute renal failure, gangrenous digits, hypertension, infarctions (e.g., bowel, cerebral, myocardial, or spinal cord), pancreatitis, "purple toe" syndrome, renal artery occlusion.

ANTIDOTE

Notify physician of all side effects. Note even the most minute bleeding tendency. Oozing at IV sites is expected. Control minor bleeding by local pressure. For severe bleeding in a critical location, discontinue second dose of reteplase if it has not been given and any heparin therapy immediately. Whole blood, packed RBCs, cryoprecipitate, fresh-frozen plasma, platelets, desmopressin, tranexamic acid, and aminocaproic acid may all be indicated. Topical preparations of aminocaproic acid may stop minor bleeding. Consider protamine if heparin has been used. Treat bradycardia with atropine, reperfusion arrhythmias with lidocaine or procainamide; VT or VF may require cardioversion. Treat minor allergic reactions symptomatically. Discontinue drug and treat anaphylaxis as indicated; resuscitate as necessary. Discontinue therapy if any symptoms of cholesterol embolism occur.

Rh_o(D) IMMUNE GLOBULIN INTRAVENOUS (HUMAN)

(im-myoun′ gloh′byou-lin in′trah-ve-nes)

Immunizing agent (passive)
Platelet count stimulator

Rh_o(D)-IGIV, WinRho SD

pH 6.5 to 7.6

USUAL DOSE

Treatment of immune thrombocytopenic purpura (ITP); Adults and children: Confirm Rh_o(D) positive status of patient. Must be given IV. Hemoglobin should be greater than 10 Gm/dl. Give 250 IU (50 mcg)/kg of body weight as the initial dose. May be given as a single dose or divided in half and given on two consecutive days. If response to the initial dose is adequate, maintenance doses of 125 to 300 IU (25 to 60 mcg)/kg may be given. If response to the inital dose is inadequate; see Dose Adjustments. Dose and frequency based on patient's clinical response (e.g., RBC, hemoglobin, reticulocyte levels, and platelet counts); see Dose Adjustments.

Pregnancy, predelivery: Confirm Rh_o(D) negative status of patient. May be given IV or IM. 1,500 IU (300 mcg) at 28 weeks' gestation. If administered early in the pregnancy, it should be repeated at 12-week intervals to maintain an adequate level of passively acquired anti-Rh.

Pregnancy, postdelivery: Confirm Rh_o(D) negative status of patient. May be given IV or IM. 600 IU (120 mcg) as soon as possible after delivery of a confirmed Rh_o(D)-positive baby. Usually given no later than 72 hours postdelivery. If the Rh status of the infant is unknown at 72 hours, administer to the mother at that time. Should be given as soon as possible up to 28 days after delivery. This second dose postdelivery (first dose given predelivery; see above) can reduce treatment failure to 0.1%.

Postabortion, amniocentesis (after 34 weeks' gestation), or any other manipulation late in pregnancy (after 34 weeks' gestation): Confirm Rh_o(D) negative status of patient. May be given IV or IM. 600 IU (120 mcg) immediately after abortion or procedure associated with increased risk of Rh isoimmunization. Must be given within 72 hours. One half of a dose (a mini-dose [IM product]) may be given if a pregnancy terminates before 13 weeks gestation, administration within 3 hours is preferred. According to the literature, this mini-dose can provide 100% effectiveness in preventing Rh immunization.

Postamniocentesis before 34 weeks' gestation or after chorionic villus sampling: Confirm Rh_o(D) negative status of patient. May be given IV or IM. 1,500 IU (300 mcg) immediately after the procedure. Repeat every 12 weeks during the pregnancy.

Threatened abortion: Confirm Rh_o(D) negative status of patient. May be given IV or IM. 1,500 IU (300 mcg) as soon as possible.

Transfusion or fetal hemorrhage: Confirm Rh_o(D) negative status of patient. Administer within 72 hours of an incompatible event involving Rh_o(D) positive blood such as exposure to incompatible blood transfusions (Rh+ whole blood or Rh+ red blood cells) or massive fetal hemorrhage. Give up to 3,000 IU (600 mcg) every 8 hours IV or every 12 hours IM until the total dose is administered. Total dose is 45 IU (9 mcg) for every milliliter of Rh+ whole blood exposure or 90 IU (18 mcg) for every milliliter of Rh+ red blood cells exposure.

PEDIATRIC DOSE

Treatment of ITP: See Usual Dose and Dose Adjustments.

DOSE ADJUSTMENTS

Treatment of ITP: Adults and children: If the hemoglobin level is less than 10 Gm/dl before or after the initial dose reduce the initial dose and/or maintenance doses to 125 to 200 IU (25 to 40 mcg)/kg to minimize the risk of increasing the severity of anemia in the patient. ■ In patients with adequate platelet response to the initial dose, adjust maintenance doses based on platelet and hemoglobin levels. ■ If response to the initial dose is inadequate adjust subsequent doses as follows:

Hemoglobin above 10 Gm/dl, redose with 250 to 300 IU (50 to 60 mcg)/kg.

Hemoglobin is 8 to 10 Gm/dl, redose with 125 to 200 IU (25 to 40 mcg)/kg.

Hemoglobin below 8 Gm/dl, use with caution, may increase severity of anemia.

Continued

Pregnancy and obstetrical conditions: Protection must be maintained throughout pregnancy once Rh_o(D) immune globulin is administered. Level of passively acquired anti-Rh_o(D) should not fall below levels required to prevent an immune response to Rh_o(D)+ blood. Additional doses should be given every 12 weeks during pregnancy and at delivery unless the previous dose was administered within 3 weeks and there is less than 15 ml of fetomaternal red blood cell hemorrhage during delivery. **Suppression of Rh isoimmunization:** A large fetomaternal hemorrhage may cause an incorrect evaluation by standard tests of the amount of Rh_o(D) IGIV required. Assess the amount of hemorrhage and adjust dose accordingly.

DILUTION

Each 600 or 1,500 IU vial must be reconstituted with 2.5 ml of NS, provided by manufacturer. Reconstitute the 5,000 IU vial with 8.5 ml of NS. Direct diluent slowly onto the inside wall of the vial and gently swirl until dissolved. Avoid foaming, do not shake. Should dissolve within 10 minutes. Use as many vials as are required to achieve desired dose. In all dilutions 5 IU equals 1 mcg.

Storage: Store unopened vials in refrigerator. Note expiration date. Do not freeze. Reconstituted vials can be stored in the refrigerator but must be used within 12 hours of reconstitution. Discard unused portion.

COMPATIBILITY

Manufacturer states, "Should be administered separately from other drugs." Dilute only with NS.

RATE OF ADMINISTRATION

A single dose as an IV injection over 3 to 5 minutes.

ACTIONS

A specialty immunoglobulin containing human plasma protein fraction, consisting primarily of IgG. Reduces the incidence of Rh immunization of an Rh_o(D)-negative mother by an Rh_o(D)-positive infant before, during and after delivery; reduces the likelihood of hemolytic disease in an Rh_o(D)-positive infant in present and future pregnancies. Has also been shown to increase platelet counts in nonsplenectomized Rh_o(D)-positive patients with immune thrombocytopenic purpura (ITP). A 1,500-IU vial contains 300 mcg of anti-Rh_o(D), which can effectively suppress the immunizing potential of approximately 17 ml of Rh_o(D)-positive blood cells, and, in addition, contains 25 to 40 mg of nonspecific gammaglobulin. Pooled from source plasma selected for high titers of Rh_o(D) antibody. Purified and standardized by several specific methods (e.g., solvent-detergent viral inactivation process to decrease the possibility of transmission of blood-borne pathogens [e.g., HIV, hepatitis]). Similar to native IgG that normally circulates in human plasma and has a similar half-life (23 to 26 days). Platelet counts usually begin to rise in 1 to 2 days with peak effect in 7 to 14 days. Some effects last about 30 days. Crosses the blood-brain barrier.

INDICATIONS AND USES

Treatment of nonsplenectomized Rh_o(D)-positive children with acute or chronic immune thrombocytopenic purpura (ITP), adults with chronic ITP, or children and adults with ITP secondary to HIV infection in clinical situations requiring an increase in platelet counts to prevent excessive hemorrhage. ■ Suppression of Rh isoimmunization in nonsensitized

Rh_o(D)-negative women during the normal course of pregnancy, within 72 hours after spontaneous or induced abortions, amniocentesis, chorionic villus sampling, ruptured tubal pregnancy, abdominal trauma or transplacental hemorrhage, unless the blood type of the fetus or father is known to be Rh_o(D)-negative (prophylaxis and Rh hemolytic disease of the newborn). ■ Suppression of Rh isoimmunization in Rh_o(D)-negative female children and female adults in their childbearing years transfused with Rh_o(D)-positive red blood cells or blood components containing Rh_o(D)-positive RBCs.

CONTRAINDICATIONS

All uses: History of a prior severe hypersensitivity reaction to human immune globulin preparations or their component (may contain thiomerosol); patient with isolated IgA deficiency or pre-existing IgA antibodies. **Treatment of ITP:** Not recommended for use in Rh_o(D)-negative or splenectomized individuals.

Suppression of Rh isoimmunization in pregnancy: For suppression of Rh isoimmunization in the mother. ***Do not administer to the infant.*** Not recommended for use in Rh_o(D)-negative individuals shown to be Rh immunized by standard screening tests.

PRECAUTIONS

All uses: Confirm vial label—must state for IV or IV/IM use; several similar products are for IM use only (e.g., RhoGam). ■ May risk transmission of infectious agents (e.g., hepatitis, HIV, possibly the Creutzfeldt-Jakob disease [CJD] agent); see Actions. ■ Contains trace amounts of anti-A, anti-B, anti-C, and anti-E blood group antibodies.

Treatment of ITP: IV route required for ITP. ■ If the hemoglobin level is less than 8 Gm/dl, use with extreme caution; may increase severity of anemia. ■ Trace amounts of anti-A, anti-B, anti-C, and anti-E blood group antibodies may be detectable in direct and indirect antiglobulin (Coombs) tests following treatment with Rh_o(D).

Suppression of Rh isoimmunization in pregnancy: More than 1 dose of Rh_o(D) immune globulin may be required. A fetal RBC count can be done on maternal blood to determine the required dose. ■ If a large fetomaternal hemorrhage occurs late in pregnancy or after delivery Rh_o(D) IGIV should be administered in sufficient doses if there is any doubt about the mother's blood type (e.g., presence of passively administered anti-Rh_o(D) in maternal or fetal blood [positive Coombs test]). ■ See Monitor. ■ Manufacturer recommends IM or IV use. Another source recommends IM injection when Rh_o(D) is used as an immunizing agent. ■ Not effective in Rh_o(D) negative females who have already been sensitized to the Rh_o(D) erythrocyte factor, however if administered, the risk of side effects are not increased.

Monitor: ***All uses:*** See Precautions.

Treatment of ITP: Obtain baseline RBC, hemoglobin, reticulocyte levels, and platelet counts. Monitor during therapy to determine clinical response. ■ Given to Rh_o(D)-positive patients, in this situation, interaction with RBC usually cause some degree of RBC hemolysis; observe carefully. Monitor for S/S of intravascular hemolysis (IVH), clinically compromising anemia, and renal insufficiency. ■ If transfusion is required, use Rh_o(D)-negative RBC's to avoid exacerbating ongoing IVH. Platelet products may contain RBC's, use caution if platelets from an Rh_o(D)+ donor are used.

Suppression of Rh isoimmunization in pregnancy: Maintain accurate records of Rh factor and Rh_o(D)-IGIV. ■ Obtain CBC and other appropriate lab work based on procedure or situation. ■ Monitor vital signs if indicated.

Patient Education: ***ITP:*** May cause a considerable drop in hemoglobin; follow-up testing important. ■ Report feelings of dizziness, tiredness, weakness.

Maternal/Child: Category C: use only if clearly needed. ■ Specific information not available on safety during breast-feeding. ■ For the suppression of Rh isoimmunization in the mother; do not administer to the infant.

Elderly: No specific information available.

DRUG/LAB INTERACTIONS

Interaction with other drugs has not been evaluated. ■ Antibodies contained in Rh_o(D) immune globulin may interfere with the body's immune response to certain live virus vaccines. Do not administer live virus vaccines (e.g., measles, mumps, polio or rubella) for at least 3 months after Rh_o(D) administration.

SIDE EFFECTS

All uses: Chills, discomfort at the injection site, fever, and headache occur most frequently.

ITP: Destruction of Rh_o(D) red cells resulting in decreased hemoglobin (range was 0.4 to 6.1 Gm/dl). IVH (back pain, shaking chills, hemoglobinuria), acute onset and exacerbation of anemia, and renal insufficiency have been reported in Rh_o(D)-positive patients. Has rarely resulted in death.

Suppression of Rh isoimmunization in pregnancy: Only 26 out of 9,905 women had treatment failures resulting in development of Rh_o(D) antibodies.

ANTIDOTE

Keep physician informed of side effects; may require symptomatic treatment. ***ITP:*** Treatment may have to be discontinued if drop in hemoglobin too severe. Transfusion may be required.

RIFAMPIN

(rih-fam′pin)

Rifadin

Antibacterial (antituberculosis)

pH 7.8 to 8.8

USUAL DOSE

Dose and schedule may vary depending on treatment regimen selected. IV doses are the same as oral. Use oral dose form as soon as practical.

Tuberculosis: 10 mg/kg once a day. Do not exceed 600 mg/day. Another source suggests 600 mg once a day or 10 mg/kg not to exceed 600 mg/dose two or three times a week. Prescribed concurrently with at least one other antituberculin drug (e.g., ethambutol [Myambutol], isoniazid, pyrazinamide, or streptomycin).

Meningococcal carriers: 600 mg daily as a single dose for 4 days or 600 mg every 12 hours for 2 days.

Leprosy (unlabeled): 600 mg once a month for a minimum of 2 years or until smear is negative, whichever is longer. Given in combination with other antileprosy agents.

PEDIATRIC DOSE

Children 1 month of age and older.

Tuberculosis: 10 to 20 mg/kg of body weight either once a day or two or three times a week depending on regimen. Do not exceed 600 mg. Prescribed concurrently with at least one other antituberculin drug (e.g., ethambutol [Myambutol], isoniazid, pyrazinamide, or streptomycin).

Meningococcal infection (prophylaxis): 10 mg/kg every 12 hours for 2 days.

NEONATAL DOSE

Tuberculosis: 10 to 20 mg/kg either once a day or two or three times a week depending on regimen. Prescribed concurrently with at least one other antituberculin drug (e.g., ethambutol [Myambutol], isoniazid, pyrazinamide, or streptomycin).

Meningococcal infection (prophylaxis); ***under 1 month of age:*** 5 mg/kg every 12 hr for 2 days. ***Over 1 month of age:*** 10 mg/kg every 12 hr for 2 days.

DOSE ADJUSTMENTS

Dose reduction to 10 mg/kg/day may be required in the debilitated or elderly. ■ Reduced dose required in impaired hepatic function. A 50% reduction in dose may be required in severe impaired hepatic function. ■ No dose adjustment is necessary in impaired renal function; serum concentrations do not change. ■ See Drug/Lab Interactions.

DILUTION

Each 600-mg vial must be initially diluted in 10 ml of SW for injection (60 mg/ml). Swirl gently to dissolve. Withdraw desired dose and further dilute in 500 ml (preferred) or 100 ml of D5W. If dextrose is contraindicated, NS may be used. 100-ml dilution used only in selected situations.

Storage: Use solution diluted in D5W within 4 hours; solution diluted in NS stable for 24 hours. Protect from light before dilution.

COMPATIBILITY

Manufacturer states, "May form a precipitate with diltiazem (Cardizem) at the Y-site."

RATE OF ADMINISTRATION

A single dose equally distributed as an infusion over 3 hours. In selected situations a single dose diluted in 100 ml may be administered over 30 minutes.

ACTIONS

A semisynthetic, antituberculosis antibiotic. Has a bactericidal or bacteriostatic action that is effective in susceptible cells during cell division or at the resting stage and average levels are maintained for 8 to 12 hours based on dose. Rapidly distributed throughout the body and present in many organs and body fluids including CSF. Metabolized in the liver and excreted in bile and urine. Half-life following repeated dosing is 2 to 3 hours. Crosses the placental barrier. Secreted in breast milk.

INDICATIONS AND USES

Treatment or retreatment of tuberculosis when the drug cannot be taken by mouth. ■ Treatment of asymptomatic carriers of *Neisseria* meningitis. Not indicated for treatment of meningococcal infection because of rapid emergence of resistant meningococci. ■ Used in combination with other agents in the treatment of certain atypical mycobacterial infections (e.g., *Mycobacterium avium*). Used in combination with other antistaphylococcal agents to treat serious staphylococcal infections.

Unlabeled uses: Leprosy.

CONTRAINDICATIONS

Hypersensitivity to any rifamycins; individuals with liver disease are at higher risk for complications.

PRECAUTIONS

For IV use only. Do not administer IM or SC. ■ Risk of liver damage is markedly increased if impaired liver function is present. Hepatotoxicity, hepatic encephalopathy, and death associated with jaundice have occurred in patients with liver disease and when rifampin is given with other hepatotoxic agents (e.g., isoniazid, halothane). Discontinue one or both drugs if signs of hepatocellular damage occur. ■ Obtain cultures before starting therapy to confirm susceptibility of the organism to rifampin. Repeat cultures periodically during therapy to monitor for the emergence of resistance. ■ Susceptibility tests also required before use as treatment for asymptomatic carriers of *Neisseria* meningitis. ■ May exacerbate porphyria. ■ Urine, feces, saliva, sputum, sweat, and tears may be colored red-orange. Soft contact lenses may be permanently stained. CSF may be light yellow. ■ Pseudomembranous colitis has been reported. May range from mild to life-threatening. Consider in patients that present with diarrhea during or after treatment with rifampin.

Monitor: Obtain baseline measurements of hepatic enzymes (e.g., ALT [SGPT] and AST [SGOT]), bilirubin, SrCr, CBC, and platelet count. Routine lab monitoring in patients with normal baseline labs is generally not necessary. However, patients should be seen monthly and questioned about symptoms that may indicate adverse reactions. ■ Notify physician immediately if flu-like symptoms develop; may be due to hepatotoxicity. ■ Thrombocytopenia has occurred. Reversible if rifampin is discontinued as soon as purpura occurs. Cerebral hemorrhage has occurred when rifampin has been continued or resumed after the appearance of purpura. Contact physician immediately if purpura occurs. ■ Confirm patency of IV; avoid extravasation. Restart IV at a new site for any signs of inflammation or irritation. ■ Do all lab tests and affected radiology studies before daily dose of medication. ■ See Drug/Lab Interactions.

Patient Education: Use of nonhormonal contraceptives recommended. ■ Avoid use of alcohol or other hepatotoxic agents (e.g., acetaminophen [Anacin-3, Tylenol], NSAIDs [ibuprofen (Advil, Motrin) naproxen (Aleve, Naprosyn)], phenothiazines [e.g., promethazine (Phenergan)], some antineoplastic agents, sulfonamides). ■ May cause reddish-orange discoloration of feces, saliva, sputum, sweat, urine, and tears. ■ May discolor soft contact lenses.

Maternal/Child: Category C: has teratogenic potential. Safety for use during pregnancy not established. Benefit must outweigh risk. See literature for best combinations with least known risk. ■ Administration during the last few weeks of pregnancy may cause postnatal hemorrhages in mother and infant; treatment with vitamin K may be required. ■ Closely monitor neonates of rifampin-treated mothers for adverse effects. ■ Discontinue breast-feeding if mother requires treatment.

Elderly: Differences in response between elderly and younger patients have not been identified. ■ Risk of hepatitis increased after age 50 years. ■ See Dose Adjustments.

DRUG/LAB INTERACTIONS

Interactions are numerous and potentially life threatening. Review of drug profile by pharmacist imperative. ■ Hepatotoxicity, hepatic encephalopathy, and death associated with jaundice have occurred when rifampin is given with other hepatotoxic agents (e.g., alcohol, isoniazid, halothane). Discontinue one or both drugs for signs of hepatocellular damage. ■ Rifampin increases metabolism and clearance and decreases serum levels and effectiveness of acetaminophen (Tylenol), amiodarone (Cordarone), amprenavir (Agenerase), analgesics (e.g., narcotics), antifungals (e.g., fluconazole [Diflucan], itraconazole [Sporanox], Ketoconazole [Nizoral]), barbiturates (e.g., phenobarbital), benzodiazepines (e.g., diazepam [Valium], midazolam [Versed]), beta-blockers (e.g., propranolol [Inderal]), buspirone [BuSpar], calcium channel blockers (e.g., diltiazem [Cardizem], nifedipine [Procardia], verapamil [Isoptin]), chloramphenicol, clofibrate (Atromid-S), clozapine (Clozaril), corticosteroids (e.g., prednisone), cyclosporine (Sandimmune), dapsone, digoxin and digitoxin, disopyramide (Norpace), doxycycline (Vibramycin), estrogens, fluoroquinolones (e.g., ciprofloxacin [Cipro], gatifloxacin [Tequin]), haloperidol (Haldol), hydantoins (e.g., phenytoin [Dilantin]), lamotrigine (Lamictal), levothyroxine (Synthroid), losartan (Cozaar), methadone, mexiletine (Mexitil), oral antidiabetics (glyburide [DiaBeta], tolbutamide [Orinase]), oral anticoagulants (warfarin [Coumadin]), ondansetron (Zofran), oral contraceptives, progestins (e.g., megestrol [Megace], progesterone), propafenone (Rythmol), quinidine, quinine, sildenafil (Viagra), tacrolimus (Prograf), theophyllines (e.g., aminophylline), tocainide (Tonocard), tricyclic antidepressants (e.g., amitriptyline [Elavil], nortriptyline [Aventyl]), zidovudine (AZT), and zolpidem (Ambien). Increased doses of these drugs may be required. Monitor carefully; obtain prothrombin daily when used with anticoagulants (e.g., warfarin); use of nonhormonal contraceptives recommended during rifampin therapy; and diabetes may be more difficult to control. ■ May reduce analgesic effects of morphine and methadone. Monitor carefully; an alternate analgesic may be required (see statement above). ■ Treatment failure of ketoconazole (Nizoral) or rifampin may occur when given concomitantly. ■ Concomitant use of rifampin and macrolide antibiotics (e.g., clarithromycin) may decrease the metabolism of rifampin and increase the metabolism of the macrolide antibiotic. ■ Concomitant use of rifampin and protease inhibitors (e.g., amprenavir [Agenerase], indinavir [Crixivan], nelfinavir [Viracept], ritonavir [Norvir], saquinavir [Fortovase]) may decrease the metabolism of rifampin and increase the metabolism of the protease inhibitors. See CDC guidelines for possible concomitant use. ■ Concurrent use with nonnucleoside reverse transcriptase inhibitors (NNRTIs) (e.g., delavirdine [Rescriptor], efavirenz [Sustiva], nevirapine [Viramune]) may decrease the metabolism of rifampin and increase the metabolism of the NNRTIs. ■ Inhibited by clofazimine (Lamprene). Decreases rate of absorption and delays peak plasma levels of rifampin. ■ Potentiated by probenecid. ■ May cause hypertension with enalapril (Vasotec). ■ Para-aminosalicylic acid (PAS) will decrease serum levels of rifampin. Drugs should be taken at least 8 hours apart. ■ Pyrazinamide may also reduce rifampin serum levels. ■ When taken concomitantly, decreased concentrations of atovaquone (Mepron) and increased concentration of rifampin have been observed. ■ May induce metabolism of endogenous substrates including adrenal hormones, thyroid hormones, and vitamin D. Reduced levels of vitamin D may be accompanied by decreased serum calcium and phosphate and increased parathyroid hormone. ■ Cross-reactivity and false-positive urine screening tests for opiates have been reported when using certain assays. Gas chromatography or mass spectrometry will distinguish rifampin from opiates. ■ May cause an early rise in bilirubin during initial days of treatment; should subside. Throughout treatment transient abnormalities in liver function tests will occur. ■ Therapeutic levels inhibit assays of serum folate and vitamin B_{12}. ■ Reduced biliary excretion of contrast media for gallbladder studies may occur. Perform test prior to dose of rifampin.

SIDE EFFECTS

Average dose: Anaphylaxis may occur even with repeat doses. Abnormal liver function tests, anorexia, ataxia, behavioral changes, conjunctivitis (exudative), cramps, diarrhea, dizziness, edema of face and extremities, epigastric distress, eosinophilia, fatigue, flushing, flu-like symptoms (e.g., chills, fever, headache, malaise, muscle and bone pain), gas, heartburn, hematuria, hemolytic anemia, hepatic reactions, hepatitis, hypotension, leukopenia, menstrual disturbances, mental confusion, myopathy (rare), muscle weakness, nausea, numbness (generalized), pain in extremities, pseudomembranous colitis, psychosis purpura, pruritus, rash, renal failure (acute), shortness of breath, sore mouth and tongue, thrombocytopenia, urticaria, visual disturbances, vomiting, wheezing.

Overdose: Abdominal pain, bilirubin levels and/or liver enzymes may increase rapidly; brown-red discoloration of feces, skin, sweat, tears, and urine is proportional to amount of overdose; headache, lethargy, nausea, and vomiting are immediate; liver enlargement and tenderness; pruritis, unconsciousness. Arrhythmias, cardiac arrest, hypotension, and seizures have been reported in fatal overdoses.

ANTIDOTE

With increasing severity of any side effect, alterations in liver function tests, flu-like symptoms, purpura, thrombocytopenia, or symptoms of overdose, discontinue the drug and notify the physician immediately. Antiemetics (e.g., ondansetron [Zofran], prochlorperazine [Compazine]) may be required to control nausea and vomiting. Forced diuresis will promote excretion. Bile drainage may be indicated in the presence of seriously impaired hepatic function lasting more than 24 to 48 hours. Hemodialysis may be useful. Treat anaphylaxis and resuscitate as necessary.

RITUXIMAB

(rih-tuks′ih-mab)

Rituxan

Recombinant monoclonal antibody
Antineoplastic

pH 6.5

USUAL DOSE

Premedication: Acetaminophen (Tylenol) and diphenhydramine (Benadryl) should be considered as premedication before each dose to prevent or attenuate severe hypersensitivity reactions.

Single agent: *Initial therapy:* 375 mg/M^2 as an infusion once a week for four or eight doses. See Drug/Lab Interactions.

Single agent: *Retreatment therapy:* Patients who subsequently develop progressive disease may be retreated with 375 mg/M^2 as an IV infusion once each week for four doses. Data on more than 2 courses are limited.

Therapeutic regimen with ibritumomab tiuxetan: 250 mg/M^2 as an IV infusion. Given in a specific protocol in combination with ibritumomab tiuxetan (Zevalin [In-111 ibritumomab and Y-90 ibritumomab]); see ibritumomab monograph.

PEDIATRIC DOSE

Safety and effectiveness for use in children not established.

DOSE ADJUSTMENTS

No dose adjustments recommended. See Rate of Administration.

DILUTION

Each single dose must be further diluted to a final concentration of 1 to 4 mg/ml with NS or D5W. 500 mg (50 ml) in 450 ml will yield 1 mg/ml; 500 mg (50 ml) in 75 ml will yield 4 mg/ml. Gently invert to mix solution. Contains no preservatives; discard any unused portion left in vial.

Storage: Refrigerate vials at 2° to 8° C (36° to 46° F) and protect from light. Do not use beyond expiration date. Diluted solutions may be refrigerated for 24 hours and are stable at room temperature for an additional 24 hours.

COMPATIBILITY

Manufacturer states, "Rituximab should not be mixed or diluted with other drugs." No incompatibilities with polyvinylchloride or polyethylene bags have been observed.

RATE OF ADMINISTRATION

Must be given as an infusion. ***Do not administer as an IV push or bolus.*** Hypersensitivity reactions are a common occurrence and may be prevented or lessened with premedication and a reduced rate of infusion.

First infusion: Begin with an initial rate of 50 mg/hr (at this rate a 500-mg dose would be infused over 10 hours). If no discomfort or adverse effects occur, may be gradually increased by 50-mg/hr increments at 30-minute intervals to a maximum rate of 400 mg/hr. At any time that discomfort or adverse effects occur, reduce the rate of infusion. Discontinue the infusion for severe reactions and treat as indicated; see Antidote. When symptoms have completely resolved, the infusion can be restarted at half the previous rate.

Subsequent infusions: If the patient did not tolerate the first infusion well, follow instructions under first infusion. If no discomfort or adverse effects occurred with the first infusion, subsequent infusions may begin with an initial rate of 100 mg/hr and increased by 100-mg/hr increments at 30-minute intervals to a maximum rate of 400 mg/hr. See all precautionary measures under First Infusion (see p. 991).

ACTIONS

An antineoplastic agent. A humanized (Ig)G_1 monoclonal antibody produced by recombinant DNA technology. Designed to bind to the CD20 antigen found on the surface of normal and malignant B lymphocytes. CD20 is also expressed on more than 90% of B-cell non-Hodgkin's lymphomas but is not expressed on hematopoietic stem cells. CD20 regulates an early step(s) in the activation process for cell cycle initiation and differentiation. Rituximab binds to lymphoid cells in the thymus, the white pulp of the spleen, and a majority of B lymphocytes in peripheral blood and lymph nodes. There is little or no binding to non-lymphoid tissue. Results in a rapid and sustained depletion (cytotoxity) of circulating and tissue-based B cells. Cell lysis may be the result of complement-dependent cytotoxicity and antibody-dependent cellular cytotoxicity. May sensitize drug-resistant human B-cell lymphoma cell lines to cytotoxic chemotherapy. Detected in serum for 3 to 6 months after completion of therapy. Depletion was sustained for 6 to 9 months posttreatment in 83% of patients. B-cell recovery begins at approximately 6 months, and most levels return to normal by 12 months following completion of treatment. Average serum half-life was 76.3 hours (range 31.5 to 152.6 hours) after the first infusion and 205.8 hours (range 83.9 to 407 hours) after the fourth infusion. Wide range may reflect variable tumor burdens and decreasing numbers of CD20–positive B-cells with repeated infusions. Peak and trough serum levels were inversely correlated with baseline values for the number of circulating CD20–positive B-cells and measures of disease burden. Serum concentrations were found to be higher in responders than in non-responders. IgG antibodies may cross the placental barrier. May be secreted in breast milk.

INDICATIONS AND USES

As a single agent in the treatment of patients with relapsed or refractory low-grade or follicular CD20–positive B-cell non-Hodgkin's lymphoma. ■ In combination with ibritumomab tiuxetan as part of a therapeutic regimen for the treatment of patients with relapsed or refractory low-grade, follicular, or transformed B-cell non-Hodgkin's lymphoma, including patients with rituximab-refractory follicular non-Hodgkin's lymphoma.

CONTRAINDICATIONS

Known hypersensitivity or anaphylactic reactions to murine proteins, rituximab, or any of its components.

PRECAUTIONS

Has been given on an outpatient basis; however, rituximab should be administered by or under the direction of the physician specialist in facilities equipped to monitor the patient and respond to any medical emergency. ■ Severe infusion reactions and hypersensitivity reactions have occurred, and some have been fatal. Most severe reactions occur within 30 min to 2 hr of beginning the first infusion. S/S of severe reactions may include hypotension, angioedema, hypoxia, or bronchospasm. More severe manifestations may include pulmonary infiltrates, acute respiratory distress syndrome, myocardial infarction, ventricular fibrillation, and cardiogenic shock. ■ Use caution in patients who either have or develop HAMA/HACA titers; may have allergic reactions when treated with rituximab or other murine or chimeric monoclonal antibodies. ■ Tumor lysis syndrome (TLS) has been reported within 12 to 24 hours after the first rituximab infusion. S/S are rapid reduction in tumor volume, renal insufficiency, hyperkalemia, hypocalcemia, hyperuricemia, or hyperphosphatasemia. May cause acute renal failure requiring dialysis and has been fatal. ■ TLS occurs more often in patients with high numbers of circulating malignant cells or high tumor burden. Consider prophylactic measures; see Monitor. ■ Renal toxicity occurs more frequently in patients with high numbers of circulating malignant cells, high tumor burden, and/or TLS. ■ Safety of immunization with vaccines, particularly live viral vaccines, and the ability of the patient to respond to vaccines following rituximab therapy has not been studied. ■ Mucocutaneous reactions, some with fatal outcomes, have been reported. ■ See Rate of Administration, Drug/Lab Interactions, and Antidote.

Monitor: Obtain baseline CBC and platelet count and repeat at regular intervals. Repeat more frequently in patients who develop cytopenias (e.g., leukopenia, neutropenia, thrombocytopenia). Duration of cytopenias may extend beyond the treatment period. ■ Observe patient continuously for symptoms of allergic reactions; more frequent during the first infusion, but can occur at any time. ■ Monitor HR and BP frequently. ■ ECG and pulmonary monitoring required during and in the immediate posttreatment period in patients with pre-existing cardiac or pulmonary conditions and in any patient who develops or has previously developed a clinically significant cardiopulmonary adverse event during treatment. ■ Monitor patients with high numbers of circulating malignant cells (greater than or equal to $25{,}000/mm^3$) with or without other evidence of high tumor burden for infusion reaction and tumor lysis syndrome. Monitoring of serum electrolytes and renal function indicated. ■ Prevention and treatment of hyperuricemia due to TLS may be accomplished with adequate hydration and, if necessary, allopurinol (Aloprim, Zyloprim) and alkalinization of urine. ■ Prevention and/or treatment of hyperphosphatemia, hyperkalemia, and hypercalcemia due to TLS is also indicated. ■ Observe closely for signs of infection. Prophylactic antibiotics may be indicated pending results of C/S in a febrile neutropenic patient. ■ Use prophylactic antiemetics to reduce nausea and vomiting and increase patient comfort. ■ Monitor for thrombocytopenia (platelet count less than $50{,}000/mm^3$). Initiate precautions to prevent excessive bleeding (e.g., inspect IV sites, skin, and mucous membranes; use extreme care during invasive procedures; test urine, emesis, stool, and secretions for occult blood). ■ See Premedication in Usual Dose, Rate of Administration, Drug/Lab Interactions; and Antidote.

Patient Education: Avoid pregnancy; nonhormonal birth control recommended. See Maternal/Child. ■ Review monitoring requirements and potential side effects before therapy. ■ Report any unusual or unexpected symptoms or side effects promptly. ■ See Appendix D, p. 1148.

Maternal/Child: Category C: avoid pregnancy; women of childbearing age should use birth control during treatment and for up to 12 months after completion of treatment. Could potentially cause fetal B-cell depletion. Use only if clearly needed. ■ Discontinue breast-feeding until circulating drug levels are no longer detectable. ■ Safety and effectiveness in children not established.

Elderly: In patients older than 65 years of age, response rates were higher, duration of response was shorter, and incidence, type, and severity of side effects were similar when compared to younger patients.

DRUG/LAB INTERACTIONS

Transient hypotension may occur during rituximab infusion; consider withholding antihypertensive medications 12 hours before rituximab infusion. ■ May inhibit the generation of an anamnestic (immunologic memory) or humoral (development of antibodies in the blood) response to any vaccine. ■ Pharmacokinetics of rituximab remained similar to rituximab alone when given in combination with CHOP chemotherapy (cyclophosphamide, doxorubicin, vincristine, prednisone). ■ Risk of renal toxicity increased in patients receiving concomitant therapy with cisplatin.

SIDE EFFECTS

Major side effects include: Infusion reactions, tumor lysis syndrome (may occur within 12 to 24 hours), mucocutaneous reactions (e.g., lichenoid dermatitis, paraneoplastic pemphigus, Stevens-Johnson syndrome, toxic epidermal necrolysis, and vesiculobullous dermatitis), hypersensitivity reactions (e.g., hypotension, bronchospasm, and angioedema), cardiac arrhythmias (e.g., supraventricular and ventricular tachycardia, ventricular fibrillation), angina, and renal failure. Hypersensitivity or infusion-related side effects generally occur within 30 minutes to 2 hours of beginning of first infusion. Fever and chills are most common. Other side effects include abdominal pain, anorexia, anxiety, arthralgia, asthenia, back pain, bone marrow depression (e.g., anemia, leukopenia, neutropenia, thrombocytopenia, prolonged pancytopenia, and marrow hypoplasia), cough, depression, diarrhea, dizziness, dyspnea, elevated LDH, fatigue, flushing, headache, hyperglycemia, hypertension, hypotension, infections (with or without neutropenia), myalgia, nausea, night sweats, pain at disease sites, peripheral edema, pruritus, rash, respiratory symptoms (e.g., acute infusion-related bronchospasm, acute pneumonitis 1 to 4 weeks post-rituximab infusion, bronchiolitis obliterans [one case ended in death]), rhinitis, sinusitis, tachycardia, throat irritation, urticaria, and vomiting.

ANTIDOTE

Keep physician informed of all side effects. May constitute a medical emergency or will be treated symptomatically as indicated. Hypersensitivity or infusion-related side effects generally resolve with slowing or interruption of the rituximab infusion and with supportive care (IV saline; diphenhydramine; bronchodilators such as albuterol [Ventolin], terbutaline [Brethaire], or aminophylline; and acetaminophen). Most patients who have had non–life-threatening reactions have been able to complete the full course of therapy. Restart the infusion at half the previous rate after symptoms have resolved completely. Discontinue the infusion immediately for any life-threatening side effect (e.g., clinically significant bronchospasm, cardiac arrhythmias, or hypotension; tumor lysis syndrome). Treat anaphylaxis with oxygen, antihistamines (diphenhydramine), epinephrine, and corticosteroids. Maintain a patent airway. Treat arrhythmias if indicated and monitor ECG until recovery and with subsequent doses. Treat hypotension with IV fluids, Trendelenburg position, and, if necessary, vasopressors (e.g., norepinephrine [Levophed], dopamine [Intropin]). Blood modifiers (e.g., darbepoetin alfa [Aranesp], epoetin alfa [Epogen, Procrit], filgrastim [Neupogen], pegfilgrastim [Neulasta], sargramostim [Leukine], oprelvekin [Neumega]) may be indicated to treat bone marrow toxicity. Tumor lysis syndrome requires correction of electrolyte abnormalities, monitoring of renal function and fluid balance, and supportive care including dialysis. Following complete resolution of all symptoms and their complications, rituximab has been tolerated when readministered with prophylactic therapy for TLS in a limited number of cases. Resuscitate if indicated.

SARGRAMOSTIM

(sar-gram′oh-stim)

Colony-stimulating factor
Antineutropenic

GM-CSF, Human Granulocyte-Macrophage Colony-Stimulating Factor, Leukine

pH 7.1 to 7.7

USUAL DOSE

Myeloid reconstitution after allogenic or autologous bone marrow transplantation: 250 mcg/M^2/day as a 2-hour infusion daily for 21 days. Initial infusion must begin 2 to 4 hours after bone marrow infusion and not less than 24 hours after the last dose of chemotherapy and 12 hours after the last dose of radiation. Post–marrow infusion absolute neutrophil count (ANC) should be less than 500 cells/mm^3.

Engraftment delay or failure of bone marrow transplantation: 250 mcg/M^2/day as a 2-hour infusion daily for 14 days. Wait for 7 days; if engraftment has not occurred, repeat 14-day course of 250 mcg/M^2. Wait an additional 7 days; if engraftment has still not occurred, give a 14-day course of 500 mcg/M^2. If engraftment does not occur, further courses or dose increases are not indicated. Note time restrictions on chemotherapy and radiation above and in Drug/Lab Interactions.

Neutrophil recovery following chemotherapy in acute myelogenous leukemia (AML) in adults 55 years of age or older: 250 mcg/M^2/day as an infusion over 4 hours. Begin on day 11 or 4 days after induction chemotherapy is complete. Day 10 bone marrow should be hypoplastic with fewer than 5% blasts. Repeat sargramostim daily until absolute neutrophil count (ANC) is greater than 1,500/mm^3 for three consecutive days or a maximum of 42 days. Use same criteria if a second cycle of induction chemotherapy is indicated.

Mobilization of peripheral blood progenitor cells: 250 mcg/M^2/day as a 24-hour continuous infusion (or give SC once daily). Continue at the same dose until adequate numbers of progenitor stem cells are collected. Collection of progenitor cells (apheresis) usually begins about day 5 and is repeated daily. All cells are stored until predetermined targets are achieved. After immunosuppression with selected antineoplastic bone marrow depressant agents to neutralize remaining tumor cells or ineffective leukocytes, the collected progenitor stem cells are reinfused into the patient by IV infusion. This process has been used primarily in patients who were not candidates for bone marrow transplant; however, it is increasingly being used instead of bone marrow transplant.

Post–peripheral blood progenitor cell transplantation: 250 mcg/M^2/day as a 24-hour continuous infusion (or give SC once daily). Begin immediately following infusion of harvested progenitor cells and continue until an ANC is greater than 1,500/mm^3 for three consecutive days. Neutrophil recovery occurs somewhat sooner in patients receiving sargramostim stimulation. Results in a shorter time to platelet and RBC transfusion independence.

DOSE ADJUSTMENTS

May require reduced dose in impaired renal or hepatic function. Based on individual patient response. ■ For an ANC above 20,000 cells/mm^3, WBC above 50,000 cells/mm^3, or a platelet count above 500,000/mm^3, reduce dose by one half or temporarily discontinue. ■ See Antidote.

DILUTION

Now available in liquid form (reconstituted) or each 250- or 500-mcg vial of the dry product must be reconstituted with 1 ml SW for injection with or without preservative. Confirm expiration date to ensure valid product. Direct diluent to the side of the vial and swirl gently. Avoid foaming or vigorous agitation. Do not shake. Either product must be further diluted in NS for infusion. If the final concentration of sargramostim will be below 10 mcg/ml, albumin (human) must be added to the NS before addition of the sargramostim (1 ml of 5% albumin to each 50 ml NS). This will prevent adsorption of the drug into the components of the IV delivery system. Liquefied product contains benzyl alcohol. Use sterile technique; enter vial only to dilute and/or to withdraw a single dose. Discard any unused portion. Should be clear and colorless.

Storage: Must be refrigerated in all forms; do not freeze or shake. Reconstituted with SW without preservatives or any diluted solution should be used within 6 hours. Reconstituted with bacteriostatic SW (benzyl alcohol preservative) or the new liquid preparation can be refrigerated for up to 20 days.

INCOMPATIBLE WITH

Manufacturer recommends that no medication other than albumin be added to the infusion solution until specific compatibility data are available.

COMPATIBLE WITH **(Underline Indicates Conflicting Compatibility Information)**

Consult pharmacist; specific conditions may apply; see Compatibilities, p. xvi.

Y-site: Amikacin (Amikin), aminophylline, <u>amphotericin B (Fungizone)</u>, aztreonam (Azactam), bleomycin (Blenoxane), butorphanol (Stadol), calcium gluconate, carboplatin (Paraplatin), carmustine (BiCNU), cefazolin (Kefzol), cefepime (Maxipime), cefotaxime (Claforan), cefotetan (Cefotan), <u>ceftazidime (Fortaz)</u>, ceftizoxime (Cefizox), ceftriaxone (Rocephin), cefuroxime (Zinacef), cimetidine (Tagamet), cisplatin (Platinol), clindamycin (Cleocin), cyclophosphamide (Cytoxan), cyclosporine (Sandimmune), cytarabine (ARA-C), dacarbazine (DTIC), dactinomycin (Cosmegen), dexamethasone (Decadron), diphenhydramine (Benadryl), dopamine (Intropin), doxorubicin (Adriamycin), doxycycline (Vibramycin), droperidol (Inapsine), etoposide (VePesid), famotidine (Pepcid IV), fentanyl (Sublimaze), fluconazole (Diflucan), fluorouracil (5-FU), furosemide (Lasix), gentamicin (Garamycin), granisetron (Kytril), heparin, idarubicin (Idamycin), ifosfamide (Ifex), immune globulin IV (IGIV), magnesium sulfate, mannitol, mechlorethamine (nitrogen mustard), meperidine (Demerol), mesna (Mesnex), methotrexate (Folex), metoclopramide (Reglan), metronidazole (Flagyl IV), minocycline (Minocin), mitoxantrone (Novantrone), pentostatin (Nipent), piperacillin/tazobactam (Zosyn), potassium chloride (KCl), prochlorperazine (Compazine), promethazine (Phenergan), ranitidine (Zantac), sulfamethoxazole-trimethoprim (Bactrim), teniposide (Vumon), ticarcillin (Ticar), ticarcillin/clavulanate (Timentin), <u>vancomycin (Vancocin)</u>, vinblastine (Velban), vincristine (Oncovin), zidovudine (AZT, Retrovir).

RATE OF ADMINISTRATION

See Usual Dose. Each single dose must be evenly distributed over 2, 4, or 24 hours. Do not use an in-line membrane filter. Reduce rate or temporarily discontinue for onset of any side effects that cause concern (e.g., allergic reaction).

ACTIONS

Colony-stimulating factors are glycoproteins that bind to specific hematopoietic cell surface receptors and stimulate proliferation, differentiation commitment, and some end-cell functional activation. Utilizing recombinant DNA technology, sargramostim is produced in a yeast *(Saccharomyces cerevisiae)*. It differs slightly from endogenous G-CSF. It induces partially committed progenitor cells to divide and differentiate in the granulocyte-macrophage pathways. Can also activate mature granulocytes and macrophages. It is a multilineage factor and has dose-dependent effects. It increases the cytotoxicity of monocytes toward certain neoplastic cell lines and activates polymorphonuclear neutrophils to inhibit the growth of tumor cells. It significantly improves the time to neutrophil recovery (engraftment), decreases length of hospitalization, shortens the duration of infectious episodes, and decreases antibiotic usage. Patients with fewer impaired organs have the best opportunity for improvement in survival. Detected in the serum in 5 minutes; peak levels are reached 2 hours after injection and last at least 6 hours.

INDICATIONS AND USES

Acceleration of hematopoietic recovery (myeloid engraftment) in patients undergoing allogenic or autologous bone marrow transplantation. ■ Bone marrow transplantation failure or engraftment delay. ■ Neutrophil recovery following chemotherapy in acute myelogenous leukemia (AML); safety for use in adults under 55 years not established. ■ Mobilization of peripheral blood progenitor cells. ■ Stimulate neutrophil recovery post–peripheral blood progenitor cell transplantation.

Unlabeled uses: Increase WBC in myelodysplastic syndromes and in AIDS patients receiving zidovudine. ■ Correct neutropenia in aplastic anemia. ■ Decrease transplantation-associated organ system damage, especially in kidney and liver transplants.

CONTRAINDICATIONS

Hypersensitivity to any components of sargramostim or yeast products; patients with leukemic myeloid blasts in the bone marrow or peripheral blood equal to 10% or more.

PRECAUTIONS

Should be administered under the direction of a physician knowledgeable about appropriate use. ■ Use caution if considered for use in any malignancy with myeloid characteristics. Can act as a growth factor for any tumor type, particularly myeloid malignancies. ■ Can be effective in patients receiving purged bone marrow if the purging process preserves a sufficient number of progenitors. ■ Effects may be limited in patients previously exposed to intensive chemotherapy or radiation therapy. ■ Neutralizing antibodies may form after receiving sargramostim and may inhibit therapeutic effect.

Monitor: Obtain a CBC with differential before administration and twice weekly thereafter to monitor for excessive leukocytosis (WBC above 50,000 cells/mm^3; or an absolute neutrophil count [ANC] above 20,000 cells/mm^3). ■ If blast cells appear or disease progression occurs, treatment should be discontinued. ■ Anemia, leukocytopenia, and thrombocytopenia occur as side effects of various procedures; monitor carefully. ■ Observe for fluid retention; may cause peripheral edema, pleural effusion, and/or pericardial effusion. May occur more frequently in individuals with pre-existing lung disease or cardiac disease, including a history of arrhythmias. Use with caution. ■ Use with caution in patients with pre-existing renal or hepatic dysfunction; an increased SrCr or increased bilirubin and hepatic enzymes may occur. Reversible if drug discontinued. Monitor renal and hepatic function biweekly. ■ Flushing, hypotension, and syncope may occur, especially with the initial dose. Reduce rate or stop temporarily.

Patient Education: Promptly report any symptoms of infection (e.g., fever) or allergic reaction (e.g., itching, swelling, redness at the injection site).

Maternal/Child: Has been used in more than 100 children from 4 months to 18 years of age with similar experience to the adult population, even though literature says safety not established. ■ Category C: safety for use in pregnancy and breast-feeding not established; use only if clearly needed. ■ Liquefied product contains benzyl alcohol; do not use in premature infants.

DRUG/LAB INTERACTIONS

Do not administer within 24 hours preceding or following chemotherapy or within 12 hours preceding or following radiotherapy. Rapidly dividing cells and the success of the treatment would be adversely affected by chemotherapy and radiation. ■ Myeloproliferative effects may be potentiated by lithium or corticosteroids; use with caution.

SIDE EFFECTS

Asthenia, diarrhea, malaise, peripheral edema, rash, and urinary tract disorders are most common. Allergic reactions, including anaphylaxis, are possible; arthralgia, capillary leak syndrome, dyspnea, fever, headache, hypoxia, local injection site reactions, myalgia, pericardial effusion, peripheral edema, pleural effusion, and supraventricular arrhythmias have been reported.

ANTIDOTE

Discontinue sargramostim for anaphylaxis, if blast cells appear, or there is progression of underlying disease. A maximum dose limit has not been determined; for accidental overdose, discontinue and monitor for WBC increase and respiratory symptoms. For an ANC above 20,000 cells/mm^3, WBC above 50,000 cells/mm^3, or a platelet count above 500,000/mm^3, reduce dose by one half or temporarily discontinue. Blood cell count should return to baseline level in 3 to 7 days. For any side effect that causes concern, reduce dose or temporarily discontinue. Keep physician informed. Treat anaphylaxis and resuscitate as necessary.

SECRETIN

(si-kret′in)

Diagnostic agent

SecreFlo

pH 3 to 6.5

USUAL DOSE

IV test dose for all indications: 0.2 mcg (0.1 ml). If no allergic reaction occurs in 1 minute, administer diagnostic dose.

Secretin stimulation testing: ***Aid in the diagnosis of exocrine pancreas dysfunction:*** 0.2 mcg/kg by IV injection over 1 minute.

Aid in the diagnosis of gastrinoma: 0.4 mcg/kg by IV injection over 1 minute.

Aid in cannulation of the pancreatic ducts: 0.2 mcg/kg by IV injection over 1 minute.

PEDIATRIC DOSE

Safety and effectiveness for use in pediatric patients not established.

DILUTION

Reconstitute vial containing 16 mcg of secretin with 8 ml of NS (2 mcg/ml). Shake vigorously to ensure dilution. Use diluted solution immediately and discard unused portion.

Storage: Store unreconstituted product in the freezer at approximately 20° C.

COMPATIBILITY

Specific information not available. Should be considered incompatible with any drug in a syringe because of specific use.

RATE OF ADMINISTRATION

A single dose as an IV injection evenly distributed over 1 minute.

ACTIONS

A gastrointestinal peptide hormone. Has an amino acid sequence identical to the naturally occurring porcine secretin. It acts to increase the bicarbonate content and volume of pancreatic secretions. A volume response of less than 2 ml/kg/hr, bicarbonate concentration of less than 80 mEq/L, and bicarbonate output of less than 0.2 mEq/kg/hr are consistent with impaired pancreatic function. Also acts to stimulate gastrin release in patients with gastrinoma (an increase from basal levels of 110 pg/ml or greater indicates a positive test, whereas little or no change in gastrin levels is seen in normal subjects or in patients with peptic ulcer disease). Also facilitates the identification of the ampulla of Vater and the accessory papilla during endoscopic retrograde cholangio-pancreatography (ERCP) to assist in cannulation of the pancreatic ducts. After a bolus injection, concentration rapidly declines to baseline secretin levels within 60 to 90 minutes. Elimination half-life is 27 minutes.

INDICATIONS AND USES

Stimulation of pancreatic secretions, including bicarbonate, to aid in the diagnosis of pancreatic exocrine dysfunction. ■ Stimulation of gastrin secretion to aid in the diagnosis of gastrinoma. ■ Stimulation of pancreatic secretions to facilitate the identification of the ampulla of Vater and accessory papilla during ERCP.

CONTRAINDICATIONS

Known hypersensitivity to secretin, acute pancreatitis until attack subsided.

PRECAUTIONS

Use of a test dose is recommended. ■ Use with caution in patients with a history of allergy and/or asthma. ■ Emergency equipment, medications, and supplies for treatment of hypersensitivity reactions must be readily available. Use with extreme caution in pancreatitis; note Contraindications. ■ Patients who have undergone a vagotomy, are receiving anticholinergic agents (e.g., atropine, glycopyrrolate), or have inflammatory bowel disease may be hyporesponsive to secretin test; response not indicative of pancreatic disease. ■ A greater than normal volume response to secretin stimulation, which can mask coexisting pancreatic disease, may be seen in some patients with alcoholic or other liver diseases.

Monitor: ***All situations:*** Monitor for S/S of hypersensitivity reactions; have not been reported when the desired dose of secretin is administered after a negative test dose.

Diagnosis of exocrine pancreatic dysfunction: A specific double-lumen tube is inserted through the mouth after a 12- to 15-hour fast. Correct positioning under fluoroscopic guidance is required. Intermittent negative pressure of 25 to 40 mm Hg is applied to both lumens throughout the test. When duodenal contents have a pH of 6 or greater, a baseline sample of duodenal fluids is collected over 10 minutes. Administer test dose and, if no untoward reaction after 1 minute, the dose of secretin (usually done by physician). All duodenal fluid is collected for the next 60 minutes at 15-minute intervals. The lumen of the tube is cleared with air after collection of each sample. Volume of aspirate in each 15-minute period should be similar; if it is not, aspiration could be incomplete. Samples should be chilled and sent to the laboratory to be analyzed for volume and bicarbonate concentration.

Diagnosis of gastrinoma: Fasting for 12 hours prior to the test is required. Draw two blood samples for fasting (baseline) serum gastrin levels. Administer test dose and, if no untoward reaction after 1 minute, the dose of secretin. Collect blood samples at 1, 2, 5, 10, and 30 minutes for serum gastrin concentrations.

Cannulation of the pancreatic ducts during ERCP: Administration of secretin will result in visible excretion of pancreatic fluid from the orifices of the accessory papilla. With their identification, cannulation is facilitated.

Maternal/Child: Category C: use during pregnancy only if clearly needed. Safety not established, and fluoroscopy may be required. ■ Use caution during breast-feeding; effect not known.

Elderly: Safety, pharmacologic response, and diagnostic effectiveness similar to younger patients. Greater sensitivity cannot be ruled out.

DRUG/LAB INTERACTIONS

Concurrent use of anticholinergic agents (e.g., atropine, glycopyrrolate) may make patients hyporesponsive (may produce a false-positive result).

SIDE EFFECTS

A protein product; hypersensitivity reactions, including anaphylaxis, can occur. Other mild side effects, including abdominal discomfort, diaphoresis, flushing, hypotension, and nausea have been reported.

ANTIDOTE

Discontinue drug immediately if any signs of allergic reaction. Treat anaphylaxis with epinephrine, antihistamines (e.g., diphenhydramine [Benadryl]), vasopressors (e.g., dopamine [Intropin]), aminophylline, and corticosteroids as indicated. Maintain a patent airway and resuscitate as necessary.

SODIUM ACETATE
(so'de-um as'ah-tat)

Electrolyte replenisher
Antihyponatremic
Alkalizing agent

pH 6 to 7

USUAL DOSE
Determined by nutritional needs, evaluation of electrolytes, and degree of hyponatremia. Some solutions may contain aluminum; see Precautions. Available in 2 mEq and 4 mEq/ml concentrations. Each ml provides 2 or 4 mEq each of sodium and acetate.

DOSE ADJUSTMENTS
Lower-end initial doses may be appropriate in the elderly based on the potential for decreased organ function and concomitant disease or drug therapy.

DILUTION
Must be added to larger volumes of IV infusion solutions including total parenteral nutrition. Use only clear solutions. Check labels for aluminum content; see Precautions.

Storage: Store at room temperature. Discard unused portion.

COMPATIBLE WITH
Consult pharmacist; specific conditions may apply; see Compatibilities, p. xvi.

Syringe: Cimetidine (Tagamet).

Y-site: Enalaprilat (Vasotec IV), esmolol (Brevibloc), labetalol (Normodyne), ondansetron (Zofran).

RATE OF ADMINISTRATION
Administer at prescribed rate for infusion solutions. Rapid or excessive administration may produce sodium overload, water retention, alkalosis, or hypokalemia.

ACTIONS
An alkalizing agent and sodium salt. Sodium is the predominant cation of extracellular fluid. It controls water distribution throughout the body. Hypothalamus osmoreceptors, sensitive to osmolarity changes in the blood, control serum sodium concentration (142 mEq/L). Body fluid is lost when sodium content decreases and retained when sodium content increases. Sodium is excreted by the kidney. The acetate ion is metabolized to bicarbonate, thus providing a source of bicarbonate. It also acts as a hydrogen ion receptor.

INDICATIONS AND USES
To prevent or correct hyponatremia in patients with restricted intake, especially in individualized IV formulations when basic needs are not met by standard solutions. ■ Treatment of mild to moderate acidotic states. ■ Source of sodium ions in hemodialysis and peritoneal dialysis.

CONTRAINDICATIONS
Patients with hypernatremia or water retention.

PRECAUTIONS
Use with caution in impaired renal function, congestive heart failure, hypertension, peripheral or pulmonary edema, any condition resulting in salt retention, and in patients receiving corticosteroids. ■ Use acetate-containing solutions with extreme caution in patients with metabolic or

respiratory alkalosis and/or impaired hepatic function. ■ Temporary therapy in acidosis. Treatment of primary condition must be instituted. ■ Sodium bicarbonate is the drug of choice for use in severe acidosis that requires immediate correction. ■ Some solutions of sodium acetate contain aluminum. In impaired kidney function, aluminum may reach toxic levels. Premature neonates are particularly at risk because of their immature kidneys and requirement for calcium and phosphate, which also contain aluminum. Research indicates that patients with impaired renal function who receive more than 4 to 5 mcg/kg/day of parenteral aluminum are at risk for developing CNS or bone toxicity associated with aluminum accumulation.

Monitor: Evaluate electrolytes frequently during treatment. ■ Evaluate fluid balance. ■ Rapid or excessive administration may produce alkalosis or hypokalemia. Cardiac arrhythmias may result from an intracellular shift of potassium. Many other complications may arise from electrolyte imbalance.

Maternal/Child: Category C: safety not established; use only if clearly needed.

Elderly: Differences in response between elderly and younger patients have not been identified. Lower-end initial doses may be appropriate in the elderly; see Dose Adjustments.

SIDE EFFECTS

Hypernatremia, sodium level over 147 mEq/L, is most common (congestive heart failure, delirium, dizziness, edema, fever, flushing, headache, hypotension, oliguria, pulmonary edema, reduced salivation and lacrimation, respiratory arrest, restlessness, swollen tongue, tachycardia, thirst, weakness). Alkalosis and fluid or solute overload can occur.

ANTIDOTE

Notify the physician of any side effect. Reduce rate and notify physician at first sign of congestion or fluid overload. May be treated by sodium restriction and/or use of diuretics (e.g., furosemide [Lasix]) or dialysis. Resuscitate as necessary.

SODIUM BICARBONATE

(so′de-um bi-kahr′bon-nat)

Electrolyte replenisher
Alkalizing agent

pH 7 to 8.5

USUAL DOSE

Adjusted according to pH, $Paco_2$, calculated base deficit, clinical response, and fluid limitations of the patient. In the presence of a low CO_2 content, adjust gradually to avoid unrecognized alkalosis. Correction to a CO_2 of 20 mEq/L within 24 hours will most likely result in a normal pH if the cause of acidosis is controlled and normal kidney function is present. Average dose for most indications is 2 to 5 mEq/kg/24 hr in adults and children.

Cardiac arrest: 1 mEq/kg of body weight, only when appropriate (see Precautions; evidence supports little benefit and use may be detrimental). Repeat half dose in 10 minutes if indicated by blood pH and $Paco_2$.

Continued

PEDIATRIC DOSE

For neonates and children up to 2 years of age, dose must never exceed 8 mEq/kg/24 hr of a 4.2% or more dilute solution; see Usual Dose, Monitor, and Maternal/Child.

DILUTION

Available as:

4.2% sodium bicarbonate solution: 5 mEq/10 ml (0.5 mEq/ml).

5% sodium bicarbonate solution: 297.5 mEq/500 ml (0.595 mEq/ml).

7.5% sodium bicarbonate solution: 44.6 mEq/50 ml or 8.9 mEq/10 ml (0.892 mEq/ml).

8.4% sodium bicarbonate solution: 50 mEq/50 ml or 10 mEq/10 ml (1 mEq/ml).

neut (4% sodium bicarbonate solution): 2.4 mEq/5 ml (0.48 mEq/ml). Use limited to a buffering solution. Will raise pH of IV fluids and medications. Never used as a systemic alkalinizer.

May be given in prepared solutions. 7.5% and 8.4% solutions should be diluted with equal amount of water for injection, or diluted with compatible IV solutions, depending on desired dosage and desired rate of administration. 4.2% or a more dilute solution is preferred for infants and children. Use only clear solutions.

INCOMPATIBLE WITH

Will form a precipitate with many drugs, including epinephrine. ***If coadministration with epinephrine is indicated, give at separate sites.***

COMPATIBLE WITH

(Underline Indicates Conflicting Compatibility Information)

Consult pharmacist; specific conditions may apply; see Compatibilities, p. xvi.

Additive: Amikacin (Amikin), aminophylline, amphotericin B (Fungizone), atropine, bretylium (Bretylate), calcium chloride, cefoxitin (Mefoxin), ceftazidime (Fortaz), chloramphenicol (Chloromycetin), chlorothiazide (Diuril), cimetidine (Tagamet), clindamycin (Cleocin), cytarabine (ARA-C), ergonovine maleate (Ergotrate), erythromycin lactobionate (Erythrocin), esmolol (Brevibloc), furosemide (Lasix), heparin, hydrocortisone (Hydrocortone, Solu-Cortef), kanamycin (Kantrex), lidocaine, mannitol, meperidine (Demerol), methotrexate (Folex), methyldopate (Aldomet), multivitamins (M.V.I.), nafcillin (Nafcil), nalmefene (Revex), ofloxacin (Floxin IV), oxacillin (Bactocill), oxytocin (Pitocin), penicillin G potassium, pentobarbital (Nembutal), phenobarbital (Luminal), phenylephrine (Neo-Synephrine), phenytoin (Dilantin), phytonadione (Aquamephyton), potassium chloride (KCl), prochlorperazine (Compazine), thiopental (Pentothal), vancomycin (Vancocin), verapamil (Isoptin).

Syringe: Lidocaine, milrinone (Primacor), pentobarbital (Nembutal).

Y-site: Acyclovir (Zovirax), alatrofloxacin (Trovan IV), amifostine (Ethyol), asparaginase (Elspar), aztreonam (Azactam), cefepime (Maxipime), ceftriaxone (Rocephin), ciprofloxacin (Cipro IV), cisatracurium (Nimbex), cladribine (Leustatin), cyclophosphamide (Cytoxan), cytarabine (ARA-C), daunorubicin (Cerubidine), dexamethasone (Decadron), diltiazem (Cardizem), docetaxel (Taxotere), doxorubicin (Adriamycin), etoposide (Etopophos, VePesid), famotidine (Pepcid IV), filgrastim (Neupogen), fludarabine (Fludara), gatifloxacin (Tequin), gemcitabine (Gemzar), granisetron (Kytril), heparin, ifosfamide (Ifex), indomethacin (Indocin), insulin (regular), levofloxacin (Levaquin), linezolid (Zyvox), melphalan (Alkeran), mesna (Mesnex), methylprednisolone (Solu-Medrol), milrinone (Primacor), morphine, paclitaxel (Taxol), piperacillin/

tazobactam (Zosyn), potassium chloride (KCl), propofol (Diprivan), remifentanil (Ultiva), tacrolimus (Prograf), teniposide (Vumon), thiotepa (Thioplex), vancomycin (Vancocin).

RATE OF ADMINISTRATION

Flush IV line thoroughly before and after administration. Usual rate of administration of any solution is 2 to 5 mEq/kg over 4 to 8 hours. Do not exceed 50 mEq/hr. Decrease rate for children. See Pediatric Dose. Rapid or excessive administration may produce alkalosis, hypernatremia, hypokalemia, and hypocalcemia. Cardiac arrhythmias may result from an intracellular shift of potassium. Will also produce pain and irritation along injection site.

Cardiac arrest: Up to 1 mEq/kg of body weight properly diluted over 1 to 3 minutes.

ACTIONS

An alkalizing agent and sodium salt. Helps to maintain osmotic pressure and ion balance. It is the buffering agent in blood. Bicarbonate ion elevates blood pH promptly. 99% reabsorbed with normal kidney function. Only 1% is excreted in the urine.

INDICATIONS AND USES

Metabolic acidosis (blood pH below 7.2 or plasma bicarbonate of 8 mEq/L or less) caused by circulatory insufficiency resulting from shock or severe dehydration, extracorporeal circulation of blood, severe renal disease, cardiac arrest (see Precautions), uncontrolled diabetes with ketoacidosis (low-dose insulin preferred), and primary lactic acidosis. ■ Hyperkalemia. ■ Hemolytic reactions requiring alkalinization of urine to reduce nephrotoxicity. ■ Severe diarrhea. ■ Barbiturate, methyl alcohol, or salicylate intoxication. ■ Buffering solution to raise pH of IV fluids and medications.

CONTRAINDICATIONS

Diuretics known to produce hypochloremic alkalosis (e.g., thiazides), edema, hypertension, hypocalcemia (alkalosis may produce CHF, convulsions, hypertension, and tetany), hypochloremia (from vomiting, GI suction, or diuretics), impaired renal function, metabolic alkalosis, respiratory alkalosis or acidosis, and any situation in which the administration of sodium could be clinically detrimental.

PRECAUTIONS

Temporary therapy in metabolic acidosis. Treatment of primary condition must be instituted. Best to partially correct acidosis and allow compensatory mechanisms to complete the correction. ■ Use with caution in cardiac, liver, or renal disease; CHF, fluid/solute overload, elderly and postoperative patients with renal or cardiovascular insufficiency, and in patients receiving corticosteroids. ■ Use in cardiac arrest indicated only if prolonged resuscitation with effective ventilation or after return of spontaneous circulation after a long arrest interval. ■ Adequate alveolar ventilation should control acid-base balance in most arrest situations except prolonged cardiac arrest, arrested patients with pre-existing metabolic acidosis, hyperkalemia, or tricyclic or barbiturate overdose.

Monitor: Confirm absolute patency of vein. Extravasation may cause chemical cellulitis, necrosis, ulceration, or sloughing. ■ Flush IV line thoroughly before and after administration; many incompatibilities. ■ Determine blood pH, Po_2, Pco_2, and electrolytes several times daily during intensive treatment and daily in most other situations. Determine base excess or deficit in infants and children (dose = 0.3 × kg × base deficit). Notify physician of all results. ■ Rapid or excessive administration may produce alkalosis, hypokalemia, and hypocalcemia. Cardiac arrhythmias may result from an intracellular shift of potassium. Many other complications may arise from electrolyte imbalance. ■ Use only 50-ml ampules in cardiac arrest to prevent accidental overdose. Recent practice indicates smaller doses may be appropriate when indicated in cardiac arrest and may prevent secondary alkalosis. Adequate alveolar ventilation is imperative. Evaluate patient response and blood gases.

Maternal/Child: Category C: safety for use in pregnancy not established; use only if clearly needed. ■ Use caution in breast-feeding. ■ Doses in excess of 8 mEq/kg/24 hr and/or given too rapidly (10 ml/min) may cause intracranial hemorrhage, hypernatremia, and decrease in cerebrospinal fluid pressure in neonates and children under 2 years.

Elderly: Contains sodium; use caution in the elderly with renal or cardiovascular insufficiency with or without CHF; see Precautions.

DRUG/LAB INTERACTIONS

Inhibits tetracyclines, chlorpropamide, lithium carbonate, methotrexate, and salicylates. ■ Potentiates anorexiants (e.g., amphetamines), sympathomimetics (e.g., ephedrine, dopamine [Intropin]), flecainide, mecamylamine, and quinidine.

SIDE EFFECTS

Rare when used with caution: alkalosis (hyperirritability and tetany), hypernatremia (edema, CHF), hypokalemia, local site pain with venous irritation.

ANTIDOTE

Discontinue the drug and notify the physician of any side effect. Hypokalemia usually occurs with alkalosis. Sodium and potassium chloride must be supplemented as indicated for correction. Treatment of alkalosis often results in more alkalosis. Rebreathing expired air from a paper bag may help to control beginning symptoms of alkalosis. Calcium gluconate may help in severe alkalosis. Administration of a balanced hypotonic electrolyte solution (Isolyte H, Normosol-M, Plasma-lyte 56) with sodium and potassium chloride added may help to excrete the bicarbonate ion in the urine. Ammonium chloride may be indicated. Treat tetany as indicated (calcium gluconate). For extravasation, discontinue infusion; aspirate fluid, drug, and/or 3 to 5 ml of blood through the in-place needle, then remove the needle. Elevate the extremity and apply warm moist compresses. Resuscitate as necessary.

SODIUM CHLORIDE
(so'de-um klor'id)

Electrolyte replenisher
Antihyponatremic

pH 4.8

USUAL DOSE

Highly individualized and related to specific condition, concentration of salts in the plasma, and/or loss of body fluids.

Hypotonic: (0.45% [½NS], 4.5 Gm of sodium chloride/L or 77 mEq of sodium and 77 mEq of chloride [approximately 155 mOsm/L]) 2 to 4 L/24 hr.

Isotonic: (0.9% [NS], 9 Gm of sodium chloride/L or 154 mEq of sodium and 154 mEq of chloride [approximately 310 mOsm/L]), 1.5 to 3 L/24 hr. ***Bacteriostatic isotonic NS*** contains benzyl alcohol as a preservative. It is used in small amounts (usually 1 to 2 ml) as a diluent for injectable drugs (IV, IM, SC) or to flush peripheral lines. Do not exceed 30 ml/24 hr in adults. Never used in neonates.

Hypertonic: Calculate sodium deficit. Total body water [TBW] is 45% to 50% in females and 50% to 60% in males.

Na deficit in mEq = TBW [desired – observed plasma Na]

Hypertonic (3%, 30 Gm of sodium chloride/L or 513 mEq of sodium and 513 mEq of chloride [approximately 1,030 mOsm/L] or 5%, 50 Gm of sodium chloride/L or 855 mEq of sodium and 855 mEq of chloride [approximately 1,710 mOsm/L]), 200 to 400 ml/24 hr. Continue until serum sodium is 130 mEq/L or neurologic symptoms improve. Occasionally may have to be repeated within the 24-hour period. See Precautions.

Concentrated: To be used only as an additive in parenteral fluid therapy (14.6% contains 2.5 mEq of sodium and chloride/ml; 23.4% contains 4 mEq of sodium and chloride/ml).

DOSE ADJUSTMENTS

Dose selection should be cautious in the elderly, especially with hypertonic or concentrated solutions. Start at the lower end of the desired dosing range.

DILUTION

Available as ***hypotonic*** 25 ml, 50 ml, 150 ml, 250 ml, 500 ml, 1 L; ***isotonic*** (2 ml, 3 ml, 5 ml, 10 ml, 20 ml, 25 ml, 30 ml, 50 ml, 100 ml, 150 ml, 250 ml, 500 ml, 1 L); or ***hypertonic*** (500 ml) solution in vials and/or bottles for injection or infusion and ready for use. Isotonic and hypotonic sodium chloride are frequently combined with 5% or 10% dextrose. ***Concentrated*** must be diluted before use. Used only as an additive in parenteral fluids. Permits specific mEq for mEq replacement of sodium and chloride without contributing to fluid overload. Available in 14.6% strength in 20 ml, 40 ml, and 200 ml; 23.4% strength in 30 ml, 50 ml, 100 ml, and 200 ml.

Bacteriostatic isotonic available in 2-ml, 10-ml, and 30-ml vials ready for use as a diluent. Never use in neonates.

Storage: Store at CRT. Do not freeze.

COMPATIBLE WITH

Consult pharmacist; specific conditions may apply; see Compatibilities, p. xvi.

Syringe: Cimetidine (Tagamet).

Y-site: Ciprofloxacin (Cipro IV).

RATE OF ADMINISTRATION

Isotonic and hypotonic: A single daily dose equally distributed over 24 hours. Rate is dependent on age, weight, and clinical condition of the patient.

Hypertonic: One-half the calculated dose over at least 8 hours. Do not exceed 100 ml over 1 hour. Too-rapid infusion may cause local pain and venous irritation; reduce rate for tolerance.

Concentrated: Properly diluted in parenteral fluids and equally distributed over 24 hours. Never exceed hypertonic rate (see above) based on actual mEq of sodium chloride.

ACTIONS

Sodium is the predominant cation of extracellular fluid. It controls water distribution throughout the body. Hypothalamus osmoreceptors, sensitive to osmolarity changes in the blood, control serum sodium concentration (142 mEq/L). Body fluid is lost when sodium content decreases and retained when sodium content increases. Readily absorbed in kidney tubules. Frequently exchanged for hydrogen and potassium ions. Excess excreted in urine.

INDICATIONS AND USES

Replace lost sodium and chloride ions in the body (e.g., hyponatremia or low salt syndrome). ■ Maintain electrolyte balance.

Hypotonic: Water replacement without increase of osmotic pressure or serum sodium levels; treatment of hyperosmolar diabetes requiring considerable fluid without excess sodium.

Isotonic: To replace sodium and chloride lost from vomiting because of obstructions and/or aspiration of GI fluids; treatment of metabolic alkalosis with fluid loss and sodium depletion. ■ Diluent in parenteral preparations. ■ To initiate and terminate blood transfusions without hemolyzing RBCs. ■ Maintain patency and perform routine irrigations of many types of intravascular devices (e.g., catheters, implanted ports). ■ Antidote for drug-induced hypercalcemia. Given concurrently with furosemide (Lasix). ■ Priming solution in hemodialysis procedures.

Hypertonic: Used only when high sodium and/or chloride content without large amounts of fluid is required (e.g., electrolyte and fluid loss replaced with sodium-free fluids, excessive water intake resulting in drastic dilution of body water, emergency treatment of severe salt depletion, addisonian crisis, diabetic coma).

Concentrated: Used to meet the specific requirements of patients with unusual fluid and electrolyte needs (e.g., special problems of sodium electrolyte intake or excretion).

CONTRAINDICATIONS

Hypernatremia; fluid retention; situations where sodium or chloride could be detrimental. 3% and 5% sodium chloride solutions are contraindicated with elevated, normal, or slightly decreased serum sodium and chloride levels. Bacteriostatic sodium chloride is contraindicated in newborns.

PRECAUTIONS

Use caution in circulatory insufficiency, congestive heart failure, edema with sodium retention, kidney dysfunction, hepatic disease, hypoproteinemia, in the elderly or debilitated individuals, and in patients receiving corticosteroids. ■ Use with caution in surgical patients; see Monitor. ■ More than 1 liter of NS may cause hypernatremia, which can result in loss of bicarbonate ions and acidosis. ■ Change IV tubing at least every 48 hours. ■ All uses require preservative-free solutions except the limited use of bacteriostatic NS as a diluent or flushing agent. ■ Inadvertent direct injection or absorption of concentrated sodium chloride may cause sudden hypernatremia, cardiovascular shock, CNS disorders, extensive hemolysis, cortical necrosis of the kidneys, and severe local tissue necrosis with extravasation. Use extreme caution.

Monitor: Maintain accurate intake and output; monitor electrolytes and acid-base balance, especially in prolonged therapy. ■ Monitor vital signs as indicated. ■ Monitor for signs of hyponatremia (sodium less than 135 mEq/L [e.g., disorientation, headache, lethargy, nausea, weakness]). May progress to coma and seizures. ■ NS can cause sodium retention resulting in fluid retention, edema, and circulatory overload during or immediately after surgery. Observe closely. Rarely used unless salt depletion factors are present. ■ Excessive administration of potassium-free solutions may cause hypokalemia. ■ Before and during use of hypertonic or concentrated sodium chloride, determine osmolar concentrations and chloride and bicarbonate content of the serum. Observe patient continuously to prevent pulmonary edema. ■ With hypertonic or concentrated solutions, use a small needle and a large vein to reduce venous irritation and avoid extravasation; see Precautions.

Maternal/Child: Category C: safety for use during pregnancy not established; use only if clearly needed. ■ Use caution in breast-feeding. ■ Benzyl alcohol preservative in bacteriostatic sodium chloride has caused toxicity in newborns. Do not use. ■ Safety for use in children not established.

Elderly: Lower-end initial doses may be indicated in the elderly; see Dose Adjustments. ■ Incidence of adverse reactions may be increased; monitor carefully, especially with renal or cardiac insufficiency with or without CHF. ■ See Precautions.

SIDE EFFECTS

Due to sodium excess: aggravation of existing acidosis, anorexia, cellular dehydration, deep respiration, disorientation, distention, edema, hydrogen loss, hyperchloremic acidosis, hypertension, increased BUN, nausea, oliguria, potassium loss, pulmonary edema, water retention, weakness. Excessive excretion of crystalloids to maintain normal osmotic pressure will increase excretion of potassium and bicarbonate and further increase acidosis. Other salts (e.g., iodide and bromide) used for therapy will also be excreted rapidly.

ANTIDOTE

Discontinue or decrease the rate of infusion and notify the physician of side effects. Sodium excess can be treated by sodium restriction and/or use of diuretics or hemodialysis to remove excessive amounts. Observe the patient carefully and treat symptomatically. Save balance of fluid for examination.

SODIUM FERRIC GLUCONATE COMPLEX

(so′de-um fer′ik glu-ko-nat com′pleks)

Ferrlecit

Antianemic
Iron supplement

pH 7.7 to 9.7

USUAL DOSE

Dose is represented in terms of mg of elemental iron. Given as an infusion and may be administered during the dialysis session.

Test dose: 25 mg (2 ml) as a test dose is recommended before initiating therapeutic doses. If no adverse reactions, full dose may be given.

Treatment of iron deficiency in hemodialysis patients: 125 mg (10 ml)/dose. A minimum cumulative dose of 1 Gm of elemental iron is required by most patients. May be administered over eight sessions at sequential dialysis treatments to achieve a favorable hemoglobin or hematocrit response. Additional doses as necessary are indicated to maintain target levels of hemoglobin, hematocrit, and laboratory parameters of iron storage within acceptable limits. Use the lowest dose that achieves this goal.

DOSE ADJUSTMENTS

Begin at the low end of the dosing range in elderly patients.

DILUTION

Available in ampules containing 62.5 mg/5 ml (12.5 mg/1 ml) of elemental iron.

Test dose: 25-mg (2-ml) dose should be diluted in 50 ml NS.

Therapeutic dose: 125-mg (10-ml) dose should be diluted in 100 ml NS.

Storage: Store ampules at CRT. Use immediately after dilution in NS.

COMPATIBILITY

Manufacturer states, "Do not mix with other medications or add to parenteral nutrition solutions." Known to be compatible only with NS.

RATE OF ADMINISTRATION

Too-rapid administration may cause hypotension associated with fatigue; flushing; light-headedness; malaise; severe pain in the chest, back, flanks, or groin; and weakness.

Test dose and therapeutic dose: A single dose as an infusion over 60 minutes. Do not exceed a rate of 2.1 mg/min.

ACTIONS

A stable macromolecular complex in sucrose injection. Contains elemental iron as the sodium salt of a ferric ion carbohydrate complex. Free of ferrous ion and dextran polysaccharides. Used to replete the total body content of iron. Iron is critical for normal hemoglobin synthesis to maintain oxygen transport and necessary for metabolism and synthesis of DNA and various other processes. Total body iron content of an adult ranges from 2 to 4 Gm. Approximately two thirds is in hemoglobin and one third in reticuloendothelial storage (bone marrow, spleen, liver) and ferritin. Doses of 1 mg/day are adequate to replenish losses in healthy nonmenstruating adults. Iron complex is not dialyzable.

INDICATIONS AND USES

Treatment of iron deficiency anemia in patients undergoing chronic hemodialysis who are receiving supplemental erythropoietin therapy (e.g., EPO, Epogen, Procrit).

CONTRAINDICATIONS

All anemias not associated with iron deficiency. Hypersensitivity to sodium ferric gluconate complex or any of its components.

PRECAUTIONS

Use only when truly indicated to avoid excess storage of iron. Not recommended for use in patients with iron overload. ■ Too-rapid administration may cause hypotension; see Rate of Administration and Side Effects. ■ Studies included five chronic hemodialysis patients with a history of anaphylaxis to iron dextran who received up to 1 g of sodium ferric gluconate complex without an allergic reaction. ■ Serum iron levels greater than 300 mcg/dl combined with transferrin oversaturation may indicate iron poisoning; see Side Effects.

Monitor: Recumbent position during and after injection may help to prevent postural hypotension. Hypotensive effects may be additive to transient hypotension during dialysis and/or from too-rapid rate of infusion; monitor closely. ■ Observe continuously for an allergic reaction during an infusion. Monitor vital signs. ■ Periodic monitoring of hemoglobin and hematocrit and iron storage levels recommended. Doses in excess of iron needs may lead to accumulation of iron in iron storage sites and iatrogenic hemosiderosis.

Patient Education: Report S/S of allergic reaction (e.g., difficulty breathing, rash, shortness of breath) promptly. Report pain at injection site.

Maternal/Child: Category B: use during pregnancy only if potential benefit justifies potential risk to fetus. ■ Safety for use during breast-feeding and in children not established. ■ Contains benzyl alcohol; should not be used in neonates.

Elderly: No age differences identified. Caution in the elderly suggested; see Dose Adjustments. ■ Consider decreased cardiac, hepatic, or renal function, and concomitant disease or other drug therapy.

DRUG/LAB INTERACTIONS

Specific information not available.

SIDE EFFECTS

Hypotension associated with fatigue; flushing; light-headedness; malaise; severe pain in the chest, back, flanks, or groin; and weakness may be caused by too-rapid infusion. Severe hypersensitivity reactions (e.g., angioedema, bronchospasm, cardiac arrest, cardiovascular collapse, dyspnea, edema [oral or pharyngeal], muscle spasm, pain [back or chest], pruritus, urticaria) have been reported rarely. Many side effects occurred in less than 1% of patients and may or may not be attributable to sodium ferric gluconate complex.

Overdose: Abdominal pain, diarrhea, or vomiting progressing to pallor or cyanosis, lassitude, drowsiness, hyperventilation due to acidosis, iatrogenic hemosiderosis, and cardiovascular collapse.

ANTIDOTE

Reduce rate or temporarily discontinue infusion for hypotension; volume expanders (e.g., albumin, dextran, hetastarch [Hespan]) may be indicated. Restart when resolved. Discontinue drug and treat allergic reaction or resuscitate as necessary; notify physician. Epinephrine (Adrenalin) and diphenhydramine (Benadryl) should always be available. Iron complex is not dialyzable.

SODIUM NITRITE AND SODIUM THIOSULFATE

(so′de-um ni′trat, so′de-um thi′o-sul′fat)

Antidote

pH 7 to 9 ▪ pH 6 to 9.5

USUAL DOSE

Cyanide poisoning and treatment of nitroprusside sodium–induced cyanide toxicity: Following administration of amyl nitrite inhalant or immediately if an IV line is in place, give 300 mg (10 ml) 3% sodium nitrite IV followed by sodium thiosulfate 12.5 Gm IV (125 ml 10% solution or 50 ml 25%). 150 to 200 mg/kg is an alternate dosing schedule for sodium thiosulfate. One half of the initial dose of both drugs may be repeated in 2 hours if signs of toxicity persist.

Prophylaxis against nitroprusside sodium–induced cyanide toxicity (sodium thiosulfate only): Co-administration of sodium thiosulfate in doses 5 to 10 times that of nitroprusside sodium has been used to avoid toxicity with larger doses or necessary long-term therapy. May potentiate hypotensive action; use with caution.

Arsenic poisoning (sodium thiosulfate only [unlabeled use]): 100 mg (1 ml 10% solution, 0.4 ml 25%) on the first day. Increase dose by 100 mg each day until 500-mg dose is reached. Thereafter, give 500 mg every other day as needed.

Prophylaxis against cisplatin-induced nephrotoxicity (sodium thiosulfate only [unlabeled]): A standard dose has not been established. A common recommendation is a bolus dose of 4 Gm/M^2 (range is 3 to 7.5 Gm/M^2) before cisplatin administration followed by an infusion of 2 Gm/M^2/hr for 5 to 12 hours as cisplatin is being instilled.

PEDIATRIC DOSE

Cyanide poisoning or treatment of nitroprusside sodium–induced cyanide toxicity: Following administration of amyl nitrite inhalant, or immediately if an IV line is in place, give 180 to 240 mg (6 to 8 ml) of 3% sodium nitrite/M^2 (or 4 to 6 mg/kg [0.2 ml/kg]) followed by sodium thiosulfate 7 Gm/M^2 (70 ml of 10% solution/M^2 or 28 ml of 25% solution/M^2). Do not exceed adult doses.

DILUTION

Both may be given undiluted.

Storage: Ampule must be airtight for storage. Store at CRT.

COMPATIBILITY

Specific information not available. Consider specific use; consult pharmacist.

RATE OF ADMINISTRATION

Cyanide poisoning: Sodium nitrite at 2.5 ml/min; sodium thiosulfate, a single dose equally distributed over 10 minutes or longer.

Arsenic poisoning: Each 100 mg or fraction thereof equally distributed over at least 2 minutes.

ACTIONS

Sodium nitrite produces methemoglobinemia that combines with the cyanide ion to make cyanmethemoglobin. It dissociates to make free cyanide, which is then converted to thiocyanate by sodium thiosulfate. The end product is excreted in urine.

INDICATIONS AND USES

A cyanide antidote kit containing sodium thiosulfate, sodium nitrate and amyl nitrite is used to facilitate the removal of cyanide in intoxication and in nitroprusside-induced cyanide toxicity. ■ Sodium thiosulfate is also used for prophylaxis against nitroprusside sodium–induced cyanide toxicity and as an injection into tissue infiltrated by extravasation of mechlorethamine.

Unlabeled use: Sodium thiosulfate may be used in the treatment of arsenic poisoning and for prophylaxis against cisplatin-induced nephrotoxicity in the intraperitoneal treatment of ovarian cancer.

CONTRAINDICATIONS

None when used for specific indication.

PRECAUTIONS

Read instructions supplied in kit thoroughly. ■ Dimercaprol (BAL) IM is more commonly used as an antidote for arsenic poisoning. ■ If there is reasonable suspicion of cyanide toxicity, initiate treatment immediately (usually before lab results are known).

Monitor: Monitor the patient very carefully, maintain a patent airway, and provide oxygen. ■ Control BP with IV fluids and vasopressors (e.g., dopamine [Intropin]), and correct acidosis if indicated (may not appear until more than 1 hour after dangerous cyanide levels occur). Measurement of cyanide levels and arterial blood gases to determine venous hyperoxemia and acidosis may be indicated. Measurement of methemoglobin concentrations may be indicated.

Maternal/Child: Category C: use only when clearly needed.

SIDE EFFECTS

Abdominal pain, angina, apprehension, dizziness, headache (severe), hypotension, involuntary passing of urine and feces, nausea and vomiting, paradoxical bradycardia, restlessness, tachycardia, weakness, vertigo.

ANTIDOTE

Keep physician informed of all side effects; will be treated symptomatically. Rapid infusion of sodium nitrite may cause excessive vasodilation and hypotension. A decrease in rate of administration may be necessary. Resuscitate as indicated.

STREPTOKINASE

(strep-toe-kye′nase)

Thrombolytic agent

Kabikinase, Streptase

pH 6 to 8

USUAL DOSE

Some clinicians suggest premedication with hydrocortisone (Solu-Cortef) or methylprednisolone (Solu-Medrol) 100 mg IV and diphenhydramine 50 mg IV to decrease the risk of severe hypersensitivity and febrile reactions.

Coronary artery thrombi: 1.5 million IU direct IV within 6 hours of onset of symptoms of acute transmural myocardial infarction. An alternative is 20,000 IU given directly into coronary artery within 6 hours of onset of symptoms of acute transmural myocardial infarction. Follow with 2,000 IU/min for 1 hour. Total dose equals 140,000 IU. Other protocols are in use. Recent studies suggest that other thrombolytics (e.g., alteplase [tPA]) may be preferred.

Deep vein thrombosis, pulmonary or arterial embolism, arterial thrombosis: ***Loading dose:*** 250,000 IU. ***Maintenance dose:*** 100,000 IU/hr for 24 to 72 hours depending on diagnosis. May be increased based on thrombin time evaluations.

Arteriovenous cannula occlusion: 100,000 to 250,000 IU into each occluded limb of cannula. See Contraindications.

PEDIATRIC DOSE

Thromboembolism or acute arterial thrombosis: 1,000 IU (up to 3,000 IU)/kg of body weight over 5 to 30 minutes. Follow with 1,000 IU (up to 1,500 IU)/kg/hr for 12 to 24 hours. See Maternal/Child.

DILUTION

All uses except cannula occlusion: Each vial (250,000, 600,000, 750,000, or 1,500,000 IU) must be diluted with 5 ml of NS (preferred) or D5W. Add diluent slowly, direct to sides of vial, roll and tilt gently. Do not shake. Further slowly dilute each vial to a total volume of 45 ml (preferred). May be diluted to a maximum of 500 ml in 45-ml increments. Discard solution with large amounts of flocculation or any solution remaining after 24 hours. Can be infused through a 0.8-micron or larger pore filter.

Arteriovenous cannula occlusion: Each vial (250,000 IU) must be diluted with 2 ml NS. Use care in dilution as above.

Storage: Refrigerate after initial dilution. Discard after 24 hours.

INCOMPATIBLE WITH

Manufacturer states, "Do not add other medications to the container of streptokinase." Another source recommends not administering other medications through the same IV line.

COMPATIBLE WITH

See Incompatible With. Consult pharmacist; specific conditions may apply; see Compatibilities, p. xvi.

Y-site: Dobutamine (Dobutrex), dopamine (Intropin), heparin, lidocaine, nitroglycerin (Nitro-Bid IV).

RATE OF ADMINISTRATION

Volumetric or syringe infusion pump required. Reconstituted streptokinase will alter drop size and impact correct dosage with drop size mechanisms.

IV injection for coronary artery thrombi: 1.5 million IU-dose evenly distributed over 60 minutes.

Coronary artery thrombi: Bolus dose over 15 to 30 seconds via coronary catheter placed by Judkins or Sones technique directly to thrombosed site verified by selective coronary angiography. Follow with 2,000 IU/min for 60 minutes.

Deep vein thrombosis, pulmonary arterial embolism, arterial thrombi: ***Loading dose:*** A single dose equally distributed over 25 to 30 minutes.

Maintenance dose: 100,000 IU or more as ordered equally distributed every hour for 24 to 72 hours. Dissolution of arterial thrombi may occur in 24 hours or less; deep vein thrombi may take up to 72 hours.

Arteriovenous cannula occlusion: A single dose slowly (do not force) into each occluded limb of cannula. Clamp for 2 hours, then aspirate contents, flush with saline, and reconnect.

ACTIONS

An enzyme prepared from filtrates of beta-hemolytic streptococci. It combines with plasminogen and converts it to plasmin, which degrades fibrin clots, fibrinogen, and other plasma proteins. This activation takes place within a thrombus as well as on the surface. Onset of action is prompt and may last up to 12 to 24 hours. End products of this activity possess an anticoagulant effect. Bleeding may be very difficult to control.

INDICATIONS AND USES

Lysis of coronary artery thrombi. AHA standards identify thrombolytic agents as Class I therapy in patients younger than 70 years with chest pain consistent with acute MI and at least 0.1 mV of ST segment elevation in at least two ECG leads. Use in all other patients based on age, accurate diagnosis, and time from onset of chest pain. ■ Lysis of acute massive pulmonary emboli if one or more lobes are involved or if hemodynamics are unstable. ■ Lysis of an equivalent amount of thrombi in other vessels (deep veins). ■ Lysis of acute arterial thrombi and arterial emboli. ■ Clearing of occluded arteriovenous cannulae as an alternative to surgical revision.

CONTRAINDICATIONS

Active internal bleeding, cerebral vascular accident within 2 months, intracranial or intraspinal surgery, intracranial neoplasm, hypersensitivity to streptokinase. ***Not indicated for restoration of patency of intravenous catheters.***

PRECAUTIONS

Administered only in the hospital under the direction of a physician knowledgeable in its use and with appropriate emergency drugs (e.g., antihistamines, glucocorticoids), diagnostic and laboratory facilities immediately available. ■ For coronary catheter procedure, diagnosis of acute myocardial infarction must be confirmed and the site of the coronary thrombosis confirmed with selective angiography. Concurrent heparin therapy may be required in this situation. ■ Diagnosis of pulmonary or other emboli should be confirmed. Best results obtained if started within 5 to 7 days of onset of pulmonary emboli; 3 to 4 days of onset of DVT, and 3 days of onset of arterial thrombi. Discontinue streptokinase if thrombin time or other lysis parameters are not above 1½ times normal in 4 hours. Excessive resistance may be present. ■ Use extreme caution in presence of atrial fibrillation or mitral stenosis with atrial fibrillation; very high risk of stroke from dislodged emboli. ■ May cause severe hypersensitivity reactions. Prior sensitization to streptokinase increases risk of allergic reaction in subsequent courses of treatment. Antigenic (promotes antibody formation); incidence of allergic reaction greater than with alteplase (tPA). Use of an alternate agent (e.g., alteplase) may be indicated if repeat thrombolytic therapy required. ■ Use extreme caution in the following situations: any surgical procedure, biopsy, lumbar puncture, thoracentesis, paracentesis, multiple cutdowns, or intraarterial diagnostic procedures within 10 days; ulcerative wounds; recent trauma with possible internal injury; visceral malignancy; pregnancy and first 10 days postpartum; any lesion of GI or GU tract with a potential for bleeding (e.g., diverticulitis, ulcerative colitis); severe hypertension; acute or chronic hepatic or renal insufficiency; uncontrolled hypocoagulable state; chronic lung disease with cavitation; rheumatic valvular disease; subacute bacterial endocarditis; and any condition where bleeding might be hazardous or difficult to manage because of location. ■ See Contraindications; not indicated for restoration of patency in IV catheters. May cause life-threatening hypotension, hypersensitivity reactions, apnea, and bleeding.

Monitor: Establish a separate IV line for streptokinase. ■ Observe patient continuously. Obtain hematocrit, platelet count, activated PTT, thrombin time, PT, and CPK before therapy. ■ Diphenhydramine (Benadryl) 50 mg IV prophylactically is recommended. ■ In 4 hours and during therapy thrombin time or PT changes are monitored and will reflect effectiveness of treatment. Keep physician continuously informed. Request specific parameters for notifying physician after initial supervised injection. ■ Coronary thrombi may lyse in 1 hour; continue treatment to ensure complete lysis. ■ Monitor ECG and record strips with greatest ST segment elevation initially and every 15 minutes for at least 4 hours. ■ Monitor BP frequently. ■ When thrombin time is less than twice the normal control value, initiate heparin infusion to keep PTT at 60 seconds. Prompt, easy treatment of IV injection a distinct advantage over catheter procedure. ■ Maintain strict bed rest and apply pressure dressings to any recently invaded site. ■ A greater alteration of hemostatic status than with heparin; use care in handling patient; avoid arterial puncture, venipuncture, and IM injection. Use extreme precautionary methods (use of radial artery, not femoral; extended pressure application of up to 30 minutes) if above procedures absolutely necessary. Minor bleeding occurs often at streptokinase insertion sites. Do not reduce or stop streptokinase as lytic activity will be increased and cause more bleeding. ■ Monitor for hypotension and arrhythmias during therapy; atrial and ventricular arrhythmias can occur. ■ Intensive follow-up therapy with continuous infusion of heparin (without a loading dose) is indicated in all situations to prevent recurrent thrombosis. Begin in about 3 to 4 hours of completion of streptokinase, when the thrombin time or aPTT is reduced to less than twice the normal control value. ■ Do not take BP in lower extremities; thrombi may be dislodged. ■ Attempt to clear arteriovenous cannulae occlusions with good syringe technique and heparinized saline before using streptokinase. Allow effect of heparin to diminish. Instruct patient to exhale and hold his breath any time the catheter is not connected to the IV tubing or a syringe to prevent air from entering the open catheter and thus the circulatory system.

Patient Education: Report any signs of allergic reaction promptly (e.g., itching, rash, shortness of breath). ■ Compliance with all measures to minimize bleeding (e.g., strict bed rest) is very important. ■ Avoid use of razors, toothbrushes, and other sharp items. ■ Use caution while moving to avoid excessive bumping. ■ Report all episodes of bleeding and apply local pressure if indicated.

Maternal/Child: Category C: use only if clearly needed. Safety for use in pregnancy, breast-feeding, or children not established. ■ Use in children based on anecdotal reports in patients from less than 1 month to 16 years of age.

Elderly: See Indications and Precautions. ■ May have poorer prognosis following MI and pre-existing conditions that may increase risk of intracranial bleeding. Select patients carefully to maximize benefits.

DRUG/LAB INTERACTIONS

Risk of bleeding may be increased by any medicine that affects blood clotting including anticoagulants (e.g., heparin, lepirudin [Refludan], warfarin [Coumadin]); glycoprotein GPIIb/IIIa receptor antagonists (e.g., abciximab [ReoPro], eptifibatide [Integrilin], tirofiban [Aggrastat]); any medication that may cause hypoprothrombinemia, thrombocytopenia, or GI ulceration or bleeding (e.g., selected antibiotics such as cefamandole [Mandol], cefoperazone [Cefobid], cefotetan [Cefotan], ticarcillin [Ticar], aspirin, NSAIDs [e.g., ibuprofen (Advil, Motrin), naproxen (Aleve, Naprosyn), phenylbutazone (Butazolidin)]); and/or any other medication that inhibits platelet aggregation (e.g., clopidogrel [Plavix], dipyridamole [Persantine], plicamycin [Mithracin], sulfinpyrazone [Anturane], ticlopidine [Ticlid], valproic acid [Depacon]). Concurrent use not recommended with the exception of heparin and aspirin (in AMI) to reduce the risk of rethrombosis. If concurrent or subsequent use indicated (e.g., management of acute coronary syndrome, percutaneous coronary intervention) monitor PT and aPTT closely. ■ Coagulation tests will be unreliable; specific procedures can be used; notify the lab of streptokinase use.

SIDE EFFECTS

Allergic reactions, including anaphylaxis, are not uncommon with streptokinase. Arrhythmias, hypotension. Fever increase of 1° to 2° F is common. Bleeding can be life threatening.

ANTIDOTE

Notify physician of all side effects. Note even the most minute bleeding tendency. Therapy may have to be discontinued with serious blood loss and bleeding not controlled by local pressure. Whole blood, packed RBCs, cryoprecipitate, fresh-frozen plasma, platelets, desmopressin, tranexamic acid, and aminocaproic acid may all be indicated. Do not use dextran. Topical preparations of aminocaproic acid may stop minor bleeding. Consider protamine if heparin has been used. Treat bradycardia with atropine, reperfusion arrhythmias with lidocaine or procainamide; VT or VF may require cardioversion. If hypotension occurs, reduce rate promptly. If not resolved, vasopressors (e.g., dopamine [Intropin]), Trendelenburg position, and suitable plasma expanders (e.g., albumin, plasma protein fraction [Plasmanate], or hetastarch) may be indicated. Treat minor allergic reactions symptomatically. Discontinue drug and treat anaphylaxis as indicated; resuscitate as necessary.

STREPTOMYCIN SULFATE

(strep-toe-mye′sin sul′fat)

Antibacterial (aminoglycoside) Antituberculosis

pH 5 to 8

USUAL DOSE

***Mycobacterium* tuberculosis (unlabeled):** 12 to 15 mg/kg daily. Calculation based on ideal body weight, not actual weight. 12 to 27 mg/kg has been used safely. Doses over 20 mg/kg are usually given every other day. Used in combination with isoniazid (INH), rifampin (Rifadin), and pyrazinamide. Maximum suggested total cumulative dose over course of therapy is 120 Gm.

***Mycobacterium avium* complex (unlabeled):** 11 to 13 mg/kg daily. Part of a multiple drug regimen of three to five agents.

DOSE ADJUSTMENTS

Reduced dose required in renal impairment and/or nitrogen retention. ■ Reduce dose in patients over 60 years based on age, renal function, and eighth nerve impairment. ■ Elevated peak drug concentrations require a reduced dose. ■ See Drug/Lab Interactions.

DILUTION

Prepared solution equals 400 mg/ml. Further dilute total daily dose to a volume of 100 ml with D5W or D5NS.

Storage: Refrigerate undiluted ampules. Diluted solution is stable for 24 hours at room temperature. According to the National Jewish Center guidelines, the current formulation from Pfizer is stable for up to 30 days after dilution if refrigerated.

INCOMPATIBLE WITH

Inactivated in solution with beta-lactam antibiotics (e.g., cephalosporins, penicillins) and vancomycin. Do not mix in the same solution. Appropriate spacing required because of physical incompatibilities. See Drug/Lab Interactions.

COMPATIBLE WITH

See Incompatible With. Consult pharmacist; specific conditions may apply; see Compatibilities, p. xvi.

Additive: Bleomycin (Blenoxane).

Y-site: Esmolol (Brevibloc).

RATE OF ADMINISTRATION

Total daily dose, properly diluted, as an infusion over 30 minutes. Slow rate to 60 minutes if any tingling or dizziness occurs during administration or if elevated peak drug concentrations occur.

ACTIONS

An aminoglycoside antibiotic with potential neuromuscular blocking action. Inhibits protein synthesis in bacterial cells. Bactericidal against specific gram-negative organisms and bacilli. Well distributed through all organ tissues except the brain (unless meninges inflamed). Peak serum levels of 25 to 50 mcg/ml occur promptly and gradually decrease to 12.5 to 25 mcg/ml over 5 to 6 hours. Usual half-life is 2.5 hours. Half-life is prolonged in infants, postpartum females, liver disease and ascites, spinal cord injury, cystic fibrosis, and the elderly. May be prolonged up to 100 hours in end-stage renal disease. Half-life is shorter in anemia, severe burns, and fever. Crosses the placental barrier. 30% to 90% excreted in urine within 24 hours.

INDICATIONS AND USES

All IV uses are unlabeled. Treatment of *Mycobacterium* tuberculosis when one or more of the following drugs (ethambutol [Myambutol], isoniazid [INH], rifampin [Rifadin], or pyrazinamide) is contraindicated because of toxicity, intolerance, or drug resistance. Increased rates of drug resistance and/or concomitant HIV infection are more common than in previous times. Usual four-drug regimen is either ethambutol or streptomycin with isoniazid, rifampin, and pyrazinamide. IV administration is especially useful in cachectic patients or those needing prolonged streptomycin therapy. ■ *Mycobacterium avium* complex, a common infection in AIDS patients. ■ Prophylactically after coronary artery bypass surgery.

CONTRAINDICATIONS

Known streptomycin sensitivity. Known aminoglycoside sensitivity may be a contraindication due to cross-sensitivity.

PRECAUTIONS

Labeled for IM use only; probably due to impurities in early preparations. New formulations are being given safely IV; check your hospital's policy in case an informed consent or release is required. ■ Handle with care; may cause skin sensitivity reactions. ■ Used only when other, less hazardous agents are ineffective or contraindicated. ■ Adequate laboratory and audiometric testing facilities must be available. ■ Sensitivity studies necessary to determine susceptibility of causative organism to streptomycin. ■ Risk of neurotoxicity (e.g., auditory and vestibular ototoxicity) increased in patients with pre-existing renal damage or in normal renal function with prolonged use. Partial or total irreversible deafness may continue to develop after streptomycin is discontinued. ■ Superinfection may occur from overgrowth of nonsusceptible organisms. ■ Pseudomembranous colitis has been reported. May range from mild to life-threatening. Consider in patients that present with diarrhea during or after treatment with streptomycin. ■ May contain sulfites; use caution in patients with asthma. ■ For additional questions, consultations may be obtained from the Division of Infectious Disease at National Jewish Center (800-423-8891, ext. 1279).

Monitor: Monitor serum BUN, creatinine, calcium, magnesium, potassium, and sodium before therapy and weekly. ■ Calcium, magnesium, potassium, and sodium levels may decline and require replacement. ■ Observe for any adverse effects including at the infusion site. ■ High serum levels increase risk of ototoxicity and neurotoxicity. Assess adequacy of dose and clearance of drug with serum streptomycin concentrations (2 to 6 hours after a timed dose) initially and every 2 to 4 weeks. Peak therapeutic levels are between 20 and 30 mcg/ml. Serum levels over 50 mcg/ml may be toxic. ■ Watch for decrease in urine output, rising BUN and SrCr, and declining CrCl levels. Dose may require decreasing; serum levels should not exceed 25 mcg/ml if any kidney damage is present. ■ Assess vestibular function toxicity weekly (Romberg test, past point, heel-to-toe, and lateral nystagmus). ■ Assess ototoxicity with audiograms every 2 to 4 weeks. ■ All of the above monitoring may be done more frequently if indicated. Permanently implanted central venous catheters allow treatment on an outpatient basis. Blood work may be done every 2 weeks and all other tests every 4 weeks when stable enough to be treated as an outpatient. ■ Maintain good hydration. Dehydration may increase risk of nephrotoxicity; monitor closely if vomiting, diarrhea, or other events that may cause dehydration occur. ■ Closely monitor patients with impaired renal function for nephrotoxicity and neurotoxicity (e.g., auditory and vestibular ototoxicity); nephrotoxicity may be reversible. ■ National Jewish Center uses chromatographic assay to determine streptomycin serum levels; concomitantly administered antibiotics do not have to be withheld when collecting samples for analysis. ■ Usual length of treatment for tuberculosis is 1 year. Discontinue streptomycin therapy whenever toxic symptoms appear, impending toxicity is feared, organisms become resistant, or full therapeutic effect is achieved. ■ In long-term therapy, alkalinization of urine may minimize renal irritation. ■ See Drug/Lab Interactions.

Patient Education: Report promptly any changes in balance, dizziness, hearing loss or weakness. ■ Consider birth control options.

Maternal/Child: Category D: avoid pregnancy; has caused total, irreversible, bilateral deafness in infants whose mothers received streptomycin during pregnancy. ■ Discontinue breast-feeding. ■ Has caused CNS depression, including stupor, flaccidity, coma, and deep respiratory depression in very young infants.

Elderly: Risk of toxicity increased; see Dose Adjustments.

DRUG/LAB INTERACTIONS

Synergistic when used in combination with beta-lactam antibiotics (e.g., cephalosporins, penicillins) and vancomycin. Synergism may be inconsistent; see Incompatible With. ■ Concurrent use with any other neurotoxic, ototoxic, or nephrotoxic agents should be avoided. May have dangerous additive effects with other aminoglycosides (e.g., gentamicin, tobramycin), diuretics (e.g., furosemide [Lasix], mannitol), beta-lactam antibiotics (e.g., cephalosporins), colistin (Coly-Mycin S), polymyxin B (Aerosporin), vancomycin, cyclosporine, and many others. ■ May be antagonized by bacteriostatic antibiotics (e.g., chloramphenicol, erythromycin, and tetracycline); bactericidal action may be affected. ■ Magnesium sulfate may reduce antibiotic activity of streptomycin. ■ Anesthetics (e.g., enflurane) and neuromuscular blocking muscle relaxants (e.g., doxacurium [Nuromax], succinylcholine) are potentiated by aminoglycosides. Respiratory paralysis and ***apnea can occur.*** ■ Aminoglycosides are potentiated by anticholinesterases (e.g., edrophonium), antineoplastics (e.g., nitrogen mustard, cisplatin). ■ See Side Effects.

SIDE EFFECTS

Occur more frequently with impaired renal function, higher doses, prolonged administration, dehydration, in the elderly, and in patients receiving other ototoxic or nephrotoxic drugs. Allergic reactions (e.g., angioneurotic edema, anaphylaxis, itching, rash, urticaria), apnea, azotemia, cochlear ototoxicity (hearing loss and deafness), eosinophilia, exfoliative dermatitis, hemolytic anemia, facial paresthesias, fever, leukopenia, muscular weakness, neuromuscular blockade, pancytopenia, pseudomembranous colitis, roaring in the ears, seizures, thrombocytopenia, tinnitus, vestibular ototoxicity (nausea and vomiting, vertigo). Least nephrotic of the aminoglycosides but nephrotoxicity does occur. Has caused severe chilling (rigors) with penicillins if spacing is not adequate.

ANTIDOTE

Notify the physician of all side effects. Discontinue streptomycin with any evidence of renal impairment, ototoxicity, or vestibular toxicity. Tinnitus, roaring noises, or a sense of fullness in the ears indicate a need for audiometric examination. Auditory changes are usually irreversible and bilateral and may be partial or total. Vestibular symptoms are reversible if detected early. A reduction in dose may be required or an alternate drug used. In overdose hemodialysis may be indicated. Monitor fluid balance, CrCl, and plasma levels carefully. Complexation with ticarcillin may be as effective as hemodialysis. Calcium salts or neostigmine may reverse neuromuscular blockade. Resuscitate as necessary.

STREPTOZOCIN

(strep-toe-zoe′sin)

Antineoplastic (alkylating agent/nitrosurea)

Zanosar

pH 3.5 to 4.5

USUAL DOSE

500 mg/M^2 for 5 consecutive days; see Monitor. Repeat every 6 weeks until maximum benefit or treatment-limiting toxicity observed. May also give 1,000 mg/M^2 weekly for 2 doses. May then increase up to 1,500 mg/M^2 to achieve therapeutic response if significant toxicity not observed. Overall cumulative dose to onset of response is 2,000 mg/M^2. Maximum response is usually achieved with 4,000 mg/M^2 total cumulative dose.

DOSE ADJUSTMENTS

Reduce dose in impaired renal function; see Precautions/Monitor. ■ Reduce dose or discontinue drug if mild proteinuria occurs. ■ Can be used with other antineoplastic drugs in reduced doses to achieve tumor remission.

DILUTION

Specific techniques required; see Precautions. Each 1-Gm vial must be diluted with 9.5 ml NS or D5W (100 mg/ml). Usually further diluted in larger amounts (50 to 250 ml) of the same solutions.

Storage: Store in refrigerator before and after dilution. Discard within 12 hours of dilution. Contains no preservatives. Protect from light.

COMPATIBLE WITH

Consult pharmacist; specific conditions may apply; see Compatibilities, p. xvi.

Y-site: Amifostine (Ethyol), etoposide phosphate (Etopophos), filgrastim (Neupogen), gemcitabine (Gemzar), granisetron (Kytril), melphalan (Alkeran), ondansetron (Zofran), teniposide (Vumon), thiotepa (Thioplex), vinorelbine (Navelbine).

RATE OF ADMINISTRATION

A single dose in minimum diluent given over 5 to 15 minutes is recommended. Increase injection time somewhat if additional diluent used or if indicated for patient comfort. Has been given as a continuous infusion over 5 days. Some side effects may be reduced, but CNS side effects (e.g., confusion, depression, lethargy) may be increased.

ACTIONS

An alkylating agent of the nitrosurea group with antitumor activity, cell cycle phase nonspecific. Has a diabetogenic (hyperglycemic) effect resulting from selective uptake into and toxicity to pancreatic islet beta cells. Disappears from the blood serum rapidly. Concentrates in the liver and kidneys. Excreted primarily in urine.

INDICATIONS AND USES

Suppress or retard neoplastic growth in metastatic pancreatic islet cell carcinoma. Use limited by renal toxicity to those with symptomatic or progressive metastatic disease.

Unlabeled uses: Treatment of adrenocortical and colon cancers and Hodgkin's lymphoma.

CONTRAINDICATIONS

Hypersensitivity to streptozocin. Severely impaired liver or renal function may be a contraindication.

PRECAUTIONS

Follow guidelines for handling cytotoxic agents. See Appendix A, p. 1142. ■ Administered by or under the direction of the physician specialist. ■ Marked decrease in leukocyte and platelet counts has occurred and may be fatal. ■ Risk of nephrotoxicity may be reduced by decreasing renal and urinary concentration of streptozocin and its metabolites with adequate hydration.

Monitor: Renal toxicity is dose related, cumulative, and can be fatal. Monitor renal function before, weekly, and for 4 weeks after each course of therapy (serial urinalysis, BUN, plasma creatinine, serum electrolytes, CrCl). Reduce dose or discontinue drug if mild proteinuria occurs. Further deterioration of renal function may occur; see Precautions. ■ Determine absolute patency and quality of vein and adequate circulation of extremity. Local inflammation (e.g., burning, edema, erythema, tenderness), severe cellulitis, and/or necrosis may result from extravasation. If extravasation occurs, discontinue injection; use another vein. ■ Have IV dextrose available especially with the first dose. Sudden release of insulin may precipitate hypoglycemia. Monitor serum glucose at periodic intervals. ■ Monitor CBC and liver function tests weekly. ■ Nausea and vomiting have occurred in all patients and can be severe. Prophylactic administration of antiemetics recommended. ■ Observe for any signs of infection. Use of prophylactic antibiotics may be indicated pending results of C/S in a febrile neutropenic patient. ■ Maintain hydration; see Precautions. ■ Monitor for thrombocytopenia (platelet count less than $50{,}000/mm^3$). Initiate precautions to prevent excessive bleeding (e.g., inspect IV sites, skin, and mucous membranes; use extreme care during invasive procedures; test urine, emesis, stool, and secretions for occult blood). ■ See Drug/Lab Interactions.

Patient Education: Avoid pregnancy; nonhormonal birth control recommended. ■ Report IV site burning or stinging promptly. ■ Use caution in tasks that require alertness, such as driving or using complex machinery. ■ See Appendix D, p. 1148.

Maternal/Child: Category D: avoid pregnancy. Produces teratogenic effects in rats. Has mutagenic potential. ■ Discontinue breast-feeding.

DRUG/LAB INTERACTIONS

Do not administer live vaccines to patients receiving antineoplastic drugs. ■ Concurrent use with hepatotoxic or nephrotoxic medications and radiation therapy may increase toxicity and could be fatal. ■ Toxicity may be additive when used in combination with other cytotoxic drugs (e.g., cyclophosphamide [Cytoxan], doxorubicin [Adriamycin, Doxil]). ■ May prolong the elimination half-life of doxorubicin and lead to severe bone marrow suppression. A reduced dose of doxorubicin may be indicated. ■ Concurrent use with phenytoin (Dilantin) may decrease therapeutic effects of streptozocin.

SIDE EFFECTS

Anemia, decreased platelet count (precipitous), diarrhea, elevated AST (SGOT) and LDH, hepatic toxicity (usually reversible), hypoalbuminemia, hypoglycemia, insulin shock, leukopenia (precipitous), nausea and vomiting (severe), proteinuria, thrombocytopenia. Two cases of diabetes insipidus have been reported.

ANTIDOTE

Notify physician of all side effects. Nausea and vomiting, hematologic changes, and renal toxicity (proteinuria) may require dose reduction or discontinuation of the drug. There is no specific antidote. Supportive therapy as indicated will help sustain the patient in toxicity. Administration of whole blood products (e.g., packed RBCs, platelets, leukocytes) and/or blood modifiers (e.g., darbepoetin alfa [Aranesp], epoetin alfa [Epogen, Procrit], filgrastim [Neupogen], pegfilgrastim [Neulasta], sargramostim [Leukine], oprelvekin [Neumega]) may be indicated to treat bone marrow toxicity. For extravasation, elevate extremity, consider injection of long-acting dexamethasone (Decadron LA) throughout extravasated tissue. Use a 27- or 25-gauge needle. Apply warm, moist compresses.

SUCCINYLCHOLINE CHLORIDE

(suk-sin-ill-koe′leen klor′id)

Neuromuscular blocking agent (depolarizing)
Anesthesia adjunct

Anectine, Quelicin PF

pH 3 to 4.5

USUAL DOSE

A test dose of 0.1 mg is sometimes used to test patient sensitivity and recovery time.

0.3 to 1.1 mg/kg of body weight initially for short-term muscle relaxation (average is 0.6 mg/kg). Should be administered after unconsciousness induced to reduce patient discomfort. If muscle relaxation must be sustained over a long period of time, maintain with intermittent IV injections of 0.04 to 0.07 mg/kg at appropriate intervals or with a continuous infusion of 0.5 to 10 mg/min (average is 2.5 to 4.3 mg/min). Monitoring with a peripheral nerve stimulator advisable to avoid overdose, especially with a continuous infusion. Highly individualized, depending on response and degree of relaxation required. 1 mg/kg of body weight is sufficient to cause respiratory paralysis. Never exceed 150 mg total dose.

Electroshock therapy: 10 to 30 mg 1 minute before shock.

PEDIATRIC DOSE

Infants and small children: 1 to 2 mg/kg (most sources say 2 mg/kg).

Older children and adolescents: 1 mg/kg. To sustain muscle relaxation in all pediatric patients maintain with intermittent injections of 0.3 to 0.6 mg/kg/dose at 5- to 10-minute intervals. Monitoring with a peripheral nerve stimulator advisable. Continuous infusion not recommended; increased risk of malignant hyperpyrexia.

DOSE ADJUSTMENTS

Minimal doses with extreme care are required in patients with low plasma pseudocholinesterase (e.g., abnormal body temperatures, anemia, burns, cancer, collagen diseases, dehydration, exposure to neurotoxic insecticides, malnutrition, myxedema, patients with a recessive hereditary trait, pregnancy, severe liver disease or cirrhosis, and patients receiving antimalarials, antineoplastics, chlorpromazine [Thorazine], echothiophate iodide [Phospholine], irradiation, MAO inhibitors [e.g., selegiline (Eldepryl)], neostigmine, oral contraceptives, or pancuronium). Use a test dose of 5 to 10 mg or cautiously administer a 0.1% infusion. ■ Lower-end initial doses may be indicated in the elderly based on potential for decreased organ function and concomitant disease or drug therapy.

DILUTION

May be given undiluted if short-term muscle relaxation is desired. For intermittent or continuous infusion during anesthesia add 1 Gm of succinylcholine to 500 ml or 1 L of D5W, D5NS, or NS. 1 ml of diluted solution delivers 2 mg (1 mg) of succinylcholine. For all other uses, 100 mg in 1 L delivers 0.1 mg succinylcholine. Use only freshly prepared solutions.

Storage: Store in refrigerator after dilution. Multidose vials stable at room temperature for up to 14 days. Powder for infusion may be stored at room temperature before preparation.

INCOMPATIBLE WITH

Manufacturer states, "Acidic; should not be mixed with alkaline solutions having a pH greater than 8.5" (e.g., barbiturates [e.g., thiopental (Pentothal)]).

COMPATIBLE WITH (Underline Indicates Conflicting Compatibility Information)

Consult pharmacist; specific conditions may apply; see Compatibilities, p. xvi.

Additive: Amikacin (Amikin), isoproterenol (Isuprel), meperidine (Demerol), methyldopate (Aldomet), morphine, norepinephrine (Levophed), <u>pentobarbital (Nembutal)</u>, scopolamine.

Syringe: Heparin.

Y-site: Etomidate (Amidate), hetastarch in electrolytes (Hextend), potassium chloride (KCl), propofol (Diprivan).

RATE OF ADMINISTRATION

Too-rapid rate may cause profound bradycardia and rarely asystole. Incidence of bradycardia higher with a second dose.

IV injection: Single initial dose over 30 seconds.

Intermittent or continuous infusion: Variable, depending on individual response and muscle relaxation required. Use an infusion pump or microdrip (60 gtt/ml) for accuracy. Never exceed 10 mg/min.

ACTIONS

An ultra-short-acting depolarizing skeletal muscle relaxant. Causes paralysis by interfering with neural transmission at the myoneural junction. Onset of action is within 0.5 to 1 minute. Duration of peak effect is 4 to 10 minutes. Metabolized to succinic acid and choline. Only a small amount is excreted by the kidneys. Crosses placental barrier in small amounts.

INDICATIONS AND USES

Skeletal muscle relaxation during operative and manipulative procedures. ■ Facilitate management of patients undergoing mechanical ventilation. ■ Termination or prevention of convulsive episodes resulting from drug toxicity or electroshock therapy.

CONTRAINDICATIONS

Hypersensitivity to succinylcholine, family history of malignant hyperthermia, genetic disorders of plasma pseudocholinesterase, myopathies associated with elevated CPK values, acute narrow-angle glaucoma, penetrating eye injuries.

PRECAUTIONS

Primarily used by or under the direct observation of the anesthesiologist. ■ Small doses of nondepolarizing muscle relaxants (e.g., tubocurarine) will reduce severity of muscle fasciculations and incidence of myoglobinuria (occurs more frequently in children) but may cause a prolonged mixed block. ■ Incidence of bradycardia increased with repeat dosing; more pronounced in children. Pretreatment with anticholinergic agents (e.g., atropine) may reduce the occurrence of bradyarrhythmias. ■ May cause prolonged blockade with hypocalcemia, hypokalemia, and cardiovascular, hepatic, or pulmonary disorders. ■ May cause serious cardiac arrhythmias, including cardiac arrest in patients who are digitalized or on quinidine, as well as those with electrolyte imbalance, hyperkalemia, or severe trauma. Use extreme caution. ■ Patients with pre-existing hyperkalemia, or those with spinal cord injuries, paralysis, or degenerative or dystrophic neuromuscular disease may become severely hyperkalemic with succinylcholine; use caution. ■ Prolonged respiratory paralysis may occur in patients with low plasma pseudocholinesterase (see Dose Adjustments; decreased plasma cholinesterase activity potentiates this drug). ■ Muscle fasciculation may cause additional trauma in patients with fractures or muscle spasm. ■ May cause cardiac arrest in children with undiagnosed skeletal muscle myopathy (e.g., Duchenne's muscular dystrophy); see Monitor. ■ Patients with myasthenia gravis may be resistant to succinylcholine. ■ May increase intraocular pressure. ■ May convert to a nondepolarizing block during repeated or prolonged administration. Respiratory depression and apnea are common. Use a peripheral nerve stimulator to confirm diagnosis before treating with anticholinergic agents and atropine; see Antidote.

Monitor: This drug may produce apnea. Controlled artificial ventilation must be available and under direct observation at all times. ■ Observe for early signs of malignant hyperthermic crisis (jaw muscle spasm, lack of laryngeal relaxation, rigidity, and unresponsive tachycardia). ■ Continuous ECG monitoring recommended. Observe for peaked T-waves; may be an early sign of skeletal muscle myopathy. Occurs more often in males under 8 years. ■ Monitor for increased intragastric pressure; avoid regurgitation and possible aspiration. ■ See Precautions and Drug/Lab Interactions.

Maternal/Child: Category C: use extreme caution in pregnancy. There is greater potential for prolonged apnea because of increased sensitivity to succinylcholine in pregnant women. If used during cesarean section, apnea and flaccidity may occur in the neonate, depending on mother's dose. ■ Use caution in breast-feeding. ■ A few occurrences of hyperkalemia-induced cardiac arrest have been noted in male pediatric patients.

Elderly: Lower-end initial doses may be indicated; see Dose Adjustments. ■ Response of older vs. younger patients not documented. ■ Delay in onset time may be caused by slower circulation time in cardiovascular disease, old age, or edematous states; allow more time for drug to achieve maximum effect.

DRUG/LAB INTERACTIONS

May cause a prolonged mixed block with nondepolarizing muscle relaxants (e.g., atracurium, tubocurarine). ■ May cause cardiac arrhythmias in digitalized patients resulting from a sudden loss of potassium from muscle cells. ■ Potentiated by neuromuscular blocking antibiotics (e.g., aminoglycosides [e.g., kanamycin, neomycin]), selected nonpenicillin antibiotics (e.g., bacitracin, colistimethate, polymyxins, tetracyclines, vancomycin), beta-adrenergic blocking agents (e.g., propranolol [Inderal]), furosemide (Lasix), procainamide (Pronestyl), organic phosphate compounds (insecticides), anticholinesterase drugs (e.g., neostigmine, edrophonium), cimetidine (Tagamet), cyclophosphamide (Cytoxan), isoflurane, lidocaine, lithium carbonate, quinine, quinidine, and magnesium salts. ■ Increased neuromuscular blockade and prolonged respiratory depression may occur for several days after cyclophosphamide therapy is stopped. Potentiated by amphotericin B and thiazide diuretics in patients with electrolyte imbalance (e.g., hypocalcemia, hypokalemia); reduced dose indicated. ■ Incidence of cardiac arrhythmias and/or malignant hyperthermia may be increased with inhalation anesthetics (e.g., cyclopropane, halothane). ■ Incidence of cardiac arrhythmias may be increased by narcotic analgesics. ■ May cause muscle paralysis and respiratory collapse with vancomycin. ■ Capable of innumerable other drug interactions. ■

Inhibited by previous administration of diazepam (Valium). See Dose Adjustments.

SIDE EFFECTS

Bradycardia, or other cardiac arrhythmias, histamine release, hyperkalemia, muscular twitching, myoglobinemia, myoglobinuria, rash, respiratory depression, salivation (excessive).

Major: Cardiac arrhythmias, hyperthermia, malignant hyperthermic crisis, prolonged apnea with progression to a phase II block (usually results from repeated or prolonged administration).

ANTIDOTE

Discontinue drug with onset of any major side effect. An anesthesiologist should be present. Controlled artificial ventilation must be continuous. Endotracheal intubation or tracheostomy is considered prophylactic if necessary for adequate respiratory exchange. Confirm diagnosis of phase II block by using a peripheral nerve stimulator; presence of muscle twitch must also have returned for at least 20 minutes. Both of these are necessary before reversal with anticholinesterase drugs (e.g., neostigmine) is attempted. Whole blood transfusion may restore absent cholinesterase activity and stimulate voluntary respiration in unresponsive cases. Atropine should help to control bradycardia. Treat malignant hyperthermic crisis symptomatically with cooling measures, restoration of electrolyte balance, IV fluids, and maintenance of urinary output. Sodium bicarbonate may be indicated. Dantrolene may be indicated. IV calcium, bicarbonate, and glucose with insulin concurrent with hyperventilation have been used to resuscitate children with skeletal muscle myopathy. Resuscitate as necessary.

SULFAMETHOXAZOLE-TRIMETHOPRIM

(sul-fa-meth-ox′a-zole-tri-meth′o-prim)

Antibacterial
Antiprotozoal

Bactrim, Septra, SMZ-TMP, TMP-SMZ

pH 10

USUAL DOSE

Doses listed are based on the trimethoprim component of the drug.

Severe urinary tract infections and shigellosis in adults and children over 2 months of age: 8 to 10 mg/kg of body weight in equally divided doses every 6, 8, or 12 hours for 14 days (urinary tract infections) or 5 days (shigellosis).

***Pneumocystis carinii* pneumonitis in adults and children over 2 months of age:** 15 to 20 mg/kg in equally divided doses every 6 or 8 hours for up to 14 days.

DOSE ADJUSTMENTS

Reduce dose by one half for CrCl between 15 and 30 ml/min; see Contraindications. ▪ Reduced dose may be indicated in the elderly. ▪ See Monitor and Drug/Lab Interactions.

DILUTION

Each 5-ml ampule must be diluted in 125 ml D5W and given as an infusion. Reduce diluent to 75 ml for each ampule only if fluid restriction required. Standard dilution must be used within 6 hours; fluid restriction dilution must be used within 2 hours. Available in 5-, 10-, 20-, and 30-ml vials. Concentration per ml same as 5-ml ampule. Discard if cloudiness or crystallization is present.

Storage: Store at room temperature; do not refrigerate.

INCOMPATIBLE WITH

Manufacturer states, "Do not mix with other drugs or solutions."

COMPATIBLE WITH

(Underline Indicates Conflicting Compatibility Information)

Consult pharmacist; specific conditions may apply; see Compatibilities, p. xvi.

Syringe: ***Not recommended by manufacturer.*** Heparin.

Y-site: Acyclovir (Zovirax), aldesleukin (Proleukin, IL-2), allopurinol (Aloprim, Zyloprim), amifostine (Ethyol), amphotericin B cholesteryl (Amphotec), atracurium (Tracrium), aztreonam (Azactam), cefepime (Maxipime), cisatracurium (Nimbex), cyclophosphamide (Cytoxan), diltiazem (Cardizem), docetaxel (Taxotere), doxorubicin liposome (Doxil), enalaprilat (Vasotec IV), esmolol (Brevibloc), etoposide phosphate (Etopophos), filgrastim (Neupogen), fludarabine (Fludara), foscarnet (Foscavir), gatifloxacin (Tequin), gemcitabine (Gemzar), granisetron (Kytril), hetastarch in electrolytes (Hextend), hydromorphone (Dilaudid), labetalol (Normodyne), linezolid (Zyvox), lorazepam (Ativan), magnesium sulfate, melphalan (Alkeran), meperidine (Demerol), morphine, pancuronium (Pavulon), perphenazine (Trilafon), piperacillin/tazobactam (Zosyn), remifentanil (Ultiva), sargramostim (Leukine), tacrolimus (Prograf), teniposide (Vumon), thiotepa (Thioplex), vecuronium (Norcuron), zidovudine (AZT, Retrovir).

RATE OF ADMINISTRATION

A single dose must be infused over 60 to 90 minutes. When administered by an infusion device, thoroughly flush all lines used to remove any residual sulfamethoxazole-trimethoprim. Avoid rapid infusion or bolus injection.

ACTIONS

A broad-spectrum antibacterial and antiprotozoal combination agent with bactericidal action effective against gram-positive and gram-negative organisms. Blocks sequential steps in the folic acid pathway, preventing the synthesis of nucleic acids and proteins essential to many bacteria. Combination contains 400 mg sulfamethoxazole and 80 mg trimethoprim per each 5 ml. Widely distributed in all body fluids and tissues, including cerebrospinal fluid, sputum, and bile. Onset of action is prompt and serum levels are maintained up to 10 hours. Metabolized in the liver and up to 60% is excreted in urine in 24 hours. Crosses placental barrier. Secreted in breast milk. Partially removed by hemodialysis.

INDICATIONS AND USES

Severe urinary tract infections. ■ *Pneumocystis carinii* pneumonia. ■ Shigellosis. ■ Prophylaxis in neutropenic patients. ■ Used orally in HIV and other immunocompromised patients to prevent pneumonia.

Unlabeled uses: Treatment of cholera and salmonella type infections. ■ An alternative agent in the treatment of meningitis caused by susceptible organisms.

CONTRAINDICATIONS

CrCl less than 15 ml/min, hypersensitivity to trimethoprim or sulfonamides, megaloblastic anemia resulting from folate deficiency, nursing mothers, pregnancy at term and infants less than 2 months of age (may cause hemolytic anemia, jaundice, and kernicterus), streptococcal pharyngitis.

PRECAUTIONS

Sensitivity studies indicated to determine susceptibility of the causative organism to sulfamethoxazole-trimethoprim. ■ Not for IM use. ■ Use caution in impaired liver or renal function, possible folate deficiency, allergic individuals, bronchial asthma, porphyria, glucose 6-phosphate dehydrogenase (G-6PD) deficiency, and in the elderly. ■ A sulfonamide drug; allergic reactions can occur. Use caution in patients with a history of hypersensitivity to furosemide (Lasix), thiazide diuretics (e.g., chlorothiazide), sulfonylureas (e.g., tolbutamide), or carbonic anhydrase inhibitors (e.g., acetazolamide). ■ Some products contain bisulfites; use caution in patients with allergies. ■ Incidence of side effects markedly increased in AIDS patients. May not tolerate or respond to this drug. ■ Pseudomembranous colitis has been reported. May range from mild to life-threatening. Consider in patients that present with diarrhea during or after treatment with sulfamethoxazole-trimethoprim.

Monitor: Maintain adequate hydration to prevent crystalluria and stone formation. ■ CBC required before and during therapy. Discontinue for any significant reduction in a blood-forming element. Urinalysis and renal function tests also indicated. ■ If extravasation occurs, discontinue and restart at a new site. May cause phlebitis. ■ Monitor closely if any signs of rash appear or have appeared in previous infusions. Several cases of life-threatening reactions have occurred. ■ See Precautions and Drug/Lab Interactions.

Patient Education: Maintain adequate hydration. ■ Report bruising or bleeding, fever, rash, or sore throat promptly. ■ Possible skin photosensitivity. Avoid unprotected exposure to sunlight.

Maternal/Child: Category C: no adequate studies. May interfere with folic acid metabolism in mother and fetus. Benefits must outweigh risks. ■ May contain benzyl alcohol. ■ See Contraindications. ■ Discontinue breast-feeding. ■ Two infants who developed a rash had life-threatening reactions when sulfamethoxazole-trimethoprim was restarted.

Elderly: See Dose Adjustments. ■ Increased risk of severe side effects (e.g., bone marrow depression, decrease in platelets with or without purpura, skin reactions), especially in impaired renal or liver function or with other drugs (e.g., diuretics).

DRUG/LAB INTERACTIONS

May be potentiated by probenecid. ■ May inhibit cyclosporine (Sandimmune) and increase nephrotoxicity. ■ May potentiate warfarin (Coumadin), phenytoin (Dilantin), oral hypoglycemics, dapsone, and zidovudine (Retrovir, AZT). ■ The sulfa component may displace methotrexate from its binding sites, increasing free fraction of methotrexate and its potential for toxicity. The trimethoprim component inhibits methotrexate metabolism and increases toxicity. ■ May decrease effectiveness of tricyclic antidepressants (e.g., amitriptyline [Elavil]). ■ Concurrent use with folate antagonists (e.g., hydantoins [e.g., phenytoin], methotrexate), is not recommended. May increase possibility of megaloblastic anemia. ■ Concurrent use with leucovorin calcium may cause treatment failure and increased morbidity in HIV-infected patients being treated for *Pneumocystis carinii* pneumonia. ■ Concurrent use with bone marrow depressants (e.g., antineoplastics [e.g., busulfan, cisplatin], amphotericin B [all formulations], ganciclovir [Cytovene]) may increase leukopenic or thrombocytopenic effects. Monitor differential blood count. ■ Serum levels of digoxin may be increased with concurrent use, monitor digoxin levels. ■ Concurrent use with hemolytics (e.g., doxapram [Dopram], methyldopate [Aldomet], procainamide [Pronestyl], quinidine) may increase potential for toxic side effects. ■ Concurrent use with hepatotoxic agents (e.g., alatrofloxacin [Trovan], amiodarone [Cordarone], erythromycins, fluconazole [Diflucan]) may increase incidence of hepatotoxicity. Risk increased with prolonged use or in patients with a history of liver disease. ■ May form an insoluble precipitate in acid urine or cause crystalluria with methenamine (Mandelamine), concurent use not recommended. ■ May decrease clearance and increase serum concentrations of N-acetylprocainamide (NAPA) and procainamide (Pronestyl). ■ Concurrent use with rifampin (Rifadin) will increase elimination, reduce serum concentrations, and shorten half-life of trimethoprim. ■ Concurrent use with thiazide diuretics (e.g., chlorothiazide) in the elderly may result in an increased incidence of thrombocytopenia with purpura. ■ May interfere with serum methotrexate assay and Jaffe assay for creatinine. ■ See Precautions.

SIDE EFFECTS

All side effects of sulfonamides including allergic reaction are possible. Nausea, vomiting, and rash occur most frequently. Ataxia, convulsions, tremors, and respiratory depression are symptoms of major toxicity. With high doses or administration over an extended period of time, bone marrow depression (leukopenia, megaloblastic anemia, thrombocytopenia) may occur. Pseudomembranous colitis has been reported.

ANTIDOTE

Notify the physician of any side effect. Discontinue the drug at any sign of major toxicity or bone marrow depression. Some sources recommend leucovorin calcium 5 to 15 mg daily for treatment of bone marrow depression. Peritoneal dialysis is not effective in toxicity; hemodialysis may be moderately effective in reducing serum levels. Acidification of urine may increase excretion. Treat anaphylaxis with epinephrine, corticosteroids, antihistamines, and vasopressors as indicated.

TACROLIMUS

(tak-roe-leem′us)

Immunosuppressant

Prograf

USUAL DOSE

See Precautions. IV route used for patients unable to take oral medications; risk of anaphylaxis increased with IV administration.

Prophylaxis of organ rejection in kidney or liver transplant: ***Adults and children:*** 0.03 to 0.05 mg/kg/day as a continuous infusion is the recommended starting dose. (Dose recommendations have been lowered by the manufacturer [were 0.05 to 0.1] and dose regimens vary among transplant centers and approved or investigational use [range 0.01 to 0.05].) Begin no sooner than 6 hours after transplantation. Adults usually receive doses at the lower end of the range. Children usually require doses at the upper end of the range. Individualized adjustment based on clinical assessment of rejection (e.g., trough blood concentrations) or patients' tolerance is imperative and may be required on a daily basis. Adjunctive adrenal corticosteroid therapy early posttransplant is recommended. Initiate oral tacrolimus therapy as soon as feasible. Oral doses vary with specific organ transplant and in adults and children (see literature). Total dose in mg/kg/day is given in equally divided doses every 12 hours. Begin 8 to 12 hours after IV tacrolimus is discontinued.

Treatment of organ rejection in kidney or liver transplants and prophylaxis or treatment of other solid organ transplants (unlabeled): 0.01 to 0.05 mg/kg/day. See all comments and protocol above.

Prophylaxis of graft-versus-host disease (unlabeled): 0.04 mg/kg/day as a continuous infusion started the day before bone marrow transplant. See all comments and protocol above.

Treatment of graft-versus-host disease (unlabeled): 0.1 mg/kg/day as an infusion in equally divided doses every 12 hours. Administer each infusion over 4 hours. See all comments and protocol above and on page 1030.

PEDIATRIC DOSE

Used in children, but safety and efficacy not established. See Usual Dose for mg/kg/day dose recommendations. Studies indicate that higher doses may be required to maintain blood trough concentrations similar to adults. See Dilution and Maternal/Child.

DOSE ADJUSTMENTS

Use lowest dosing range initially for patients with impaired renal or hepatic function (pretransplant or posttransplant). Nephrotoxicity may be increased and further reductions may be required; should be based on tacrolimus trough levels in blood. ■ Delay tacrolimus therapy up to 48 hours in patients with postoperative oliguria. ■ Lower doses may be appropriate for maintenance. ■ See Monitor and Drug/Lab Interactions.

DILUTION

A 24-hour dose must be diluted with an appropriate amount of NS or D5W. Desired concentration is between 4 and 20 mcg/ml. May leach phthalate from polyvinylchloride containers; use diluents in glass or polyethylene infusion bottles. Use PVC-free IV tubing in pediatric patients. The following chart provides some dose and dilution examples.

Tacrolimus Dose and Dilution Examples

Desired Dose (mg/kg)	Wt (kg)	Total Dose	Amount of Diluent (ml)	mcg/ml
0.08	20	1.6 mg/24 hr	250	6.4
			100	16
0.05	60	3 mg/24 hr	500	6
			250	12
0.04	100	4 mg/24 hr	1,000	4

Storage: Store at CRT before dilution. Discard diluted solution in 24 hours.

INCOMPATIBLE WITH

Manufacturer states, "Should not be mixed with solutions of pH 9 or greater (e.g., acyclovir [Zovirax], ganciclovir [Cytovene]). See Dilution.

COMPATIBLE WITH **(Underline Indicates Conflicting Compatibility Information)**

Consult pharmacist; specific conditions may apply; see Compatibilities, p. xvi.

Additive: Cimetidine (Tagamet).

Y-site: ***See Incompatible With.*** Acyclovir (Zovirax), aminophylline, amphotericin B (Fungizone), ampicillin, ampicillin/sulbactam (Unasyn), benztropine (Cogentin), calcium gluconate, cefazolin (Kefzol), cefotetan (Cefotan), ceftazidime (Fortaz), ceftriaxone (Rocephin), cefuroxime (Zinacef), chloramphenicol (Chloromycetin), cimetidine (Tagamet), ciprofloxacin (Cipro IV), clindamycin (Cleocin), dexamethasone (Decadron), digoxin (Lanoxin), diphenhydramine (Benadryl), dobutamine (Dobutrex), dopamine (Intropin), doxycycline (Vibramycin), erythromycin lactobionate (Erythrocin), esmolol (Brevibloc), fluconazole (Diflucan), furosemide (Lasix), ganciclovir (Cytovene), gentamicin (Garamycin), haloperidol (Haldol), heparin, hydrocortisone sodium succinate (Solu-Cortef), hydromorphone (Dilaudid), imipenem-cilastatin (Primaxin), insulin (regular), isoproterenol (Isuprel), leucovorin calcium, lorazepam (Ativan), methylprednisolone (Solu-Medrol), metoclopramide (Reglan), metronidazole (Flagyl IV), morphine, multivitamins (M.V.I.), nitroglycerin (Nitro-Bid IV), nitroprusside sodium, oxacillin (Bactocill), penicillin G potassium, perphenazine (Trilafon), phenytoin (Dilantin), piperacillin (Pipracil), potassium chloride (KCl), propranolol (Inderal), ranitidine (Zantac), sodium bicarbonate, sulfamethoxazole-trimethoprim (Bactrim), tobramycin (Nebcin), vancomycin (Vancocin).

RATE OF ADMINISTRATION

A single dose properly diluted and equally distributed over 24 hours as a continuous infusion. Use of a metriset (60 gtt/min) or infusion pump suggested.

ACTIONS

A potent immunosuppressive agent. Prolongs survival of allogeneic kidney and liver transplants. Suppresses some humoral immunity (within the body fluids) but suppresses cell-mediated reactions to a greater extent (e.g., allograft rejection, delayed type hypersensitivity, collagen-induced arthritis, experimental allergic encephalomyelitis, graft-versus-host disease). Inhibition of T-lymphocyte activation results in immunosuppression. Highly protein bound. Metabolized primarily by the P_{450} enzyme system to up to 10 metabolites. Minimal excretion in urine. Crosses the placental barrier. Secreted in breast milk.

INDICATIONS AND USES

Prophylaxis of organ rejection in allogeneic kidney and liver transplants in conjunction with adrenal corticosteroids. Studies show a reduction in rejection episodes as compared to other immunosuppressants and a reduced use of steroids and antilymphocytes (e.g., antilymphocyte globulin, antithymocyte globulin) to reduce rejection and retain some resistance to infection.

Unlabeled uses: Treatment of organ rejection in kidney or liver transplants. Prophylaxis and treatment of organ rejection in bone marrow, heart, pancreas, pancreatic island cell, and small bowel transplants. ■ Treatment of autoimmune diseases and severe recalcitrant psoriasis.

CONTRAINDICATIONS

Hypersensitivity to tacrolimus or polyoxyl 60 hydrogenated castor oil.

PRECAUTIONS

For IV use only. Oral dosing preferred; begin as soon as feasible. ■ Usually administered in the hospital by or under the direction of a physician experienced in immunosuppressive therapy and management of organ transplant patients. ■ Adequate laboratory and supportive medical resources must be available. ■ Risk of anaphylaxis increased by IV route versus oral route; use caution. ■ Use caution in impaired renal function; increases in SrCr may require dose reduction or use of an alternate immunosuppressant. ■ Use caution in severe hepatic dysfunction (mean Pugh score: greater than 10), clearance decreased. ■ May cause lymphomas and other malignancies (especially of skin), and has been associated with a lymphoproliferative disorder (LPD) related to Epstein-Barr virus. ■ Antiviral prophylaxis (e.g., acyclovir, ganciclovir, immune globulin) may be advisable in some patients.

Monitor: Obtain baseline CBC, differential, platelets, electrolytes, BUN, and SrCr. Monitor regularly during therapy. ■ Contains a castor oil derivative and alcohol; observe continuously for signs of an allergic reaction for the first 30 minutes of the infusion and frequently thereafter. A source of oxygen and epinephrine must always be available. ■ Monitor urine output and SrCr carefully. Overt nephrotoxicity occurs more frequently early after transplant, resulting in increased SrCr and decreased urine output. ■ Monitor tacrolimus blood levels to evaluate rejection, toxicity, need for dose reduction, and patient compliance. Whole blood median trough concentrations (measured by ELISA) may vary considerably during the first week but then stabilize; rejection is minimized with median ranges from 9.8 ng/ml to 19.4 ng/ml, but target ranges will depend on indication and protocol. ■ Monitor all parameters to evaluate possibility of organ rejection. ■ Monitor BP; antihypertensives may be indicated. ■ Monitor serum potassium and magnesium levels. May cause hyperkalemia or hypomagnesemia. ■ May cause hyperglycemia. Monitor carefully; treatment may be required. ■ Observe for signs of infection (e.g., fever, sore throat, tiredness) or unusual bleeding or bruising. ■ Use of prophylactic antibiotics may be indicated pending results of C/S in a febrile neutropenic patient. ■ See Precautions and Drug/Lab Interactions.

Patient Education: Nonhormonal birth control preferred to oral contraceptives to reduce complications of drug interactions. ■ Emphasize need for frequent routine lab work; compliance imperative. ■ Interacts with many medications. Discuss any changes in drug regimen (prescription or nonprescription) with doctor or pharmacist. ■ Promptly report any side effects. ■ Inform of increased risk of neoplasia. ■ See Appendix D, p. 1148.

Maternal/Child: Category C: use only if necessary; benefits must outweigh risk to fetus. Has been associated with hyperkalemia and renal dysfunction in the fetus. ■ Discontinue breast-feeding. ■ Appears to be an increased risk for LPD and primary Epstein-Barr virus infection in immunosuppressed children.

Elderly: Consider age-related organ impairment.

DRUG/LAB INTERACTIONS

May be used concurrently only with adrenocorticosteroids. ***Do not use simultaneously with cyclosporine (Sandimmune).*** If a change of immunosuppressants is indicated (tacrolimus to cyclosporine or cyclosporine to tacrolimus), avoid additive nephrotoxicity by waiting for at least 24 hours before starting the alternate drug. If elevated blood concentrations are present, further extend the interval between the two drugs. ■ Concurrent use with sirolimus (Rapamune) has been associated with an excess rate of death and graft loss in liver transplant patients. ■ Use extreme caution with other nephrotoxic agents (e.g., aminoglycosides [gentamicin, tobramycin], amphotericin B [Fungizone], cisplatin [Platinol]). ■ Do not use potassium-sparing diuretics (e.g., spironolactone [Aldactone]); increases risk of hyperkalemia. ■ Calcium channel blockers (e.g., diltiazem [Cardizem], nicardipine [Cardene], verapamil [Isoptin]), antifungal agents (e.g., clotrimazole [Mycelex], fluconazole [Diflucan], itraconazole [Sporanox], ketoconazole [Nizoral]), bromocriptine (Parlodel), cimetidine (Tagamet), clarithromycin (Biaxin), cyclosporine (Sandimmune), danazol (Cyclomen), erythromycin, methylprednisone (Medrol), metoclopramide (Reglan), metronidazole (Flagyl), nelfinavir (Viracept), and theophylline (e.g., TheoDur) may inhibit the P_{450} enzyme system and increase tacrolimus blood levels, increasing toxicity potential. Tacrolimus toxicity may also be increased if given concurrently with nefazodone (Serzone). ■ Anticonvulsants (e.g., carbamazepine [Tegretol], phenobarbital, phenytoin [Dilantin]), and rifamycins (e.g., rifabutin [Mycobutin], rifampin [Rifadin]) may induce the P_{450} enzyme system, decreasing effectiveness and leading to decreased tacrolimus blood levels and organ rejection. ■ Tacrolimus may increase serum concentrations of mycophenolate (CellCept), phenytoin, and St. John's wort. ■ Grapefruit juice may affect certain enzymes of the P_{450} system and should be avoided. ■ Avoid vaccinations and do not use live vaccines in patients receiving tacrolimus.

SIDE EFFECTS

Occur in a majority of patients and are more pronounced at higher doses. May improve somewhat over time. Nephrotoxicity (abnormal renal function with increased SrCr and BUN, oliguria), and neurotoxicity (delirium, headache, insomnia, paresthesia, tremor, seizures) may be dose limiting. Abdominal pain, abnormal liver function tests, anemia, anorexia, ascites, asthenia, atelectasis, back pain, blood dyscrasias, coma, constipation, diarrhea, dyspnea, fever, gastroenteritis, hyperglycemia, hyperkalemia or hypokalemia, hypertension, hypomagnesemia, leukocytosis, nausea, peripheral edema, pleural effusion, pruritus, rash, seizures, thrombocytopenia, urinary tract infections, vomiting. Many other side effects have occurred in less than 3% of patients.

ANTIDOTE

Notify the physician of all side effects. Most will be treated symptomatically. Tacrolimus may be decreased or discontinued or alternate immunosuppressive agents substituted. Nephrotoxicity, neurotoxicity, or hematopoietic depression may require temporary reduction of dose or discontinuation of therapy. Dialysis is not effective in overdose. Discontinue immediately if anaphylaxis occurs and treat with oxygen, epinephrine, corticosteroids, and/or antihistamines (e.g., diphenhydramine [Benadryl]). Resuscitate as necessary.

TENECTEPLASE

(ten-ek'ta-place)

Thrombolytic agent (recombinant)

TNKase

pH 7.3

USUAL DOSE

Initiate therapy as soon as possible after the onset of acute myocardial infarction (AMI) symptoms. Total dose is based on patient weight and should not exceed 50 mg. See the chart below.

Tenecteplase Dosing Guidelines

Patient Weight (kg)	Tenecteplase (mg)	Volume of Tenecteplase* to be Administered (ml)
<60	30	6
>60 to <70	35	7
>70 to <80	40	8
>80 to <90	45	9
>90	50	10

*From one vial of tenecteplase reconstituted with 10 ml of SW.

Concurrent administration of heparin and aspirin has been used in MI patients receiving tenecteplase therapy. In the ASSENT-2 trial, the following doses were used.

Aspirin: 150 to 325 mg as soon as possible was followed by 150 to 325 mg daily.

Heparin IV: Was administered based on weight. ***Patients weighing 67 kg or less*** received a heparin loading dose of 4,000 units followed by an infusion at 800 units/hr. ***Patients weighing more than 67 kg*** received a heparin loading dose of 5,000 units followed by an infusion at 1,000 units/hr. Heparin was continued for 48 to 72 hours with the infusion rate adjusted to maintain the aPPT at 50 to 75 seconds.

DOSE ADJUSTMENTS

None noted.

DILUTION

Remove the shield assembly from the manufacturer-supplied B-D® 10 ml syringe with TwinPak™ dual Cannula Device. Aseptically withdraw 10 ml of SW from the supplied diluent vial using the red hub cannula syringe filling device. Do not use bacteriostatic water for injection. Do not discard the shield assembly. Inject the 10 ml of SW into the tenecteplase vial, directing the diluent stream into the powder. Slight foaming may occur. Allow product to stand for several minutes. Gently swirl until contents are completely dissolved. Do not shake. The reconstituted preparation is colorless to pale yellow and contains tenecteplase 50 mg/10 ml. Withdraw the desired dose from the vial using the syringe. Once the appropriate dose is drawn into the syringe, stand the shield vertically on a flat surface with the green side down and passively recap the red hub cannula. Remove the entire shield assembly, including the red hub cannula, by twisting counterclockwise. Note: The shield assembly also contains the clear-ended blunt plastic cannula; retain for split septum IV access. The supplied syringe is compatible with a conventional needle and with needleless IV systems. See package insert for complete instructions for administration.

Storage: Store unopened vial at CRT or under refrigeration (at 2° to 8° C [(36° to 46° F]). Reconstitution immediately before use preferred, or may be refrigerated for up to 8 hours.

COMPATIBILITY

Manufacturer states, "Precipitation may occur when tenecteplase is administered in an IV line containing dextrose. Dextrose-containing lines should be flushed with a saline-containing solution prior to and following single bolus administration of tenecteplase."

RATE OF ADMINISTRATION

A single bolus dose over 5 seconds. Flush line with saline-containing solution to ensure delivery of entire dose.

ACTIONS

A tissue plasminogen activator and enzyme produced by recombinant DNA technology. Binds to fibrin in a thrombus and converts plasminogen to plasmin. Plasmin digests fibrin and dissolves the clot. Onset of action is prompt. Cleared via hepatic metabolism. Terminal half-life is 90 to 130 minutes.

INDICATIONS AND USES

For use in the reduction of mortality associated with acute myocardial infarction (AMI). Treatment should be initiated as soon as possible after the onset of AMI symptoms.

CONTRAINDICATIONS

Active internal bleeding, history of cerebrovascular accident, intracranial or intraspinal surgery or trauma within the past 2 months, intracranial neoplasm, arteriovenous malformation, or aneurysm, known bleeding diathesis, and severe uncontrolled hypertension.

PRECAUTIONS

Administered under the direction of a physician knowledgeable in its use and with appropriate emergency drugs and diagnostic and laboratory facilities available. ■ Most common complication is bleeding. May be internal bleeding or superficial or surface bleeding. Strict bed rest indicated to reduce risk of bleeding. Use extreme care with the patient; avoid any excessive or rough handling or pressure; avoid invasive procedures (e.g., arterial puncture, venipuncture, IM injection). If these procedures are absolutely necessary, use extreme precautionary methods (use radial artery instead of femoral; use small-gauge catheters and needles, and sites that are easily observed and compressible where bleeding can be controlled; avoid handling catheter sites; and use extended pressure application of up to 30 minutes). Minor bleeding occurs often at catheter insertion sites. Avoid use of razors and toothbrushes. If serious bleeding (not controlled by local pressure) occurs, discontinue any concomitant heparin or antiplatelet agents immediately. ■ Use extreme caution in the following situations: recent major surgery (e.g., CABG), previous puncture of noncompressible vessels, organ biopsy, or trauma, cerebrovascular disease, recent GI or GU bleeding, hypertension (systolic BP above 180 and/or diastolic BP above 110), high likelihood of left heart thrombus (e.g., mitral stenosis with atrial fibrillation), acute pericarditis, subacute bacterial endocarditis, hemostatic defects (including those secondary to severe hepatic or renal disease), severe hepatic dysfunction, pregnancy or recent childbirth, diabetic hemorrhagic retinopathy, septic thrombophlebitis or occluded AV cannula at a seriously infected site, advanced age, patients currently receiving oral anticoagulants (e.g., warfarin), recent administration of GPIIb/IIIa inhibitors (e.g., abciximab [ReoPro], eptifibatide [Integrilin]), any other condition in which bleeding constitutes a significant hazard or would be particularly difficult to manage because of its location. In the presence of any of these situations, the risk versus benefit of tenecteplase therapy must be evaluated. ■ Cholesterol embolism has been reported rarely in patients treated with all types of thrombolytic agents. See Side Effects. ■ Reperfusion arrhythmias (e.g., sinus bradycardia, accelerated idioventricular rhythm, ventricular premature depolarization, ventricular tachycardia) may occur following coronary thrombolysis. Manage with standard antiarrhythmic measures. Have antiarrhythmic meds readily available. ■ Standard management of MI should be implemented concomitantly with tenecteplase therapy. Simultaneous therapy with heparin and aspirin is used to reduce the risk of rethrombosis. Increases risk of bleeding; see Usual Dose. ■ Readministration of tenecteplase to patients who have received prior plasminogen activator therapy has not been studied. Use caution if deemed necessary, and monitor for signs of allergic or anaphylactic reactions.

Monitor: Obtain appropriate clotting studies (e.g., PT, PTT, aPTT, fibrinogen levels), CBC, and platelet count. ■ Diagnosis-specific baseline studies (e.g., ECG, CPK with isoenzymes, troponin) are indicated. Baseline assessment (patient condition, pain, hematomas, petechiae, or recent wounds) should be completed before administration. ■ Type and cross-match may also be ordered. ■ Maintain strict bed rest; monitor the patient carefully and frequently for pain and signs of bleeding; observe catheter sites at least every 15 minutes and apply pressure dressings to any recently invaded site; watch for hematuria, hematemesis, bloody stool, petechiae, hematoma, flank pain, muscle weakness; and do neuro checks every hour (or more frequently if indicated). Continue until normal clotting function returns. ■ Monitor ECG continuously. ■ See Precautions and Drug/Lab Interactions.

Patient Education: Compliance with all measures to minimize bleeding (e.g., strict bed rest) is very important. ■ Avoid use of razors, toothbrushes, and other sharp items. Use caution while moving to avoid excessive bumping. ■ Report all episodes of bleeding and apply local pressure if indicated. Expect oozing from IV sites.

Maternal/Child: Category C: safety for use in pregnancy, breast-feeding and children not established.

Elderly: See Indications and Precautions. May have poorer prognosis following AMI and pre-existing conditions that may increase risk of adverse events, including bleeding. Select patients carefully to maximize benefits.

DRUG/LAB INTERACTIONS

Formal studies have not been performed. ■ Risk of bleeding may be increased by any medicine that affects blood clotting including anticoagulants (e.g., heparin, lepirudin [Refludan], warfarin [Coumadin]); glycoprotein GPIIb/IIIa inhibitors (e.g., abciximab [ReoPro], eptifibatide [Integrilin], tirofiban [Aggrastat]); any medication that may cause hypoprothrombinemia, thrombocytopenia, or GI ulceration or bleeding (e.g., selected antibiotics such as cefamandole [Mandol], cefoperazone [Cefobid], cefotetan [Cefotan], ticarcillin [Ticar], aspirin, NSAIDs [e.g., ibuprofen (Advil, Motrin), naproxen (Aleve, Naprosyn), phenylbutazone (Butazolidin)]); and/or any other medication that inhibits platelet aggregation (e.g., clopidogrel [Plavix], dipyridamole [Persantine], plicamycin [Mithracin], sulfinpyrazone [Anturane], ticlopidine [Ticlid], valproic acid [Depacon, Depakene]). Concurrent use not recommended with the exception of heparin and aspirin to reduce the risk of rethrombosis. If concurrent or subsequent use indicated (e.g., management of acute coronary syndrome, percutaneous coronary intervention) monitor PT and aPTT closely. ■ Coagulation test will be unreliable; specific procedures can be used; notify the lab of tenecteplase use.

SIDE EFFECTS

Bleeding is most common: internal (GI tract, GU tract, retroperitoneal, or intracranial), epistaxis, gingival, and superficial or surface bleeding (venous cutdowns, arterial punctures, sites of recent surgical intervention). Allergic reactions (e.g., anaphylaxis, angioedema, laryngeal edema, rash and urticaria) have been reported rarely. Fever, hypotension, nausea and vomiting, and reperfusion arrhythmias have occurred. Cholesterol embolization can occur with thrombolytic therapy, but has been reported rarely. Clinical features may include livedo reticularis, "purple toe" syndrome, acute renal failure, gangrenous digits, hypertension, pancreatitis, MI, cerebral, spinal cord or bowel infarction, retinal artery occlusion, and rhabdomyolysis. Several other adverse events have been reported. These reactions are frequently sequelae of the underlying disease, and the effect of tenecteplase on the incidence of these events is unknown.

ANTIDOTE

Notify physician of all side effects. Note even the minutest bleeding tendency. Oozing at IV sites is expected. Control minor bleeding by local pressure. For severe bleeding in a critical location or suspected intracranial bleeding, discontinue any heparin therapy immediately. Obtain PT, aPTT, platelet count, and fibrinogen. Draw blood for type and cross-match. Platelets and cryoprecipitate are most commonly used but whole blood, packed red blood cells, fresh-frozen plasma, desmopressin, tranexamic acid, or aminocaproic acid may be indicated. Topical preparations of aminocaproic acid may stop minor bleeding. Consider protamine if heparin has been used. Treat bradycardia with atropine, reperfusion arrhythmias with lidocaine, procainamide, or other standard antiarrhythmic therapy; VT or VF may require cardioversion. If hypotension occurs, vasopressors (e.g., dopamine [Intropin]), Trendelenburg position, and suitable plasma expanders (e.g., albumin, plasma protein fraction [Plasmanate], or hetastarch) may be indicated. Treat minor allergic reactions symptomatically. Discontinue drug and treat anaphylaxis as indicated; resuscitate as necessary.

TENIPOSIDE
(ten-uh-po′sid)

VM-26, Vumon

Antineoplastic (mitotic inhibitor)

pH 4 to 6.5

USUAL DOSE

Non-Hodgkin's lymphoma (unlabeled): ***Single agent:*** 30 mg/M²/day for 10 days, 30 mg/M²/day every 5 days, or 50 to 100 mg/M² once each week as a single agent. ***Combination therapy:*** 60 to 70 mg/M² once each week. Used in combination with other antineoplastic agents.

Small-cell lung cancer (unlabeled): 80 to 90 mg/M² daily for 5 days.

PEDIATRIC DOSE

Acute lymphocytic leukemia (ALL): 165 mg/M² in combination with cytarabine 300 mg/M² twice weekly for 8 to 9 doses. An alternate regimen includes 250 mg/M² in combination with vincristine 1.5 mg/M² once each week for 4 to 8 weeks plus predisone 40 mg/M² PO for 28 days.

Neuroblastoma (unlabeled): ***Single agent:*** 130 to 180 mg/M² once each week as a single agent. ***Combination therapy:*** 100 mg/M² once every 21 days. Used in combination with other antineoplastic agents.

DOSE ADJUSTMENTS

Reduce dose by one half in patients with Down syndrome and leukemia (increased sensitivity to myelosuppressive chemotherapy). Higher doses may be used in subsequent courses based on degree of myelosuppression and mucositis. Must be individualized. ▪ Reduced dose may be necessary in severe renal or hepatic impairment. ▪ Reduced dose may be indicated in combination therapy. Withhold dose if platelets less than 50,000/mm³ or absolute neutrophil count less than 500/mm³. Do not restart until adequate recovery.

DILUTION

Specific techniques required; see Precautions. Must be diluted and given as an infusion. May leach the toxic plasticizer DEHP from PVC infusion bags or sets; prepare and store in bottles (glass, polypropylene) or plastic bags (polypropylene, polyolefin) and administer through polyethylene-lined administration sets (e.g., lipid administration sets or low DEHP–containing nitroglycerin sets). Undiluted tenoposide has caused acrylic or ABS plastic devices to crack and leak; handle carefully during dilution process. Compatible with NS or D5W. Final concentration of 0.1, 0.2, 0.4, or 1 mg/ml desired. Contains 10 mg/ml. 100 mg (10 ml) in 990 ml yields 0.1 mg/ml, in 490 ml yields 0.2 mg/ml, in 240 ml yields 0.4 mg/ml, in 90 ml yields 1 mg/ml. Precipitation may occur at recommended concentrations, especially with excessive agitation. Avoid contact of diluted solution with any other drugs or fluids; flush IV line with D5W or NS before and after administration.

Storage: Refrigerate unopened ampules in original packaging. Do not refrigerate diluted solutions; 1 mg/ml should be administered within 4 hours; all other dilutions are stable at CRT for up to 24 hours.

INCOMPATIBLE WITH

Manufacturer states, "Heparin solution can cause precipitation of teniposide; flush IV line thoroughly with D5W or NS before and after administration of teniposide. Because of potential for precipitation, compatibility with other drugs, infusion materials, or IV pumps cannot be ensured." See Dilution, Rate of Administration, and Precautions/Monitor.

COMPATIBLE WITH

See Incompatible With. Consult pharmacist; specific conditions may apply; see Compatibilities, p. xvi.

Y-site: Acyclovir (Zovirax), allopurinol (Aloprim, Zyloprim), amifostine (Ethyol), amikacin (Amikin), aminophylline, amphotericin B (Fungizone), ampicillin, ampicillin/sulbactam (Unasyn), aztreonam (Azactam), bleomycin (Blenoxane), bumetanide (Bumex), buprenorphine (Buprenex), butorphanol (Stadol), calcium gluconate, carboplatin (Paraplatin), carmustine (BiCNU), cefazolin (Kefzol), cefoperazone (Cefobid), cefotaxime (Claforan), cefotetan (Cefotan), cefoxitin (Mefoxin), ceftazidime (Fortaz), ceftizoxime (Cefizox), ceftriaxone (Rocephin), cefuroxime (Zinacef), chlorpromazine (Thorazine), cimetidine (Tagamet), ciprofloxacin (Cipro IV), cisplatin (Platinol), cladribine (Leustatin), clindamycin (Cleocin), cyclophosphamide (Cytoxan), cytarabine (ARA-C), dacarbazine (DTIC), dactinomycin (Cosmegen), daunorubicin (Cerubidine), dexamethasone (Decadron), diphenhydramine (Benadryl), doxorubicin (Adriamycin), doxycycline (Vibramycin), droperidol (Inapsine), enalaprilat (Vasotec IV), etoposide (Etopophos, VePesid), famotidine (Pepcid IV), fluconazole (Diflucan), fludarabine (Fludara), fluorouracil (5-FU), furosemide (Lasix), ganciclovir (Cytovene), gemcitabine (Gemzar), gentamicin (Garamycin), granisetron (Kytril), haloperidol (Haldol), hydrocortisone (Hydrocortone, Solu-Cortef), hydromorphone (Dilaudid), ifosfamide (Ifex), imipenem-cilastatin (Primaxin), leucovorin calcium, lorazepam (Ativan), mannitol, mechlorethamine (nitrogen mustard), melphalan (Alkeran), meperidine (Demerol), mesna (Mesnex), methotrexate (Folex), methylprednisolone (Solu-Medrol), metoclopramide (Reglan), metronidazole (Flagyl IV), minocycline (Minocin), mitomycin (Mutamycin), mitoxantrone (Novantrone), morphine, nalbuphine (Nubain), ondansetron (Zofran), piperacillin (Pipracil), plicamycin (Mithracin), potassium chloride (KCl), prochlorperazine (Compazine), promethazine (Phenergan), ranitidine (Zantac), sargramostim (Leukine), sodium bicarbonate, streptozocin (Zanosar), sulfamethoxazole-trimethoprim (Bactrim), thiotepa (Thioplex), ticarcillin (Ticar), ticarcillin/clavulanate (Timentin), tobramycin (Nebcin), vancomycin (Vancocin), vinblastine (Velban), vincristine (Oncovin), vinorelbine (Navelbine), zidovudine (AZT, Retrovir).

RATE OF ADMINISTRATION

Total desired dose, properly diluted and evenly distributed over at least 30 to 60 minutes. Infusion time may be extended. Flush IV line with D5W or NS before and after administration to avoid precipitation of teniposide in IV catheter. Rapid infusion may cause marked hypotension or increased nausea and vomiting.

ACTIONS

An antineoplastic agent. A semisynthetic derivative of podophyllotoxin related to etoposide. Cell cycle–specific for the late S or early G_2 phase. Cytotoxic effects are related to the relative number of single- and double-strand DNA breaks produced in cells. Active against certain murine leukemias with acquired resistance to cisplatin, doxorubicin, amsacrine, daunorubicin, mitoxantrone, or vincristine. Highly protein bound; limits distribution within the body (a beneficial effect). Plasma levels increase with dose. Distribution half-life is approximately 1 hour, terminal half-life

5 hours. Method of metabolism is not known. Only about 10% excreted as unchanged drug in urine.

INDICATIONS AND USES

Induction therapy in refractory childhood acute lymphoblastic leukemia. Used in combination with other antineoplastic agents.

Unlabeled uses: A second-line single agent or combination therapy in neuroblastoma in patients who have not responded or who have relapsed on other regimens. ■ A second-line single agent or combination therapy in non-Hodgkin's lymphoma in patients who are refractory to other regimens. ■ Small-cell lung cancer.

CONTRAINDICATIONS

Hypersensitivity to teniposide, etoposide (no cross-sensitivity to date), or a history of prior severe hypersensitivity reactions to other drugs formulated in Cremophor EL (e.g., cyclosporine, paclitaxel).

PRECAUTIONS

Follow guidelines for handling cytotoxic agents. See Appendix A, p. 1142. ■ Usually administered by or under the direction of the physician specialist. ■ Adequate diagnostic and treatment facilities must be readily available. ■ Use caution in patients with impaired hepatic or renal function; may reduce plasma clearance and increase toxicity. ■ Incidence of hypersensitivity may be increased in patients with brain tumors or neuroblastoma. ■ Acute CNS depression and hypotension occurred in patients receiving high-dose teniposide pretreated with antiemetic drugs; use caution. ■ Children with ALL in remission on teniposide maintenance therapy have shown an increased risk of developing secondary acute nonlymphocytic leukemia (ANLL). ■ Plasma drug levels decline following IV infusion in children; in adults levels increase with dose. No cumulative toxicity has been reported.

Monitor: Use caution to prevent bone marrow depression; occurs early with indicated doses and can be profound. Obtain baseline hemoglobin, WBC count with differential, and platelet count. Monitor frequently during therapy, before each dose, and after therapy. See Dose Adjustments. ■ Severe hypersensitivity reactions can occur with the first dose of teniposide and may be life-threatening. Epinephrine, oxygen, and other emergency supplies must be at the bedside. Monitor patient continuously and take vital signs very frequently during the first hour and at intervals thereafter. ■ Monitor renal and hepatic function tests before and during therapy. ■ Determine absolute patency and quality of vein and adequate circulation of extremity. Avoid extravasation; can cause local tissue necrosis and thrombophlebitis. ■ Precipitation sufficient to occlude central venous access catheters has occurred; monitor infusion closely, and flush thoroughly before and after administration. ■ Use prophylactic antiemetics to increase patient comfort. ■ Steady-state volume of distribution increases with a decrease in plasma albumin levels; monitor children with hypoalbuminemia carefully. ■ If severe myelosuppression occurs, bone marrow examination should be repeated before a decision to continue therapy is made. ■ Monitor for thrombocytopenia (platelet count less than 50,000/mm^3). Initiate precautions to prevent excessive bleeding (e.g., inspect IV sites, skin, and mucous membranes; use extreme care during invasive procedures; test urine, emesis, stool, and secretions for occult blood). ■ Observe closely for signs of infection. Prophylactic antibiotics may be indicated pending results of C/S in a febrile neutropenic patient.

Patient Education: Report IV site burning or stinging promptly. ■ Avoid pregnancy; nonhormonal birth control recommended. ■ Report any signs of hypersensitivity promptly (e.g., chills, difficult breathing, fever, flushing, rapid heartbeat, rash). ■ Secondary acute nonlymphocytic leukemia (ANLL) has been reported (see Precautions). ■ Interacts with many medications. Discuss all drugs (prescription or nonprescription) with doctor or pharmacist. ■ See Appendix D, p. 1148.

Maternal/Child: Category D: avoid pregnancy. May cause fetal harm. ■ Potential for serious adverse reactions in nursing infants; discontinue breast-feeding. ■ Contains benzyl alcohol; not recommended for use in premature infants. ■ Intended for use in children, but see Precautions/Monitor. ■ When used as a single agent, side effects in pediatric patients from 2 weeks to 20 years of age are similar to other age-groups.

Elderly: Monitor renal, hepatic, and hematologic function closely.

DRUG/LAB INTERACTIONS

Sodium salicylate, sulfamethizole, and tolbutamide displace teniposide from protein-binding sites. Can cause substantial increases in free drug levels and increase toxicity of teniposide. ■ May result in clinically significant drug interactions with other drugs highly bound to protein (e.g., buprenorphine, calcium channel blocking agents [e.g., diltiazem, verapamil], phenothiazines [e.g., prochlorperazine (Compazine)]). ■ May increase plasma clearance and increase intracellular levels of methotrexate. ■ Phenobarbital and phenytoin (Dilantin) increase clearance of teniposide; may reduce effectiveness. ■ Depressant and hypotensive effects of antiemetics may be additive with alcohol in teniposide. ■ May cause additive effects with bone marrow-depressing agents or agents that cause blood dyscrasias (e.g., amphotericin B, antithyroid agents [Methimazole (Tapazole)], azathioprine [Imuran], chloramphenicol, ganciclovir [Cytovene], interferon, plicamycin [Mithracin], zidovudine [AZT]) and radiation therapy. ■ Do not administer live virus vaccines.

SIDE EFFECTS

Most are reversible if detected early. Hypersensitivity reactions (e.g., bronchospasm, chills, dyspnea, facial flushing, fever, hypertension, hypotension, tachycardia, urticaria) have occurred in 5% of patients and can be fatal if not treated promptly. Myelosuppression (anemia [88%], leukopenia [89%], neutropenia [95%], thrombocytopenia [85%]) occurs early, can be profound, and recovery can be delayed. Alopecia (9%), bleeding (5%), diarrhea (33%), fever (3%), hypotension/cardiovascular (2%), infection (12%), mucositis (76%), nausea and vomiting (29%), rash (3%), thrombophlebitis. Hepatic dysfunctions, metabolic abnormalities, neurotoxicity, and renal dysfunction have occurred in less than 1% of patients.

ANTIDOTE

Keep physician informed of all side effects. Symptomatic treatment is often indicated. Discontinue teniposide and treat hypersensitivity reactions immediately (epinephrine [Adrenalin], antihistamines [e.g., diphenhydramine (Benadryl)], cimetidine [Tagamet], corticosteroids [e.g., dexamethasone (Decadron)], bronchodilators [e.g., theophylline (Aminophylline)], IV fluids). Consider risk/benefit before rechallenging any patient who has had a severe hypersensitivity reaction. Pretreatment with corticosteroids and antihistamines and constant observation are imperative. For other severe side effects (e.g., myelosupression), drug dose may be reduced or it may be discontinued. Administration of whole blood products (e.g., packed RBCs, platelets, leukocytes) and/or blood modifiers (e.g., darbepoetin alfa [Aranesp], epoetin alfa [Epogen, Procrit], filgrastim [Neupogen], pegfilgrastim [Neulasta], sargramostim [Leukine], oprelvekin [Neumega]) may be indicated to treat bone marrow toxicity. Consider diazepam (Valium) or phenytoin (Dilantin) for seizures. Hypotension is usually due to a rapid infusion rate; discontinue temporarily. Trendelenburg position and IV fluids should reverse the hypotension; vasopressors (e.g., dopamine [Intropin]) may be required. In addition to antiemetics (e.g., ondansetron [Zofran]), rate reduction may reduce nausea and vomiting. For extravasation, discontinue the drug immediately and administer into another site. Consider injection of long-acting dexamethasone (Decadron LA) throughout extravasated tissue. Use a 27- or 25-gauge needle. Elevate extremity; moist heat may be helpful. Resuscitate as necessary.

THIAMINE HYDROCHLORIDE

Nutritional supplement (vitamin)

(thy′a-min hye-droe-klor′id)

Vitamin B_1 **pH 2.5 to 4.5**

USUAL DOSE

Intradermal test dose (1/100 of actual dose) recommended in suspected sensitivity. Observe for 30 minutes.

Wet beriberi with myocardial failure: 5 to 30 mg 3 times daily.

Wernicke's encephalopathy: 100 mg daily for 3 days. Up to 500 mg may be required in the first 24 hours with extreme caution.

PEDIATRIC DOSE

Infantile beriberi with myocardial failure: 10 to 25 mg/24 hr.

DILUTION

May be given by IV injection or added to most IV solutions and given as an infusion. See chart on inside back cover.

Storage: Can be refrigerated; protect from freezing and from light.

INCOMPATIBLE WITH

Manufacturer states, "Unstable in neutral or alkaline solutions. Do not use in combination with alkaline solutions (e.g., acetates, barbiturates [e.g., phenobarbital (Luminal)], carbonates, citrates, copper ions). Incompatible with solutions containing sulfites and other oxidizing and reducing agents."

COMPATIBLE WITH

Consult pharmacist; specific conditions may apply; see Compatibilities, p. xvi.

Syringe: Doxapram (Dopram).

Y-site: Famotidine (Pepcid IV).

RATE OF ADMINISTRATION

100 mg or fraction thereof over 5 minutes. For 100 mg or larger doses, equal distribution over an extended time as an infusion is preferred.

ACTIONS

A water-soluble vitamin, thiamine is necessary to most metabolic processes in humans, especially carbohydrate metabolism. Widely distributed in all body tissues, metabolized in the liver, and excreted in urine.

INDICATIONS AND USES

Prophylaxis or treatment of thiamine deficiency syndromes including beriberi (wet or dry), Wernicke's encephalopathy, or peripheral neuritis.

CONTRAINDICATIONS

Known hypersensitivity to thiamine hydrochloride.

PRECAUTIONS

Not commonly administered IV; PO or IM is preferred. ■ Rarely used alone, it is more often administered as a multiple B vitamin. ■ In thiamine deficiency, administer thiamine before giving any glucose load to prevent the sudden onset of Wernicke's encephalopathy or add 100 mg to each of the first few liters of IV fluid to avoid precipitating heart failure. ■ Requirements may be increased in certain conditions (e.g., alcoholism, burns, GI disease or malabsorption). ■ Supplementation is necessary in patients receiving total parenteral nutrition (usually administered as a multivitamin).

Patient Education: Dietary consultation indicated to prevent relapse.

Maternal/Child: Category A: use only if clearly needed. ■ Use caution in breast-feeding.

SIDE EFFECTS

Anaphylaxis and death caused by sensitivity reaction can occur with IV administration. Recent studies have shown that allergic reactions can occur with equal frequency by any route. Incidence after IV administration is less than 0.1%. May increase in frequency with repeat injections. Other reactions include feeling of warmth, nausea, pruritus, pain, sweating, urticaria, and weakness.

ANTIDOTE

Discontinue the drug, treat allergic reaction or resuscitate as necessary, and notify the physician.

THIOPENTAL SODIUM

(thi′o-pen-tal so′de-um)

Barbiturate
General anesthetic
Anticonvulsant

Pentothal Sodium

pH 10 to 11

USUAL DOSE

Administer a test dose of 25 to 75 mg. Wait at least 1 minute and assess patient reaction and sensitivity.

Convulsions: 75 to 125 mg. Up to 250 mg may be required. Use only enough medication to achieve desired effect.

Increased intracranial pressure in neurosurgical patients: 1.5 to 5 mg/kg intermittently as needed to reduce ICP.

Narcoanalysis: 100 mg/min with patient counting backward from 100. Discontinue when counting confused and before sleep.

DOSE ADJUSTMENTS

Reduce dosage and use caution in the elderly, in cardiovascular disease, hypotension, shock, medication potentiation, impaired renal or liver function, Addison's disease, myxedema, elevated blood urea, elevated intracranial pressure, asthma, severe anemia, and myasthenia gravis. ■ See Drug/Lab Interactions.

DILUTION

Each 500 mg of sterile thiopental powder must be reconstituted with at least 20 ml of SW for injection (supplied) to make a 2.5% solution. Each 1 ml equals 25 mg. The 20 ml of 2.5% solution may be further diluted to 125 to 250 ml in NS or D5W to provide a 0.2% to 0.4% solution for infusion. Solutions stronger than a 2.5% concentration will cause hemolysis. Prepared solutions also available. Use only freshly prepared, clear solutions. Discard unused portion after 24 hours.

INCOMPATIBLE WITH

Manufacturer states, "Do not mix solutions of succinylcholine, tubocurarine (Curare), or other drugs that have an acid pH with thiopental solutions."

COMPATIBLE WITH (Underline Indicates Conflicting Compatibility Information)

Consult pharmacist; specific conditions may apply; see Compatibilities, p. xvi.

Additive: Chloramphenicol (Chloromycetin), ephedrine, hydrocortisone sodium succinate (Solu-Cortef), oxytocin (Pitocin), pentobarbital (Nembutal), phenobarbital (Luminal), potassium chloride (KCl), sodium bicarbonate.

Syringe: Aminophylline, hydrocortisone sodium succinate (Solu-Cortef), neostigmine (Prostigmin), pentobarbital (Nembutal), propofol (Diprivan), scopolamine, tubocurarine (Curare).

Y-site: Cisatracurium (Nimbex), doxacurium (Nuromax), fentanyl (Sublimaze), heparin, hetastarch in electrolytes (Hextend), lorazepam (Ativan), milrinone (Primacor), mivacurium (Mivacron), morphine, nitroglycerin (Nitro-Bid IV), propofol (Diprivan), ranitidine (Zantac), remifentanil (Ultiva).

RATE OF ADMINISTRATION

Each 25 mg or fraction thereof over 1 minute. Titrate slowly to desired effect. Rapid injection rate may cause symptoms of overdose (e.g., serious respiratory depression).

ACTIONS

An ultra-short-acting barbiturate and CNS depressant that produces hypnosis and anesthesia without analgesia. Has potent anticonvulsant effects. Onset of action is prompt and lasts about 15 to 30 minutes. Rapidly distributes into all body tissues. Some is retained in fatty tissue, causing sustained or delayed effect. Excreted in changed form in the urine. Crosses the placental barrier. Secreted in breast milk.

INDICATIONS AND USES

Administration generally limited to the anesthesiologist. ■ Control of convulsive states during or after anesthesia. ■ Decrease intracranial pressure in neurosurgical patients (adequate ventilation required). ■ Narcoanalysis or narcosynthesis.

CONTRAINDICATIONS

History of porphyria, known hypersensitivity to barbiturates, status asthmaticus, suitable veins not available.

PRECAUTIONS

Usually administered by or under direct observation of a physician. One-time use is most common (e.g., anesthesia). ■ See Dose Adjustments. **Monitor:** Record vital signs every 3 to 5 minutes. Keep patient under constant observation. ■ Treat the cause of the convulsion. ■ Maintain a patent airway and have equipment for artificial ventilation available. ■ Highly alkaline; determine absolute patency of vein. Extravasation will cause necrosis and sloughing; intraarterial injection can cause gangrene. ■ See Drug/Lab Interactions.

Patient Education: Avoid alcohol or other CNS depressants (e.g., antihistamines, diazepam [Valium]) for 24 hours. ■ Possibility of psychomotor impairment for 24 hours. Use caution in any task requiring alertness.

Maternal/Child: Category C: safety for use in pregnancy not established. Benefits must outweigh risks. ■ Only small amounts appear in breast milk; delay breast-feeding. ■ May cause paradoxical excitement in children.

Elderly: See Dose Adjustments. ■ May have increased sensitivity to barbiturates; may cause marked excitement, depression, confusion, and increased risk of barbiturate-induced hypothermia. ■ Recovery of cognitive and psychomotor functions may be slower. ■ Consider reduced hepatic function.

DRUG/LAB INTERACTIONS

Use with extreme caution if any other CNS depressants have been given, such as alcohol, narcotic analgesics, anesthetics, antidepressants, antihistamines, hypnotics, MAO inhibitors, phenothiazines, sedatives, neuromuscular blocking antibiotics, or tranquilizers. Potentiation with respiratory depression and/or increased excitability may occur. ■ Anesthesia extended with probenicid; reduced dose may be indicated. ■ Anesthetic effects may be increased with sulfisoxazole. ■ Monitor phenytoin and barbiturate levels when both drugs are used concurrently. ■ A single dose may affect BSP and liver function studies.

SIDE EFFECTS

Average dose: Depression, dermatitis, facial edema, fever, hypotension, neonatal apnea, respiratory depression (hypoventilation), thrombocytopenic purpura. Anaphylactic reactions can occur.

Overdose: Apnea, cardiac arrhythmias, coma, cough reflex depression, flat EEG (reversible unless hypoxic damage has occurred), hypotension, hypothermia, laryngospasm, pulmonary edema, renal shutdown, respiratory depression, sluggish or absent reflexes.

ANTIDOTE

Call any side effect to the physician's attention. Symptomatic and supportive treatment is most important in overdosage. Keep the patient warm. IV volume expanders (dextran) and IV fluids will help maintain adequate circulation. Diuretics and ventilation will promote the elimination of the drug. Vasopressors (e.g., dopamine [Intropin]) will maintain BP. For extravasation, local injection of 1% procaine will relieve pain and promote vasodilation. Local heat application may be helpful.

THIOTEPA
(thi′o-te-pah)

Antineoplastic (alkylating agent/nitrosurea)

Thioplex, TSPA

pH 7.6

USUAL DOSE

0.3 to 0.4 mg/kg of body weight every 1 to 4 weeks. An alternate dosing regimen is 0.2 mg/kg for 4 to 5 days every 2 to 4 weeks. Maintenance dose and frequency adjusted according to blood cell counts before and after treatment. Dose based on average weight in presence of ascites or edema.

DOSE ADJUSTMENTS

Reduce dose or discontinue if WBC or platelet count falls rapidly. ■ Usually contraindicated but can be used with extreme caution and in low doses in patients with existing hepatic, renal, or bone marrow damage if benefits outweigh risks.

DILUTION

Specific techniques required; see Precautions. Each 15 mg of drug is reconstituted with 1.5 ml of SW for injection (10 mg/ml). Shake solution gently and allow to stand until clear. A hypotonic solution, it should be filtered through a 0.22-micron filter and further diluted with NS before administration. May then be given through Y-tube or three-way stopcock of a free-flowing IV infusion. Final solution should be clear; do not use if hazy, opaque, or a precipitate is present. Thioplex is a newer formulation with a longer shelf-life.

Storage: Must be refrigerated before and after reconstitution. Protect from light at all times. Use reconstituted solution within 8 hours. Use diluted solution immediately.

COMPATIBLE WITH

Consult pharmacist; specific conditions may apply; see Compatibilities, p. xvi.

Y-site: Acyclovir (Zovirax), allopurinol (Aloprim, Zyloprim), amifostine (Ethyol), amikacin (Amikin), aminophylline, amphotericin B (Fungizone), ampicillin, ampicillin/sulbactam (Unasyn), aztreonam (Azactam), bleomycin (Blenoxane), bumetanide (Bumex), buprenorphine (Buprenex), butorphanol (Stadol), calcium gluconate, carboplatin (Paraplatin), carmustine (BiCNU), cefazolin (Kefzol), cefepime (Maxipime), cefoperazone (Cefobid), cefotaxime (Claforan), cefotetan (Cefotan), cefoxitin (Mefoxin), ceftazidime (Fortaz), ceftizoxime (Cefizox), ceftriaxone (Rocephin), cefuroxime (Zinacef), chlorpromazine (Thorazine), cimetidine (Tagamet), ciprofloxacin (Cipro IV), clindamycin (Cleocin), cyclophosphamide (Cytoxan), cytarabine (ARA-C), dacarbazine (DTIC), dactinomycin (Cosmegen), daunorubicin (Cerubidine), dexamethasone (Decadron), diphenhydramine (Benadryl), dobutamine (Dobutrex), dopamine (Intropin), doxorubicin (Adriamycin), doxycycline (Vibramycin), droperidol (Inapsine), enalaprilat (Vasotec IV), etoposide (Etopophos, VePesid), famotidine (Pepcid IV), fluconazole (Diflucan), fludarabine (Fludara), fluorouracil (5-FU), furosemide (Lasix), ganciclovir (Cytovene), gemcitabine (Gemzar), gentamicin (Garamycin), granisetron (Kytril), haloperidol (Haldol), heparin, hydrocortisone (Hydrocortone, Solu-Cortef), hydromorphone (Dilaudid), idarubicin (Idamycin), ifosfamide (Ifex), imipenem-cilastatin (Primaxin), leucovorin calcium, lorazepam (Ativan), magnesium sulfate, mannitol, melphalan (Alkeran), meperidine (Demerol), mesna (Mesnex), methotrexate (Folex), methylprednisolone (Solu-Medrol), metoclopramide (Reglan), metronidazole (Flagyl IV), mitomycin (Mutamycin), mitoxantrone (Novantrone), morphine, nalbuphine (Nubain), ofloxacin (Floxin IV), ondansetron (Zofran), paclitaxel (Taxol), piperacillin (Pipracil), piperacillin/tazobactam (Zosyn), plicamycin (Mithracin), potassium chloride (KCl), prochlorperazine (Compazine), promethazine (Phenergan), ranitidine (Zantac), sodium bicarbonate, streptozocin (Zanosar), sulfamethoxazole-trimethoprim (Bactrim), teniposide (Vumon), ticarcillin (Ticar), ticarcillin/clavulanate (Timentin), tobramycin (Nebcin), vancomycin (Vancocin), vinblastine (Velban), vincristine (Oncovin), zidovudine (AZT, Retrovir).

RATE OF ADMINISTRATION

60 mg or fraction thereof over 1 minute by IV injection.

ACTIONS

An alkylating agent of the nitrosurea group with antitumor activity. Cell cycle phase–nonspecific. Thought to have a radiomimetic action, which releases ethylenimine radicals that disrupt DNA bonds and destroy actively dividing cells. Well distributed, it is metabolized in the liver and excreted as metabolites in the urine.

INDICATIONS AND USES

To suppress or retard neoplastic growth in adenocarcinomas of the breast and ovary. ■ Treatment of Hodgkin's lymphomas. ■ Also used intracavitary to treat some bladder cancers and to control intracavitary effusions (pericardial or pleural) secondary to neoplastic disease (toxicity still occurs from systemic absorption).

CONTRAINDICATIONS

Hepatic, renal, or bone marrow damage unless need is greater than the risk; known hypersensitivity to thiotepa.

PRECAUTIONS

Follow guidelines for handling cytotoxic agents. See Appendix A, p. 1142. ■ Administered by or under the direction of the physician specialist. ■ Use caution in leukopenia, thrombocytopenia, recent radiation therapy, and infection. ■ See Dose Adjustments and Side Effects.

Monitor: Daily blood cell and platelet counts are necessary during initial treatment and weekly thereafter until 3 weeks after therapy is discontinued. Very toxic to hematopoietic system. ■ Be alert for signs of bone marrow depression or infection. Use of prophylactic antibiotics may be indicated pending results of C/S in a febrile neutropenic patient. ■ May induce hyperuricemia, increased doses of antigout agents may be necessary (e.g., allopurinol, probenecid). Allopurinol preferred to reduce risk of uric acid nephropathy associated with uricosuric antigout agents. ■ Prophylactic antiemetics may increase patient comfort. ■ Monitor for thrombocytopenia (platelet count less than 50,000/mm^3). Initiate precautions to prevent excessive bleeding (e.g., inspect IV sites, skin, and mucous membranes; use extreme care during invasive procedures; test urine, emesis, stool, and secretions for occult blood). ■ See Drug/Lab Interactions.

Patient Education: Nonhormonal birth control recommended for patient and partner. ■ See Appendix D, p. 1148.

Maternal/Child: Category D: avoid pregnancy. Will produce teratogenic effects on the fetus. Has a mutagenic potential. ■ Discontinue breast-feeding. ■ Safety for use in children up to 12 years of age not established. **Elderly:** Consider possibility of impaired organ function.

DRUG/LAB INTERACTIONS

May cause irreversible bone marrow damage with other antineoplastic drugs, radiation therapy, or any drugs that cause bone marrow depression (e.g., amphotericin B [all formulations], ganciclovir [Cytovene]). Allow complete recovery verified by WBC count before using a second agent. ■ Potentiates succinylcholine. May cause prolonged apnea. ■ Do not administer live virus vaccines to patients receiving antineoplastic drugs.

SIDE EFFECTS

Amenorrhea, anorexia, dizziness, fever, headache, hives, hyperuricemia, nausea, pain at injection site, skin rash, throat tightness, vomiting.
Major: Anaphylaxis, hemorrhage, intestinal perforation, septicemia. Bone marrow depression (anemia, leukopenia, thrombocytopenia) may be life threatening, is dose related, and does occur with usual doses.

ANTIDOTE

Minor side effects will be treated symptomatically if necessary. Discontinue the drug and notify the physician of major side effects. If platelet count below 150,000/mm^3 or WBCs below 3,000/mm^3, discontinue use and notify physician. Administration of whole blood products (e.g., packed RBCs, platelets, or leukocytes) and/or blood modifiers (e.g., darbepoetin alfa [Aranesp], epoetin alfa [Epogen, Procrit], filgrastim [Neupogen], pegfilgrastim [Neulasta], sargramostim [Leukine], oprelvekin [Neumega]) may be indicated to treat bone marrow toxicity. Treat allergic reaction as indicated.

TICARCILLIN DISODIUM

(tye-kar-sill'in di-so'de-um)

Ticar

Antibacterial (extended-spectrum penicillin)

pH 6 to 8

USUAL DOSE

150 to 300 mg/kg of body weight/24 hr in divided doses every 3, 4, or 6 hours (18.75 to 37.5 mg/kg every 3 hours, 25 to 50 mg/kg every 4 hours, or 37.5 to 75 mg/kg every 6 hours). All doses vary depending on the severity of the infection. Maximum dose is 24 Gm/24 hr.

PEDIATRIC DOSE

Under 40 kg (88 lb): 50 to 300 mg/kg of body weight/24 hr in divided doses every 4, 6, or 8 hours (8.3 to 50 mg/kg every 4 hours, 12.5 to 75 mg/kg every 6 hours, or 16.67 to 100 mg/kg every 8 hours). Do not exceed adult dose.

Cystic fibrosis: 300 to 600 mg/kg/24 hr equally divided and given every 4 to 6 hours (50 to 100 mg/kg every 4 hours or 75 to 150 mg/kg every 6 hours). Maximum dose is 24 Gm/24 hr.

NEONATAL DOSE

Under 1,200 Gm; age up to 4 weeks: 75 mg/kg of body weight every 12 hours.
Under 2,000 Gm; age up to 7 days: 75 mg/kg every 12 hours. **Over 7 days of age:** 75 mg/kg every 8 hours.

Over 2,000 Gm; age up to 7 days: 75 mg/kg every 8 hours. **Over 7 days of age:** 75 mg/kg every 6 hours.

DOSE ADJUSTMENTS

Reduce daily dose commensurate with amount of renal or hepatic impairment. Intervals between injections should also be increased.

DILUTION

Each 1 Gm or fraction thereof is reconstituted with 4 ml of SW for injection. Further dilution of each gram with an additional 20 to 50 ml or more of SW for injection, D5W, NS, or sodium lactate ⅙ M is required for IV injection or intermittent piggyback infusion to decrease vein irritation. May be added to larger volumes and given as a continuous infusion.

Storage: Stable at room temperature for at least 48 hours.

INCOMPATIBLE WITH

Inactivated in solution with aminoglycosides (e.g., amikacin [Amikin], gentamicin [Garamycin]). Do not mix in the same solution. Appropriate spacing and/or separate sites required. See Drug/Lab Interactions.

COMPATIBLE WITH

(Underline Indicates Conflicting Compatibility Information)

Consult pharmacist; specific conditions may apply; see Compatibilities, p. xvi.

Additive: Ranitidine (Zantac), verapamil (Isoptin).

Y-site: Acyclovir (Zovirax), aldesleukin (Proleukin, IL-2), allopurinol (Aloprim, Zyloprim), amifostine (Ethyol), aztreonam (Azactam), cisatracurium (Nimbex), cyclophosphamide (Cytoxan), diltiazem (Cardizem), docetaxel (Taxotere), doxorubicin liposome (Doxil), etoposide phosphate (Etopophos), famotidine (Pepcid IV), filgrastim (Neupogen), fludarabine (Fludara), gatifloxacin (Tequin), gemcitabine (Gemzar), granisetron (Kytril), heparin, hetastarch in electrolytes (Hextend), hydromorphone (Dilaudid), insulin (regular), linezolid (Zyvox), magnesium sulfate, melphalan (Alkeran), meperidine (Demerol), morphine, ondansetron (Zofran), perphenazine (Trilafon), propofol (Diprivan), remifentanil (Ultiva), sargramostim (Leukine), teniposide (Vumon), theophylline, thiotepa (Thioplex), vancomycin (Vancocin), verapamil (Isoptin), vinorelbine (Navelbine).

RATE OF ADMINISTRATION

Too-rapid injection may cause seizures. Slow infusion rate for pain along venipuncture site.

IV injection: 1 Gm or fraction thereof over 5 minutes or more to reduce vein irritation.

Intermittent infusion: A single dose over 30 minutes to 2 hours. In neonate give over 10 to 20 minutes.

Continuous infusion: At specified rate not to exceed rate and concentration of intermittent infusion.

ACTIONS

An extended-spectrum penicillin. Bactericidal for many gram-negative, gram-positive, and anaerobic organisms. Large doses with high blood levels are well tolerated. Distributes into cerebrospinal fluid only if inflammation is present. Crosses the placental barrier. Excreted in the urine. Secreted in breast milk.

INDICATIONS AND USES

Bacterial septicemia; acute and chronic infections of the respiratory tract, skin and soft tissue, intraabdominal area, female pelvis, genital tract, and urinary tract. ■ Useful in infections complicated by impaired renal functions or in patients receiving immunosuppressive or oncolytic drugs.

CONTRAINDICATIONS

Known penicillin or cephalosporin sensitivity (not absolute).

PRECAUTIONS

Sensitivity studies indicated to determine susceptibility of the causative organism to ticarcillin. ■ Superinfection caused by overgrowth of nonsusceptible organisms can occur. ■ Incidence of side effects increased in patients with cystic fibrosis. ■ Continue for at least 2 days after symptoms of infection have disappeared. ■ Pseudomembranous colitis has been reported. May range from mild to life-threatening. Consider in patients that present with diarrhea during or after treatment with ticarcillin.

Monitor: Periodic evaluation of renal, hepatic, hematopoietic systems and serum potassium is recommended in prolonged therapy. Observe for hypokalemia and increased bleeding tendencies. ■ Observe for electrolyte imbalance and cardiac irregularities. Contains 4.7 to 5 mEq sodium/Gm. May aggravate CHF. ■ May cause thrombophlebitis; observe carefully and rotate infusion sites. ■ Test patients with syphilis for HIV. ■ See Drug/Lab Interactions.

Patient Education: May require alternate birth control.

Maternal/Child: Category B: use only if clearly needed. ■ May cause diarrhea, candidiasis, or allergic response in nursing infants. ■ Elimination rate markedly reduced in neonates.

Elderly: No problems documented. Age-related decrease in renal or hepatic function may require decrease in dose.

DRUG/LAB INTERACTIONS

Probenecid decreases rate of ticarcillin elimination resulting in higher and more prolonged blood levels. May be desirable or may cause toxicity. ■ Synergistic when used in combination with aminoglycosides (e.g., amikacin [Amikin], gentamicin [Garamycin]). Synergism may be inconsistent; see Incompatible With. ■ May be antagonized by bacteriostatic antibiotics (e.g., chloramphenicol, erythromycin, and tetracyclines); may interfere with bactericidal action. ■ Concomitant use with beta-adrenergic blockers (e.g., propranolol [Inderal]) may increase risk of anaphylaxis and inhibit treatment. ■ May increase risk of bleeding; monitoring of coagulation tests may be indicated. Use caution with anticoagulants (e.g., heparin). ■ May inhibit effectiveness or oral contraceptives; breakthrough bleeding or pregnancy could result. ■ Monitoring of serum lithium indicated with concurrent use. Sodium may alter renal excretion. ■ May decrease clearance and increase toxicity of methotrexate. ■ May cause false urine protein reactions with various tests. See Side Effects and/or literature.

SIDE EFFECTS

Abnormal clotting time or PT, anaphylaxis, anemia, convulsions, elevated SrCr, alkaline phosphatase, LDH, serum bilirubin, AST (SGOT) and ALT (SGPT), eosinophilia, fever, hypokalemia, leukopenia, nausea, neutropenia, phlebitis, pruritus, pseudomembranous colitis, skin rash, thrombocytopenia, urticaria, vomiting. Hypersensitivity myocarditis can occur (fever, eosinophilia, rash, sinus tachycardia, ST-T changes and cardiomegaly). Higher than normal doses may cause neurologic adverse reactions, including convulsions, especially with impaired renal function.

ANTIDOTE

Notify the physician immediately of any adverse symptoms. For severe symptoms, discontinue the drug, treat allergic reaction (epinephrine, antihistamines, corticosteroids), and resuscitate as necessary. Hemodialysis is effective in overdose.

TICARCILLIN DISODIUM AND CLAVULANATE POTASSIUM

(tye-kar-sill′in dye-so′de-um and klav-you-lan′ate poe-tass′ee-um)

Timentin

Antibacterial (extended-spectrum penicillin and beta-lactamase inhibitor)

pH 5.5 to 7.5

USUAL DOSE

3.1 Gm of preparation available contains 3 Gm ticarcillin to 0.1 Gm clavulanate. Doses vary depending on the severity of the infection, susceptibility of the organism, and condition of the patient. Treatment usually continued for 10 to 14 days; may be extended if required.

Over 60 kg (130 lb): 3.1 Gm every 4 to 6 hours.

Under 60 kg: 200 to 300 mg/kg of body weight/24 hr in equally divided doses every 4 to 6 hours (33.3 to 50 mg/kg every 4 hours or 50 to 75 mg/kg every 6 hours).

Surgical prophylaxis (unlabeled): 3.1 Gm 30 to 60 minutes before start of surgery or as soon as the umbilical cord is clamped in cesarean section. Repeat at 4-hour intervals for 3 doses.

PEDIATRIC DOSE

Infants and children 3 months to 12 years of age and less than 60 kg: 50 mg/kg every 6 hours. Base dose on the ticarcillin component. In serious infections, increase to 50 mg/kg every 4 hours. See Contraindications.

Children with cystic fibrosis: 350 to 450 mg ticarcillin and 11.7 to 17 mg clavulanate/kg/24 hr. Give in equally divided doses every 4 to 6 hours (58.3 to 75 mg/kg every 4 hours or 87.5 to 112.5 mg/kg every 6 hours).

NEONATAL DOSE

Safety for use in infants under 3 months of age not established but has been used. Base dose on ticarcillin component. See Contraindications.

Under 1,200 Gm; age up to 4 weeks: 75 mg/kg of body weight every 12 hours.

Under 2,000 Gm; age up to 7 days: 75 mg/kg every 12 hours. **Over 7 days of age:** 75 mg/kg every 8 hours.

Over 2,000 Gm; age up to 7 days: 75 mg/kg every 8 hours. **Over 7 days of age:** 75 mg/kg every 6 hours.

DOSE ADJUSTMENTS

Reduce dose in impaired renal function according to the chart below.

Ticarcillin/Clavulanate Dose in Impaired Renal Function

Creatinine Clearance (mL/min)	Dosage
>60	3.1 Gm q 4 hr
30-60	2 Gm q 4 hr
10-30	2 Gm q 8 hr
<10	2 Gm q 12 hr
<10 with hepatic dysfunction	2 Gm q 24 hr
Patients on peritoneal dialysis	3.1 Gm q 12 hr
Patients on hemodialysis	2 Gm q 12 hr supplemented with 3.1 Gm after each dialysis

■ Reduce dose in impaired hepatic function. ■ Reduced dose may be indicated in the elderly.

DILUTION

Each 3.1 Gm or fraction thereof is reconstituted with 13 ml of SW or NS (200 mg/ml). Shake well. A single dose must be further diluted in 50 to 100 ml or more of D5W, NS, or LR and given as an intermittent infusion. Also available prediluted and frozen and in ADD-Vantage vials for use with ADD-Vantage infusion containers.

Storage: Stable at room temperature for at least 6 hours or for 72 hours under refrigeration. Stability extended after further dilution (see literature).

INCOMPATIBLE WITH

May be inactivated in solution with aminoglycosides (e.g., amikacin [Amikin], gentamicin [Garamycin]). Do not mix in the same solution. Appropriate spacing and/or separate sites required. See Drug/Lab Interactions. Manufacturer lists as incompatible with sodium bicarbonate.

COMPATIBLE WITH **(Underline Indicates Conflicting Compatibility Information)**

Consult pharmacist; specific conditions may apply; see Compatibilities, p. xvi.

Y-site: Allopurinol (Aloprim, Zyloprim), amifostine (Ethyol), aztreonam (Azactam), cefepime (Maxipime), <u>cisatracurium (Nimbex)</u>, cyclophosphamide (Cytoxan), diltiazem (Cardizem), docetaxel (Taxotere), doxorubicin liposome (Doxil), etoposide phosphate (Etopophos), famotidine (Pepcid IV), filgrastim (Neupogen), fluconazole (Diflucan), fludarabine (Fludara), foscarnet (Foscavir), gatifloxacin (Tequin), gemcitabine (Gemzar), granisetron (Kytril), heparin, hetastarch in electrolytes (Hextend), insulin (regular), melphalan (Alkeran), meperidine (Demerol), morphine, ondansetron (Zofran), perphenazine (Trilafon), propofol (Diprivan), remifentanil (Ultiva), sargramostim (Leukine), teniposide (Vumon), theophylline, thiotepa (Thioplex), topotecan (Hycamtin), vancomycin (Vancocin), vinorelbine (Navelbine).

RATE OF ADMINISTRATION

Intermittent infusion: A single dose over 30 minutes. May be given through Y-tube or three-way stopcock of infusion set. Discontinue primary IV during administration. Too-rapid injection may cause seizures. Slow infusion rate for pain along venipuncture site.

ACTIONS

An extended-spectrum penicillin. Bactericidal for many gram-negative, gram-positive, and anaerobic organisms. This specific formulation extends activity by protecting ticarcillin from degradation by beta-lactamase enzymes. Large doses with high blood levels are well tolerated. Widely distributed in all body fluids and tissues. Distributes into cerebrospinal fluid only if inflammation is present. Peak serum levels achieved by end of infusion. Crosses the placental barrier. Excreted in the urine. Secreted in breast milk.

INDICATIONS AND USES

Bacterial septicemia, acute and chronic infections of the respiratory tract, skin and skin structure, bone and joint, endometrium, and urinary tract caused by beta-lactamase–producing organisms. Useful in infections complicated by impaired renal functions or in patients receiving immunosuppressive or oncolytic drugs.

Unlabeled use: Surgical prophylaxis.

CONTRAINDICATIONS

Known sensitivity to penicillins, cephalosporins, or beta-lactamase inhibitors (not absolute). ▪ Not recommended in infants and children under 16 years of age for the treatment of septicemia or infections where the suspected or proven pathogen is *Haemophilus influenzae* type B.

PRECAUTIONS

Specific process sensitivity studies indicated to determine susceptibility of the causative organism to ticarcillin and clavulanate. ▪ Superinfection caused by overgrowth of nonsusceptible organisms can occur. ▪ Use caution in patients with CHF or those with a history of bleeding disorders or GI disease (e.g., colitis). ▪ Incidence of side effects increased in patients with cystic fibrosis. ▪ Continue for at least 2 days after signs and symptoms of infection have disappeared. ▪ Pseudomembranous colitis has been reported. May range from mild to life-threatening. Consider in patients that present with diarrhea during or after treatment with ticarcillin/clavulanate.

Monitor: Periodic evaluation of renal, hepatic, and hematopoietic systems and serum potassium is recommended in prolonged therapy. Observe for electrolyte imbalance and cardiac irregularities. Observe for hypokalemia. Contains 4.75 mEq sodium/Gm. May aggravate CHF. ▪ Observe for increased bleeding tendencies in all patients but especially those with impaired renal function. ▪ May cause thrombophlebitis; observe carefully and rotate infusion sites. ■ Test patients with syphilis for HIV. ■ See Drug/Lab Interactions.

Patient Education: Report promptly: fever, rash, sore throat, unusual bleeding or bruising, severe stomach cramps and/or diarrhea, seizures. ■ May require alternate birth control.

Maternal/Child: Category B: use only if clearly needed. Studies in rats have not shown adverse effects on the fetus. ■ May cause diarrhea, candidiasis, or allergic response in nursing infants. ■ Has been used in infants under 3 months of age but safety for use not established.

Elderly: No problems documented; age-related decrease in renal or hepatic function may require decreased dose.

DRUG/LAB INTERACTIONS

Probenecid decreases rate of ticarcillin elimination, resulting in higher and more prolonged blood levels of ticarcillin; will not affect clavulanate levels. May be desirable or may cause toxicity. ■ Synergistic when used in combination with aminoglycosides (e.g., amikacin [Amikin], gentamicin [Garamycin]). Synergism may be inconsistent; see Incompatible With. ■ May be antagonized by bacteriostatic antibiotics (e.g., chloramphenicol, erythromycin, tetracyclines); may interfere with bactericidal action. ■ Concomitant use with beta-adrenergic blockers (e.g., propranolol [Inderal]) may increase risk of anaphylaxis and inhibit treatment. ■ Use caution with anticoagulants (e.g., heparin), thrombolytic agents (e.g., alteplase [tPA], anistreplase [Eminase]), platelet aggregation inhibitors (e.g., aspirin, NSAIDs, dextran, dipyridamole, plicamycin). Risk of bleeding may be increased. Monitoring of coagulation tests may be indicated. Concurrent use with thrombolytic agents is not recommended; may increase risk of severe hemorrhage. ■ May inhibit effectiveness of oral contraceptives; breakthrough bleeding or pregnancy could result. ■ Monitoring of serum lithium indicated with concurrent use; increased sodium may alter renal excretion. ■ May decrease clearance and increase toxicity of methotrexate. ■ Clavulanic acid may cause a false-positive Coombs' test. ■ May cause false urine protein reactions with various tests; see Side Effects and/or literature.

SIDE EFFECTS

Anaphylaxis; anemia; arthralgia; chest discomfort; chills; convulsions; diarrhea; disturbances of taste and smell; elevated alkaline phosphatase, BUN, LDH, serum bilirubin, AST (SGOT), and ALT (SGPT); eosinophilia; fever; flatulence; epigastric pain; headache; hypernatremia; hypokalemia; increased bleeding time; leukopenia; myalgia; nausea; neutropenia; phlebitis; prolonged clotting time or PT; pruritus; pseudomembranous colitis; skin rash; stomatitis; thrombocytopenia; urticaria; vomiting. Hypersensitivity myocarditis can occur (fever, eosinophilia, rash, sinus tachycardia, ST-T changes, and cardiomegaly). Higher than normal doses may cause neurologic adverse reactions including convulsions; especially with impaired renal function.

ANTIDOTE

Notify the physician immediately of any adverse symptoms. For severe symptoms, discontinue the drug; treat allergic reaction (epinephrine, antihistamines, corticosteroids), and resuscitate as necessary. Hemodialysis may be indicated in overdose.

TIROFIBAN HYDROCHLORIDE

Platelet aggregation inhibitor

(tye-roe-fye'ban hye-droe-klor'id)

Aggrastat

pH 5.5 to 6.5

USUAL DOSE

Tirofiban: A ***loading infusion*** of 0.4 mcg/kg/min for 30 minutes, followed by a ***maintenance infusion*** of 0.1 mcg/kg/min. Unless contraindicated, give in conjunction with ***aspirin*** and ***heparin.***

Aspirin: 325 mg/day.

Heparin: Administer a heparin bolus of 5,000 units, followed by an infusion titrated to maintain an aPTT of 2 times control. Heparin and tirofiban may be administered through the same intravenous catheter. Duration of therapy will vary depending on patient condition and procedures performed. In one major study, infusion was continued for 48 to 108 hours. The infusion should be continued through angiography and for 12 to 24 hours after angioplasty or arthrectomy.

DOSE ADJUSTMENTS

Patients with severe renal insufficiency (CrCl less than 30 ml/min) should receive half the usual rate of infusion. See Rate of Administration. ■ Differences in plasma clearance based on age, race, gender, or mild to moderate hepatic insufficiency do not require dose adjustment.

DILUTION

Available premixed in a plastic container in a 50 mcg/ml concentration (5 mg/100 ml or 12.5 mg/250 ml). Remove overwrap. Plastic may be somewhat opaque due to sterilization process. Opacity should diminish. Squeeze inner container to check for leak. Discard if leakage noted; sterility is impaired. Also available in vials containing 6.25 mg/25 ml or 12.5 mg/50 ml (both equal a 250 mcg/ml concentration). Vials must be diluted to the same concentration as a premixed solution before administration (50 mcg/ml). Manufacturer suggests three methods for dilution. One is to withdraw 100 ml from a 500-ml bag of NS or D5W and replace this volume with 100 ml of tirofiban (four 25-ml vials or two 50-ml vials). A second choice is to withdraw 50 ml from a 250-ml bag of NS or D5W and replace this volume with 50 ml of tirofiban (two 25-ml vials or one 50-ml vial). A third choice is to add the contents of one 25-ml vial to 100 ml of NS or D5W. Mix well. Concentration of all three of these solutions is 50 mcg/ml. Do not use plastic containers in a series connection.

Storage: Store unopened or premixed containers at 25° C (77° F). Variations from 15° to 30° C (59° to 86° F) are acceptable for short periods. Protect from light during storage. Do not freeze. Discard unused solution.

INCOMPATIBLE WITH

Manufacturer states, "Do not add other drugs or remove solution directly from the bag with a syringe. Should not be administered in the same IV line as diazepam (Valium).

COMPATIBLE WITH

Manufacturer indicates compatibility at the **Y-site** with atropine, dobutamine (Dobutrex), dopamine (Intropin), epinephrine (Adrenalin), famotidine (Pepcid IV), furosemide (Lasix), lidocaine, midazolam (Versed), morphine, nitroglycerin (Nitro-Bid IV), potassium chloride, propranolol (Inderal). Another source adds heparin.

RATE OF ADMINISTRATION

Loading infusion: 0.4 mcg/kg/min for 30 minutes.
Maintenance infusion: 0.1 mcg/kg/min.

Tirofiban Infusion Rates				
	Most Patients		Severe Renal Impairment	
Patient Weight (kg)	30-Min Loading Infusion Rate (ml/hr)	Maintenance Infusion Rate (ml/hr)	30-Min Loading Infusion Rate (ml/hr)	Maintenance Infusion Rate (ml/hr)
30-37	16	4	8	2
38-45	20	5	10	3
46-54	24	6	12	3
55-62	28	7	14	4
63-70	32	8	16	4
71-79	36	9	18	5
80-87	40	10	20	5
88-95	44	11	22	6
96-104	48	12	24	6
105-112	52	13	26	7
113-120	56	14	28	7
121-128	60	15	30	8
129-137	64	16	32	8
138-145	68	17	34	9
146-153	72	18	36	9

ACTIONS

A non-peptide antagonist of the platelet glycoprotein GPIIb/IIIa receptor. It inhibits platelet aggregation by preventing the binding of fibrinogen to the receptor site on activated platelets. Inhibits platelet aggregation in a dose- and concentration-dependent manner. When given according to the recommended regimen, greater than 90% inhibition is attained by the end of the 30-minute infusion. Bleeding time is prolonged. Inhibition is reversible, with aggregation returning to baseline in more than 90% of patients within 4 to 8 hours following cessation of the infusion. Has been shown to decrease the rate of a combined endpoint of death, new myocardial infarction, or refractory ischemia/repeat cardiac procedure (see literature). Half-life is approximately 2 hours. Cleared from the plasma primarily by renal excretion, with about 65% of the unchanged drug appearing in the urine and about 25% appearing in feces. Metabolism is limited.

INDICATIONS AND USES

Used in combination with heparin and aspirin for the prevention of acute cardiac ischemic complications in patients with acute coronary syndrome (characterized by prolonged [more than 10 minutes] or repetitive symptoms of cardiac ischemia occurring at rest or with minimal exertion, associated with either ischemic ST-T wave changes on electrocardiogram [ECG] or elevated cardiac enzymes. Includes "unstable angina" and "non–Q-wave myocardial infarction" but excludes myocardial infarction that is associated with Q-waves or nontransient ST-segment elevation). May be used in patients who are being medically managed and in those undergoing percutaneous coronary intervention (PCI) or arthrectomy.

CONTRAINDICATIONS

Known hypersensitivity to any component of the product; active internal bleeding or history of bleeding diathesis within the previous 30 days (a second source indicates within the previous year); a history of intracranial hemorrhage, intracranial neoplasm, arteriovenous malformation, or aneurysm; a history of thrombocytopenia following prior exposure to tirofiban; a history of stroke within 30 days or any history of hemorrhagic stroke, major surgical procedure or severe physical trauma within the previous month; history, symptoms, or findings suggestive of aortic dissection; severe hypertension (systolic BP above 180 mm Hg and/or diastolic BP above 110 mm Hg); concomitant use of another parenteral GPIIb/IIIa inhibitor (e.g., abciximab [ReoPro]); acute pericarditis; liver disease.

PRECAUTIONS

Use with caution in patients with platelet count less than 150,000/mm^3, in patients with hemorrhagic retinopathy, and in patients with a history of cerebrovascular disease. ■ Use caution when given with drugs that affect hemostasis (e.g., warfarin [Coumadin]). Safety when used in combination with thrombolytic agents (e.g., alteplase [tPA, Activase], reteplase [Retavase], urokinase [Abbokinase], streptokinase [Streptase]) has not been established. See Drug/Lab Interactions. ■ Use with caution in patients with renal insufficiency. See Dose Adjustments. ■ Bleeding is the most common complication encountered during therapy. Incidence may be slightly higher in females and the elderly. ■ Most major bleeding occurs at the arterial access site for cardiac catheterization. Care should be taken when attempting vascular access that only the anterior wall of the femoral artery is punctured.

Monitor: Obtain platelet count, hemoglobin, and hematocrit before therapy, within 6 hours following the loading infusion, and at least daily thereafter. More frequent monitoring may be indicated. ■ If platelet count drops to below 90,000/mm^3, additional platelet counts should be performed to exclude pseudothrombocytopenia. If thrombocytopenia is confirmed, heparin and tirofiban should be discontinued and appropriate therapy initiated. ■ Obtain an aPTT 6 hours after the start of the heparin infusion. Adjust heparin infusion rate to maintain an aPTT 2 times control. ■ Patients receiving percutaneous coronary intervention who have a sheath in place should be maintained on complete bed rest with the head of the bed elevated 30 degrees and the affected limb restrained in a straight position. Monitor sheath insertion site(s) and distal pulses of affected leg(s) frequently while sheath is in place and for 6 hours after removal. Measure any hematoma and monitor for enlargement. ■ Monitor the patient for signs of bleeding; take vital signs (avoiding automatic BP cuffs), observe any invaded sites at least every 15 minutes (e.g., sheaths, IV sites, cutdowns, punctures, Foleys, NGs); watch for hematuria, hematemesis, bloody stool, petechiae, hematoma, flank pain, muscle weakness. Perform neuro checks frequently. If during therapy bleeding cannot be controlled with pressure, tirofiban and heparin infusions should be discontinued. ▪ Use care in handling patient; minimize use of urinary catheters, nasotracheal intubation, and nasogastric tubes. Avoid arterial puncture, venipuncture, epidural procedures, and IM injection. Use extreme precautionary methods and only compressible sites if these procedures are absolutely necessary (i.e., avoid subclavian or jugular veins). Apply pressure for 30 minutes to any invaded site and then apply pressure dressings. Saline or heparin locks suggested to facilitate blood draws. ▪ In patients receiving percutaneous coronary intervention, heparin should be discontinued 3 to 4 hours before pulling the sheath and an activated clotting time (ACT) less than 180 seconds or an aPTT less than 45 seconds should be documented. ▪ Care should be taken to obtain proper hemostasis after removal of the sheath using standard compressive techniques followed by close observation. Sheath hemostasis should be achieved at least 4 hours before hospital discharge.

Patient Education: Compliance with all measures to minimize bleeding (e.g., strict bed rest, positioning) is imperative. ▪ Avoid use of razors, toothbrushes, and other sharp items. ▪ Use caution while moving to avoid excessive bumping. ▪ Report all episodes of bleeding and apply local pressure if indicated. ▪ Expect oozing from IV sites.

Maternal/Child: Category B: safety for use in pregnancy not established. Benefits must outweigh risks. ▪ Discontinue breast-feeding until 24 hours after completion of tirofiban therapy. ▪ Safety and efficacy have not been established for children.

Elderly: Clearance is reduced in the elderly, possibly due to age-related renal impairment. Dose adjustment is not necessary unless renal impairment severe; see Dose Adjustments. Incidence of bleeding complications increase somewhat but are similar to use of heparin as a single agent. Incidence of non-bleeding side effects also increased.

DRUG/LAB INTERACTIONS

All studies with tirofiban included the use of aspirin and heparin. Concomitant use, although indicated, increases the risk of bleeding. ▪ Use caution when given with drugs that affect hemostasis (e.g., thrombolytics [e.g., alteplase (tPA, Activase), reteplase (Retavase), urokinase (Abbokinase), streptokinase (Streptase)], oral anticoagulants [e.g., warfarin (Coumadin)], NSAIDs [e.g., ibuprofen (Advil, Motrin), naproxen (Aleve, Naprosyn)], dipyridamole [Persantine], ticlopidine [Ticlid], selected antibiotics [e.g., cefamandole (Mandol), cefoperazone (Cefobid)]). ▪ Patients receiving omeprazole (Prilosec) or levothyroxine (Synthroid) concurrently with tirofiban had a higher clearance of tirofiban. Clinical significance of this observation is not known. ▪ The following drugs were coadministered with tirofiban in clinical trials: acebutolol (Monitan), acetaminophen (Tylenol), alprazolam (Xanax), amlodipine, aspirin, atenolol (Tenormin), bromazepam, captopril (Capoten), diazepam (Valium), digoxin, diltiazem (Cardizem), docusate sodium, enalapril (Vasotec), furosemide (Lasix), glyburide, heparin, insulin, isosorbide, lorazepam (Ativan), lovastatin (Mevacor), metoclopramide (Reglan), metoprolol (Lopressor), morphine, nifedipine (Procardia), nitrate preparations (e.g., nitroglycerin), oxazepam (Serax), potassium chloride, propranolol (Inderal), ranitidine (Zantac), simvastatin (Zocor), sucralfate (Sulcrate), and temazepam (Restoril). Plasma clearance of tirofiban was not affected by co-administration.

SIDE EFFECTS

Bleeding is the most frequent adverse event and is usually reported as mild oozing. In post-marketing experience, intracranial bleeding, retroperitoneal bleeding, spinal-epidural hematoma, and hemopericardium have been reported. Laboratory findings related to bleeding include decrease in hemoglobin, hematocrit, and platelet count and occult blood in urine and feces. Decreased platelet count may be associated with chills and fever. In post-marketing experience, acute decreases in platelet counts have been reported. Other side effects that occur at an incidence of greater than 1%, regardless of drug relationship, are bradycardia, dissection of the coronary artery, dizziness, edema, fever, headache, hypersensitivity reactions (e.g., hives, rash), leg pain, nausea, pelvic pain, sweating, thrombocytopenia, and vasovagal reflex.

ANTIDOTE

Keep physician informed of laboratory values and side effects. Discontinue the infusion of tirofiban and heparin if any serious bleeding not controllable with pressure occurs. If platelet count drops to below 90,000 mm^3, obtain additional platelet counts to exclude pseudothrombocytopenia. If thrombocytopenia is confirmed, discontinue tirofiban and heparin. Platelet transfusion may be required. If a hypersensitivity reaction should occur, discontinue the infusion and treat as indicated by severity (e.g., epinephrine, dopamine [Intropin], theophylline, antihistamines [e.g., diphenhydramine (Benadryl)], and/or corticosteroids as necessary).

No specific antidote is available. Overdosage should be treated by assessment of the patient's clinical condition and cessation or adjustment of the drug infusion as appropriate. Hemodialysis may be useful in an overdose situation.

TOBRAMYCIN SULFATE

(toe-bra-mye'sin sul'fat)

Nebcin

Antibacterial (aminoglycoside)

pH 3 to 6.5

USUAL DOSE

3 mg/kg of body weight/24 hr equally divided into 3 doses and given every 8 hours (1 mg/kg every 8 hours). Up to 5 mg/kg equally divided into 3 or 4 doses may be given in life-threatening infections (1.25 mg/kg every 6 hours or 1.67 mg/kg every 8 hours). Reduce to usual dose as soon as feasible. Dose based on lean body weight plus 40% for obese patients. Do not exceed 5 mg/kg/day unless serum levels are monitored.

Recent studies suggest that a single daily dose of 5 to 7 mg/kg (instead of divided into 2 to 3 doses) may provide higher peak levels and enhance drug effectiveness while actually reducing or having no adverse effects on risk of toxicity. Various procedures for monitoring blood levels are in use. Some health facilities are monitoring with trough levels; others may draw levels at predetermined times and plot the concentration on nomograms. Depending on the protocol in place, doses or intervals may be adjusted. See Precautions.

Patients with cystic fibrosis: 5 to 7.5 mg/kg/24 hr equally divided into 3 doses and given every 8 hours for 7 to 21 days (1.67 to 2.5 mg/kg every 8 hours).

PEDIATRIC DOSE

In pediatric and neonatal patients, monitor serum levels. Wide interpatient variability; see Monitor.

Over 1 week of age: 6 to 7.5 mg/kg of body weight/24 hr in 3 or 4 equally divided doses (1.5 to 1.89 mg/kg every 6 hours or 2 to 2.5 mg/kg every 8 hours). Another source suggests the same as adult dose.

A single daily dose is also being used in children. See comments under Usual Dose.

Severe cystic fibrosis: 10 mg/kg/day in equally divided doses every 6 hours (2.5 mg/kg every 6 hours).

NEONATAL DOSE

1 week of age or less: Up to 4 mg/kg of body weight/24 hr in two equal doses every 12 hours (up to 2 mg/kg every 12 hours). Lower doses may be safer because of immature kidney function. 2.5 mg/kg every 18 hours or 3 mg/kg every 24 hours may provide acceptable peak and trough levels in neonates weighing less than 2,000 Gm.

DOSE ADJUSTMENTS

Reduce daily dose commensurate with amount of renal impairment and/or increase intervals between injections. Measurement of serum concentrations following a loading dose of 1 mg/kg is suggested. Adjust dose accordingly. ■ Reduced doses or extended intervals may be required in the elderly. ■ See Drug/Lab Interactions.

DILUTION

Prepared solutions equal 10 or 40 mg/ml. Further dilute each single dose in 50 to 100 ml of NS or D5W and administer through an additive tubing. Also available in ADD-Vantage vials for use with ADD-Vantage infusion containers. Reduce volume of diluent proportionately for children.

INCOMPATIBLE WITH

Manufacturer states, "Do not physically premix with other drugs; administer separately." Inactivated in solution with beta-lactam antibiotics (e.g., cephalosporins, penicillins) and vancomycin; do not mix in the same solution. Appropriate spacing required because of physical incompatibilities. See Drug/Lab Interactions.

COMPATIBLE WITH

See Incompatible With. Consult pharmacist; specific conditions may apply; see Compatibilities, p. xvi.

Additive: ***Not recommended by manufacturer.*** Aztreonam (Azactam), bleomycin (Blenoxane), calcium gluconate, cefoxitin (Mefoxin), ciprofloxacin (Cipro IV), clindamycin (Cleocin), furosemide (Lasix), linezolid (Zyvox), metronidazole (Flagyl IV), ofloxacin (Floxin IV), ranitidine (Zantac), verapamil (Isoptin).

Syringe: Doxapram (Dopram).

Y-site: Acyclovir (Zovirax), alatrofloxacin (Trovan IV), aldesleukin (Proleukin, IL-2), amifostine (Ethyol), amiodarone (Cordarone), aztreonam

(Azactam), ciprofloxacin (Cipro IV), cisatracurium (Nimbex), cyclophosphamide (Cytoxan), diltiazem (Cardizem), docetaxel (Taxotere), doxorubicin liposome (Doxil), enalaprilat (Vasotec IV), esmolol (Brevibloc), etoposide phosphate (Etopophos), filgrastim (Neupogen), fluconazole (Diflucan), fludarabine (Fludara), foscarnet (Foscavir), furosemide (Lasix), gatifloxacin (Tequin), gemcitabine (Gemzar), granisetron (Kytril), hetastarch in electrolytes (Hextend), hydromorphone (Dilaudid), insulin (regular), labetalol (Normodyne), linezolid (Zyvox), magnesium sulfate, melphalan (Alkeran), meperidine (Demerol), midazolam (Versed), morphine, perphenazine (Trilafon), remifentanil (Ultiva), tacrolimus (Prograf), teniposide (Vumon), theophylline, thiotepa (Thioplex), vinorelbine (Navelbine), zidovudine (AZT, Retrovir).

RATE OF ADMINISTRATION

Each single dose, properly diluted, over a minimum of 20 and a maximum of 60 minutes.

ACTIONS

An aminoglycoside antibiotic with potential neuromuscular blocking action. Inhibits protein synthesis in bacterial cells. Bactericidal against specific gram-negative and bacilli, including *Escherichia coli*, *Klebsiella*, *Proteus*, and *Pseudomonas*. Well distributed through all body fluids. Usual half-life is 2 to 2.5 hours. Half-life is prolonged in infants, postpartum females, fever, liver disease and ascites, spinal cord injury, cystic fibrosis, and the elderly; shorter in severe burns. Crosses the placental barrier. Excreted in the kidneys.

INDICATIONS AND USES

Short-term treatment of serious infections caused by susceptible organisms (e.g., septicemia, meningitis [concentration low, combine with intrathecal], peritonitis). ■ Primarily used when penicillin and other less toxic antibiotics ineffective or contraindicated. ■ Concurrent therapy with a penicillin or cephalosporin sometimes indicated.

CONTRAINDICATIONS

Known tobramycin or aminoglycoside sensitivity. Sulfite sensitivity may be a contraindication.

PRECAUTIONS

Use extreme caution if therapy is required over 7 to 10 days. ■ Sensitivity studies necessary to determine susceptibility of causative organism to tobramycin. ■ Superinfection may occur from overgrowth of nonsusceptible organisms. ■ Use caution in infants, children, and the elderly. ■ May contain sulfites; use caution in patients with asthma. ■ Risk of neurotoxicity (e.g., auditory and vestibular ototoxicity) increased in patients with pre-existing renal damage or in normal renal function with prolonged use. Partial or total irreversible deafness may continue to develop after tobramycin discontinued. ■ Single daily dosing has been used effectively in abdominal, pelvic inflammatory, and GU infections in patients with normal renal function. Not recommended in bacteremia caused by *Pseudomonas aeruginosa*, endocarditis, meningitis, during pregnancy, or in patients less than 6 weeks postpartum. Limited data available for use in all other situations (e.g., burns, children or the elderly, cystic fibrosis, renal impairment). ■ Pseudomembranous colitis has been reported. May range from mild to life-threatening. Consider in patients that present with diarrhea during or after treatment with tobramycin.

Monitor: Watch for decrease in urine output, rising BUN and SrCr, and declining CrCl levels. Dose may require decreasing. ■ Routine evaluation of hearing is recommended. ■ Narrow range between toxic and therapeutic levels. Periodically monitor peak and trough concentrations to avoid peak serum concentrations above 12 mcg/ml and trough concentrations above 2 mcg/ml. Therapeutic levels are between 4 and 8 mcg/ml. ■ Maintain good hydration. ■ Monitor serum calcium, magnesium, potassium, and sodium; levels may decline. ■ Closely monitor patients with impaired renal function for nephrotoxicity and neurotoxicity (e.g., auditory and vestibular ototoxicity); nephrotoxicity may be reversible. ■ In extended treatment, monitoring of serum levels, electrolytes, renal, auditory, and vestibular functions daily is recommended. ■ See Drug/Lab Interactions.

Patient Education: Report promptly dizziness, hearing loss, weakness, or any changes in balance. ■ Consider birth control options.

Maternal/Child: Category D: avoid pregnancy; use during pregnancy and breast-feeding only when absolutely necessary. Potential hazard to fetus. ■ Peak concentrations are generally lower in infants and young children. ■ Use extreme caution in premature infants and neonates; immature kidney function will result in prolonged half-life. ■ See Precautions.

Elderly: Consider less toxic alternatives. ■ Monitor renal function and drug levels carefully. Measurement of CrCl more useful than BUN or SrCr to assess renal function. ■ Half-life prolonged; longer intervals between doses may be more important than reduced doses. ■ See Precautions, Dose Adjustments, and Side Effects.

DRUG/LAB INTERACTIONS

Synergistic when used in combination with beta-lactam antibiotics (e.g., cephalosporins, penicillins) and vancomycin. Synergism may be inconsistent; see Incompatible With. ■ Concurrent use topically or systemically with any other ototoxic or nephrotoxic agents should be avoided. May have dangerous additive effects with anesthetics (e.g., enflurane), other neuromuscular blocking antibiotics (e.g., kanamycin), diuretics (e.g., furosemide [Lasix]), beta-lactam antibiotics (e.g., cephalosporins), vancomycin, and many others. ■ Neuromuscular blocking muscle relaxants (e.g., doxacurium [Nuromax], succinylcholine) are potentiated by aminoglycosides. ***Apnea can occur.*** ■ May be antagonized by bacteriostatic antibiotics (e.g., chloramphenicol, erythromicin, and tetracycline); bactericidal action may be affected. Magnesium sulfate may reduce the antibiotic activity of tobramycin. ■ Aminoglycosides are potentiated by anticholinesterases (e.g., edrophonium), antineoplastics (e.g., nitrogen mustard, cisplatin). ■ See Side Effects.

SIDE EFFECTS

Occur more frequently with impaired renal function, higher doses, prolonged administration, dehydration, in the elderly, and in patients receiving other ototoxic or nephrotoxic drugs.

Dizziness; fever; headache; increased AST (SGOT), ALT (SGPT), and serum bilirubin; itching; lethargy; rash; roaring in the ears; seizures; urticaria; vomiting.

Major: Apnea; blood dyscrasias; cylindruria; elevated BUN, nonprotein nitrogen (NPN), and creatinine; hearing loss; leukocytosis, neuromuscular blockade; oliguria; proteinuria; pseudomembranous colitis; seizures (large doses); tinnitus; vertigo.

ANTIDOTE

Notify the physician of all side effects. If minor side effects persist or any major symptom appears, discontinue the drug and notify the physician. Treatment is symptomatic or a reduction in dose may be required. In overdose hemodialysis may be indicated. Monitor fluid balance, CrCl, and plasma levels carefully. Complexation with ticarcillin may be as effective as hemodialysis. Consider exchange transfusion in the newborn. Calcium salts or neostigmine may reverse neuromuscular blockade. Resuscitate as necessary.

TOPOTECAN HYDROCHLORIDE

(toh-poh-tee′kan hye-droe-klor′id)

Antineoplastic (topoisomerase I inhibitor)

Hycamtin

pH 2.5 to 3.5

USUAL DOSE

Before giving the initial dose, the baseline neutrophil count must be at least 1,500/mm^3 and baseline platelet count must be at least 100,000/mm^3.

Ovarian cancer: 1.5 mg/M^2/day as an infusion each day for 5 consecutive days (days 1 through 5 of a 21-day course). Begin the second course on day 22. A minimum of four courses is recommended; median time to response has been 9 to 12 weeks. See Dose Adjustments.

Small-cell lung cancer: 1.5 mg/M^2/day (range 1.25 to 2 mg/M^2) as an infusion each day for 5 consecutive days. Repeat every 21 days.

Non–small-cell lung cancer (unlabeled): 1.5 mg/M^2/day as an infusion each day for 5 consecutive days. Repeat every 21 days.

Myelodysplastic syndrome/chronic myelomonocytic leukemia (unlabeled): 2 mg/M^2/day as a continuous 24-hour infusion. Repeat every day for 5 consecutive days. Repeat every 3 to 4 weeks until remission, then repeat once a month.

DOSE ADJUSTMENTS

Do not begin subsequent courses of topotecan until neutrophils recover to more than 1,000/mm^3, platelets recover to 100,000/mm^3, and hemoglobin recovers to 9 mg/dl (with transfusion if necessary). ■ If severe neutropenia occurs (neutrophils less than or equal to 500/mm^3) during any course, either reduce dose for all subsequent courses by 0.25 mg/M^2 or, before resorting to dose reduction, give G-CSF (filgrastim) starting with day 6 (must be at least 24 hours after the final dose of that course). ■ If platelet count falls below 25,000/mm^3, reduce dose for all subsequent courses by 0.25 mg/M^2. ■ Reduce dose to 0.75 mg/M^2 in patients with moderate impaired renal function (CrCl 20 to 39 ml/min). There are inadequate data at this time to recommend a dose in severe renal impairment. ■ Dose adjustment may be required in the elderly because of age related renal impairment. ■ No dose adjustment required in patients with impaired hepatic function (bilirubin more than 1.5 to less than 10 mg/dl).

DILUTION

Specific techniques required; see Precautions. Reconstitute each 4-mg vial with 4 ml of SW (1 mg/ml). Withdraw the calculated dose and further dilute in 50 to 100 ml of NS or D5W.

Storage: Store unopened vials in cartons protected from light at CRT. Reconstituted solutions contain no preservative; use immediately. Solutions diluted for infusion are stable at room temperature in soft light for 24 hours.

COMPATIBLE WITH (Underline Indicates Conflicting Compatibility Information)

Consult pharmacist; specific conditions may apply; see Compatibilities, p. xvi.

Y-site: Carboplatin (Paraplatin), cimetidine (Tagamet), cisplatin (Platinol), cyclophosphamide (Cytoxan), doxorubicin (Adriamycin), etoposide (VePesid), gemcitabine (Gemzar), granisetron (Kytril), ifosfamide (Ifex), methylprednisolone (Solu-Medrol), metoclopramide (Reglan), ondansetron (Zofran), paclitaxel (Taxol), prochlorperazine (Compazine), <u>ticarcillin/clavulanate (Timentin)</u>, vincristine (Oncovin).

RATE OF ADMINISTRATION

A single dose as an infusion evenly distributed over 30 minutes.

Myelodysplastic syndrome/chronic myelomonocytic leukemia: See Usual Dose.

ACTIONS

A new class of antineoplastic agent that inhibits the enzyme topoisomerase I required for DNA replication. A topoisomerase I inhibitor, it is a semisynthetic derivative of camptothecin. Metabolized through a specific process to its active lactone form. Causes cell death by damaging DNA produced during the S-phase of cell synthesis. Distributes evenly between plasma and blood cells and is found in significant quantities in CSF. Minor additional metabolism occurs in the liver. Terminal half-life is from 2 to 3 hours. Moderately bound to plasma protein (35%). Some excretion in urine and bile.

INDICATIONS AND USES

Treatment of metastatic carcinoma of the ovary after failure of initial or subsequent chemotherapy. ■ Treatment of small-cell lung cancer sensitive disease after failure of first-line chemotherapy.

Unlabeled uses: Treatment of non–small-cell lung cancer. ■ Treatment of myelodysplastic syndrome and chronic myelomonocytic leukemia (CMML).

CONTRAINDICATIONS

Hypersensitivity to topotecan or any of its components. Not recommended for use during pregnancy, breast-feeding, or in patients with severe bone marrow depression.

PRECAUTIONS

Follow guidelines for handling cytotoxic agents. See Appendix A, p. 1142. ■ Administered by or under the direction of the physician specialist. ■ Adequate diagnostic and treatment facilities must be available to meet any medical emergency. ■ Must have adequate bone marrow reserves. An 80% to 90% decrease in WBC count at nadir is typical after the first cycle of therapy. Neutropenia is not cumulative over time. ■ Use with caution in patients who have received previous cytotoxic drug therapy or radiation therapy. ■ Use with caution in impaired renal function; clearance decreased. ■ Use caution in patients with a history of allergies.

Monitor: Baseline neutrophil count must be at least 1,500 cells/mm^3 and platelets at least 100,000 cell/mm^3 before the initial dose. ■ Obtain a baseline CBC with differential and platelets. ■ Monitor before each course and frequently during treatment. Platelet count must be 100,000/mm^3, neutrophils 1,000/mm^3, and hemoglobin 9 mg/dl before a course of therapy can be repeated. Anemia is frequent and transfusion is often indicated. ■ Baseline CrCl and BUN suggested. ■ Monitor vital signs. ■ Maintain adequate hydration. ■ Nausea and vomiting are frequent and may be severe; use prophylactic administration of antiemetics to increase patient comfort. ■ Observe closely for S/S of infection. Prophylactic antibiotics may be indicated pending results of C/S in a febrile or nonfebrile neutropenic patient. ■ Not a vesicant, but monitor injection site for inflammation and/or extravasation. ■ Expected nadir for neutrophils is 11 days, 15 days for platelets and hemoglobin. ■ Monitor for thrombocytopenia (platelet count less than 50,000/mm^3). Initiate precautions to prevent excessive bleeding (e.g., inspect IV sites, skin, and mucous membranes; use extreme care during invasive procedures; test urine, emesis, stool, and secretions for occult blood).

Patient Education: Nonhormonal birth control recommended. ■ Report any unusual or unexpected symptoms or side effects as soon as possible (e.g., signs of infection [e.g., chills, fever, night sweats] or signs of bleeding [e.g., bruising, black tarry stools]). ■ See Appendix D, p. 1148.

Maternal/Child: Category D: avoid pregnancy; may cause fetal harm. ■ Discontinue breast-feeding. ■ Safety and effectiveness for use in children not established. One study showed that severe myelotoxicity may occur at lower doses in children than in adults.

Elderly: No dose adjustment necessary except in age-related renal impairment.

DRUG/LAB INTERACTIONS

May cause severe prolonged myelosuppression and grade 3 or 4 nonhematologic effects (e.g., diarrhea, lethargy, nausea, vomiting) with cisplatin. ■ Concurrent administration of G-CSF (filgrastim) can prolong the duration of neutropenia. If used, do not administer before day 6, at least 24 hours after the final dose of topotecan. ■ Concurrent or consecutive administration of other bone marrow depressants (e.g., cyclophosphamide [Cytoxan], paclitaxel [Taxol]), radiation therapy or agents that cause blood dyscrasias (e.g., amphotericin B, anticonvulsants [e.g., phenytoin, valproic acid], NSAIDs [e.g., ibuprofen (Advil, Motrin), naproxen (Aleve, Naprosen)]) may produce additive bone marrow depression. Dose reduction may be required based on blood cell counts. ■ Concurrent use of immunosuppressants (e.g., tacrolimus [Prograf], corticosteroids, muromonab CD-3 [Orthoclone]) may increase the risk of infection. ■ Probenecid may decrease renal clearance and increase the risk of toxicity. ■ Do not administer live or killed virus vaccines.

SIDE EFFECTS

Bone marrow depression, primarily neutropenia, is the dose-limiting toxicity of topotecan. Abdominal pain, alopecia, anorexia, bone marrow toxicity such as anemia (less than 10 mg/dl [96%], less than 8 mg/dl [40%]), leukopenia (less than 3,000/mm^3 [98%], less than 1,000/mm^3 [32%]), neutropenia (less than 1,500/mm^3 [98%], less than 500/mm^3 [81%]), thrombocytopenia (less than 75,000/mm^3 [63%], less than 25,000/mm^3 [26%]), constipation, diarrhea, dyspnea, fatigue, fever, headache, infection with neutropenia less than 500/mm^3 (26%), nausea (77%), paresthesia, stomatitis, transient increases in AST (SGOT) and ALT (SGPT), vomiting (58%), weakness.

ANTIDOTE

Keep physician informed of all side effects. Withhold topotecan until myelosuppression has improved to minimum requirements. Neutropenia recovery may be aided by G-CSF (filgrastim, pegfilgrastim [Neulasta]) under specific conditions; see Dose Adjustments or Drug/Lab Interactions. Anemia required RBC or whole blood tranfusions in 50% of patients. Thrombocytopenia may require platelet transfusion. Death can result from the progression of many side effects. No known antidote for overdose. Symptomatic and supportive treatment is indicated. Treat allergic reactions with oxygen, epinephrine, corticosteriods, and antihistamines.

TORSEMIDE INJECTION

(tor′se-mide in-jek′shun)

Diuretic (loop)
Antihypertensive

Demadex

pH over 8.3

USUAL DOSE

IV and oral doses are therapeutically equivalent. Oral dose can replace an IV dose at any time. If diuretic response is not adequate, titrate the recommended dose upward by doubling the dose until desired response achieved or maximum suggested dose reached.

Edema of congestive heart failure: 10 to 20 mg once daily. See general instructions above; single doses over 200 mg have not been adequately studied.

Edema of chronic renal failure: 20 mg once daily. See general instructions above; single doses over 200 mg have not been adequately studied.

Hepatic cirrhosis with ascites: 5 to 10 mg once daily. To prevent hypokalemia and metabolic alkalosis give in combination with an aldosterone antagonist (e.g., spironolactone [Aldactone]) or a potassium-sparing diuretic (e.g., dyazide). See general instructions above; single doses over 40 mg have not been adequately studied.

Hypertension: 5 mg once daily. May be increased to 10 mg in 4 to 6 weeks if BP reduction is inadequate. If response is still inadequate, the addition of other antihypertensive agents is recommended instead of larger doses of torsemide. Usually given PO.

Continuous infusion: Studies used a 100-mg dose divided as follows. A ***loading dose*** of 25 mg (2.5 ml) as an IV injection over 2 minutes (25% of total daily dose). Follow with an infusion at 3.1 mg/hr (10 ml/hr) or 75% of total daily dose equally distributed over 24 hours.

DOSE ADJUSTMENTS

Higher doses may be required in renal failure. See Drug/Lab Interactions.

DILUTION

Available as 10 mg/ml. May be given undiluted. May be given through Y-tube or three-way stopcock of infusion set. May be further diluted in NS, ½NS, or D5W. For a 75-mg dose (75% of the 100-mg total daily dose), dilute 7.5 ml to a total volume of 240 ml. 200 mg in 250 ml diluent yields 0.8 mg/ml. 50 mg in 500 ml diluent yields 0.1 mg/ml.

Storage: Store at CRT. Do not freeze.

INCOMPATIBLE WITH

Manufacturer recommends flushing the IV line before and after torsemide injection to avoid incompatibilities caused by alkaline pH.

COMPATIBLE WITH

Consult pharmacist; specific conditions may apply; see Compatibilities, p. xvi.

Y-site: Milrinone (Primacor).

RATE OF ADMINISTRATION

Ototoxicity (usually reversible) has occurred with too-rapid injection and doses over 200 mg. Flush IV line with NS before and after administration.

IV injection: Each 200 mg or fraction thereof over 2 minutes.

Continuous infusion: Balance of daily dose after loading dose equally distributed over 24 hours. For a 75-mg dose, the rate would be 3.1 mg (10 ml/hr) for 24 hours.

ACTIONS

A sulfonamide type loop diuretic. Acts from within the ascending portion of the loop of Henle to excrete water, sodium, chlorides, and some potassium. Diuretic action correlates better with the rate of drug excretion in urine than with plasma concentration. Will produce diuresis in alkalosis or acidosis. Effects begin within 10 minutes and peak within 1 hour. Diuresis lasts 6 to 8 hours. Highly protein bound. Metabolized by the liver (80%). 20% eliminated via urinary excretion. Other loop diuretics cross the placental barrier and are secreted in breast milk; specific information not available for torsemide.

INDICATIONS AND USES

Treatment of edema associated with congestive heart failure, cirrhosis of the liver with ascites, and chronic renal failure. Used when a rapid onset of diuresis is desired or when oral administration is impractical. ■ Treatment of hypertension.

CONTRAINDICATIONS

Known hypersensitivity to torsemide or to sulfonylureas and in anuric patients.

PRECAUTIONS

Tests to determine serum levels of torsemide not widely available. ■ In patients with congestive heart failure and/or renal failure, a smaller dose is actually delivered to the ascending loop of Henle, resulting in less response at any given dose. ■ Use caution and improve basic condition first in hepatic coma, electrolyte depletion, and advanced cirrhosis of the liver. Initiation of therapy in the hospital is preferred. ■ Use extreme caution in patients sensitive to bumetanide (Bumex), furosemide (Lasix), or sulfonamides (including thiazide diuretics); may also be sensitive to torsemide. ■ In patients with hepatic disease with cirrhosis and ascites use a potassium-sparing diuretic (e.g., dyazide) or an aldosterone antagonist (e.g., spironolactone) concurrently to prevent hypokalemia and metabolic alkalosis. ■ Use caution in acute MI; excessive diuresis may precipitate shock. ■ In nonanuric renal failure, may cause marked increases in water and sodium excretion without impacting steady-state fluid retention. High doses (500 to 1,200 mg) have caused seizures. ■ May activate or exacerbate systemic lupus erythematosus. Chronic use in renal or hepatic disease has not been adequately studied. ■ Antihypertensive effects greater in black patients.

Monitor: Monitor BP frequently, especially during initial therapy. May precipitate excessive diuresis with water and electrolyte depletion. Dehydration, electrolyte imbalance, hypovolemia, prerenal axotemia, embolism, or thrombosis can occur. Routine checks on electrolyte panel, CO_2, and BUN are necessary during therapy. Potassium chloride and/or magnesium replacement may be required. ▪ Risk of hypokalemia greatest in patients with cirrhosis of the liver, during brisk diuresis, with inadequate oral electrolyte intake, or with concurrent administration of corticosteroids (e.g., prednisone). ▪ May increase blood glucose, serum cholesterol, and triglycerides. ▪ Slight increases in BUN, SrCr, and uric acid may occur, usually reverse when therapy discontinued. Sudden changes in fluid and electrolyte balance may precipitate hepatic coma in patients with hepatic disease and ascites. ▪ Rarely precipitates an attack of gout. ▪ See Drug/Lab Interactions.

Patient Education: Hypotension may cause dizziness; request assistance with ambulation. ▪ May cause a decrease in potassium levels and require a supplement. ▪ Possible skin photosensitivity. Avoid unprotected exposure to sunlight. ▪ Report cramps, dizziness, muscle weakness, or nausea promptly.

Maternal/Child: Category B: use only if clearly needed during pregnancy; safety for use not established. ▪ Safety for use during breast-feeding not established; other loop diuretics suggest discontinuing breast-feeding. ▪ Safety and effectiveness in children under 18 not established. Administration of other loop diuretics to premature infants with edema due to patent ductus arteriosus and hyaline membrane disease may have caused renal calcifications; also other loop diuretics may have increased the risk of persistent patient ductus arteriosus in premature infants with hyaline membrane disease. Torsemide has not been studied in these situations.

Elderly: No specific age-related differences; dose adjustment not indicated. May be more susceptible to dehydration; observe carefully. ▪ Avoid rapid contraction of plasma volume and hemoconcentration. May cause thromboembolic episodes (e.g., CVA, pulmonary emboli).

DRUG/LAB INTERACTIONS

Concurrent administration with high-dose salicylates may cause salicylate toxicity. ▪ Probenicid decreases the diuretic activity of torsemide. ▪ May reduce renal clearance of spironolactone, but dose adjustment not required. ▪ Has been administered with beta-blockers (e.g., atenolol), ACE inhibitors (e.g., captopril), calcium-channel blockers (e.g., diltiazem), cimetidine (Tagamet), digoxin, and nitrates (e.g., nitroglycerin) without new or unexpected adverse events; however, torsemide has caused severe hypotension with ACE inhibitors in sodium- or volume-depleted patients. ▪ Does not affect protein binding of glyburide (DiaBeta) or coumarin derivatives (e.g., warfarin). ▪ May cause excessive potassium depletion with amphotericin B (Fungizone, Abelcet), corticosteroids, thiazide diuretics (e.g., hydrochlorothiazide [HydroDiuril]). Monitor electrolytes closely. ▪ May cause cardiac arrhythmias with digitalis and other antiarrhythmic agents secondary to potassium and magnesium depletion. ▪ NSAIDs (e.g., indomethacin [Indocin], ibuprofen [Advil, Motrin], naproxen [Aleve, Naprosyn]) or salicylates (e.g., aspirin) may cause retention of sodium and water and may decrease diuretic and antihypertensive effects. ▪ Antihypertensive effects may be increased by any hypotension-producing agent (e.g., lidocaine, nitroglycerin, nitroprusside sodium, paclitaxel); reduced dose of the antihypertensive agent or both drugs may be indicated. ▪ May potentiate propranolol (Inderal), salicylates, muscle relaxants (e.g., mivacurium [Mivacron]), and hypotensive effect of other diuretics. ▪ May increase ototoxicity in doses exceeding the usual or in conjunction with ototoxic drugs (e.g., cisplatin, aminoglycosides [e.g., amikacin, streptomycin, gentamicin], ethacrynic acid [Edecrin]). ■ May increase nephrotoxicity if given concurrently with any other nephrotoxic agent (e.g., amphotericin B, aminoglycosides [e.g., gentamicin], foscarnet [Foscavir], rifampin [Rifadin]). Concurrent use with amphotericin B is not recommended, especially in patients with some impaired renal function. ■ Anticoagulants (e.g., coumarin, heparin, streptokinase) may require dose adjustment; effects reduced by decreased plasma volumes and/or increased metabolism. ■ May be inhibited by phenytoin (Dilantin). ■ May reduce excretion of lithium and cause lithium toxicity. ■ May increase or decrease effectiveness of theophyllines.

SIDE EFFECTS

Arthralgia, constipation, cough, diarrhea, dizziness, dyspepsia, ECG abnormalities, edema, electrolyte imbalance, esophageal hemorrhage, excessive thirst, excessive urination, headache, hyperglycemia, hyperuricemia, hypokalemia, impotence, insomnia, myalgia, nervousness, ototoxicity (usually reversible), rhinitis, sore throat, and tinnitus have all been reported. Allergic reactions can occur. Hypocalcemia and hypomagnesemia have been minimal with usual doses.

Major: Anorexia, dizziness, drowsiness, dryness of the mouth, hypotension, increased BUN, lethargy; mental confusion, muscle cramps, fatigue, or pain; nausea and vomiting, oliguria, restlessness, tachycardia, thirst, or weakness may indicate severe electrolyte imbalance, hypovolemia, or prerenal azotemia.

Overdose: Circulatory collapse, dehydration, excessive diuresis, hemoconcentration, hypochloremic alkalosis, hyperchloremia or hypochloremia, hyperkalemia or hypokalemia, hypomagnesemia, hypernatremia or hyponatremia, hypotension, hypovolemia, vascular thrombosis, and embolism.

ANTIDOTE

Notify the physician of any side effect. Depending on severity the physician may treat the side effects symptomatically and either continue or discontinue torsemide. Fluid and electrolyte replacement may be indicated. If side effects are progressive or any major side effects or signs of overdose appear, discontinue the drug immediately and notify the physician. Treatment of overdose is symptomatic and aggressive. Hemodialysis is not effective in overdose. Resuscitate as necessary. Torsemide may be restarted at a lower dose after the patient is stable.

TRACE METALS

Nutritional supplement

(tras met′al)

Chromium
ConTE-Pak-4
Copper
Iodine
Manganese
Molybdenum,
M.T.E.-4, 5, 6, & 7
M.T.E.-4, 5, & 6 Concentrated
MulTE-PAK-4,
MulTE-PAK-5
Multiple Trace Element
Multiple Trace Element Concentrated
Multiple Trace Element With Selenium
Multiple Trace Element With Selenium Concentrated
Selenium
T.E.C.
Trace Metals Additive in 0.9% NaCl
Zinc

Multiple Trace Element Neonatal, Neotrace-4, Pediatric Multiple Trace Element, PedTE-PAK-4, Pedtrace-4, P.T.E.-4

USUAL DOSE

Available as single elements, selected combined elements in various strengths, and in combination with electrolytes. Some preparations may contain aluminum; see Precautions. Selection of correct product based on minimum daily requirement and individual needs.

Zinc: 2.5 to 4 mg/day; add 2 mg in acute catabolic states. Increase to 12.2 mg/L of total parenteral nutrition (TPN) if there is fluid loss from the small bowel. May contain aluminum.

Copper: 0.5 to 1.5 mg/day.

Manganese: 0.15 to 0.8 mg/day. May contain up to 100 mcg/L of aluminum; see Precautions.

Molybdenum: 20 to 120 mcg/day. Increase to 163 mcg/day for 21 days in deficiency states resulting from prolonged TPN.

Chromium: 10 to 15 mcg/day. Increase to 20 mcg/day with intestinal fluid loss.

Selenium: 20 to 40 mcg/day. Increase to 100 mcg/day for 31 days in deficiency states resulting from prolonged TPN.

Iodine: 1 to 2 mcg/kg of body weight/day. Increase to 2 to 3 mcg/kg/day in growing children, pregnant and lactating women.

PEDIATRIC DOSE

Zinc: 100 mcg/kg/day for full-term infants and children up to 5 years of age. 300 mcg/kg/day for premature infants with birth weights from 1,500 Gm to 3 kg. May contain aluminum.

Copper: 20 mcg/kg/day.

Manganese: 2 to 10 mcg/kg/day. May contain up to 100 mcg/L of aluminum; see Precautions.

Molybdenum: Dosage must be calculated by extrapolation; consult pharmacist.

Chromium: 0.14 to 0.2 mcg/kg/day.

Selenium: 3 mcg/kg/day.

DOSE ADJUSTMENTS

Reduce or omit dose in impaired renal function.

DILUTION

Must be added to daily volume of IV infusion fluids including TPN. Check labels for aluminum content; see Precautions.

COMPATIBILITY

Specific trace metals may present compatibility problems. Check incompatibilities of each agent to be admixed or delivered to Y-site.

RATE OF ADMINISTRATION

Administer properly diluted at rate prescribed for IV infusion fluids or TPN.

ACTIONS

All are basic elements present in the human body. Specific amounts required to initiate, facilitate, or maintain appropriate body systems.

INDICATIONS AND USES

Nutritional supplement to IV solutions given for total parenteral or central nutrition.

CONTRAINDICATIONS

Do not give direct IV; hypersensitivity to any component (especially iodides). Manganese contraindicated in presence of high manganese levels. Molybdenum without copper supplementation contraindicated in copper-deficient patients.

PRECAUTIONS

Selenium enhances vitamin E and decreases the toxicity of mercury, cadmium, and arsenic. ■ Patients with biliary tract obstruction may retain copper and manganese. ■ Avoid copper in patients with Wilson's disease (genetic disorder of copper metabolism). ■ Assess possibility of diabetes mellitus when giving chromium supplements to maintain normal glucose metabolism. ■ Some solutions may contain aluminum (e.g., manganese, zinc). In impaired kidney function, aluminum may reach toxic levels. Premature neonates are particularly at risk because of their immature kidneys and requirement for calcium and phosphate, which also contain aluminum. Research indicates that patients with impaired renal function who receive more than 4 to 5 mcg/kg/day of parenteral aluminum are at risk for developing CNS or bone toxicity associated with aluminum accumulation.

Monitor: Monitor serum trace metal concentration to avoid accumulation. Results will also determine use of a single element or a combined product.

Maternal/Child: Category C: use in pregnancy only if clearly indicated. Use manganese with caution in the nursing mother. ■ May contain benzyl alcohol; may cause fatal "gasping" syndrome in premature infants.

DRUG/LAB INTERACTIONS

Therapeutic serum levels of copper and zinc will decrease if not given together.

SIDE EFFECTS

Toxicity is rare at recommended doses. Iodine may cause anaphylaxis.

ANTIDOTE

Dosage will be adjusted based on serum levels. Keep physician informed. Resuscitate as necessary.

TRANEXAMIC ACID

(tran-eks-am-ik as′id)

Cyklokapron

Antifibrinolytic
Antihemorrhagic

pH 6.5 to 7.5

USUAL DOSE

Dental extraction in adults and children with hemophilia:

Preoperative: Normal renal function required. 10 mg/kg IV immediately before surgery. Another regimen suggests 25 mg/kg PO every 6 to 8 hours beginning 1 day before surgery. Other sources suggest that a single factor VIII infusion (e.g., ReFacto) of 40 IU/kg or a coagulation factor IX infusion (e.g., AlphaNine) of 60 IU/kg at least 8 hours before surgery is often enough to attain normal hemostasis; see Drug/Lab Interactions.

Postoperative: Follow with 25 mg/kg PO every 6 to 8 hours after surgery for 2 to 8 days; another source says 7 to 10 days. If unable to take oral medicine, use 10 mg/kg IV every 6 to 8 hours for 2 to 8 days (7 to 10 days).

Hemorrhage, hyperfibrinolysis-induced (unlabeled): 15 mg/kg or 1 Gm every 6 to 8 hours. Continue until bleeding stops or lab tests indicate treatment may be stopped.

Postsurgical hemorrhage following prostatectomy or bladder surgery (unlabeled): 1 Gm during the surgical procedure. Repeat 1 Gm every 8 hours for 3 days. Continue treatment with 1 Gm PO every 8 hours until macroscopic hematuria is no longer present.

Replacement of oral doses for all indications: If unable to take oral medicine, use 10 mg/kg IV according to the dosing schedule for that indication.

DOSE ADJUSTMENTS

Lower-end initial and/or reduced doses may be indicated in the elderly based on the potential for decreased organ function and concomitant disease or drug therapy. ■ Reduce dose in impaired renal function according to the following chart.

Tranexamic Dose Guidelines in Impaired Renal Function

Serum Creatinine (mg/dl)	Dose
1.36-2.83	10 mg/kg two times per day
2.83-5.66	10 mg/kg once per day
<5.66	10 mg/kg every 48 hours or 5 mg/kg every 24 hours

DILUTION

100 mg equals 1 ml of prepared solution. Further dilute a single dose with at least 50 ml compatible infusion solutions (e.g., NS, dextrose solutions in water or various concentrations of NS, Ringer's solution; see Compatible With. Prepare solution immediately before use; discard any unused solution.

INCOMPATIBLE WITH

Manufacturer states, "Do not mix with blood and do not mix with solutions containing penicillins."

COMPATIBLE WITH

Consult pharmacist; specific conditions may apply; see Compatibilities, p. xvi.

Solutions: May be mixed with IV solutions, including solutions containing electrolytes, carbohydrates, amino acids, or dextran.

Additive: Heparin.

RATE OF ADMINISTRATION

100 mg or fraction thereof over at least 1 minute. Too-rapid infusion may cause hypotension.

ACTIONS

A synthetic amino acid with the specific action of inhibiting plasminogen activator substances; to a lesser degree inhibits plasmin activity. Increases fibrinogen activity in clot formation by inhibiting the enzyme required for destruction of formed fibrin. More potent than aminocaproic acid. Onset of action is prompt. Half-life approximately 2 hours. Readily excreted in the urine. Crosses the placental barrier. Secreted in breast milk.

INDICATIONS AND USES

Reduce or prevent hemorrhage and reduce the need for replacement therapy in hemophilia patients during and following tooth extraction.

Unlabeled uses: Treatment of severe hemorrhage caused by antifibrinolytic agents (e.g., alteplase [tPA], reteplase [r-PA]), postsurgical hemorrhage following prostatectomy or bladder surgery. Also used with NS as a bladder irrigation following bladder surgery.

CONTRAINDICATIONS

Acquired defective color vision, active intravascular clotting, subarachnoid hemorrhage.

PRECAUTIONS

For short-term use only (2 to 8 days). ■ Use extreme caution; retinal changes, leukemia, hyperplasia of the biliary tract, cholangioma, and adenocarcinoma of the intrahepatic biliary system have been found in animal studies. ■ Rapid administration in any form may cause hypotension. ■ Whole blood transfusions may be given if necessary but must be given through a second infusion site. ■ In patients with upper urinary tract bleeding, ureteral obstruction due to clot formation has been reported. ■ Risk of venous or arterial thrombosis increased in patients with a previous history of thromboembolic disease. ■ Thromboembolic events (e.g., central retinal artery and vein obstruction, cerebral thrombosis, deep vein thrombosis, pulmonary embolism) have been reported rarely in patients receiving transexamic acid for indications other than hemorrhage prevention in patients with hemophilia. ■ Patients with DIC being treated with tranexamic acid require the strict supervision of a physician specialist.

Monitor: Use only in conjunction with general and specific tests to determine the amount of fibrinolysis present. ■ In repeated treatment or if treatment will last more than several (2 to 3) days, a complete ophthalmologic examination (visual acuity, color vision, eyeground, visual fields) should be done before and at regular intervals during treatment. Discontinue use if changes are found.

Maternal/Child: Category B: use caution and only if clearly needed in pregnancy and breast-feeding.

Elderly: Lower-end initial or reduced doses may be indicated; see Dose Adjustments. ■ Monitoring of renal function suggested.

DRUG/LAB INTERACTIONS

Concomitant use with factor IX complex (e.g., AlphaNine, Mononine, Konyne) or anti-inhibitor coagulant complex (e.g., Autoplex-T, Feiba VH) is not recommended; may increase the risk for venous or arterial thrombosis. One reference suggests that administration of tranexamic acid should be delayed for 8 hours after factor IX complex or anti-inhibitor coagulant complex.

SIDE EFFECTS

Diarrhea, giddiness, hypotension, nausea and vomiting. Thromboembolic events (e.g., central retinal artery and vein obstruction, cerebral thrombosis, deep vein thrombosis, pulmonary embolism), have been reported rarely.

ANTIDOTE

All side effects may subside with reduced dosage or rate of administration. Discontinue use of drug if any changes are found during follow-up ophthalmologic examinations. Resuscitate as necessary.

TRASTUZUMAB

(tras-tuz′uh-mab)

Herceptin

Monoclonal antibody
Antineoplastic

pH 6

USUAL DOSE

Premedication: Pretreatment with antihistamines (e.g., diphenhydramine [Benadryl]) and/or corticosteroids (e.g., dexamethasone [Decadron]) may be indicated and is suggested for patients being retreated after a hypersensitivity reaction or a severe infusion reaction; see Precautions. Pretreatment may not be successful; hypersensitivity reaction and/or infusion reaction may recur. Preassessment required; see Monitor.

Loading dose: 4 mg/kg. Follow with a ***maintenance dose*** of 2 mg/kg at weekly intervals.

Combination therapy with paclitaxel: Trastuzumab dose as above.

Paclitaxel dose: 175 mg/M^2 over 3 hours every 21 days for at least 6 cycles.

DOSE ADJUSTMENTS

No recommendations for dose adjustments are provided.

DILUTION

Manufacturer supplies a 30-ml vial of bacteriostatic water for injection (BWFI). ***To obtain the correct concentration, use only 20 ml of this vial of BWFI to reconstitute trastuzumab. New supplies will contain only 20 ml of diluent (BWFI).*** Inject diluent slowly directed at the lyophilized cake. Swirl gently; ***do not shake*** (is sensitive to agitation or rapid expulsion from a syringe). Allow vial to stand for 5 minutes, slight foaming is permissible. Will yield a multidose solution containing 21 mg/ml. Label vial immediately with a "do not use after" date 28 days from date of reconstitution. SW may be used to reconstitute trastuzumab for patients with a known hypersensitivity to benzyl alcohol, but the calculated dose must be withdrawn, used immediately, and the balance of the reconstituted solution discarded. Reconstituted solution must be further diluted and given as an infusion. Withdraw the calculated dose from the reconstituted vial (21 mg/ml) and add it to an infusion bag containing 250 ml of NS. Gently invert to mix the solution. A loading dose for a 70-kg patient would be 280 mg or 13.33 ml; a maintenance dose would be 140 mg or 6.67 ml of reconstituted solution.

Storage: Refrigerate unopened and reconstituted vials at 2° to 8° C (36° to 46° F). Vials reconstituted in supplied diluent are stable for 28 days after reconstitution. Discard remaining diluent. Discard reconstituted trastuzumab after expiration date written or stamped on vial. Solutions diluted in NS may be refrigerated for 24 hours before use. Do not freeze reconstituted trastuzumab.

COMPATIBILITY

Manufacturer states, "Do not reconstitute with drugs other than BWFI or SW. Further dilute infusion with NS. Infusions should not be administered or mixed with dextrose solutions." Is compatible with polyethylene and polyvinylchloride infusion bags and tubing.

RATE OF ADMINISTRATION

Use of a microdrip (60 gtt/min) or other IV controller suggested. Inline filters are not necessary but may be used (0.2-micron filters were evaluated). For infusion only, ***do not administer*** as an IV push or bolus.

Loading dose: A single dose must be given as an infusion over a minimum of 90 minutes. Observe for chills, fever, or other infusion-associated symptoms; see Precautions/Monitor.

Maintenance dose: A single dose as an infusion over a minimum of 30 minutes if the initial loading dose was well tolerated.

Paclitaxel dose: See Usual Dose.

ACTIONS

A recombinant DNA–derived humanized monoclonal antibody that selectively binds with high affinity to the extracellular domain of the human epidermal growth factor receptor 2 (HER2) protein that is overexpressed in selected breast cancer cells. Inhibits proliferation and mediates an antibody-dependent cellular toxicity in cancer cells that overexpress the HER2 protein. HER2 overexpression is observed in 25% to 30% of primary breast cancers, determined by using an immunohistochemistry-based assessment of fixed tumor blocks. Half-life increases and clearance decreases with increasing doses. With recommended loading and maintenance doses a mean half-life of 5.8 days was observed (range of 1 to 32 days). May cross the placental barrier. May be secreted in breast milk.

INDICATIONS AND USES

As a single agent for treatment of patients with metastatic breast cancer whose tumors overexpress the HER2 protein and who have received one or more chemotherapy regimens for their metastatic disease. ■ In combination with paclitaxel (Taxol), for the treatment of patients with metastatic breast cancer whose tumors overexpress the HER2 protein and who have not received chemotherapy for their metastatic disease.

CONTRAINDICATIONS

None known when used as indicated; see Precautions.

PRECAUTIONS

Trastuzumab should be used only in patients whose tumors have HER2 overexpression. Beneficial treatment effects were largely limited to patients with the highest level of HER2 protein overexpression (3+). Recent studies suggest that FISH (fluorescence in situ hybridization) may be an effective testing method for HER2 overexpression. ■ Administered by or under the direction of the physician specialist. May be given on an outpatient basis. ■ Adequate laboratory and supportive medical resources must be available. ■ Emergency equipment and drugs for treatment of left ventricular dysfunction and/or hypersensitivity reactions must be immediately available; see Antidote. ■ Use with caution in patients with known hypersensitivity to trastuzumab, Chinese hamster ovary cell proteins, benzyl alcohol, or any component of this product. ■ Hypersensitivity reactions and infusion reactions (including some with a fatal outcome) and pulmonary events (including ARDS and death) have occurred. Retreatment after full recovery from a hypersensitivity reaction has been tried following pretreatment with antihistamines and/or corticosteroids. Some tolerated treatment, and others had another severe hypersensitivity reaction. ■ Congestive heart failure may be severe; has been associated with disabling cardiac failure, mural thrombosis leading to stroke, and death. ■ Incidence of cardiac dysfunction was highest in patients who received trastuzumab concurrently with anthracyclines (e.g., doxorubicin [Adriamycin]) and cyclophosphamide, and in elderly patients. ■ Use extreme caution in treating patients with pre-existing cardiac dysfunction or pulmonary compromise. Pre-existing cardiac disease or prior cardiotoxic therapy (e.g., anthracyclines), radiation therapy to the chest or pre-existing pulmonary compromise secondary to intrinsic lung disease and/or malignant pulmonary involvement may decrease the ability to tolerate trastuzumab. ■ Low titers of human anti-human antibodies (HAHA) were detected in one patient who had no symptoms of allergic reaction. ■ Little information is available on the effect of dexrazoxane in patients treated with trastuzumab. ■ No experience is available to compare liposomal doxorubicin to traditional doxorubicin.

Monitor: Treatment with trastuzumab can result in the development of ventricular dysfunction and CHF. All patients should have a thorough baseline cardiac assessment to evaluate left ventricular function, including history and physical exam and one or more of the following: ECG, echocardiogram, and/or MUGA scan. Monitoring and assessment may not identify all patients at risk for developing cardiotoxicity. ■ Monitor all vital signs before and during therapy. Obtain baseline CBC with differential and platelet count and repeat as needed. ■ Chills and/or fever occur in 40% of patients during the first infusion. May be treated with acetaminophen (Tylenol), diphenhydramine (Benadryl), and meperidine (Demerol) with or without reduction in the rate of infusion. During infusion, monitor closely; asthenia, bronchospasm, dizziness, dyspnea, headache, hypotension (may be severe), hypoxia, nausea, pain (may be at tumor site), rash, rigors, and vomiting have also occurred. Recurrence of this syndrome is infrequent with subsequent infusions. ■ Monitor closely; in addition to the symptoms of infusion reaction noted above, severe and sometimes fatal hypersensitivity reactions (e.g., anaphylaxis, angioedema, bronchospasm, hypotension, urticaria) have occurred during and after the infusion. ■ Monitor closely throughout treatment for S/S of deteriorating cardiac function (e.g., cough, dyspnea, paroxysmal nocturnal dyspnea, peripheral edema, S_3 gallop, or reduced ejection fraction [symptomatic or asymptomatic]). ■ Monitor for thrombocytopenia (platelet count less than $50,000/mm^3$). Initiate precautions to prevent excessive bleeding (e.g., inspect IV sites, skin, and mucous membranes; use extreme care during invasive procedures; test urine, emesis, stool, and secretions for occult blood). ■ Not a vesicant; if extravasation occurs, discontinue infusion and restart using another vein.

Patient Education: During infusion, report chills and/or fever and other S/S of infusion reaction promptly. ■ Report cough, difficulty breathing, and swelling of extremities promptly. ■ Avoid pregnancy; nonhormonal birth control preferred. ■ See Appendix D, p. 1148.

Maternal/Child: Category B: use during pregnancy only if clearly needed. No evidence of impaired fertility or harm to the fetus in monkeys but HER2 protein expression is high in many embryonic tissues including cardiac and neural tissues. Discontinue breast-feeding during trastuzumab therapy and for 6 months after the last dose. ■ Safety and effectiveness for use in children not established.

Elderly: Advanced age may increase the risk of cardiac dysfunction.

DRUG/LAB INTERACTIONS

No formal drug interaction studies have been done. Use with paclitaxel may decrease trastuzumab clearance and increase serum levels. ■ Use in combination with cisplatin, doxorubicin, epirubicin, or cyclophosphamide did not suggest any interactions; however, risk of cardiotoxicity increased with concurrent use or previous use of anthracyclines (e.g., doxorubicin, epirubicin). ■ Bone marrow toxicity may be additive with other antineoplastic agents (e.g., anthracyclines, cyclophosphamide).

SIDE EFFECTS

Congestive heart failure and left ventricular dysfunction are dose-limiting side effects. Anemia and leukopenia, diarrhea, increased incidence of URIs or catheter infections, and infusion-related syndrome (e.g., chills, fever) are most common. Abdominal pain, accidental injury, acne, allergic reactions, anorexia, arthralgia, asthenia, back pain, bone pain, cough, depression, dizziness, dyspnea, edema, flu syndrome, headache, herpes simplex, hypotension, insomnia, nausea and vomiting, neuropathy, pain (may be at tumor site), paresthesia, peripheral edema, peripheral neuritis, pharyngitis, rash, rhinitis, sinusitis, and tachycardia have been reported in more than 5% of patients. Many other serious side effects have been reported in some patients (e.g., cardiac arrest, coagulation disorder, death; hypersensitivity reactions [e.g., angioedema, bronchospasm, dyspnea, urticaria, wheezing]; hypotension, non-cardiogenic pulmonary edema, pancytopenia, pericardial or pleural effusion, pulmonary infiltrates, pulmonary insufficiency and hypoxemia requiring O_2 and/or ventilatory support, shock arrhythmia, syncope, vascular thrombosis). Post-marketing reports of serious adverse events have included hypersensitivity reactions and infusion reactions, including some with a fatal outcome; and pulmonary events including ARDS and death. Symptoms occurred most commonly during the infusion, but some occurred 24 hours or more after the infusion.

ANTIDOTE

Notify physician of all side effects. Most will be treated symptomatically. Temporarily discontinue infusion if dyspnea or clinically significant hypotension occurs. Discontinue infusion, and strongly consider discontinuing trastuzumab therapy in patients who develop anaphylaxis, angioedema, ARDS, and/or a clinically significant decrease in left ventricular function. Strongly consider discontinuation of trastuzumab therapy in patients who develop clinically significant congestive heart failure. Safety of continuation or resumption of therapy has not been studied. Treatment may include diuretics, ACE inhibitors (e.g., lisinopril [Prinivil, Zestril], enalaprilat [Vasotec]), inotropic agents (e.g., digoxin, inamrinone [Inocor], isoproterenol [Isuprel]), beta-blockers (e.g., atenolol [Tenormin], propranolol [Inderal]), and/or supplemental oxygen. Infusion reaction is treated with acetaminophen, diphenhydramine, and meperidine. Administration of whole blood products (e.g., packed RBCs, platelets, leukocytes) and/or blood modifiers (e.g., darbepoetin alfa [Aranesp], epoetin alfa [Epogen, Procrit], filgrastim [Neupogen], pegfilgrastim [Neulasta], sargramostim [Leukine], oprelvekin [Neumega]) may be indicated to treat bone marrow toxicity from concurrent antineoplastics. Treat allergic reactions (may be more frequent with coadministration of paclitaxel) with epinephrine, antihistamines, corticosteroids, bronchodilators, and oxygen. To treat extravasation, apply cold compresses and elevate extremity. Resuscitate as indicated.

TRIMETREXATE GLUCURONATE

(tri-mi-trek′sat glu-kyur′uh-nat)

Antiprotozoal (folate antagonist)

Neutrexin

USUAL DOSE

See Monitor.

45 mg/M^2 once daily by IV infusion for 21 days. Must be given with concurrent leucovorin calcium 20 mg/M^2 every 6 hours (total dose of 80 mg/M^2/day) to avoid potentially serious or life-threatening toxicities. Leucovorin calcium must be given every day of trimetrexate treatment and for 72 hours after the last trimetrexate dose. Leucovorin calcium solution may be given before or following trimetrexate, but they cannot be mixed together. Flushing of line before and after leucovorin calcium with at least 10 ml of D5W is mandatory; see Incompatible With. See leucovorin calcium monograph for appropriate IV administration information.

PEDIATRIC DOSE

Unlabeled: Same as Usual Dose. See Maternal/Child.

DOSE ADJUSTMENTS

Reduce dose based on the worst hematologic toxicity.

Trimetrexate Dose Modification for Hematologic Toxicity				
Toxicity Grade	Neutrophils/mm^3	Platelets/mm^3	Trimetrexate Dose (mg/M^2)	Leucovorin Dose (mg/M^2)
1	>1,000	>75,000	45 mg/M^2 once daily	20 mg/M^2 every 6 hr
2	750-1,000	50,000-75,000	45 mg/M^2 once daily	40 mg/M^2 every 6 hr
3	500-749	25,000-49,999	22 mg/M^2 once daily	40 mg/M^2 every 6 hr
4	<500	<25,000	Day 1-9 any mg/M^2 discontinue Day 10-21 any mg/M^2 interrupt up to 96 hours	40 mg/M^2 every 6 hr

With grade 4 toxicity before day 10, discontinue trimetrexate and give leucovorin calcium 40 mg/M^2 every 6 hours for 72 hours. After day 10, trimetrexate dose may be withheld for up to 96 hours to allow counts to recover; continue leucovorin calcium. If counts recover to grade 3 in 96 hours administer that specific dose as above. When counts recover to grade 2 administer that specific dose as above and maintain increased leucovorin calcium dose for remainder of treatment. ■ Leucovorin calcium may be given PO if dose does not exceed 25 mg. Each dose should be rounded up to the next higher 25-mg increment. ■ Interrupt trimetrexate if transaminase levels or alkaline phosphatase levels increase to more than 5 times the upper limit of normal range. Interrupt trimetrexate if SrCr levels increase to more than 2.5 mg/dl and the increase is thought to be secondary to trimetrexate. ■ Interrupt trimetrexate if severe mucosal toxicity interferes with oral intake. ■ Discontinue trimetrexate for an oral temperature over 40.5° C (105° F) not responsive to antipyretics. ■ In all the above situations, continue leucovorin calcium every 6 hours for 72 hours after trimetrexate is discontinued. ■ See Drug/Lab Interactions.

DILUTION

Specific techniques required; see Precautions. Reconstitute each 25-mg vial with 2 ml D5W or SW (12.5 mg/ml). A pale greenish-yellow solution; must be clear and free from precipitation. Further dilute by using a 0.22-micron filter to add to D5W. Desired concentration range is 0.25 mg/ml to 2 mg/ml. A 100-mg dose in 50 ml diluent yields 2 mg/ml, in 400 ml diluent 0.25 mg/ml.

Storage: Store vials at CRT; protect from light. Reconstituted solution is stable at CRT for 6 hours or refrigerated for 24 hours. Do not freeze. Diluted solution is stable for 24 hours at CRT or refrigerated.

INCOMPATIBLE WITH

Will cause immediate precipitation with leucovorin calcium or any solution containing chloride ion (e.g., metronidazole [Flagyl IV], potassium chloride). See Usual Dose or Rate of Administration; flushing of line required.

COMPATIBLE WITH **(Underline Indicates Conflicting Compatibility Information)**

Consult pharmacist; specific conditions may apply; see Compatibilities, p. xvi.

Y-site: Amifostine (Ethyol), <u>zidovudine (AZT, Retrovir)</u>; see Monitor.

RATE OF ADMINISTRATION

A single dose as an infusion over 60 to 90 minutes. Flush IV line before and after administration with 10 ml D5W. See Precautions.

ACTIONS

A nonclassic folate antagonist and synthetic inhibitor of the enzyme dihydrofolate reductase (DHFR). Results in the disruption of DNA, RNA, and protein synthesis and causes cell death. Trimetrexate but not leucovorin calcium is selectively transported into the *P. carinii* organism. The concurrent administration of leucovorin calcium protects normal host cells from the cytotoxicity of trimetrexate without inhibiting trimetrexate's cytotoxicity to *P. carinii*. In one study distribution half-life ranged from 29 to 85 minutes and terminal half-life ranged from 13 to 19 hours. Metabolism in man is probably hepatic but has not been defined; does utilize the P_{450} enzyme system. 10% to 30% excreted unchanged in urine. Increased urine flow may increase clearance. Some excretion in feces. Crosses the placental barrier.

INDICATIONS AND USES

Alternative therapy with concurrent leucovorin calcium to treat moderate-to-severe *Pneumocystis carinii* pneumonia (PCP) in immunocompromised patients, including those with AIDS, who are intolerant of or refractory to sulfamethoxazole-trimethoprim (Bactrim) or pentamidine therapy or for whom either or both drugs are contraindicated.

Unlabeled uses: Treatment of *Pneumocystis carinii* pneumonia in children under 18 years of age. ■ Treatment of non–small-cell lung, prostate, and colorectal cancer.

CONTRAINDICATIONS

Clinically significant hypersensitivity to trimetrexate, leucovorin calcium, or methotrexate.

PRECAUTIONS

Follow guidelines for handling cytotoxic agents. See Appendix A, p. 1142. ■ Administered by or under the direction of the physician specialist, with facilities for monitoring the patient and responding to any medical emergency. ■ Must be used with concurrent leucovorin calcium to avoid potentially serious or life-threatening complications, including bone marrow suppression, oral and GI mucosal ulceration, and renal and hepatic dysfunction. ■ A known inhibitor of histamine metabolism. Allergic reactions, including anaphylaxis, have been reported. Most occurred following too-rapid injection, administration of higher than recommended doses, or when given in combination with fluorouracil (5-FU) and leucovorin calcium. ■ Pharmacokinetics of trimetrexate have not been determined in patients with impaired renal or hepatic dysfunction. Use with caution; see Dose Adjustments. ■ Use with caution in patients with impaired hematologic function. ■ See Monitor and Drug/Lab Interactions.

Monitor: CBC, including an absolute neutrophil count (ANC), and platelets, SrCr, BUN, AST, ALT and alkaline phosphatase should be monitored at least twice weekly throughout therapy. Carefully monitor patients who require concomitant therapy with nephrotoxic agents (e.g., aminoglycosides, antineoplastics, NSAIDs [e.g., ibuprofen (Advil, Motrin), naproxen (Aleve, Naprosyn)]), myelosuppressive (e.g., antineoplastics, ganciclovir), or hepatotoxic (e.g., IV fat emulsion [prolonged use], NSAIDs, phenytoin [Dilantin]). ■ Discontinue treatment with zidovudine during trimetrexate therapy to allow for full therapeutic doses of trimetrexate. ■ Monitor for symptoms of clinical deterioration; may have concurrent pulmonary conditions (e.g., bacterial, viral, or fungal pneumonia or mycobacterial diseases). ■ Prophylactic antiemetics may be indicated. ■ See Dose Adjustments, Precautions, and Drug/Lab Interactions.

Patient Education: Avoid pregnancy; nonhormonal birth control recommended. ■ Leucovorin calcium must be taken every 6 hours for a full 24 days; failure to do so can lead to fatal toxicity. ■ Zidovudine will be discontinued during trimetrexate therapy. ■ See Appendix D, p. 1148.

Maternal/Child: Category D: avoid pregnancy. Can cause significant maternal and fetotoxicity, as well as skeletal, visceral, ocular, and cardiovascular abnormalities. ■ Has caused degeneration of the testes and arrest of sperm formation in rats. ■ Discontinue breast-feeding. ■ Safety and effectiveness in children under age 18 have not been established. Has been used under Compassionate Use Protocol in children with no serious or unexpected adverse effects.

Elderly: Consider age-related organ impairment (e.g., bone marrow reserve, renal, hepatic).

DRUG/LAB INTERACTIONS

Plasma concentrations may be altered by any other agent metabolized by a P_{450} enzyme system (e.g., cimetidine [Tagamet], erythromycin, fluconazole [Diflucan], ketoconazole [Nizoral], rifabutin [Mycobutin], rifampin [Rifadin]). ■ Cimetidine may cause a significant reduction in trimetrexate metabolism and result in increased serum levels and toxicity. ■ Acetaminophen may compete for metabolites and alter concentration of trimetrexate metabolites. ■ Triazole antifungal agents (e.g., clotrimazole, ketoconazole, itraconazole [Sporanox], miconazole [Monistat]) may decrease metabolism and increase serum levels of trimetrexate; monitor carefully. ■ Additive bone marrow depression may occur when used concurrently or consecutively with other bone marrow depressants (e.g., antineoplastics) or radiation. Reduced doses may be indicated.

SIDE EFFECTS

Myelosuppression from hematologic toxicity (e.g., anemia, neutropenia, thrombocytopenia) is the usual dose-limiting side effect. Allergic reactions, including anaphylaxis; confusion; elevated serum alkaline phosphatase, ALT, AST, bilirubin, and creatinine; fatigue, fever, GI and oral mucosal ulceration, hypocalcemia, hyponatremia, nausea/vomiting, rash, pruritus, seizures (rare), and stomatitis can occur. May be difficult to distinguish from symptoms of underlying medical condition.

Overdose: Severe bone marrow suppression, oral and GI mucosal ulceration, renal and hepatic dysfunction.

ANTIDOTE

For accidental overdose, discontinue trimetrexate and give leucovorin calcium 40 mg/M^2 every 6 hours for 3 days. Keep physician informed of all side effects. Myelosuppression, stomatitis, and GI toxicities can generally be managed by increasing the dose of leucovorin calcium. Temporarily or permanently interrupt treatment for renal, hepatic, and mucosal toxicity and fever. Parameters described in Dose Adjustments.

TROMETHAMINE

(troe-meth′a-meen)

Tham

Alkalizing agent

pH 10 to 11.5

USUAL DOSE

Limit dose to amount needed to increase blood pH to normal limits (7.35 to 7.45) and to correct acid-base derangements. Evaluate the need for repeat doses by serial determinations of existing base deficit, pH, and clinical observations. Tham-E contains electrolytes.

Acidosis: Required dose (ml of 0.3 molar solution) equal to body weight in kilograms × base deficit in mEq/L × 1.1.

Acidosis in cardiac bypass surgery: 9 ml/kg of body weight. 500 ml (18 Gm) is an average adult dose. Up to 1,000 ml has been used. Never exceed 500 mg/kg in any individual dose over less than 1 hour.

Correct acidity of ACD priming blood: Stored blood has a pH of 6.22 to 6.8. An average of 60 ml (15 to 77 ml) tromethamine to each 500 ml of stored blood is required to correct pH to 7.4.

Acidosis in cardic arrest: Use only if indicated. Never inject into cardiac muscle. Initial dose in an open chest is 62 to 185 ml (2 to 6 Gm). Additional doses should be based on evaluation of base deficit. If the chest is not open, give 111 to 333 ml (3.6 to 10.8 Gm); use a large peripheral vein. After arrest is reversed, additional amounts may be needed to control persistent acidosis.

PEDIATRIC DOSE

Correction of metabolic acidosis associated with RDS in neonates and infants: 1 ml/kg of body weight for each pH unit below 7.4. Repeat doses may be given according to changes in $Pa{O_2}$, pH, and $P{CO_2}$.

DOSE ADJUSTMENTS

Lower-end initial doses may be appropriate in the elderly based on the potential for decreased organ function and concomitant disease or drug therapy.

DILUTION

Supplied as a 0.3 molar solution. Each 100 ml contains tromethamine 3.6 Gm in water for injection. May be given undiluted as an infusion or added to pump oxygenator blood, other priming fluid, or ACD blood.

Storage: Store at CRT. Single use container, discard unused solution.

COMPATIBILITY

Specific information not available. Consider specific use; consult pharmacist.

RATE OF ADMINISTRATION

Slow IV infusion recommended. 5 ml or less/min would deliver up to 300 ml in 1 hour. Rate dictated by patient's condition and intended use; see Usual Dose and Precautions. Reduced rate may control venospasm.

ACTIONS

Acts as a proton acceptor and actively binds hydrogen ions in metabolic acids and carbonic acid. Releases bicarbonate anions. Rapidly excreted in the urine, it has an osmotic diuretic effect, increases urine output, urine pH, and excretion of fixed acids, CO_2 and electrolytes. Also capable of neutralizing acidic ions of the intracellular fluid.

INDICATIONS AND USES

Prevention and correction of systemic acidosis; particularly metabolic acidosis associated with cardiac bypass surgery, correction of acidity of ACD blood in cardiac bypass surgery, and cardiac arrest.

CONTRAINDICATIONS

Hypersensitivity to tromethamine, anuria, and uremia. In neonates it is also contraindicated in chronic respiratory acidosis and salicylate intoxication.

PRECAUTIONS

Intended for short-term use only (1 day). ■ Sodium bicarbonate or sodium lactate is effective in most acidotic situations and has fewer side effects. ■ Use extreme caution in impaired renal function or decreased urine output.

Monitor: Determine blood pH, PCO_2, bicarbonate, glucose, and electrolytes before, during, and after administration. ■ Avoid overdose (total drug or too-rapid rate). Severe alkalosis and/or prolonged hypoglycemia may result. May cause fluid and/or solute overload, resulting in dilution of serum electrolyte concentrations, overhydration, congested states, or pulmonary edema. ■ Use a large peripheral vein. Determine absolute patency of vein; necrosis may result from extravasation. ■ May severely depress respiration. Incidence may be increased in patients who have chronic hypoventilation or those who have been treated with drugs that depress respiration. Oxygen and controlled ventilation equipment must always be available. ■ ECG monitoring and frequent serum potassium measurements are required to rule out hyperkalemia in impaired renal function or decreased urine output. Decreased excretion of tromethamine may also occur, resulting in toxicity.

Maternal/Child: Category C: safety for use not established. Benefits must outweigh risks. ■ Has been used to treat severe cases of metabolic acidosis with concurrent respiratory acidosis because it does not raise PCO_2 as bicarbonate does in neonates and infants with respiratory failure. It has also been used in neonates and infants with hypernatremia and metabolic acidosis to avoid the additional sodium given with the bicarbonate. However, because the osmotic effects of tromethamine are greater and large continuous doses are required, bicarbonate is preferred to tromethamine in the treatment of acidotic neonates and infants with RDS. ■ Severe hypoglycemia or severe hemorrhagic liver necrosis may occur in premature or full-term infants. ■ Infusion via low-lying umbilical venous catheters has been associated with hepatocellular necrosis. ■ Discontinue breast-feeding.

Elderly: Lower-end initial doses may be appropriate in the elderly; see Dose Adjustments. Differences in response between elderly and younger patients have not been identified.

DRUG/LAB INTERACTIONS

Potentiates amphetamines, ephedrine, and quinidine. ■ Inhibits lithium, methotrexate, and salicylates. ■ Incidence of respiratory depression may be increased in patients receiving drugs that depress respiration (e.g., narcotic analgesics [morphine]).

SIDE EFFECTS

Hyperkalemia, hypoglycemia, phlebitis, respiratory depression, and thrombosis.

Overdose: Alkalosis, overhydration, severe prolonged hypoglycemia, solute overload. May be due to total drug or too-rapid rate of administration.

ANTIDOTE

Notify physician of all side effects. Reduced rate of infusion may prevent hypoglycemia. Use glucose if indicated. Discontinue drug immediately for hyperkalemia or extravasation. Local infiltration with 1% procaine with phentolamine may reduce tissue necrosis. Use a number 25 needle. Symptomatic treatment is indicated. Alternate drugs are indicated (sodium bicarbonate, sodium lactate).

VALPROATE SODIUM

Anticonvulsant

(val-proe′ate so′de-um)

Depacon

pH 7.6

USUAL DOSE

Adults and children 10 years of age or older: For all indications optimal clinical response is usually achieved with doses less than 60 mg/kg/24 hr. Usual therapeutic range of plasma levels is 50 to 100 mcg/ml. A total daily dose exceeding 250 mg should be given in divided doses every 6 hours (studies used an every-6-hour regimen). See Precautions, Monitor, and Drug/Lab Interactions. Transfer to oral dosing as soon as practical. Oral and IV doses are considered to be equivalent and should be given at previously established intervals (e.g., every 6 or 8 hours).

Complex partial seizures (monotherapy): Begin with an initial dose of 10 to 15 mg/kg/24 hr. May be increased by 5 to 10 mg/kg/week until desired clinical response achieved or side effects are dose limiting.

Complex partial seizures (conversion to monotherapy): Begin with an initial dose of 10 to 15 mg/kg/24 hr. May be increased by 5 to 10 mg/kg/week until desired clinical response achieved. Concomitant antiepilepsy drug (AED) dosage can usually be reduced by 25% every 2 weeks. Dose of AEDs may be decreased at the beginning of valproate therapy or decrease may be delayed for 1 to 2 weeks to avoid unwanted seizures.

Complex partial seizures (adjunctive therapy): Begin with an initial dose of 10 to 15 mg/kg/24 hr. May be increased by 5 to 10 mg/kg/week until desired clinical response achieved.

Simple and complex absence seizures: Begin with an initial dose of 15 mg/kg/24 hr. May be increased by 5 to 10 mg/kg/week until seizures are controlled or side effects are dose limiting.

PEDIATRIC DOSE

No IV dose recommendations available for children under 10 years of age.

DOSE ADJUSTMENTS

Monitor plasma concentrations when transferring from oral to IV or IV to oral; dose increases or decreases may be indicated. ■ Reduce initial dose in the elderly; base subsequent doses on clinical response and/or development of side effects. ■ Reduced dose or discontinuation of therapy may be indicated if there is evidence of bruising, hemorrhage, or a disorder of hemostasis/coagulation. ■ Reduced doses and increased monitoring are indicated in hyperammonemia with or without lethargy or coma. Reduce dose further or discontinue if clinically significant symptoms occur (e.g., abnormal liver function tests, lethargy, coma). ▪ No dose adjustments required for impaired renal function, gender, or race. ▪ See Maternal/Child.

DILUTION

Each single dose should be diluted with at least 50 ml of D5W, NS, or LR. **Storage:** Store vials at CRT. Diluted solutions stable at CRT for 24 hours. No preservative added; discard unused contents of vial.

COMPATIBILITY

Specific information not available. Consider specific use; consult pharmacist.

RATE OF ADMINISTRATION

A single dose as an infusion over 60 minutes. Manufacturer has recommended that a rate of 20 mg/minute not be exceeded; however, a recent labeling change suggests that selected patients tolerated rates up to 3 mg/kg/min, allowing administration of up to 15 mg/kg/dose over 5 to 10 minutes. Incidence of side effects may be increased with too-rapid infusion.

ACTIONS

An anticonvulsant. A sodium salt of valproic acid. Therapeutic effect in epilepsy may result from increased brain concentrations of gamma-aminobutyric acid (GABA). Peak effect occurs at the end of a 60-minute infusion or 4 hours after an oral dose. Plasma protein binding is high and is concentration dependent. Concentration in CSF is similar to unbound concentrations in plasma (10%). Half-life range is 9 to 16 hours. The half-life will be in the lower part of the range in patients receiving other enzyme-inducing antiepileptic agents (e.g., carbamazepine [Tegretol], phenobarbital [Luminal], phenytoin [Dilantin]). Metabolized in the liver. 30% to 50% excreted in changed form in urine. Crosses placental barrier. Secreted in breast milk.

INDICATIONS AND USES

Use of IV product indicated in the following specific conditions when oral administration of valproate products (e.g., divalproex sodium [Depakote]) is temporarily not feasible. ▪ Treatment of complex partial seizures occurring in isolation or with other seizures (monotherapy or adjunctive therapy). ▪ Treatment of simple and complex absence seizures (monotherapy or adjunctive therapy). ▪ Adjunctive treatment of multiple seizure types that include absence seizures.

Unlabeled uses: Used alone or in combination with other antiepileptic drugs for treatment of absence, myoclonic and grand mal seizures and for treatment of patients with intractable status epilepticus who have not responded to other therapies.

CONTRAINDICATIONS

Known hypersensitivity to valproate products, patients with hepatic disease or significant hepatic dysfunction, and patients with known urea cycle disorders. ▪ Not recommended for use in patients with acute head trauma or for the prophylaxis of posttraumatic seizures.

PRECAUTIONS

Use of IV valproate for more than 14 days has not been studied. ▪ Use caution in patients with a history of hepatic disease. ▪ Has caused fatal hepatic failure. Risk further increased in patients who are on multiple anticonvulsants or have congenital metabolic disorders, severe seizure disorders with mental retardation, or organic brain disease. Children under 2 years of age are at greatest risk. Incidence of fatal hepatotoxicity decreases in progressively older patient groups. If valproate is used in patients with these increased risk factors or in children under 2 years of age with or without these increased risk factors, benefits must outweigh risks; use only as a sole agent with extreme caution. ■ Cases of life-threatening pancreatitis have been reported in both children and adults receiving valproate. Some of the cases have been described as hemorrhagic with rapid progression from initial symptoms to death. May occur at any time from shortly after initiation of therapy to years later. If pancreatitis is diagnosed, valproate should be discontinued. ■ Hyperammonemic encephalopathy has been reported in patients with urea cycle disorders (UCD); has been fatal. Before starting valproate, consider a possible diagnosis of UCD in patients with a history of unexplained encephalopathy or coma, encephalopathy associated with a protein load, pregnancy-related or postpartum encephalopathy, unexplained mental retardation, a history of elevated plasma ammonia or glutamine, cyclical vomiting or lethargy, episodic extreme irritability, ataxia, low BUN, protein avoidance, a family history of UCD or unexplained infant deaths, or any other S/S of UCD. ■ Some adverse effects (e.g., elevated liver enzymes and thrombocytopenia) appear to be dose-related. Must weigh benefit of improved therapeutic effect with higher doses against the possibility of an increased incidence of adverse effects. ■ Incidence of thrombocytopenia increases at total trough concentrations greater than 110 mcg/ml in females and greater than 135 mcg/ml in males. ■ Plasma protein binding is decreased and free fraction is increased in the elderly, in hyperlipidemic patients, in chronic hepatic disease, in impaired renal function, and in the presence of other drugs; see Drug/Lab Interactions. Total plasma concentrations may be normal, but free concentrations may be substantially elevated in these patients. ■ Reduce AED doses gradually to prevent status epilepticus in patients treated for major seizure activity. ■ In vitro studies suggest that valproate may stimulate the replication of the HIV and CMV viruses under certain experimental conditions. The clinical significance of this is unknown but should be kept in mind when evaluating patients with HIV or CMV.

Monitor: Thrombocytopenia, inhibition of the secondary phase of platelet aggregation, and abnormal coagulation parameters have been reported. Obtain baseline platelet counts and coagulation tests and monitor during therapy. Repeat before planned surgery. ■ Obtain baseline liver function tests and monitor frequently during therapy, especially during the first 6 months. ■ Observe closely for S/S of hepatotoxicity (e.g., anorexia, facial edema, lethargy, loss of seizure control, malaise, weakness, vomiting). ■ Abdominal pain, anorexia, nausea, and vomiting may be symptoms of pancreatitis and should be evaluated promptly. ■ Therapeutic serum levels for most patients will range from 50 to 100 mcg/ml; however, a good correlation has not been established between daily dose, serum levels, and therapeutic effect. ■ Monitor antiepileptic concentrations more frequently whenever concomitant AEDs are being introduced or withdrawn and observe closely for seizure activity. ■ Monitor serum concentrations more frequently if an asymptomatic elevation of ammonia occurs; may need to discontinue valproate sodium if hyperammonemia appears. ■ Monitor serum concentrations more frequently if any of the risk factors listed in Dose Adjustments or Precautions are present, and when any drugs that affect hepatic enzymes are introduced or discontinued; see Drug/Lab Interactions. ■ Evaluate for S/S of UCD; see Precautions and Antidote. ■ Total serum valproic acid concentration is affected by variable free-fractions of drug; consider hepatic metabolism and protein binding when interpreting valproic acid concentrations. ■ See Dose Adjustments, Precautions, and Drug/Lab Interactions for additional monitoring requirements.

Patient Education: May cause drowsiness; determine effects before driving or operating any machinery. ■ Consider birth control options. ■ Report symptoms such as abdominal pain, anorexia, jaundice, nausea, or vomiting promptly.

Maternal/Child: Category D: avoid pregnancy. Known to produce birth defects (e.g., spina bifida). Use during pregnancy only if essential for seizure management. Appropriate testing to detect birth defects is indicated. See package insert for additional information. ■ When used during pregnancy, valproate has caused clotting abnormalities, including afibrinogenemia in a newborn; monitor clotting parameters carefully. Has also caused hepatic failure in a newborn and an infant. ■ Effects on testicular development and sperm production not known. ■ Discontinue breast-feeding. ■ Neonates under 2 months have a markedly decreased ability to eliminate valproate compared to older children and adults. ■ Children 3 months to 10 years have 50% higher clearance rates based on weight. ■ Younger pediatric patients, especially those receiving enzyme-inducing drugs (e.g., carbamazepine, phenobarbital, phenytoin) will require larger maintenance doses to achieve therapeutic valproic acid concentrations. ■ IV product has not been studied in children under 2 years of age. ■ See Precautions and Monitor.

Elderly: May be more prone to adverse events. Initial dose should be lower, and dosage should be increased slowly. Rate of clearance decreased, free fraction increased; see Dose Adjustments. ■ Monitor for fluid, nutritional intake, dehydration, somnolence, and other adverse events.

DRUG/LAB INTERACTIONS

Clearance increased and effectiveness reduced by drugs that induce hepatic enzymes (e.g., phenytoin [Dilantin], carbamazepine [Tegretol], phenobarbital [Luminal], primidone [Mysoline]); increased monitoring of valproate and concomitant drug concentrations indicated. ■ Aspirin decreases protein binding, inhibits metabolism, and increases free concentration of valproate; use caution and monitor valproate concentrations if administered concomitantly. ■ Peak concentrations increased if coadministered with felbamate (Felbatol); reduced dose of valproate indicated. ■ Metabolism may be decreased and serum levels increased when given concurrently with chlorpromazine (Thorazine), cimetidine (Tagamet), or erythromycin. ■ Meropenem (Merrem) may reduce serum levels of valproate to subtherapeutic levels. ■ Rifampin (Rifadin) may increase clearance of valproate and require dose adjustment. ■ Inhibits metabolism of barbiturates (e.g., phenobarbital) and primidone, increasing their effects. Monitor for neurologic toxicity; obtain barbiturate serum levels and reduce barbiturate dose as indicated. ■ May increase or decrease serum levels of carbamazepine. ■ Concomitant use with clonazepam (Klonopin) may induce absence status in patients with a history of absence-type seizures. ■ Displaces some protein-bound drugs, inhibits their metabolism, and increases their effects (e.g., carbamazepine, diazepam [Valium], phenytoin, tolbutamide [Orinase], warfarin [Coumadin]). Dose adjustments and serum concentrations may be indicated. Phenytoin with valproate has caused breakthrough seizures in patients with epilepsy; adjust dose of phenytoin as indicated by serum concentrations. ■ Monitor coagulation tests if administered with anticoagulants (e.g., warfarin). ■ CNS effects may be increased when given concurrently with CNS depressants (e.g., benzodiazepines [e.g., diazepam (Valium)] and tricyclic antidepressants [e.g., amitriptyline (Elavil)]). ■ May decrease clearance and increase effects of amitriptyline (Elavil) and nortriptyline (Aventyl). Dose reduction of these drugs may be required. ■ Inhibits metabolism of ethosuximide (Zarontin); monitor serum concentrations of both drugs with concomitant administration. ■ Concurrent administration of lamotrigine (Lamictal) and valproate may decrease valproate levels and increase lamotrigine levels. Dose adjustments may be required. ■ Decreases clearance and may increase toxicity of zidovudine (AZT). ■ May decrease serum levels of cisplatin (Platinol) and doxorubicin (Adriamycin). ■ See package insert for additional information about many drugs that do not present significant clinical interactions. ■ May alter thyroid function tests. ■ May cause false-positive urine ketone test.

SIDE EFFECTS

Abdominal pain, abnormal gait, acute pancreatitis, anaphylaxis, chest pain, diarrhea, dizziness, elevated serum amylase, euphoria, hallucinations, headache, hyperesthesia, injection site reaction, insomnia, nausea, nervousness, parkinsonism, pharyngitis, pneumonia, taste perversion, somnolence, thrombocytopenia, tremor, vasodilation, vomiting. Frequency of elevated liver enzymes and thrombocytopenia may be dose related. Fatal hepatotoxicity (anorexia, facial edema, lethargy, loss of seizure control, malaise, sweating, weakness, vasodilation, vomiting) has occurred.

Overdose: Somnolence, deep coma, heart block. Some fatalities have been reported.

ANTIDOTE

Keep physician informed of all side effects. Some may respond to a decrease in the rate of administration. Discontinue immediately if signs of suspected or apparent significant hepatic dysfunction appear (e.g., hyperammonemia, elevated liver function tests) or S/S of underlying UCD. Hepatic dysfunction may progress after valproate is discontinued. Reduce dose or discontinue if bruising, hemorrhage, or abnormal coagulation parameters occur (e.g., thrombocytopenia). Maintain a patent airway and resuscitate as indicated. Support patient as required in treatment of overdose; monitor and maintain adequate urine output. Hemodialysis is effective in overdose. Naloxone (Narcan) may reverse CNS depressant effects in overdose but may also reverse antiepilepsy effects of valproate.

VANCOMYCIN HYDROCHLORIDE

(van-koe-mye′sin hye-droe-klor′id)

Antibacterial (tricylic-glycopeptide)

Vancocin, Vancoled

pH 2.4 to 4.5

USUAL DOSE

7.5 mg/kg or 500 mg every 6 hours or 15 mg/kg or 1 Gm every 12 hours for 7 to 10 days. Maximum dosage or 3 to 4 Gm/24 hr used only in extreme situations. Normal renal function required.

Prevention of bacterial endocarditis in selected penicillin-allergic patients having GI, biliary, or GU surgery or instrumentation (unlabeled use):
Adults and adolescents: 1 Gm IV before the procedure. Give gentamicin 1.5 mg/kg IV concurrently in high-risk patients (not to exceed 120 mg). Infusion must be administered over at least 60 minutes and should be complete within 30 minutes of starting the procedure. Gentamicin may not be necessary in moderate-risk patients. Both doses may be repeated in 8 to 12 hours for high-risk patients. Vancomycin alone may be indicated in selected patients having dental procedures or upper respiratory tract surgery or instrumentation. No longer recommended for standard use by the American Heart Association or the American Dental Association.

Treatment of patients with methicillin-resistant or methicillin-susceptible staphylococcal endocarditis who have a prosthetic valve or other prosthetic material: 30 mg/kg/24 hr equally divided into 2 doses (15 mg/kg every 12 hours) or 4 doses (7.5 mg/kg every 6 hours) for 6 weeks or longer. If more than 2 Gm/day are required, monitoring of serum concentrations of vancomycin is recommended. Given in conjunction with oral rifampin 300 mg every 8 hours for 6 weeks or longer and IM or IV gentamicin 1 mg/kg every 8 hours during the first 2 weeks of vancomycin therapy.

Treatment of endocarditis caused by viridans streptococci or Streptococcus bovis: 30 mg/kg/24 hr equally divided into 2 doses (15 mg/kg every 12 hours) for 4 weeks. If more than 2 Gm/day are required, monitoring of serum concentrations of vancomycin is recommended.

Treatment of enterococcal endocarditis: 30 mg/kg/24 hr equally divided into 2 doses (15 mg/kg every 12 hours) for 4 to 6 weeks. If more than 2 Gm/day are required, monitoring of serum concentrations of vancomycin is recommended. Given in conjunction with IM or IV gentamicin 1 mg/kg every 8 hours for 4 to 6 weeks.

Perioperative prophylaxis in selected surgeries (e.g., cardiac, prosthetic valve, coronary artery bypass, joint replacement, craniotomy) when a cephalosporin cannot be used or there is a high incidence of methicillin-resistant staphylococci at the institution (unlabeled use): 1 Gm IV 30 minutes before the start of surgery. May be repeated one or more times if surgery is prolonged or major blood loss occurs. Postoperative doses are considered generally unnecessary and are not recommended.

PEDIATRIC DOSE

Children and infants 1 month of age or older: 40 mg/kg of body weight/24 hr equally divided and given every 6 to 8 hours (10 mg/kg every 6 hours or 13.33 mg/kg every 8 hours) for 7 to 10 days. Up to 60 mg/kg/24 hr (15 mg/kg every 6 hours or 20 mg/kg every 8 hours) has been used if there is CNS involvement. Do not exceed 2 Gm in 24 hours.

Prevention of bacterial endocarditis in selected penicillin-allergic patients having GI, biliary, or GU surgery or instrumentation: 20 mg/kg before the procedure. Give gentamicin 1.5 mg/kg concurrently in high-risk patients (not to exceed 120 mg). Gentamicin may not be necessary in moderate-risk patients. Infusion must be administered over at least 60 minutes and should be complete within 30 minutes of starting the procedure. Both doses may be repeated in 8 to 12 hours for high-risk patients. Note comments about dental and upper respiratory surgery or instrumentation under Usual Dose.

NEONATAL DOSE

15 mg/kg as an initial dose. See Maternal/Child. Follow with 10 mg/kg. Adjust interval based on age and/or weight as follows:

Infants up to 1 week of age: Give every 12 hours.

Infants up to 1 month of age: Give every 8 hours.

Neonates under 7 days of age and under 1 kg: Give every 24 hours.

Neonates under 7 days of age and between 1 kg and 2 kg: Give every 18 hours.

Neonates over 7 days of age and under 1 kg: Give every 18 hours.

Another source suggests:

Low-birthweight neonates (weight less than 1.2 kg) and under 4 weeks of age: 15 mg/kg once every 24 hours.

Low-birthweight neonates (weight less than 1.2 kg at birth) over 4 weeks of age: 15 mg/kg once every 18 to 24 hours.

Under 1 week of age and weighing 2 kg or less: 10 to 15 mg/kg every 12 to 18 hours.

Under 1 week of age and weighing more than 2 kg: 10 to 15 mg/kg every 8 to 12 hours.

1 week of age or older and weighing 2 kg or less: 10 to 15 mg/kg every 8 to 12 hours.

1 week of age or older and weighing more than 2 kg: 10 to 15 mg/kg every 6 hours or 15 to 20 mg/kg every 8 hours.

DOSE ADJUSTMENTS

Reduce total daily dose in premature infants and the elderly. Greater dose reductions than expected may be necessary in these patients because of impaired renal function. ■ Dose reduction required in impaired renal function. In all renal impaired patients (including functionally anephric and anuric patients), the initial dose should be no less than 15 mg/kg. See product insert; dose is reduced for every decrease of 10 ml/min in the CrCl. Subsequent doses of 250 to 1,000 mg every several days are suggested for functionally anephric patients. Subsequent doses of 1,000 mg every 7 to 10 days are suggested for anuric patients. Monitoring of serum levels is recommended.

DILUTION

Available premixed, premixed and frozen, or reconstitute each 500-mg vial with 10 ml of SW for injection. Each 500 mg must be further diluted with 100 ml of NS or D5W and given as an intermittent infusion. Also compatible in D5NS, LR, D5LR, D5 Normosol-M, Isolyte E, and acetated Ringer's injection. Concentrations greater than 5 mg/ml are not recommended. If absolutely necessary, 1 to 2 Gm may be further diluted in sufficient amounts of the same infusion fluids and given over 24 hours. Not recommended. Also available in ADD-Vantage vials for use with ADD-Vantage infusion containers.

Storage: Store in refrigerator after initial dilution. Maintains potency for 2 weeks in D5W or NS, 96 hours for other infusion solutions. Solutions prepared from ADD-Vantage vials stable at room temperature for 24 hours.

INCOMPATIBLE WITH

Several sources recommend not admixing with other drugs. They suggest it is incompatible with alkaline solutions (e.g., aminophylline, aztreonam [Azactam], barbiturates [e.g., pentobarbital (Nembutal)], chloramphenicol [Chloromycetin], dexamethasone [Decadron], sodium bicarbonate) and may form a precipitate with heavy metals. May inactivate aminoglycosides; should also not be combined in the same solution with albumin, selected cephalosporins, foscarnet (Foscavir), or selected penicillins; if administered concurrently, administer at separate sites or separate intervals (flush IV line with a compatible solution before and after administration).

COMPATIBLE WITH **(Underline Indicates Conflicting Compatibility Information)**

Consult pharmacist; specific conditions may apply; see Compatibilities, p. xvi.

Additive: Amikacin (Amikin), aminophylline, atracurium (Tracrium), aztreonam (Azactam), calcium gluconate, cefepime (Maxipime), cimetidine (Tagamet), dimenhydrinate (Dinate), famotidine (Pepcid IV), heparin, hydrocortisone sodium succinate (Solu-Cortef), meropenem (Merrem IV), ofloxacin (Floxin IV), potassium chloride (KCl), ranitidine (Zantac), sodium bicarbonate, verapamil (Isoptin).

Y-site: Acyclovir (Zovirax), alatrofloxacin (Trovan IV), allopurinol (Aloprim, Zyloprim), amifostine (Ethyol), amiodarone (Cordarone), ampicillin, ampicillin/sulbactam (Unasyn), atracurium (Tracrium), aztreonam (Azactam), cefazolin (Kefzol), cefotaxime (Claforan), cefotetan (Cefotan), cefoxitin (Mefoxin), ceftazidime (Fortaz), ceftizoxime (Cefizox), ceftriaxone (Rocephin), cefuroxime (Zinacef), cisatracurium (Nimbex), cyclophosphamide (Cytoxan), diltiazem (Cardizem), docetaxel (Taxotere), doxorubicin liposome (Doxil), enalaprilat (Vasotec IV), esmolol (Brevibloc), etoposide phosphate (Etopophos), filgrastim (Neupogen), fluconazole (Diflucan), fludarabine (Fludara), foscarnet (Foscavir), gemcitabine (Gemzar), granisetron (Kytril), hetastarch in electrolytes (Hextend), hydromorphone (Dilaudid), insulin (regular), labetalol (Normodyne), levofloxacin (Levaquin), linezolid (Zyvox), lorazepam (Ativan), magnesium sulfate, melphalan (Alkeran), meperidine (Demerol), meropenem (Merrem IV), methotrexate (Folex), midazolam (Versed), morphine, nafcillin (Nafcil), ondansetron (Zofran), paclitaxel (Taxol), pancuronium (Pavulon), perphenazine (Trilafon), piperacillin (Pipracil), piperacillin/tazobactam (Zosyn), propofol (Diprivan), remifentanil (Ultiva), sargramostim (Leukine), sodium bicarbonate, tacrolimus (Prograf), teniposide (Vumon), theophylline, thiotepa (Thioplex), ticarcillin (Ticar), ticarcillin/clavulanate (Timentin), vecuronium (Norcuron), vinorelbine (Navelbine), warfarin (Coumadin), zidovudine (AZT, Retrovir).

RATE OF ADMINISTRATION

Severe hypotension, with or without red blotching of the face, neck, chest, and extremities, and cardiac arrest can occur with too-rapid injection.

A single dose properly diluted (concentration of no more than 5 mg/ml) at a rate not to exceed 10 mg/min or 60 minutes, whichever is longer. Another reference suggests infusion over 1 to 2 hours. This intermittent infusion is the preferred route of administration because of high incidence of thrombophlebitis.

Pediatric rate: A single dose over a minimum of 60 minutes.

ACTIONS

A very potent tricyclic glycopeptide antibiotic, it is bactericidal against gram-positive organisms. Well distributed in all body tissues and fluids including spinal fluid if the meninges are inflamed. Vancomycin is excreted in biologically active form in the urine. Crosses the placental barrier. Secreted in breast milk.

INDICATIONS AND USES

Serious gram-positive infections (e.g., staphylococcal) infections including endocarditis, septicemia, bone, lower respiratory tract, and skin and skin structure infections that do not respond or are resistant to other less toxic antibiotics, such as penicillins or cephalosporins. ■ To substitute for contraindicated penicillin therapy if absolutely necessary. ■ Treatment of endocarditis caused by *Streptococcus viridans* or *S. bovis* concurrently with an aminoglycoside antibiotic; endocarditis caused by diphtheroids or *S. epidermidis* concurrently with rifampin and/or an aminoglycoside. ■ Parenteral form used orally for pseudomembranous colitis/staphylococcal enterocolitis caused by *C. difficile.*

Unlabeled uses: Prophylaxis against bacterial endocarditis in moderate or high-risk (prosthetic heart valves, congenital or rheumatic heart disease) penicillin-allergic patients undergoing GI, biliary or GU surgery or instrumentation. Given in combination with gentamicin (Garamycin) in GI or GU procedures.

CONTRAINDICATIONS

Known hypersensitivity to vancomycin.

PRECAUTIONS

Sensitivity studies necessary to determine susceptibility of the causative organism to vancomycin. ■ Prolonged use of drug may result in superinfection caused by overgrowth of nonsusceptible organisms. ■ May be ototoxic and nephrotoxic. Some clinicians feel the risk of ototoxicity and nephrotoxicity is minimal in patients with normal renal function who receive vancomycin as a single agent. ■ Use caution in impaired hearing, impaired renal function, pregnancy, breast-feeding, neonates, and the elderly. ■ Pseudomembranous colitis has been reported. May range from mild to life-threatening. Consider in patients that present with diarrhea during or after treatment with vancomycin. ■ Oral vancomycin has a local effect only (e.g., in the bowel); not for systemic use.

Monitor: Monitoring of serum levels and SrCr may be indicated in patients at increased risk for developing nephrotoxicity and/or ototoxicity (e.g., underlying renal dysfunction, or receiving concomitant aminoglycosides [e.g., gentamicin]). ■ Determine absolute patency of vein. Necrosis and sloughing will result from extravasation. Rotate injection sites every 2 to 3 days. ■ Observe for furry tongue, diarrhea, and foul-smelling stools. ■ Severe hypotension, with or without red blotching of the face, neck, chest, and extremities, and cardiac arrest can occur with too-rapid injection (red man or red neck syndrome). ■ Monitor BP continuously during infusion to prevent a precipitous drop. ■ Auditory testing indicated with prolonged use. ■ Periodic monitoring of leukocyte count recommended in prolonged therapy. ■ See Drug/Lab Interactions.

Maternal/Child: Category C: studies not conclusive. Use only if clearly needed. ■ Safety for use in breast-feeding not established; discontinue breast-feeding. ■ Neonates have immature renal function; blood levels may be excessive. Confirmation of desired serum concentrations suggested in premature and full-term neonates.

Elderly: Systemic and renal clearance may be reduced; dosage reduction required.

DRUG/LAB INTERACTIONS

Use caution with dimenhydrinate (Dramamine), which can mask ototoxicity. ■ May potentiate nephrotoxicity of neuromuscular blocking antibiotics (e.g., gentamicin, tobramycin). ■ May be potentiated by other nephrotoxic, neurotoxic, or ototoxic drugs (e.g., cisplatin, ethacrynic acid [Edecrin], furosemide [Lasix]). ■ May enhance neuromuscular blockade with nondepolarizing muscle relaxants (e.g., pancuronium [Pavulon], mivacurium [Mivacron]). ■ May cause muscle paralysis and respiratory collapse with succinylcholine. ■ May cause erythema and histamine-like flushing in children with anesthetics. ■ May inhibit methotrexate excretion and increase methotrexate toxicity. May occur even if 10 days have elapsed since vancomycin administered. Adjust methotrexate dose as indicated.

SIDE EFFECTS

Chills, dizziness, fever, macular rashes, pain at injection site, pruritus, tinnitus, urticaria.

Major: Anaphylaxis, cardiac arrest, dyspnea, eosinophilia, hearing loss, hypotension, interstitial nephritis, neutropenia, pseudomembranous colitis, red neck or red man syndrome, renal failure, Stevens-Johnson syndrome (erythema multiforme [flu-like symptoms that can be fatal]), thrombophlebitis, wheezing.

ANTIDOTE

Notify the physician of all side effects. Hearing loss may progress even if drug is discontinued. If minor side effects are progressive or any major side effect occurs, discontinue the drug, treat allergic reaction, or resuscitate as necessary. Prevent severe hypotension by slowing infusion rate to 2 hours. Fluids, antihistamines, corticosteroids, and vasopressors (e.g., dopamine [Intropin]) may be required. Hemodialysis or CAPD will not decrease blood levels in toxicity.

VASOPRESSIN INJECTION

(vay-soe-press′in in-jek′shun)

Hormone
Antidiuretic
Vasopressor (unlabeled)

Pitressin, ✤ Pressyn

pH 2.5 to 4.5

USUAL DOSE

IV use is unlabeled. AHA Emergency Cardiovascular Care recommends 40 units by IV push or through the endotracheal tube for 1 dose only.

PEDIATRIC DOSE

Use in adults as a vasopressor is unlabeled; safety or effectiveness for IV use in pediatric patients not established, and use is not recommended.

DILUTION

AHA Guidelines do not mention the use of a diluent, which suggests that vasopressin may be given undiluted. Another source recommends dilution for IV use to a 0.1 to 1 unit/ml dilution with NS or D5W. 38 ml diluent to 2 ml vasopressin (40 units) yields 1 unit/ml.

Storage: Store unopened vials at CRT.

COMPATIBILITY

Specific information not available. Consider specific use and unlabeled IV use; consult pharmacist. One source lists it as compatible as an additive with verapamil (Isoptin).

RATE OF ADMINISTRATION

A single dose IV push; see Precautions.

ACTIONS

Synthetic vasopressin of the posterior pituitary gland standardized to 20 units/ml. An antidiuretic. Also a potent vasoconstrictor. Causes smooth muscle contraction of all parts of the vascular bed (e.g., capillaries, small arterioles, and venules). Has a lesser effect on the smooth muscles of larger arteries and veins. This direct contractile effect on the smooth muscle of the vascular system is not antagonized by adrenergic blocking agents (e.g., atenolol [Tenormin], metoprolol [Lopressor]) and is not prevented by vascular denervation (loss of nerve impulse to the vascular system). Its IV use is as an alternative pressor agent to epinephrine. Rapidly metabolized and destroyed in the liver and kidneys. Plasma half-life is 10 to 20 minutes. A small amount is excreted unchanged in the urine.

INDICATIONS AND USES

Used IM or SC as an antidiuretic in central diabetes insipidus or as a diagnostic aid in diabetes insipidus.

Unlabeled uses: The AHA Handbook of Emergency Cardiovascular Care recommends use in the treatment of adult shock-refractory ventricular fibrillation (class IIb) (an alternative pressor agent to epinephrine) and for hemodynamic support in vasodilatory shock (e.g., septic shock). ***IV uses are unlabeled.***

CONTRAINDICATIONS

Hypersensitivity to vasopressin or any of its components; see Precautions. AHA Guidelines state "not recommended for responsive patients with coronary heart disease."

PRECAUTIONS

IV uses are unlabeled. ■ Precautions listed are for the approved use of this medication and may not be as applicable to the unlabeled IV use. ■ Use with extreme caution in patients with vascular disease, especially coronary artery disease; may cause cardiac ischemia. Small doses may precipitate anginal pain, and larger doses may cause myocardial infarction. ■ May produce water intoxication; use with caution in patients with asthma, epilepsy, heart failure, migraine, or any conditions in which a rapid addition to extracellular water could be hazardous.

Monitor: Used only during emergency cardiac care in non-responsive patients. In addition to management of airway, oxygenation, and blood gas determinations, the continuous monitoring of ECG, vital signs, and fluid and electrolyte status is mandatory. ■ Use an indwelling urinary catheter to confirm urine output. ■ Fluid restriction may be indicated; initial signs of water intoxication include drowsiness, listlessness, and headache, which can rapidly progress to terminal coma and convulsions.

Maternal/Child: Category C: safety for use during pregnancy not established; use only if clearly needed. ■ Safety for use during breast-feeding not established.

Elderly: See Precautions; elderly may be more sensitive to adverse effects.

DRUG/LAB INTERACTIONS

Additive pressor response with ganglionic blocking agents (e.g., trimethaphan [Arfonad (rarely used antihypertensive)]). ■ Antidiuretic effect may be increased with concurrent use of carbamazepine (Tegretol), chlorpropamide (Diabinese), clofibrate (Atromid-S), fludrocortisone (Florinef), tricyclic antidepressants (e.g., amitriptyline [Elavil]), urea. ■ Antidiuretic effect may be decreased with concurrent use of alcohol, demeclocycline (Declomycin), heparin, lithium (Carbolith), norepinephrine (Levophed).

SIDE EFFECTS

Abdominal cramps, anaphylaxis, angina, arrhythmias, bronchial constriction, cardiac arrest, circumoral pallor, cutaneous gangrene, decreased cardiac output, diaphoresis, flatus, gangrene, headache (pounding), myocardial ischemia, nausea, peripheral vasoconstriction, shock, sweating, tremor, urticaria, vertigo, and vomiting.

Overdose: Water intoxication.

ANTIDOTE

In an emergency cardiac care situation, all side effects can present life-threatening additional problems. Monitor the patient closely and observe all S/S that may indicate further deterioration. Treat symptomatically according to AHA Guidelines. Treat water intoxication with water restriction and discontinue vasopressin. If severe, may require osmotic diuresis with mannitol, hypertonic dextrose, or urea alone or with furosemide (Lasix).

VECURONIUM BROMIDE

(vek′u-ro′ne-um bro′mid)

Neuromuscular blocking agent (nondepolarizing)
Anesthesia adjunct

Norcuron — **pH 4**

USUAL DOSE

Adjunct to general anesthesia: Must be individualized, depending on previous drugs administered and degree and length of muscle relaxation required. 0.08 to 0.1 mg/kg (80 to 100 mcg/kg) of body weight initially as an IV bolus. Must be used with adequate anesthesia and/or sedation and after unconsciousness induced. Determine need for ***maintenance dose*** based on beginning symptoms of neuromuscular blockade reversal determined by a peripheral nerve stimulator. ***IV bolus:*** 0.01 to 0.015 mg/kg (10 to 15 mcg/kg) will be required in approximately 25 to 40 minutes and every 12 to 20 minutes thereafter to maintain muscle relaxation. Higher doses (0.15 to 0.28 mg/kg) at longer intervals have been given with proper ventilation without causing adverse cardiac effects. ***Continuous infusion:*** 1 mcg/kg/min. Begin in 20 to 40 minutes after initial bolus dose.

Support of intubated, mechanically ventilated, or respiratory-controlled adult ICU patients (unlabeled): IV bolus injection: 0.1 to 0.2 mg/kg (100 to 200 mcg/kg) every 1 hour. ***Continuous infusion:*** Begin with a loading dose of 0.1 mg/kg (100 mcg/kg) followed by a ***maintenance dose*** of 0.05 to 0.1 mg/kg/hr (50 to 100 mcg/kg/hr). A lower-end or reduced dose may be indicated if administered more than 5 minutes after the start of an inhalation agent, when steady-state has been achieved, or in patients with organ dysfunction (e.g., impaired liver function). Adjust dose according to clinical assessment of the patient's response. Use of a peripheral nerve stimulator is recommended. Vecuronium may be the preferred agent for patients with renal failure.

PEDIATRIC DOSE

Adjunct to general anesthesia: 1 to 10 years of age: May require high end of initial adult dose, and maintenance dose may be required on a more frequent basis.

DOSE ADJUSTMENTS

Reduce dose by 15% if administered more than 5 minutes after inhalation general anesthetics. ■ Reduce dose to 0.04 to 0.06 mg/kg if following succinylcholine administration. Succinylcholine must show signs of wearing off before vecuronium is given. Use caution. ■ Reduced dose required with numerous drugs; see Drug/Lab Interactions. ■ Reduced dose may be required in renal or hepatic impairment. Preparation by dialysis before surgery is recommended for patients with renal failure. In an emergency surgery when dialysis cannot be accomplished, consider a lower initial dose. ■ Infants between 7 weeks and 1 year may require a slightly lower dose, and recovery time will be extended.

DILUTION

Each 10 mg must be diluted with 5 ml SW for injection (supplied). May be given by IV injection or 10 (20) mg may be further diluted in up to 100 ml NS, D5W, D5NS, or LR and given as an infusion 0.1 (0.2) mg/ml concentration. Titrated to symptoms of neuromuscular blockade reversal. **Storage:** Stable at room temperature before reconstitution. Store under refrigeration. Discard after 24 hours except if reconstituted with bacteriostatic water; stable refrigerated up to 5 days.

COMPATIBLE WITH

Consult pharmacist; specific conditions may apply; see Compatibilities, p. xvi.
Y-site: Aminophylline, cefazolin (Kefzol), cefuroxime (Zinacef), cimetidine (Tagamet), diltiazem (Cardizem), dobutamine (Dobutrex), dopamine (Intropin), epinephrine (Adrenalin), esmolol (Brevibloc), fentanyl (Sublimaze), fluconazole (Diflucan), gatifloxacin (Tequin), gentamicin (Garamycin), heparin, hetastarch in electrolytes (Hextend), hydrocortisone sodium succinate (Solu-Cortef), hydromorphone (Dilaudid), isoproterenol (Isuprel), labetalol (Normodyne), linezolid (Zyvox), lorazepam (Ativan), midazolam (Versed), milrinone (Primacor), morphine, nicardipine (Cardene IV), nitroglycerin (Nitro-Bid IV), nitroprusside sodium, norepinephrine (Levophed), propofol (Diprivan), ranitidine (Zantac), sulfamethoxazole-trimethoprim (Bactrim), vancomycin (Vancocin).

RATE OF ADMINISTRATION

Adjunct to general anesthesia: A single dose as an IV bolus over 30 to 60 seconds. If maintenance dose is given as an infusion, adjust rate to specific dose desired, usually 1 mcg/kg/min. See chart, Guidelines for Vecuronium Infusion.

Vecuronium Guidelines for Infusion During General Anesthesia		
Desired Vecuronium Delivery Rate (mcg/kg/min)	Vecuronium Infusion Delivery Rate (mL/kg/min)	
	0.1 mg/ml*	**0.2 mg/ml****
0.7	0.007	0.0035
0.8	0.008	0.0040
0.9	0.009	0.0045
1.0	0.010	0.0050
1.1	0.011	0.0055
1.2	0.012	0.0060
1.3	0.013	0.0065

*10 mg of Norcuron® in 100 ml solution
**20 mg of Norcuron® in 100 ml solution

Mechanical ventilation support in ICU: Dose must be calculated, chart is for use during general anesthesia only. See Usual Dose for specific rates and criteria.

ACTIONS

A nondepolarizing skeletal muscle relaxant about one-third more potent than pancuronium with a shorter duration of neuromuscular blockade. Acts by competing for cholinergic receptors at the motor end-plate. Onset of action is within 30 seconds, is dose dependent, produces maximum neuromuscular blockade (paralysis) within 3 to 5 minutes, and lasts about 25 minutes. It may take up to 60 minutes or more before complete recovery occurs. Up to three times the therapeutic dose has been given without significant changes of hemodynamic parameters in good-risk surgical patients. Excreted as metabolites in bile and urine. Crosses the placental barrier.

INDICATIONS AND USES

Adjunctive to general anesthesia, to facilitate endotracheal intubation and to relax skeletal muscles during surgery or mechanical ventilation.

Unlabeled uses: Support of intubated, mechanically ventilated, or respiratory-controlled patients in ICU.

CONTRAINDICATIONS

Known hypersensitivity to vecuronium.

PRECAUTIONS

For IV use only. ■ Administered by or under the direct observation of the anesthesiologist. ■ Repeated doses have no cumulative effect if recovery is allowed to begin before administration. ■ Use extreme caution in patients with cirrhosis, cholestasis, obesity, or circulatory insufficiency. ■ Myasthenia gravis and other neuromuscular diseases increase sensitivity to drug. Can cause critical reactions. ■ Acid base and/or electrolyte imbalance, debilitation, hypoxic episodes, and/or the use of other drugs (e.g., broad-spectrum antibiotics, narcotics, steroids) may prolong the effects of vecuronium.

Monitor: ***All uses:*** This drug produces apnea. Controlled artificial ventilation with oxygen must be continuous and under direct observation at all times.

Maintain a patent airway. ■ Use a peripheral nerve stimulator to monitor response to vecuronium and avoid overdose. Have reversal agents available (e.g., edrophonium, neostigmine, pyridostigmine with atropine or glycopyrrolate); see Antidote. ■ Patient may be conscious and completely unable to communicate by any means. Has no analgesic or sedative properties. Respiratory depression with morphine may be preferred in some patients requiring mechanical ventilation. ■ Action is altered by dehydration, electrolyte imbalance, body temperatures, and acid-base imbalance. ■ Recovery time extended in infants 7 weeks to 1 year. ■ See Drug/Lab Interactions. ***Mechanical ventilation support in ICU:*** Physical therapy is recommended to prevent muscular weakness, atrophy, and joint contracture. Muscular weakness may be first noticed during attempts to wean patients from the ventilator.

Maternal/Child: Category C: use in pregnancy only if use justifies potential risk to fetus. Has been used during cesarean section; monitor infant carefully. Action may be enhanced by magnesium administered for the management of toxemia of pregnancy. ■ Use caution during breast-feeding. ■ Safety for use in infants under 7 weeks of age not established. ■ Some preparations contain benzyl alcohol; do not use in premature infants. ■ See Dose Adjustments.

DRUG/LAB INTERACTIONS

Potentiated by acidosis, hypokalemia, some carcinomas, general anesthetics (e.g., enflurane, isoflurane, halothane), many antibiotics (e.g., clindamycin [Cleocin], kanamycin [Kantrex], gentamicin [Garamycin]), polypeptide antibiotics (e.g., bacitracin, colistimethate), tetracyclines, diuretics, diazepam (Valium) and other muscle relaxants, magnesium sulfate, quinidine, morphine, meperidine, succinylcholine, verapamil, and others. May need to reduce dose of vecuronium. Use with caution. ■ Effects may be decreased by acetylcholine, alkalosis, anticholinesterases, azathioprine, carbamazepine, phenytoin, and theophylline. ■ Succinylcholine must show signs of wearing off before vecuronium is given. Use caution.

SIDE EFFECTS

No side effects have occurred except with overdose: prolonged action resulting in respiratory insufficiency or apnea, airway closure caused by relaxation of epiglottis, pharynx, and tongue muscles. Hypersensitivity reactions including anaphylaxis are possible. Muscular weakness and atrophy may occur with long-term use (1 to 3 weeks).

ANTIDOTE

All side effects are medical emergencies. Treat symptomatically. Controlled artificial ventilation must be continuous until full muscle control returns. Edrophonium (Enlon), pyridostigmine (Mestinon) or neostigmine (Prostigmin) given with atropine or glycopyrrolate will probably reverse the muscle relaxation but should not be required because of short time of effectiveness. Not effective in all situations; may aggravate severe overdose. Resuscitate as necessary.

VERAPAMIL HYDROCHLORIDE

(ver-ap′a-mill hye-droe-klor′id)

Isoptin

Calcium channel blocker
Antiarrhythmic

pH 4.1 to 6

USUAL DOSE

5 to 10 mg initially (0.075 to 0.15 mg/kg of body weight). May cause transient bradycardia or hypotension. 10 mg (0.15 mg/kg) may be repeated in 30 minutes if needed to achieve appropriate response. Maximum total dose is 20 mg. AHA recommendation is 2.5 to 5 mg as an initial dose. Repeat 5 to 10 mg in 15 to 30 min. Maximum dose 20 mg or give 5 mg every 15 min to a total dose of 30 mg. Sometimes given as an infusion after initial bolus dose ***(unlabeled).***

PEDIATRIC DOSE

Infants up to 1 year of age: 0.1 to 0.2 mg/kg of body weight (usually 0.75 to 2 mg). Repeat in 30 minutes if indicated.

1 to 15 years of age: 0.1 to 0.3 mg/kg (usually 2 to 5 mg). Do not exceed 5 mg. Repeat in 30 minutes if response not adequate. Repeat dose should not exceed 10 mg as a single dose.

DOSE ADJUSTMENTS

Reduced dose may be required in hepatic or renal disease, especially with repeat dosing. ■ See Drug/Lab Interactions.

DILUTION

IV injection: May be given undiluted through Y-tube or three-way stopcock of tubing containing D5W, NS, or Ringer's solution for infusion or further diluted for infusion (1 mg/ml).

Infusion (unlabeled): Verapamil 100 mg (40 ml) diluted in 60 ml D5W equals 1 mg/ml. More diluent may be used (100 mg in 360 ml diluent equals 0.25 mg/ml). Use with extreme caution.

Storage: Protect from light. Do not use if discolored or particulate matter present. Discard unused solution.

INCOMPATIBLE WITH

Manufacturer states, "Forms a precipitate with nafcillin (Nafcil) or sodium bicarbonate in ½NS and will precipitate in any solution with a pH greater than 6." Lists as incompatible with albumin, aminophylline, amphotericin B (Fungizone), hydralazine, sulfamethoxazole-trimethoprim (Bactrim).

COMPATIBLE WITH

(Underline Indicates Conflicting Compatibility Information)

See Incompatible With. Consult pharmacist; specific conditions may apply; see Compatibilities, p. xvi.

Additive: Amikacin (Amikin), aminophylline, amiodarone (Cordarone), ampicillin, ascorbic acid (Cenolate), atropine, bretylium (Bretylate), calcium chloride, calcium gluconate, cefamandole (Mandol), cefazolin (Kefzol), cefotaxime (Claforan), cefoxitin (Mefoxin), chloramphenicol (Chloromycetin), cimetidine (Tagamet), clindamycin (Cleocin), dexamethasone (Decadron), diazepam (Valium), digoxin (Lanoxin), dobutamine (Dobutrex), dopamine (Intropin), epinephrine (Adrenalin), erythromycin lactobionate (Erythrocin), furosemide (Lasix), gentamicin (Garamycin), heparin, hydrocortisone (Hydrocortone, Solu-Cortef), hydromorphone (Dilaudid), insulin (regular), isoproterenol (Isuprel), lidocaine, magnesium sulfate, mannitol, meperidine (Demerol), methyldopate (Aldomet), methylprednisolone (Solu-Medrol), metoclopramide (Reglan), morphine, multivitamins (M.V.I.), nafcillin (Nafcil), naloxone (Narcan), nitroglycerin (Nitro-Bid IV), nitroprusside sodium, norepinephrine (Levophed), oxacillin (Bactocill), oxytocin (Pitocin), pancuronium (Pavulon), penicillin G potassium and sodium, pentobarbital (Nembutal), phenobarbital (Luminal), phentolamine (Regitine), phenytoin (Dilantin), piperacillin (Pipracil), potassium chloride (KCl), potassium phosphate, procainamide (Pronestyl), propranolol (Inderal), protamine sulfate, quinidine gluconate, sodium bicarbonate, theophylline, ticarcillin (Ticar), tobramycin (Nebcin), vancomycin (Vancocin), vasopressin (Pitressin).

Syringe: Heparin, inamrinone (Inocor), milrinone (Primacor).

Y-site: Ciprofloxacin (Cipro IV), dobutamine (Dobutrex), dopamine (Intropin), famotidine (Pepcid IV), gatifloxacin (Tequin), hetastarch in electrolytes (Hextend), hydralazine, inamrinone (Inocor), linezolid (Zyvox), meperidine (Demerol), milrinone (Primacor), penicillin G potassium, piperacillin (Pipracil), ticarcillin (Ticar).

RATE OF ADMINISTRATION

IV injection: A single dose over 2 minutes for adults and children. Extend to 3 minutes in the elderly.

Infusion: Infusion pump required; separate IV line preferred to ensure accuracy and prevent accidental bolusing during addition of other fluids. Rate may be constant (e.g., 5 to 10 mg/hr) or titrated to HR.

ACTIONS

A calcium (and possibly sodium) ion inhibitor through slow channels. Slows conduction through SA and AV nodes, prolongs effective refractory period in the AV node, and reduces ventricular rates. Prevents reentry phenomena through the AV node. Reduces myocardial contractility, afterload, arterial pressure, vascular tone, and oxygen demand. Effective within 1 to 5 minutes. Hemodynamic effects last about 20 minutes, but antiarrhythymic effects may last up to 6 hours. Does not alter total serum calcium levels. Metabolized in the liver. Crosses the placental barrier. Excreted in urine and feces. Secreted in breast milk.

INDICATIONS AND USES

Treatment of supraventricular tachyarrhythmias including conversion to normal sinus rhythm of paroxysmal supraventricular tachycardia (includes Wolff-Parkinson-White and Lown-Ganong-Levine syndromes). ■ Temporary control of rapid ventricular rate in atrial flutter or atrial fibrillation. ■ Narrow-complex PSVT not responsive to adenosine.

CONTRAINDICATIONS

Atrial fibrillation or flutter when associated with an accessory bypass tract (e.g., Wolff-Parkinson-White or Lown-Ganong-Levine syndromes), cardiogenic shock, congestive heart failure (severe) unless secondary to supraventricular tachyarrhythmia treatable with verapamil, known sensitivity to verapamil, second- or third-degree AV block, severe hypotension, sick sinus syndrome (unless functioning artificial pacemaker in place), patients receiving IV beta-adrenergic blocking drugs (e.g., propranolol [Inderal]) within 2 to 4 hours, and ventricular tachycardia.

PRECAUTIONS

Valsalva maneuver recommended before use of verapamil in all paroxysmal supraventricular tachycardias if clinically appropriate. ■ Caution required in hepatic and renal disease, especially if repeated dosing is required. ■ Use extreme caution in patients with hypertrophic cardiomyopathy. ■ May cause ventricular fibrillation in patients with wide-complex ventricular tachycardia. ■ May precipitate respiratory muscle failure in patients with muscular dystrophy or increase intracranial pressure during anesthesia induction in patients with supratentorial tumors. Use caution. ■ Reduction of myocardial contractility may worsen CHF in patients with severe left ventricular dysfunction. ■ Continue regular dosing on day of surgery and thereafter unless otherwise specified by physician. May cause severe angina or MI if discontinued. ■ Recent studies indicate that verapamil inhibits thrombus formation and platelet aggregation.

Monitor: ECG monitoring during administration mandatory for infants and children, and during an infusion; recommended for all others. ■ Document cardiac rhythm before therapy, with any significant change in type or rate, and at least every 4 hours. See PR interval. ■ Monitor BP very closely, every 5 minutes times 3 or until reasonably stabilized, every 15 minutes times 4 and hourly thereafter. May need more frequent checks with increased drip rate. ■ Emergency resuscitation drugs and equipment must always be available. ■ Treat heart failure with digitalis and diuretics before using verapamil. ■ Pulmonary wedge pressure above 20 mm Hg and/or ejection fraction below 20% to 30% indicates acute heart failure. ■ Maintain bed rest until effects on HR, BP, and potential dizziness evaluated. ■ Monitor for side effects (AV block) and digoxin levels when used concurrently with digitalis. ■ Monitor for any unusual bleeding or bruising. ■ See Drug/Lab Interactions.

Maternal/Child: Category C: safety for use in pregnancy not yet established; use only when clearly indicated. ■ Discontinue breast-feeding. ■ Children under 6 months of age may not respond to treatment with verapamil. ■ Severe hemodynamic side effects (e.g., bradycardia, hypotension, or a rapid ventricular rate in atrial flutter/fibrillation) can occur in infants and neonates. Use caution and monitor closely.

Elderly: May have an increased hypotensive effect; see Rate of Administration. ■ Consider reduced renal function; half-life may be prolonged. ■ May cause drug-induced tinnitus.

DRUG/LAB INTERACTIONS

Potentiates digoxin; lower dose may be appropriate. ■ Do not give comcomitantly (within a few hours) with oral, opthalmic, or IV beta-adrenergic blocking drugs (e.g., propranolol [Inderal]); see Contraindications. Both drugs depress myocardial contractility and AV node conduction. ■ Do not administer disopyramide (Norpace) within 48 hours before or 24 hours after verapamil. ■ Potentiates cyclosporine, carbamazepine, and theophyllines. ■ Potentiates nondepolarizing muscle relaxants (e.g., vecuronium [Norcuron]); use lower doses of muscle relaxant and extreme caution. ■ Serum concentrations may be increased by itraconazole (Sporanox). ■ May cause excessive hypotension with other antihypertensive drugs (vasodilators and diuretics). ■ Serum concentrations and effectiveness of verapamil may be decreased by barbiturates (e.g., phenobarbital), calcium salts, phenytoin (Dilantin), sulfinpyrazone (Anturane), vitamin D. ■ Hyperkalemia and myocardial depression may result from concurrent administration of dantrolene (Dantrium). ■ Use with quinidine may cause AV block, bradycardia, hypotension, ventricular tachycardia, and pulmonary edema. ■ May cause severe hypotension with fentanyl (Sublimaze). ■ May inhibit other highly protein-bound drugs (e.g., oral hypoglycemics, warfarin). Use caution. ■ In two case reports AV block and severe hypotension occurred with clonidine. ■ Grapefruit juice may affect certain enzymes of the P_{450} enzyme system and should be avoided.

SIDE EFFECTS

Abdominal discomfort, allergic reactions including anaphylaxis, asystole, bradycardia, dizziness, headache, second- and third-degree heart block, heart failure, hypotension (symptomatic), increased ventricular response in atrial flutter, fibrillation (Wolff-Parkinson-White and Lown-Ganong-Levine syndromes), nausea, PVCs, tachycardia.

ANTIDOTE

Discontinue verapamil and notify physician promptly if hypotension, bradycardia, or second- or third-degree heart block occurs. Keep physician informed of all side effects. Treatment will depend on clinical situation. Calcium chloride may reverse effects of verapamil and can be used in toxicity. Glucagon may also be used in toxicity; see Glucagon monograph. Rapid ventricular response in atrial flutter/fibrillation should respond to cardioversion, procainamide, and/or lidocaine. Treat bradycardia, AV block, and asystole with standard AHA protocol (atropine, pacing). Levarterenol or dopamine will reverse hypotension. Treat allergic reactions or resuscitate as necessary.

VERTEPORFIN

(ver-tee-poor′fin)

Visudyne

Photosensitizing agent
Macular degeneration therapy adjunct

USUAL DOSE

A course is a ***two-stage process*** requiring administration of both drug and light. Each course may be repeated every 3 months as indicated. Body surface area, lesion size determination, and spot size determination of the choroidal neovascularization (CNV) are used by the retina specialist to calculate dosing of verteporfin. The greatest linear dimension of the lesion is estimated by fluorescein angiography and color fundus photography. The treatment spot size should be 1000 microns larger than the greatest linear dimension of the lesion on the retina to allow a 500 micron border. The nasal edge of the treatment spot must be positioned at least 200 microns from the temporal edge of the optic disc.

First stage: 6 mg/M^2 of verteporfin as a single IV infusion.

Second stage: Activation of verteporfin using a recommended light dose of 50 J/cm^2 of neovascular lesion administered at an intensity of 600 mW/cm^2 over 83 seconds. Initiate 689 $\pm$ 3 nm wavelength laser light delivery 15 minutes after the start of the verteporfin infusion. Light is delivered to the retina as a single circular spot via a fiber optic and a slit lamp, using a suitable ophthalmic magnification lens. Light dose, light intensity, ophthalmic lens magnification factor, and zoom lens setting are important parameters for the appropriate delivery of light to the predetermined treatment spot. Follow the laser system manuals for procedure set up and operation.

Concurrent bilateral treatment: In patients who present with eligible lesions in both eyes without prior verteporfin therapy, treat only one eye (the most aggressive lesion) during the first course. One week after the first course, if no significant safety issues are identified, the second eye can be treated, using the same treatment regimen including a verteporfin infusion and light activation. Approximately 3 months later, both eyes can be evaluated and concurrent treatment following a new verteporfin infusion can be started if both lesions still show evidence of leakage. When treating both eyes concurrently, the more aggressive lesion should be treated first, at 15 minutes after the start of infusion. Immediately at the end of light application to the first eye, the laser settings should be adjusted to introduce the treatment parameters for the second eye, with the same light dose and intensity as for the first eye, starting no later than 20 minutes from the start of the infusion.

PEDIATRIC DOSE

Safety and effectiveness for use in children not established.

DOSE ADJUSTMENTS

No adjustments required. See Precautions.

DILUTION

Specific techniques required; see Precautions. Reconstitute each vial of verteporfin with 7 ml of SW to provide 7.5 ml of opaque, dark green solution containing 2 mg/ml. Withdraw the desired dose from the vial and further dilute with D5W to a total infusion volume of 30 ml.

Storage: Store at CRT (20° to 25° C [68° to 77° F]). Reconstituted solution must be protected from light and used within 4 hours.

COMPATIBILITY

Specific information not available. Consider specific use; consult pharmacist. Do not mix with solutions other than those listed under Dilution.

RATE OF ADMINISTRATION

A 30 ml infusion equally distributed over 10 minutes (3 ml/min), using an appropriate syringe pump and an in-line filter (pore size 0.22 to 1.2 micron).

ACTIONS

A light activated drug (photosensitizing agent) for use in photodynamic therapy (PDT). Transported in the plasma by lipoproteins. Endothelial cells of the abnormal choroidal blood vessels which have high concentrations of lipoprotein receptors take up the lipoprotein-verteporfin complex. Light activation in the presence of O_2, induces a photochemical reaction, generating highly reactive singlet oxygen and reactive oxygen radicals that cause local damage to the neovascular endothelium. The damaged endothelium releases procoagulant and vasoactive factors through the lipo-oxygenase (leukotriene) and cyclo-oxygenase (eicosanoids such as thromboxane) pathways, resulting in platelet aggregation, fibrin clot formation, vasoconstriction, and ultimately, vessel occlusion. Verteporfin appears to preferentially accumulate in neovasculature, including chorioidal neovasculature. However, animal models indicate that the drug is also present in the retina. Therefore there may be collateral damage to retinal structures following photoactivation. Terminal elimination half-life of verteporfin is 5 to 6 hours. It is metabolized to a small extent by liver and plasma esterases and is eliminated primarily by the fecal route as unchanged drug.

INDICATIONS AND USES

Treatment of patients with predominantly classic subfoveal choroidal neovascularization due to age-related macular degeneration, pathologic myopia, or presumed ocular histoplasmosis. Slows retinal damage, does not reverse loss of vision in eyes damaged by AMD. ■ Not recommended for use in treatment of predominantly occult subfoveal choroidal neovascularization; evidence insufficient.

Unlabeled uses: Treatment of psoriasis, psoriatic arthritis, and rheumatoid arthritis.

CONTRAINDICATIONS

Patients with porphyria or a known hypersensitivity to any component of this preparation.

PRECAUTIONS

Use rubber gloves and eye protection during preparation and administration. Avoid any skin or eye contact since that area will become photosensitive. Wipe up spills with a damp cloth. Dispose of all contaminated materials in a polyethylene bag to avoid accidental contact by others. Protection from light will be necessary if accidental exposure or overexposure occurs. Note process in Patient Education. ■ Administered by or under the direction of the physician specialist with appropriate knowledge of the selected laser system. Facilities for monitoring the patient and responding to any medical emergency must be available. ■ Requires laser systems and a fiber-optic diffuser to activate. *Coherent Opal Photoactivator Laser Console and LaserLink Adapter and Zeiss VISULAS 690s laser and VISILINK PDT adapter* are two laser systems that have been tested for compatibility with verteporfin and are approved for delivery of a stable power output at a wavelength of 689 ± 3 nm. Use of incompatible lasers that do not provide the required characteristics of light could result in incomplete treatment due to partial photoactivation, overtreatment due to overactivation, or damage to surrounding normal tissue. ■ Following verteporfin administration, care should be taken to avoid exposure of skin or eyes to direct sunlight or bright indoor light for 5 days. If emergency surgery is necessary within 48 hours after treatment, as much of the internal tissue as possible should be protected from intense light. ■ Patients who experience severe decrease of vision of 4 lines or more within 1 week after treatment should not be retreated, at least until their vision completely recovers to pretreatment levels. Potential risk versus benefit of any subsequent treatment should be considered. ■ Use with caution in patients with moderate to severe hepatic impairment or biliary obstruction, and in anesthetized patients. There is no clinical experience with these patient populations. ■ Older patients, patients with dark irides, patients with occult lesions or patients with less than 50% classic CNV may be less likely to benefit from verteporfin therapy. ■ Safety and efficacy of verteporfin beyond two years have not been demonstrated.

Monitor: Standard precautions should be taken to avoid extravasation (e.g., establish a free-flowing IV line in a large arm vein, preferably the antecubital vein). If extravasation occurs, the infusion should be stopped immediately and cold compresses applied. The extravasation area must be thoroughly protected from direct light until the swelling and discoloration have faded in order to prevent the occurrence of a local burn which could be severe. ■ Patient should be reevaluated every 3 months and if choroidal neovascular leakage is detected on fluorescein angiography, therapy should be repeated. ■ See Usual Dose, Precautions, Patient Education, and Drug/Lab Interactions.

Patient Education: ■ Must observe precautions to avoid exposure of skin and eyes to direct sunlight or bright indoor light for 5 days. Photosensitivity is due to residual drug, which is present in all parts of the skin. Ambient indoor light is beneficial as it gradually inactivates the remaining drug through a photobleaching reaction. Do not remain in a darkened room. Do expose skin to ambient indoor light. Avoid bright indoor light from examination lamps, dental lamps, operating room lamps, bright halogen lighting, and unshaded light bulbs. Limit time outdoors to necessary excursions and completely cover body with clothing and shade face before going out. Ultraviolet sunscreens are of no value because photoactivation is caused by visible light, not UV rays. Eyes will be sensitive to sun, bright lights, and car headlights; wear dark sunglasses with an average white light transmittance of less than 4%.

Maternal/Child: Category C: use during pregnancy only if benefits justify potential risk to fetus. Effective contraception necessary for women of childbearing age. Has caused maternal and fetal toxicity in rats and rabbits. ■ Discontinue breast-feeding; not known if it is secreted in breast milk. ■ Safety and effectiveness in children not established.

Elderly: Reduced treatment effect was seen with increasing age (75 years of age or older).

DRUG/LAB INTERACTIONS

Formal drug interaction studies have not been performed. Based on the mechanism of action of verteporfin, many drugs used concomitantly could influence the effect of verteporfin therapy. ■ Calcium channel blockers (e.g., diltiazem [Cardizem], verapamil [Isoptin], nicardipine [Cardene]), polymyxin B, or radiation therapy could enhance the rate of verteporfin uptake by the vascular endothelium. ■ Use with other photosensitizing agents (e.g., griseofulvin, phenothiazines [e.g., prochlorperazine (Compazine)], sulfonamides [sulfisoxazole (Gantrisin)], ophthalmic solutions (AK-Sulf)], sulfonylurea hypoglycemic agents [tolbutamide (Orinase)], tetracyclines [doxycycline (Vibramycin)], thiazide diuretics [chlorothiazide (Diuril)]) could increase the photosensitivity reaction. ■ Compounds that quench active oxygen species or scavenge radicals (e.g., dimethyl sulfoxide (DMSO), beta-carotene, ethanol, formate, mannitol) would be expected to decrease verteporfin activity. ■ Effectiveness may be reduced by drugs that decrease clotting (e.g., heparin, alteplase [tPA]), vasoconstriction (e.g., nicardipine [Cardene]), or platelet aggregation (e.g., clopidogrel (Plavix), dipyradamole [Persantine], ticlopidine [Ticlid]). ■ Glucocorticoid hormones (e.g., dexamethasone [Decadron]) given before or with PDT may reduce the effectiveness of verteporfin by inhibiting the production of thromboxane A_2.

SIDE EFFECTS

The most frequently reported side effects are headache, injection site reactions (e.g., extravasation and rashes), visual disturbances (e.g., blurred vision, decreased visual acuity and visual field defects), and self-resolving photosensitivity. Less frequently reported side effects include abnormal white blood cell count (decreased or increased), albuminuria, anemia, arthralgia, arthrosis, asthenia, atrial fibrillation, back pain (primarily during infusion), cataracts, conjunctivitis, constipation, decreased hearing, diplopia, dry eyes, elevated liver function tests, eye hemorrhage (subconjunctival, subretinal, or vitreous), eczema, fever, flu-like syndrome, hypertension, hyperesthesia, increased creatinine, lacrimation disorder, myasthenia, nausea, ocular itching, peripheral vascular disorder, pharyngitis, photosensitivity, pneumonia, prostatic disorder, severe vision loss (equivalent of 4 lines or more within 7 days of treatment), sleep disturbance, varicose veins, and vertigo.

Overdose: Overdose of drug and/or light may result in nonperfusion of normal retinal vessels with the possibility of severe decrease in vision that could be permanent. May also result in prolongation of the time during which the patient will be photosensitive.

ANTIDOTE

Keep the physician informed of all side effects; most will be treated symptomatically. In the event of an overdose of drug and/or light, extend the photosensitivity precautions for a time proportional to the overdose.

VINBLASTINE SULFATE

(vin-blas′ten sul′fat)

Velban, ✦Velbe, VLB

Antineoplastic
(mitotic inhibitor-vinca alkaloid)

pH 3.5 to 5

USUAL DOSE

Auxiliary labeling required; see Precautions.

3.7 mg/M^2 initially. Administered once every 7 days, increasing the dose to specific amounts (5.5, 7.4, 9.25, 11.1 mg/M^2) a single step each week until the WBC count is decreased to 3,000 cells/ml, remission is achieved, or a maximum dose of 18.5 mg/M^2 is reached. Maintenance dose is one step below any dose that causes leukopenia (3,000 cells/ml or less), once every 7 to 14 days. Usually 5.5 to 7.4 mg/M^2. Continue treatment for 4 to 6 weeks. Up to 12 weeks often necessary.

PEDIATRIC DOSE

One source suggests 2.5 mg/M^2 initially. Use same procedure as for adult dose using steps to 3.75, 5, 6.25, and 7.5 mg/M^2. Maximum dose is 12.5 mg/M^2. Maintenance dose is calculated by same parameters as Usual Dose (above). Usually differs with each individual. Other sources suggest that initial doses vary depending on the schedule used, use of vinblastine as a single agent, or in a combination regimen. Some suggested doses are:

Letterer-Siwe disease (unlabeled): As a single agent, an initial dose of 6.5 mg/M^2.

Hodgkin's disease: An initial dose of 6 mg/M^2 in combination with other chemotherapeutic agents.

Testicular cancer: An initial dose of 3 mg/M^2 in combination with other chemotherapeutic agents.

DOSE ADJUSTMENTS

Reduce dose by 50% if serum bilirubin above 3 mg/dl. ■ Often used with other antineoplastic drugs and corticosteroids in reduced doses and/or extended intervals to achieve tumor remission.

DILUTION

Specific techniques required; see Precautions. Each 10 mg is diluted with 10 ml of NS for injection. 1 mg equals 1 ml. Also available in liquid form (1 mg/ml). May be given by IV injection or through Y-tube or three-way stopcock of a free-flowing IV infusion.

Storage: Store in refrigerator before and after dilution. Potency maintained for 28 days after dilution if reconstituted with bacteriostatic NS.

INCOMPATIBLE WITH

Manufacturer suggests that the pH not be altered from between 3.5 to 5 by an additive or a diluent, and it recommends NS as a diluent and not admixing with other drugs in the same container.

COMPATIBLE WITH

(Underline Indicates Conflicting Compatibility Information)

Consult pharmacist; specific conditions may apply; see Compatibilities, p. xvi.

Additive: ***Not recommended by manufacturer.*** Bleomycin (Blenoxane), dacarbazine (DTIC), doxorubicin (Adriamycin), metoclopramide (Reglan).

Syringe: Bleomycin (Blenoxane), cisplatin (Platinol), cyclophosphamide (Cytoxan), doxorubicin (Adriamycin), droperidol (Inapsine), fluorouracil (5-FU), heparin, leucovorin calcium, methotrexate (Folex), metoclopramide (Reglan), mitomycin (Mutamycin), vincristine (Oncovin).

Y-site: Allopurinol (Aloprim, Zyloprim), amifostine (Ethyol), amphotericin B cholesteryl (Amphotec), aztreonam (Azactam), bleomycin (Blenoxane), cisplatin (Platinol), cyclophosphamide (Cytoxan), doxorubicin (Adriamycin), doxorubicin liposome (Doxil), droperidol (Inapsine), etoposide phosphate (Etopophos), filgrastim (Neupogen), fludarabine (Fludara), fluorouracil (5-FU), gatifloxacin (Tequin), gemcitabine (Gemzar), granisetron (Kytril), heparin, leucovorin calcium, melphalan (Alkeran), methotrexate (Folex), metoclopramide (Reglan), mitomycin (Mutamycin), ondansetron (Zofran), paclitaxel (Taxol), piperacillin/tazobactam (Zosyn), sargramostim (Leukine), teniposide (Vumon), thiotepa (Thioplex), vincristine (Oncovin), vinorelbine (Navelbine).

RATE OF ADMINISTRATION

IV injection: Total desired dose, properly diluted, over 1 minute.

ACTIONS

An alkaloid of the periwinkle plant with antitumor activity. Cell cycle–specific for M phase. Thought to interfere with the metabolic pathways of amino acids. Sometimes pharmacologically effective without any noticeable improvement in symptoms of malignancy. Cell energy production and synthesis of nucleic acid may also be inhibited. Half-life is 24.8 hours. Metabolism mediated by the hepatic cytochrome P_{450} isoenzymes in the CYP 3A subfamily. Some excretion through bile and urine.

INDICATIONS AND USES

To suppress or retard neoplastic growth. Remission and probable cure has been achieved with bleomycin and cisplatin in testicular malignancies. Response has been noted in Hodgkin's disease, non-Hodgkin's lymphomas, choriocarcinoma, Kaposi's sarcoma, mycosis fungoids, breast and renal cell malignancies. ■ Used to treat many other malignancies.

CONTRAINDICATIONS

Bacterial infection or leukopenia below 3,000 cells/ml.

PRECAUTIONS

Follow guidelines for handling cytotoxic agents. See Appendix A, p. 1142. ■ Usually administered by or under the direction of the physician specialist. ■ Manufacturer provides an auxillary sticker labeled "Fatal if given intrathecally, for IV use only" and an overwrap labeled "Do not remove covering until moment of injection. Fatal if given intrathecally. For Intravenous use only." Each and every syringe(s) containing a specific dose and prepared in advance of actual administration must be labeled with the provided auxiliary sticker and packaged in this overwrap. If intrathecal injection should occur, immediate neurosurgical intervention is required, consult package insert for immediate steps to be taken. ■ May cause corneal ulceration with accidental contact to the eye. ■ Use caution in presence of ulcerated skin areas, cachexia, or impaired liver function. ■ Leukocyte and platelet counts have fallen precipitously in patients with malignant-cell infiltration of the bone marrow following moderate doses of vinblastine. Further administration is not recommended. ■ Acute pulmonary reactions including acute shortness of breath and severe bronchospasm have been reported in patients receiving vinca alkaloids. Occurs most frequently when given in combination with mitomycin C. Onset of reaction may occur minutes to hours after vinca administration and up to 2 weeks following the mitomycin dose.

Monitor: Determine absolute patency, quality of vein, and adequate circulation of extremity. Severe cellulitis may result from extravasation.

Rinse syringe and needle with venous blood before withdrawal from the vein. ■ Leukopenia is dose-limiting toxicity. Nadir occurs 5 to 10 days after therapy. Recovery occurs within another 7 to 14 days. ■ WBC count must be checked before each dose. Must be above 4,000 cells/ml. ■ Be alert for signs of bone marrow depression or infection. ■ Prophylactic antibiotics may be indicated pending results of C/S in a febrile neutropenic patient. ■ Thrombocytopenia is rare, but may occur in patients whose bone marrow has been impaired by prior radiation therapy or other bone marrow depressants. If platelet count is less than 50,000/mm^3, initiate precautions to prevent excessive bleeding (e.g., inspect IV sites, skin, and mucous membranes; use extreme care during invasive procedures; test urine, emesis, stool, and secretions for occult blood). ■ Observe for increased uric acid levels; may require increased doses of antigout agents; allopurinol (Zyloprim) preferred. ■ Maintain adequate hydration. ■ Prophylactic antiemetics may increase patient comfort. ■ See Drug/Lab Interactions.

Patient Education: Avoid pregnancy; nonhormonal birth control recommended. ■ Report IV site burning or stinging promptly. ■ Report chills, fever, sore mouth, or throat promptly. ■ Maintain adequate hydration; avoid constipation. ■ See Appendix D, p. 1148.

Maternal/Child: Category D: avoid pregnancy. May produce teratogenic effects on the fetus. Has a mutagenic potential. ■ Discontinue breast-feeding. ■ Do not use diluents containing benzyl alcohol in premature infants.

Elderly: Leukopenic response may be increased in malnutrition or with skin ulcers.

DRUG/LAB INTERACTIONS

Inhibited by some amino acids, glutamic acid, and tryptophan. ■ Potentiated by other bone marrow depressants (e.g., antineoplastics, radiation therapy). ■ Do not administer live-virus vaccines to patients receiving antineoplastic drugs. ■ Acute pulmonary reactions can occur with Mitomycin-C; see Precautions. ■ May inhibit effects of phenytoin (Dilantin); increased doses of phenytoin may be needed. ■ Erythromycin decreases metabolism and increases toxicity of vinblastine. ■ Use caution with any drug that inhibits P_{450} enzymes (e.g., calcium channel blockers [e.g., diltiazem (Cardizem), nicardipine (Cardene), verapamil (Isoptin)], antifungal agents [e.g., fluconazole (Diflucan), itraconazole (Sporanox), ketoconazole (Nizoral)], bromocriptine [Parlodel], cimetidine [Tagamet], clarithromycin [Biaxin], cyclosporine [Sandimmune], danazol [Medrol], metoclopramide [Reglan]); may increase vinblastine blood levels and increase toxicity. ■ Effect of bleomycin is significantly enhanced if vinblastine is administered 6 to 8 hours prior to bleomycin administration.

SIDE EFFECTS

Usually dose related and not always reversible: abdominal pain, alopecia, anorexia, cellulitis, constipation, convulsions, diarrhea, dizziness, extravasation, gonadal suppression, headache, hemorrhage, ileus, leukopenia (severe), malaise, mental depression, myelosuppression, nausea, numbness, oral lesions, paresthesias, peripheral neuritis, pharyngitis, Raynaud's syndrome, reflex depression (deep tendon), skin lesions, thrombophlebitis, tumor site pain, vomiting, weakness.

ANTIDOTE

For extravasation, discontinue the drug immediately and administer into another vein. Hyaluronidase should be injected locally into extravasated area. Use a fine hypodermic needle. Elevate extremity. Moist heat may be helpful. Notify the physician of all side effects; symptomatic treatment is often indicated. Administration of whole blood products (e.g., packed RBCs, platelets, leukocytes) and/or blood modifiers (e.g., darbepoetin alfa [Aranesp], epoetin alfa [Epogen, Procrit], filgrastim [Neupogen], pegfilgrastim [Neulasta], sargramostim [Leukine], oprelvekin [Neumega]) may be indicated to treat bone marrow toxicity. Glutamic acid blocks toxicity of vinblastine but also blocks its antineoplastic activity.

VINCRISTINE SULFATE

(vin-kris′teen sul′fat)

Antineoplastic (mitotic inhibitor-vinca alkaloid)

Oncovin, VCR, Vincasar PFS

pH 3.5 to 5.5

USUAL DOSE

Auxiliary labeling required; see Precautions.

Neurotoxicity appears to be dose related. Use extreme care in calculating and administering vincristine. Overdose may be fatal.

1.4 mg/M^2 administered once every 7 days. Various dosage schedules have been used with caution.

PEDIATRIC DOSE

1.5 to 2 mg/M^2. For children weighing less than 10 kg (22 lb) or with a body surface area less than 1 M^2, give 0.05 mg/kg of body weight once a week. See comments under Usual Dose.

DOSE ADJUSTMENTS

In impaired hepatic function, reduce initial doses to 0.05 to 1 mg/M^2 or by 50% if direct bilirubin above 3 mg/dl. May be increased gradually based on individual response. ■ Usually given with other antineoplastic drugs and corticosteroids in reduced doses to achieve tumor remission. ■ See Drug/Lab Interactions.

DILUTION

Specific techniques required; see Precautions. Available in preservative-free solutions (1 mg/ml). May be given by IV injection or through Y-tube or three-way stopcock of a free-flowing IV infusion. Occasionally further diluted in 50 ml or more NS or D5W and given as an infusion.

Storage: Store in refrigerator before and after dilution. Potency maintained for 14 days after dilution. Label vial pertaining to mg/ml.

INCOMPATIBLE WITH

Manufacturer suggests that the pH not be altered from between 3.5 to 5.5 by an additive or a diluent, and it recommends NS or D5W as a diluent and not admixing with other drugs in the same container.

COMPATIBLE WITH

Consult pharmacist; specific conditions may apply; see Compatibilities, p. xvi.

Additive: *Not recommended by manufacturer.* Bleomycin (Blenoxane), cytarabine (ARA-C), doxorubicin (Adriamycin), fluorouracil (5-FU), methotrexate (Folex), metoclopramide (Reglan).

Syringe: ***Not recommended by manufacturer.*** Bleomycin (Blenoxane), cisplatin (Platinol), cyclophosphamide (Cytoxan), doxapram (Dopram), doxorubicin (Adriamycin), droperidol (Inapsine), fluorouracil (5-FU), heparin, leucovorin calcium, methotrexate (Folex), metoclopramide (Reglan), mitomycin (Mutamycin), vinblastine (Velban).

Y-site: Allopurinol (Aloprim, Zyloprim), amifostine (Ethyol), amphotericin B cholesteryl (Amphotec), aztreonam (Azactam), bleomycin (Blenoxane), cisplatin (Platinol), cladribine (Leustatin), cyclophosphamide (Cytoxan), doxorubicin (Adriamycin), doxorubicin liposome (Doxil), droperidol (Inapsine), etoposide phosphate (Etopophos), filgrastim (Neupogen), fludarabine (Fludara), fluorouracil (5-FU), gatifloxacin (Tequin), gemcitabine (Gemzar), granisetron (Kytril), heparin, leucovorin calcium, linezolid (Zyvox), melphalan (Alkeran), methotrexate (Folex), metoclopramide (Reglan), mitomycin (Mutamycin), ondansetron (Zofran), paclitaxel (Taxol), piperacillin/tazobactam (Zosyn), sargramostim (Leukine), teniposide (Vumon), thiotepa (Thioplex), topotecan (Hycamtin), vinblastine (Velban), vinorelbine (Navelbine).

RATE OF ADMINISTRATION

IV injection: Total desired dose, properly diluted, over 1 minute.

Infusion: A single dose over 20 to 30 minutes or as a continuous infusion prolonged over up to 96 hours.

ACTIONS

An alkaloid of the periwinkle plant with antitumor activity. Cell cycle–specific for the M phase. Well distributed except in spinal fluid, it is primarily excreted through bile and feces.

INDICATIONS AND USES

To suppress or retard neoplastic growth; good response experienced in leukemia, Hodgkin's disease, lymphosarcoma, oat cell, Wilms' tumor and others.

Unlabeled uses: Treatment of idiopathic thrombocytopenic purpura; treatment of Kaposi's sarcoma, breast and bladder cancer.

CONTRAINDICATIONS

Demyelinating form of Charcot-Marie-Tooth syndrome.

PRECAUTIONS

Follow guidelines for handling cytotoxic agents. See Appendix A, p. 1142. ■ Administered by or under the direction of the physician specialist. ■ Manufacturer provides an auxiliary sticker labeled "Fatal if given intrathecally, for IV use only" and an overwrap labeled "Do not remove covering until moment of injection. Fatal if given intrathecally. For Intravenous use only." Each and every infusion bag(s) or syringe(s) containing a specific dose and prepared in advance of actual administration must be labeled with the provided auxiliary sticker and packaged in this overwrap. If intrathecal injection should occur, immediate neurosurgical intervention is required, consult package insert for immediate steps to be taken. ■ Use extreme caution in combination with radiation therapy. ■ May cause corneal ulceration with accidental contact to the eye; flush eyes with water immediately. ■ Use caution in pre-existing neuromuscular disease or impaired liver function. ■ Not recommended for use in patients receiving radiation therapy that involves the liver.

Monitor: Determine absolute patency and quality of vein and adequate circulation of extremity. Severe cellulitis may result from extravasation. ■ Monitor CBC, platelets and evaluate neuro status before therapy and at frequent intervals. ■ Be alert for signs of bone marrow depression or infection. ■ Prophylactic antibiotics may be indicated pending results of C/S in a febrile neutropenic patient. ■ Observe for increased uric acid levels; may require increased doses of antigout agents; allopurinol (Zyloprim) preferred. ■ Maintain adequate hydration. ■ Prophylactic antiemetics may increase patient comfort. ■ Monitor for hyponatremia and inappropriate secretion of antidiuretic hormone (ADH); may require fluid limitation. ■ Use a laxative to prevent constipation. ■ Monitor for thrombocytopenia (platelet count less than 50,000/mm^3). Initiate precautions to prevent excessive bleeding (e.g., inspect IV sites, skin, and mucous membranes; use extreme care during invasive procedures; test urine, emesis, stool, and secretions for occult blood). ■ See Drug/Lab Interactions.

Patient Education: Avoid pregnancy; nonhormonal birth control recommended. ■ Report IV site burning or stinging promptly. ■ See Appendix D, p. 1148. ■ Use laxatives to avoid constipation.

Maternal/Child: Category D: avoid pregnancy. May produce teratogenic effects on the fetus. Has a mutagenic potential. ■ Discontinue breast-feeding.

Elderly: Neurotoxicity may be more severe (observe closely for constipation, ileus, and urinary retention).

DRUG/LAB INTERACTIONS

May cause severe bone marrow depression with other antineoplastic drugs or radiation therapy. ■ Use with asparaginase or doxorubicin not recommended. Asparaginase inhibits the elimination of vincristine and increases its toxicity. The manufacturer suggests giving vincristine 12 to 24 hours before asparaginase; use caution. ■ Concurrent use with itraconazole (Sporanox) may increase vincristine toxicity. ■ Acute pulmonary reactions can occur with mitomycin-C. ■ Inhibited by glutamic acid. ■ Do not administer live-virus vaccines to patients receiving antineoplastic drugs. ■ Inhibits digoxin and phenytoin. Monitor serum levels of digoxin and phenytoin; increased doses of these drugs may be required. ■ Use with filgrastim may induce a severe atypical neuropathy (foot pain, severe motor weakness). ■ Use caution with concurrent use of drugs known to inhibit drug metabolism by hepatic cytochrome P_{450} isoenzymes such as azole antifungals (e.g., fluconazole [Diflucan], itraconazole [Sporanox], ketoconazole [Nizoral]), cimetidine (Tagamet), diltiazem (Cardizem), verapamil (Isoptin), macrolide antibiotics (e.g., erythromycin), omeprazole (Prilosec), and ranitidine (Zantac).

SIDE EFFECTS

Frequently dose related and not always reversible: abdominal pain, alopecia, anaphylaxis, ataxia, bronchospasm, cellulitis, constipation, convulsions, cranial nerve damage, diarrhea, dysuria, extravasation, fever, foot-drop, gonadal suppression, headache, hypertension, hypotension, leukopenia (rare), muscle wasting, nausea, neuritic pain, oral lacerations, paralytic ileus, paresthesias, polyuria, reflex changes, sensory impairment, shortness of breath, SIADH, tingling and numbness of extremities, thrombocytopenia (rare), thrombophlebitis, upper colon impaction, uric acid nephropathy, vomiting, weakness, weight loss.

ANTIDOTE

For extravasation, discontinue the drug immediately and administer into another vein. Hyaluronidase or hydrocortisone sodium succinate (Solu-

Cortef) may be injected locally into extravasated area. Use a fine hypodermic needle. Elevate extremity; moist heat may be helpful. Notify the physician of all side effects; symptomatic treatment is often indicated. Will probably reduce dose at earliest signs of neurologic toxicity (tingling and numbness of extremities). Discontinue for inappropriate ADH secretion or hyponatremia. Treat with fluid restriction and diuretics. Phenobarbital may be needed for convulsions. Use enemas or cathartics to treat constipation or prevent ileus. Glutamic acid blocks toxicity of vincristine, but also blocks its antineoplastic activity. Folinic acid, 100 mg IV every 3 hours for 24 hours and then every 6 hours for at least 48 hours, may be helpful in overdose. Supportive measures still required. Administration of whole blood products (e.g., packed RBCs, platelets, leukocytes) and/or blood modifiers (e.g., darbepoetin alfa [Aranesp], epoetin alfa [Epogen, Procrit], filgrastim [Neupogen], pegfilgrastim [Neulasta], sargramostim [Leukine], oprelvekin [Neumega]) may be indicated to treat bone marrow toxicity.

✦VINDESINE SULPHATE

(vin′dah-sen sul′fat)

Antineoplastic (mitotic inhibitor-vinca alkaloid)

✦Eldisine

pH 4.2 to 4.5

USUAL DOSE

Auxiliary labeling required; see Precautions.

3 mg/M^2 administered once every 7 to 10 days. Repeat for 8 cycles. May be adjusted upward if necessary. Do not exceed 4 mg/M^2. Calculate carefully in presence of edema or ascites; overdose may be fatal. Decreased bone marrow function induced by disease will require full doses to restore marrow function. Will require constant monitoring.

PEDIATRIC DOSE

4 mg/M^2 administered once every 7 to 10 days. Repeat for 8 cycles. 2 mg/M^2/day for 2 consecutive days may be given as an alternate regimen. Follow by 5 to 7 days without the drug and repeat for 8 cycles.

DOSE ADJUSTMENTS

Decrease dose in significant hepatic disease and in patients with bone marrow depression from previous treatment. May be increased gradually based on clinical response. ■ Reduced dose may be required in the elderly (over 60 years of age). ■ See Precautions/Monitor.

DILUTION

Specific techniques required; see Precautions. Each 5-mg vial must be diluted with 5 ml of bacteriostatic NS. 1 mg equals 1 ml. Do not add to IV solutions. Must be given by IV injection or through Y-tube or three-way stopcock of a free-flowing IV infusion.

Storage: Store in refrigerator. Stable after dilution at room temperature for 24 hours and up to 14 days if refrigerated. Label vial pertaining to mg/ml.

COMPATIBILITY

May precipitate in any solution with a pH above 6. Manufacturer suggests not mixing with any other drug in syringe or solution.

RATE OF ADMINISTRATION

Total desired dose, properly diluted, over 1 to 3 minutes.

ACTIONS

An antineoplastic agent; a vinca alkaloid with properties similar to but more potent than vincristine and vinblastine. Cell cycle–specific for the M phase. Can prevent invasion of normal tissue by malignant cells. Has been effective in patients who have relapsed on multiple-agent treatment that included vincristine. Well distributed through plasma and body tissues. Half-life is 24 hours. It is primarily excreted through bile and feces.

INDICATIONS AND USES

Treatment of acute lymphocytic leukemia of childhood resistant to vincristine and non–oat cell lung cancer.

CONTRAINDICATIONS

Drug-induced severe granulocytopenia or thrombocytopenia; serious bacterial infections.

PRECAUTIONS

Follow guidelines for handling cytotoxic agents. See Appendix A, p. 1142. Avoid contact with eye. Will cause severe irritation or ulceration. Contaminated eye should be washed immediately with H_2O or saline. ■

Administered by or under the direction of the physician specialist. ■ This is a Canadian product and may not adhere to FDA labeling requirements but the manufacturer should provide an auxillary sticker labeled "Fatal if given intrathecally, for IV use only" and an overwrap labeled "Do not remove covering until moment of injection. Fatal if given intrathecally. For Intravenous use only." Each and every syringe(s) containing a specific dose and prepared in advance of actual administration must be labeled with the provided auxiliary sticker and packaged in this overwrap. If intrathecal injection should occur, immediate neurosurgical intervention is required, consult package insert for immediate steps to be taken or look at the package insert of a vinca alkaloid manufactured in the U.S. (e.g., vinblastine [Velban]). ■ Use extreme caution in patients with impaired liver function, Charcot-Marie-Tooth Syndrome, severe drug-induced granulocytopenia or thrombocytopenia, pre-existing neuromuscular disease, or those taking other neurotoxic drugs (e.g., antineoplastics [cisplatin], phenothiazines [prochlorperazine]). Neurotoxicity may require dose reduction or discontinuation of vindesine. ■ Prior radiation therapy or treatment with other antineoplastic agents may cause thrombocytopenia (platelets below 200,000/mm^3). Not common in patients with normal bone marrow function receiving once-a-week dosage.

Monitor: Monitor CBC with differential and platelet count 1 or 2 times weekly. Temporary leukopenia is an expected effect and is directly related to the dose. Discontinue or reduce dosage if abnormal depression of the bone marrow occurs (sustained WBC count below 2,500/mm^3). Maximum depression usually occurs in 3 to 5 days, and recovery of bone marrow should occur 7 to 10 days after each dose. ■ Monitor liver function before initiating therapy and periodically as indicated. ■ Strict adherence to recommended dose schedule is very important. Changes may result in increased side effects. ■ Determine absolute patency and quality of vein and adequate circulation of extremity. Severe cellulitis and phlebitis with sloughing can result from extravasation. After administration elevate extremity to above the level of the heart to reduce intravenous pressure and prevent post-injection leakage. ■ Be alert for any sign of infection. Infections must be brought under control before beginning therapy with vindesine. ■ Prophylactic antibiotics may be indicated pending results of C/S in a febrile neutropenic patient. ■ Maintain adequate hydration. ■ Observe for increased uric acid levels; may require increased doses of antigout agents; allopurinol (Zyloprim) preferred. ■ Prophylactic antiemetics may increase patient comfort. ■ Use a stool softener to prevent impaction. Monitor bowel sounds to prevent obstipation. ■ Inappropriate secretion of antidiuretic hormone (ADH) may require fluid limitation and diuretics (e.g., furosemide [Lasix]). ■ Monitor for thrombocytopenia (platelet count less than 50,000/mm^3). Initiate precautions to prevent excessive bleeding (e.g., inspect IV sites, skin, and mucous membranes; use extreme care during invasive procedures; test urine, emesis, stool, and secretions for occult blood). ■ See Drug/Lab Interactions.

Patient Education: Report IV site burning or stinging promptly. ■ Emphasize adherence to dose schedule. ■ Avoid pregnancy, nonhormonal birth control recommended. ■ See Appendix D, p. 1148.

Maternal/Child: Embryotoxic and may be teratogenic. Must be given with caution in men and women capable of conception. ■ Discontinue breast-feeding.

DRUG/LAB INTERACTIONS

Neurotoxicity increased by other neurotoxic drugs (e.g., antineoplastics [cisplatin], phenothiazines [prochlorperazine]); may require dose reduction or discontinuation of vindesine. ■ Mitomycin-C may cause or aggravate acute pulmonary reactions (e.g., acute shortness of breath, bronchospasm). May require oxygen, bronchodilators, and/or corticosteroids. ■ Additive bone marrow depression may occur with radiation therapy and/or other bone marrow depressing agents (e.g., azathioprine [Imuran], chloramphenicol, melphalan [Alkeran]); dose reductions may be required. ■ Leukopenic effects may be increased by agents that cause similar blood dyscrasias (e.g., anticonvulsants, antidepressants, phenothiazines). ■ May decrease phenytoin concentration, increasing risk of seizure. Monitor levels and adjust dose if needed. ■ Do not administer vaccine or chloroquine to patients receiving antineoplastic drugs. ■ Use caution with concurrent use of drugs known to inhibit drug metabolism by hepatic cytochrome P_{450} isoenzymes, such as azole antifungals (e.g., fluconazole [Diflucan], itraconazole [Sporanox], ketoconazole [Nizoral]), cimetidine (Tagamet), diltiazem (Cardizem), verapamil (Isoptin), macrolide antibiotics (e.g., erythromycin), omeprazole (Prilosec), and ranitidine (Zantac).

SIDE EFFECTS

Frequently dose related and not always reversible: abdominal pain; alopecia; anorexia; cellulitis; constipation; convulsions; cortical blindness; depression; diarrhea; epilation, chills, and fever; extravasation; generalized musculoskeletal pain; granulocytopenia; headache; jaw pain; leukopenia (rare); loss of deep tendon reflexes; macular skin rash; malaise; nausea; neuritic pain; neurotoxicity; oral lacerations; pain in tumor site; paralytic ileus; peripheral neuritis; thrombocytopenia (rare); thrombophlebitis; tingling and numbness of extremities (paresthesias); upper colon impaction; vomiting.

Overdose: Cardiovascular collapse, ileus, syndrome of inappropriate antidiuretic hormone (SIADH), seizures, serious bone marrow depression, death.

ANTIDOTE

For extravasation, discontinue the drug immediately and administer into another vein. Hyaluronidase should be injected locally into extravasated area. Use a fine hypodermic needle. Moist heat may be helpful. Notify the physician of all side effects; symptomatic and supportive treatment is often indicated. Will probably reduce dose at earliest signs of neurologic toxicity (tingling and numbness of extremities). Discontinue or reduce dose with abnormal depression of bone marrow. Administration of whole blood products (e.g., packed RBCs, platelets, leukocytes) and/or blood modifiers (e.g., darbepoetin alfa [Aranesp], epoetin alfa [Epogen, Procrit], filgrastim [Neupogen], pegfilgrastim [Neulasta], sargramostim [Leukine], oprelvekin [Neumega]) may be indicated to treat bone marrow toxicity. Discontinue for SIADH or hyponatremia. Glutamic acid blocks toxicity of vindesine but also blocks its antineoplastic activity. Diuretics and fluid restriction may be required for SIADH. Diazepam (Valium) or phenobarbital may be required for seizures. Administer cathartics to prevent ileus if needed.

VINORELBINE TARTRATE

(vi-nor′el-ben tahr′trat)

Antineoplastic
(mitotic inhibitor-vinca alkaloid)

Navelbine, NVB

pH 3.5

USUAL DOSE

Auxiliary labeling required; see Precautions.

30 mg/M^2 administered once each week until disease progression or dose-limiting toxicity. Calculate carefully in presence of edema or ascites. Vinorelbine 25 mg/M^2 weekly has been used in combination with cisplatin 100 mg/M^2 every 4 weeks. Vinorelbine 30 mg/M^2 weekly has also been used in combination with cisplatin 120 mg/M^2 on days 1 and 29 and then once every 6 weeks. Premedication with dexamethasone (Decadron) may be beneficial in patients who experience acute or subacute pulmonary reactions.

PEDIATRIC DOSE

Safety and effectiveness for use in pediatric patients not established; see Maternal/Child.

DOSE ADJUSTMENTS

Reduce or withhold dose based on hematologic toxicity or hepatic insufficiency (e.g., hyperbilirubinemia) on the day of treatment. For patients with both hematologic toxicity and hepatic insufficiency, administer the lower of the doses determined appropriate from the following charts.

Vinorelbine Dose Adjustments for Hematologic Toxicity

Granulocytes (cells/mm^3) on Day of Treatment	Dose of Vinorelbine
≥1,500	100%
1,000 to 1,499	50%
<1,000	Do not administer. Repeat count in 1 week. If 3 consecutive weekly doses are held because granulocyte count is <1,000 cells/mm^3, discontinue vinorelbine
For patients who during treatment with vinorelbine have experienced fever and/or sepsis while granulocytopenic or had 2 consecutive weekly doses held due to granulocytopenia, subsequent doses of vinorelbine should be:	
≥1,500	75%
1,000 to 1,499	37.5%
<1,000	Same as <1,000 above

Vinorelbine Dose Adjustments for Impaired Hepatic Function

Total Bilirubin (mg/dl)	Dose of Vinorelbine
≤2	100%
2.1 to 3	50%
>3	25%

Appropriate dose reductions for cisplatin should be made when vinorelbine is used in combination. During studies, most patients required a 50% dose reduction of vinorelbine by day 15 and a 50% dose reduction of cisplatin by cycle 3. ■ No dose adjustment is required for impaired renal function. ■ If grade 2 or greater neurotoxicity develops, discontinue vinorelbine.

DILUTION

Specific techniques required; see Precautions.

IV injection: Each 10 mg (1 ml) must be further diluted with a minimum of 2 to 5 ml NS or D5W. Desired concentration is 1.5 to 3 mg/ml (2 ml diluent yields 3 mg/ml concentration, 5 ml yields 1.5 mg/ml concentration). Must be given into the side-arm port of a free-flowing IV infusion.

Intermittent infusion: Each 10 mg (1 ml) must be further diluted with 4 to 19 ml NS or D5W, ½NS, D5/½NS, R, or LR. Desired concentration is 0.5 to 2 mg/ml (4 ml diluent yields 2 mg/ml concentration, 19 ml yields 0.5 mg/ml concentration). Other references recommend diluting a single dose to a minimum total volume of 100 ml. Must be given into the side-arm port of a free-flowing IV infusion or may be given directly into a large central vein.

Storage: Refrigerate vials and protect from light; are stable at room temperature for up to 72 hours. Diluted solution stable for 24 hours at 5° to 30° C.

INCOMPATIBLE WITH

Manufacturer recommends mixing only with solutions listed under Dilution.

COMPATIBLE WITH **(Underline Indicates Conflicting Compatibility Information)**

Consult pharmacist; specific conditions may apply; see Compatibilities, p. xvi.

Y-site: Amikacin (Amikin), aztreonam (Azactam), bleomycin (Blenoxane), bumetanide (Bumex), buprenorphine (Buprenex), butorphanol (Stadol), calcium gluconate, carboplatin (Paraplatin), carmustine (BiCNU), cefotaxime (Claforan), ceftazidime (Fortaz), ceftizoxime (Cefizox), chlorpromazine (Thorazine), cimetidine (Tagamet), cisplatin (Platinol), clindamycin (Cleocin), cyclophosphamide (Cytoxan), cytarabine (ARA-C), dacarbazine (DTIC), dactinomycin (Cosmegen), daunorubicin (Cerubidine), dexamethasone (Decadron), diphenhydramine (Benadryl), doxorubicin (Adriamycin), doxorubicin liposome (Doxil), doxycycline (Vibramycin), droperidol (Inapsine), enalaprilat (Vasotec IV), etoposide (VePesid), famotidine (Pepcid IV), filgrastim (Neupogen), fluconazole (Diflucan), fludarabine (Fludara), gatifloxacin (Tequin), gemcitabine (Gemzar), gentamicin (Garamycin), granisetron (Kytril), haloperidol (Haldol), <u>heparin</u>, hydrocortisone (Hydrocortone, Solu-Cortef), hydromorphone (Dilaudid), idarubicin (Idamycin), ifosfamide (Ifex), imipenem-cilastatin (Primaxin), lorazepam (Ativan), mannitol, mechlorethamine (nitrogen mustard), melphalan (Alkeran), meperidine (Demerol), mesna (Mesnex), methotrexate (Folex), metoclopramide (Reglan), metronidazole (Flagyl IV), minocycline (Minocin), mitoxantrone (Novantrone), morphine, nalbuphine (Nubain), ondansetron (Zofran), plicamycin (Mithracin), streptozocin (Zanosar), teniposide (Vumon), ticarcillin (Ticar), ticarcillin/clavulanate (Timentin), tobramycin (Nebcin), vancomycin (Vancocin), vinblastine (Velban), vincristine (Oncovin), zidovudine (AZT, Retrovir).

RATE OF ADMINISTRATION

Inadequate flushing of the vein after administration may increase the risk of phlebitis.

IV injection: Total desired dose, properly diluted over 6 to 10 minutes through the side-arm port of a free-flowing IV. After administration, flush with at least 75 to 125 ml of diluent solution over 10 minutes or more. Up to 300 ml has been used as a flush.

Intermittent infusion: Total desired dose, properly diluted over 6 to 10 minutes. Other references recommend over 20 minutes. Must be given into the side-arm port of a free-flowing IV infusion or may be given directly into a large central vein. Flush according to directions for IV injection.

ACTIONS

An antineoplastic agent. A semisynthetic vinca alkaloid with chemical differences from other vinca alkaloids that may provide unique clinical benefits with a lower incidence of clinical neurotoxicity. Causes depolymerization of microtubules and inhibits microtubule assembly. May be more specific to mitotic microtubules. Cell cycle–specific and produces a blockade in the cell-cycle progression in G_2 and M phase. Widely distributed in the body. Elimination half-life is 27 to 43 hours. Metabolized in the liver by hepatic cytochrome P_{450} isoenzymes in the CYP3A subfamily. Excreted in bile, feces, and urine.

INDICATIONS AND USES

Treatment of unresectable advanced non–small-cell lung cancer (ANSCLC), in ambulatory patients. Used as a single agent or in combination with cisplatin. ■ Indicated as a single agent or in combination with cisplatin in patients with Stage IV NSCLC and in combination with cisplatin in patients with Stage III NSCLC.

Unlabeled uses: Treatment of breast, cervical, and epithelial ovarian cancers; treatment of desmoid tumors and fibromatosis, and advanced Kaposi's sarcoma.

CONTRAINDICATIONS

Patients with pretreatment granulocyte counts less than 1,000 cells/mm^3.

PRECAUTIONS

Follow guidelines for handling cytotoxic agents. See Appendix A, p. 1142. Severe irritation of the eye has been reported with accidental exposure to another vinca alkaloid. If exposure occurs, thoroughly flush eye with water immediately. ■ Administered by or under the direction of the physician specialist. ■ Manufacturer provides an auxillary sticker labeled "Fatal if given intrathecally, for IV use only" and an overwrap labeled "Do not remove covering until moment of injection. Fatal if given intrathecally. For Intravenous use only." Each and every syringe(s) containing a specific dose and prepared in advance of actual administration must be labeled with the provided auxiliary sticker and packaged in this overwrap. If intrathecal injection should occur, immediate neurosurgical intervention is required, consult package insert for immediate steps to be taken. ■ Adequate diagnostic and treatment facilities must be readily available. ■ Use extreme caution in patients with hepatic impairment, pre-existing neuromuscular disease, pre-existing peripheral neuropathies, or those taking other neurotoxic drugs (e.g., antineoplastics [cisplatin], phenothiazines [prochlorperazine]). ■ Acute SOB and severe bronchospasm have been reported, most commonly when vinorelbine was used with mitomycin. May require treatment with oxygen, bronchodilators (e.g., albuterol), and/or corticosteroids (e.g., hydrocortisone). Incidence may be increased when there is pre-existing pulmonary dysfunction. ▪ Prior radiation therapy or treatment with other antineoplastic agents may cause an increase in myelotoxicity; use with extreme caution. ▪ Administration to patients with prior radiation therapy may result in radiation recall reactions. ▪ See Monitor and Drug/Lab Interactions.

Monitor: Monitor CBC, differential, platelets, and bilirubin on each day of treatment to determine correct dose and 1 or 2 times weekly, granulocytopenia is dose-limiting. Temporary leukopenia is an expected effect. Maximum depression usually occurs in 7 to 10 days after the dose, and recovery should occur within the following 7 to 14 days. ▪ Cases of interstitial pulmonary changes and Adult Respiratory Distress Syndrome (ARDS), most of which were fatal, have been reported. Onset of symptoms has occurred in 3 to 8 days. Promptly evaluate patients with alterations in their baseline pulmonary symptoms or with new onset of cough, dyspnea, hypoxia, or other symptoms. ▪ Monitor AST (SGOT) frequently. ▪ Evaluate neurologic status frequently (e.g., constipation, decreased deep tendon reflexes, paresthesia). ▪ Closely monitor patients who have had symptoms of neuropathy with previous drug regimens (e.g., paclitaxel [Taxol]) for new or worsening neuropathy. ▪ Determine absolute patency and quality of vein and adequate circulation of extremity. Cellulitis and phlebitis with sloughing can result from extravasation. ▪ Be alert for any sign of infection. Infections must be brought under control before beginning therapy with vinorelbine. ▪ Use of prophylactic antibiotics may be indicated pending results of C/S in a febrile neutropenic patient. ▪ Maintain adequate hydration. ▪ Prophylactic antiemetics may increase patient comfort; haloperidol and oral dexamethasone have benefited some patients. ▪ May cause severe (grade 3-4) constipation, paralytic ileus, intestinal obstruction, necrosis, and/or perforation. Use a laxative to prevent constipation. Monitor bowel sounds. ▪ Monitor for hyponatremia and syndrome of inappropriate secretion of antidiuretic hormone (SIADH). ▪ Monitor for thrombocytopenia (platelet count less than 50,000/mm^3). Initiate precautions to prevent excessive bleeding (e.g., inspect IV sites, skin, and mucous membranes; use extreme care during invasive procedures; test urine, emesis, stool, and secretions for occult blood). ▪ See Precautions and Drug/Lab Interactions.

Patient Education: Report burning or stinging at IV site promptly. ▪ Report chills, fever, difficulty breathing, or shortness of breath promptly. ▪ Avoid pregnancy; nonhormonal birth control recommended. ▪ Take laxatives consistently to avoid constipation. ▪ See Appendix D, p. 1148.

Maternal/Child: Category D: avoid pregnancy; may cause fetal harm. ▪ Discontinue breast-feeding. ▪ Safety and effectiveness for use in children has been investigated. In one study, vinorelbine was considered to be ineffective when used in doses similar to those used in adults in a limited number of pediatric patients with recurrent solid malignant tumors (e.g., rhabdomyosarcoma/undifferentiated sarcoma, neuroblastoma, and CNS tumors). Toxicities were similar to those reported in adults.

Elderly: The pharmacokinetics of vinorelbine in elderly and younger adult patients are similar. No relationship between age, systemic exposure, and hematologic toxicity has been observed.

DRUG/LAB INTERACTIONS

Neurotoxicity may be increased by other neurotoxic drugs (e.g., antineoplastics [such as cisplatin, paclitaxel (Taxol)] and phenothiazines [prochlorperazine]); may require dose reduction or discontinuation of vinorelbine. Vestibular and auditory deficits have been observed, usually when vinorelbine is used in combination with cisplatin. ▪ Do not administer live vaccines to patients receiving antineoplastic drugs. ▪ Mitomycin-C may cause or aggravate acute pulmonary reactions (e.g., acute shortness of breath, bronchospasm). May require oxygen, bronchodilators, and/or corticosteroids. ▪ Granulocytopenia significantly higher when used in combination with cisplatin. ▪ Additive bone marrow depression may occur with radiation therapy and/or other bone marrow depressing agents (e.g., azathioprine [Imuran], chloramphenicol, melphalan [Alkeran]); dose reductions may be required. ▪ Leukopenic effects may be increased by agents that cause similar blood dyscrasias (e.g., anticonvulsants, antidepressants, phenothiazines). ▪ Drugs that inhibit the cytochrome P_{450} isoenzymes in the CYP3A subfamily (e.g., azole antifungals [e.g., itraconazole (Sporanox)], macrolides [e.g., erythromycin (Erythrocin), troleandomycin (TAO)]) may inhibit the metabolism of vinorelbine and increase its toxicity. ***Other vinca alkaloids cause interactions with the following drugs; vinorelbine has not been studied.*** ▪ Use with asparaginase or doxorubicin may not be recommended or require specific scheduling. ▪ May be potentiated by calcium channel blockers (e.g., verapamil). ▪ May inhibit digoxin and phenytoin; increased doses of these drugs may be required. ▪ See Precautions.

SIDE EFFECTS

Granulocytopenia is the major dose-limiting toxicity and may be significantly greater in combination regimens. Alopecia (12%, mild); anemia (87%, mild to moderate); ARDS, auditory deficits, bronchospasm, chest pain (7%); constipation (35%); diarrhea; dyspnea [2%] (acute and reversible shortness of breath may occur within a few hours); elevated total bilirubin and AST (SGOT); fatigue; hematologic toxicity [99%] (leukopenia and neutropenia are the most frequent and are dose-limiting); hemorrhagic cystitis (rare); hypertension; hypotension; intestinal obstruction, necrosis, and/or perforation; jaw pain; loss of deep tendon reflexes (5%); nausea and vomiting (50% [23%]); pain and redness at injection site (38%); pancreatitis, paralytic ileus (less than 2%); peripheral neuropathy (31%), mild to moderate paresthesia and hypesthesia, phlebitis (10%); pulmonary edema; radiosensitizing effects in patients with prior or concomitant radiation therapy; SIADH (few); subacute pulmonary reactions (4%, e.g., cough, dyspnea, hypoxemia, and interstitial infiltrates on chest x-ray); thrombocytopenia (rare), thrombocytosis (asymptomatic), tumor pain, vestibular deficits. Pattern of side effects similar when vinorelbine is used as a single agent or in combination.

ANTIDOTE

For severe reactions, discontinue vinorelbine or reduce subsequent doses. If grade 2 or greater neurotoxicity develops, discontinue vinorelbine. For extravasation, discontinue the drug immediately and administer into another vein. Elevate the extremity. Moist heat may be helpful. Notify the physician of all side effects; symptomatic treatment is often indicated. Discontinue for hyponatremia or SIADH, may require fluid limitation and diuretics (e.g., furosemide [Lasix]). Bone marrow toxicity is reversible after discontinuing vinorelbine. Administration of whole blood products (e.g., packed RBCs, platelets, leukocytes) may be indicated. Filgrastim (Neupogen), pegfilgrastim (Neulasta), sargramostim (Leukine), oprelvekin (Neumega), darbepoetin alfa [Aranesp], or epoetin alfa (Epogen) may be used to promote bone marrow recovery but may not be given within 24 hours of a dose of cytotoxic therapy or until 24 hours after a dose of cytotoxic therapy. Acute or chronic pulmonary reactions may be an allergic phenomena, corticosteroids (e.g., hydrocortisone [Solu Cortef]), oxygen and bronchodilators (e.g., albuterol [Ventolin, Proventil]) may be helpful. Neurologic toxicity may be reversible.

VORICONAZOLE

Antifungal

(vor-i-koh′na-zohl)

VFEND IV

USUAL DOSE

IV and oral doses are therapeutically equivalent. Oral dose can replace an IV dose as soon as practical; see Precautions. Duration of treatment is based on severity of the underlying disease, recovery from immunosuppression, and clinical response. Pretesting required; see Monitor. Obtain baseline electrolytes and correct calcium, magnesium, and potassium deficiencies before initiating voriconazole.

Loading dose: Begin with 6 mg/kg. Repeat 6 mg/kg in 12 hours. Follow with a **maintenance dose** of 4 mg/kg every 12 hours; see Dose Adjustments.

PEDIATRIC DOSE

Safety and effectiveness for use in pediatric patients less than 12 years of age not established; see Maternal/Child.

DOSE ADJUSTMENTS

Reduce the maintenance dose to 3 mg/kg every 12 hours in patients unable to tolerate treatment. ■ Increase the maintenance dose to 5 mg/kg every 12 hours if phenytoin (Dilantin) is being administered concurrently; see Drug/Lab Interactions. ■ No dose adjustment is indicated based on age or gender or in patients with baseline liver function tests (ALT, AST) up to 5 times the upper limit of normal (see Precautions and Monitor). ■ In patients with mild to moderate hepatic cirrhosis (Child-Pugh Class A and B), use the standard loading dose but reduce the maintenance dose by one half and administer every 12 hours based on tolerance of treatment and/or concurrent medication. ■ No dose adjustment is required in patients with a CrCl of 50 ml/min or greater; however, the intravenous vehicle, sulfobutyl ether beta-cyclodextrin sodium (SBECD), accumulates in patients with a CrCl of less than 50 ml/min. Use of oral voriconazole is recommended in these patients; see Precautions and Monitor. ■ A 4-hour hemodialysis session does not remove a sufficient amount of voriconazole to warrant dose adjustment.

DILUTION

Reconstitute each vial with exactly 19 ml SW. Use of a standard 20-ml (nonautomated) syringe is recommended to facilitate exact measurement.

Volume will be 20 ml (10 mg/ml). Discard the vial if a vacuum is not present to pull the diluent into the vial. Shake until all powder is dissolved. Calculate the required dose based on patient weight (see chart below). Must be further diluted for infusion in D5W, D5LR, LR, NS, D5/½NS, D5NS, ½NS, or D5W with 20 mEq KCl. Withdraw a volume equal to the calculated dose of voriconazole from an infusion bag or bottle (30 ml in the following example). The volume of diluent left in the infusion bag or bottle should be enough to allow a final concentration of not less than 0.5 mg/ml or greater than 5 mg/ml after voriconazole is added. Withdraw the required volume of reconstituted drug and add to the infusion bag or bottle. For example, a patient weighing 50 kg will require a loading dose of 300 mg (6 mg/kg × 50 kg), which equals 30 ml of reconstituted drug (1½ vials). Withdraw and discard 30 ml of solution from a 100-ml infusion bag and add the 30 ml of reconstituted drug. Final concentration equals 3 mg/ml.

Required Volumes of 10 mg/ml Voriconazole Concentrate			
	Volume of Voriconazole Concentrate (10 mg/ml) required for:		
Body Weight (kg)	3 mg/kg dose (number of vials)	4 mg/kg dose (number of vials)	6 mg/kg dose (number of vials)
30	9 ml (1)	12 ml (1)	18 ml (1)
35	10.5 ml (1)	14 ml (1)	21 ml (2)
40	12 ml (1)	16 ml (1)	24 ml (2)
45	13.5 ml (1)	18 ml (1)	27 ml (2)
50	15 ml (1)	20 ml (1)	30 ml (2)
55	16.5 ml (1)	22 ml (2)	33 ml (2)
60	18 ml (1)	24 ml (2)	36 ml (2)
65	19.5 ml (1)	26 ml (2)	39 ml (2)
70	21 ml (2)	28 ml (2)	42 ml (3)
75	22.5 ml (2)	30 ml (2)	45 ml (3)
80	24 ml (2)	32 ml (2)	48 ml (3)
85	25.5 ml (2)	34 ml (2)	51 ml (3)
90	27 ml (2)	36 ml (2)	54 ml (3)
95	28.5 ml (2)	38 ml (2)	57 ml (3)
100	30 ml (2)	40 ml (2)	60 ml (3)

Storage: Store unopened vials at CRT. Immediate use of reconstituted vials is preferred; however, they may be refrigerated up to 24 hours at 2° to 8° C (37° to 46° F). Discard partially used vials.

COMPATIBILITY

Manufacturer states, "Must not be infused into the same line or cannula concomitantly with other drug infusions, and infusions of blood products must not occur simultaneously with voriconazole." Infusions of total parenteral nutrition can occur simultaneously. Manufacturer lists voriconazole as incompatible with Aminofusin 10% Plus and states that it should not be diluted with 4.2% sodium bicarbonate solution. Compatibility with other concentrations of sodium bicarbonate is unknown; do not use.

RATE OF ADMINISTRATION

A single dose as an infusion over 1 to 2 hours. Do not exceed a rate of 3 mg/kg/hr.

ACTIONS

A triazole antifungal agent. Inhibits a fungal cytochrome P_{450}-mediated essential step in fungal ergosterol biosynthesis. With a loading dose, peak plasma concentrations (steady state) and trough concentrations are achieved within the first 24 hours. Extensively distributed into tissues. Plasma protein binding (estimated at 58%) is not affected by varying degrees of hepatic and renal insufficiency. Metabolized by cytochrome P_{450} enzymes (CYP2C19 is significantly involved). Terminal half-life is dose dependent and is not useful in predicting accumulation or elimination. Eliminated via hepatic metabolism; less than 2% is excreted unchanged in urine.

INDICATIONS AND USES

Treatment of invasive aspergillosis caused by *Aspergillus fumigatus* and other species of *Aspergillus.* ■ Treatment of serious fungal infections caused by *Scedosporium apiospermum* and *Fusarium* species, including *Fusarium solani*, in patients intolerant of or refractory to other therapy.

CONTRAINDICATIONS

Hypersensitivity to voriconazole or any of its components. Use caution in patients exhibiting hypersensitivity to other azoles (e.g., fluconazole [Diflucan], itraconazole [Sporanox], ketoconazole [Nizoral]); see Precautions. ■ Co-administration is specifically contraindicated with CYP3A4 substrates (e.g., cisapride [Propulsid], pimozide [Orap], and quinidine [astemizole and terfenadine would be included but are no longer commercially available]); increased plasma concentrations of these drugs may result in QT prolongation and torsades de pointes. ■ Co-administration is contraindicated with the following drugs: barbiturates (long acting [e.g., phenobarbital (Luminal)]), carbamazepine (Tegretol), ergot alkaloids (ergotamine and dihydroergotamine [D.H.E. 45]), rifabutin (Mycobutin), rifampin (Rifadin), and sirolimus (Rapamune); see Drug Interactions.

PRECAUTIONS

Do not give as an IV bolus, for infusion only. ■ Infusion-related hypersensitivity reactions, including anaphylaxis, chest tightness, dyspnea, faintness, fever, flushing, nausea, pruritus, rash, sweating, and tachycardia have occurred. Usually appear at the beginning of the infusion. If a hypersensitivity reaction occurs, discontinue the infusion. ■ Consider use in patients with severe hepatic insufficiency only if the benefit outweighs potential risk; monitor carefully for drug toxicity. ■ Serious hepatic reactions (including clinical hepatitis, cholestasis, and fulminant hepatic failure, including fatalities) have occurred. Usually occur in patients with serious underlying medical conditions (e.g., hematologic malignancy); however, hepatic reactions, including hepatitis and jaundice, have occurred in patients with no other identifiable risk factors. Liver function usually improves with discontinuation of voriconazole. ■ Consider use of IV formulation in patients with a CrCl less than 50 ml/min only if the benefit outweighs potential risk. Accumulation of SBECD may occur with the IV formulation; use of the oral formulation is recommended. ■ Acute renal failure has been reported, usually in patients receiving concomitant nephrotoxic drugs; see Drug/Lab Interactions. ■ May cause prolongation of the QT interval on ECG and rarely torsades de pointes. Use with caution in patients with proarrhythmic conditions (e.g., cardiotoxic chemotherapy, cardiomyopathy, hypokalemia, and concomitant medications that may also prolong the QT interval). ■ Because of the enzymes involved in metabolism, Asian populations may be poor metabolizers, and serum concentrations may be elevated from 2 to 4 times higher than normal metabolizers. Some Caucasians and Blacks are also poor metabolizers. ■ Blurred vision, color vision changes, and/or photophobia are common but may be associated with higher serum concentrations and/or doses. Usually resolves within 2 weeks of the end of voriconazole therapy. ■ Fungi with reduced susceptibility to one azole antifungal agent may also be less susceptible to other azole derivatives. Cross-resistance may occur and may require alternative antifungal therapy. ■ Oral maintenance doses adjusted based on weight (above or below 40 kg); see product literature.

Monitor: Specimens for fungal culture, serology, and histopathology should be obtained before therapy to isolate and identify causative organisms. Therapy may begin as soon as all specimens are obtained and before results are known. Reassess after test results are known. ■ Obtain baseline electrolytes and make rigorous attempts to correct calcium, magnesium, and potassium before initiating voriconazole. Monitor electrolytes during therapy; may cause hypocalcemia, hypokalemia, and hypomagnesemia. ■ Obtain baseline liver function tests (e.g., alkaline phosphatase, ALT, AST, bilirubin), serum creatinine, and electrolytes in all patients. Monitor liver function tests during therapy, more frequently in patients with increasing or pre-existing elevated liver function tests and/or impaired hepatic function, and any time S/S suggestive of liver dysfunction develop (e.g., jaundice, lethargy). ■ Monitor serum creatinine during therapy, more frequently in patients with a CrCl less than 50 ml/min. If increases occur, consider changing to the oral formulation. ■ Monitor for S/S of hypersensitivity reactions; see Precautions and Antidote. ■ Monitor visual acuity, visual field, and color perception if treatment continues beyond 28 days. ■ If a rash develops, serious cutaneous reactions (e.g., Stevens-Johnson syndrome) may develop; monitor closely and consider discontinuing voriconazole. ■ See Precautions, Drug/Lab Interactions, and Antidote.

Patient Education: Avoid pregnancy; nonhormonal birth control recommended. Should pregnancy occur, notify physician immediately and discuss potential hazards. ■ Do not drive at night; changes to vision, including blurring and/or photophobia, may occur. ■ If a change in vision occurs, avoid hazardous tasks, such as driving or operating machinery. ■ Avoid strong, direct sunlight. ■ Promptly report S/S of a hypersensitivity reaction (e.g., itching, hives, shortness of breath).

Maternal/Child: Category D: avoid pregnancy; may cause fetal harm. Teratogenic in rats and embryotoxic in rabbits. Use of effective contraception is required in women of childbearing age. ■ Discontinue breast-feeding. ■ Twenty-two pediatric patients between 12 and 18 years of age with invasive aspergillosis were included in studies.

Elderly: Safety profile similar to younger adults. ■ Peak plasma concentrations slightly higher in elderly males; however, dose adjustment is not indicated. ■ Use caution; consider decreased cardiac, hepatic, or renal function and effects of concomitant disease or other drug therapy. ■ Monitor liver and renal function closely.

DRUG/LAB INTERACTIONS

Interactions are numerous and potentially life threatening. Review of drug profile by pharmacist is imperative.

Contraindicated with CYP3A4 substrates (e.g., cisapride [Propulsid], pimozide [Orap], and quinidine [astemizole and terfenadine would be included but are no longer commercially available]); increased plasma concentrations of these drugs may result in QT prolongation and torsades de pointes. ■ **Contraindicated** with long-acting barbiturates (e.g., phenobarbital [Luminal]), carbamazepine (Tegretol), and rifampin (Rifadin); these drugs may significantly increase metabolism and decrease serum concentrations of voriconazole. ■ **Contraindicated** with sirolimus (Rapamune); metabolism of sirolimus is decreased, and serum concentrations are significantly increased by voriconazole. ■ **Contraindicated** with rifabutin (Mycobutin); voriconazole significantly increases the serum concentrations of rifabutin, and rifabutin significantly decreases voriconazole serum concentrations.

Contraindicated with ergot alkaloids (e.g., ergotamine and dihydroergotamine (D.H.E. 45); serum concentrations of ergot alkaloids may be increased and may lead to ergotism. ■ May decrease the metabolism and increase serum levels of cyclosporine (Sandimmune). If concurrent administration with voriconazole is indicated, reduce the dose of cyclosporine by one half and monitor cyclosporine serum levels frequently. When voriconazole is discontinued, monitor cyclosporine levels frequently and increase the dose as necessary. ■ May decrease the metabolism and increase serum levels of tacrolimus (Prograf). If concurrent administration with voriconazole is indicated, reduce the dose of tacrolimus by one third and monitor tacrolimus serum levels frequently. When voriconazole is discontinued, monitor tacrolimus levels frequently and increase the dose as necessary. ■ Concurrent use with warfarin (Coumadin) or oral coumarin preparations may cause a significant increase in PT or INR. Monitor PT or INR closely and adjust warfarin dose as necessary. ■ May decrease the metabolism and increase serum concentrations of CYP3A4 substrates, such as selected HMG-CoA reductase inhibitors (statins such as lovastatin [Mevacor]), selected benzodiazepines (e.g., alprazolam [Xanax], midazolam [Versed], triazolam [Halcion]), selected calcium channel blockers (e.g., felodipine [Plendil]), vinca alkaloids (e.g., vinblastine [Velban], vincristine [Oncovin]), and CYP2C9 substrates such as sulfonylureas (e.g., glipizide [Glucotrol XL], glyburide [DiaBeta], tolbutamide [Orinase]). To reduce the potential for toxic effects that may be caused by these drugs (e.g., rhabdomyolysis, prolonged sedative effect, cardiac toxicity, neurotoxicity, hypoglycemia), close monitoring of serum levels of all of these drugs is indicated, and in most cases dose reduction is indicated during concomitant administration of voriconazole. ■ Concurrent use with phenytoin (Dilantin) may require dose adjustments of both drugs. Phenytoin increases metabolism and decreases serum concentrations of voriconazole. An increased dose of voriconazole is indicated; see Dose Adjustments. Voriconazole decreases the metabolism of phenytoin and increases serum concentrations. Monitor phenytoin serum concentrations and reduce dose as necessary to avoid toxicity. ■ May decrease the metabolism and increase serum levels of selected HIV protease inhibitors (e.g., amprenavir [Agenerase], nelfinavir [Viracept], saquinavir [Invirase]). Selected HIV protease inhibitors (e.g., amprenavir, ritonavir [Norvir], saquinavir) may decrease the metabolism of voriconazole and increase its serum levels. Monitor frequently for drug toxicity with co-administration of voriconazole and HIV protease inhibitors. No dose adjustment is required with indinavir (Crixivan). ■ May decrease the metabolism and increase serum levels of omeprazole (Prilosec). If concurrent administration with voriconazole is indicated, reduce a dose of omeprazole of 40 mg or more by one half. The metabolism of other selected proton pump inhibitors may react similarly. ■ Non-nucleoside reverse transcriptase inhibitors (NNRTIs) such as delavirdine (Rescriptor) and efavirenz (Sustiva) may decrease the metabolism of voriconazole and increase its serum concentrations. Voriconazole may inhibit the metabolism of the same NNRTIs and increase their serum levels. Monitor frequently for drug toxicity with co-administration of voriconazole and NNRTIs. ■ Concurrent use with other nephrotoxic drugs (e.g., aminoglycosides, cyclosporine) may result in decreased renal function or acute renal failure. ■ May have minor interactions with cimetidine (Tagamet), macrolide antibiotics (e.g., azithromycin, erythromycin), and ranitidine (Zantac); however, no dose adjustments are required. ■ No significant interactions have been observed with indinavir (Crixivan), prednisolone, digoxin (Lanoxin), and mycophenolate mofetil (CellCept).

SIDE EFFECTS

Abdominal pain, diarrhea, dyspnea, fever, headache, hypokalemia, increases in liver function tests, nausea, peripheral edema, rash, sepsis, visual disturbances, and vomiting occur most frequently. Blurred vision, color vision change, and/or photophobia are common but may be associated with higher serum concentrations and/or doses. Hypersensitivity reactions, including anaphylaxis, have been reported. Rarely, Stevens-Johnson syndrome and photosensitivity skin reactions have been reported. Numerous other side effects may occur, including QT prolongation and rarely torsades de pointes.

ANTIDOTE

Notify physician of all side effects; most will be treated symptomatically. If a hypersensitivity reaction (e.g., an infusion reaction) occurs, discontinue the infusion and treat with oxygen, epinephrine, antihistamines (e.g., diphenhydramine [Benadryl]), corticosteroids (e.g., dexamethasone [Decadron]), or bronchodilators (e.g., albuterol [Ventolin]) as indicated. Consider discontinuation of voriconazole if liver function tests are elevated and/or clinical S/S of liver disease attributable to voriconazole develop, if visual disturbances occur, if an increase in serum creatinine occurs, or if a rash develops (may be the first sign of an exfoliative skin disorder). No known specific antidote. Hemodialysis may assist in the removal of some voriconazole in accidental overdose and in the removal of SBECD. Resuscitate as indicated.

WARFARIN SODIUM

(war′far-in so′de-um)

Anticoagulant

Coumadin

pH 8.1 to 8.3

USUAL DOSE

Used primarily for patients on Coumadin when oral dosing is not feasible. IV and oral doses are the same. Dose must be individualized and adjusted based on PT/International Normalized Ratio (INR). An INR of greater than 4 appears to provide no additional benefit in most patients and is associated with a higher risk of bleeding. Loading doses may increase the incidence of complications and do not offer greater prompt anticoagulation protection. Heparin is preferred in situations requiring prompt anticoagulation because the anticoagulant actions for warfarin are not effective for at least 60 hours after initial dosing begins (60 hours is the half-life of the last clotting factor [II] to be affected by warfarin).

Maintenance dose: 2 to 10 mg/day. Adjust dose to maintain desired INR.

Atrial fibrillation, prophylaxis and treatment of venous thromboembolism, prophylaxis and treatment of pulmonary embolism: Adjust dose to maintain an INR of 2 to 3.

Postmyocardial infarction: Usually initiated 2 to 4 weeks postinfarction and maintained long term. Adjust dose to maintain an INR of 2.5 to 3.5.

Mechanical heart valves: Adjust dose to maintain an INR of 2.5 to 3.5. Maintained long term.

Bioprosthetic heart valves: Adjust dose to maintain an INR of 2 to 3 for 12 weeks after valve insertion. Longer-term therapy may be required in patients with additional risk factors (e.g., atrial fibrillation, prior thromboembolism).

PEDIATRIC DOSE

Safety for use in children under age 18 not established, but is used. Usually given PO.

Prophylaxis and treatment of thromboembolic events: 0.1 mg/kg/24 hr. Adjust to desired PT/INR.

Maintenance dose: 0.05 to 0.34 mg/kg/24 hr.

DOSE ADJUSTMENTS

Use low initial doses in the elderly, debilitated, and those with expected increased PT/INR responses. ■ Use lower end of dose range in patients at increased risk of bleeding or those on aspirin therapy. ■ Reduced dose is required in impaired hepatic function. ■ No dose adjustment is required in impared renal function. ■ Higher doses may be required in selected situations (e.g., patients with recurrent systemic embolism or mechanical prosthetic valves). The American College of Chest Physicians (ACCP) and the National Heart, Lung, and Blood Institute (NHLBI) suggest maintaining an INR of 3 to 4.5.

DILUTION

Reconstitute the 5-mg vial with 2.7 ml of SW (2 mg/ml).

Storage: Protect from light by storing in carton at CRT. Store reconstituted solution at room temperature and use within 4 hours. Do not refrigerate; discard any unused solution.

INCOMPATIBLE WITH

One source lists amikacin (Amikin), epinephrine (Adrenalin), oxytocin (Pitocin), and vancomycin (Vancocin). Some adsorption may occur in PVC containers and tubing when diluted in D5W or NS.

COMPATIBLE WITH (Underline Indicates Conflicting Compatibility Information)

Consult pharmacist; specific conditions may apply; see Compatibilities, p. xvi.

Y-site: Amikacin (Amikin), ammonium chloride, ascorbic acid (Cenolate), cefazolin (Kefzol), ceftriaxone (Rocephin), dopamine (Intropin), epinephrine (Adrenalin), heparin, lidocaine, morphine, nitroglycerin (Nitro-Bid IV), oxytocin (Pitocin), potassium chloride (KCl), ranitidine (Zantac), vancomycin (Vancocin).

RATE OF ADMINISTRATION

A single dose as an injection over 1 to 2 minutes.

ACTIONS

An anticoagulant that acts by inhibiting vitamin K–dependent coagulation factors (e.g., Factor II, VII, IX, and X) and the anticoagulant proteins C and S in the liver, resulting in a depression of their activities. An anticoagulant effect occurs within 24 hours; however, peak anticoagulant effect may be delayed for 72 to 96 hours. Effective half-life ranges from 20 to 60 hours. Effects may be more pronounced as daily maintenance doses overlap. Well-established clots are not dissolved, but growth is prevented. Metabolized by the liver to inactive metabolites and reduced metabolites. Excreted primarily in urine with small amounts excreted in bile. Crosses the placental barrier. Secreted in breast milk in an inactive form.

INDICATIONS AND USES

Prophylaxis and/or treatment of venous thrombosis and pulmonary embolism. ■ Prophylaxis and/or treatment of the thromboembolic complications of atrial fibrillation and/or cardiac valve replacement. ■ Reduce the risk of death, recurrent myocardial infarction, and thromboembolic events such as stroke or systemic embolization after myocardial infarction. ■ Treatment of patients receiving oral warfarin who are unable to take oral medication.

CONTRAINDICATIONS

Localized or general physical condition or circumstance in which the hazard of hemorrhage might be greater than the potential clinical benefits of anticoagulation (e.g., bleeding tendencies associated with active ulceration or overt bleeding of GI, GU, or respiratory tracts, CVA, aneurysms [cerebral or aortic], pericarditis, pericardial effusions, bacterial endocarditis; hemorrhagic tendencies or blood dyscrasias, inadequate laboratory facilities; major regional or lumbar block anesthesia; malignant hypertension; pregnancy; spinal puncture or other procedures with potential for uncontrollable bleeding; threatened abortion, eclampsia, preeclampsia; unsupervised patients who would find it difficult to cooperate [e.g., senility, alcoholism, or psychosis]; and recent or contemplated surgery of the CNS, eye, or traumatic surgery resulting in large open surfaces).

PRECAUTIONS

For IV use only; do not administer IM. ■ Determinations of whole blood clotting and bleeding times are not an accurate measurement to adjust dose. ■ A severe aPTT elevation (greater than 50 seconds) with a PT/INR in the normal range is an indicator of increased risk of postoperative hemorrhage. ■ Use caution in the elderly or debilitated, severe to moderate impaired hepatic or renal function, severe to moderate hypertension, severe diabetes, with indwelling catheters, infectious diseases or disturbances of intestinal flora (e.g., sprue, antibiotic therapy), surgery or trauma involving large raw surfaces or that may result in internal bleeding, patients with a history of allergic problems, polycythemia vera, vasculitis, and known or suspected deficiency in protein C anticoagulant response. ■ Increased PT/INR response may occur in patients with blood dyscrasias (see Contraindications), cancer, collagen vascular disease, congestive heart failure, diarrhea, elevated temperature, hyperthyroidism, infectious hepatitis, jaundice, poor nutritional state, steatorrhea, or vitamin K deficiency. ■ Decreased PT/INR response may occur in patients with edema, hereditary coumarin resistance, hyperlipidemia, hypothyroidism, or nephrotic syndrome. Patients who are protein C or S deficient (inherited thrombotic conditions) must be covered with heparin and warfarin. ■ If dental procedures or surgery or other minor surgical procedures are necessary, the PT/INR should be adjusted to the lower end of the therapeutic range. Monitor PT/INR just before treatment. Operative site should be limited so local procedures for hemostasis can be used. Warfarin therapy may have to be interrupted; consider risks versus benefits.

Monitor: PT/INR must be done before initial injection. Frequent monitoring of PT/INR required (bedside monitoring units are now available that are very accurate). Usually repeated daily during initiation of therapy, every 1 to 4 weeks after PT/INR has stabilized in the therapeutic range. Monitor with any change in patient regimen that may affect treatment (e.g., diet, illness, change in drug regimen). Draw blood for prothrombin just before a heparin dose being given concomitantly. If heparin is given as a continuous infusion, PT/INR may be drawn at any time. ■ See Precautions. ■ Has a narrow therapeutic range that can be affected by other drugs and dietary vitamin K. See Drug/Lab Interactions. ■ Decrease dose gradually over 3 to 4 weeks.

Patient Education: Nonhormonal birth control recommended. ■ Adhere to dose schedule; do not take or discontinue any prescription or over-the-counter medication, including herbal products, without physician's approval. ■ Confirm procedure for missed dose. ■ Avoid alcohol. ■ Avoid any activity or sport that may result in traumatic injury. ■ Regular PT/INR testing and physician visits are imperative. ■ Notify physician of any illness (e.g., diarrhea, infection, fever) or unusual bleeding (e.g., increased menstrual flow, nosebleeds, tarry stools), headache, dizziness, or weakness. ■ Carry an ID stating that warfarin is being taken.

Maternal/Child: Category X: avoid pregnancy. May cause fatal hemorrhage to the fetus, has caused birth deformities, and may cause abortion and/or stillbirth. ■ In mothers requiring warfarin, consider alternative methods of infant feeding, or use extreme caution if decision is made to breast-feed. Prolonged PTs have been reported in breast-fed infants. Careful monitoring of coagulation tests and vitamin K status in the breast-fed infant and the mother's PT/INR is required.

Elderly: Less warfarin is required to produce a therapeutic level of anticoagulation in patients over 60 years of age; may have a greater-than-expected PT/INR response; see Dose Adjustments. ■ Not recommended for use in an unsupervised patient with senility.

DRUG/LAB INTERACTIONS

Monitor PT/INR carefully when drugs are added or discontinued. ***Interactions are numerous and potentially life threatening. Review of drug profile by pharmacist is imperative.*** ▪ Listed are some of the most significant. ▪ Not recommended for concurrent use with streptokinase or urokinase; may be hazardous. ▪ **Increased PT/INR response** (risk of bleeding increased) may occur with amiodarone (Cordarone), antifungal agents (e.g., fluconazole [Diflucan], itraconazole [Sporanox], miconazole [Monistat (intravaginal or systemic)]), aspirin, capecitabine (Xeloda), celecoxib (Celebrex), cimetidine (Tagamet), cisapride (Propulsid), clofibrate (Atromid-S), cyclophosphamide (Cytoxan), erythromycin, fenofibrate (Tricor), fluoroquinolones (e.g., levofloxacin [Levaquin]), fluvastatin (Lescol), heparin, herbal medicines (e.g., bromelains, danshen, dong quai, garlic, ginkgo biloba, and ginseng), isoniazid (Nydrazid), metronidazole (Flagyl), NSAIDs (e.g., ibuprofen [Advil, Motrin], naproxen [Aleve, Naprosyn, phenylbutazone [Butazolidin]), omeprazole (Prilosec), propafenone (Rhythmol), propranolol (Inderal), rofecoxib (Vioxx), sulfinpyrazone (Anturane), sulfonamides (e.g., SMX-TMP [Bactrim]), ticlopidine (Ticlid), tolterodine (Detrol), tramadol (Ultram). ▪ **Decreased PT/INR response** (anticoagulant effects decreased and risk of blood clots increased) may occur with barbiturates (e.g., phenobarbital), carbamazepine (Tegretol), cholestyramine (Questran), griseofulvin (Fulvicin), nevirapine (Viramune), penicillins (e.g., nafcillin [Nafcil]), rifampin (Rifadin), ritonavir (Norvir), sucralfate (Carafate), and increased oral vitamin K intake (e.g., leafy greens, supplements). ▪ Atorvastatin (Lipitor) and pravastatin (Pravachol) may increase or decrease PT/INR. ▪ May inhibit metabolism and increase effects of nifedipine (Adalat), oral antidiabetic agents (e.g., tolbutamide [Orinase]), phenytoin (Dilantin); may cause toxicity.

SIDE EFFECTS

Bleeding when the PT/INR is within the therapeutic range (may unmask an unsuspected lesion [e.g., tumor, ulcer]), hemorrhage in any tissue or organ, necrosis and/or gangrene of skin and other tissues. Complications from systemic cholesterol microembolization (e.g., "purple toes syndrome") from release of atheromatous plaque emboli. Allergic reactions do occur. Protein C deficiency may occur if not covered by heparin long enough.

ANTIDOTE

Keep physician informed of all side effects; some may be life threatening. Discontinue if warfarin is suspected to be the cause of developing necrosis (e.g., "purple toes syndrome"); consider heparin therapy if anticoagulation required. Phytonadione (Aquamephyton) is a specific antagonist and indicated in overdose or desired warfarin reversal (e.g., severe bleeding). In one small study, IV vitamin K (Phytonadione) decreased the INR more rapidly in 24 hours than SC phytonadione; however, within 72 hours, results were similar. Will impede subsequent anticoagulant therapy. Fresh whole blood, fresh frozen plasma, Factor IX complex (not purified Factor IX preparations, they increase PT levels) may be indicated.

ZIDOVUDINE

Antiviral

(zye-doh'vyou-deen)

Azidothymidine, AZT, Compound S, Retrovir

pH 5.5

USUAL DOSE

Treatment of HIV infection (symptomatic or asymptomatic): 1 mg/kg every 4 hours (5 or 6 times daily) is the most frequent dose used in the United States. Dose recommendation in Canada is 1 to 2 mg/kg every 4 hours. Initiate oral therapy as soon as possible (100 mg PO approximately equal to 1 mg/kg IV). Impaired renal or hepatic function may increase toxicity. Usually part of a multi-drug regimen (e.g., zidovudine, zalcitabine [HIVID], saquinavir [Invirase]); see Drug/Lab Interactions.

Prevention of maternal-fetal HIV transmission: 2 mg/kg of total body weight over 1 hour when labor begins. Follow with an infusion of 1 mg/kg/hr (of total body weight) until umbilical cord is clamped.

PEDIATRIC DOSE

Treatment of HIV infections in children 3 months to 12 years of age: 120 mg/M^2 every 6 hours as an intermittent infusion or a continuous infusion of 20 mg/M^2/hr. Reduce 120 mg/M^2 dose to 90 mg/M^2 in pediatric patients with granulocytopenia. Follow with oral therapy; see comments in Usual Dose.

NEONATAL DOSE

Prevention of maternal-fetal HIV transmission: 1.5 mg/kg infused over 30 minutes every 6 hours. Oral dosing preferred. Consider impaired hepatic or renal function. Begin within 12 hours of birth and continue until 6 weeks of age. Another source suggests 1.5 mg/kg/dose every 12 hours in premature infants from birth to 2 weeks of age, then increase to 2 mg/kg/dose every 8 hours.

DOSE ADJUSTMENTS

Dose selection should be cautious in the elderly based on the potential for decreased organ function and concomitant disease or drug therapy. ■ Reduce dose to 1 mg/kg every 6 to 8 hours in patients with ESRD. ■ Reduce the 120 mg/M^2 dose to 90 mg/M^2 in pediatric patients with granulocytopenia. ■ May be required in anemia and/or with other drugs. See Monitor, Drug/Lab Interactions, and Antidote.

DILUTION

Each 1 mg of the calculated dose must be diluted in at least 0.25 ml of D5W (4 mg/ml). For a 70-kg patient at 1 mg/kg, a 70-mg dose would be diluted in 17.5 ml (equals 4 mg/ml [70 mg in 35 ml equals 2 mg/ml]). More dilute solutions are preferred (e.g., 1 mg/ml).

Infusion: Dilute 1 Gm in 1,000 ml D5W (1 mg/ml), 500 mg in 500 ml (1 mg/ml), 1 Gm in 500 ml (2 mg/ml), or 1 Gm in 250 ml (4 mg/ml).

Storage: Store undiluted vials at 15° to 25° C (59° to 77° F). Protect from light. Stable after dilution for 8 hours at room temperature, 24 hours if refrigerated.

INCOMPATIBLE WITH

Manufacturer states, "Admixture in biologic or colloidal fluids (e.g., blood products, protein solutions) is not recommended."

COMPATIBLE WITH (Underline Indicates Conflicting Compatibility Information)

Consult pharmacist; specific conditions may apply; see Compatibilities, p. xvi.

Additive: Meropenem (Merrem IV).

Y-site: Acyclovir (Zovirax), allopurinol (Aloprim, Zyloprim), amifostine (Ethyol), amikacin (Amikin), amphotericin B (Fungizone), amphotericin B cholesteryl (Amphotec), aztreonam (Azactam), cefepime (Maxipime), ceftazidime (Fortaz), ceftriaxone (Rocephin), cimetidine (Tagamet), cisatracurium (Nimbex), clindamycin (Cleocin), dexamethasone (Decadron), dobutamine (Dobutrex), docetaxel (Taxotere), dopamine (Intropin), doxorubicin liposome (Doxil), erythromycin lactobionate (Erythrocin), etoposide phosphate (Etopophos), filgrastim (Neupogen), fluconazole (Diflucan), fludarabine (Fludara), gatifloxacin (Tequin), gemcitabine (Gemzar), gentamicin (Garamycin), granisetron (Kytril), heparin, imipenem-cilastatin (Primaxin), linezolid (Zyvox), lorazepam (Ativan), melphalan (Alkeran), meropenem (Merrem IV), metoclopramide (Reglan), morphine, nafcillin (Nafcil), ondansetron (Zofran), oxacillin (Bactocill), paclitaxel (Taxol), pentamidine, phenylephrine (Neo-Synephrine), piperacillin (Pipracil), piperacillin/tazobactam (Zosyn), potassium chloride (KCl), ranitidine (Zantac), remifentanil (Ultiva), sargramostim (Leukine), sulfamethoxazole-trimethoprim (Bactrim), teniposide (Vumon), thiotepa (Thioplex), tobramycin (Nebcin), trimetrexate (Neutrexin), vancomycin (Vancocin), vinorelbine (Navelbine).

RATE OF ADMINISTRATION

Intermittent infusion: Each single dose properly diluted must be delivered at a constant rate over 1 hour. Avoid rapid infusion or IV bolus.

Continuous infusion: Prevention of maternal-fetal HIV transmission: 2 mg/kg equally distributed over 1 hour, followed by 1 mg/kg/hr until umbilical cord clamped.

Pediatric continuous infusion: 0.5 to 1.8 mg/kg/hr.

Neonatal in prevention of maternal-fetal HIV transmission: A single dose infused over 30 min.

ACTIONS

An antiviral agent. Through a specific process this thymidine analog inhibits the in vitro replication and terminates the DNA chain of some retroviruses, including HIV (HTLV III, LAV, or ARV). May also have antiviral activity against the Epstein-Barr virus. Metabolized by glucuronidation in the liver and excreted through the kidneys. Crosses the placental barrier. Secreted in breast milk.

INDICATIONS AND USES

Treatment of HIV infection in combination with other anti-retroviral agents. ■ Prevention of maternal-fetal HIV transmission. Protocol includes oral zidovudine beginning with week 14 to week 34 of gestation, continuing until labor begins, IV dosing during labor, and zidovudine syrup or IV dosing to the newborn.

CONTRAINDICATIONS

Life-threatening allergic reactions to any of the components.

PRECAUTIONS

Do not give IM. ■ Zidovudine has not been shown to reduce the risk of transmission to others. ■ Use with extreme caution in patients with bone marrow compromise as indicated by a granulocyte count of less than 1,000/mm^3 or hemoglobin below 9.5/dl. ■ Zidovudine resistance seems to develop more quickly in patients with advanced disease. ■ Decrease in

CD4 count or clinical deterioration may be reversed with a switch to didanosine. ■ Prolonged use of zidovudine has been associated with myopathy and myositis with pathological changes similar to those produced by HIV disease. ■ Rare cases of potentially fatal lactic acidosis (without hypoxemia) and severe hepatomegaly with steatosis have been reported with the use of some antiretroviral nucleoside analogs. Lactic acidosis should be considered, and therapy suspended, in patients who develop unexplained tachypnea, dyspnea, or a fall in serum sodium bicarbonate. ■ Use with caution in any patient (especially obese women) with hepatomegaly, hepatitis, or other risk factors for liver disease. Suspend therapy with rapidly elevating aminotransferase levels (ALT), progressive hepatomegaly, or metabolic/lactic acidosis of unknown etiology. ■ See Drug/Lab Interactions.

Monitor: Observe closely; not a cure for HIV infections. Patients may acquire illnesses associated with AIDS or ARC, including opportunistic infections. ■ Frequent blood cell counts are required. Hematologic toxicity, including granulocytopenia, severe anemia, and occasionally reversible pancytopenia are common. Anemia occurs most commonly after 4 to 6 weeks of therapy; dosage adjustments and/or transfusions may be required. ■ Monitor liver function. ■ See Drug/Lab Interactions.

Patient Education: Report abdominal pain, jaundice, muscle weakness, shortness of breath, or rapid breathing promptly. ■ Requires close follow-up with physician; keep all appointments. ■ Check with physician before taking any other meds.

Maternal/Child: Category C: safety for use during pregnancy has been evaluated. Risk versus benefit appears justified only in HIV-infected mothers. Congenital deformities not increased in studies. ■ Discontinue breast-feeding to reduce incidence of HIV transmission and potential for serious adverse reactions in nursing infants. ■ Safety for use in children under 12 years of age not established but has been used. Consider impaired hepatic and renal function.

Elderly: Dose selection should be cautious; see Dose Adjustments.

DRUG/LAB INTERACTIONS

Toxicity may be increased by nephrotoxic and/or cytotoxic drugs and/or drugs that interfere with RBC or WBC number and function (e.g., amphotericin B [Fungizone], dapsone, doxorubicin [Adriamycin], flucytosine, interferons, pentamidine, vinblastine [Velban], vincristine [Oncovin], vindesine [Eldesine]). ■ ***Do not use in combination with other products that contain zidovudine (e.g., lamivudine/zidovudine [Combivir], abacavir/lamivudine/zidovudine [Trizivir]).*** ■ Use caution with any drug metabolized by glucuronidation (e.g., acetaminophen, diazepam [Valium], morphine); toxicity of both drugs may be increased. ■ Probenicid may inhibit glucuronidation or reduce renal excretion of zidovudine, increasing zidovudine toxicity. ■ Use with atovaquone (Mepron), fluconazole (Diflucan), or sulfamethoxazole-trimethoprim (Bactrim) may increase zidovudine serum levels. Acetaminophen (Anacin-3, Tylenol), aspirin, or indomethacin (Indocin), and rifamycins (e.g., rifampin [Rifadin], rifabutin [Mycobutin]) may reduce zidovudine serum levels, increase clearance, and reduce effectiveness. ■ Acetaminophen has increased the incidence of granulocytopenia. ■ Hematologic toxicity may be increased by nucleoside analogs being evaluated in AIDS and ARC patients (e.g., didanosine [DDI]) because of their effect on RBC or WBC numbers or function. The same analogs can affect DNA replication and may antagonize effects of zidovudine. Avoid concomitant administration. ■ Hematologic toxicity increased with ganciclovir (Cytovene) and interferons. ■ Phenytoin levels may increase or decrease; monitor carefully to assure proper dosing. ■ Phenytoin may also increase zidovudine levels by decreasing clearance. ■ Use with acyclovir may cause neurotoxicity (drowsiness, lethargy).

SIDE EFFECTS

Directly related to pretreatment bone marrow reserve, dose and duration and inversely related to T4 lymphocyte numbers. Anaphylaxis, anemia (severe), anorexia, asthenia, constipation, diaphoresis, diarrhea, dizziness, dyspepsia, dysphagia, dyspnea, fever, flatulence, GI pain, granulocytopenia, gynecomastia, headache, hepatomegaly (severe), insomnia, malaise, mouth ulcers, myalgia, myopathy and myositis, nausea, neutropenia, pancytopenia (reversible), paresthesia, rash, somnolence, taste perversion, vomiting. Suspect lactic acidosis if dyspnea, a fall in serum bicarbonate level, or tachypnea occurs.

ANTIDOTE

Notify physician of all side effects; most will be treated symptomatically. Moderate anemia or granulocytopenia may respond to a reduction in dose. Discontinue zidovudine for severe anemia (less than 7.5 Gm/dl or a 25% reduction from baseline) or severe granulocytopenia (less than 750/mm^3 or 50% reduction from baseline). Transfusions may be required. Rash may be the first sign of anaphylaxis; notify physician and treat with diphenhydramine (Benadryl), epinephrine (Adrenalin), and corticosteriods as indicated. Sulfamethoxazole-trimethoprim (Bactrim), pyrimethamine (Daraprim), and acyclovir (Zovirax) may be indicated to treat opportunistic infections.

ZOLEDRONIC ACID

(zoh′leh-dron-ick as′id)

Antihypercalcemic (bisphosphonate)

Zometa

pH 2

USUAL DOSE

Prehydration required. Always used in conjunction with adequate hydration and appropriate monitoring. See Dose Adjustments, Precautions, and Monitor.

Hypercalcemia of malignancy (corrected serum calcium equal to or greater than 12 mg/dl [3 mmol/L]): One dose of 4 mg as an infusion over no less than 15 minutes.

Experience is limited, but retreatment with the same dose may be considered if serum calcium does not return to normal or remain normal after initial treatment. Wait at least 7 days from completion of the first infusion to allow full response.

Multiple myeloma and metastatic bone lesions from solid tumors: 4 mg as an infusion over no less than 15 minutes every 3 or 4 weeks. Concurrent daily administration of PO calcium 500 mg and a multivitamin with 400 units vitamin D is recommended.

PEDIATRIC DOSE

Safety and effectiveness for use in pediatric patients not established.

DOSE ADJUSTMENTS

In patients who experience a decrease in renal function after receiving the initial dose of zoledronic acid, delayed dosing is required before retreatment as follows:

Normal serum creatinine (SrCr) before treatment: If SrCr has increased 0.5 mg/dl within 2 weeks of planned retreatment, withhold retreatment dose until recovery to within 10% of baseline SrCr value.

Abnormal SrCr before treatment: If SrCr has increased 1 mg/dl within 2 weeks of planned retreatment, withhold retreatment dose until the SrCr is within 10% of baseline value.

Dose adjustment is not indicated based on age or race. Studies have not been conducted in patients with hepatic or severe renal impairment; see Precautions.

DILUTION

Reconstitute each 4-mg dose with 5 ml of SW. Dissolve completely. Must be further diluted in 100 ml of NS or D5W.

Storage: Store vials in carton at CRT. Use immediately after reconstitution and dilution is preferred. Reconstituted solution may be refrigerated but must be used and the infusion completed within 24 hours of initial reconstitution.

COMPATIBILITY

Manufacturer states, "Must not be mixed with calcium-containing infusion solutions (e.g., LR). Should be administered as a single IV solution in a line separate from all other drugs."

RATE OF ADMINISTRATION

A 4-mg dose equally distributed over no less than 15 minutes. An increase in renal toxicity that can progress to renal failure can result from shorter infusion times.

ACTIONS

A bisphosphonate hypocalcemic agent. Reduces serum calcium concentrations by inhibiting bone resorption. Inhibits osteoclastic (destructive to bone) activity and induces osteoclast apoptosis (fragmentation of a cell into particles for elimination). Blocks the osteoclastic resorption of mineralized bone and cartilage through its binding to bone and inhibits the increased osteoclastic activity and skeletal calcium release induced by various tumors. Decreases serum calcium and phosphorus and increases urinary calcium and phosphorus excretion. Reduction in calcium levels seen in 24 to 48 hours, but maximal response may take up to 7 days. Most bound to bone and slowly released back into the systemic circulation. Primarily excreted intact via the kidney. Half-life is triphasic with a terminal half-life of 167 hours.

INDICATIONS AND USES

Treatment of hypercalcemia of malignancy (HCM). ▪ Treatment of patients with multiple myeloma and patients with documented bone metastases from solid tumors in conjunction with chemotherapy. ▪ Safety for use in the treatment of hypercalcemia associated with hyperparathyroidism or with other non–tumor related conditions has not been established.

Unlabeled uses: Prevent or decrease bone loss in women undergoing chemotherapy.

CONTRAINDICATIONS

Hypersensitivity to zoledronic acid, any of its components, or other bisphosphonates (e.g., pamidronate [Aredia], etidronate [Didronel]).

PRECAUTIONS

Calcium is bound to serum protein; concentration fluctuates with changes in blood volume. Changes in serum calcium (especially during rehydration) may not reflect true plasma levels. Measurement with ionized calcium levels is preferred. If unavailable, all calcium measurement should be corrected for albumin to establish a basis for treatment and evaluation of treatment. ■ Mild or asymptomatic hypercalcemia will be treated with conservative measures (e.g., saline hydration, with or without diuretics [after correcting hypovolemia]). Consider patient's cardiovascular status. Corticosteroids may be indicated if the underlying cancer is sensitive (e.g., hematologic cancers). ■ Bisphosphonates have been associated with deterioration of renal function and potential renal failure. Doses over 4 mg and a rate of administration less than 15 minutes increased this risk. ■ Use with caution in patients with aspirin-sensitive asthma. ■ Use in patients with severe renal impairment has not been studied (e.g., SrCr equal to or greater than 4.5 mg/dl [400 mmol/L]). After considering other treatment options, use only if benefit outweighs risk of renal failure. ■ Retreatment may increase potential for renal failure; before retreatment, consider other available treatment options and risk versus benefit; evaluate serum creatinine before each dose. ■ May be used adjunctively with chemotherapy, radiation, or surgery. ■ See Monitor.

Monitor: Obtain baseline measurements of serum calcium (corrected for serum albumin), electrolytes, phosphate, magnesium, creatinine, and CBC with differential and hematocrit/hemoglobin. Monitor all closely as indicated by baseline results (may be daily). ■ Patients with cancer-related hypercalcemia are often dehydrated. Must be adequately hydrated orally and/or IV before treatment is initiated. Hydration with saline is preferred to facilitate the renal excretion of calcium and correct dehydration. A pretreatment urine output of 2 L/day is recommended. Maintain adequate hydration and urine output throughout treatment. ■ Correct hypovolemia before using diuretics. ■ Avoid overhydration in patients with compromised cardiovascular status. Observe frequently for signs of fluid overload. ■ Serum phosphate levels will decrease (hypophosphatemia) and may require treatment. Short-term supplemental therapy may also be required for hypocalcemia or hypomagnesemia. ■ Monitor patients with pre-existing anemia, leukopenia, or thrombocytopenia very carefully during treatment and the first 2 weeks following treatment. ■ See Precautions and Drug/Lab Interactions.

Patient Education: Regular visits and assessment of lab tests imperative. ■ Dietary restriction of calcium and vitamin D may be required. ■ Take only prescribed medications. ■ Report abdominal cramps, chills, confusion, fever, muscle spasms, sore throat, and/or any new medical problems promptly.

Maternal/Child: Category C: use in pregnancy has not been studied. Caused an increase in stillbirths in rats. Use only if benefit justifies the potential risk to the fetus. ■ Safety for use during breast-feeding not established; use with extreme caution.

Elderly: Response similar to that seen in younger patients. ■ Use with caution based on age-related impaired organ function and concomitant disease or other drug therapy; monitor renal function closely. ■ Monitor fluid and electrolyte status carefully to avoid overhydration.

DRUG/LAB INTERACTIONS

Concurrent use with loop diuretics (e.g., furosemide [Lasix]) may increase risk of hypocalcemia. ■ Concurrent use with aminoglycosides (e.g., gentamicin [Garamycin]) may have an additive hypocalcemic effect that may persist for a prolonged period. ■ Does not interfere with any known primary cancer therapy. ■ Effects may be antagonized by calcium-containing preparations or vitamin D; avoid use. ■ Thought not to inhibit CYP_{450} enzymes; however, no specific drug interaction studies have been completed.

SIDE EFFECTS

Fever is the most common side effect. Abdominal pain, agitation, anemia, anorexia, anxiety, chest pain, confusion, conjunctivitis, constipation, cough, dehydration, diarrhea, dyspnea, dysphagia, edema, flu-like syndrome (e.g., fever, chills, bone pain and/or arthralgias, and myalgias), granulocytopenia, headache, hypocalcemia (abdominal cramps, confusion, muscle spasms), hypokalemia, hypomagnesemia, hypophosphatemia, hypotension, increased serum creatinine, injection site reactions, nausea, pancytopenia, pleural effusion, pruritus, rash, somnolence, thrombocytopenia, urinary tract infection, vomiting, and weakness occurred in 10% or more of patients. Fluid overload, hypokalemia, hypomagnesemia, and hypophosphatemia may occur more often with the use of concurrent fluid and diuretics.

Overdose: Clinically significant hypocalcemia, hypophosphatemia, and hypomagnesemia may occur. Elevated SrCr levels and renal tubular necrosis may occur with excessive dose or rate of administration.

ANTIDOTE

Keep physician informed of side effects. According to the manufacturer, no specific treatment was required in most cases of flu-like syndrome, GI symptoms, and infusion site reactions, and the symptoms subsided in 24 to 48 hours. Some side effects may respond to symptomatic treatment. Magnesium, phosphorus, and potassium may require replacement if depletion is too severe. If mild, all will probably return toward normal in 7 to 10 days. For asymptomatic or mild to moderate hypocalcemia (6.5 to 8 mg/100 ml [1 dl] corrected for serum albumin), short-term calcium therapy (e.g., calcium gluconate) may be indicated. Discontinue drug for any symptoms of hypersensitivity or overdose. Monitor serum calcium and use vigorous IV hydration, with or without diuretics, for 2 to 3 days. Monitor intake and output to ensure adequacy and balance. Use short-term IV calcium therapy if indicated. Potassium or sodium phosphate and/or magnesium sulfate may be required to treat hypophosphatemia and hypomagnesemia. High fever may respond to steroids. RBC transfusions may be required in anemia. Treat anaphylaxis and resuscitate as indicated.

Recommendations for the Safe Handling of Cytotoxic Drugs

INTRODUCTION

Cytotoxic drugs are toxic compounds and are known to have carcinogenic, mutagenic, and/or teratogenic potential. With direct contact they may cause irritation to the skin, eyes, and mucous membranes, and ulceration and necrosis of tissue. The toxicity of cytotoxic drugs dictates that the exposure of health care personnel to these drugs should be minimized. At the same time, the requirement for maintenance of aseptic conditions must be satisfied.

POTENTIAL ROUTES OF EXPOSURE

This brochure reviews the routes through which exposure may occur and presents recommendations for the safe handling of parenteral cytotoxic drugs by pharmacists, nurses, physicians and other personnel who participate in the preparation and administration of these drugs to patients. These guidelines apply in any setting where cytotoxic drugs are prepared—including pharmacies, nursing units, clinics, physicians' offices and the home health care environment. The primary routes of exposure during the preparation and administration phases are through the inhalation of aerosolized drug or by direct skin contact.

During drug preparation, a variety of manipulations are used which may result in aerosol generation, spraying, and splattering. Examples of these manipulations include: the withdrawal of needles from drug vials; the use of syringes and needles or filter straws for drug transfer; the opening of ampules; and the expulsion of air from the syringe when measuring the precise volume of a drug. Pharmaceutical practice calls for the use of aseptic techniques and a sterile environment. Many pharmacies provide this sterile environment by using a horizontal laminar flow work bench. However, while this type of unit provides product protection, it may expose the operator and other room occupants to aerosols generated during drug preparation procedures. Therefore, a Class II laminar flow (vertical) biological safety cabinet that provides both product and operator protection is needed for the preparation of cytotoxic drugs. This is accomplished by filtering incoming and exhaust air through a high-efficiency particulate air (HEPA) filter. It should be noted that these filters are not effective for volatile materials because they do not capture vapors and gases. Personnel should be familiar with the capabilities, limitations and proper utilization of the biological safety cabinet selected.

During administration, clearing air from a syringe or infusion line and leakage at tubing, syringe, or stopcock connections should be avoided to prevent opportunities for accidental skin contact and aerosol generation. Dispose of syringes and unclipped needles into a leakproof and puncture-resistant container.

The disposal of cytotoxic drugs and trace contaminated materials (e.g., gloves, gowns, needles, syringes, vials) presents a possible source of exposure to pharmacists, nurses and physicians as well as to ancillary personnel,

From U.S. Department of Health and Human Services, Public Health Service, National Institutes of Health: NIH Publication No. 92-2621. Prepared by the NIH Division of Safety and the NIH Clinical Center Pharmacy Department and Cancer Nursing Service. Updated March, 1999.

especially the housekeeping staff. Excreta from patients receiving cytotoxic drug therapy may contain high concentrations of the drug. All personnel should be aware of this source of potential exposure and should take appropriate precautions to avoid accidental contact.

The potential risks to pharmacists, nurses and physicians from repeated contact with parenteral cytotoxic drugs can be effectively controlled by using a combination of specific containment equipment and certain work techniques which are described in the recommendations sections. For the most part, the techniques are merely an extension of good work practices by health care and ancillary personnel, and similar in principle and practice to *Universal Precautions*.[1] These may be supplemented as deemed appropriate for the work being performed. By using these precautions, personnel are better able to minimize possible exposure to cytotoxic drugs.

SAFE PREPARATION OF CYTOTOXIC DRUGS

A. Part 1—All procedures involved in the preparation of cytotoxic drugs should be performed in a Class II, Type A or Type B laminar flow biological safety cabinet. The cabinet exhaust should be discharged to the outdoors in order to eliminate the exposure of personnel to drugs that may volatilize after retention on filters of the cabinet. The cabinet of choice is a Class II, Type B which discharges exhaust to the outdoors and can be obtained with a bag-in/bag-out filter to protect the personnel servicing the cabinet and to facilitate disposal.
   Part 2—Alternatively, a Class II, Type A cabinet can be equipped with a canopy or thimble unit which exhausts to the outdoors. For detailed information about the design, capabilities and limitations of various types of biological safety cabinets, refer to the National Sanitation Foundation Standard 49.[2]
B. The work surface of the safety cabinet should be covered with plastic-backed absorbent paper. This will reduce the potential for dispersion of droplets and spills and facilitate cleanup. This paper should be changed after any overt spill and at the end of each work shift.
C. Personnel preparing the drugs should wear unpowdered latex surgical gloves and a disposal gown with knit cuffs. Gloves should be changed regularly and immediately if torn or punctured. Protective clothing should not be worn outside of the drug preparation area. Overtly contaminated gowns require immediate removal and replacement. In case of skin contact with any cytotoxic drug, thoroughly wash the affected area with soap and water. However, do not abrade the skin by using a scrub brush. Flush the affected eye(s), while holding back the eyelid(s), with copious amounts of water for at least 15 minutes. Then seek medical evaluation by a physician.
D. Vials containing drugs requiring reconstitution should be vented to reduce the internal pressure with a venting device using a 0.22 micron hydrophobic filter or other appropriate means such as a chemo-

---

1. Centers for Disease Control. 1988. Update: Universal precautions for prevention of transmission of human immunodeficiency virus, hepatitis B virus, and other blood-borne pathogens in health-care settings. *Morbidity and Mortality Weekly Report*, 37(24): 377-382, 387-388.
2. National Science Foundation. Standard 49 for Class II (Laminar Flow) Biohazard Cabinetry.

therapy dispensing pin. This reduces the probability of spraying and spillage.

E. If a chemotherapy dispensing pin is not used, a sterile alcohol pad should be carefully placed around the needle and vial top during withdrawal from the septum.

F. The external surfaces contaminated with a drug should be wiped clean with an alcohol pad before transfer or transport.

G. When opening the glass ampule, wrap it and then snap it at the break point using an alcohol pad to reduce the possibility of injury and to contain the aerosol produced. Use a 5 micron filter needle or straw when removing the drug solution.

H. Syringes and I.V. bottles containing cytotoxic drugs should be labeled and dated. Before these items leave the preparation area, an additional label reading, *"Caution—Chemotherapy, Dispose of Properly"* is recommended.

I. After completing the drug preparation process, wipe down the interior of the safety cabinet with water (for injection or irrigation) followed by 70% alcohol using disposable towels. All wastes are considered contaminated and should be disposed of properly.

J. Contaminated needles and syringes, I.V. tubing, butterfly clips, etc., should be disposed of intact to prevent aerosol generation and injury. *Do not recap needles.* Place these items in a puncture-resistant container along with any contaminated bottles, vials, gloves, absorbent paper, disposable gowns, gauze and other waste. The container should then be placed in a box labeled, *"Cytotoxic waste only,"* sealed and disposed of according to Federal, state and local requirements. Linen contaminated with drugs, patient excreta or body fluids should be handled separately.

K. Hands should be washed between glove changes and after glove removal.

L. Cytotoxic drugs are categorized as regulated wastes and therefore, should be disposed of according to Federal, state and local requirements.

RECOMMENDED PRACTICES FOR PERSONNEL ADMINISTERING PARENTERAL CYTOTOXIC DRUGS

A. A protective outer garment such as a closed-front surgical-type gown with knit cuffs should be worn. Gowns may be of the disposable or washable variety.

B. Disposable latex surgical gloves should be worn during those procedures where exposure to the drugs may result and when handling patient body fluids or excreta. When bubbles are removed from syringes or I.V. tubing, an alcohol pad should be placed carefully over the tip of such items in order to collect any of the cytotoxic drugs which may be inadvertently discharged. Discard gloves after each use and wash hands.

C. Contaminated needles and syringes and I.V. apparatus should be disposed of intact into a labeled, puncture-resistant container in order to minimize aerosol generation and risk of injury. ***Do not recap needles.*** The container, as well as contaminated materials should be placed in a box labeled, ***"Cytotoxic waste only."*** Linen overtly contaminated with any cytotoxic agent or excreta from a patient within 48 hours following drug administration, may be safely handled by using the procedures prescribed for isolation cases. For example, place the contaminated articles in a "yellow" cloth bag lined with a water-soluble plastic bag and then place into the washing machine. Linen without overt contamination can be handled by routine laundering procedures.

D. In case of skin contact with an cytotoxic drug, thoroughly wash the affected area with soap and water. However, do not abrade the skin by using a scrub brush. Flush affected eye(s), while holding back the eyelid(s), with copious amounts of water for at least 15 minutes. Then seek evaluation by a physician. Always wash hands after removing gloves.

Pictures illustrating each of the prescribed actions and accompanied by this text may be found at the NIH website http://www.nih.gov/od/ors/ds/pubs/cyto/index.htm

APPENDIX B

FDA Pregnancy Categories

No drug should be used during pregnancy unless clearly needed and the risks to the fetus are outweighed by the benefits to the mother.

Category A Adequate studies have not demonstrated a risk to the fetus in any trimester.

Category B May have caused adverse effects in animals, but no adverse effects have been demonstrated in humans in any trimester or no demonstrated risk in animals but there are no adequate studies in pregnant women.

Category C Animal studies have shown an adverse effect but there are no adequate studies in pregnant women or no animal studies and no studies in pregnant women.

Category D Definite fetal risks. May be given in spite of risks if needed in life-threatening conditions.

Category X Will cause fetal abnormalities. Risk of use outweighs benefits. Not recommended for use at any time during pregnancy. Consider alternatives before treating a pregnant woman.

Consider all men and women capable of conception when any drug in Category D or Category X is to be administered. Discuss birth control options to avoid pregnancy if a specific drug in these categories must be administered. Some drugs require birth control for months after all dosing is complete. Research complete information and keep patient informed.

Alternate Choices for Infrequently Used Drugs

Many new drugs have been included each year in *Intravenous Medications.* Although the goal has always been to make this reference as complete as possible, this rapid increase in new drugs requires some deletions to prevent *Intravenous Medications* from becoming too cumbersome to be useful. After extensive consultation, the following drugs have been deleted. They were generally selected because they were rarely used and newer, sometimes more effective, drugs are now preferred for intravenous use for the same indications. The following chart includes the deleted drugs and suggested alternates. After thorough review and updating, they will be accessible on the Elsevier website.

Infrequently Used Drugs		
Deleted Drug	**Category**	**Suggested Alternate(s)**
*15 ammonium chloride	acidifying agent	consult pharmacist
*15 benztropine (Cogentin)	antidyskinetic	diphenhydramine (Benadryl), p. 378
*12 betamethasone	corticosteroid	dexamethasone (Decadron), p. 342
*15 calcium gluceptate	electrolyte replenisher	calcium gluconate, p. 200 calcium chloride, p. 196
*13 chlorothiazide (Diuril)	diuretic	loop diuretics (e.g., furosemide [Lasix]), p. 536
*8 colistimethate sodium (Coly-Mycin M)	antibacterial organism-specific	aminoglycosides (e.g., gentamicin [Garamycin]), p. 562
*15 cysteine hydrochloride	amino acid	consult pharmacist
*13 dexpanthenol (Ilopan)	GI stimulant	no equivalent; see 13th edition
*13 dimenhydrinate	antihistamine/ antiemetic	diphenhydramine (Benadryl), p. 378, prochlorperazine (Compazine), p. 929, ondansetron (Zofran), p. 834

*Information can be found in this previous edition of *Intravenous Medications.*

Infrequently Used Drugs—cont'd		
Deleted Drug	**Category**	**Suggested Alternate(s)**
*13 eflornithine (Ornidyl)	antiprotozoal Tx of sleeping sickness	no equivalent; see 13th edition
*13 ethacrynic acid (Edecrin)	diuretic	loop diuretics (e.g., furosemide [Lasix]), p. 536
*13 fentanyl citrate with droperidol (Innovar)	narcotic analgesic	fentanyl (Sublimaze), p. 499
*13 mezlocillin sodium	antibacterial	ticarcillin (Ticar), p. 1050
*8 minocycline HCl (Minocin)	tetracycline antibacterial	ampicillin, p. 98 erythromycin, p. 472 doxycycline (Vibramycin), p. 415
*8 nicotinic acid (Niacin) and nicotinamide (Niacinamide)	water-soluble B vitamin	well absorbed via other routes
*15 scopolamine hydrochloride	anticholinergic	atropine sulfate, p. 154
*8 sodium lactate	alkalinizing agent	sodium bicarbonate, p. 1003
*13 theophylline & 5% dextrose	bronchodilator	aminophylline, p. 76

*Information can be found in this previous edition of *Intravenous Medications.*

mation for Patients Receiving Immunosuppressive Agents

- Report allergic or sensitivity reactions you may have had to drugs or food.
- Report other medical problems you may have (e.g., exposure to chickenpox, herpes zoster, infections, bone marrow, heart, kidney, or liver problems).
- Provide a complete list of all medications you take, prescription and over the counter.
- In most situations birth control is essential and may be required for both patient and partner. Nonhormonal birth control reduces the possibility of drug interactions, but compliance is imperative. If there is any possibility you or your partner may be pregnant, inform your physician promptly.
- Discontinue breast-feeding.
- Take only prescribed medication(s) in the exact amounts prescribed and at the times prescribed. This will help to maintain correct blood levels and avoid drug interactions.
- Confirm procedure if you should miss a dose. If any questions, notify physician.
- Confirm procedure for correct storage of your medication(s).
- Close monitoring by your physician is very important; keep all appointments and have all required lab work done on schedule. Your medications may interfere with some test results. Discuss with your physician.
- Do not take any immunizations without your physician's approval. Polio vaccine is especially virulent in your condition; request family members to defer immunization and either avoid friends who have been immunized or wear a protective mask covering your nose and mouth while visiting.
- Dental procedures may need to be completed before starting therapy or deferred until therapy is completed. Use caution with your toothbrush, toothpicks, or dental floss. Alternate methods of dental hygiene may be necessary should your gums become tender, inflamed, or bleed.
- Review all side effects with your physician. Confirm those that may be a special problem for you and discuss solutions and expectations.
- Avoid anyone with an infection or fever. Report symptoms such as: chills, fever, cough, hoarseness, lower back or side pain, painful or difficult urination.
- Wash hands before touching your eyes or the inside of your nose.
- Report unusual bleeding, bruising, black tarry stools, blood in urine, or pinpoint red spots on your skin (petechiae).
- Report redness, swelling, or soreness in the mouth (symptoms of stomatitis).
- Report mild hair loss, nausea and vomiting, rash, tiredness, weakness.
- Avoid accidental cuts whenever possible (e.g., razors, fingernail and toenail clippers).
- Avoid contact sports where you might be bruised or injured.
- Drink adequate amounts of fluids to prevent increases in serum uric acid concentrations. Allopurinol (Zyloprim) and/or alkalinization of urine may be required.
- Anesthesia during dental, surgical, or emergency treatment may be a problem. Best to consult with your physician, but inform all health professionals of the medications you are taking before they treat you in any way.

National Cancer Institute Common Toxicity Grading Criteria

	Grade				
Toxicity	0	1	2	3	4
WBC	≥4	3-3.9	2-2.9	1-1.9	<1
Plt	WNL	75-normal	50-74.9	25-49.9	<25
HgB	WNL	10-normal	8-10	6.5-7.9	<6.5
Granulocytes/bands	≥2	1.5-1.9	1-1.4	0.5-0.9	<0.5
Lymphocytes	≥2	1.5-1.9	1-1.4	0.5-0.9	<0.5
Hemorrhage (clinical)	None	Mild, no transfusion	Gross, 1-2 units transfusion per episode	Gross, 3-4 units transfusion per episode	Massive, ≥4 units transfusion per episode
Infection	None	Mild	Moderate	Severe	Life-threatening
Nausea	None	Able to eat reasonable intake	Intake significantly decreased but can eat	No significant intake	—
Vomiting	None	1 episode in 24 hrs	2-5 episodes in 24 hrs	6-10 episodes in 24 hrs	≥10 episodes in 24 hrs, or requiring parenteral support
Diarrhea	None	Increase of 2-3 stools/day over pre-Rx	Increase of 4-6 stools/day, or nocturnal stools, or moderate cramping	Increase of 7-9 stools/day, or incontinence, or severe cramping	Increase of ≥10 stools/day or grossly bloody diarrhea or need for parenteral support
Stomatitis	None	Painless ulcers, erythema, or mild soreness	Painful erythema, edema, or ulcers, but can eat	Painful erythema, edema, or ulcers, and cannot eat	Requires parenteral or enteral support
Bilirubin	WNL	—	<1.5 × N	1.5-3 × N	>3 × N

N, Normal, *WNL*, within normal limits.

Continued

National Cancer Institute Common Toxicity Grading Criteria—cont'd

	Grade				
Toxicity	0	1	2	3	4
Transaminase (SGOT, SGPT)	WNL	≤2.5 × N	2.6-5 × N	5.1-20 × N	>20 × N
Alk Phos or 5′nucleotidase	WNL	≤2.5 × N	2.6-5 × N	5.1-20 × N	>20 × N
Liver (clinical)	No change from base-line	—	—	Pre-coma	Hepatic coma
Creatinine	WNL	<1.5 × N	1.5-3.0 × N	3.1-6 × N	>6 × N
Proteinuria	No change	1+ or <0.3-1 Gm% or <3 Gm/L	2-3+ or 0.3-1 Gm% or 3-10 Gm/L	4+ or >1 Gm% or >10 Gm/L	Nephrotic syndrome
Hematuria	Negative	Micro only	Gross, no clots	Gross + clots	Requires transfusion
Alopecia	No loss	Mild hair loss	Pronounced or total hair loss	—	—
Pulmonary	None or no change	Asymptomatic, with abnormality in PFTs	Dyspnea or significant exertion	Dyspnea at normal level of activity	Dyspnea at rest
Cardiac arrhythmias	None	Asymptomatic, transient, requiring no therapy	Recurrent or persistent, no therapy required	Requires treatment	Requires monitoring, or hypotension, or ventricular tachycardia, or fibrillation
Cardiac function	None	Asymptomatic, decline of resting ejection fraction by >20% of baseline value	Asymptomatic, decline of resting ejection fraction by >20% of baseline value	Mild CHF, responsive to therapy	Severe or refractory CHF

Cardiac ischemia	None	Non-specific T-wave flattening	Asymptomatic, ST and T-wave changes suggesting ischemia	Angina without evidence of infarction	Acute myocardial
Cardiac (pericardial)	None	Asymptomatic effusion, no intervention required	Pericarditis (rub, chest pain, ECG changes)	Symptomatic effusion; drainage required	Tamponade; drainage urgently required
Hypertension	None or no change	Asymptomatic, transient increase by >20 mm Hg (D) or to >150/100 if previously WNL. No treatment required	Recurrent or persistent increase by >20 mm Hg (D) or to >150/100 if previously WNL. No treatment required	Requires therapy	Hypertensive crisis
Hypotension	None or no change	Changes requiring no therapy (including transient orthostatic hypotension)	Requires fluid replacement or other therapy but not hospitalization	Requires therapy and hospitalization; resolves within 48 hr of stopping the agent	Requires therapy and hospitalization for >48 hr after stopping the agent
Neuro–Sensory	None or no change	Mild paresthesias; loss of deep tendon reflexes	Mild or moderate objective sensory loss; moderate paresthesias	Severe objective sensory loss or paresthesias that interfere with function	—
Neuro–Motor	None or no change	Subjective weakness; no objective findings	Mild objective weakness without significant impairment of function	Objective weakness with impairment of function	Paralysis
Neuro–Cortical	None	Mild somnolence or agitation	Moderate somnolence or agitation	Severe somnolence, agitation, confusion, disorientation, or hallucinations	Coma, seizures, toxic psychosis
Neuro–Cerebellar	None	Slight incoordination, dysdiadochokinesis	Intense tremor, dysmetria, slurred speech, nystagmus	Locomotor ataxia	Cerebellar necrosis

N, Normal, *WNL*, within normal limits.

Continued

National Cancer Institute Common Toxicity Grading Criteria—cont'd

	Grade				
Toxicity	0	1	2	3	4
Neuro–Mood	No change	Mild anxiety or depression	Moderate anxiety or depression	Severe anxiety or depression	Suicidal ideation
Neuro–Headache	None	Mild	Moderate or severe but transient	Unrelenting and severe	—
Neuro–Constipation	None or no change	Mild	Moderate	Severe	Ileus >96 hr
Neuro–Hearing	None or no change	Asymptomatic, hearing loss on audiometry only	Tinnitus	Hearing loss interfering with function but correctable with hearing aid	Deafness, not correctable
Neuro–Vision	None or no change	—	—	Symptomatic subtotal loss of vision	Blindness
Skin	None or no change	Scattered macular or papular eruption or erythema that is asymptomatic	Scattered macular or papular eruption or erythema with pruritus or other associated symptoms	Generalized symptomatic macular, papular, or vesicular eruption	Exfoliative dermatitis or ulcerating dermatitis
Allergy	None	Transient rash, drug fever <38°C (100.4°F)	Urticaria, drug fever = 38°C (100.4°F), mild bronchospasm	Serum sickness, bronchospasm, requires parenteral meds	Anaphylaxis
Fever in absence of infection	None	37.1-38°C (98.7-100.4°F)	38.1-40°C (100.5-104°F)	>40°C (>104°F) for <24 hr	>40°C (104°F) for >24 hr or fever accompanied by hypotension

Local	None	Pain	Pain and swelling, with inflammation or phlebitis	Ulceration	Plastic surgery indicated
Weight gain/loss	<5%	5-9.9%	10-19.9%	≥20%	—
Hyperglycemia	<116	116-160	161-250	251-500	>500 or ketoacidosis
Hypoglycemia	>64	55-64	40-54	30-39	<30
Amylase	WNL	<1.5 × N	1.5-2.0 × N	2.1-5 × N	>5.1 × N
Hypercalcemia	<10.6	10.6-11.5	11.6-12.5	12.6-13.5	≥13.5
Hypocalcemia	>8.4	8.4-7.8	7.7-7	6.9-6.1	≤6
Hypomagnesemia	>1.4	1.4-1.2	1.1-0.9	0.8-0.6	≤0.5
Fibrinogen	WNL	0.99-0.75 × N	0.74-0.5 × N	0.49-0.25 × N	≤0.24 × N
Prothrombin time	WNL	1.01-1.25 × N	1.26-1.5 × N	1.51-2 × N	>2 × N
Partial thromboplastin time	WNL	1.01-1.66 × N	1.67-2.33 × N	2.34-3 × N	>3 × N
Headache	None	Mild	Moderate or severe but transient	Unrelenting and severe	—
Aching pain (muscle or bone)	None	Mild, transient; does not interfere with casual daily activity	Moderate; interferes with usual daily activity	Severe; interrupts usual daily activity	Intractable
Chills	None	Mild, transient	Moderate	Severe	Intractable
Malaise	None	25% of time	50% of time	75% of time	100% of time
Fatigue/asthenia	None	25% of time	50% of time	75% of time	100% of time
Anorexia	None	Able to eat normal meals, loss of hunger	Able to eat 2 meals/day with loss of hunger	Able to eat 1 meal/day with loss of hunger	Unable to eat a meal, some nutritional fluids tolerated

N, Normal, *WNL*, within normal limits.

BORTEZOMIB

(bore-tez'oh-meb)

Velcade

Antineoplastic

pH 2 to 6.5

USUAL DOSE

1.3 mg/M^2/dose as an IV bolus 2 times a week for 2 weeks (days 1, 4, 8, and 11). Follow with a 10-day rest period (days 12 through 21). At least 72 hours should elapse between doses of bortezomib (e.g., days 1, 4, 8, and 11). A treatment cycle is 21 days. Up to 8 treatment cycles were administered during clinical trials (mean was 6 treatment cycles). 33% of participants required dose reduction, and 63% had at least 1 dose withheld; see Dose Adjustments.

PEDIATRIC DOSE

Safety and effectiveness for use in pediatric patients not established.

DOSE ADJUSTMENTS

Dose adjustments are based on clinical toxicities. Withhold dose if a Grade 3 nonhematologic toxicity (e.g., 6 to 10 emeses/24 hr, severe infection) or a Grade 4 hematologic toxicity (e.g., thrombocytopenia less than 25,000/mm^3) occurs. When symptoms have resolved, resume treatment with a dose reduced by 25% (1.3 mg/M^2/dose reduced to 1 mg/M^2/dose, 1 mg/M^2/dose reduced to 0.7 mg/M^2/dose). ■ Dose adjustments based on age, gender, race, or hepatic or renal impairment have not been evaluated; see Precautions. ■ Reduce dose in patients who develop bortezomib-related neuropathic pain and/or peripheral sensory neuropathy according to the following chart:

Recommended Dose Modification for Bortezomib-Related Neuropathic Pain and/or Peripheral Sensory Neuropathy

Severity of Peripheral Neuropathy Signs and Symptoms	Modification of Dose and Regimen
Grade 1 (paresthesias and/or loss of reflexes) without pain or loss of function	No action
Grade 1 with pain or Grade 2 (interfering with function but not with activities of daily living)	Reduce dose to 1 mg/M^2
Grade 2 with pain or Grade 3 (interfering with activities of daily living)	Withhold therapy until toxicity resolves. When toxicity resolves, reinitiate with a reduced dose of 0.7 mg/M^2 and change treatment schedule to once per week
Grade 4 (permanent sensory loss that interferes with function)	Discontinue bortezomib

DILUTION

Specific techniques required; see Precautions. Reconstitute each 3.5-mg vial with 3.5 ml NS. Concentration equals 1 mg/ml.

Storage: Stable until expiration date when stored at CRT in original package and protected from light. Reconstituted solution stable at CRT for up to 3 hours in a syringe or up to 8 hours in original vial. Must be given within 8 hours.

COMPATIBILITY

Specific information not available. Consider specific use; consult pharmacist.

RATE OF ADMINISTRATION

A single dose as an IV bolus injection over 3 to 5 seconds. May be given into a peripheral vein. To ensure the full dose is administered, flush with NS after injection.

May also be given through an IV port if the primary IV is temporarily discontinued. Flush with NS before and after administration.

ACTIONS

A reversible inhibitor of the 26S proteasome, which is a large protein complex that degrades ubiquitinated proteins. The blocking of this proteasome disrupts numerous biologic pathways related to the growth and survival of cancer cells and can lead to cell death. Over 80% is bound to plasma proteins. Mean elimination half-life ranges from 9 to 15 hours. Metabolized in the liver via selected cytochrome P_{450} enzymes. Pathways of elimination in humans have not been determined. Median time to response was 38 days (range 30 to 127 days).

INDICATIONS

Treatment of patients with multiple myeloma who have been treated with at least two prior therapies and continue to have disease progression.

CONTRAINDICATIONS

Hypersensitivity to bortezomib, boron, or mannitol.

PRECAUTIONS

Follow guidelines for handling cytotoxic agents. See Appendix A, p. 1142. ■ For IV use only. ■ Administered by or under the supervision of a physician experienced in the use of antineoplastic therapy in a facility equipped to monitor the patient and respond to any medical emergency. ■ Use caution in patients with pre-existing peripheral neuropathy; symptoms may worsen. Many have been treated previously with neurotoxic agents. ■ May cause orthostatic/postural hypotension. Use with caution in patients with a history of syncope, in patients receiving concomitant medications that may cause hypotension, and in patients who are dehydrated. ■ Thrombocytopenia occurred in about 40% of patients; see Monitor. Gastrointestinal and intracerebral hemorrhages have been reported. ■ Clearance may be decreased in patients with liver impairment; see Monitor. ■ No clinical information available for use in patients with a CrCl less than 13 ml/min or in patients on dialysis. ■ Response decreased in patients with greater than 50% plasma cells or abnormal cytogenetics in the bone marrow. ■ Tumor response occurred in clinical trials; however, improvement in survival has not yet been demonstrated.

Monitor: Obtain baseline CBC with differential and platelet count; monitor frequently during treatment. ■ Obtain baseline electrolytes, including serum calcium and potassium. Monitor fluid and electrolyte balance and replace as indicated. Prevent dehydration. ■ Monitor BP closely. Dehydration and/or concomitant medications may cause hypotension. Assist with ambulation. ■ Confirm patency of vein; however, tissue damage did not occur with extravasation during clinical studies. ■ Monitor patients with impaired liver and/or renal function closely for S/S of bortezomib toxicity. Baseline liver studies and CrCl may be appropriate. Repeat as indicated. ■ Use prophylactic antiemetics to reduce nausea and vomiting and increase patient comfort. ■ Antidiarrheal medication (e.g., loperamide [Imodium]) may be indicated. ■ Monitor for S/S of peripheral neuropathy (e.g., hyperesthesia [sensitivity of skin], hypoesthesia [impairment of any sense, especially touch], paresthesia [abnormal sensation such as burning, prickling]). Incidence may be increased in patients treated previously with neurotoxic agents (e.g., cisplatin [Platinol], thalidomide [Thalomid], vinca alkaloids [e.g., vincristine (Oncovin)]). See Dose Adjustments; may require change of dose or schedule. ■ Monitor for thrombocytopenia (platelet count less than 50,000/mm^3). Onset is most common in the first 2 cycles but can occur throughout therapy. Thrombocytopenia was maximal at day 11 and usually recovered by the next cycle. Initiate precautions to prevent excessive bleeding (e.g., inspect IV sites, skin, and mucous membranes; use extreme care during invasive procedures; test urine, emesis, stool, and secretions for occult blood). ■ Hypoglycemia and hyperglycemia have been reported in patients taking oral diabetic agents; see Drug/Lab Interactions.

Patient Education: Avoid pregnancy; use effective contraceptive measures. Should pregnancy occur, notify physician immediately and discuss potential hazards. ■ May cause blurred vision, dizziness, or hypotension; use caution when driving or operating machinery. ■ Review all medications with your physician and/or pharmacist; effects of medications for high blood pressure and other medications that may lower blood pressure may increase hypotension. Other agents may increase peripheral neuropathy. May interfere with medications for diabetes. ■ Review of monitoring requirements and adverse events before therapy is imperative. ■ Avoid dehydration; promptly report diarrhea, dizziness, fainting spells, lightheadedness, and vomiting. ■ Promptly report any signs of infection (e.g., chills, fever, night sweats) or signs of bleeding (e.g., bruising, tarry stools, blood in urine, pinpoint red spots on skin). ■ Promptly report symptoms of peripheral neuropathy (e.g., burning sensation, skin sensitivity, impairment of any sense [especially touch]). If these symptoms pre-existed, report if they seem to be worse. ■ See Appendix D, p. 1148.

Maternal/Child: Category D: avoid pregnancy; may cause fetal harm. Use of effective contraception required. ■ Discontinue breast-feeding.

Elderly: In clinical trials, patients over 65 years of age had a reduced response compared to younger adults (19% versus 32%) and had a slightly increased incidence of Grade 3 or 4 toxicity.

DRUG/LAB INTERACTIONS

Drug interaction studies have not been conducted. ■ A poor inhibitor of selected cytochrome P_{450} enzymes; however, concomitant administration of inhibitors or inducers of selected cytochrome P_{450} enzymes may cause toxicity or reduce effectiveness. Consult pharmacist. Examples of inhibitors may include cimetidine (Tagamet), erythromycins, grapefruit juice, antifungal agents (e.g., itraconazole [Sporanox]), nefazodone (Serzone), ritonavir (Norvir), verapamil (Isoptin). Inhibitors may reduce metabolism and increase serum levels. Examples of inducers may include carbamazepine (Tegretol), phenobarbital (Luminal), phenytoin (Dilantin), rifampin (Rifadin). Inducers may increase metabolism and decrease serum levels and effectiveness. ■ Hypotension may be increased by agents that induce hypotension (e.g., alcohol, antihypertensives [e.g., ACE inhibitors (e.g., lisinopril)], beta-blockers [e.g., atenolol (Tenormin)], opioid narcotics, sildenafil [Viagra], tricyclic antidepressants [e.g., amitryptyline (Elavil)]). ■ Peripheral neuropathy may be increased by numerous agents. Some examples are acyclovir (Zovirax), amiodarone (Cordarone), antineoplastics (e.g., cisplatin [Platinol], vinca alkaloids [e.g., vincristine (Oncovin)]), foscarnet (Foscavir), isoniazid (INH), nitrofurantoin (Furadantin), thalidomide (Thalomid), statins (e.g., lovastatin [Mevacor], simvastatin [Zocor]). ■ May increase or decrease the effects of oral antidiabetic agents (e.g., glyburide [DiaBeta], glipizide [Glucotrol]). Monitor blood glucose levels and adjust dose of antidiabetic medication as indicated.

SIDE EFFECTS

Diarrhea, fatigue, peripheral neuropathy, excessive vomiting, and thrombocytopenia may be dose limiting. Most common side effects reported include anemia, anorexia, blurred vision, constipation, dehydration, diarrhea, diplopia, dizziness, fatigue, fever, headache, malaise, nausea and vomiting, neutropenia, orthostatic/postural hypotension, peripheral neuropathy, pneumonia, syncope, thrombocytopenia, and weakness. Numerous other side effects have been reported that may or may not be related to bortezomib and may include acute pancreatitis, allergic reactions (including anaphylaxis), bacteremia, cardiac arrhythmias, CVA, disseminated intravascular coagulation (DIC), hyperbilirubinemia, hyperuricemia, hypocalcemia, hypokalemia, hyponatremia, pleural effusion, pulmonary embolism, respiratory distress, and tumor lysis syndrome.

Overdose: Profound progressive hypotension, tachycardia, and increased cardiac contractility resulted in death within 12 to 14 hours in monkeys given a dose of 3 mg/M^2 (approximately twice the recommended clinical dose).

ANTIDOTE

Keep physician informed of all side effects. Most will be treated symptomatically as indicated. Temporarily discontinue bortezomib if Grade 4 thrombocytopenia occurs (less than $25{,}000/mm^3$); may be resumed at a reduced dose after thrombocytopenia is resolved. Severe thrombocytopenia may require platelet transfusions or may be treated with oprelvekin (Neumega). Reduce dose, withhold dose, or discontinue based on S/S of peripheral neuropathy. Symptoms of peripheral neuropathy may improve or return to baseline if bortezomib is discontinued. Hypotension may respond to adjustment of antihypertensive medications, hydration, or administration of mineralocorticoids. Recovery from neutropenia may be spontaneous or may be treated with filgrastim (G-CSF, Neupogen) or pegfilgrastim (Neulasta). Treat anemia as indicated with whole blood products (e.g., packed RBCs) or blood modifiers (e.g., darbepoetin alfa [Aranesp], epoetin alfa [Epogen, Procrit]). In overdose, monitor V/S continuously and provide supportive care. Maintain BP with dopamine (Intropin), epinephrine, or norepinephrine (Levophed) as needed. Maintain body temperature. There is no specific antidote; supportive therapy will help sustain the patient in toxicity. Resuscitate as indicated.

INDEX

A

Abbokinase*
Abbokinase open-cath*
Abciximab, 1
Abelcet, 90
ACE inhibitor
enalaprilat, 435
Acetazolamide sodium, 6
Acidifying agent
ammonium chloride, 1146
Acova, 134
Acthrel*
Activase, 56
Acyclovir, 8
Adenocard, 12
Adenoscan, 12
Adenosine, 12
ADR, 408
Adrenalin chloride, 440
Adrenocortical steroids
*corticorelin ovine triflutate**
cosyntropin, 301
dexamethasone sodium phosphate, 342
hydrocortisone phosphate, 590
hydrocortisone sodium succinate, 590
methylprednisolone sodium succinate, 747
*prednisolone sodium phosphate**
Adriamycin PFS, 408
Adriamycin RDF, 408
Adrucil, 518
Aggrastat, 1056
AHF, 106
Alatrofloxacin mesylate, 16
Albumarc, 22
Albumin 5%, 22
Albumin 25%, 22
Albumin (human), 22
Albumin, normal serum, 22
Albuminar-5, 22
Albuminar-25, 22
Albunex 5%, 22
Albutein 5%, 22
Albutein 25%, 22
Aldesleukin, 26
Aldomet, 743
Alefacept, 35
Alemtuzumab, 38
Alfentanil hydrochloride, 42
Alfenta, 42
Alglucerase*
Alkalizing agents
acetazolamide, 6
sodium acetate, 1002
sodium bicarbonate, 1003
tromethamine, 1084
Alkeran, 723
Alkylating antineoplastic agents
busulfan, 183
carboplatin, 206
carmustine (BCNU), 210
cisplatin, 286
cyclophosphamide, 302
dacarbazine, 314
ifosfamide, 610
mechlorethamine, 721
melphalan, 723
streptozocin, 1021
thiotepa, 1047
Aloprim, 48
Allopurinol, 48
Alpha-adrenergic blocking agent
phentolamine, 890
Alpha-adrenoreceptor agonist
dexmedetomidine, 346
$Alpha_1$-antitrypsin, 52
$Alpha_1$ antitrypsin replenisher
$alpha_1$-proteinase inhibitor, 52
Alpha/beta-adrenergic blocking agent
labetalol, 671
Alphanate, 106
AlphaNine SD, 484
$Alpha_1$-PI, 52
$Alpha_1$-proteinase inhibitor (human), 52
Alprostadil, 54
Alteplase, recombinant, 56
Amevive, 35
AmBisome, 90
Amicar, 74
Amifostine, 64

Color type indicates generic drug name.
Italic type indicates drug categories and listings.
*See http://evolve.elsevier.com/IVMeds for detailed information.

Amikacin sulfate, 70
Amikin, 70
Aminess 5.2%, with histadine, 948
Amino acid (protein) products, 948
Aminocaproic acid, 74
Aminoglycosides
  amikacin, 70
  gentamicin, 562
  kanamycin, 664
  streptomycin, 1018
  tobramycin, 1060
Aminophylline, 76
Aminosyn 3.5%, 948
Aminosyn 3.5% M, 948
Aminosyn 5%, 948
Aminosyn 7%, 948
Aminosyn 8.5%, 948
Aminosyn 7% with electrolytes, 948
Aminosyn 8.5% with electrolytes, 948
Aminosyn 10% with electrolytes, 948
Aminosyn HBC 7%, 948
Aminosyn HF 8%, 948
Aminosyn PF 7%, 948
Aminosyn PF 10%, 948
Aminosyn (pH 6) 7%, 948
Aminosyn (pH 6) 8.5%, 948
Aminosyn (pH 6) 10%, 948
Aminosyn RF 5.2%, 948
Aminosyn II 7%, 948
Aminosyn II 8.5%, 948
Aminosyn II 10%, 948
Aminosyn II 15%, 948
Aminosyn II 3.5% in D5, 948
Aminosyn II 3.5% in D25, 948
Aminosyn II 5% in D25, 948
Aminosyn II 8.5% with electrolytes, 948
Aminosyn II 10% with electrolytes, 948
Aminosyn II 4.25% in D10, 948
Aminosyn II 4.25% in D20, 948
Aminosyn II 4.25% in D25, 948
Aminosyn II 3.5% in D25 with electrolytes and calcium, 948
Aminosyn II 4.25% in D20 with electrolytes and calcium, 948
Aminosyn II 4.25% in D25 with electrolytes and calcium, 948
Amiodarone hydrochloride, 84
Ammonium chloride, 1146
Amnestic agents
  diazepam, 358
Amnestic agents —cont'd
  lorazepam, 706
  midazolam, 760
Amobarbital sodium*
Amphotec, 90
Amphotericin B, 90
Amphotericin B lipid-based products, 90
Ampicillin sodium, 98
Ampicillin sodium and sulbactam sodium, 102
Ampicin 🍁, 98
Amytal*
Analeptics
  *caffeine and sodium benzoate**
  doxapram, 402
Analgesics, narcotic agonist/antagonists
  buprenorphine, 181
  butorphanol, 187
  *dezocine**
  nalbuphine, 799
  pentazocine, 877
Analgesics, narcotic agonist/CNS depressants
  alfentanil, 42
  fentanyl, 499
  hydromorphone, 595
  levorphanol, 689
  meperidine, 727
  morphine, 778
  oxymorphone, 845
  remifentanil, 968
Analgesic, nonnarcotic NSAID
  ketorolac tromethamine, 668
Analgesic radiopharmaceuticals
  *samarium SM**
  *strontium-89**
Ancef, 220
Anectine, 1024
Anesthesia adjuncts
  alfentanil, 42
  atracurium, 150
  buprenorphine, 181
  butorphanol, 187
  cisatracurium, 281
  *doxacurium**
  droperidol, 418
  fentanyl citrate, 499
  levorphanol, 689
  meperidine, 727

Color type indicates generic drug name.
Italic type indicates drug categories and listings.
*See http://evolve.elsevier.com/IVMeds for detailed information.

Anesthesia adjuncts—cont'd
midazolam, 760
*mivacurium**
morphine, 778
nalbuphine, 799
pancuronium, 860
pentazocine, 877
*pipecuronium**
propofol, 936
remifentanil, 968
*rocuronium**
succinylcholine, 1024
*tubocurarine**
vecuronium, 1098
Anesthetics
alfentanil, 42
fentanyl, 499
midazolam, 760
propofol, 936
remifentanil, 968
thiopental, 1044
Angiomax, 168
Anistreplase*
Antiallergic agents
diphenhydramine, 378
epinephrine, 440
Antianemic agents
darbepoetin alfa, 324
epoetin alfa, 452
folic acid, 522
iron dextran, 650
iron sucrose, 653
sodium ferric gluconate, 1010
Antianginal agents
dipyridamole, 383
nitroglycerin IV, 814
Antianxiety agents
*chlordiazepoxide**
diazepam, 358
fentanyl, 499
haloperidol, 574
lorazepam, 706
midazolam, 760
perphenazine, 884
prochlorperazine, 929
promethazine, 933
Antiarrhythmic agents
adenosine, 12
amiodarone, 84
atenolol, 146
Antiarrhythmic agents—cont'd
atropine, 154
bretylium, 176
digoxin, 368
diltiazem, 374
edetate disodium, 428
epinephrine, 440
esmolol, 474
glucagon (rDNA origin), 566
ibutilide, 604
inamrinone, 626
isoproterenol, 656
lidocaine, 694
magnesium sulfate, 714
metoprolol, 754
milrinone, 767
nicardipine, 812
phenytoin, 894
procainamide, 925
propranolol, 943
quinidine gluconate, 955
verapamil, 1102
Antibacterial agents
alatrofloxacin, 16
amikacin, 70
ampicillin, 98
ampicillin/sulbactam, 102
azithromycin, 159
aztreonam, 162
capreomycin, 204
cefamandole, 216
cefazolin, 220
cefepime, 224
cefoperazone, 229
cefotaxime, 232
cefotetan, 236
cefoxitin, 240
ceftazidime, 244
ceftizoxime, 248
ceftriaxone, 252
cefuroxime, 256
chloramphenicol, 260
ciprofloxacin, 276
clindamycin, 294
cytomegalovirus immune globulin IV (human), 312
doxycycline, 415
ertapenem, 469
erythromycin, 472

Color type indicates generic drug name.
Italic type indicates drug categories and listings.
*See http://evolve.elsevier.com/IVMeds for detailed information.

Antibacterial agents—cont'd
gatifloxacin, 548
gentamicin, 562
imipenem-cilastatin, 616
immune globulin intravenous, 619
kanamycin, 664
levofloxacin, 684
linezolid, 698
meropenem, 730
metronidazole, 757
moxifloxacin, 782
nafcillin, 796
ofloxacin, 830
oxacillin, 839
penicillin G, 872
piperacillin, 904
piperacillin/tazobactam, 907
quinupristin/dalfopristin, 958
rifampin, 986
streptomycin, 1018
sulfamethoxazole-trimethoprim, 1027
ticarcillin, 1050
ticarcillin/clavulanate, 1052
tobramycin, 1060
vancomycin, 1092
Antibiotics, see Antibacterial agents
Anticholinesterase antagonist
pralidoxime, 922
Anticholinergics/antispasmodics
atropine, 154
glycopyrrolate, 568
*L-hyoscyamine**
Anticholinesterase muscle stimulants (cholinergic)
edrophonium, 430
edrophonium and atropine, 432
neostigmine methylsulfate, 806
physostigmine, 900
*pyridostigmine bromide**
Anticoagulants
abciximab, 1
alteplase, recombinant, 56
*anistreplase**
antithrombin III, 116
argatroban, 134
bivalirudin, 168
heparin, 578
lepirudin, 674
reteplase, recombinant, 979
streptokinase, 1014
Anticoagulants—cont'd
tenecteplase, 1035
tirofiban, 1056
*urokinase**
warfarin, 1131
Anticonvulsants
acetazolamide, 6
*amobarbital**
diazepam, 358
fosphenytoin, 533
lidocaine, 694
lorazepam, 706
magnesium sulfate, 714
pentobarbital, 879
phenobarbital, 888
phenytoin, 894
thiopental, 1044
valproate, 1086
Antidiabetic agent
insulin, 636
Antidiarrheal
octreotide, 826
Antidiuretics
desmopressin, 339
vasopressin, 1096
Antidotes
amifostine, 64
antivenin (Crotalidae) polyvalent, 121
antivenin crotalidae polyvalent immune fab (ovine), 123
antivenin (Latrodectus mactans), 127
antivenin (Micrurus fulvius), 129
atropine, 154
deferoxamine, 333
dexrazoxane, 349
dextran 1, 354
digoxin immune fab, 365
edetate calcium disodium, 425
edetate disodium, 428
edrophonium, 430
edrophonium and atropine, 432
epinephrine, 440
flumazenil, 514
fomepizole, 524
glucagon (rDNA origin), 566
glycopyrrolate, 568
leucovorin calcium, 678
mesna, 734
*methylene blue**
nalmefene, 801

Color type indicates generic drug name.
Italic type indicates drug categories and listings.
*See http://evolve.elsevier.com/IVMeds for detailed information.

Antidotes—cont'd
naloxone, 804
neostigmine, 806
nitroprusside sodium, 818
physostigmine, 900
phytonadione, 902
pralidoxime, 922
protamine, 946
*pyridostigmine**
pyridoxine, 953
sodium nitrite, 1012
sodium thiosulfate, 1012
Antidyskinetics
diphenhydramine, 378
haloperidol, 574
Antiemetics
chlorpromazine, 263
dexamethasone, 342
diphenhydramine, 378
dolasetron, 396
droperidol, 418
granisetron, 571
haloperidol, 574
hydrocortisone phosphate, 590
hydrocortisone sodium succinate, 590
lorazepam, 706
metoclopramide, 751
ondansetron, 834
perphenazine, 884
prochlorperazine, 929
promethazine, 933
Antifibrinolytic agents
aminocaproic acid, 74
aprotinin, 130
tranexamic acid, 1073
Antifungals
amphotericin B, 90
amphotericin B lipid-based preparations, 90
caspofungin acetate, 213
fluconazole, 506
itraconazole, 660
voriconazole, 1125
Antiglaucoma agents
acetazolamide, 6
Antigout agents
allopurinol, 48
*colchicine**
Antihemophilic factor (human or recombinant), 106
Antihemophilic factor (porcine) Hyate: C, 106
Antihemophilic factor, von Willebrand factor, 110
Antihemophilic products
antihemophilic factor, 106
antihemophilic factor/von Willebrand factor, 110
anti-inhibitor coagulant complex, 114
factor IX (human), 484
factor IX complex (human), 484
factor IX (recombinant), 487
Antihemorrhagic agents
aminocaproic acid, 74
antihemophilic factor, 106
antihemophilic factor/von Willebrand factor, 110
anti-inhibitor coagulant complex, 114
aprotinin, 130
coagulation factor VIIa, 297
conjugated estrogens, 300
desmopressin acetate, 339
factor IX, 484
factor IX complex (human), 484
factor IX (recombinant), 487
oxytocin, 847
phytonadione, 902
tranexamic acid, 1073
Antihistamines
diphenhydramine, 378
promethazine, 933
Antihypercalcemic agents
edetate disodium, 428
etidronate, 478
furosemide, 536
gallium nitrate, 541
pamidronate, 856
plicamycin, 912
sodium chloride, 1007
zoledronic acid, 1138
Antihyperkalemic agents
calcium chloride, 196
calcium gluconate, 200
Antihypermagnesemic agents
calcium chloride, 196
calcium gluconate, 200
Antihyperparathyroid agents
calcitriol, 193
doxercalciferol, 405
paricalcitol, 866

Color type indicates generic drug name.
Italic type indicates drug categories and listings.
*See http://evolve.elsevier.com/IVMeds for detailed information.

Antihypertensives
diazoxide, 363
enalaprilat, 435
epoprostenol (pulmonary), 457
fenoldopam, 496
furosemide, 536
hydralazine, 588
labetalol, 671
methyldopate, 743
nicardipine, 812
nitroglycerin IV, 814
nitroprusside sodium, 818
phentolamine, 890
torsemide, 1067
Antihyperuricemic agent
allopurinol, 48
*colchicine**
rasburicase, 966
Antihypocalcemic agents
calcium chloride, 196
calcium gluconate, 200
Antihypoglycemic agents
glucagon (rDNA origin), 566
octreotide (unlabeled), 826
Antihypokalemic agents
potassium acetate, 919
potassium chloride, 919
potassium phosphate, 898
Antihyponatremic agents
sodium acetate, 1002
sodium chloride, 1007
Antihypophosphatemic
phosphate, 898
Anti-infectives
acyclovir, 8
alatrofloxacin, 16
amikacin, 70
amphotericin B, 90
amphotericin B lipid-based preparations, 90
ampicillin, 98
ampicillin/sulbactam, 102
azithromycin, 159
aztreonam, 162
capreomycin, 204
caspofungin, 213
cefamandole, 216
cefazolin, 220
cefepime, 224
cefoperazone, 229
Anti-infectives—cont'd
cefotaxime, 232
cefotetan, 236
cefoxitin, 240
ceftazidime, 244
ceftizoxime, 248
ceftriaxone, 252
cefuroxime, 256
chloramphenicol, 260
cidofovir, 268
ciprofloxacin, 276
clindamycin, 294
cytomegalovirus IGIV (human), 312
doxycycline, 415
ertapenem, 469
erythromycin, 472
fluconazole, 506
foscarnet, 528
ganciclovir, 544
gatifloxacin, 548
gentamicin, 562
imipenem-cilastatin, 616
immune globulin IV, 619
itraconazole, 660
kanamycin, 664
levofloxacin, 684
linezolid, 698
meropenem, 730
metronidazole, 757
moxifloxacin, 782
nafcillin, 796
ofloxacin, 830
oxacillin, 839
penicillin G, 872
pentamidine, 875
piperacillin, 904
piperacillin/tazobactam, 907
quinupristin/dalfopristin, 958
rifampin, 986
streptomycin, 1018
sulfamethoxazole-trimethoprim, 1027
ticarcillin disodium, 1050
ticarcillin/clavulanate, 1052
tobramycin, 1060
trimetrexate, 1080
vancomycin, 1092
voriconazole, 1125
zidovudine, 1135

Antiinflammatory agents
dexamethasone, 342
hydrocortisone phosphate, 590
hydrocortisone sodium succinate, 590
methylprednisolone sodium succinate, 747
*prednisolone sodium phosphate**
Anti-inhibitor coagulant complex, 114
Antilirium, 900
Antimalarial agent
doxycycline, 415
Antimyasthenic agents
neostigmine, 806
*pyridostigmine bromide**
Antineoplastics
aldesleukin, 26
alemtuzumab, 38
arsenic trioxide, 138
asparaginase, 144
bleomycin, 173
bortezomib, 1154
busulfan, 183
carboplatin, 206
carmustine (BCNU), 210
cisplatin, 286
cladribine, 290
cyclophosphamide, 302
cytarabine, 309
dacarbazine, 314
dactinomycin, 319
daunorubicin citrate, 328
daunorubicin hydrochloride, 328
denileukin diftitox, 335
docetaxel, 390
doxorubicin hydrochloride, 408
doxorubicin liposome, 408
epirubicin, 446
etoposide, 480
fludarabine, 511
fluorouracil, 518
gemcitabine, 554
gemtuzumab ozogamicin, 558
ibritumomab tiuxetan, 598
idarubicin, 607
ifosfamide, 610
interferon alfa-2b, 639
irinotecan, 642
mechlorethamine, 721
melphalan, 723
methotrexate, 738
Antineoplastics—cont'd
mitomycin, 771
mitoxantrone, 774
oxaliplatin, 841
paclitaxel, 850
pegaspargase, 869
pentostatin, 882
plicamycin, 912
porfimer sodium, 914
rituximab, 991
*samarium SM153**
sodium phosphate P_{32}*
streptozocin, 1021
*strontium-89 chloride**
teniposide, 1039
thiotepa, 1047
topotecan, 1064
trastuzumab, 1076
vinblastine, 1110
vincristine, 1113
vindesine 🍁, 1117
vinorelbine, 1120
Antineoplastic adjuncts
allopurinol, 48
amifostine, 64
dexrazoxane, 349
leucovorin calcium, 678
mesna, 734
sodium thiosulfate, 1012
Antineutropenic agents
filgrastim, 502
sargramostim, 996
Antiparkinson agent
diphenhydramine, 378
Antiplatelet agents
abciximab, 1
dipyridamole, 383
eptifibatide, 462
tirofiban, 1056
Antipolyneuropathy agent
immune globulin IV, 619
Antiprotozoal agents
AmBisome, 90
clindamycin, 294
doxycycline, 415
metronidazole, 757
pentamidine, 875
sulfamethoxazole-trimethoprim, 1027
trimetrexate, 1080

Antipsoriatic
methotrexate, 738
Antipsychotic agents
chlorpromazine, 263
haloperidol, 574
perphenazine, 884
prochlorperazine, 929
Antirheumatics
infliximab, 632
methotrexate, 738
Antithrombin III, 116
Antithrombotic agents
abciximab, 1
antithrombin III, 116
eptifibatide, 462
tirofiban, 1056
Anti-Thymocyte Globulin (Equine), 711
Anti-thymocyte globulin (rabbit), 118
Antitoxin
diphtheria antitoxin, 381
Anti-tuberculins
capreomycin, 204
kanamycin, 664
rifampin, 986
streptomycin, 1018
Antiulcer agents
cimetidine, 272
famotidine, 490
ranitidine, 962
Antivenin *(Crotalidae)* polyvalent, 121
Antivenin Crotalidae polyvalent immune fab (ovine), 123
Antivenin *(Latrodectus mactans),* 127
Antivenin *(Micrurus fulvius),* 129
Antivenins
antivenin (Crotalidae) *polyvalent,* 121
antivenin crotalidae polyvalent immune fab (ovine), 123
antivenin (Latrodectus mactans), 127
antivenin (Micrurus fulvius), 129
Antivertigo agent
diphenhydramine, 378
Antiviral agents
acyclovir, 8
cidofovir, 268
cytomegalovirus immune globulin IV (human), 312
foscarnet, 528
ganciclovir, 544
Antiviral agents—cont'd
immune globulin IV, 619
zidovudine, 1135
Antizol, 524
Anzemet, 396
APD, 856
Aprotinin injection, 130
APSAC*
Aquamephyton, 902
ARA-C, 309
Aralast, 52
Aranesp, 324
Arduan*
Aredia, 856
Argatroban, 134
Arginine hydrochloride*
Arsenic trioxide, 138
Ascorbic acid, 142
Asparaginase, 144
Astramorph PF, 778
Atenolol, 146
Atgam, 711
Ativan, 706
Atracurium besylate, 150
Atracurium besylate PF, 150
Atropine sulfate, 154
AT-III, 116
Autoplex-T, 114
Avelox, 782
Azactam, 162
Azathioprine sodium, 157
Azidothymidine, 1135
Azithromycin, 159
AZT, 1135
Aztreonam, 162

B

Bactocill, 839
Bactrim, 1027
Barbiturates
*amobarbital**
pentobarbital, 879
phenobarbital, 888
thiopental, 1044
Basiliximab, 165
Bebulin VH, 484
Benadryl, 378
BeneFIX, 487
Benzodiazepine antagonist
flumazenil, 514

Color type indicates generic drug name.
Italic type indicates drug categories and listings.
*See http://evolve.elsevier.com/IVMeds for detailed information.

Benzodiazepines
*chlordiazepoxide**
diazepam, 358
lorazepam, 706
midazolam, 760
Benztropine mesylate, 1146
Beta-adrenergic blocking agents
atenolol, 146
esmolol, 474
metoprolol, 754
propranolol, 943
Beta-lactamase inhibitors
ampicillin/sulbactam, 102
piperacillin/tazobactam, 907
ticarcillin/clavulanate, 1052
Betamethasone sodium phosphate, 1146
Bicarbonate sodium, 1003
BiCNU, 210
Bioclate (recombinant), 106
Biological response modifiers
aldesleukin, 26
denileukin diftitox, 335
interferon alfa-2b, 639
Bisphosphonates
etidronate, 478
pamidronate, 856
zoledronic acid, 1138
Bivalirudin, 168
Black Widow Spider Species Antivenin, 127
Blenoxane, 173
Bleomycin sulfate, 173
Blood modifiers
abciximab, 1
albumin normal serum, 22
alteplase (recombinant), 56
aminocaproic acid, 74
*anistreplase**
antihemophilic factor, 106
antihemophilic factor, von Willebrand factor, 110
anti-inhibitor coagulant, 114
antithrombin III, 116
aprotinin, 130
argatroban, 134
bivalirudin, 168
coagulation factor VIIa, 297
conjugated estrogens, 300
darbepoetin alfa, 324
Blood modifiers—cont'd
dextran high molecular weight, 351
dextran low molecular weight, 352
dextran 1, 354
dipyridamole, 383
drotrecogin alfa, 421
epoetin alfa, 452
eptifibatide, 462
factor IX, 484
factor IX complex (human), 484
factor IX (recombinant), 487
filgrastim, 502
folic acid, 522
hemin, 577
heparin, 578
hetastarch, 585
immune globulin IV, 619
iron dextran, 650
iron sucrose, 653
lepirudin, 674
leucovorin calcium, 678
phytonadione, 902
plasma protein fraction, 910
protamine sulfate, 946
reteplase (recombinant), 979
sargramostim, 996
sodium ferric gluconate, 1010
streptokinase, 1014
tenecteplase, 1035
tirofiban, 1056
tranexamic acid, 1073
*urokinase**
warfarin, 1131
Bortezomib, 1154
Branch Amin 4%, 948
Bretylate ♣, 176
Bretylium tosylate, 176
Bretylium tosylate PF, 176
Brevibloc, 474
Bronchial dilating agents (smooth muscle relaxants)
aminophylline, 76
ephedrine, 438
epinephrine, 440
isoproterenol, 656
Bumetanide, 178
Bumex, 178
Buminate 5%, 22
Buminate 25%, 22
Buprenex, 181

Buprenorphine hydrochloride, 181
Busulfan, 183
Busulfex, 183
Butorphanol tartrate, 187

C

Cafcit, 190
Caffeine citrate, 190
Caffeine and sodium benzoate*
Calcijex, 193
Calcitriol, 193
Calcium channel blocking agents
diltiazem, 374
nicardipine, 812
verapamil, 1102
Calcium chelating agents
edetate disodium, 428
Calcium chloride, 196
Calcium disodium edetate, 425
Calcium disodium versenate, 425
Calcium EDTA, 425
Calcium gluceptate, 1146
Calcium gluconate, 200
Calcium leucovorin, 678
Campath, 38
Camptosar, 642
Cancidas, 213
Capastat, 204
Capreomycin, 204
Carbapenems
ertapenem, 469
impenem-cilastatin, 616
meropenem, 730
Carboplatin, 206
Cardene IV, 812
Cardiac glycoside
digoxin, 368
Cardiac stimulants
digoxin, 368
dobutamine, 385
dopamine, 398
epinephrine, 440
inamrinone, 626
isoproterenol, 656
Cardioprotective agent
dexrazoxane, 349
Cardiotonic agents
calcium chloride, 196
calcium gluconate, 200
nesiritide, 808
Cardizem, 374
Carmustine (BCNU), 210
L-carnitine, 681
Carnitor, 681
Caspofungin acetate, 213
Cathflo Activase, 56
CDDP, 286
Cefamandole nafate, 216
Cefazolin sodium, 220
Cefepime hydrochloride, 224
Cefizox, 248
Cefobid, 229
Cefoperazone sodium, 229
Cefotan, 236
Cefotaxime sodium, 232
Cefotetan disodium, 236
Cefoxitin sodium, 240
Ceftazidime, 244
Ceftizoxime sodium, 248
Ceftriaxone sodium, 252
Cefuroxime sodium, 256
CellCept intravenous, 792
Cenolate, 142
Cephalosporins
cefamandole, 216
cefazolin, 220
cefepime, 224
cefoperazone, 229
cefotaxime, 232
cefotetan, 236
cefoxitin, 240
ceftazidime, 244
ceftizoxime, 248
ceftriaxone, 252
cefuroxime, 256
Ceptaz, 244
Cerebyx, 533
Ceredase*
Cerezyme, 613
Cernevit, 786
Cernevit-12, 786
Cerubidine, 328
Chelating agents
deferoxamine (iron), 333
dexrazoxane, 349
edetate calcium disodium (lead), 425
edetate disodium (calcium), 428
Chloramphenicol sodium succinate, 260

Color type indicates generic drug name.
Italic type indicates drug categories and listings.
*See http://evolve.elsevier.com/IVMeds for detailed information.

Chemotherapy agents
aldesleukin, 26
alemtuzumab, 38
arsenic trioxide, 138
asparaginase, 144
bleomycin, 173
bortezomib, 1154
busulfan, 183
carboplatin, 206
carmustine (BCNU), 210
cisplatin, 286
cladribine, 290
cyclophosphamide, 302
cytarabine, 309
dacarbazine, 314
dactinomycin, 319
daunorubicin citrate, 328
daunorubicin hydrochloride, 328
denileukin diftitox, 335
docetaxel, 390
doxorubicin hydrochloride, 408
doxorubicin liposome, 408
epirubicin, 446
etoposide, 480
fludarabine, 511
fluorouracil, 518
gemcitabine, 554
gemtuzumab ozogamicin, 558
ibritumomab tiuxetan, 598
idarubicin, 607
ifosfamide, 610
interferon alfa-2b, 639
irinotecan, 642
mechlorethamine, 721
melphalan, 723
methotrexate, 738
mitomycin, 771
mitoxantrone, 774
oxaliplatin, 841
paclitaxel, 850
pegaspargase, 869
pentostatin, 882
plicamycin, 912
porfimer sodium, 914
rituximab, 991
*samarium SM 153**
sodium phosphate P_{32}*
streptozocin, 1021
*strontium-89 chloride**
teniposide, 1039
Chemotherapy agents—cont'd
thiotepa, 1047
topotecan, 1064
trastuzumab, 1076
vinblastine, 1110
vincristine, 1113
vindesine ♣, 1117
vinorelbine, 1120
Chlordiazepoxide hydrochloride*
Chloromycetin, 260
Chlorothiazide sodium, 1146
Chlorpromazine hydrochloride, 263
Cholinergic agents
edrophonium, 430
edrophonium and atropine, 432
neostigmine, 806
physostigmine, 900
*pyridostigmine**
Cholinesterase inhibitors
edrophonium, 430
edrophonium and atropine, 432
neostigmine, 806
physostigmine, 900
*pyridostigmine**
Chromium, 1071
Cidofovir injection, 268
Cidomycin ♣, 562
Cimetidine, 272
Ciprofloxacin, 276
Cipro IV, 276
Cisatracurium besylate, 281
Cisplatin, 286
Citrovorum factor, 678
Cladribine, 290
Claforan, 232
Cleocin phosphate, 294
Clindamycin phosphate, 294
Clinimix 2.75% SF in D5, 948
Clinimix 2.75% SF in D10, 948
Clinimix 2.75% SF in D25, 948
Clinimix 4.25% SF in D5, 948
Clinimix 4.25% SF in D10, 948
Clinimix 4.25% SF in D20, 948
Clinimix 4.25% SF in D25, 948
Clinimix 5% SF in D10, 948
Clinimix 5% SF in D15, 948
Clinimix 5% SF in D20, 948
Clinimix 5% SF in D25, 948
Clinimix 5% SF in D35, 948

Color type indicates generic drug name.
Italic type indicates drug categories and listings.
*See http://evolve.elsevier.com/IVMeds for detailed information.

Clinimix E 2.75% SF in D5 with electrolytes and calcium, 948
Clinimix E 2.75% SF in D10 with electrolytes and calcium, 948
Clinimix E 2.75% SF in D25 with electrolytes and calcium, 948
Clinimix E 4.25% SF in D5 with electrolytes and calcium, 948
Clinimix E 4.25% SF in D10 with electrolytes and calcium, 948
Clinimix E 4.25% SF in D20 with electrolytes and calcium, 948
Clinimix E 4.25% SF in D25 with electrolytes and calcium, 948
Clinimix E 5% SF in D10 with electrolytes and calcium, 948
Clinimix E 5% SF in D15 with electrolytes and calcium, 948
Clinimix E 5% SF in D20 with electrolytes and calcium, 948
Clinimix E 5% SF in D25 with electrolytes and calcium, 948
Clinimix E 5% SF in D35 with electrolytes and calcium, 948
Clinisol 15% SF, 948
CMV-IGIV, 312
CNS stimulants
  caffeine citrate, 190
  *caffeine and sodium benzoate**
  doxapram, 402
Coagulation factor VIIa, 297
Cogentin, 1146
Colchicine*
Colistimethate sodium, 1146
Colony stimulating factors
  filgrastim, 502
  sargramostim, 996
Coly-Mycin M, 1146
Compazine, 929
Compound S, 1135
Conjugated estrogens, 300
ConTE-Pak-4, 1071
Copper, 1071
Cordarone, 84
Corlopam, 496
Coronary vasodilators
  adenosine, 12
  dipyridamole, 383
Corticorelin ovine triflutate*
Cortrosyn, 301
Corvert, 604
Cosmegen, 319
Cosyntropin, 301
Coumadin, 1131
CPT-11, 642
CroFab, 123
Crohn's disease agent
  infliximab, 632
Crystalline amino acid infusions, 948
Curare*
Cyclophosphamide, 302
Cyclosporine, 306
Cyklokapron, 1073
Cysteine hydrochloride, 1146
Cytarabine, 309
CytoGam, 312
Cytomegalovirus immune globulin intravenous (human), 312
Cytoprotective agent
  amifostine, 64
Cytosar ♣, 309
Cytosar-U, 309
Cytovene IV, 544
Cytoxan lyophilized, 302

D

Dacarbazine, 314
Daclizumab, 316
Dactinomycin, 319
Dalgan*
Dantrium intravenous, 322
Dantrolene sodium, 322
Darbepoetin alfa, 324
Daunorubicin hydrochloride, 328
Daunorubicin citrate liposome injection, 328
Daunoxome, 328
DDAVP, 339
1-Deamino-8-D-Arginine vasopressin, 339
Decadron, 342
Decadron phosphate, 342
Deferoxamine mesylate, 333
Demadex, 1067
Demerol, 727
Demerol hydrochloride, 727
Denileukin diftitox, 335
2-Deoxycoformycin, 882
Depacon, 1086

Color type indicates generic drug name.
Italic type indicates drug categories and listings.
*See http://evolve.elsevier.com/IVMeds for detailed information.

Depolarizing neuromuscular blocker
succinylcholine chloride, 1024
Desferal, 333
Desmopressin acetate, 339
Dexamethasone sodium phosphate, 342
DexFerrum, 650
DexIron ✦, 650
Dexmedetomidine hydrochloride, 346
Dexpanthenol, 1146
Dexrazoxane, 349
Dextran adjunct
dextran 1, 354
Dextran, high molecular weight, 351
Dextran 40, 352
Dextran, low molecular weight, 352
Dextran 1, 354
Dextran 70, 351
Dextran 75, 351
Dextrose, 356
Dextrose USP 2½%, 356
Dextrose USP 5%, 356
Dextrose USP 10%, 356
Dextrose USP 20%, 356
Dextrose USP 30%, 356
Dextrose USP 38.5%, 356
Dextrose USP 40%, 356
Dextrose USP 50%, 356
Dextrose USP 60%, 356
Dextrose USP 70%, 356
Dezocine*
D.H.E. 45, 372
DHPG, 544
Diagnostic agents
adenosine, 12
*arginine**
*corticorelin ovine triflutate**
cosyntropin, 301
dexamethasone, 342
dipyridamole, 383
edrophonium, 430
ergonovine maleate, 467
glucagon (rDNA origin), 566
*gonadorelin hydrochloride**
*L-hyoscyamine sulfate**
mannitol, 718
*methylene blue**
*protirelin**
*secretin** and 1000
*sermorelin acetate**
Diagnostic agents—cont'd
*sincalide**
*teriparatide acetate**
*tolbutamide sodium**
Diagnostic radiopharmaceutical
*indium In-111 pentetreotide**
Diamox, 6
Diazemuls ✦, 358
Diazepam, 358
Diazoxide, 363
Didronel IV, 478
Diflucan, 506
Digibind, 365
DigiFab, 365
Digoxin immune fab (ovine), 365
Digoxin injection, 368
Dihydroergotamine mesylate, 372
Dilantin, 894
Dilantin sodium, 894
Dilaudid, 595
Diltiazem hydrochloride, 374
Dimenhydrinate, 1146
Diphenhydramine hydrochloride, 378
Diphtheria antitoxin, 381
Diprivan, 936
Dipyridamole, 383
Direct thrombin inhibitors
argatroban, 134
bivalirudin, 168
lepirudin, 674
Disodium cefotetan, 236
Disodium edetate, 428
Disodium endrate, 428
Disodium etidronate, 478
Disodium pamidronate, 856
Disodium ticarcillin, 1050
Disodium ticarcillin and clavulanate potassium, 1052
Diuretics
acetazolamide, 6
bumetanide, 178
dextrose, 356
furosemide, 536
mannitol, 718
torsemide, 1067
Diuril, 1146
Dobutamine hydrochloride, 385
Dobutrex, 385
Docetaxel, 390
Dolasetron mesylate, 396

Color type indicates generic drug name.
Italic type indicates drug categories and listings.
*See http://evolve.elsevier.com/IVMeds for detailed information.

Dopamine hydrochloride, 398
Dopram, 402
Doxacurium chloride*
Doxapram hydrochloride, 402
Doxercalciferol, 405
Doxil, 408
Doxorubicin hydrochloride, 408
Doxorubicin hydrochloride liposome injection, 408
Doxy 100, 415
Doxy 200, 415
Doxycycline hyclate, 415
Droperidol, 418
Drotrecogin alfa (activated), 421
DTIC, 314
DTIC-Dome, 314
Ductus arteriosus patency adjunct
alprostadil, 54
Duramorph, 778

E

Edecrin ✤, 1147
Edetate calcium disodium, 425
Edetate disodium, 428
Edrophonium chloride, 430
Edrophonium chloride and atropine sulfate, 432
EDTA disodium, 428
Eflornithine hydrochloride, 1147
Eldisine ✤, 1117
Electrolyte (replenishers)
calcium chloride, 196
calcium gluconate, 200
magnesium sulfate, 714
phosphate, 898
potassium acetate, 919
potassium chloride, 919
sodium acetate, 1002
sodium bicarbonate, 1003
sodium chloride, 1007
Elitek, 966
Ellence, 446
Eloxatin, 841
Elspar, 144
Eminase*
Enalaprilat, 435
Endrate, 428
Enlon, 430
Enlon-Plus, 432
Enzyme inhibitors
hemin, 577
pentostatin, 882
Enzyme replenisher (glucocerebrosidase)
*alglucerase**
imiglucerase, 613
Enzymes, thrombolytic
alteplase, recombinant, 56
*anistreplase**
reteplase, recombinant, 979
streptokinase, 1014
tenecteplase, 1035
*urokinase**
Ephedrine sulfate, 438
Epinephrine hydrochloride, 440
Epirubicin hydrochloride, 446
EPO, 452
Epoetin alfa, 452
Epogen, 452
Epoprostenol sodium, 457
Eprex ✤, 452
Eptifibatide, 462
Ergonovine maleate, 467
Ergot alkaloid
dihydroergotamine, 372
Ergotrate maleate, 467
Ertapenem, 469
Erythrocin IV, 472
Erythromycin lactobionate, 472
Erythropoietin, 452
Esmolol hydrochloride, 474
Ethacrynic acid, 1147
Ethyol, 64
Etidronate disodium, 478
Etopophos, 480
Etoposide, 480
Etoposide phosphate, 480
Extended-spectrum penicillins
piperacillin, 904
piperacillin/tazobactam, 907
ticarcillin, 1050
ticarcillin/clavulanate, 1052

F

Factor VIII, 106
Factor IX complex (human), 484
Factor IX (human), 484
Factor IX (recombinant), 487
Factrel*
Famotidine, 490

Color type indicates generic drug name.
Italic type indicates drug categories and listings.
*See http://evolve.elsevier.com/IVMeds for detailed information.

Fat emulsion, intravenous, 492
Fatty acid
fat emulsion, intravenous, 492
Feiba VH, 114
Fenoldopam mesylate, 496
Fentanyl, 499
Fentanyl citrate, 499
Fentanyl citrate PF, 499
Fentanyl citrate with droperidol, 1147
Ferrlecit, 1010
Filgrastim, 502
Flagyl IV, 757
Flagyl IV RTU, 757
Flolan, 457
Floxin I.V., 830
Fluconazole, 506
Fludara, 511
Fludarabine phosphate, 511
Flumazenil, 514
Fluoroquinolones
alatrofloxacin, 16
ciprofloxacin, 276
gatifloxacin, 548
levofloxacin, 684
moxifloxacin, 782
ofloxacin, 830
Fluorouracil, 518
5-Fluorouracil, 518
Folate antagonists
methotrexate, 738
trimetrexate, 1080
Folic acid, 522
Folinic acid, 678
Folvite, 522
Fomepizole injection, 524
Fortaz, 244
Foscavir, 528
Foscarnet sodium, 528
Fosphenytoin sodium, 533
FreAmine HBC 6.9%, 948
FreAmine III 8.5%, 948
FreAmine III 10%, 948
FreAmine III 3% with electrolytes, 948
FreAmine III 8.5% with electrolytes, 948
5-FU, 518
Fungizone, 90
Furosemide, 536

G
Gallium nitrate, 541
Gamimune N, 619
Gammagard SD, 619
Gammar P-IV, 619
Ganciclovir sodium, 544
Ganite, 541
Garamycin, 562
Gastric acid inhibitors
cimetidine, 272
famotidine, 490
pantoprazole, 862
ranitidine, 962
Gastric sphincter relaxants
glucagon, 566
metoclopramide, 751
Gatifloxacin, 548
Gaucher's disease
*alglucerase**
imiglucerase, 613
G-CSF, 502
Gemcitabine hydrochloride, 554
Gemtuzumab ozogamicin, 558
Gemzar, 554
General anesthetics
alfentanil, 42
propofol, 936
remifentanil, 968
thiopental, 1044
Gentamicin sulfate, 562
Gentran 40, 352
Gentran 75, 351
Geref*
GI antispasmodic
*L-hyoscyamine**
G.I. stimulant
metoclopramide hydrochloride, 751
GlucaGen, 566
Glucagon for injection, 566
Glucagon (rDNA origin), 566
Glucocerebrosidase* and 613
Glucose, 356
Glucose elevating agents
glucagon (rDNA origin), 566
octreotide (unlabeled), 826
Glycoprotein GPIIb/IIIa receptor antagonists
abciximab, 1
eptifibatide, 462
tirofiban, 1056

Color type indicates generic drug name.
Italic type indicates drug categories and listings.
*See http://evolve.elsevier.com/IVMeds for detailed information.

Glycopyrrolate, 568
GM-CSF, 996
Gonadorelin hydrochloride*
Granulocyte colony stimulating factor (human)
filgrastim, 502
Granulocyte-macrophage colony stimulating factor (human)
sargramostim, 996
Granisetron hydrochloride, 571
Growth hormone suppressant
octreotide, 826

H

5 HT_3 receptor antagonists
dolasetron, 396
granisetron, 571
ondansetron, 834
H_2 antagonists
cimetidine, 272
famotidine, 490
ranitidine, 962
Haldol, 574
Haloperidol lactate, 574
Hectoral injection, 405
Helixate (recombinant), 106
Helixate FS (recombinant), 106
Hematinic agents
iron dextran, 650
iron sucrose, 653
sodium ferric gluconate, 1010
Hemin, 577
Hemofil M, 106
Hemorrhagic cystitis (prophylactic)
mesna, 734
Hemostatics, systemic
aminocaproic acid, 74
antihemophilic factor, 106
antihemophilic factor/von Willebrand factor, 110
anti-inhibitor coagulant, 114
conjugated estrogen, 300
factor IX, 484
factor IX complex (human), 484
factor IX (recombinant), 487
tranexamic acid, 1073
HepaAmine 8%, 948
Hepalean ♣, 578
Heparin antagonist
protamine sulfate, 946
Heparin Lock-Flush, 578
Heparin sodium, 578
Heparin sodium-PF, 578
Hepatosol 8%, 948
Hep-Flush 10, 578
Hep-Lock, 578
Hep-Lock U/P, 578
Hep-Pak Lock Flush, 578
Herceptin, 1076
Herpes simplex virus encephalitis
acyclovir, 8
Hespan, 585
Hetastarch, 585
Hextend, 585
Histamine antagonists
cimetidine, 272
famotidine, 490
ranitidine, 962
HN_2, 721
Hormones
conjugated estrogens, 300
*corticorelin ovine triflutate**
desmopressin, 339
dexamethasone sodium phosphate, 342
*gonadorelin hydrochloride**
hydrocortisone phosphate, 590
hydrocortisone sodium succinate, 590
insulin injection (regular), 636
levothyroxine, 692
liothyronine, 703
methylprednisolone sodium succinate, 747
octreotide, 826
oxytocin, 847
*prednisolone phosphate**
*sermorelin acetate**
*teriparatide acetate**
vasopressin, 1096
Human granulocyte colony stimulating factor, 502
Human granulocyte-macrophage colony stimulating factor, 996
Humate-P, 110
Humulin R, 636
Hyate: C Porcine AHF, 106
Hycamtin, 1064
Hydantoins
fosphenytoin, 533
phenytoin, 894
Hydralazine hydrochloride, 588

Color type indicates generic drug name.
Italic type indicates drug categories and listings.
*See http://evolve.elsevier.com/IVMeds for detailed information.

Hydrocortisone sodium phosphate, 590
Hydrocortisone sodium succinate, 590
Hydrocortone phosphate, 590
Hydromorphone hydrochloride, 595
Hyoscyamine sulfate*
L-Hyoscyamine sulfate*
Hyperalimentation, 948
Hyperstat IV, 363
Hypnotic/sedatives, CNS depressants
*amobarbital**
*chlordiazepoxide**
dexmedetomidine, 346
diazepam, 358
diphenhydramine, 378
haloperidol, 574
lorazepam, 706
midazolam, 760
pentobarbital, 879
phenobarbital, 888
promethazine, 933
propofol, 936
thiopental, 1044

I

Ibritumomab tiuxetan, 598
Ibutilide fumarate, 604
Idamycin, 607
Idamycin PFS, 607
Idarubicin hydrochloride, 607
IDR, 607
Ifex, 610
Ifosfamide, 610
IGIV, 619
Ilopan, 1146
Imiglucerase, 613
Imipenem-cilastatin, 616
Immune globulin intravenous, 619
Immunizing agents
cytomegalovirus IGIV (passive), 312
diphtheria antitoxin (active), 381
immune globulin IV (passive), 619
lymphocyte immune globulin, 711
respiratory syncytial virus immune globulin intravenous (passive), 976
Rh_o(D) IGIV (passive), 982
Immunomodulator
aldesleukin, 26
Immunosuppressive agents
alefacept, 35
anti-thymocyte globulin, 118
azathioprine sodium, 157
basiliximab, 165
cyclosporine, 306
daclizumab, 316
dexamethasone, 342
lymphocyte immune globulin, 711
muromonab-CD3, 789
mycophenolate mofetil, 792
*prednisolone sodium phosphate**
tacrolimus, 1030
Imuran, 157
Inamrinone lactate, 626
Inapsine, 418
Inderal, 943
Indium In-111 pentetreotide*
Indocin IV, 629
Indomethacin sodium trihydrate, 629
InFed, 650
Inflammatory bowel disease agent
infliximab, 632
Infliximab, 632
Infufer 🍁, 650
Infuvite, 786
Infuvite pediatric, 786
Innovar, 1147
Inocor, 626
Inotropic agents
digoxin, 368
dobutamine, 385
dopamine, 398
inamrinone, 626
isoproterenol, 656
milrinone, 767
Insulin injection (regular), 636
Integrilin, 462
Interferon alfa-2b recombinant, 639
Interleukin-2 recombinant, 26
Intralipid 10%, 492
Intralipid 20%, 492
Intralipid 30%, 492
Intravenous fat emulsion, 492
Intron A, 639
Intropin, 398
Invanz, 469
Iodine, 1071
Irinotecan hydrochloride, 642
Iron dextran injection, 650

Color type indicates generic drug name.
Italic type indicates drug categories and listings.
*See http://evolve.elsevier.com/IVMeds for detailed information.

Iron sucrose, 653
Iron supplements
iron dextran, 650
iron sucrose, 653
sodium ferric gluconate, 1010
Isoproterenol hydrochloride, 656
Isoptin, 1102
Isuprel hydrochloride, 656
Itraconazole, 660
Iveegam, 619

K

Kabikinase, 1014
Kanamycin sulfate, 664
Kantrex, 664
Kefurox, 256
Kefzol, 220
Ketorolac tromethamine, 668
Kidrolase 🍁, 144
Kinevac*
Koate DVI, 106
Kogenate (recombinant), 106
Kogenate FS (recombinant), 106
Konyne 80, 484
Kytril, 571

L

Labetalol hydrochloride, 671
Lanoxin, 368
Lanoxin pediatric, 368
Lasix, 536
Lead mobilization
edetate calcium disodium, 425
Lepirudin, 674
Leucovorin calcium, 678
Leukine, 996
Leustatin, 290
Levaquin, 684
Levarterenol bitartrate, 822
Levocarnitine, 681
Levo-Dromoran, 689
Levofloxacin, 684
Levophed, 822
Levorphanol tartrate, 689
Levothyroxine sodium, 692
Levsin*
Librium*
Lidocaine hydrochloride, 694
Lidocaine PF, 694
Linezolid, 698
Liothyronine sodium, 703
Lipid-based products
amphotericin B, 90
daunorubicin, 328
doxorubicin, 408
Liposyn II 10%, 492
Liposyn II 20%, 492
Liposyn III 10%, 492
Liposyn III 20%, 492
Liposyn III 30%, 492
L.M.D. 10%, 352
Loop diuretics
bumetanide, 178
furosemide, 536
torsemide, 1067
Lopressor, 754
Lorazepam, 706
Luminal sodium, 888
Lymphocyte immune globulin, 711

M

Macrodex, 351
Macular degeneration therapy adjunct
verteporfin, 1106
Manganese, 1071
Magnesium sulfate, 714
Mandol, 216
Mannitol, 718
Maxeran 🍁, 751
Maxipime, 224
Mechlorethamine hydrochloride, 721
Mefoxin, 240
Melphalan hydrochloride, 723
Meperidine hydrochloride, 727
Meperidine HCl PF, 727
Meropenem, 730
Merrem I.V., 730
Mesna, 734
Mesnex, 734
Mestinon*
Metastron*
Methergine, 745
Methocarbamol, 735
Methotrexate PF, 738
Methotrexate sodium, 738
Methyldopate hydrochloride, 743
Methylene blue*
Methylergonovine maleate, 745
Methylprednisolone sodium succinate, 747

Color type indicates generic drug name.
Italic type indicates drug categories and listings.
*See http://evolve.elsevier.com/IVMeds for detailed information.

Methylthionine chloride*
Metoclopramide hydrochloride, 751
Metoprolol tartrate, 754
Metronidazole hydrochloride, 757
Metronidazole RTU, 757
Mezlocillin sodium, 1147
Midazolam hydrochloride, 760
Migraine agent
  dihydroergotamine, 372
Milrinone lactate, 767
Minocin, 1147
Minocycline hydrochloride, 1147
Mithracin, 912
Mitomycin, 771
Mitoxantrone hydrochloride, 774
Mivacron*
Mivacurium chloride*
Molybdenum, 1071
Monarc-M, 106
Monoclate P, 106
Monoclonal antibodies
  abciximab, 1
  alemtuzumab, 38
  basiliximab, 165
  daclizumab, 316
  gemtuzumab, 558
  ibritumomab tiuxetan, 598
  infliximab, 632
  muromonab-CD3, 789
  rituximab, 991
  trastuzumab, 1076
Mononine, 484
Morphine sulfate, 778
Moxifloxacin hydrochloride, 782
MTC, 771
M.T.E.-4, 1071
M.T.E.-5, 1071
M.T.E.-6, 1071
M.T.E.-7, 1071
M.T.E.-4 concentrated, 1071
M.T.E.-5 concentrated, 1071
M.T.E.-6 concentrated, 1071
MTX, 738
MulTE-Pak-4, 1071
MulTE-Pak-5, 1071
Multiple trace element, 1071
Multiple trace element concentrated, 1071
Multiple trace element neonatal, 1071
Multiple Trace Element with Selenium, 1071
Multiple Trace Element with Selenium Concentrated, 1071
Multivitamin infusion, 786
Muromonab-CD3, 789
Muscle relaxants
  atracurium, 150
  cisatracurium, 281
  dantrolene, 322
  diazepam, 358
  *doxacurium**
  lorazepam, 706
  methocarbamol, 735
  *mivacurium**
  orphenadrine, 837
  pancuronium, 860
  *pipecuronium**
  *rocuronium**
  succinylcholine, 1024
  *tubocurarine**
  vecuronium, 1098
Mustargen, 721
Mutamycin, 771
M.V.I.-12, 786
M.V.I. Pediatric, 786
Mycophenolate mofetil hydrochloride, 792
Mylotarg, 558

N

Nafcil, 796
Nafcillin sodium, 796
Nalbuphine hydrochloride, 799
Nallpen, 796
Nalmefene hydrochloride, 801
Naloxone hydrochloride, 804
Narcan, 804
Narcotic analgesics, agonist/antagonists
  buprenorphine, 181
  butorphanol, 187
  *dezocine**
  nalbuphine, 799
  pentazocine, 877
Narcotic analgesics, agonists/CNS depressants
  alfentanil, 42
  fentanyl, 499
  hydromorphone, 595
  levorphanol, 689

Color type indicates generic drug name.
Italic type indicates drug categories and listings.
*See http://evolve.elsevier.com/IVMeds for detailed information.

Narcotic analgesics, agonists/CNS depressants—cont'd
meperidine, 727
morphine, 778
oxymorphone, 845
remifentanil, 968
Narcotic antagonists
nalmefene, 801
naloxone, 804
Natrecor, 808
Navelbine, 1120
Nebcin, 1060
Nembutal sodium, 879
Neosar, 302
Neostigmine methylsulfate, 806
Neo-Synephrine, 892
Neotrace-4, 1071
Nephramine 5.4%, 948
Nesiritide, 808
Neupogen, 502
Neuromuscular blocking agents (nondepolarizing)
atracurium, 150
cisatracurium, 281
*doxacurium**
*mivacurium**
pancuronium, 860
*pipecuronium**
*rocuronium**
*tubocurarine**
vecuronium, 1098
Neuromuscular blocking agent (depolarizing)
succinylcholine, 1024
Neutrexin, 1080
Niacin, 1147
Niacinamide, 1147
Nicardipine hydrochloride, 812
Nicotinamide, 1147
Nicotinic acid, 1147
Nimbex, 281
Nipent, 882
Nitro-Bid IV, 814
Nitrogen mustard, 721
Nitroglycerin IV, 814
Nitroprusside sodium, 818
Nondepolarizing neuromuscular blocker antagonists
edrophonium, 430
edrophonium and atropine, 432
Nondepolarizing neuromuscular blocker antagonists—cont'd
neostigmine, 806
*pyridostigmine**
Nondepolarizing neuromuscular blocking agents
atracurium, 150
cisatracurium, 281
*doxacurium**
*mivacurium**
pancuronium, 860
*pipecuronium**
*rocuronium**
*tubocurarine**
vecuronium, 1098
Nonsteroidal anti-inflammatory agent
ketorolac, 668
Norcuron, 1098
Norepinephrine, 822
Norflex, 837
Normal saline, 1007
Normal serum albumin (human), 22
Normodyne, 671
North American coral snake antivenin, 129
Novamine 11.4%, 948
Novamine 15%, 948
Novantrone, 774
Novolin-ge-Toronto 🍁, 636
NovoSeven, 297
NSAID
ketorolac, 668
Nubain, 799
Numorphan, 845
Nuromax*
Nutritional products (supplements)
ascorbic acid, 142
calcium chloride, 196
calcium gluconate, 200
cysteine hydrochloride, 1146
dextrose, 356
fat emulsion, intravenous, 492
folic acid, 522
levocarnitine, 681
magnesium sulfate, 714
multivitamin infusion, 786
potassium acetate, 919
potassium chloride, 919
potassium phosphate, 898
protein (amino acid) products, 948

Color type indicates generic drug name.
Italic type indicates drug categories and listings.
*See http://evolve.elsevier.com/IVMeds for detailed information.

Nutritional products (supplements)—cont'd
pyridoxine hydrochloride, 953
sodium acetate, 1002
sodium bicarbonate, 1003
sodium chloride, 1007
sodium phosphate, 898
thiamine hydrochloride, 1043
trace metals, 1071
NVB, 1120

O

Octreo Scan*
Octreotide acetate, 826
Ofloxacin, 830
OKT3, 789
Omnipen-N, 98
Oncaspar, 869
Oncovin, 1113
Ondansetron hydrochloride, 834
Ontak, 335
Onxol, 850
Orinase diagnostic*
Ornidyl, 1147
Orphenadrine citrate, 837
Orthoclone OKT3, 789
Osmitrol, 718
Oxacillin sodium, 839
Oxaliplatin, 841
Oxazolidinone
linezolid, 698
Oxymorphone hydrochloride, 845
Oxytocics
ergonovine, 467
methylergonovine, 745
oxytocin, 847
Oxytocin injection, 847

P

Paclitaxel, 850
L-PAM, 723
Pamidronate disodium, 856
Pancuronium bromide, 860
Panglobulin, 619
Panhematin, 577
Pantoprazole sodium, 862
Papaverine hydrochloride, 865
Paraplatin, 206
Paraplatin-AQ 🍁, 206
Parathar*
Paricalcitol, 866
Patent ductus arteriosus agent
indomethacin sodium trihydrate, 629
Pavulon, 860
Pediatric multiple trace element, 1071
PedTE-Pak-4, 1071
Pedtrace-4, 1071
Pegaspargase, 869
Peg-L-asparaginase, 869
Penicillin and beta-lactamase inhibitors
ampicillin/sulbactam, 102
piperacillin/tazobactam, 907
ticarcillin/clavulanate, 1052
Penicillin G, 872
Penicillin G, aqueous, 872
Penicillin G, potassium, 872
Penicillin G sodium, 872
Penicillins
ampicillin sodium, 98
ampicillin/sulbactam, 102
nafcillin sodium, 796
oxacillin sodium, 839
penicillin G potassium and sodium, 872
piperacillin sodium, 904
piperacillin/tazobactam, 907
ticarcillin disodium, 1050
ticarcillin/clavulanate, 1052
Pentacarinat 🍁, 875
Pentamidine isethionate, 875
Pentazocine lactate, 877
Pentobarbital sodium, 879
Pentostatin, 882
Pentothal sodium, 1044
Pepcid IV, 490
Perphenazine, 884
Persantine IV, 383
Pfizerpen, 872
Pharmorubicin PFS 🍁, 446
Phenergan, 933
Phenobarbital sodium, 888
Phenothiazines
chlorpromazine, 263
perphenazine, 884
prochlorperazine, 929
promethazine, 933
Phentolamine mesylate, 890
Phenylalanine mustard, 723
Phenylephrine hydrochloride, 892
Phenytoin sodium, 894

Color type indicates generic drug name.
Italic type indicates drug categories and listings.
*See http://evolve.elsevier.com/IVMeds for detailed information.

Phosphate, 898
Phosphate replacement products
potassium phosphate, 898
sodium phosphate, 898
Photofrin, 914
Photosensitizing agent
porfimer sodium, 914
verteporfin, 1106
Physostigmine salicylate, 900
Phytonadione, 902
Pipecuronium bromide*
Piperacillin sodium, 904
Piperacillin sodium and tazobactam sodium, 907
Pipracil, 904
Pitocin, 847
Pitressin, 1096
Plasbumin-5, 22
Plasbumin-20, 22
Plasbumin-25, 22
Plasmanate, 910
Plasma protein fraction, 910
Plasma protein fractions
albumin, normal serum, 22
plasma protein fraction, 910
Plasma proteins
albumin, 22
antithrombin III (human), 116
plasma protein fraction, 910
Plasmatein, 910
Plasma volume expanders
albumin, 22
dextran high molecular weight, 351
dextran, low molecular weight, 352
hetastarch, 585
plasma protein fraction, 910
Platelet aggregation inhibitors
abciximab, 1
dipyridamole, 383
eptifibatide, 462
tirofiban, 1056
Platelet count stimulator
immune globulin IV, 619
Rh_o(D) IGIV, 982
Platinol ♣, 286
Platinol-AQ, 286
Plicamycin, 912
Polycillin N, 98
Polygam SD, 619
Porfimer sodium, 914
Porphyrin inhibitor
hemin, 577
Potassium acetate, 919
Potassium chloride, 919
Potassium penicillin G, 872
Potassium phosphate, 898
Potassium replacement products
potassium acetate, 919
potassium chloride, 919
potassium phosphate, 898
Pralidoxime chloride, 922
Precedex, 346
Prednisolone phosphate*
Prednisolone sodium phosphate*
Premarin intravenous, 300
Pressyn ♣, 1096
Primacor, 767
Primaxin, 616
Procainamide hydrochloride, 925
ProcalAmine, 948
Prochlorperazine edisylate, 929
Procrit, 452
Procytox ♣, 302
Profinine SD, 484
Prograf, 1030
Prolastin, 52
Proleukin, 26
Promethazine hydrochloride, 933
Promit, 354
Pronestyl, 925
Proplex T, 484
Propofol injection, 936
Propranolol hydrochloride, 943
ProSol 20% SF, 948
Prostaglandin
alprostadil, 54
Prostaglandin E_1, 54
Prostaglandin inhibitor
indomethacin, 629
Prostaphlin, 839
Proteasome inhibitor
bortezomib, 1154
Prostigmin, 806
Prostin VR pediatric, 54
Protamine sulfate, 946
Protein (amino acid) products, 948
Protein hydrolysates, 948
Protein inhibitors
$alpha_1$-proteinase inhibitor (human), 52
aprotinin, 130

Color type indicates generic drug name.
Italic type indicates drug categories and listings.
*See http://evolve.elsevier.com/IVMeds for detailed information.

Protenate, 910
Protirelin*
Protonix IV, 862
Proton pump inhibitor
pantoprazole, 862
Protopam chloride, 922
P.T.E.-4, 1071
Pulmonary antihypertensives
epoprostenol, 457
Pulmonary edema (adjunct)
morphine, 778
Pyridostigmine bromide*
Pyridoxine hydrochloride, 953

Q

Quadramet*
Quelicin PF, 1024
Quinidine gluconate injection, 955
Quinupristin/dalfopristin, 958

R

Radiopharmaceuticals
ibritumomab tiuxetan, 598
*indium In-111 pentetreotide**
*samarium SM 153 lexidronam**
*sodium phosphate P_{32}**
*strontium-89 chloride**
Ranitidine, 962
Rasburicase, 966
Recombinant agents
abciximab, 1
aldesleukin, 26
alemtuzumab, 38
alteplase, 56
antihemophilic factor, 106
antihemophilic factor/von Willebrand factor, 110
basiliximab, 165
coagulation factor VIIa, 297
daclizumab, 316
denileukin diftitox, 335
epoetin alfa, 452
factor IX, 487
filgrastim, 502
gemtuzamab, 558
glucagon (rDNA origin), 566
imiglucerase, 613
infliximab, 632
insulin, 636
Recombinant agents—cont'd
interferon alfa-2b, 639
lepirudin, 674
muromonab-CD3, 789
rasburicase, 966
reteplase, 979
rituximab, 991
sargramostim, 996
tenecteplase, 1035
trastuzumab, 1076
Recombinant human erythropoietin
epoetin alfa, 452
Recombinant interleukin-2, 26
Recombinate, 106
Recombinant tPA, 56
Redoxon 🍁, 142
ReFacto, 106
Refludan, 674
Regitine, 890
Reglan, 751
Regular Iletin II (pork), 636
Regular Iletin II (purified pork), 636
Regular insulin (pork), 636
Regular insulin (purified pork), 636
Relaxants, skeletal muscle
atracurium, 150
cisatracurium, 281
dantrolene, 322
diazepam, 358
*doxacurium**
lorazepam, 706
methocarbamol, 735
midazolam, 760
*mivacurium**
orphenadrine, 837
pancuronium, 860
*pipecuronium**
*rocuronium**
succinylcholine, 1024
*tubocurarine**
vecuronium, 1098
Relaxants, smooth muscle
*L-hyoscyamine sulfate**
Relaxants, smooth muscle (uterine)
magnesium sulfate, 714
Relaxants, smooth muscle (vascular)
alprostadil, 54
inamrinone, 626
milrinone, 767
Remicade, 632

Color type indicates generic drug name.
Italic type indicates drug categories and listings.
*See http://evolve.elsevier.com/IVMeds for detailed information.

Remifentanil hydrochloride, 968
RenAmin without electrolytes, 948
ReoPro, 1
RespiGam, 976
Respiratory stimulant adjuncts
aminophylline, 76
caffeine citrate, 190
*caffeine and sodium benzoate**
doxapram hydrochloride, 402
Respiratory syncytial virus immune globulin intravenous, 976
Retavase, 979
Reteplase, recombinant, 979
Retrovir, 1135
Reversol, 430
Revex, 801
Revimine ♣, 398
R-Gene 10*
Rheomacrodex, 352
Rh_o(D)-IGIV, 982
Rh_o(D) immune globulin intravenous (human), 982
Rifadin, 986
Rifampin, 986
Rituxan, 991
Rituximab, 991
Robaxin, 735
Rocephin, 252
Rocuronium bromide*
Romazicon, 514
r-PA, 979
RSV-IGIV, 976
rt-PA, 56
Rubex, 408

S

Salt replacement products
sodium acetate, 1002
sodium chloride, 1007
Samarium SM 153 lexidronam injection*
Sandimmune, 306
Sandoglobulin, 619
Sandostatin, 826
L-Sarcolysin, 723
Sargramostim, 996
Scopolamine hydrochloride, 1147
SecreFlo 1000 and *
Secretin 1000 and *
Sedative/hypnotic CNS depressants
*amobarbital**
*chlordiazepoxide**
dexmedetomidine, 346
diazepam, 358
diphenhydramine, 378
haloperidol, 574
lorazepam, 706
midazolam, 760
pentobarbital, 879
phenobarbital, 888
promethazine, 933
propofol, 936
thiopental, 1044
Selenium, 1071
Septra, 1027
Sermorelin acetate*
Serum albumin, 22
Simulect, 165
Sincalide*
SM 153*
SMZ-TMP, 1027
Sleeping sickness
eflornithine, 1147
Sodium acetate, 1002
Sodium acetazolamide, 6
Sodium amobarbital*
Sodium ampicillin, 98
Sodium ampicillin/sodium sulbactam, 102
Sodium amytal*
Sodium ascorbate, 142
Sodium azathioprine, 157
Sodium bicarbonate, 1003
Sodium cefazolin, 220
Sodium cefoperazone, 229
Sodium cefotaxime, 232
Sodium cefoxitin, 240
Sodium ceftizoxime, 248
Sodium ceftriaxone, 252
Sodium cefuroxime, 256
Sodium chloride, 1007
Sodium dilantin, 894
Sodium epoprostenol, 457
Sodium ferric gluconate complex, 1010
Sodium foscarnet, 528
Sodium fosphenytoin, 533
Sodium ganciclovir, 544
Sodium heparin, 578

Color type indicates generic drug name.
Italic type indicates drug categories and listings.
*See http://evolve.elsevier.com/IVMeds for detailed information.

Sodium lactate, 1147
⅙ molar sodium lactate, 1147
Sodium levothyroxine, 692
Sodium liothyronine, 703
Sodium luminal, 888
Sodium methotrexate, 738
Sodium nafcillin, 796
Sodium nembutal, 879
Sodium nitrite, 1012
Sodium nitroprusside, 818
Sodium oxacillin, 839
Sodium pantoprazole, 862
Sodium penicillin G, 872
Sodium pentobarbital, 879
Sodium pentothal, 1044
Sodium phenobarbital, 888
Sodium phenytoin, 894
Sodium phosphate, 898
Sodium phosphate P_{32}*
Sodium piperacillin, 904
Sodium porfimer, 914
Sodium thiopental, 1044
Sodium thiosulfate, 1012
Sodium tolbutamide*
Sodium valproate, 1086
Solu-Cortef, 590
Solu-Medrol, 747
Sporanox, 660
Stadol, 187
Stadol PF, 187
Stemetil ♣, 929
Stimulants, anticholinesterase (cholinergic) muscle
edrophonium, 430
edrophonium and atropine, 432
neostigmine, 806
physostigmine, 900
*pyridostigmine**
Stimulants, central nervous system
caffeine citrate, 190
*caffeine and sodium benzoate**
doxapram, 402
Stimulants, smooth muscle
metoclopramide, 751
Streptase, 1014
Streptokinase, 1014
Streptomycin sulfate, 1018
Streptozocin, 1021
Strontium-89 chloride injection*
Sublimaze, 499
Succinylcholine chloride, 1024
Sulfamethoxazole-trimethoprim, 1027
Sulfonamides
sulfamethoxazole-trimethoprim, 1027
Sympathomimetic bronchodilators
ephedrine, 438
epinephrine, 440
isoproterenol, 656
Synercid, 958
Synthroid, 692
Syntocinon, 847

T

T_3, 703
T_4, 692
Tacrolimus, 1030
Tagamet, 272
Talwin, 877
Taxol, 850
Taxotere, 390
Tazicef, 244
Tazidime, 244
T.E.C., 1071
Tenecteplase, 1035
Teniposide, 1039
Tenormin, 146
Tensilon, 430
Tequin, 548
Teriparatide acetate*
Tetracylines
doxycycline, 415
Tham, 1084
79% theophylline (aminophylline), 76
Theophylline and dextrose 5%, 1147
Theophylline ethylenediamine, 76
Thiamine hydrochloride, 1043
Thiopental sodium, 1044
Thioplex, 1047
Thiotepa, 1047
Thorazine, 263
Thrombate III, 116
Thrombolytic agents
alteplase, 56
*anistreplase**
drotrecogin alfa, 421
reteplase, 979
streptokinase, 1014
tenecteplase, 1035
*urokinase**
Thymoglobulin, 118

Color type indicates generic drug name.
Italic type indicates drug categories and listings.
*See http://evolve.elsevier.com/IVMeds for detailed information.

Thypinone*
Thyrel-TRH*
Thyroid agents
levothyroxine, 692
liothyronine, 703
L-thyroxine, 692
Ticar, 1050
Ticarcillin disodium, 1050
Ticarcillin disodium and clavulanate potassium, 1052
Timentin, 1052
Tirofiban hydrochloride, 1056
Tissue plasminogen activators
alteplase, 56
reteplase, 979
tenecteplase, 1035
TMP-SMZ, 1027
TNKase, 1035
Tobramycin sulfate, 1060
Tolbutamide sodium*
Toposar, 480
Topotecan hydrochloride, 1064
Toradol, 668
Torsemide injection, 1067
Totacillin-N, 98
Total parenteral nutrition, 948
tPA, 56
Trace metals, 1071
Trace metals additive in NS, 1071
Tracrium, 150
Trandate, 671
Tranexamic acid, 1073
Trastuzumab, 1076
Trasylol, 130
Travasol 2.75% in D5, 948
Travasol 2.75% in D10, 948
Travasol 2.75% in D15, 948
Travasol 2.75% in D20, 948
Travasol 2.75% in D25, 948
Travasol 4.25% in D5, 948
Travasol 4.25% in D10, 948
Travasol 4.25% in D15, 948
Travasol 4.25% in D20, 948
Travasol 4.25% in D25, 948
Travasol 2.75% SF in D5 with electrolytes, 948
Travasol 2.75% SF in D10 with electrolytes, 948
Travasol 2.75% SF in D15 with electrolytes, 948
Travasol 2.75% SF in D20 with electrolytes, 948
Travasol 2.75% SF in D25 with electrolytes, 948
Travasol 4.25% SF in D5 with electrolytes, 948
Travasol 4.25% SF in D10 with electrolytes, 948
Travasol 4.25% SF in D15 with electrolytes, 948
Travasol 4.25% SF in D20 with electrolytes, 948
Travasol 4.25% SF in D25 with electrolytes, 948
Travasol 5.5% with electrolytes, 948
Travasol 8.5% with electrolytes, 948
Travasol 5.5% without electrolytes, 948
Travasol 8.5% without electrolytes, 948
Travasol 10% without electrolytes, 948
Travasol SF 3.5% with electrolytes, 948
Travasol SF 5.5% with electrolytes, 948
Travasol SF 10% with electrolytes, 948
Tridil, 814
Trilafon, 884
Trimethoprim-sulfamethoxazole, 1027
Trimetrexate glucuronate, 1080
Triostat, 703
Trisenox, 138
Tromethamine, 1084
TrophaAmine 6%, 948
TrophaAmine 10%, 948
Trovan IV, 16
TSPA, 1047
Tubarine 🍁*
Tubocurarine chloride*

U

Ultiva, 968
Unasyn, 102
Uric acid reduction
allopurinol, 48
*colchicine**
Urinary alkalinizer
acetazolamide, 6
Uritol 🍁, 536
Urokinase*
Uromitexan 🍁, 734
Urticaria adjunct
cimetidine, 272

Color type indicates generic drug name.
Italic type indicates drug categories and listings.
*See http://evolve.elsevier.com/IVMeds for detailed information.

Uterine smooth muscle relaxant
magnesium sulfate, 714
Uterine stimulants
ergonovine, 467
methylergonovine, 745
oxytocin, 847

V

Valium, 358
Valproate sodium, 1086
Vancocin, 1092
Vancoled, 1092
Vancomycin hydrochloride, 1092
Vasodilators
adenosine, 12
amiodarone, 84
diazoxide, 363
dipyridamole, 383
enalaprilat, 435
epoprostenol, 457
fenoldopam, 496
hydralazine, 588
inamrinone, 626
milrinone, 767
nesiritide, 808
nicardipine, 812
nitroglycerin IV, 814
nitroprusside sodium, 818
papaverine, 865
phentolamine, 890
Vasopressin, 1096
Vasopressors
dopamine, 398
ephedrine, 438
epinephrine, 440
isoproterenol, 656
norepinephrine, 822
phenylephrine, 892
vasopressin, 1096
Vasotec IV, 435
VCR, 1113
Vecuronium bromide, 1098
Velban, 1110
Velbe ♣, 1110
Velcade, 1154
Venofer, 653
Venoglobulin-S, 619
VePesid, 480
Verapamil hydrochloride, 1102
Versed, 760
Verteporfin, 1106
Vesicants
carmustine, 210
dacarbazine, 314
dactinomycin, 319
daunorubicin, 328
doxorubicin, 408
epirubicin, 446
idarubicin, 607
mechlorethamine, 721
mitomycin, 771
plicamycin, 912
streptozocin, 1021
vinblastine, 1110
vincristine, 1113
vindesine ♣, 1117
vinorelbine, 1120
VFEND IV, 1125
Vibramycin IV, 415
Vinblastine sulfate, 1110
Vinca alkaloids
vinblastine, 1110
vincristine, 1113
vindesine ♣, 1117
vinorelbine, 1120
Vincasar PFS, 1113
Vincristine sulfate, 1113
Vindesine sulphate ♣, 1117
Vinorelbine tartrate, 1120
Vistide, 268
Visudyne, 1106
Vitamin B_1, 1043
Vitamin B_6, 953
Vitamin C, 142
Vitamin D, 193
Vitamin D analogs
calcitriol, 193
doxercalciferol, 405
paricalcitol, 866
Vitamin K_1, 902
Vitamins
ascorbic acid, 142
folic acid, 522
multivitamin infusion, 786
phytonadione, 902
pyridoxine, 953
thiamine, 1043

Color type indicates generic drug name.
Italic type indicates drug categories and listings.
*See http://evolve.elsevier.com/IVMeds for detailed information.

VLB, 1110
VM-26, 1039
Von Willebrand factor complex (human), 110
Voriconazole, 1125
VP-16-213, 480
Vumon, 1039

W

Warfarin sodium, 1131
WinRho SD, 982

X

Xanthine bronchodilators
theophylline ethylenediamine (aminophylline), 76
Xigris, 421
Xylocaine PF, 694
Xylocard ✱, 694

Z

Zanosar, 1021
Zantac, 962
Zemplar, 866
Zemuron*
Zenapax, 316
Zevalin, 598
Zidovudine, 1135
Zinacef, 256
Zinc, 1071
Zinecard, 349
Zithromax, 159
Zofran, 834
Zoledronic acid, 1138
Zometa, 1138
Zosyn, 907
Zovirax, 8
Zyloprim for injection, 48
Zyvox, 698

Solution Compatibility Chart

Intravenous Medication	D2½W	D5W	D10W	D5/¼NS	D5/½NS	D5NS	NS	½NS	R	LR	D5R	D5LR	Dextran 6%/D5W/NS	Fruc 10%/W/NS	Invert sug 10%/W/NS	Na Lactate ⅙ M
Acetazolamide	C	C	C	C	C	C	C	C	C	C	C	C	C	C	C	C
Acyclovir		C		C	C	C	C			C						
Aminophylline	C	C	C	C	C	C	C	C	C	C	C	C	C			C
Antithymocyte Globulin	C	C	C	C	C	C	C	C								
Ascorbic Acid	C	C	C	C	C	C	C	C	C	C	C	C	C	C	C	C
Aztreonam		C	C	C	C	C	C		C	C		C				C
Calcium Chloride		C	C	C	C	C	C		C	C	C	C				
Calcium Gluconate		C	C			C	C			C		C		W		C
Cefazolin Na		C	C	C	C	C	C		C	C		C			W	
Cefoperazone Na		C	C	C		C	C			C		C				
Cefotaxime Na		C	C	C	C	C	C			C					W	C
Cefotetan		C					C									
Cefoxitin Na		C	C	C	C	C	C		C	C		C			C	C
Ceftazidime		C	C	C	C	C	C		C	C					W	C
Ceftizoxime Na		C	C	C	C	C	C		C	C					W	
Ceftriaxone Na		C	C		C		C								W	C
Cefuroxime Na		C	C	C	C	C	C		C	C					W	C
Cimetidine		C	C	C	C	C	C		C	C		C			W	
Clindamycin		C	C		C	C	C			C	C					
Dexamethasone		C					C									
Dobutamine HCl		C	C		C	C	C	C		C		C				C
Dopamine HCl		C	C		C	C	C			C		C				C
Doxycycline		C					C		C						W	
Epinephrine	C	C	C	C	C	C	C		C	C	C	C	C	C	C	C
Famotidine		C	C				C			C						
Fentanyl		C					C									
Folic Acid		C					C									
Furosemide		C	C			C	C			C		C				C
Gentamicin		C	C				C		C	C						
Heparin Na	C	C		C	C	C	C	C	C		C	C	C	C	C	
Hydrocortisone Phosphate		C	C				C	C								
Hydrocortisone Na Succinate	C	C	C	C	C	C	C	C	C	C	C	C	C	C	C	C
Hydromorphone HCl		C	C		C	C	C	C	C	C	C	C		W		C
Imipenem-Cilastatin		C[4]	C[4]	C[4]	C[4]	C[4]	C[10]									
Insulin (Regular)		C[P]	C		C		C[P]			C	C					
Isoproterenol	C	C[P]	C	C	C	C	C[P]		C	C	C	C	C	C	C	
Kanamycin		C	C			C	C			C						
Labetalol		C		C		C	C		C	C	C	C				
Lidocaine		C[P]			C	C	C	C		C		C				
Magnesium Sulfate		C					C			C						
Meperidine HCl	C	C	C	C	C	C	C	C	C	C	C	C	C	C	W	C
Meropenem		C[1]	C[1]	C[1]		C[1]	C[4]		C[4]	C[4]		C[1]				C[2]